To David, my husband and soulmate,
who has believed in me from the day we met nearly 40 years ago.
Thank you for your unwavering support and your daily cheers of "Write, write!"
which kept me focused and resolute through the peaks and valleys of this project.

To Kay, whose friendship is a rare gemstone. Thank you for keeping me sane.

To all my students, past and future.
Thank you for inspiring me to decipher our crazy world of healthcare
and make it comprehensible.
Hopefully this book is a beginning.

Preface

ICD-10-CM/PCS Coding: A Map for Success is a comprehensive text on the healthcare industry's new coding system, intended for students studying coding at career colleges, community colleges, and universities. They may be planning to become dedicated coders or may be preparing for a related role such as clinician or administrator. The book is also useful for professional coders and providers, as well as billers, claims examiners, and medical assistants seeking to learn ICD-10-CM/PCS.

The text is written to be friendly to those with basic exposure to, but not mastery of, medical terminology and limited or no experience in the medical field. The flexibility of the text allows experienced professionals to skim the basics and concentrate on new information pertaining to ICD-10-CM/PCS. The text is designed to be both student-friendly and instructor-friendly.

Coding examples and answer keys are based on the 2012 Draft ICD-10-CM/PCS code sets.

When the final rule requiring adoption of ICD-10-CM/PCS was issued in 2009, the Department of Health and Human Services (DHHS) established October 1, 2013, as the implementation date for all HIPAA-covered entities. As this text went to press in 2012, DHHS announced its intention to reevaluate the implementation date. Please refer to **http://www.cms.gov/ICD10** for current details.

Welcome to ICD-10-CM/PCS

The implementation of ICD-10-CM/PCS marks one of the greatest changes the medical coding field has ever experienced. Diagnosis codes used by all providers are greatly expanded and follow a new format; hospital inpatient procedure codes comprise an entirely new approach to coding. While the industry spent years fine-tuning the code sets and preparing for the many systemic changes they require, learning how to utilize the code sets is a formidable challenge in itself. All coders, including college instructors, are faced with the largest learning curve of their careers. A text must be welcoming to students and uncomplicated for instructors to adopt. This requires not simply a substitution of new codes for old, but an original approach to teaching a coding system that has a very new and different structure.

Development Story

I love to teach because I love to learn, and every time I teach, I learn. For those in healthcare, the learning challenge of ICD-10-CM/PCS is formidable. When I first heard of ICD-10-CM/PCS many years ago, I knew that I wanted to be on the leading edge of its implementation. When Pearson asked me to write this text, I eagerly set forth on a mission to learn and to teach. The time had come to communicate coding in a way that made it easier for instructors to teach and students to learn.

My driving passion is to take complex technical subjects and break them down into practical, understandable pieces that others can apply. When teaching, I obsessively search for new ways of explaining this ever-evolving field of coding. Drawing on years of trial and error, listening to students, and collaborating with fellow instructors, I wanted to create a text that would approach coding in a fresh way. Students needed to not just learn a list of rules, but to get inside the mind of an experienced coder and grasp the rationale behind coding. They also needed to be able to relate new concepts to familiar experiences. Instructors needed material they could use "out of the box" and hit on the points where students need the most support. I assembled my many original handouts, short-cut tools, and visual aids; created new charts and tables; and proceeded to craft a text that I hope stands out from the crowd.

ORGANIZATION OF THE TEXT

I have always believed it is important to know why you are learning something before you start learning it. I also appreciate that students want to know where they are going to end up before they begin. Therefore, this text is organized to give the student a context and framework for coding, before jumping into the technical skills.

Section One, Foundations of Coding, establishes the basis of the coding career, reimbursement process, and ICD-10-CM/PCS transition. Students enter coding class with many questions about their future careers, so those questions are addressed up front. Then, by walking students through the claims and reimbursement process, they gain a contextual understanding of how codes are used and how they impact an organization's success. The transition from ICD-9-CM to ICD-10-CM/PCS is discussed to help students understand the context in which they enter this field. Section One may be taught at the end of the course for those preferring a more traditional approach.

Section Two, Diagnosis Coding, arranges ICD-10-CM chapters based on ease of student learning and/or frequency of use, rather than following the strict order of the manual itself. This is because the sequencing of topics in the coding manual is based on the logic of a classification system, not on student needs. Therefore, this text organizes the chapters in a nontraditional sequence, placing four chapters that apply across all body systems before the individual body system chapters on diagnosis coding. (The Instructor's Manual provides a crosswalk for those who wish to teach chapters in the traditional order of the coding manual.)

- After an introduction to diagnosis coding, neoplasms are introduced, because students encounter them in every body system. General neoplasm coding is addressed here, and neoplasms related to each body system appear within each body system chapter.
- Coding for symptoms and signs appears next so that students can begin by learning when and when not to assign these codes, a common point of confusion.
- Coding for factors influencing health status and contact with health services enables students to learn the basics of these codes and apply them to case scenarios in each body system throughout the course.
- Coding for external causes is also addressed so that these codes, which have been expanded and restructured in ICD-10-CM, can be integrated into all subsequent chapters.
- Body system chapters are sequenced based on ease of learning and frequency of use, rather than in strict coding manual order. The digestive system appears first because it is easier for students to understand and relate to. Chapters on obstetrics, perinatal, and congenital conditions are placed last because students and instructors frequently find these to be the most challenging.

Each ICD-10-CM chapter is covered in one textbook chapter. No chapters are combined or split, which allows great flexibility to adapt the book to any curriculum format. The chapters can be taught in any order that best suits the curriculum. A variety of crosswalks appear in the accompanying Instructor's Manual.

Section Three, Inpatient Procedure Coding, provides an introduction to a completely new coding system for inpatient hospitals. ICD-10-PCS is developed based on the type of Root Operation rather than body system. Medical and surgical Root Operations, which account for 85% of all PCS codes, are covered in greatest detail to help the student learn the structure and use of ICD-10-PCS. These skills are then applied to the other sections of PCS in subsequent chapters. Consistent definitions, internal to the PCS system, and a methodical structure should be welcomed by both instructors and students. This section may be surveyed or omitted by physician-based coding programs or programs with accelerated calendars.

Section Four, Putting It All Together, introduces students to coding from chart notes and operative reports, as well as using electronic coding tools. Annotated report examples help students make the transition from basic to advanced coding. An overview of health information technology introduces the student to current and developing technology in the field. This section may be surveyed or omitted by programs with accelerated calendars.

Each chapter in the text provides in-chapter exercises so that students can review and apply material as they learn it. Additional end-of-chapter exercises enable students to recall, synthesize, and solidify content from the entire chapter. Coding chapters provide over 50 coding exercises in each chapter.

CONCEPTUAL APPROACH

The goal of this text is not only to create one of the first comprehensive ICD-10-CM texts, but to approach coding in a way that gives instructors new tools to communicate successfully and gives students new skills to learn effectively. Four concepts are the focus of each chapter.

Abstracting, Assigning, and Arranging Codes

Students need a simple and methodical approach to the complex coding process. This text organizes coding around the learning mnemonic for an **A**ce Coder: "**A**bstract, **A**ssign, and **A**rrange (Sequence)" codes. The Official Guidelines for Coding and Reporting (OGCR) are integrated into each chapter's discussion, rather than being reprinted in their entirety with minimal explanation. Guided examples walk students through the three steps of coding and reveal the critical thinking process of applying OGCR. By focusing on these basic skills consistently and repeatedly, the outcome is students who can tackle a variety of coding scenarios with confidence.

Application of Medical Terminology

Students need to apply what they learned in medical terminology and anatomy courses to coding. To support the increased emphasis on anatomy in ICD-10-CM/PCS, the body system diagram that begins each Section Two body system chapter is dually labeled with the English word and the medical combining form, such as **stomach** and **gastr/o**. This helps students make both visual and verbal connection with medical terms. Commonly used prefixes and suffixes are presented, as well as easily confused medical terms, within each body system. Terminology exercises and examples in each chapter show students how to continue building terminology skills and apply them to coding. The outcome is students who understand the terminology they encounter in coding exercises and, as a result, code more accurately.

Relationship of Diagnoses and Procedures

Students need to understand how diagnoses and procedures relate to each other. In traditional texts, exercises present a list of diagnoses but no treatments, or a list of procedures but no diagnoses. In this text, every chapter highlights diagnoses and the related treatments together, so students learn the relationship between the two. Exercises describe both diagnoses and services, even though the coding focus is on one or the other. The outcome is students who comprehend the full coding picture and, as a result, make a smooth transition into coding cases.

Context of the Patient Encounter

Students need to abstract information from a patient encounter rather than code solely from isolated statements that are five to ten words in length. In this text, exercises utilize an original "mini-medical-record," which presents excerpts of patient, diagnostic, and procedural information. "Tips" accompany difficult exercises to help students interpret the information. The outcome is students who learn abstracting skills in every exercise and are better prepared for advanced coding courses and the workplace.

FEATURES

Consistent pedagogical elements appear in each chapter to facilitate instruction and learning.

Learning Objectives—Each chapter begins with a list of the primary skills students should have after completing the chapter.

Key Terms and Abbreviations—A list of the important terms students need to know but may not have learned in previous classes appears at the beginning of each chapter. These terms appear in green boldface type and are defined upon first appearance in the chapter. They also appear in the Glossary at the end of the book.

Chapter Outline—A list of the major topics covered in the chapter appears at the beginning.

Introduction—The text utilizes the theme of a road trip to take the student through the challenges of coding. The theme, which is highlighted in chapter introductions, creates a consistent and familiar frame of reference for analogies and provides a lighthearted perspective for relating to new information.

Supplemental Terms and Abbreviations—Additional terms or abbreviations that some students may be unfamiliar with appear in **bold** type and are defined only in the Glossary, for reference.

Success Step—Short tips throughout the chapter help students abstract, assign, and sequence codes.

Coding Caution—Short warnings throughout the chapter alert students to coding situations that can be tricky or confusing.

Coding Practice—Coding exercises throughout the chapter consist of three to five patient scenarios related to a specific chapter topic. The first exercise in the coding chapters reviews medical terms related to the body system or type of procedure and introduces students to simple coding for the body system. Subsequent exercises walk students through the skills of abstracting, assigning, and sequencing codes. Exercises increase in difficulty as the chapter progresses, while remaining appropriate for an introductory course. Most chapters have 20 to 30 coding questions in this feature. Answers to odd-numbered exercises appear in the Appendix.

Guided Examples—Step-by-step demonstrations allow students to experience the thinking process of a seasoned coder as they observe a coder abstract, assign, and sequence codes from a mini-medical-record.

Figures—Anatomical illustrations show English names and medical terms for major body parts and organs; illustrations annotate sample pages from the coding manuals; photographs and diagrams portray key points.

Tables—Tables throughout the text provide definitions of terms, conditions, and treatments, as well as comparative information that highlights key concepts.

Summary—Each chapter ends with a brief restatement of key points in the chapter.

Special typefaces—Distinct fonts and color-coding enable students to visually identify various types of information, as follows:

- **Key terms and abbreviations**
- **Supplemental terms and abbreviations**
- *Simulated content in a patient's medical record*
- **Codes, code titles, and instructional notes from the ICD-10-CM/PCS coding manuals**

End-of-Chapter Material

A review section at the end of each chapter reinforces key concepts, provides opportunity for additional skills practice, and offers resources for additional learning.

Concept Quiz—Definitions and key concepts are reviewed using ten completion and ten multiple choice questions.

Coding Challenge—Ten coding scenarios drawn from all sections of the chapter review coding skills learned in the chapter. The Coding Challenge in procedure coding (PCS) chapters requires both diagnosis and procedure codes.

Keep on Coding—Twenty-five coding exercises in one-line-statement format provide additional student practice.

Coder's Toolbox—A list of Internet resources and reference material related to chapter content appears at the end of each chapter. Active links appear online in MyHealthProfessionsLab and in the Instructor's Manual.

End-of-Book Material

Appendix—Answer Key to Coding Practice Exercises (Odd-numbered)—The answers for odd-numbered Coding Practice Exercises allow students to check their progress as they work through the chapter. Each coding answer also provides one coding path—the series of Main Terms and subterms required to locate the code in the Index.

Glossary—The Glossary defines key terms, supplemental terms, and abbreviations and indicates the chapter in which the term was introduced.

Index—An alphabetic crosswalk identifies page references for major topics discussed in this text.

Coder's Index—Alphabetic lists of ICD-10-CM and ICD-10-PCS provide cross-references to the pages on which all specific codes are discussed. The Coder's Index can be found at MyHealthProfessionsKit and MyHealthProfessionsLab.

Supplement Package/Ancillary Materials

A robust supplement package accompanies *ICD-10-CM/PCS Coding: A Map for Success*:

- MyHealthProfessionsLab™: Your online medical coding workbook. Practice, practice, practice and test your retention of key concepts.
- **MyHealthProfessionsKit:** Includes the Coder's Index, a link to a trial encoder, active web links to Coder's Toolbox resources, and any code updates.

- **Access your free trial of Pearson's SpeedECoder at http://sec.pearsonhighered.com.**
- **Instructor's Manual**
- **PowerPoint Slides**
- **Image Library**
- **MyTest**

ABOUT THE AUTHOR

Lorraine M. Papazian-Boyce, MS, CPC
AHIMA-Approved ICD-10-CM/PCS Trainer

Lorraine M. Papazian-Boyce holds an M.S. in Health Systems Management from Rush University in Chicago, Illinois; the Certified Professional Coder (CPC) credential from AAPC; and is an AHIMA-Approved ICD-10-CM/PCS Trainer. She was named Educator of the Year—Instruction (2010–11) by Career Education Corporation (CEC).

Lorraine has over 30 years of experience in healthcare administration as a biller and coder; office manager; business owner of a medical billing and coding service; management consultant to hospitals, nursing homes, and physicians; author and speaker; college instructor; externship coordinator; and board of directors officer. She has taught at Colorado Technical University-Online (Career Education Corporation), Everest College (Corinthian Colleges), Pioneer Pacific College (Clackamas, Oregon), and University of Phoenix.

In addition to teaching, Lorraine works with Pearson as a subject matter expert and trains college instructors in ICD-10-CM/PCS. She has contributed to several Pearson texts including *Guide to Medical Billing and Coding,* 3rd edition (Brown/Tyler); *A Coding Journey: A Comprehensive Guide to Coding Diagnoses, Services, and Procedures* (Rich-Martin); *Medical Assisting: Foundations and Practices* (Frazier/Malone); *Comprehensive Health Insurance: Billing, Coding, and Reimbursement* (Vines/Braceland); *and Mastering Medisoft* (Flom).

Lorraine writes a blog for coders and billers at http://luvtocode.blogspot.com/.

ACKNOWLEDGMENTS

Publishing a textbook is a collaborative process that requires the skills of many talented people. I am truly grateful to everyone at Pearson who accompanied me on this journey.

- First and foremost, I wish to thank Joan Gill, my tireless Executive Editor, for embracing my vision and bringing it to fruition. Your ability to transform my concept into a useful text is remarkable, and your concern for the learner's experience is unmatched. Thank you for this opportunity to realize a long-time aspiration.
- Alexis Breen Ferraro, Developmental Editor, who skillfully and patiently guided the development process and ensured that we met all deadlines, so the text could reach the hands of its users as quickly as possible.
- Bronwen Glowacki, Associate Editor, who shepherded the project through production and confirmed that my goals for the student were met at every step of the process.
- Carrie Fox, Assistant Managing Editor at Electronic Publishing Services, and the production team, who painstakingly transformed 1,500 pages of manuscript into a stunning text; and especially the artists, who meticulously rendered each figure in order to enhance student comprehension.
- Margie Stackhouse, who contributed hundreds of Keep on Coding exercises, so that students can practice their new-found coding skills.
- Lori Tyler, who contributed the clinical details of selected exercises, so that students can have a more realistic coding experience.
- Allison Murray, who diligently researched photographs, that enrich students' understanding of abstract topics, and tackled the arduous task of preparing the final art manuscript, allowing me to maintain a laser-like focus on writing.
- Kristy Rodecker, Pauline Newton, Karen Weiss, and Marie Schanbacher, who graciously shared their inspirational stories for the section-opener profiles.
- Mary Ellen Ruitenberg and Stephanie Kiel, Editorial Assistants, whose follow-up and attention to detail I always appreciate.

REVIEWERS

The invaluable feedback and direction provided by the following educators and healthcare professionals is deeply appreciated:

Lurrean Bentley, RMA, CMRS
Instructor for Medical Assisting and Medical Coding Programs
Remington College, TN

Becky Buegel, RHIA, CHP, CHC, AHIMA-Certified ICD-10-CM/PCS
Trainer
Health Information Technology Program Director
Brookline College
Avondale, AZ

Rhoda Cooper, CPC, RMC, NCICS
Director of Health Information Management, Instructor
Piedmont Virginia Community College, VA

Melissa Hibbard, BS, CEHRS, CMRS, CPC, CPhT
Program Director, Medical Business
Miami Jacobs Career College, OH

Susan Holler, MSEd, CMRS
Allied Health Faculty
Bryant and Stratton College, NY

Kristin Knox, CCS, CMA, AS
Allied Health Instructor
Techskills, FL

Aimee Michaelis, Med., CPC
Lead Instructor, Medical Administrative Assisting
Pima Medical Institute, CO

Sandra Miller-Davis, BS, CPC, CCS
Medical Billing and Coding Program Coordinator
Southeastern Institute—Nashville Campus, TN

Amy D. Lawrence, MBA/HR, CPC, CCA
Program Chair, Medical Administrative Assistant and Medical Office Billing Specialist Online Programs
Ultimate Medical Academy
Brandon, FL

Trasey Pfluger, RMA, CMAA, CBCS, NCICS
Program Director, Health Information Technology
Fortis College
Winter Park, FL

Fannie Sue Martin, CPC
Instructor
YTI Career Institute, PA

Le'Cheryl Purnell, CCS-P, CPI
Medical Billing and Coding Coordinator
Centura College, SC

Jerri Rowe, MA, CPC
Program Director, Medical Billing and Coding
MedVance Institute, FL

Tiffiny J. Stewart, CPC, NRCCS, CAHI, CMBS
Medical Coding Instructor/Externship/Job Placement Coordinator
Delta Technical College, TN

Contents in Brief

Contents

Road Map

This Road Map acquaints users with the text and shows them how to use the pedagogical features to their greatest advantage.

Learning Objectives—Each chapter begins with a list of the primary skills students should have after completing the chapter.

> **Learning Objectives**
>
> After completing this chapter, you should have the skills to:
>
> - Spell and define the key words, medical terms, and abbreviations related to the respiratory system.
> - Discuss the structure, function, and common conditions of the respiratory system.
> - Identify the main characteristics of coding for the respiratory system.

Key Terms and Abbreviations—A list of the important terms students need to know but may not have learned in previous classes appears at the beginning of each chapter. These terms appear in **green** boldface type and are defined upon first appearance in the chapter.

> **Key Terms and Abbreviations**
>
> acute exacerbation
> acute rhinitis
> aerosol therapy
> airway obstruction
> chronic bronchitis
> chronic obstructive pulmonary disease (COPD)
>
> **Chronic Obstructive Pulmonary Disease**
>
> Chronic obstructive pulmonary disease (COPD), one of the most common lung diseases, is the combination of chronic bronchitis and emphysema as comorbidities. An airway obstruction is a reduction in the amount of inhaled air in each breath, most commonly caused by a reduction in the diameter of the bronchioles due to inflammation.

Introduction—The text utilizes the theme of a road trip to take the student through the challenges of coding. The theme is highlighted in chapter introductions to create a consistent and familiar frame of reference for analogies and provides a lighthearted perspective for relating to new information.

> **INTRODUCTION**
>
> When your road trip takes you through a mountainous area, you probably notice the difference in the air surprisingly quickly. Even at 4,000 or 5,000 feet of elevation above sea level, breathing becomes more difficult for many people. The higher you go, the more difficult breathing becomes, not because there is less oxygen in the air, but because a decrease in air pressure causes us to inhale less air with each breath. Breathing is a body function you probably take for granted until it becomes difficult.
>
> In your tour of the respiratory system in this chapter you will learn more about how the respiratory system works, why sometimes it does not work as it should, and how physicians treat these conditions. Most importantly, you will practice coding for patient encounters related to respiratory diseases and conditions, a skill that requires you to abstract information from the mini-medical-record, assign correct codes, and arrange (sequence) the codes in the proper order.

Chapter Outline—Each chapter of the text includes a list of the major topics covered in the chapter.

> **Chapter Outline**
>
> - **Respiratory System Refresher**
> - **Coding Overview of the Respiratory System**
> - **Abstracting for the Respiratory System**
> - **Assigning Codes for the Respiratory System**
> - **Arranging Codes for the Respiratory System**
> - **Coding Neoplasms of the Respiratory System**

Supplemental Terms and Abbreviations—Additional terms or abbreviations that some students may be unfamiliar with are highlighted with bold type and defined only in the Glossary, for reference.

> Instructional notes in the Tabular List also instruct coders to assign additional codes for lung abscess, **pleural effusion**, perforated **tympanic membrane**, sinusitis, the type of pneumonia, and any additional manifestations.

Success Step—Short tips throughout the chapter help students to abstract, assign, and sequence codes.

Coding Caution—Short warnings throughout the chapter alert students to coding situations that can be tricky or confusing.

SUCCESS STEP

ICD-9-CM provided a chapter-wide note to assign an additional code to identify the infectious organism. Because ICD-10-CM has many combination codes that describe the condition and the organism, this chapter-wide note was eliminated. However, you still see a similar note in certain categories that do not provide a combination code.

CODING CAUTION

In ICD-9-CM asthma codes were divided based on whether asthma was extrinsic or intrinsic. In ICD-10-CM, these terms lead you to default codes for unspecified asthma. Instead, you need to locate asthma based on the severity level as mild intermittent, moderate intermittent, moderate persistent, and severe persistent.

Coding Practice—Coding exercises within each chapter consist of three to five patient scenarios related to a specific chapter topic. The first exercise in the coding chapters reviews medical terms related to the body system or type of procedure and introduces students to simple coding for the body system.

Coding Practice

Refresh your knowledge of terminology related to the respiratory system. Use a medical terminology text or a website such as GlobalRph.com > Medical Terminology **http://www.globalrph.com/medterm.htm** to identify the meaning of word parts that may not be familiar.

Exercise 16.1 Respiratory System Refresher

Instructions: Use your medical terminology skills and resources to define the following conditions related to the respiratory system, then assign the diagnosis code. Follow these steps:

- Use slash marks "/" to break down each term into its root(s) and suffix.
- Define the meaning of the word, based on the meaning of each word part.
- Assign the default ICD-10-CM diagnosis code (CM) for the condition usi[...]ndex and Tabular List.

Example: tonsillitis tonsil/itis Meaning: *inflammation of the tonsils*

1. pneumatocele Meaning ____________________
2. bronchiolitis Meaning ____________________

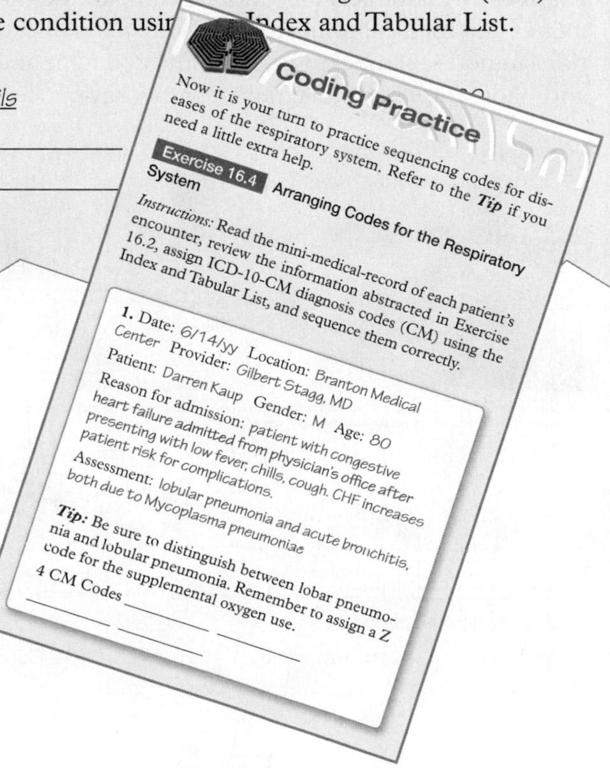

Coding Practice

Now it is your turn to practice sequencing codes for diseases of the respiratory system. Refer to the *Tip* if you need a little extra help.

Exercise 16.4 Arranging Codes for the Respiratory System

Instructions: Read the mini-medical-record of each patient's encounter, review the information abstracted in Exercise 16.2, assign ICD-10-CM diagnosis codes (CM) using the Index and Tabular List, and sequence them correctly.

1. Date: 6/14/yy Location: Branton Medical Center Provider: Gilbert Stagg, MD
Patient: Darren Kaup Gender: M Age: 80
Reason for admission: patient with congestive heart failure admitted from physician's office after presenting with low fever, chills, cough. CHF increases patient risk for complications.
Assessment: lobular pneumonia and acute bronchitis, both due to Mycoplasma pneumoniae

Tip: Be sure to distinguish between lobar pneumonia and lobular pneumonia. Remember to assign a Z code for the supplemental oxygen use.

4 CM Codes ________ ________ ________ ________

Subsequent exercises walk students through the skills of abstracting, assigning, and sequencing codes. Exercises increase in difficulty as the chapter progresses, while remaining appropriate for an introductory course.

Guided Examples—Step-by-step demonstrations of abstracting, assigning, and sequencing codes allow students to experience the thinking process of a seasoned coder. Information from the medical record appears in its own typeface so it is easy to identify. Codes numbers, code titles, and instructional notes from the ICD-10-CM/PCS manuals appears in a special typeface throughout the chapter.

Guided Example of Abstracting for the Respiratory System

Refer to the following example throughout this chapter to practice skills for abstracting, assigning, and sequencing respiratory system codes. Leanne Riehl, CCS, is a fictional coder who guides you through the coding process.

Date: 6/16/yy Location: Branton Medical Center
Provider: Gilbert Stagg, MD
Patient: Jared Hershman Gender: M Age: 73
Reason for admission: dehydration, started IV fluids
Assessment: Patient who previously smoked cigarettes for 50 years (nicotine dependence) was placed on ventilator due to COPD exacerbation. Patient acquired ventilator associated pneumonia (VAP) due to Pseudomonas. Hospital stay was prolonged due to the VAP.
Plan: discharged home after 10 days, continue antibiotics, start supplemental O_2

After he was admitted, the patient experienced an acute exacerbation of the COPD. Patient also developed VAP.

- ❑ *Does the patient use supplemental oxygen or a ventilator?* Yes, patient was placed on ventilator.
- ❑ *What is the infectious organism?* Pseudomonas. *Is it a virus or bacteria?* Bacteria
- ❑ *Is the condition the result of an external cause or procedural complication?* Yes, the pneumonia is ventilator associated.
- ❑ *Does the record document any current or past tobacco use?* Previously smoked cigarettes for 50 years (nicotine dependence).

➩ Leanne reviews all the information she has gathered about this case.

- ❑ The patient was admitted for dehydration.
- ❑ He has COPD.
- ❑ He experienced an acute exacerbation of COPD.
- ❑ He has a history of cigarette smoking.

Figures—Anatomical illustrations compare English names and medical terms for key body parts; illustrations annotate sample pages from the coding manuals; and photographs and diagrams portray key concepts.

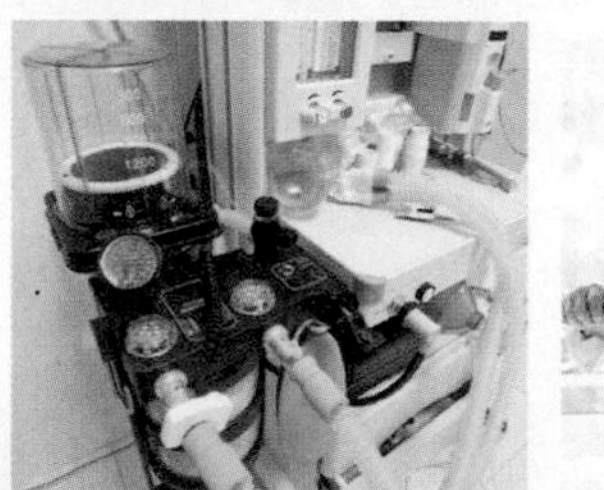

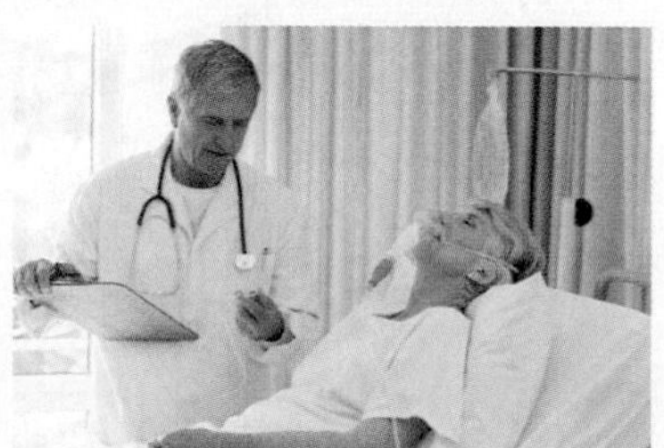

Figure 16-10 ■ Ventilators assist patients with breathing, but can also create an opportunity for pneumonia. *Sources: Paul Vinten/Shutterstock.com (left) and wavebreakmedia ltd/Shutterstock (right).*

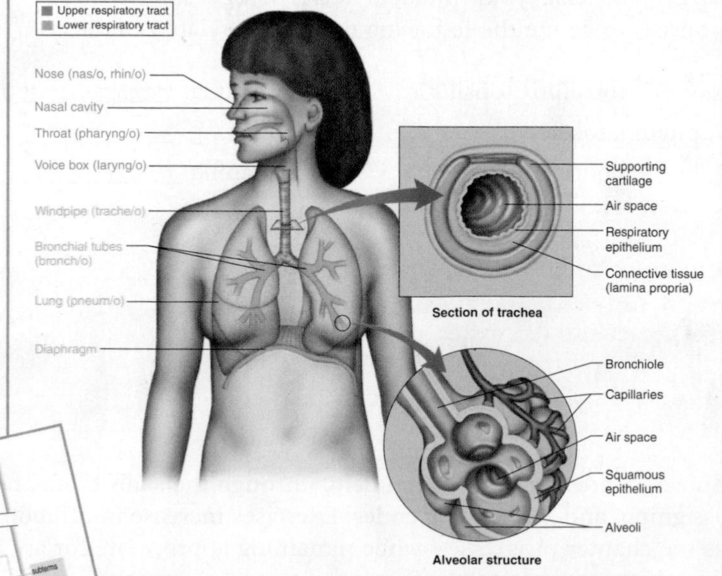

Tables—Tables provide definitions of terms, conditions, and treatments. Tables also provide comparative information that highlight key points.

Table 16-2 ■ **CONDITIONS OF THE RESPIRATORY SYSTEM**

Condition	Definition
Acute respiratory distress syndrome (ARDS)	Acute respiratory failure that result for widespread injury to the endothelium in the lung, caused by sepsis, massive blood transfusion, **aspiration** of gastric contents, or pneumonia
Acute respiratory failure (ARF)	Insufficient oxygen passing from the lungs to the blood, due to **hypercapnia** (*high carbon dioxide level*), **hypoxemia** (*low oxygen level*), or both

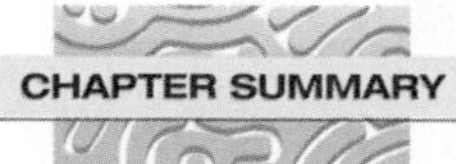

CHAPTER SUMMARY

In this chapter you learned that:

- The function of the respiratory system is to obtain oxygen from the air and deliver it to the lungs and blood for distribution to tissue cells, and to remove the gaseous waste product carbon dioxide from the blood and lungs and expel it.
- ICD-10-CM Chapter 10, Diseases of the Respiratory System (J00-J99), contains 11 blocks or subchapters that are divided by type of disorder and anatomic site.
- Coders should become familiar with chapter-wide coding considerations as well as information specifically for asthma, COPD, and influenza.
- OGCR provides specific instructions regarding sequencing codes for ventilator associated pneumonia and acute re
- Codes for n in the block the most co
- ICD-10-CM Reporting (OGCR secti chronic obst acute respira associated p

Summary—Each chapter ends with a brief restatement of key points in the chapter.

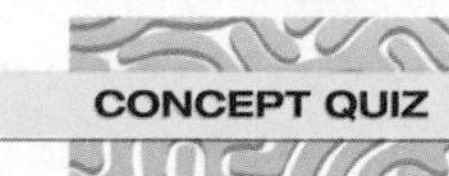

CONCEPT QUIZ

Take a moment to look back at your trip through external causes and solidify your skills. This is your opportunity to pull together everything you have learned.

Completion

Instructions: Write the term that answers each question based on the information you learned in this chapter. Choose from the following list. Some choices may be used more than once and some choices may not be

Multiple Choice

Instructions: Circle the letter of the best answer to each question based on the information you learned in this chapter. Refer to the discussion in this chapter and the Glossary at the end of this book if you need a little extra help.

1. What healthcare setting uses external cause codes?
   A. Outpatient setting only
   B. Emergency department only
   C. Inpatient setting only

End of Chapter Material

A review section at the end of each chapter reinforces key concepts, provides opportunity for additional skills practice, and offers resources for additional learning.

Concept Quiz—A review of theory in the chapter, this section consists of ten completion and ten multiple choice questions related to definitions and key concepts in the chapter.

Coding Challenge—A review of coding skills in the chapter, this section consists of ten coding scenarios drawn from all sections of the chapter for which students will assign codes.

Keep on Coding—Twenty-five coding exercises in one-line-statement format provide additional student practice.

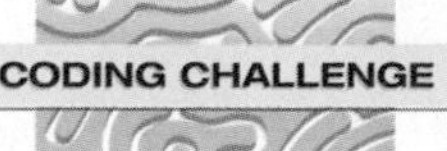

CODING CHALLENGE

Now it is your turn to demonstrate coding all aspects of diseases of the respiratory system. Refer back to the examples and discussion in this chapter when you need a little extra help. Use your medical dictionary and anatomy references when needed.

Instructions: Read the mini-medical-record of each patient's encounter, then abstract, assign, and sequence ICD-10-CM diagnosis codes (CM) using the Index and Tabular List. Write the code(s) on the line provided.

1. Date: 6/19/yy Location: North Side Pulmonology Provider: Gilbert Stagg, MD
Patient: Emilia Weyandt Gender: F Age: 1
Reason for encounter: productive cough, SOB, fever

3. Date: 6/19/yy Location: Branton Medical Center Provider: Gilbert Stagg, MD
Patient: Brad Matchett Gender: M Age: 82
Reason for admission: pneumonococcal pneumonia
Assessment: COPD with acute exacerbation required ventilation
Plan: discharged to skilled nursing facility with oxygen

Tip: One of the codes is a Z code.
3 CM Codes __________ __________ __________

KEEP ON CODING

As a coder, you can never have too much experience. Apply everything you have learned in this chapter to code the following diagnostic statements. Use the OGCR and instructional notes in the Tabular List to help determine how many codes are required.

Instructions: Read the diagnostic statement, then use the Index to External Causes and Tabular List to assign and sequence ICD-10-CM (CM) diagnosis codes. Write the code(s) on the line provided.

1. Burn of the hand while onboard a sailboat, initial encounter: CM Code(s) __________
2. Injury occurred while cheerleading (activity code): CM Code(s) __________

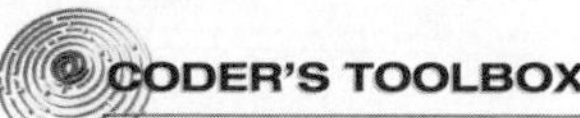

CODER'S TOOLBOX

The following resources are a starting point for learning more about diseases of the respiratory system. The > symbol indicates a menu selection within the website in order to navigate to a specific page.

American Lung Association http://www.lungusa.org/

Cancer Care http://www.lungcancer.org/

Family Allergy and Asthma > Diseases http://www.familyallergy.com/diseases/default.asp

National Heart Blood and Lung Institute (NHBLI) http://www.nhlbi.nih.gov/

The American College of Allergy, Asthma, and Immunology (ACAAI) http://www.acaai.org/allergist/Pages/default.aspx

Healthline > Videos http://www.healthline.com/vpvideo/

Coder's Toolbox—A list of Internet resources and reference material related to chapter content appears at the end of each chapter.

SECTION ONE

Foundations of Coding

Welcome to your new career in coding! You are in for the trip of a lifetime, one that is sure to take you to new and unknown places, a few familiar ones, and perhaps some that seem a little scary. This text is your road map, complete with navigational tips and warnings about potentially dangerous curves. Fasten your seat belts, here we go!

Section One: Foundations of Coding acquaints you with the medical coding field, potential career opportunities, how coding relates to reimbursement and payment, and gives you an overview of the new ICD-10-CM/PCS system.

PROFESSIONAL PROFILE

MEET...

Kristy Rodecker, CPC, CPC-H, CMA

Home-Based Medical Coder

I have been in the medical billing and coding field for ten years. I was certified as a CPC five years ago and have been coding from home since then. I started out as a front desk receptionist in a busy, multi-physician neurology office and worked my way through school to be an administrative medical assistant.

When the opportunity arose, I took a data entry position at a small billing company that was a one-and-a-half hour drive (one way) and paid peanuts! The experience I gained was priceless and it was the stepping stone for the rest of my career. The company allowed coders to work from home once they worked at the facility for six to twelve months. They wanted coders to understand the way the company worked to make sure the coders knew what they were doing before they worked independently. Once I could pass all of their milestones I began to code remotely. Eventually, I took on assignments for other coding companies as well, including Nicka, MRSI, Med Data, and Summit—sometimes coding for several companies at once. For some companies I am a regular employee and for others I work as an independent contractor.

As a home-based medical coder, I log in remotely to the customer's database to access the medical records, code them, and submit the claims to insurance companies. I enjoy reading the interesting medical records, learning about new procedures, and the challenge of finding an accurate code. I also enjoy the flexibility of setting my own hours.

The most challenging aspect of my job is isolation. Working from home can give you a good dose of cabin fever. I find it important to attend my local AAPC chapter meetings and I also volunteer at the hospital so that I can stay involved in our local medical community.

I am frequently asked by aspiring coders how to work from home, so I created a free, informational website (**www.medicalbillingandmedicalcoding.com**) to help them avoid unscrupulous get-rich-quick schemes and find ways to be successful.

My advice to coding students is to set an achievable goal and go for it! Be willing to take an entry-level position, ask lots of questions, and go the extra mile to prove you are an asset.

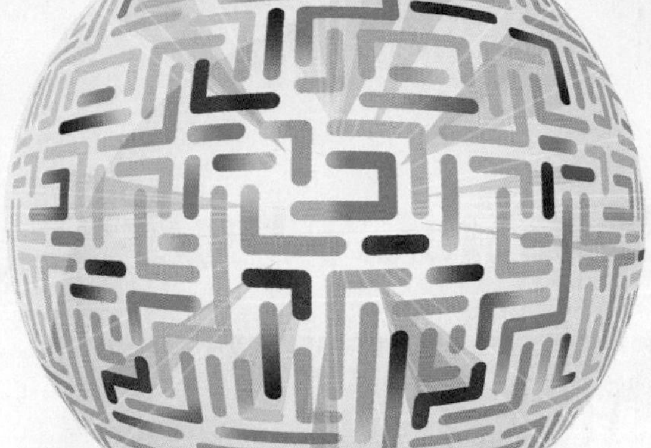

1

Your Career and Coding

Learning Objectives

After completing this chapter, you should have the skills to:

- Spell and define the key words, medical terms, and abbreviations related to your career and coding.
- Define coding, HIPAA-mandated code sets, and coding skills.
- Describe how patient encounters relate to coding.
- Identify the types of coding certification.
- Understand the career path and performance expectations for a coding career.

Key Terms and Abbreviations

AAPC
abstract
admitting privileges
advanced-level job
American Health Information Management Association (AHIMA)
ancillary
attending physician
assign
arrange
career path
case production
certification
code set
code
coding
diagnosis
document
encounter
entry-level job
Health Insurance Portability and Accountability Act (HIPAA)
International Classification of Diseases, 10th Revision, Clinical Modification (ICD-10-CM)
International Classification of Diseases, 10th Revision, Procedure Coding System (ICD-10-PCS)
inpatient encounter
mid-level job
outpatient encounter
payers
procedure
query
sequence

In addition to the key terms listed here, students should know the terms defined within tables in this chapter.

Chapter Outline

- **What Is Coding?**
- **Understanding Patient Encounters**
- **Certification**
- **Coding Careers**

CPT codes in this chapter are from the CPT 2014 code set. CPT is a registered trademark of the American Medical Association.

ICD-9-CM codes in this chapter are from the ICD-9-CM 2014 code set from the Department of Health and Human Services, Centers for Disease Control and Prevention.

ICD-10-CM codes in this chapter are from the ICD-10-CM 2014 Draft code set from the Department of Health and Human Services, Centers for Disease Control and Prevention.

ICD-10-PCS codes in this chapter are from the ICD-10-PCS 2014 Draft code set from the Department of Health and Human Services, Centers for Medicare and Medicaid Services.

INTRODUCTION

When starting on a trip, you are more likely to get where you want to go when you have a destination in mind. In this chapter you will learn about your ultimate destination: the coding profession. By understanding what coding is, the relationship between physicians and coders, and potential career opportunities, you will formulate ideas on your career goals and the steps needed to reach them.

Many jobs in the healthcare field work with codes even though they may not have a job title of Coder. For example, medical assistants, billers, schedulers, and medical secretaries may use codes as part of their jobs. This text uses the term *coder* to refer to anyone who assigns, reads, or uses codes as part of their job.

Many healthcare professionals provide patient services and use codes to bill for their services in addition to medical doctors (MDs). For example, dentists (DDSs or DMDs), osteopaths (DOs), chiropractors (DCs), and nurse practitioners (NPs) also bill their services with the same codes as physicians. This text uses the terms *physician* and *provider* interchangeably to refer to any healthcare professional who provides services that are billed with ICD-10 codes.

As you read this chapter, open up your medical terminology book and keep a medical dictionary handy to refresh your memory of any unfamiliar terms. This way, you have the information you need at your fingertips.

WHAT IS CODING?

Coding is the process of accurately assigning codes to verbal descriptions of patients' conditions and the healthcare services provided to treat those conditions. Medical **codes** are a combination of letters and numbers, three to seven characters in length. **Diagnosis** codes describe patient illnesses, diseases, conditions, injuries, or other reasons for seeking healthcare services. **Procedure** codes describe the services healthcare professionals provide to patients, such as evaluation, consultation, testing, treatments, and surgery.

Code Sets

The healthcare system in the United States uses several distinct systems of medical codes, called **code sets**, for different purposes. The various systems were developed by different organizations and follow different guidelines for their use. The **Health Insurance Portability and Accountability Act (HIPAA)**, a federal law passed in 1996, has numerous provisions relating to consumer health insurance and electronic health transactions. HIPAA defines the seven code sets that **covered entities** must use for electronic health transactions and the purpose of each (■ TABLE 1-1, page 4). This text discusses the first two code sets, **International Classification of Diseases, 10th Revision, Clinical Modification (ICD-10-CM)** and **International Classification of Diseases, 10th Revision, Procedure Coding System (ICD-10-PCS)**.

Three Skills of an Ace Coder

Coding is more than looking up numbers in a manual or software program. Accurate coding requires three major skills, which are described next: abstracting, assigning, and arranging (sequencing).

Abstracting

Before coders can assign codes, they **abstract** information from the medical record. To abstract, coders read the medical record and determine which elements of the encounter require codes. They identify the reason for the encounter, diagnostic statements from the physician, complications and co-existing conditions, and the services provided. If the medical record is not properly abstracted, it is impossible to assign the correct codes. ICD-10-CM/PCS has many rules for abstracting and some rules are specific to a particular condition or procedure. Patient encounters are discussed in this chapter.

SUCCESS STEP

The term *abstract* also describes a task in health information management in which inpatient coders review the medical record and cull data required for reporting, such as patient demographics and length of stay.

Assigning

The codes a coder selects or **assigns** must accurately describe the information documented in the medical record and must accurately describe the patient's condition and services. Each character of the code must be correct. Diagnosis codes must reflect the highest level of specificity possible and contain the correct number of characters for that code, which is between three and seven characters. Inpatient procedure codes must contain seven characters, with each character describing a specific aspect of the procedure.

Table 1-1 ■ **HIPAA-MANDATED CODE SETS**

Code Set Name	Purpose	Developed By	Code Format/Examples
ICD-10-CM International Classification of Diseases, 10th Revision, Clinical Modification	Diagnosis coding (replacement system for ICD-9-CM)	National Center for Health Statistics (NCHS) based on ICD-10 from the World Health Organization (WHO)	3 to 7 alphanumeric characters • I10 • A52.15 • T50.A11D
ICD-10-PCS International Classification of Diseases, 10th Revision, Procedure Coding System	Hospital inpatient procedure coding (replacement system for ICD-9-CM, Volume 3)	Centers for Medicare and Medicaid Services (CMS)	7 alphanumeric characters • 0B7B8DZ • 4A04XB1 • 01500ZZ
CPT® Current Procedural Terminology	Hospital outpatient and physician procedure coding	American Medical Association (AMA)	5 numbers • 99213 • 36415
HCPCS Healthcare Common Procedure Coding System	Supplies, items, and services not covered by CPT, physician and non-physician services, Medicare services, supplies	CMS	1 letter + 4 numbers • A1234 • G9874
CDT® Codes on Dental Procedures and Nomenclature	Dental services (occupies section D of HCPCS codes)	American Dental Association (ADA)	letter D + 4 numbers • D7230
ICD-9-CM International Classification of Diseases, 9th Revision, Clinical Modification	Diagnosis coding, implemented 1979	NCHS	3 to 5 numbers; supplemental codes that begin with V or E • 123 • 123.45 • V10.23 • E987.4
ICD-9-CM procedure codes	Hospital inpatient procedure coding, implemented 1979	National Center for Health Statistics (NCHS)	3 or 4 numbers • 12.3 • 12.34
NDC National Drug Codes	Identifies the manufacturer, product, and package size of all drugs and biologics recognized by the Food and Drug Administration (FDA)	Department of Health and Human Services (HHS)	10 numbers divided into 3 segments • 1234-5678-90 • 12345-678-90 • 12345-6789-0

Arranging

When more than one diagnosis or procedure code is required for an encounter, coders must **arrange**, or **sequence**, the codes in a specific order. Official coding guidelines dictate the proper sequencing, which varies depending on the codes assigned and the circumstances of the patient encounter. Codes that are not sequenced properly are not considered to be correct.

SUCCESS STEP

Memorize the definitions of the three coding skills: abstracting, assigning, and arranging. Remind yourself of these each time you sit down to code.

Coding Practice

Now it is your turn to demonstrate your understanding of the basics of coding. Try to answer the questions from memory first, then refer back to the information in this section if you need a little extra help.

Exercise 1.1 What Is Coding?

Instructions: Write the answers to the following questions in the space provided.

1. Define coding. ______________________________
____
____

2. What is the difference between diagnosis coding and procedure coding? ______________________________
____
____

3. List and briefly define the three skills of an "ace" coder. ______________________________
____
____
____

UNDERSTANDING PATIENT ENCOUNTERS

Coders assign diagnosis and procedure codes to a patient encounter (*a specific interaction between a patient and healthcare provider*) after an encounter has been completed. The provider documents the reason(s) for the encounter and the services provided in the patient's medical record. Coders read the medical record and other information the physician provides to identify the main reason for the encounter, any additional reasons for the service, the main service provided, and any additional services provided. The following sections provide an overview of patient encounters with the healthcare system, including the types of encounters and the process of an encounter. This helps coders better understand their role.

Types of Encounters

Patient encounters are generally classified by the location of the encounter because different coding and billing rules apply to each. The two basic types of locations are outpatient and inpatient, which are described next.

Outpatient Encounters

Outpatient encounters are physician interactions with patients who receive services and have not been formally admitted to a healthcare institution, such as an acute-care hospital, long-term care facility, or rehabilitation facility. Patients request outpatient encounters when they have particular health problems, need preventive services, or for follow up or ongoing treatment for known problems. ■ TABLE 1-2 (page 6) lists examples of outpatient encounters.

Inpatient Encounters

Inpatient encounters are physician interactions with patients who have been formally admitted to a healthcare facility, such as an acute-care hospital, long-term care facility, or rehabilitation facility. Patients cannot admit themselves to a facility; a physician must admit a patient for a specific medical reason, which is to either diagnose or treat a health problem. Physicians contract with hospitals for admitting privileges, meaning they have authority to admit patients and care for them in a specific hospital. They write admitting orders, conduct an admitting history and physical, and complete paperwork required by the institution. One physician, usually the one who admits the patient, is the attending physician who oversees and coordinates all aspects of the patient's care while an inpatient. Other physicians also may be involved in the diagnosis or treatment of the patient. A patient may also receive ancillary services, such as laboratory, radiology, or physical therapy, as an inpatient.

The facility codes and bills for the room, board, nursing care, use of the operating room, and most ancillary services. Physicians code and bill for services they person[illegible] provide, such as hospital visits, surgical procedur[illegible] terpretation of laboratory or radiology tests[illegible] company may contract with the facility [illegible] such as radiology or physical thera[illegible] company codes and bills its ow[illegible]

Therefore, coders do no[illegible] to a specific patient. T[illegible] by their employer [illegible] physical ther[illegible] describe [illegible] vices, bu[illegible]

Table 1-2 ■ **EXAMPLES OF OUTPATIENT ENCOUNTERS**

Setting	Purpose	Examples
Ambulatory surgery	Surgical procedure that does not require an overnight stay in the hospital	Tonsillectomy, cataract removal
Cardiology lab	Testing to evaluate a heart problem	EKG, echocardiogram, cardiac catheterization
Diagnostic radiology	Imaging study to evaluate or diagnose a health problem	X-ray, MRI, CT, PET
Emergency department	Treatment of an injury or health problem that cannot be delayed without harm to the patient	Broken leg, chest pain
Laboratory	Specimen collection	Blood draw
Observation	Extended monitoring which may require an overnight stay but does not meet the requirements for a formal inpatient admission	Chest pain
Physical therapy	Treatment of a musculoskeletal problem	Therapeutic exercises, electrical muscle stimulation
Physician office	Evaluation and management of new or existing health problem; preventive care services	Back pain, diabetes check-up, immunization
Therapeutic radiology	Receive a treatment using radiation	Anti-cancer radiation therapy

Steps in the Encounter

While each encounter is unique to the patient's situation, it generally involves three steps: diagnosis, treatment, and documentation.

Diagnosis

When a patient presents to a physician with a health problem, the physician needs to establish a diagnosis. If a diagnosis was established in a previous encounter, the physician reviews the patient's progress and updates the diagnosis. Establishing or updating a diagnosis involves a history, a physical examination, and testing.

History. A physician takes a patient's medical history, which includes questions about current symptoms and past medical problems. Because most symptoms can be caused by several different conditions, the physician asks a series of questions to narrow the possibilities. If a diagnosis was established in a previous encounter, the physician updates the history based on what has hap-ened since the last encounter.

e.

tie ***l Examination.*** The physician conducts a physical or in to further identify and evaluate abnormali- visua ination may focus on a specific body system various he entire body. Examinations include

Testing. hysical touching, and listening to such as bloc y.

s or orders diagnostic tests, sies, and physical function

tests, such as EKGs, based on the patient's situation. In some cases, the patient's condition does not require any tests.

Based on the findings from these sources, the physician identifies the most likely diagnosis and the rationale for it. Depending on the complexity of the problem, the physician may determine the diagnosis in a single encounter or it may take multiple patient encounters and multiple rounds of testing to arrive at a conclusion.

Guided Example of Physician Diagnosis. Refer to the following example throughout this chapter to learn more about patient encounters. The first portion of the example demonstrates how physicians diagnose conditions.

➩ Patient Norman Markowitz, age 41, schedules an office appointment to see Dr. Kristen Conover, a family practice physician, on January 5, due to back pain.

- ❑ Dr. Conover takes a history by asking Mr. Markowitz when the pain started, how severe it is, what makes it better or worse, and if it has occurred before.
- ❑ She performs a physical examination to see if she can detect abnormalities such as tightness, lumps, knots, or protrusions.
- ❑ She asks Mr. Markowitz to perform specific maneuvers, such as standing, sitting, and leaning forward or backward, to determine his physical abilities.

- ❑ She uses a reflex hammer to test his reflexes.
- ❑ She takes an X-ray in the office, which is negative for a fracture.
- ❑ She orders blood tests, which come back negative for arthritis on January 12.
- ❑ She then schedules Mr. Markowitz for an MRI examination on January 17, which reveals a displaced intervertebral disc.

⇨ Next, Dr. Conover will provide a treatment plan.

Treatment Plan

After establishing the diagnosis, the physician formulates a treatment plan. The treatment plan may include medication, surgery, lifestyle changes, or therapy. For complicated problems that take time to diagnose, the physician may treat symptoms to provide relief to the patient until the underlying cause is determined.

Guided Example of a Treatment Plan. Continue with the example of patient Norman Markowitz, who saw Dr. Conover due to back pain, to learn more about the treatment plan.

⇨ Dr. Conover prescribes medication to relieve Mr. Markowitz's back pain while waiting for results of the blood tests and MRI.

- ❑ After she receives the MRI results of a displaced disc, she asks Mr. Markowitz to schedule another appointment for follow up.
- ❑ On January 24, they discuss treatment options and decide to continue medication and refer Mr. Markowitz for physical therapy.
- ❑ They also discuss the possibility of surgery if physical therapy does not provide adequate relief.

⇨ Next, Dr. Conover will document the encounter.

Documentation

After each patient encounter, the physician documents the encounter, recording the reason for the encounter, the diagnostic techniques used, tests or treatments planned, and the overall assessment of the patient. This documentation is the basis from which coders assign diagnostic and procedure codes for each encounter. Coders do not do the following:

- determine what is wrong with the patient
- determine what condition(s) the patient has based on the symptoms
- code for services provided prior to the current encounter
- code for services planned, but not provided during the current encounter
- code for services delivered by other providers
- code for past conditions that are resolved
- code for current conditions that the physician does not document as relevant to the current encounter

When the documentation is unclear, coders do not make assumptions about missing information. They query (*ask*) the physician for clarification and the physician amends (*adds information to*) the medical record, if necessary.

Guided Example of Documentation. Continue with the example of Norman Markowitz, who saw Dr. Conover due to back pain, to learn more about documentation. Sherry Whittle, CPC, is a fictitious certified coder who guides you through documentation and coding.

⇨ Sherry Whittle, CPC, codes for two outpatient encounters for Mr. Markowitz, January 5 and January 24, because those were the two dates that Dr. Conover saw him in the office.

- ❑ For the January 5 encounter, Sherry assigns the ICD-10-CM diagnosis code **M54.5, Low back pain**, because Dr. Conover had not yet determined the cause of the back pain.
- ❑ She assigns CPT procedure codes for the office visit and the X-ray that was performed in the office. (CPT codes are not discussed in this text.)
- ❑ She does not assign procedure codes for the blood test or the MRI because Dr. Conover did not provide those services.

⇨ For the January 24 encounter, Sherry assigns the ICD-10-CM diagnosis code **M51.26, Other intervertebral disc displacement, lumbar region** because Dr. Conover established the diagnosis based on the MRI results.

- ❑ She also assigns a CPT code for the office visit.
- ❑ She does not assign procedure codes for physical therapy because Mr. Markowitz will go to a physical therapy clinic for the service.
- ❑ She does not assign procedure codes for surgery because surgery was not performed.

⇨ Finally, the codes and billing information will be entered into the computer and submitted to the patient's insurance company for payment.

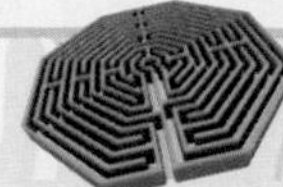

Coding Practice

Now it is your turn to demonstrate your understanding of patient encounters. Try to answer the questions from memory first, then refer back to the information in this section if you need a little extra help.

Exercise 1.2 Understanding Patient Encounters

Instructions: Write the answers to the following questions in the space provided.

1. When do coders assign codes to patient encounters?

____

2. What are the three steps in a patient encounter?

____

____

____

3. What are the three elements involved in establishing a diagnosis? _______________

____

____

CERTIFICATION

Certification is a voluntary achievement that documents that a coder has attained a certain level of proficiency by passing a rigorous examination. Certification is offered by professional organizations and is an additional step beyond a formal educational degree. It does not replace a degree and a degree is not required in order to become certified. Certification began as a form of recognition before there were many educational degrees in this area. Today, certification plus education enhances a coder's professional standing and often results in higher compensation.

Certification is not mandated by the government and is not a legal requirement. Whether or not certification is required, and which certification is acceptable, is determined by individual employers.

Most large clinics and hospitals require coders to be nationally certified. Two primary organizations offer coding certifications that are recognized by most employers: **AAPC** (formerly known as the American Academy of Professional Coders) and the **American Health Information Management Association (AHIMA)**. Both organizations offer several certification credentials, each with a unique focus.

AAPC

Founded in 1988, AAPC has historically focused on physician-based and outpatient coders (■ FIGURE 1-1). Current membership is approximately 111,000 with more than 80,000 holding certification. AAPC has local chapters in many cities which hold monthly meetings, workshops, and provide networking opportunities for members.

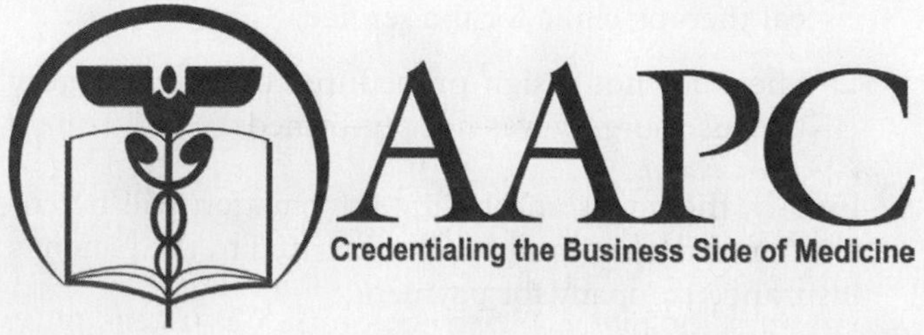

Figure 1-1 ■ AAPC Logo. *Source: AAPC. Reprinted with permission.*

The primary certification is Certified Professional Coder (CPC®), which focuses on coding of services, procedures, and diagnoses for physician offices. The Certified Professional Coder-Hospital (CPC-H®) certification focuses on outpatient hospital services, while the Certified Professional Coder-Payer (CPC-P®) focuses on coding and reimbursement skills needed by **payers** (*insurance companies or public programs that pay for healthcare services*). The Certified Professional Coder-Apprentice (CPC-A®) is earned by coders with less than two years' professional experience. AAPC also offers specialty coding certifications that enable coders to demonstrate superior levels of expertise in a medical specialty, such as orthopedics, obstetrics, or cardiology. Coders take a separate examination to achieve each type of certification.

AHIMA

Founded in 1928, AHIMA has historically focused on hospital coders and has more than 63,000 members. AHIMA has 52 Component State Associations (CSA) that provide professional education and networking opportunities for members.

The primary certification is Certified Coding Specialist (CCS), which focuses on hospital inpatient and outpatient coding. The Certified Coding Specialist-Physician (CCS-P) certification focuses on physician-based coding. The Certified Coding Apprentice (CCA) credential is geared toward entry-level coders with little or no job experience. Additional certifications are offered in more specialized functions such as the administration of privacy and security programs in healthcare organizations; data analysis; and medical records administration. Each type of certification requires coders to take a separate examination.

AHIMA and AAPC certifications are accepted in all states. When considering which certification to pursue, it is helpful to know if one particular credential is preferred over another in the local geographic area. Research this information by reviewing job postings, talking to the human resources department at area employers, and asking experienced coders in the community. As their careers progress, some coders choose to obtain certification in more than one area of expertise, such as physician and inpatient, and may become certified by both AAPC and AHIMA. Refer to the organizations' websites, provided in the Coder's Toolbox at the end of this chapter, to determine the current requirements for earning each certification.

SUCCESS STEP

When you become a member of a local AAPC or AHIMA chapter, you have the opportunity to meet coders in other companies, share helpful information, and potentially learn about job openings.

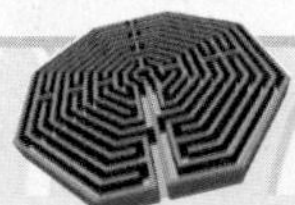

Coding Practice

Now it is your turn to demonstrate your understanding of certification. Try to answer the questions from memory first, then refer back to the information in this section if you need a little extra help.

Exercise 1.3 **Certification**

Instructions: Write the answers to the following questions in the space provided.

1. What is certification?

2. List and define three certifications offered by AAPC.

3. List and define three certifications offered by AHIMA.

CODING CAREERS

Most coding students are seeking a long-term coding career. In addition to learning the mechanics of coding, students are wise to begin learning about their career path and job performance expectations for accuracy and productivity.

Career Path

A **career path** is the progression of jobs and responsibilities throughout one's working life. In coding, like most careers, new graduates do not start at the top; they start at a basic level and work their way up with greater responsibility and more skills at each level. The career options, compensation, and benefits generally increase at each level of advancement. Advancement may come from within the same organization or it may come by moving to a new organization. In order to plan a possible career path, coding students want to learn about the job market, levels of advancement, and internal and external jobs.

Understanding the Job Market

Coders have many career options regarding where they work and what type of job they perform. While many students imagine themselves working in a hospital, the healthcare field offers many other types of organizations as well. Potential employers include all types of healthcare providers, payers, and third-party service organizations such as medical billing services. Sometimes it is best to start out in a small medical or dental office to get basic experience and then move to a larger organization later in your career. Working for a health insurance company or medical billing service can give coders a broad range of experience that will open up many career options later on. ■ TABLE 1-3 (page 10) lists examples of various types of healthcare employers.

There are many job titles in the field of medical coding (■ TABLE 1-4, page 10). The same job might be called by different titles in two different organizations, so it is good to be open minded about potential job titles.

SUCCESS STEP

Some job titles, such as Accounts Receivable or Biller, are also used by non-medical businesses. Even the job title Coder can apply to a computer engineer. When searching job postings, remember to specify a search for the healthcare field.

Table 1-3 ■ **EXAMPLES OF TYPES OF ORGANIZATIONS THAT MAY REQUIRE CODING SKILLS**

❑ Acupuncturist	❑ Medical billing service
❑ Ambulance service	❑ Naturopathic office (ND)
❑ Ambulatory surgery center	❑ Optometrist (OD)
❑ Chiropractic office (DC)	❑ Osteopath (DO)
❑ Clearinghouse	❑ Pharmacy
❑ Consulting firm	❑ Physician office (medical, surgical, all specialties)
❑ Dental office	❑ Physical therapy clinic
❑ Durable Medical Equipment supplier (DME)	❑ Self-insured employer
❑ Health insurance company	❑ Skilled nursing facility
❑ Home healthcare	❑ Temporary staffing agency
❑ Hospital	❑ Third Party Administrator (TPA)
❑ Laboratory	❑ Workers' Compensation

Table 1-4 ■ **EXAMPLES OF JOB TITLES THAT MAY REQUIRE CODING SKILLS**

❑ Accounts Receivable (A/R) Specialist	❑ Insurance Follow Up Specialist
❑ Admitting Clerk	❑ Insurance Verifier
❑ Billing Clerk	❑ Intake Specialist
❑ Charge Entry Specialist	❑ Medical Biller
❑ Claims Analyst	❑ Medical Receptionist
❑ Claims Processor	❑ Medical Records Clerk
❑ Coder I/Coder II	❑ Patient Account Specialist
❑ Coding Assistant	❑ Patient Financial Services Clerk
❑ Electronic Claims Processor	❑ Patient Service Representative
❑ Health Information Analyst	❑ Refund Specialist
❑ Insurance Biller	❑ Scheduler

Levels of Advancement

Most coders look for an **entry-level job** upon graduation in order to gain basic skills, become familiar with the healthcare field, and establish excellent work habits. When possible, coders can look for a job in healthcare that builds on previous experience in a call center, bookkeeping, customer service, or patient care. Some companies offer internships (paid training programs for those new to the field), but this is not the norm.

After a few years of experience at entry level, coders potentially become eligible for advancement to a **mid-level job**. A mid-level job allows coders to expand their skills, learn new specialties, assume more independence, and take on more responsibility.

After five or so years of proven experience, coders can progress to an **advanced-level job**. Advanced-level jobs require a solid track record of good performance in a related area. Advanced-level jobs often include management of others, but may also focus on a specialized area of expertise, such as chart auditing. Technical specialization is an excellent career path for coders who are not interested in supervision or management of others. ■ Table 1-5 shows examples of a coding career path in a physician office, a hospital, and an insurance company.

Internal and External Job Openings

When coders are ready to change jobs and advance their careers, they may seek a new job internally within their current organization, or they may choose to look externally for a job with a different company.

Many organizations post their job openings internally, available only to current employees, for a period of time before they are advertised to the public. This means that established employees can apply for a promotion or transfer to another department but stay with the same company and keep their benefits. Companies like to promote from within because they are already familiar with the employee's personality and work ethic. Therefore, one good career strategy for a coder is to identify a desired employer, secure an entry-level job in that company, perform at a high level, and take advantage of opportunities to move to another job in the same company when ready.

Coders can also move between types of organizations, such as from an insurance company to a doctor's office or hospital. When coders start in a small office that has limited advancement opportunities, they can progress by moving to a larger organization or another small one

Table 1-5 ■ **EXAMPLES OF A CODING CAREER PATH**

	Years of Experience	Physician Office	Hospital	Insurance Company
Entry Level	0–2 years	Front office receptionist Medical records file clerk Charge data entry operator	Admissions representative Cashier Billing office data entry clerk Patient account representative	Member services representative Claims representative trainee Sales assistant
Mid-Level	3–5 years	Coding specialist Insurance verifier Referral coordinator Billing specialist Home-based coder	Outpatient billing clerk Medical documentation researcher Patient accounts team leader Coding assistant	Claims analyst Provider services representative Member services team leader Hospital claims specialist
Advanced Level	More than 5 years	Billing manager Coding manager Chart auditor Collections manager	Chart auditor Medical records manager Inpatient coding specialist Home-based coder Cancer registrar Patient accounts manager	Supervisor, member services Supervisor, claims processing Claims auditor Legal researcher
	Consulting - Freelance coder - Business owner - Trainer - Author - Instructor			

that has an opening at a more advanced level. When they want to gain experience in another aspect of the healthcare industry, they can seek employment with a different type of organization. If an ultimate career goal, such as a hospital coding position, cannot be achieved in the first job, then coders can plan a career path to help get there.

SUCCESS STEP

Joining your local chapter of AAPC or AHIMA will give you the chance to get to know coders in other companies and can potentially lead to future job opportunities. Networking in this manner is an important part of your career path.

Performance Expectations

Whatever career path coders choose, or even if they are not sure where they want to end up, it is always important to demonstrate excellent job attendance, follow directions, and meet the employer's expectations for quantity and quality of work. Every job task is an opportunity to earn a good reference, and it is those recommendations that help coders get to the next step in their careers.

Performance expectations are the outcomes employers need coders to achieve in order to demonstrate competence in the job. Coding jobs have high expectations because securing payment for services from insurance companies requires a high degree of accuracy and productivity by coders. Most employers have expectations related to coding accuracy and productivity.

Coding Accuracy

Coding accuracy involves the three coding skills discussed earlier in this chapter: abstracting, assigning, and arranging (sequencing). The average expectation for coding accuracy in these three areas is 95% to 98%. New coders' work is reviewed by a mentor or supervisor until they achieve the required level of accuracy. Samples of all coders' work are reviewed by supervisors and peers on an ongoing basis to ensure that everyone maintains a high level of accuracy. High accuracy is required to be eligible for greater responsibility, advancement, or special benefits such as working from home.

Productivity

Not only is accuracy critical to a coder's job, high productivity (the amount of work accomplished in a specified timeframe) is also necessary. Productivity skills include keyboarding and case production, which are discussed next.

Keyboarding. Most coders use computers to determine or enter the codes. Therefore, high levels of speed and accuracy in keyboarding are essential. Coders must be proficient in alphanumeric (a combination of letters and numbers) keyboarding because most codes contain both letters and numbers. Many employers require that coders pass a keyboarding test before they schedule a job interview. Each employer sets its own speed requirement; 30 to 40 words per minute (wpm) or 9,000 to 12,000 keystrokes per hour (ksph) are common minimums. In keyboarding, any errors are deducted from the overall speed, so it is best to work on accuracy first, and then build up speed after the basics are mastered. With daily keyboarding drills, most students can achieve this minimum level in six months or less.

Case Production. Most coders are expected meet a **case production** standard to code a specific number of cases each day, while maintaining high accuracy. The specific production standard is based on the type of record being coded; whether coders are assigning diagnosis codes, procedure codes, or both; whether coders work from paper or electronic charts; and what other responsibilities, such as billing, coders do at the same time. For example, coders who specialize in radiology coding generally code more encounters per hour than coders who specialize in complex surgical procedures because the records they are coding from are far less complicated.

Table 1-6 ■ **EXAMPLES OF CASE PRODUCTION STANDARDS**

Specialty	Charts per Hour
Emergency Department	10–30
Inpatient Hospital	4–10
Laboratory	100–200
Radiology	100–200
Surgery	1–8

■ TABLE 1-6 provides examples of case production standards. Students do not achieve these production standards while learning, but such standards are common in the workplace.

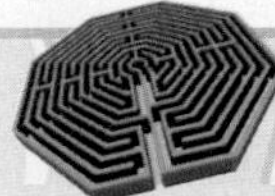

Coding Practice

Now it is your turn to demonstrate your understanding of coding careers. Try to answer the questions from memory first, then refer back to the information in this section if you need a little extra help.

Exercise 1.4 Coding Careers

Instructions: Write the answers to the following questions in the space provided.

1. List five types of organizations that may require coding skills. ____________________
2. Why do coding jobs have high performance expectations? ____________________
3. What keyboarding speed rate is commonly required by employers? ____________________

CHAPTER SUMMARY

In this chapter you learned that:

- Coding is the process of accurately assigning codes to verbal descriptions of patients' conditions and the healthcare services provided to treat those conditions.
- The three skills of an ace coder are abstracting, assigning, and arranging.
- Coders assign diagnosis and procedure codes to patient encounters after an encounter is completed.
- Certification is a voluntary achievement that documents a coder having attained a certain level of proficiency by passing a rigorous examination offered by AAPC or AHIMA.
- Students are wise to learn about their career path and job performance expectations for accuracy and productivity.

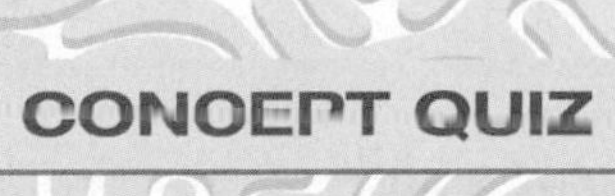

CONCEPT QUIZ

Take a moment to look back at your trip through this chapter and solidify your skills. This is your opportunity to pull together everything you have learned.

Completion

Instructions: Write the term that answers each question based on the information you learned in this chapter. Choose from the following list. Some choices may be used more than once and some choices may not be used at all. Refer to the discussion in this chapter and the Glossary at the end of this book if you need a little extra help.

abstract	diagnosis
accuracy	inpatient
amend	keyboarding
ancillary	outpatient
arrange	procedure
assign	production
assume	query
attending	testing
career path	treatment
code	

1. _______________ codes describe patient illnesses, diseases, conditions, injuries, or other reasons for seeking healthcare services.
2. The three skills of an "ace" coder are to _______________ information from the medical record; _______________ the accurate code number; and _______________ the codes in proper order.
3. _______________ encounters are physician interactions with patients who have not been formally admitted to a healthcare institution, such as an acute care hospital, long-term care facility, or rehabilitation facility.
4. _______________ encounters are physician interactions with patients who have been formally admitted to a healthcare facility, such as an acute care hospital, long-term care facility, or rehabilitation facility.
5. _______________ services include laboratory, radiology, or physical therapy.
6. The _______________ physician oversees and coordinates all aspects of the patient's care.
7. A _______________ is the progression of jobs and responsibilities throughout one's working life.
8. The _______________ plan may include medication, surgery, lifestyle changes, or therapy.
9. When the documentation is unclear, coders _______________ the physician for clarification.
10. Most coders are expected meet a case _______________ standard to code a specific number of cases each day, while maintaining high _______________.

Multiple Choice

Instructions: Circle the letter of the best answer to each question based on the information you learned in this chapter. Refer to the discussion in this chapter and the Glossary at the end of this book if you need a little extra help.

1. The replacement code set used for diagnosis coding is
   A. HCPCS.
   B. ICD-9-CM Volume 2.
   C. ICD-10-CM.
   D. ICD-10-PCS.
2. _______ is the replacement code set that is used for hospital inpatient procedure coding.
   A. CDT
   B. CPT
   C. ICD-9-CM
   D. ICD-10-PCS
3. Which of the following is NOT a HIPAA-mandated code set?
   A. ICD-10-CM
   B. DSM-IV
   C. CDT
   D. NDC
4. A specific interaction between a patient and healthcare provider is an
   A. admission.
   B. office visit.
   C. observation.
   D. encounter.
5. Which of the following is NOT an example of an outpatient encounter?
   A. Ambulatory surgery
   B. Hospital admission
   C. Emergency department
   D. Observation

6. Coders do which of the following tasks?
   A. Determine what condition(s) the patient has based on the symptoms.
   B. Assign diagnostic and procedure codes for patient encounters after an encounter is completed.
   C. Code for services planned, but not provided, during the current encounter.
   D. Code for past conditions that are resolved.
7. Which statement about certification is NOT true?
   A. All states legally mandate coder certification.
   B. Certification is a voluntary achievement.
   C. Professional organizations offer certification.
   D. Coders have a choice of which certification to pursue.
8. Most coders look for a (an) _________ job upon graduation in order to gain basic skills, become familiar with the healthcare field, and establish excellent work habits.
   A. hospital
   B. entry-level
   C. mid-level
   D. advanced-level
9. _________ is an example of an entry-level job.
   A. Data Entry Clerk
   B. Insurance Verifier
   C. Inpatient Coding Specialist
   D. Coding Assistant
10. Many organizations post their job openings _________, available only to current employees, for a period of time before they are advertised to the public.
    A. internally
    B. externally
    C. online
    D. confidentially

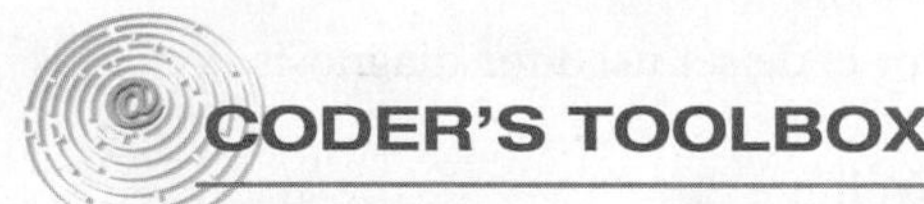

CODER'S TOOLBOX

The following resources are a starting point for learning more about the coding field. The > symbol indicates a menu selection within the website in order to navigate to a specific page.

AAPC What is Medical Coding? **http://www.aapc.com/resources/medical-coding/index.aspx**

American Health Information Management Association (AHIMA) > Medical Coding **http://www.ahima.org/coding/**

American Hospital Association (AHA) > What Is Coding? **http://www.ahacentraloffice.com/ahacentraloffice/shtml/what_is_coding.shtml**

Career Builder.com Health Care Jobs **http://health-care.careerbuilder.com/?sc_cmp2=JS_Home_SD_HC&siteid=ppc_BRD_cb_SL_HC**

Centers for Medicare and Medicaid (CMS) > Code Sets **http://www.cms.gov/TransactionCodeSetsStands/05_CodeSets.asp#TopOfPage**

Centers for Medicare and Medicaid (CMS) > Coding > ICD-10 **http://www.cms.gov/ICD10/**

Medical Billing and Coding > Remote Medical Coding Jobs **http://www.medicalbillingandmedicalcoding.com/remotemedicalcodingjobs.html**

Simply Hired **http://www.simplyhired.com/a/jobs/list/q-medical+coder**

Rapid Typing Zone **http://www.rapidtyping.com/**

Typing Web **http://www.typingweb.com/**

2

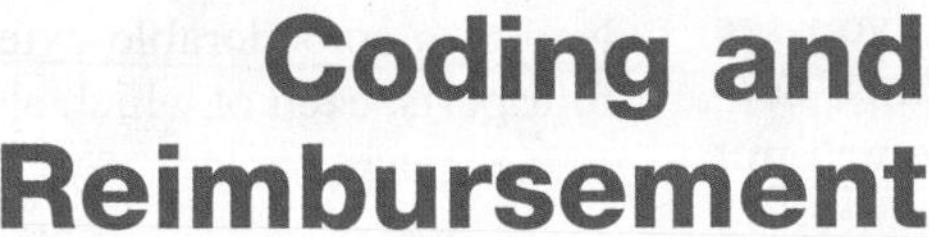

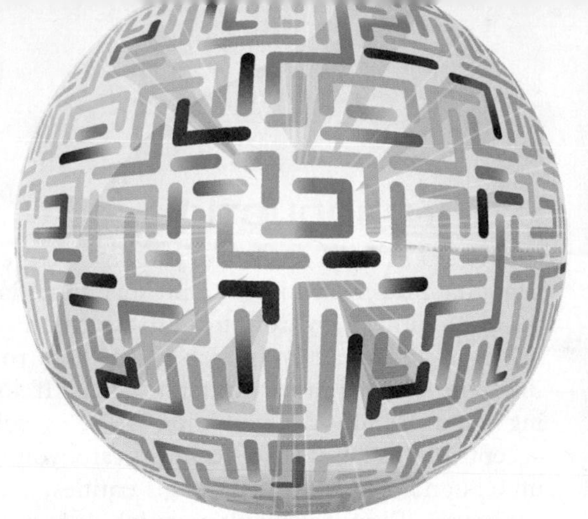

Coding and Reimbursement

Learning Objectives

After completing this chapter, you should have the skills to:

- Spell and define the key words, medical terms, and abbreviations relating to reimbursement.
- Define the types of healthcare payers.
- Discuss the importance and content of documentation.
- Describe the life cycle of an insurance claim.
- Explain the federal compliance initiatives.

Key Terms and Abbreviations

abuse
audit
automatic adjudication
beneficiaries
Centers for Medicare and Medicaid Services (CMS)
clean claims
compliance
denied
Department of Health and Human Services (DHHS)
documentation
entitlement programs
explanation of benefits (EOB)
False Claims Act (FCA)
fraud
front-end edit check
group health plan
individual health insurance
managed care plans
manual review
Medicaid (MCD)
medical necessity
medical payments
medical record
medical review
Medicare (MCR)
Medicare Administrative Contractors (MAC)
Medicare Advantage
Medigap
Office of the Inspector General (OIG)
Original Medicare
overcoding
Part A
Part B
Part C
Part D
personal injury protection (PIP)
preferred providers
private health insurance
progress notes
prompt pay
Qui Tam
reconcile
Recovery Audit Contractor (RAC)
rejected claim
self-insured health plans
State Children's Health Insurance Program (SCHIP)
supplementary medical insurance (SMI)
suspended
third-party administrator (TPA)
third-party payers
Tricare (TC)
Veteran Health Administration (VHA)
whistleblower
workers' compensation (WC)

In addition to the key terms listed here, students should know the terms defined within tables in this chapter.

Chapter Outline

- **Healthcare Payers**
- **Documentation**
- **Life Cycle of an Insurance Claim**
- **Federal Compliance**

ICD-10-CM codes in this chapter are from the ICD-10-CM 2014 Draft code set from the Department of Health and Human Services, Centers for Disease Control and Prevention.

ICD-10-PCS codes in this chapter are from the ICD-10-PCS 2014 Draft code set from the Department of Health and Human Services, Centers for Medicare and Medicaid Services.

All data regarding national health expenditures in this chapter are from the Centers for Medicare and Medicaid Services, Office of the Actuary, National Health Statistics Group, National Health Expenditures Levels, 2009.

INTRODUCTION

When you go on a road trip, you know there are driving laws that you need to obey and that some laws, such as the speed limit, vary from town to town and state to state. Even on an interstate, which is a federal road, you see different speed limits in different areas. If you miss seeing a speed limit sign, you know the state police will not accept that as an excuse. In healthcare, you also need to understand the rules of different entities, such as different payers. Even if your ultimate job does not directly involve billing, you still want to have a basic understanding of how your work as coder impacts reimbursement so you can become a valuable team member.

HEALTHCARE PAYERS

Third-party payers are entities other than the patient or physician who pay for healthcare services. They reimburse physicians and hospitals for 86% of all healthcare services in the United States. Patients pay the remaining 14% of services directly. Third-party payers include several government programs, over 1,300 private insurance companies, workers' compensation, and automobile med pay insurance. Coders need to understand the various types of third-party payers because each has separate, and sometimes conflicting, rules about coding and billing.

All healthcare payments to hospitals, physicians, and other providers are based on coding. Procedure codes describe what services were provided to patients. Physicians and hospitals assign money charges to each procedure code. Diagnosis codes justify why the services were needed. When the diagnosis code(s) does not adequately explain why the services were provided, payment may be denied or delayed.

Government Programs

Health benefit plans funded by federal or state governments pay for 47% of healthcare services. These are entitlement programs for which beneficiaries (*recipients of services*) qualify based on specific criteria. The various types of government and private insurance programs are summarized in the following sections.

Medicare

Medicare (MCR), established in 1965, is funded by the federal government and is the single largest payer of healthcare services in the United States, accounting for 24% of healthcare payments. Medicare is administered by the Centers for Medicare and Medicaid Services (CMS), which is a division of the Department of Health and Human Services (DHHS). Medicare pays for healthcare services for most people age 65 and over, people of any age with end stage renal disease (ESRD), and people with disabilities. Because it is so large, Medicare has a tremendous impact on healthcare policy and payment trends, and by extension, on coding. Other government programs and private health insurance are not required to follow Medicare rules, but it is not unusual for them to follow Medicare's lead to a considerable extent. The Medicare program has four parts, each of which also has separate rules and coding guidelines.

Part A. Medicare Part A, also called Original Medicare or traditional Medicare, is hospital insurance that covers a specific list of services for inpatient hospital care, skilled nursing facilities, hospice, and home healthcare. Most Americans who have worked as an adult, or are married to someone who has, are automatically eligible for Part A and do not pay a premium to receive benefits. They do pay deductibles and coinsurance.

Part B. Medicare Part B, also called supplementary medical insurance (SMI), covers a specific list of physician services, outpatient hospital care, and home healthcare. It was created to provide medical coverage in addition to the hospital coverage of Part A. Part B is optional and most people are required to pay a premium to enroll, as well as deductibles and coinsurance.

Medicare Part A and Part B claims are processed by private companies called Medicare Administrative Contractors (MAC). Many Medicare coding and billing rules are the same across the country, but MACs have latitude in how certain policies are interpreted and applied. Therefore, coders need to keep up to date on the national rules, as well as the MAC rules.

Part C. Medicare Part C, also called Medicare Advantage, is an optional replacement of Part A and Part B which is offered by private health insurance companies. Many Part C plans are managed care and often have a preferred or required network of providers. Private insurance companies are paid through contracts with Medicare and believe they can provide care more cost effectively than traditional Medicare, thus making a profit. Patients choose Part C when they believe they can receive more benefits for the same or slightly more cost. The amount of premium, deductible, and coinsurance varies with each plan offered by a private company.

Part D. Medicare Part D, also called prescription drug coverage, is offered by private insurance companies through contracts with Medicare and provides limited benefits for prescription drugs. Patients choose from a variety of private plans, each of which may cover different medications, and select the one that covers the majority of their most costly prescriptions. Patients pay premiums, deductibles, and coinsurance. According to Medicare, most Part C plans also include Part D.

Medigap. Medigap is a Medicare supplement insurance policy sold by private insurance companies to fill gaps in Part A and Part B coverage. In most states, patients choose from ten standardized plans labeled Plan A through Plan J. Medigap policies apply only to Original Medicare, not Part C.

CODING CAUTION

Do not confuse Medigap, which is called *Medicare supplement*, with Part B, which is called *supplementary medical insurance*. Part B is supplementary, or additional, to Part A. Medigap is a supplement, or add-on, for both Part A and Part B.

Medicaid

Medicaid (MCD), also established in 1965, is a program for low-income families that is funded two-thirds by the federal government and one-third by state governments. It accounts for 18% of national healthcare payments. CMS establishes the general plan requirements, but states have considerable latitude in determining eligibility and coverage rules. Billing and coding requirements are also determined and administered by each state.

Other Government Programs

Other government programs include:

- Tricare (TC)—health insurance coverage for family members of active duty personnel and for retired military personnel and their families.
- State Children's Health Insurance Program (SCHIP)—established in 1997 by the federal government to provide health insurance to children in families with incomes below 200% of the federal poverty level.
- Veteran Health Administration (VHA)—an integrated healthcare delivery system with more than 1,400 sites of care, including hospitals, community clinics, community living centers, and various other facilities to provide health services to veterans with service-connected disabilities.

Private Health Insurance

Private health insurance is coverage for healthcare services offered by private corporations, such as Aetna, Cigna, or UnitedHealthcare, and not-for-profit organizations, such as Blue Cross and Blue Shield. Private health insurance pays for 39% of national healthcare expenses. The three major sources of private health insurance are group health plans, self-insured plans, and individual insurance. Each insurance company and each plan offered by a company may have different requirements for coding and billing. Typically, the provider's coding and billing departments maintain files on the requirements of each plan. Most laws regarding private health insurance companies are determined by each state's legislature and implemented by the state Department of Insurance.

Group Health Plans

Approximately 60% of Americans are covered by a group health plan offered through their employer or union. The employer or union contracts with a private insurance company to provide a specific list of benefits to its employees. Often, they negotiate more than one option, each with a different set of benefits and different costs. The advantage of a group health plan is that the risk (cost of medical care) is shared by a large number of people resulting in lower premiums.

Employees choose which plan they want to enroll in based on its benefits and costs. Typically the employer pays the majority of the monthly premium and deducts a smaller portion of the premium, such as 10% or 20%, from employees' paychecks. Usually employees can cover their family members for an additional cost. In addition, employees pay deductibles and coinsurance or copays for the actual services they receive.

Self-Insured Health Plans

Self-insured health plans are offered by large employers or unions who, rather than purchasing group health insurance, set aside money in a reserve fund and pay for employees' medical expenses from the fund. States regulate how much money employers must set aside in order to ensure that they will have enough money to pay catastrophic (high cost) medical expenses.

In all other respects, a self-insured plan works similarly to a group health plan in that a specific list of benefits is covered, and, typically, employees pay a small monthly premium, deductibles, coinsurance, and copayments for medical care received. Often claims are processed by a private company called a third-party administrator (TPA).

Individual Health Insurance

Individual health insurance is a plan that people purchase directly from a health insurance company, such as those who are self-employed or do not have benefits through an employer or government program. Approximately 9% of Americans are covered by individual health insurance.

Workers' Compensation

Workers' compensation (WC) plans pay for medical costs due to employment-related injuries or illnesses. Each state establishes its own requirements for WC insurance, but must comply with federal minimums. WC may be offered by private insurance companies approved by the state, large companies who self-insure, or a statewide insurance pool. Employers pay insurance premiums to cover the costs of care injured employees receive. Federal government employees are covered by federal WC plans.

WC programs are not subject to HIPAA regulations because they do not qualify as a health insurance plan. However, states have separate privacy and security rules that govern WC. WC plans may have unique coding and billing requirements, such as their own private code sets. Coding departments need to maintain a file containing these unique requirements.

Automobile Insurance

Automobile insurance policies often include medical payments (med pay) coverage or personal injury protection (PIP), which pays for medical expenses incurred during an automobile accident. Automobile insurance is regulated by each state's Department of Insurance, not by federal or HIPAA laws that govern health insurance companies. Auto insurance companies often contract with external bill review companies to review medical claims and recommend payment amounts. Coders need to be aware of any special requirements for patients being treated for automobile accident injuries. Typically the coding or billing department maintains a file detailing these requirements for each company.

Managed Care Plans

Managed care plans are companies that attempt to control the cost of healthcare while providing better outcomes. There are many different forms of managed care, but, in general, managed care plans contract with physicians, hospitals, and other providers to offer services for a lower fee than health plans; then they contract with private health insurance companies and self-insured plans to promote an exclusive network of preferred providers. When patients use preferred providers, they are responsible for lower out-of-pocket costs for deductibles, coinsurance, and copayments than if they select a provider not on the preferred list. Managed care plans are not a separate type of insurance, but rather a way of offering services to patients who are enrolled in a group health plan, self-insured plan, or individual health plan. Managed care plans also offer services to Medicare Part C programs, Medicaid, and even WC. Managed care companies are regulated primarily by federal laws. Well-known managed care plans include Kaiser Permanente, Group Health of Seattle, WellPoint, and Humana.

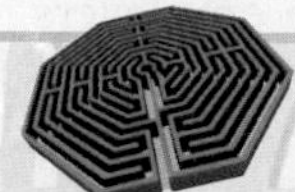

Coding Practice

Now it is your turn to demonstrate your understanding of healthcare payers. Try to answer the questions from memory first, then refer back to the information in this section if you need a little extra help.

Exercise 2.1 Healthcare Payers

Instructions: Write the answers to the following questions in the space provided.

1. Medicare pays for healthcare services for whom?

____

2. Medicaid pays for healthcare services for whom?

____

3. What are the three types of private health insurance plans? ______________________________

____

____

DOCUMENTATION

Payers have freedom to determine what services they will include in an insurance policy, but they also have a contractual obligation to pay for these services. To fulfill this obligation they may request information to determine whether the service is covered, including the site (location) of service; the medical need for and appropriateness of the diagnostic and therapeutic services provided; and the accuracy of codes for services billed on the claim based on the medical record.

Medical Necessity

The fact that a physician determines a patient needs a particular service or supply item does not mean that the insurance company or payer will agree. Medical necessity (*establishing the medical need for services*) is one of several criteria payers use to determine if, and how much, they will pay for a particular service. One of the reasons that payers establish medical necessity rules is to avoid paying unscrupulous providers who might provide a service just so they could receive payments, not because the patient

Table 2-1 ■ **EXAMPLES OF MEDICAL NECESSITY CRITERIA**

Criterion	Appropriate Example	Inappropriate Example
Improve a patient's condition	Physical therapy to treat an acute back injury	Ongoing physical therapy to maintain general back comfort
Evidence-based practice	Medications proven to benefit patients based on scientific studies	Experimental drugs or treatments
Rendered by appropriate provider	Patient going to internal medicine or family practice physician to diagnose an initial symptom stomach pain	Patient going directly to gastroenterologist and having many expensive tests performed to diagnose an initial symptom of stomach pain
Least-restrictive setting	Suture removal in physician office; outpatient cataract surgery	Suture removal in the emergency department; inpatient cataract surgery without a medical reason
Not for patient or physician convenience	Liposuction for medical reasons	Liposuction for cosmetic reasons

actually needs the service or would benefit from it. It also helps prevent patients from demanding services they do not need, such as expensive tests or cosmetic surgery.

Each of the payers discussed earlier in this chapter establishes its own definition of medical necessity and writes it into each insurance policy. ■ TABLE 2-1 lists common criteria for medical necessity and examples of each. By law, Medicare can pay only for services that are medically necessary, which is defined as services and supplies that

- are needed to diagnose or treat a medical condition or improve the functioning of a malformed body member;
- meet the standards of good medical practice in the local area; and
- are not mainly for the convenience of the patient or physician.

In addition to a general definition of medical necessity, payers may also establish criteria for specific conditions, such as limiting the number of physical therapy visits for back pain; requiring an X-ray before ordering a more expensive MRI; or restricting the age and frequency of preventive screening, such as a screening mammogram every two years for women over age 50. When providers recommend a treatment that varies from the insurance company's standard list, they may need to obtain preauthorization and provide special reports to justify the service. For some conditions, specific medical necessity criteria are not public information and patients may learn of them only after a claim is denied (*the claim was processed and found to be ineligible for payment*).

Coders should not manipulate codes in a way that distorts or alters the diagnoses and procedures as documented in the medical record. This is unethical and fraudulent. Coders do need to be certain they are accurately describing everything that was done for the patient and the reasons for which the services were provided.

The Medical Record

The medical record is the comprehensive collection of all information on a patient at a particular facility. A medical record may be paper based or electronic and provides a written, chronological record of the patient's care, including important facts, findings, and observations about an individual's health history and health status (■ FIGURE 2-1, below, and ■ FIGURE 2-2, page 20). It reports past and present illnesses, examinations, tests, treatments, and outcomes and is a legal document that verifies the care provided. The diagnosis and procedure codes reported on the health insurance claim form or billing statement must be supported by information in the medical record for each encounter. Patients have separate medical records with each physician they see and each facility to which they are admitted.

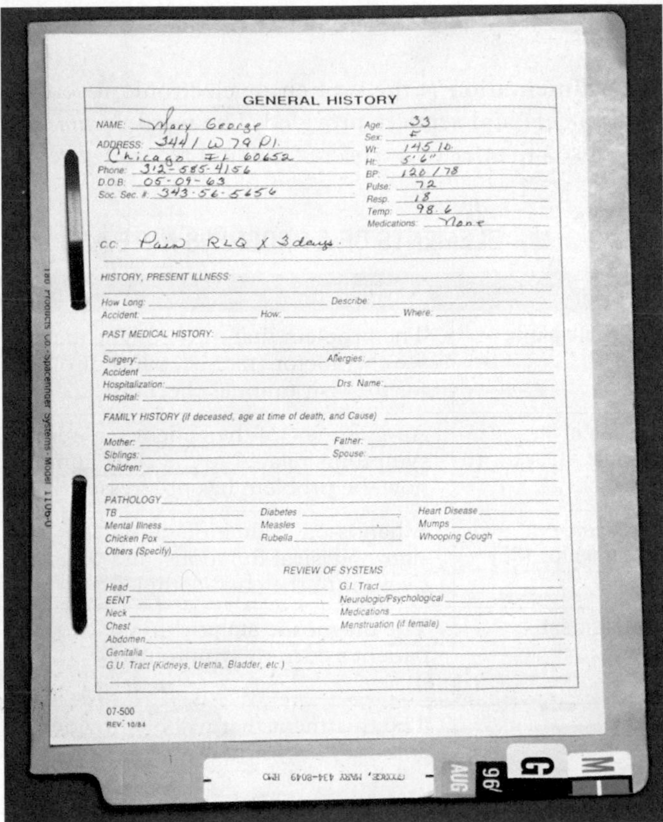

GENERAL HISTORY

NAME: Mary George
ADDRESS: 3441 W 79 Pl. Chicago Il 60652
Phone: 312-585-4156
D.O.B.: 05-09-63
Soc. Sec. #: 343-56-5656
Age: 33
Sex: F
Wt: 145 lb.
Ht: 5'6"
BP: 120/78
Pulse: 72
Resp.: 18
Temp: 98.6
Medications: None

C.C.: Pain RLQ X 3 days.

HISTORY, PRESENT ILLNESS:
How Long: Describe:
Accident: How: Where:

PAST MEDICAL HISTORY:
Surgery: Allergies:
Accident
Hospitalization: Drs. Name:
Hospital:

FAMILY HISTORY (if deceased, age at time of death, and Cause)
Mother: Father:
Siblings: Spouse:
Children:

PATHOLOGY
TB Diabetes Heart Disease
Mental Illness Measles Mumps
Chicken Pox Rubella Whooping Cough
Others (Specify)

REVIEW OF SYSTEMS
Head G.I. Tract
EENT Neurologic/Psychological
Neck Medications
Chest Menstruation (if female)
Abdomen
Genitalia
G.U. Tract (Kidneys, Uretha, Bladder, etc.)

07-500
REV. 10/84

Figure 2-1 ■ Example of a Paper-Based Medical Record

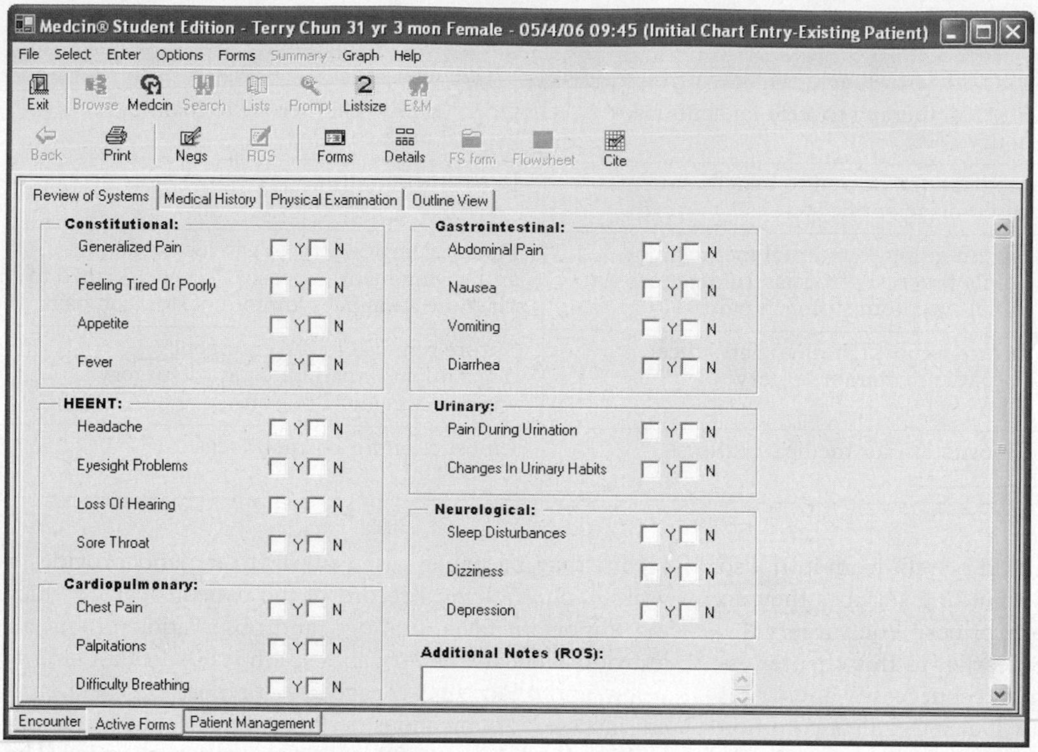

Figure 2-2 ■ Example of an Electronic Medical Record. *Source: Reprinted with permission of Medicomp, Inc.*

SUCCESS STEP

The medical record is admissible in a court of law as evidence and must be handled with the same care as any legal document.

Documentation is the written or electronic record of medical care and services provided. The word *documentation* is used to refer to the overall medical record as well as to **progress notes** (*the record of a specific patient encounter*). Thorough documentation is necessary, not only because it is the basis for delivering high-quality patient care, but also because it helps improve reimbursement. Excellent documentation can reduce the amount of time needed to code a claim, result in more accurate and complete coding, and minimize common problems associated with claims processing. ■ TABLE 2-2 shows major elements of a progress note and how coders use each type of information.

■ TABLE 2-3 shows major elements of a medical record and how coders use each type of information.

Table 2-2 ■ ELEMENTS OF A PROGRESS NOTE AND THEIR USE IN CODING

Element	Description	ICD-10-CM/PCS Application
Chief complaint (CC)	The problem that has brought the patient to see the doctor (nausea, pain) or other reason for the visit (annual checkup)	Code for symptoms if physician does not make a definitive diagnosis for an outpatient encounter.
History of the present illness (HPI)	An interview of the patient regarding symptoms related to the chief complaint and how the problem has progressed	May add details to the diagnostic statement.
Physical examination (PE)	A hands-on evaluation of patient's vital signs, physical functions, and organ systems relevant to the chief complaint	May add details to the diagnostic statement.
Assessment	The diagnostic statement; the cause of the patient's current symptoms	This is the starting point for assigning diagnosis codes. Verify the details using other areas of the medical record when necessary.
Plan	The treatment that will be provided to address the symptoms	Inpatient hospitals code for procedures performed during the stay. Do not code for future planned treatments. (Outpatient hospitals and physicians use CPT codes.)

Table 2-3 ■ **ELEMENTS OF A MEDICAL RECORD AND THEIR USE IN CODING**

Element	Description	ICD-10-CM/PCS Application
Progress notes	Description of specific encounters with the patient	Code each patient encounter based on the progress notes for that visit.
Obstetric history	Prior pregnancies, complications, and their outcomes	Use specific codes for first pregnancy, previous multiple pregnancies, and history of certain complications.
Surgical history	Date and type of past operations, operative reports (a narrative of exactly how the surgeon performed the procedure)	Assign codes for acquired absence (surgical removal) of certain organs. When an operation is performed during the current encounter, review the operative report to determine the exact procedure performed and the post-operative diagnosis.
Medications and medical allergies	Current and past medications; allergies to specific medications	Code for long-term use of certain medications.
Family history	The health status of immediate family members, causes of death (if known), diseases common in the family	Assign codes for family history of certain conditions.
Social history	Education, occupation, religious affiliation, natural support network, lifestyle habits (tobacco, alcohol, illicit drug use, sexual activity)	Assign codes for certain lifestyle habits.
Immunization history	Date and type of past vaccinations, titers (blood tests proving immunity to a specific disease)	Do not code for past vaccinations.
Lab test/Pathology results	Reports from lab tests; report from pathology regarding specimen testing	Code abnormal test results only when the physician indicates significance and makes no certain diagnosis. Review pathology reports for biopsy results (malignant neoplasm).
Ancillary reports	Narrative reports or copies of reports from additional services such as EKGs, imaging	Code abnormal results only when the physician indicates significance and makes no certain diagnosis.

Coding Practice

Now it is your turn to demonstrate your understanding of documentation. Try to answer the questions from memory first, then refer back to the information in this section if you need a little extra help.

Exercise 2.2 Documentation

Instructions: Write the answers to the following questions in the space provided.

1. What is medical necessity? ______________________

____

2. List three examples of medical necessity criteria.

____

____

____

3. What is the difference between the medical record and progress notes? ______________________

____

____

LIFE CYCLE OF AN INSURANCE CLAIM

There are many steps involved in converting a patient encounter into a paid insurance claim. Each step needs to be completed in a timely and accurate manner in order for providers to receive correct payment for their services. The exact procedures are not the same in every office and every hospital, but the general process is similar.

Before the Encounter

The life cycle of an insurance claim begins when the patient calls the physician to make an appointment, a patient arrives at the emergency department, or a physician admits a patient to the hospital. Although providers do not code or bill for scheduling an appointment, the appointment begins when providers begin collecting insurance information. When time allows, patients pre-register by completing paperwork regarding their health condition and insurance prior to the appointment. The provider verifies eligibility with the insurance company through a telephone call or secure website in order to determine if the patient is covered by insurance and what services are covered and/or require preauthorization.

During the Encounter

When patients arrive for their appointment or hospital admission, they complete registration forms or confirm the pre-registration information, provide a copy of their insurance card, and possibly make a payment, if required by the insurance. They see the physician and/or receive the treatments and procedures needed. The physician documents the patient's problem in a progress note and may check off services and diagnoses on an encounter form or charge slip. Finally, patients check out, schedule the next appointment, if needed, and may make a payment if they did not pay before they saw the physician.

After the Encounter

After the encounter is complete, the specific steps for coding and billing depend on how the encounter is recorded. In a physician's office that uses encounter forms, the physician will have already checked off the services and diagnoses for the visit. The encounter form is given to the billing department for data entry into the computer. If no encounter form is used, the chart is given to the coding department where a coder reviews the progress note, assigns diagnosis and procedure codes, and enters the codes into the computer. The billing department verifies that all information for the encounter is complete. Usually the computer system automatically inserts the charges for each procedure entered by the coder, so billers also verify that all charges are present and accurate. When they have completed their verifications, billers flag the claim in the computer as ready to be submitted to the insurance company. Most offices transmit claims electronically, usually daily or weekly depending on the volume of claims. Small offices may print out claims on paper billing forms and mail them, but this is becoming less common.

At the Insurance Company

When payers receive electronic claims, the computer system first performs a **front-end edit check**, which scans the claims for valid data including the policy number, patient name, provider number, diagnosis codes, and procedure codes. If any data was entered incorrectly by the biller or coder, such as a nonexistent code number or policy number, the computer automatically rejects the claim. A **rejected claim** is one that is not accepted into the insurance company's computer system for processing due to missing or invalid data. Providers may learn of rejected claims through an electronic or paper report. However, sometimes they may not know the claim was rejected until they notice that payment was never received. Claims submitted on paper billing forms are scanned in or data entered by the insurance company, then also go through the front-end edit.

Clean claims are those that pass the front-end edit checks and have no missing or invalid information. Most clean claims are processed using **automatic adjudication**, a process in which the computer automatically determines which procedure codes are covered, calculates how much the insurance company is obligated to pay, then triggers the payment. Medicare is required to pay clean claims within 14 days of receipt. Many private payers also pay clean claims within a few days of receipt.

The payment may be sent to the provider either electronically or on a paper check. The insurance company also sends an **explanation of benefits (EOB)**, a statement that lists all the services the provider billed, which ones were accepted for payment, how much the insurance company will pay, how much the patient owes, and how much will not be paid. If there are any services that are not eligible to be paid, the statement lists the reasons.

Some claims are **suspended** from the automatic process for **manual review**. Reasons that claims are suspended include the following:

- claims with high dollar amounts
- specific diagnoses and procedures that the payer may wish to monitor
- medical necessity review
- illogical information, such as a patient gender or age that does not match the codes
- questions about the patient's enrollment status
- any other reason the payer may want to research.

A claims analyst reviews the claim, determines if more information is needed from the provider or patient, and

Table 2-4 ■ **CODING PROBLEMS CAUSING REJECTED OR DENIED CLAIMS**

Problem	Example
Characters in a code are mistyped, creating an invalid code.	Diagnosis code **007.0** instead of **O07.0** (number *zero* instead of letter *Oh*) PCS code **0J533ZZ** instead of **0J553ZZ**
Codes have too many or too few characters.	Diagnosis code **T20.511** instead of **T20.511A** Diagnosis code **O68.10** instead of **O68.1**
Diagnosis does not match the procedure.	Diagnosis code **K28.0 Acute gastrojejunal ulcer with hemorrhage** with a procedure code for removal of gallbladder. This may happen when the code was mistyped and should have been **K82.0 Obstruction of gallbladder.**
Codes are sequenced incorrectly.	Diagnosis codes **M36.1 Arthroplasty in neoplastic disease** and **C91.A0 Mature B-cell leukemia Burkitt type not having achieved remission**. An instructional note with code M36.1 instructs the coder to "Code first underlying neoplasm."
Additional codes required by the Guidelines or Instructional Notes are missing.	Diagnosis code **I69.891 Dysphagia following other cerebrovascular disease** instructs coder to "Use additional code to identify the type of dysphagia."
Patient gender does not match the diagnosis or procedure.	Patient gender mistakenly entered as Male for a patient receiving obstetric services
Patient age does not match the diagnosis or procedure.	Diagnosis code **O09.611 Supervision of young primigravida, first trimester** used for 18 year old, but the code is defined as younger than age 16 at expected date of delivery.

sends a letter if needed. Sometimes the claims analyst may have medical questions about the claim, such as if the procedure was appropriate for the diagnosis or if all of the services were medically necessary. These claims are sent to the **medical review** department where a nurse, physician, or other clinician investigates the situation. They also may send a letter to the provider or patient requesting additional information or copies of documentation.

Clean claims may be processed within a few days of receipt, but claims that require manual review may take several weeks. Most states have **prompt pay** laws that require insurance companies to process claims within a specific period of time, such as 30 or 45 days. If the claim cannot be processed due to missing or incorrect information, insurance companies must issue any inquiry letters to providers or patients within this timeframe.

After Insurance Processing

After the payer has processed the claim, the provider receives a check or electronic deposit and an EOB. Depending on the sophistication of the provider's computer system, the payment may be automatically posted to the patient's account or a person may need to manually enter it into the computer or manual bookkeeping system. The biller or payment poster **reconciles** the EOB. They compare the EOB to the original bill to verify that each service billed was paid in the amount expected.

If payment was denied for one service or for the entire claim, an accounts receivable specialist needs to investigate the reason. Usually the reason is stated on the EOB, but the specialist may need to call the insurance company for clarification. Solutions may involve obtaining additional information from the patient, asking the coding department to review the documentation and the codes assigned, or providing copies of documentation. ■ TABLE 2-4 gives examples of coding problems that may cause claim rejections or denials. The provider needs to respond to insurance company inquiries quickly because any delay by the provider adds to the time it takes to receive payment. A new prompt payment period begins when the payer receives the requested information.

SUCCESS STEP

A student intern or new coder can bring immense value to an organization by offering to follow up on problem and unpaid claims. Positive financial results are almost always seen on neglected claims that are reactivated. In addition, new coders can learn a tremendous amount about coding and the payment process by doing insurance follow-up.

After all insurance payments are received and follow-up is complete, the office sends the patient a bill for any deductible, coinsurance, or patient-responsibility amounts that have not been paid.

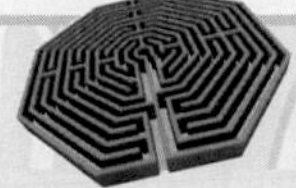

Coding Practice

Now it is your turn to demonstrate your understanding of the life cycle of an insurance claim. Try to answer the questions from memory first, then refer back to the information in this section if you need a little extra help.

Exercise 2.3 Life Cycle of an Insurance Claim

Instructions: Write the answers to the following questions in the space provided.

1. Why does the life cycle of an insurance claim begin when the patient calls the physician to make an appointment?
____
____
____

2. Define automatic adjudication.
____
____
____
____

3. List three coding problems that cause rejected or denied claims. ______________________________
____
____
____
____

FEDERAL COMPLIANCE

Not getting paid or being underpaid is not the worst impact on a provider from improper coding or billing. The worst impact is being overpaid. When providers are overpaid they are legally obligated to report the overpayment to Medicare, to refund the money, and possibly even pay interest on it.

In this era of electronic transmissions, it is much easier for payers to track patterns of billing, compare a physician to the average or norm, and target providers who deviate from the norm. If the insurance company or Medicare detects a pattern of overpayments due to **overcoding** (*coding for a more complex diagnosis or procedure than is documented*) or improper billing, they can conduct an **audit** (*an investigation of the provider's billing and coding practices*). Going through an audit is time consuming and costly, but if violations are found, severe financial penalties, loss of Medicare privileges, and even imprisonment are possible.

This should not scare coders, but make them aware of the importance of their role and the need for accuracy. Medicare places the responsibility for knowing the rules on providers (and by extension their coders). Medicare's stance is that once they publish a rule, providers should know about it and follow it.

CODING CAUTION

You already know that if an officer stops you for speeding, the excuse "I didn't see the sign" will not get you very far. It is the same with Medicare. They expect you to know and follow a multitude of rules, and the rules are usually less clear and less obvious than a speed limit sign on the side of the road.

Violating coding and billing rules can be classified as fraud or abuse. **Fraud** is knowingly billing for services that were never given or billing for a service that has a higher reimbursement than the service actually provided. **Abuse** is mistakenly accepting payment for items or services that should not be paid for by Medicare, due to improper coding and billing practices. Examples are billing for a non-covered service, assigning a more costly code to a lesser service, or coding in a way that does not follow national or local coding guidelines.

Compliance simply means following the rules. Healthcare providers must follow rules established by multiple federal, state, and country government agencies. Some rules are specific to healthcare and others pertain to any type of business. Companies and organizations establish compliance programs to actively keep informed about regulations, educate employees, and make sure that everyone in the company is cooperating. Investigation of fraud and abuse is primarily the responsibility of the Office of the Inspector General (OIG) and Recovery Audit Contractors (RAC).

Office of the Inspector General

While HIPAA is best known for its privacy rules and healthcare transaction standards, it also created several programs to further control fraud and abuse in healthcare. One of these provisions increased the amount of money the **Office of the Inspector General (OIG)** could spend to investigate fraud and abuse. It also increased the penalties for violations. The OIG is a division of DHHS that investigates fraud, abuse, and other noncompliance matters in the Medicare and Medicaid programs. As a result, healthcare fraud and abuse investigations have become a major focus, and a highly profitable one, for the government. The Health Care Fraud and Abuse Control (HCFAC) program's *Annual Report for Fiscal Year 2010* reports a three-year rolling average return on investment of $6.80 recouped for every dollar spent on enforcement activities. Over four billion dollars was recouped during fiscal year 2010 alone. OIG accomplishes its mission through the False Claims Act (FCA) and compliance programs, which are discussed next.

False Claims Act

OIG uses the False Claims Act (FCA) as the basis for much of its investigation and prosecution. FCA imposes penalties on individuals and companies who defraud government programs. It was passed in 1863, during the Civil War, to combat widespread fraud in which contractors sold the government faulty rifles and ammunition, rotten food, and sick horses. The Qui Tam provision of FCA includes a financial reward to whistleblowers, those who turn in violators. FCA has been updated several times, including 1986, 2009, and 2010.

Knowingly submitting a bill to a government healthcare program, such as Medicare, that contains incorrect codes is considered to be presenting a false claim for payment because the provider is requesting payment for a service that was not provided. If the same coding or billing error is made repeatedly, it can be considered fraud because the provider is responsible to know all the rules about how services should be billed and coded. FCA is interpreted in a broad sense to include not only intentional misrepresentation, but also errors made from ignorance. Medicare providers and their staff are obligated to know all the Medicare rules.

Compliance Programs

Also as a result of HIPAA, OIG began promoting voluntary compliance programs for the healthcare industry. OIG provided guidance to assist healthcare entities to develop effective internal controls to help them be aware of and follow the requirements of federal, state, and private health plans. The OIG believes that healthcare institutions that adopt and implement compliance programs significantly reduce fraud, abuse, and waste. Therefore, investigators tend to be more lenient with organizations that have implemented a voluntary compliance plan. The OIG issued sample compliance programs, which include seven major characteristics:

1. Develop and distribute written standards of conduct, policies, and procedures that address specific areas of potential fraud.
2. Designate a high-level manger to be the chief compliance officer who oversees compliance activities.
3. Develop and implement education and training for employees.
4. Establish a process for reporting exceptions.
5. Develop an internal system to respond to accusations or reports of improper activities, and implement disciplinary measures when appropriate.
6. Develop of an audit and monitoring system.
7. Investigate and correct system-wide problems and develop policies regarding employment or retention of sanctioned individuals.

The Patient Protection and Affordable Care Act (PPACA), passed in 2010, mandates compliance programs for providers who contract with Medicare, Medicaid, and SCHIP. The timeline for defining and implementing compliance programs has not yet been established. This rule places the greatest burden on smaller healthcare providers who never established a voluntary compliance program because now they will have to establish one in order to continue serving Medicare patients.

Recovery Audit Contractor

In the Tax Relief and Health Care Act of 2006, Congress required a permanent and national Recovery Audit Contractor (RAC) program to be in place by January 1, 2010. The national RAC program uses independent contractors to identify improper Medicare payments to healthcare providers and suppliers made on claims of healthcare services provided to Medicare beneficiaries. Improper payments may be overpayments or underpayments. Overpayments can occur when healthcare providers submit claims that do not meet Medicare's coding or medical necessity policies. Underpayments can occur when healthcare providers submit claims for a simple procedure but the medical record reveals that a more complicated procedure was actually performed. Healthcare providers that might be reviewed include hospitals, physician practices, nursing homes, home health agencies, durable medical equipment suppliers and any other provider or supplier that bills Medicare Parts A and B.

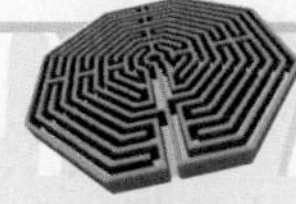

Coding Practice

Now it is your turn to demonstrate your understanding of federal compliance. Try to answer the questions from memory first, then refer back to the information in this section if you need a little extra help.

Exercise 2.4 Federal Compliance

Instructions: Write the answers to the following questions in the space provided.

1. What are the potential consequences of receiving an overpayment from Medicare? ______________________

____

____

____

____

(*continued*)

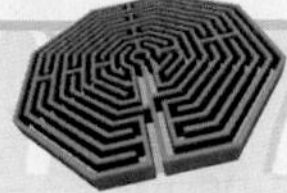

Coding Practice (continued)

2. Define overcoding. ______________________________
____
____

3. What law, passed in 1863, is the basis for much of OIG's investigation and prosecution? ______________
____

CHAPTER SUMMARY

In this chapter you learned that:

- Third-party payers reimburse physicians and hospitals for 86% of all healthcare services in the United States. Coders need to understand the different types of third-party payers because each has separate, and sometimes conflicting, rules about coding and billing.
- To fulfill their contractual obligations, payers may request information to verify whether the service is covered, including the site (location) of service; the medical need for and appropriateness of the diagnostic and therapeutic services provided; and the accuracy of codes for services billed on the claim based on the medical record.
- Each step in the life cycle of an insurance claim must be completed in a timely and accurate manner in order for providers to receive correct payment for their services.
- When providers are overpaid they are legally obligated to report the overpayment to Medicare, to refund the money, and possibly even pay interest on it.

CONCEPT QUIZ

Take a moment to look back at your trip through this chapter and solidify your skills. This is your opportunity to pull together everything you have learned. Refer to the discussion in this chapter and the Glossary at the end of this book if you need a little extra help.

Completion

Instructions: Write the term that answers each question based on the information you learned in this chapter. Choose from the following list. Some choices may be used more than once and some choices may not be used at all.

abuse	medical record	progress notes
compliance	Medigap	RCA
EOB	OIG	social history
family history	Part A	TC
FCA	Part B	VHA
fraud	Part C	
medical necessity	Part D	

1. ______________ is hospital insurance that covers a specific list of services for inpatient hospital care, skilled nursing facilities, hospice, and home healthcare.
2. ______________ is a Medicare supplement insurance policy sold by private insurance companies to fill gaps in Part A and Part B coverage.
3. ______________ is health insurance coverage for family members of active duty personnel and for retired military personnel and their families.
4. ______________ is the health status of immediate family members, causes of death (if known), and diseases common in the family.
5. Each patient encounter is coded based on the ______________ for that visit.
6. The ______________ is a statement that lists all the services the provider billed, which ones were accepted for payment, how much the insurance company will pay, how much the patient owes, and how much will not be paid.
7. ______________ is knowingly billing for services that were never given or billing for a service that has a higher reimbursement than the service provided.

8. _______________ is mistakenly accepting payment for items or services that should not be paid for by Medicare.
9. _______________ investigates fraud, abuse, and other noncompliance matters in the Medicare and Medicaid programs.
10. The OIG issued sample _______________ programs, which include seven major characteristics.

Multiple Choice

Instructions: Circle the letter of the best answer to each question based on the information you learned in this chapter. Refer to the discussion in this chapter if you need a little extra help.

1. Med pay or personal injury protection from automobile insurance policies is regulated by
   A. each state's Department of Insurance.
   B. HIPAA.
   C. CMS.
   D. each state's Department of Transportation.
2. ________ is funded two-thirds by the federal government and one-third by state governments.
   A. Medicare
   B. Medicaid
   C. Workers' compensation
   D. Self-insured health plan
3. An example of the medical necessity criterion evidence-based practice is
   A. suture removal in the emergency department.
   B. liposuction for medical reasons.
   C. a patient going to internal medicine or family practice physician to diagnose an initial symptom stomach pain.
   D. medications proven to benefit patients based on scientific studies.
4. The provider verifies eligibility with the insurance company
   A. before the encounter.
   B. during the encounter.
   C. after the encounter.
   D. after insurance company processing.
5. The chart is given to the coding department where a coder reviews the progress note, assigns diagnosis and procedure codes, and enters the codes into the computer
   A. during the encounter.
   B. after the encounter.
   C. at the insurance company.
   D. after insurance company processing.
6. The computer system first performs a front-end edit check
   A. during the encounter.
   B. after the encounter.
   C. at the insurance company.
   D. after insurance company processing.
7. Which of the following is NOT a coding problem that causes rejected or denied claims?
   A. The patient's insurance has expired.
   B. Characters in a code are mistyped, creating an invalid code.
   C. The diagnosis does not match the procedure.
   D. Additional codes required by the Guidelines or Instructional Notes are missing.
8. Knowingly submitting a bill to a government healthcare program, such as Medicare, that contains incorrect codes is considered to be presenting a
   A. medical necessity.
   B. denial.
   C. false claim.
   D. EOB.
9. The Patient Protection and Affordable Care Act (PPACA), passed in 2010, mandates ________ for providers who contract with Medicare, Medicaid, and SCHIP.
   A. front-end edit checks
   B. independent contractors
   C. compliance programs
   D. fraud and abuse
10. The RAC program uses ________ to identify Medicare overpayments and underpayments to healthcare providers and suppliers.
    A. front-end edit checks
    B. independent contractors
    C. compliance programs
    D. HIPAA

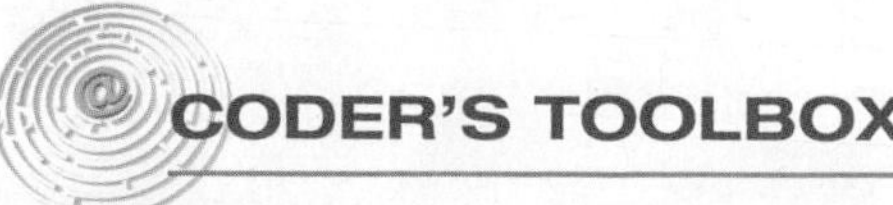

CODER'S TOOLBOX

The following resources are a starting point for learning more about coding and reimbursement.

America's Health Insurance Plans http://www.ahip.org/

Centers for Medicare and Medicaid http://www.cms.gov/

Health Care Compliance Association www.hcca-info.org

Office of the Inspector General (OIG) http://oig.hhs.gov/

Tricare http://www.tricare.mil/

Veteran Health Administration http://www.va.gov/health/aboutVHA.asp

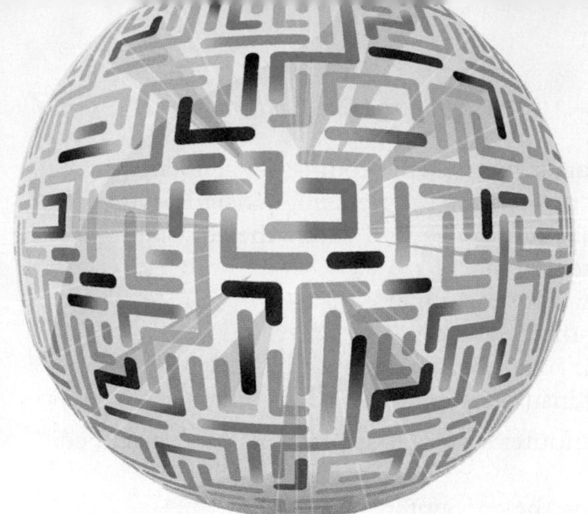

3

The Transition to ICD-10-CM/PCS

Learning Objectives

After completing this chapter, you should have the skills to:

- Spell and define the key words, medical terms, and abbreviations related to the transition to ICD-10-CM/PCS.
- Describe the history of ICD-10-CM/PCS.
- Provide an overview of the transition process.
- Discuss the impact of ICD-10-CM/PCS on healthcare information systems.
- Discuss the impact of ICD-10-CM/PCS on medical providers.
- Discuss the impact of ICD-10-CM/PCS on medical coders.

Key Terms and Abbreviations

Accredited Standards Committee (ASC) X12N Version 4010
Accredited Standards Committee (ASC) X12N Version 5010
CM
final rule
General Equivalence Mappings (GEMs)
granular
healthcare administrators
International Classification of Diseases, 10th Revision (ICD-10)
morbidity
Mortality
National Center for Health Statistics (NCHS)
PCS
transaction standards

In addition to the key terms listed here, students should know the terms defined within tables in this chapter.

Chapter Outline

- **History of ICD-10-CM/PCS**
- **Overview of the Transition Process**
- **Impact on Healthcare Information Systems**
- **Impact on Medical Providers**
- **Impact on Medical Coders**

ICD-10-CM codes in this chapter are from the ICD-10-CM 2014 Draft code set from the Department of Health and Human Services, Centers for Disease Control and Prevention.

ICD-10-PCS codes in this chapter are from the ICD-10-PCS 2014 Draft code set from the Department of Health and Human Services, Centers for Medicare and Medicaid Services.

INTRODUCTION

Have you ever driven down a road you have been on hundreds of times, only to find out that the route has changed and now you have to go a new way? As disconcerting as this may be, you soon learn the new route and come to appreciate the improvements. The healthcare industry is facing its own "re-routing" with the implementation of ICD-10-CM/PCS. For those who have worked with the old system for years, this transition may be disruptive and unnerving; those new to coding may wonder what all the fuss is about. This chapter helps you understand the reasons the change is being made, the enormity of its impact, and how to prepare for and adapt to the new environment.

HISTORY OF ICD-10-CM/PCS

The International Classification of Diseases, 10th Revision, Clinical Modification (ICD-10-CM or CM), used for diagnosis coding, and the International Classification of Diseases, 10th Revision, Procedure Coding System (ICD-10-PCS or PCS), used for procedure coding, are two separate and distinct systems that were developed by different groups. ICD-10-CM is based on ICD-10, developed by the World Health Organization (WHO) for worldwide use. ICD-10-PCS was developed by the Centers for Medicare and Medicaid (CMS) for use in the United States only. As a result, even though both code sets are called "ICD-10" and are implemented at the same time in the United States, they serve different purposes, use different and sometimes opposite conventions, and follow different guidelines. Understanding the differences in how the systems developed will help clarify their different purposes.

SUCCESS STEP

When speaking of ICD-10-CM/PCS, coding professionals often use the shorthand CM to refer to ICD-10-CM and the shorthand PCS to refer to ICD-10-PCS.

Background of ICD-10-CM

ICD-10-CM is an update and major revision to the ICD-9-CM, which has been used in the United States since 1979 for diagnosis reporting. **The International Classification of Diseases, 10th Revision (ICD-10)**, without the Clinical Modification (CM) designation, is a worldwide reporting system developed by WHO for classifying epidemiological (study of diseases in large populations) and **mortality** (*causes of death*) data. After its first full release in 1994, the system was gradually adopted by over 130 countries internationally.

The United States **National Center for Health Statistics** (NCHS) adapted and expanded ICD-10 to focus on **morbidity** (*causes of disease and illness*) in the United States. This adaptation has the phrase Clinical Modification attached to the name, creating the full name International Classification of Diseases, 10th Revision, Clinical Modification (ICD-10-CM or CM). The code set provides diagnoses for tracking and billing of patient encounters and uses terminology and detail consistent with medical practice in the United States. All modifications in ICD-10-CM must conform to WHO conventions for ICD-10. The United States has used ICD-10-CM for coding and classification of mortality data from death certificates since January 1, 1999.

Countries such as Canada and Australia have already successfully implemented ICD-10 in hospitals, but these countries do not use it in outpatient settings as the United States does. The United States' version of ICD-10 diagnosis codes is much more **granular** (*detailed*) than it is in other nations. The United States' version contains approximately 68,000 codes, compared to about 16,000 codes in the Canadian version and about 22,000 in the Australian version. ICD-10-CM is also more detailed than ICD-9-CM, which contained approximately 16,000 codes.

ICD-10-CM applies to all providers, such as hospitals, physicians, skilled nursing facilities, rehabilitation facilities, and home health agencies; payers, such as private insurance companies and government Medicare and Medicaid programs; and other HIPAA-covered entities, such as software vendors, clearinghouses, and third-party billing services.

In January 2009, CMS issued two **final rules** (*a legally required notice of final regulations which is published in the* **Federal Register**) for replacing the 30-year-old ICD-9-CM code set with ICD-10-CM/PCS. The first rule specified the compliance date for mandatory use of ICD-10-CM/PCS as October 1, 2013. In 2012, DHHS announced that it intended to reevaluate the implementation date. (As this text went to press, no changes had been announced. Refer to **www.cms.gov/ICD10** for current details.)

The second rule updated the HIPAA **transaction standards** (*programming specifications*) so software accommodates the use of the ICD-10-CM/PCS code sets. The compliance date for the second rule was January 1, 2012. Transaction standards are discussed in detail later in this chapter.

The coding process for ICD-10-CM is very similar to that of ICD-9-CM, although the organization of the manual, th format of codes, and some guidelines are different.

Background of ICD-10-PCS

ICD-10-PCS was developed by CMS f States in inpatient hospital setting

in other countries. ICD-10-PCS replaces ICD-9-CM Volume 3 procedure codes hospitals used since 1979. HIPAA requires that outpatient hospitals and physicians use Current Procedural Terminology (CPT) codes for billing. Some states may require that hospitals use ICD-10-PCS in outpatient settings, such as the emergency department, outpatient radiology, and outpatient surgery, for tracking and statistical purposes only.

ICD-9-CM contained Volume 3 for inpatient procedure codes, but ICD-10-CM does not contain any procedure codes. ICD-10-PCS is a separate system that CMS developed through a contract with 3M Health Information Systems. PCS was initially published in 1998 and has been updated annually since then. ICD-10-PCS contains over 70,000 codes compared to approximately 3,000 codes in ICD-9-CM Volume 3. ICD-10-PCS coding manual organization, code format, definitions, and guidelines are completely different from ICD-9-CM Volume 3 procedure codes and from CPT procedure codes.

PCS applies to all inpatient hospitals, including acute care hospitals, psychiatric facilities, and rehabilitation facilities; payers, such as private insurance companies and government Medicare and Medicaid programs; and other HIPAA-covered entities, such as software vendors, clearinghouses, and third-party billing services.

Benefits of ICD-10-CM/PCS

CMS and the American Health Information Management Association (AHIMA) identify numerous benefits that are expected to result from ICD-10-CM/PCS:

- Codes more accurately describe patient conditions and procedures, reducing the need for attachments to claims.
- Codes provide more detailed and higher quality data for tracking quality, safety, and effectiveness of health services.
- After users become familiar with the new system, it is expected to save time and money.
- Consistency across codes and more specific code descriptions helps reduce coding errors.
- Combined with the increased use of electronic medical records, the new code sets provide more consistent and more detailed data for physician use.
- Advancements in technology and medical practice are reflected in the organization and description of codes.
- The coding system in the United States becomes more consistent with that used in other countries.
- Public officials can better track and respond to domestic and international public health threats.
- The structure of the new code sets allows room to add codes, as needed, in the future.

Coding Practice

Now it is your turn to demonstrate your understanding of the history of ICD-10-CM/PCS. Try to answer the questions from memory first, then refer back to the information in this section if you need a little extra help.

Exercise 3.1 **History of ICD-10-CM/PCS**

Instructions: Write the answers to the following questions in the space provided.

1. What date did the 2009 final rule establish as the [illegible] date for ICD-10-CM/PCS? ____________

____

2. Name three benefits of ICD-10-CM/PCS.

____

____

____

____

3. ICD-10-PCS was developed for use by what type of provider? ____________

____

____

[illegible] THE TRANSITION

[illegible] ICD-9-CM to ICD-10- [illegible] priorities and expen- [illegible] ding changes impact many more parts of organizations than other recent changes, such as implementation of the national provider identifier (NPI) in 2005. While previous changes primarily impacted transactions with external partners, the ICD-10-CM/PCS transition impacts providers' internal operations as well.

All covered entities are affected. Everyone who is part of the healthcare system or uses its data is impacted, including providers, payers, regulators, vendors, claims clearinghouses, medical billing services, researchers, educational institutions, and support staff in each of these settings. All computer systems that collect, transmit, receive, or store diagnostic data need updating due to the expanded length, format, and structure of codes. These changes further impact the budgets of organizations and the productivity of workers.

Fortunately, patients are minimally affected because the code set is generally transparent to (unseen by) patients. However, it is likely that overall processing times may be longer at the beginning of the transition as users get used to the new systems and work out all the bugs. This may affect patients indirectly because others are taking longer to send bills, make payments, and answer questions.

Reasons for Change

The reason that the transition from ICD-9-CM to ICD-10-CM/PCS is such a major undertaking is because of the many differences between the two systems. This chapter discusses overall differences between the code sets. Some of the major differences include the following:

- ICD-10-CM/PCS contain many times the number of codes as their ICD-9-CM counterparts. This requires established coders to learn a more detailed coding process. It also requires that computer system capacity be upgraded.
- The length of diagnosis codes increased from three to five characters in ICD-9-CM to a length of three to seven characters in ICD-10-CM. Procedure codes increased from three or four characters in ICD-10-CM Volume 3 to seven characters in ICD-10-PCS. This required changes to all computer software that uses codes to accommodate a longer field size.
- Code structure changed from primarily numeric in ICD-9-CM (except for V and E codes) to all codes being alphanumeric in ICD-10-CM. This required changes to all computer software that uses codes to accept both numbers and letters for every code.
- Code formats were added in ICD-10-CM to include seventh-character extensions to describe particular circumstance. This requires established coders to learn new skills.
- ICD-10-CM terminology and disease classifications were updated to be consistent with current clinical practice. ICD-10-PCS provides unique definitions for procedures. This requires coders to learn and apply new terminology.
- ICD-10-CM codes describe greater levels of clinical detail and specificity that may have been described by a single code in ICD-9-CM. This requires established coders to learn a more detailed coding process.
- ICD-10-CM contains more combination codes that describe multiple related conditions with a single code. ICD-10-PCS requires more multiple coding than ICD-10-CM Volume 3 because most procedural combination codes were eliminated. Both of these changes require that established coders relearn certain coding rules and guidelines.

Preparing for the Change

When ICD-10 was implemented in countries such as Canada and Australia, the national, provincial, and local governments paid for software upgrades and staff training. In the United States, the costs are borne individually by each hospital, physician, and health plan. Experience in other countries demonstrated that the change requires a significant investment of time and money. Healthcare providers in other countries experienced decreased productivity for many months following the change. It is critical that healthcare organizations prepare with the information and tools they need to streamline the change process.

Healthcare administrators are the individuals in each healthcare organization responsible for managing the organization, including the transition to ICD-10-CM/PCS. This includes physicians who own their own practices as well as their managers. Administrators also include hospital and health plan managers. Others responsible for the ICD-10-CM/PCS transition include managers for clinical areas such as laboratory, radiology, and pharmacy; information systems; finance, including billing and coding; quality assurance; compliance; and public health. CMS and professional organizations published numerous rules and time schedules to aid providers in the transition. Administrators must adapt these guidelines to their own organization to ensure that the organization is able to make the transition to ICD-10-CM/PCS in a timely manner.

Planning for ICD-10-CM/PCS transition began several years in advance of implementation, in order to analyze systems; update administrative processes; coordinate activities with clearinghouses, billing services, and pay[illegible] reprint encounter forms; train staff; and establish budg[illegible] these activities. The overall process to plan for, i[illegible] and monitor the ICD-10-CM/PCS transiti[illegible] approximately five years.

The remainder of this chapter discus[illegible] on information systems, providers, [illegible]

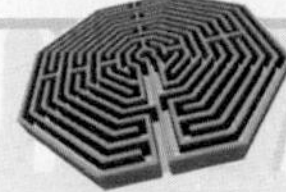

Coding Practice

Now it is your turn to demonstrate your understanding of the overview of the transition process. Try to answer the questions from memory first, then refer back to the information in this section if you need a little extra help.

Exercise 3.2 Overview of the Transition Process

Instructions: Write the answers to the following questions in the space provided.

1. What are the two final rules which were published in the Federal Register in January 2009?

____

____

2. List three examples of healthcare administrators.

____

____

____

____

3. Name three major differences between ICD-9-CM and ICD-10-CM/PCS.

____

____

____

IMPACT ON HEALTHCARE INFORMATION SYSTEMS

One of the greatest impacts of ICD-10-CM/PCS within a healthcare organization is the impact on healthcare information systems. Typically an organization has more than one electronic information system that is affected. These may include scheduling, patient registration, medical records, billing, coding, payment posting, quality, and compliance reporting (■ FIGURE 3-1). In large organizations, multiple departments are affected including laboratory, pharmacy, radiology, medical records, quality assurance, and finance. Reporting to external federal and state regulators is affected, including reporting of adverse drug events, medical devices, pay for performance, research, public health, and newborn screening. Contracts with health plans and payers with provisions related to specific diagnoses or inpatient procedures also need to be reviewed and modified to incorporate the new diagnosis codes.

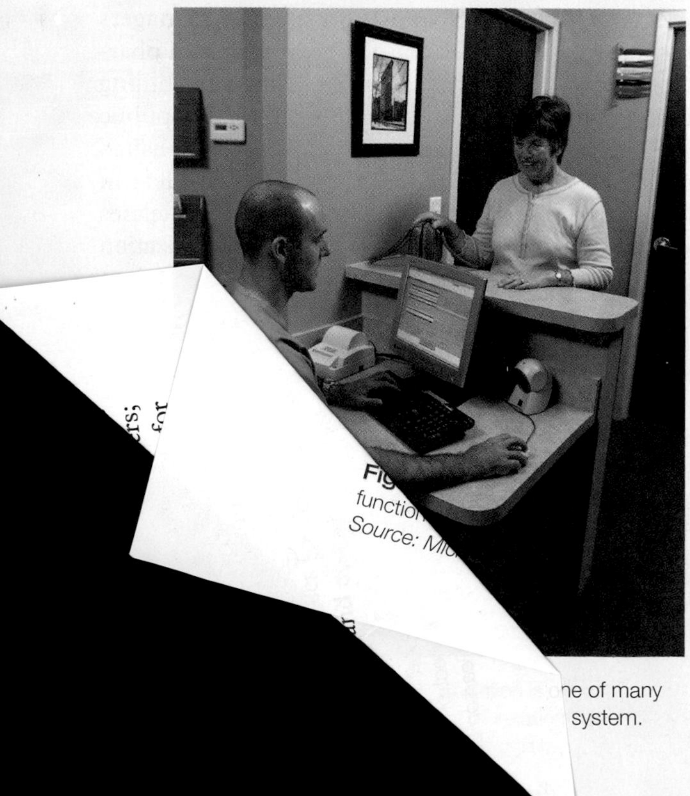

Fi... functio... Source: Mi... ne of many ... system.

Prior to ICD-10-CM/PCS the healthcare industry used an electronic transaction standard called **Accredited Standards Committee (ASC) X12N Version 4010**. This standard lacked all the functions needed, so **Accredited Standards Committee (ASC) X12N Version 5010** was developed. Version 5010 is the revised set of HIPAA transaction standards adopted to replace the current Version 4010 standards. Five types of transaction standards required updating:

- claims, encounter, and payment information
- coordination of benefits
- eligibility for a health plan
- referrals
- non-HIPAA mandated formats for Medicare Fee-for-Service (FFS)

The overall transition process from Version 4010 to Version 5010 required three years to accomplish. Providers were required to use Version 5010 on or after January 1, 2012, for HIPAA-mandated transactions. After a short grace period, electronic transactions not compliant with Version 5010 were subject to rejection. Each type of transaction required separate complex programming changes in Version 5010, such as the following:

- Modify field sizes to accommodate the longer codes.
- Change data type of fields from primarily numeric to completely alphanumeric for every character.

- Add a new field as a version indicator to distinguish between ICD-9-CM and ICD-10-CM/PCS codes.
- Increase the number of diagnosis codes allowed on a claim.
- Implement detailed rules to improve the explanations of claim corrections, reversals, recoupment of payments, and the processing of refunds.

These changes affected providers, payers, and vendors such as software companies, clearinghouses, and third-party billing services. All of these organizations needed to update their systems. In addition, they needed to communicate and work together to ensure that all parties were making the needed changes on schedule.

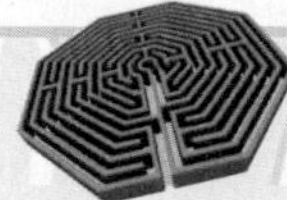

Coding Practice

Now it is your turn to demonstrate your understanding of the impact of ICD-10-CM/PCS transition on healthcare information systems. Try to answer the questions from memory first, then refer back to the information in this section if you need a little extra help.

Exercise 3.3 Impact on Healthcare Information Systems

Instructions: Write the answers to the following questions in the space provided.

1. Name the five types of electronic transactions that require updating in the Version 5010 standard. ____________________
2. What is Version 5010 and when is it mandatory? ____________________
3. Name three programming changes that Version 5010 implements. ____________________

IMPACT ON MEDICAL PROVIDERS

Physicians who own their own practices experience all the impacts to operations and budgets described earlier in this chapter:

- They are responsible for implementing the impacts on information systems.
- They need to make sure the coders they employ receive adequate training.
- They need to ensure that their own medical documentation provides the additional level of specificity needed under ICD-10-CM/PCS.
- Providers who personally assign some or all diagnostic codes themselves also need to learn the coding guidelines for ICD-10-CM.
- They must accomplish all of these changes while continuing to maintain a high patient load.

This section focuses on the specific impacts on providers' internal operations in three areas: documentation, scheduling, and treatment plans.

Impact on Documentation

One of the most concerning aspects of ICD-10-CM/PCS implementation that directly affects all clinical provid ers is the potential for increased quantity and det documentation. Because ICD-10-CM/PCS prov a greater level of granularity and specificity, pr responsible to ensure that their document the required information. Certainly a ch nitude is expected to cause a tempora ity while physicians and other cli new requirements. However, m may be permanent, such as detail. This requiremen consumes additional time each and every time a provider documents a patient encounter, even after the provider has adjusted to the initial changes.

To determine the need for documentation improvements, hospitals as well as physician practices conduct studies that evaluate random samples of various types of medical records. They determine if the documentation contains the required level of detail in new coding systems. Then they identify documentation weaknesses in order to develop a priority list of specific diagnoses and procedures that require more detail or other changes.

Physicians who perform inpatient hospital procedures need to learn about new documentation requirements for PCS in addition to CM. Recall that hospitals use PCS codes to report the facility portion of inpatient procedures that physicians perform. Even though physician offices do not report PCS codes, physicians' hospital documentation must provide the required information for hospital PCS coders. ■ TABLE 3-1 provides examples of documentation changes needed for ICD-10-CM/PCS.

Table 3-1 ■ EXAMPLES OF DOCUMENTATION CHANGES UNDER ICD-10-CM/PCS

Category	Example
Laterality	Conditions and procedures that relate to paired body parts, such as eyes, ears, and all extremities, contain laterality in both CM and PCS.
Genetic diagnoses	ICD-9-CM has one code for Down syndrome but in ICD-10-CM, the codes for Down syndrome require genetic testing results to identify the specific type of Down (meiotic nondisjunction, mitotic nondisjunction, or translocation).
Medical history	Lifestyle habits such as alcohol, tobacco, and drug abuse and dependence are required as additional codes with many diagnoses. Postmenopausal osteoporosis requires documentation of current pathological fractures.
Anatomic specificity	Throughout PCS more details regarding anatomic site are required. For example, release of a shoulder ligament requires that the specific ligament be identified.

Impact on Scheduling

Coders do not assign codes until the insurance claim is prepared, but the impact on coding begins as soon as the patient encounter is scheduled. Schedulers often select the reason or purpose for patients' planned visits from a list that is ultimately tied to diagnosis codes. When providers need to check eligibility, make a referral, or obtain preauthorization from the patient's health plan, diagnosis codes are usually required. When the patient presents for the visit, the coinsurance, copayment, or deductible payment may be affected by the expected diagnosis or visit type.

Impact on Treatment

The effect on examinations and treatment decisions is a critical and sensitive area for providers. Health plans may update coverage policies to reflect the greater specificity in ICD-10-CM/PCS coding. For example, the diagnostic criteria for coverage of a particular treatment could become more specific and, therefore, more limited. Providers may need to document additional details to support a patient's treatment plan. Providers may need to alter past treatment protocols or explain to patients why their course of treatment may change, or not be fully covered, due to new insurance company requirements. The extent of this impact will not be known until health plans review their ICD-10-CM/PCS implementation activities and determine what changes to make in their policies.

Coding Practice

Now it is your turn to demonstrate your understanding ...act of ICD-10-CM/PCS on medical providers. ...r the questions from memory first, then refer ...rmation in this section if you need a little

...ct on Medical Providers

...ers to the following questions

...ns who own their own

2. List four examples of changes needed in physician documentation under ICD-10-CM/PCS.
____
____
____
____

3. How does ICD-10-CM/PCS potentially impact scheduling? _______________
____
____
____

IMPACT ON MEDICAL CODERS

Medical coders are affected by ICD-10 CM/PCS on a daily basis. Any delays or errors in using the new code set directly impact the revenue of the organization. Therefore, coders must be trained and proficient well-before the "Go Live" date so they can be immediately effective. This involves learning the new code set, new coding guidelines, new or updated software, and updating professional certifications.

New Terminology

The added detail to ICD-10-CM/PCS codes requires additional knowledge of medical terminology, anatomy and physiology, pathophysiology, and pharmacology. Terminology used in ICD-9-CM is replaced with more current clinical terminology. ■ TABLE 3-2 shows examples of terminology differences between ICD-9-CM and ICD-10-CM.

ICD-10-PCS has numerous terminology changes because standard definitions are an integral part of the code set. ■ TABLE 3-3 shows examples of terminology differences between ICD-9-CM Volume 3 procedure codes and ICD-10- PCS.

New Abstracting Challenges

Just as providers identify areas where ICD-10-CM/PCS requires additional documentation details, coders working for those providers learn what details to abstract in order to code the case completely and accurately. ■ TABLE 3-4 (page 36) provides examples of changes in abstracting diagnoses. ■ TABLE 3-5 (page 36) provides examples of changes in abstracting procedures.

Table 3-2 ■ EXAMPLES OF TERMINOLOGY DIFFERENCES BETWEEN ICD-9-CM AND ICD-10-CM

ICD-9-CM Classification	ICD-10-CM Classification
Status asthmaticus	Mild intermittent Mild persistent Moderate persistent Severe persistent
Bleeding / Hemorrhage	Hemorrhage used when referring to ulcers Bleeding used for diseases such as gastritis, duodenitis, diverticulitis, and diverticulosis
Burns	Burns that come from a heat source, electricity, or radiation Corrosion used to describe chemical burns
Diabetes Type I or Type II; not stated as uncontrolled or stated as uncontrolled	Diabetes Type 1 or Type 2

Table 3-3 ■ EXAMPLES OF TERMINOLOGY DIFFERENCES BETWEEN ICD-9-CM VOLUME 3 AND ICD-10-PCS

ICD-9-CM Volume 3 Classification	ICD-10-PCS Classification
Number of vessels treated	Number of sites treated
Excision, resection, removal used interchangeably	Excision, resection, removal each has unique and specific definition and cannot be used interchangeably.
Ligament	Indicate the specific ligament involved

New Coding Challenges

ICD-10-CM introduces several new coding challenges, including new coding concepts, increased use of combination codes, and new guidelines. In addition, ICD-10-CM/PCS more clearly distinguishes between diagnostic and procedural descriptors for codes. Examples of each follow.

New Coding Concepts

New coding concepts are introduced in ICD-10-CM/PCS that did not exist in ICD-9-CM. Coders must identify and understand the new concepts in order to assign the correct code. Examples include the following:

- Blood type is a coding criterion in ICD-10-CM, but was non-existent in ICD-9-CM.
- Injury by **underdosing** (*taking too little*) of medication is new in ICD-10-CM.

Changes in Combination Codes

Some conditions that required multiple coding in ICD-9-CM are identified with a combination code in ICD-10-CM. Coders learn what situations are combined into a single code and what situations require separate coding.

- For example, diabetes type 2 with diabetic cataract was identified with two codes in ICD-9-CM, one for diabetes and a second for cataracts in diseases classified elsewhere. ICD-10-CM uses a combination code that includes both the type of diabetes and the specific complication.

The opposite is true in PCS. ICD-9-CM proce[illegible] codes include many combination codes for pro[illegible] commonly performed together. In ICD-10-[illegible] combination codes are eliminated and mul[illegible] more common. This preserves the purit[illegible] the system.

New Guidelines

While many of the Offici[illegible] Reporting for diagno[illegible]

Table 3-4 ■ **EXAMPLES OF CHANGES IN DIAGNOSIS ABSTRACTING**

Topic	Change	Impact
Complications	**ICD-9-CM:** Limited codes for surgical complications. **ICD-10-CM:** Codes for complications are expanded. Makes a distinction between intraoperative complications and postoperative disorders.	Coders become familiar with the expanded range of code choices and the new terminology.
External cause episode of care	**ICD-9-CM:** No codes for external cause episode of care. **ICD-10-CM:** External cause codes and injury codes require a seventh-character extension indicating if the episode of care is initial, subsequent, or for sequela.	This information should be easily determined from the medical record. Requires an additional step in code assignment.
Falls	**ICD-9-CM:** Falls, one of the leading external causes of injury, are described by about 40 codes. **ICD-10-CM:** Has codes for approximately 100 types of falls. Has three extensions to identify the episode of care as initial, subsequent, or for sequela.	Changes result in approximately 300 codes for falls. Coders become familiar with the expanded range of code choices and the new code extensions.
Laterality	**ICD-9-CM:** Codes do not distinguish laterality (right or left side) for injuries or conditions of bilateral sites such as eyes, ears, and extremities. **ICD-10-CM**: Most bilateral sites have codes for laterality.	In most cases physicians are accustomed to documenting this information. Laterality presents an added step in code selection.
Obstetrics	**ICD-9-CM:** Assign a fifth digit for the episode of care: delivered, antepartum, or postpartum, and the presence of a complication. **ICD-10-CM:** Code the trimester of pregnancy and weeks of gestation.	Easily determined from the medical record. Does not require additional documentation by physicians. Requires that coders develop a new methodology.

Table 3-5 ■ **EXAMPLES OF CHANGES IN PROCEDURE ABSTRACTING**

Topic	Change	Impact
Coronary bypass	**ICD-9-CM Vol. 3:** Defines codes based on the number of arteries bypassed. **ICD-10-PCS:** Defines codes based on the number of sites bypassed to and site bypassed from.	Coders must learn the new definitions. Coders must learn more detailed anatomy of the heart vessels.
Eponyms	**ICD-9-CM Vol. 3:** Eponyms are commonly used as the only description of a procedure. **ICD-10-PCS:** PCS does not use procedure eponyms because they can be performed with numerous variations.	When surgeons describe procedures using eponyms, coders must read the detailed operative report to determine the exact nature of what was done and assign the corresponding code.
Joint [illegible]nts	**ICD-9-CM Vol. 3:** One code for many joint replacements. **ICD-10-PCS:** As many as 18 possible codes for a joint replacement, based on laterality, the surface treated, and the type of tissue substitute.	Physicians need to document additional details. Coders must learn to locate the details.
[illegible]	[illegible]**CD-9-CM Vol. 3:** Codes do not distinguish laterality. [illegible]**-10-PCS:** Most bilateral sites have codes for [illegible]lity.	In most cases physicians are accustomed to documenting this information. Laterality presents an added step in code selection.
[illegible]	[illegible] **Vol. 3:** No standard definition of [illegible]rms. Many terms can be used [illegible] [illegible]D-10-PCS applies specific and [illegible] terms such as excision, resection, [illegible]	Physicians are not expected to adopt PCS definitions in their documentation. Coders must read the procedural documentation carefully and apply the correct PCS definitions, regardless of the terms physicians use.

ICD-9-CM and ICD-10-CM, coders must be alert for those that are different. Examples include the following:

- When coding for anemia in cancer (neoplastic disease) ICD-9-CM directed coders to sequence the codes according to the reason for the encounter. Anemia was sequenced first when it was the primary reason for the encounter.
  - ICD-10-CM guidelines direct coders to always sequence the neoplasm code first.
- ICD-9-CM defined acute myocardial infarction (AMI) as one occurring within the past eight weeks.
  - ICD-10-CM defines AMI as one occurring within the past four weeks or less.

For procedure coding, ICD-9-CM Volume 3 did not have guidelines, while ICD-10-PCS does have coding guidelines that coders must learn and follow.

Separation of Diagnostic and Procedural Descriptors

ICD-9-CM sometimes provided multiple diagnosis codes for a condition, based on the procedure that was performed. ICD-9-CM Volume 3 sometimes had multiple procedure codes based on the reason the procedure was performed. ICD-10-CM/PCS attempts to eliminate this blurring between diagnosis and procedure codes. An example of each follows.

- ICD-9-CM provided approximately 36 separate V-codes for encounters for immunization, based on the type of immunization to be administered.
  - ICD-10-CM has one code for an immunization encounter (**Z23**) with the instructional note to use a procedure code to describe the specific type of immunization given.
- ICD-9-CM Volume 3 provided separate procedure codes for a uterine repair, based on whether the repair was for a laceration, fistula, an old obstetric laceration, or a current obstetric laceration.
  - ICD-10-PCS codes only for the type of repair. The problem requiring repair is described using the diagnosis code. Only current obstetric lacerations receive a separate repair code.

Coder Training and Certification

Coders need to update their coding skills and their professional certification for ICD-10-CM/PCS. Coding professionals recommend that full training of all staff take place approximately three to six months prior to the compliance date. Managers and trainers are trained sooner, but coders benefit the most when training is provided as close to the "Go Live" date as possible, so their skills are fresh.

Professional organizations such as AAPC and AHIMA offer training in a variety of formats including distance education courses, audio seminars, web-based in-services, self-directed learning using printed materials or electronic tools, off-site workshops in a traditional classroom setting with a certified trainer, or in-house classes with a certified trainer. Experts estimate that coders need 24 to 40 hours of training, depending on their role, specialty, and type of facility.

Established coders need to demonstrate their proficiency in ICD-10-CM/PCS to maintain certification. AHIMA and AAPC have specific requirements for coders to upgrade their skills to ICD-10-CM/PCS. Coders already certified through AHIMA for ICD-9-CM/PCS must complete a specified amount of continuing education, based on their specialty and coding credential, beginning in 2011. Coders certified by AAPC must take an ICD-10-CM proficiency exam.

Coders should also upgrade keyboarding skills from what were primarily numeric data entry skills to full alphanumeric keyboarding because all ICD-10-CM/PCS codes have a random sequencing of alphabetic and numeric characters.

CODING CAUTION

Due to the large amount of code set training that is needed, there are few formal programs that focus on upgrading coders' keyboarding skills. Smart coders will take the initiative to address this skill on their own because alphanumeric keyboarding is considerably more time consuming than largely numeric keyboarding.

Appropriate Use of GEMs

CMS and the Centers for Disease Control and Prevention (CDC) needed to create a way to compare data between ICD-9-CM and ICD-10-CM/PCS and analyze long-term trends. They developed **General Equivalence Mappings (GEMs)** to be the authoritative source for comparing codes between the two code sets. Because there are more ICD-10-CM codes than ICD-9-CM codes, GEMs do not provide an exact one-to-one match between code sets but, rather, provide a general approximation of the relationship (■ TABLE 3-6). CMS publishes GEMs as

Table 3-6 ■ EXAMPLE OF GEM ONE-TO-MANY FORWARD MAPPING

ICD-9-CM	ICD-10-CM
424.1 Aortic valve disorders	I35.0 Nonrheumatic aortic (valve) sten[illegible]
	I35.1 Nonrheumatic aortic (valve) insufficiency
	I35.2 Nonrheumatic aortic ([illegible] with insufficiency
	I35.8 Other nonrheum[illegible] disorders
	I35.9 Nonrheu[illegible] unspecified

public domain electronic files available on its website. Researchers use GEMs to analyze large volumes of data over a time span that includes data both pre- and post-ICD-10-CM/PCS. Without GEMs, it would be nearly impossible to establish healthcare trends.

Coders should not use GEMs to assign codes for specific patient encounters. This means that they should not look up the ICD-9-CM code first, then use GEMs to select the ICD-10-CM/PCS code. Doing so would be misuse of data and a potentially fraudulent coding practice. All ICD-10-CM/PCS codes should be assigned using the ICD-10-CM/PCS Index and Tabular List.

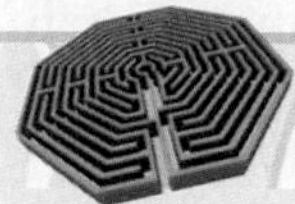

Coding Practice

Now it is your turn to demonstrate your understanding of the impact of ICD-10-CM/PCS on medical coders. Try to answer the questions from memory first, then refer back to the information in this section if you need a little extra help.

Exercise 3.5 Impact on Medical Coders

Instructions: Write the answers to the following questions in the space provided.

1. Briefly describe how abstracting will change for each of the following conditions.
   a. obstetrics ______________________
   b. falls ______________________
   c. laterality ______________________
2. Name three examples of medical terms that have new definitions under ICD-10-CM/PCS.
   ____
   ____
   ____
3. Describe an inappropriate use of GEMs by a coder.
   ____
   ____
   ____

CHAPTER SUMMARY

...er you learned that:

- ... used for diagnosis coding, and ...sed for procedure coding, are two ...nct systems that were developed by ...
- ...rt from ICD-9-CM to ... of healthcare's top priorities ...e year 2015.
- One of the greatest impacts of ICD-10-CM/PCS within a healthcare organization is the impact on healthcare information systems.
- Providers are impacted by ICD-10-CM/PCS in the areas of documentation, scheduling, and treatment plans.
- Coders must learn the new code set, new coding guidelines, new or updated software, and they must update professional certifications.

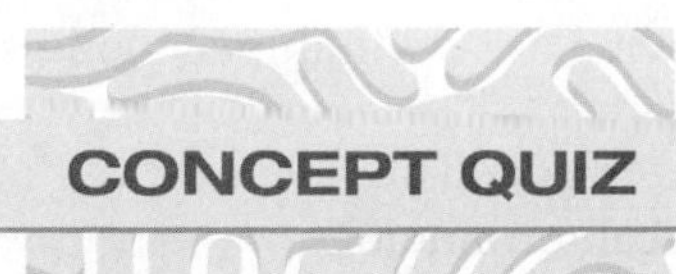

CONCEPT QUIZ

Take a moment to look back at your trip through the transition to ICD-10-CM/PCS and solidify your skills. This is your opportunity to pull together everything you have learned.

Completion

Instructions: Write the term that answers each question based on the information you learned in this chapter. Choose from following list. Some choices may be used more than once and some choices may not be used at all.

AAPC	ICD-10-PCS
AHIMA	ICD-9-CM
CDC	January 1, 2012
CMS	morbidity
complicated	mortality
five	October 1, 2014
GEMs	seven
granular	three
ICD-10	transaction standards
ICD-10-CM	Version 5010

1. ICD-10-CM codes contain ______________ to ______________ characters.
2. ICD-10-PCS codes contain ______________ characters.
3. ______________ is causes of disease and illness.
4. Version 5010 is mandatory on the date ______________.
5. The United States version of ICD-10 diagnosis codes is much more ______________ than it is in other nations.
6. The code set ______________ was developed by WHO for worldwide use.
7. The code set ______________ is used only by inpatient hospitals.
8. Coders already certified through ______________ for ICD-9-CM must complete a specified amount of continuing education, based on their specialty and coding credential.
9. ______________ uses more combination codes than ICD-9-CM.
10. Researchers use ______________ to analyze large volumes of data, but coders should not use them for code assignment.

Multiple Choice

Instructions: Circle the letter of the best answer to each question based on the information you learned in this chapter. Refer to the discussion in this chapter and the Glossary at the end of this book if you need a little extra help.

1. Which of the following is NOT a benefit of ICD-10-CM?
   A. Codes more accurately describe patient conditions and procedures, reducing the need for attachments to claims.
   B. Advancements in technology and medical practice are reflected in the organization and description of codes.
   C. The structure of the new code set allows physicians to create new codes whenever they need to, if an appropriate code is not already available.
   D. Public officials can better track and respond to domestic and international public health threats.
2. Which of the following conditions does NOT require updated terminology in ICD-10-CM?
   A. Diabetes
   B. Influenza
   C. Asthma
   D. Burns
3. Who is required to use ICD-10-CM?
   A. All physicians
   B. HIPAA-covered entities
   C. Inpatient hospitals only
   D. Patients
4. Which of the following is NOT a requirement that impacts health information systems?
   A. Create separate fields for ICD-9-CM and ICD-10-CM codes.
   B. Modify field sizes to accommodate the longer codes.
   C. Change data type of fields from primarily numeric to completely alphanumeric for every character.
   D. Add a new field as a version indicator to distinguish between ICD-9-CM and ICD-10-CM/PCS codes.

5. Which of the following is NOT an example of provider documentation changes under ICD-10-CM/PCS?
   A. Laterality
   B. Genetic diagnoses
   C. Acute vs. chronic
   D. Anatomic specificity
6. Changes in procedure abstracting under ICD-10-PCS include all of the following EXCEPT
   A. eponyms.
   B. coronary bypass.
   C. joint replacements.
   D. external causes.
7. Coding professionals recommend that full training of all staff take place approximately ________ months prior to the compliance date.
   A. one to two
   B. three to six
   C. six to 12
   D. 12 to 18
8. GEMs do not provide an exact one-to-one match between ICD-9-CM and ICD-10-CM because
   A. there are more ICD-9-CM codes than ICD-10-CM codes.
   B. there are more ICD-10-CM codes than ICD-9-CM codes.
   C. there is no way to compare ICD-9-CM and ICD-10-CM.
   D. all of the above.
9. Which of the following areas will impact coders?
   A. Learning new software
   B. Enhanced data entry skills
   C. Expanded medical terminology
   D. All of the above
10. Which is the most accurate description of GEMs?
   A. An exact one-to-one matching of the ICD-9-CM and ICD-10-CM codes
   B. An authoritative guide to assign ICD-10-CM codes to patient records for billing
   C. The authoritative source for comparing codes between ICD-10-CM/PCS and ICD-9-CM
   D. Electronic software that provides a definitive translation of ICD-9-CM codes to ICD-10-CM codes

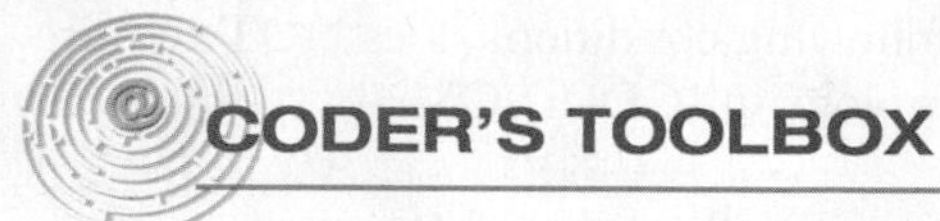

CODER'S TOOLBOX

The following resources are a starting point for learning more about the ICD-10-CM/PCS transition. The > symbol indicates a menu selection within the website in order to navigate to a specific page.

AAPC > ICD-10
http://www.aapc.com/ICD-10/index.aspx

American Health Information Management Association
http://www.ahima.org/icd10/default.aspx

Centers for Disease Control and Prevention ICD-10
http://www.cdc.gov/nchs/icd/icd10.htm

Centers for Medicare and Medicaid Services ICD-10
http://www.cms.gov/ICD10/

World Health Organization ICD **http://www.who.int/classifications/icd/en/**

SECTION TWO

Diagnosis Coding

Section Two: Diagnosis Coding guides you through the steps of diagnosis coding for each body system. You will learn how to apply the three skills of an ace coder—Abstract, Assign, and Arrange—for a broad variety of patient encounters.

PROFESSIONAL PROFILE

MEET...

Pauline T. Newton, Patient Financial Services Director
Carlisle Regional Medical Center, an HMA Facility

I have been in the billing and coding field for the past 34 years and I am continually learning something new. Even though I have a Bachelors of Arts in Business Management, I recently went back to school and earned an Associate of Science degree in medical records, coding, and billing from an accredited college to enhance my career skills. I am now working toward a Bachelor of Science in Healthcare Administration.

I went back to school in order to gain skills to address the challenges of Recovery Audit Contractor (RAC) audits I was facing in my job. I wanted to understand what the auditors are looking at and where our hospital could be lacking in documentation. Now I am able to work more closely with the clinicians to conduct random audits on medical records. Internal chart reviews help ensure that we are capturing all the revenue for services rendered and that the documentation supports what we bill. I also have a new understanding of insurance claims and reasons for denials. I worked with the case management and health information management (HIM) departments to create a proactive approach to potential denials, as well as improve our presentation of Medicare appeals to the review board and judge advocate.

I currently participate on several committees in the hospital that directly use the knowledge I gained through my formal education: Denials Management Committee, Revenue Cycle Committee, RAC Audit Committee, and Corporate Compliance Committee.

I am involved with the professional organization Healthcare Financial Management Association (HFMA), including serving as an officer of our local chapter. I was awarded the HFMA Follmer Bronze Award in 2007 for my presentations and workshops related to Revenue Cycle presented for our chapter.

My advice to new coders would be the two most important things I have learned during my career: embrace change and continue to learn and grow.

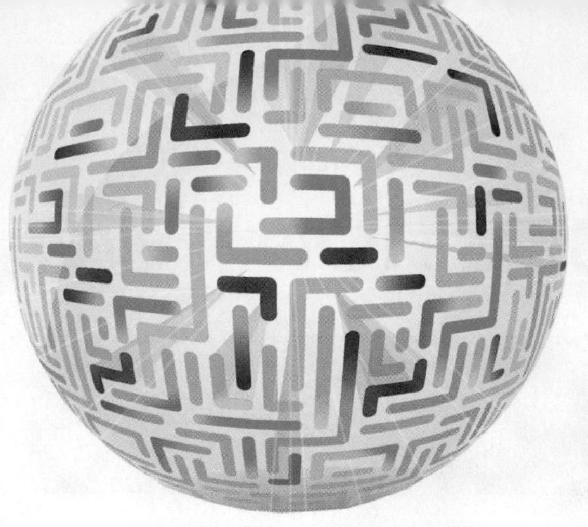

4

Introduction to ICD-10-CM Diagnosis Coding

Learning Objectives

After completing this chapter, you should have the skills to:

- Spell and define the key words, medical terms, and abbreviations related to ICD-10-CM coding.
- Identify the organization of the ICD-10-CM manual.
- Discuss ICD-10-CM Official Guidelines for Coding and Reporting.
- Name ICD-10-CM conventions.
- Demonstrate the diagnosis coding process including abstracting, assigning, and arranging codes.

Key Terms and Abbreviations

abstract
arrange
assign
block
category
chapter
circumstances of admission
clinically significant condition
code
coding path
combination code
conventions
Coordination and Maintenance Committee
default code
eponym
etiology
first-listed diagnosis
four cooperating parties
initial encounter
instructional note
late effect
Main Term
manifestations
multiple coding
nonessential modifiers
Official Guidelines for Coding and Reporting (OGCR)
principal diagnosis
relevant
sequela
sequence
subcategory
subchapter
subsequent encounter
subterm
Tabular List
uncertain diagnosis

In addition to the key terms listed here, students should know the terms defined within tables in this chapter.

Chapter Outline

- **Organization of ICD-10-CM**
- **ICD-10-CM Guidelines and Conventions**
- **How to Code Diagnoses**

ICD-10-CM codes in this chapter are from the ICD-10-CM 2014 Draft code set from the Department of Health and Human Services, Centers for Disease Control and Prevention.

INTRODUCTION

As much as we would like, no vehicle is without difficulties or breakdowns. When you take your vehicle to a mechanic for service, the mechanic needs to figure out what is wrong before he or she can fix it. They need to diagnose the problem. Similarly, when patients see physicians, physicians must diagnose the condition before they know what services to provide. In this chapter you will learn how to code for the conditions that physicians diagnose.

As you study this chapter, open up your medical terminology book and keep a medical dictionary handy to refresh your memory of any unfamiliar terms. No coder knows every detail about every condition, so the best coders consult reference materials rather than guess. Expose yourself to a variety of resources and identify the ones that work best for you.

ORGANIZATION OF ICD-10-CM

The International Classification of Diseases, 10th Revision, Clinical Modification (ICD-10-CM) is used to code diagnoses that describe patient illnesses, diseases, conditions, injuries, or other reasons for seeking healthcare services. ICD-10-CM is the United States' clinical modification of the World Health Organization's (WHO) International Classification of Diseases, 10th Revision (ICD-10). The inclusion of the term *clinical modification* in the United States' ICD-10-CM emphasizes the intent of the modification to classify and manage data related to the actual examination and treatment of patients. Uses in the United States include tracking morbidity, indexing medical records, reporting ambulatory as well as inpatient care, and reflecting advances in medical care.

Accurate coding of diagnoses is necessary in order to explain why services were provided. In order to code accurately, coders need to be familiar with the process for updating ICD-10-CM as well as overall organization of the manual, the distinct sub-levels of organization, and the significance of each.

Updates in ICD-10-CM

Because medical knowledge is constantly expanding and improving, the system for diagnosis coding must keep pace with those changes. ICD-10-CM replaces ICD-9-CM, which was used for diagnosis coding in the United States since 1979. ■ TABLE 4-1 summarizes the major differences between ICD-9-CM and ICD-10-CM.

Many of the **Official Guidelines for Coding and Reporting (OGCR)** (*rules that provide information and direction in identifying the diagnoses to be reported*) are similar between the two code sets. OGCR Section I.A. reflects new and updated conventions. Sections I.B., II, III, and IV reflect changes related to differences in code structure, such as additional characters, seventh character extensions, and laterality. Guidelines in Section C. reflect changes in chapter organization and updated clinical terminology, definitions, and practice.

Table 4-1 ■ COMPARISON OF CODES IN ICD-9-CM AND ICD-10-CM

Feature	ICD-9-CM	ICD-10-CM
Number of codes	16,000	68,000+
Code length	3 to 5 digits	3 to 7 characters
Code structure	3-digit category 4th and 5th digits for etiology, anatomic site, manifestation	3-character category 4th, 5th, 6th characters for etiology, anatomic site, severity 7th character extension for additional information
First character	Always numeric, except E codes and V codes	1st character is always alphabetic.
Subsequent characters	All numeric	2nd character is always numeric; all other characters may be alphabetic or numeric.
Decimal point	Mandatory after 3rd character, except E codes where decimal point is after 4th character	Mandatory after 3rd character on all codes
Extensions	None	Some codes use a 7th character as an extension to provide additional information.
Placeholders	None	Character "X" is used as a placeholder in certain 6- and 7-character codes.

CODING CAUTION

Coders who are familiar with ICD-9-CM OGCR must be especially alert to learn which guidelines in ICD-10-CM OGCR are similar to ICD-9-CM and which are different.

In addition to the major conversion from ICD-9-CM to ICD-10-CM, the code set is updated annually. Code definitions are revised, new codes are added, and outdated codes are deleted. Updates are effective each year on October 1, to coincide with the beginning of the federal fiscal year. Each HIPAA-covered entity must update its systems and paperwork to incorporate the changes. The ICD-10-CM **Coordination and Maintenance Committee** oversees all changes, which must be consistent with WHO's ICD-10. The Coordination and Maintenance Committee is a federal interdepartmental committee comprised of representatives from the **four cooperating parties**: the Centers for Medicare and Medicaid Services (CMS), the Centers for Disease Control and Prevention's (CDC) National Center for Health Statistics (NCHS), the American Hospital Association (AHA), and the American Health Information Management Association (AHIMA).

Overall Organization

The ICD-10-CM manual (2012 Draft) is a single volume and is not separated into three volumes as the ICD-9-CM was. Locate the Contents page near the front of the manual and become familiar with the contents and organization of the ICD-10-CM manual listed in ■Table 4-2. The purpose of each of these Contents topics is discussed later in this chapter.

Chapter Structure

The last section of the Contents page, ICD-10-CM Tabular List of Diseases and Injuries, is further subdivided into 21 chapters. Each chapter contains codes for a body system or related conditions. Coders must become acquainted with the chapter topics within ICD-10-CM as well as the internal structure within each chapter in order to locate information and follow **instructional notes**. Instructional notes are official coding directions throughout the ICD-10-CM manual. Coders are required to follow instructional notes in order to abstract, assign, and arrange codes accurately. The various types of instructional notes are discussed later in this chapter.

The location within the ICD-10-CM chapter structure where instructional notes appear dictates what codes they apply to. Each chapter is subdivided into blocks, categories, subcategories, and codes (■Table 4-3) as described below:

- A **block** or **subchapter** is a contiguous range of codes within a chapter. It is comparable to a section in ICD-9-CM.
- A **category** is three characters in length. A three-character category that has no further subdivisions is called a code.
- A **subcategory** is either four or five characters. Each level of subdivision after a category and before a code is a subcategory. A four- or five-character subcategory that has no further subdivisions is called a code.
- A **code** is the final level of subdivision. Codes may be three, four, five, six, or seven characters in length (■Table 4-4). All codes in the Tabular List of the official version of the ICD-10-CM appear in boldface type. Entries that require a seventh character extension are referred to as codes, not subcategories, even though they are not complete without the seventh character.

Any instructional notes listed at the beginning of the chapter apply to all codes within that chapter.

Table 4-2 ■ **OVERVIEW OF THE ICD-10-CM MANUAL**

Type of Information	Name of Section	Purpose
Introductory Material	Preface Introduction How to Use the ICD-10-CM (Draft 2012) ICD-10-CM Draft Conventions ICD-10-CM Draft Official Guidelines for Coding and Reporting 2012	Useful information and rules on how to use the manual.
Index	ICD-10-CM Index to Diseases and Injuries (Index) ICD-10-CM Table of Neoplasms ICD-10-CM Table of Drugs and Chemicals ICD-10-CM Index to External Causes	Alphabetical list of diseases and injuries, reasons for encounters, and external causes. Two tables provide quick look ups, one for neoplasms and one for drugs and chemicals causing injury. Coders must always reference one of these indices or tables when searching for a code.
Tabular List	ICD-10-CM Tabular List of Diseases and Injuries	Numerical list of diseases and injuries, reasons for encounters, and external causes. Provides additional instruction on how use, assign, and sequence codes. Coders must always reference the Tabular List to verify a code, after consulting the Index, and before assigning the final code.

Table 4-3 ■ ORGANIZATIONAL STRUCTURE OF ICD-10-CM CHAPTERS

Level	Example
Chapter	Chapter 15. Pregnancy, Childbirth and the Puerperium (O00-O9A)
Block	Pregnancy with abortive outcome (O00-O08)
Category	O03 Spontaneous abortion
Subcategory	O03.3 Other and unspecified complications following incomplete spontaneous abortion
Code	O03.31 Shock following incomplete spontaneous abortion

Table 4-4 ■ EXAMPLES OF ICD-10-CM CODES WITH VARYING NUMBER OF CHARACTERS

Code Length	Example
3-character code	I10
4-character code	F52.8
5-character code	K70.30
6-character code	L89.511 T50.B91
7-character code	T22.761A
7-character code with placeholder X	T51.0X1D V52.0XXS O33.4XX0

Instructional notes at the beginning of a block apply to all codes within that block, but not to other blocks. Instructional notes at the beginning of the category apply to all codes within that category, but not to previous or subsequent categories. Instructional notes at the beginning of the subcategory apply to all codes within that subcategory, but not to previous or subsequent subcategories. Instructional notes that appear under a specific code apply only to that code.

CODING CAUTION

Be on the watch for letters that can be easily confused with numbers. The letter capital I can be confused with the number 1. The letter S can be confused with the number 5. The letter capital O can be confused with the number 0. In the ICD-10-CM manual, the number zero is written as ∅ to help distinguish it from the capital letter O.

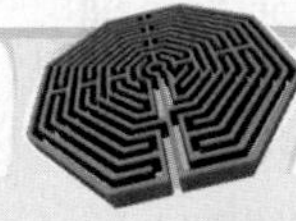

Coding Practice

Now it is your turn to demonstrate your understanding of ICD-10-CM organization. Try to answer the questions from memory first, then refer back to the information in this section if you need a little extra help.

Exercise 4.1 Organization of ICD-10-CM

Instructions: Look up the following entries in the ICD-10-CM manual. Determine if each entry is a block, category, subcategory, or code and write the answer next to each entry.

Example: F01 Vascular dementia *category*

1. D56 Thalassemia ____________
2. F20.0 Paranoid schizophrenia ____________
3. Diseases of esophagus, stomach and duodenum (K20-K31) ____________
4. O60.12 Preterm labor second trimester with preterm delivery second trimester ____________
5. O48.1 Prolonged pregnancy ____________
6. S37.0 Injury of kidney ____________
7. S67 Crushing injury of wrists, hand and fingers ____________
8. T28.1XXS Burn of esophagus, sequela ____________
9. Visual disturbances and blindness (H53-H54) ____________
10. M48.44 Fatigue fracture of vertebra, thoracic region ____________

ICD-10-CM GUIDELINES AND CONVENTIONS

ICD-10-CM is accompanied by Official Guidelines for Coding and Reporting (OGCR) and Conventions, both of which direct the coder how to use the manual.

Official Guidelines for Coding and Reporting

Refer to the Contents page of the ICD-10-CM manual to locate the sections and *ICD-10-CM Draft Official Guidelines for Coding and Reporting (OGCR)* and *ICD-10-CM Draft Conventions*.

- OGCR are rules that complement the conventions and instructional notes to provide additional information and direction in identifying the diagnoses to be reported. Health Insurance Portability and Accountability Act (HIPAA) requires that coders adhere to OGCR when assigning ICD-10-CM diagnosis codes.
- Conventions are the use of symbols, typeface, and layout features to succinctly convey interpretive information. Conventions appear in the section *ICD-10-CM Draft Conventions.* Most conventions also appear in OGCR, Section I.A.

SUCCESS STEP

Conventions are your co-pilot during your trip, helping you to avoid costly errors and pointing you in the right direction. Just as new drivers need to memorize the meaning of traffic signs, such as Stop, Yield, Do Not Enter, and Speed Limit, coders need to memorize the conventions.

Refer to the ICD-10-CM manual and locate the first page of ICD-10-CM Draft Official Guidelines for Coding and Reporting (OGCR), which contains a detailed list of contents. The topics are referenced by an alphanumeric numbering system and page numbers. An overview of each OGCR section is provided next.

Section I

Section I Conventions, General Coding Guidelines and Chapter Specific Guidelines, contains the following major divisions:

A. Conventions for the ICD-10-CM: the general rules for the use of the coding manual independent of the guidelines. Most, but not all, of the conventions listed here also appear in the separate preceding section, ICD-10-CM Draft Conventions.

B. General Coding Guidelines: overall rules that apply to all chapters in ICD-10-CM.

C. Chapter-Specific Coding Guidelines: guidelines for specific diagnoses and/or conditions, divided by ICD-10-CM chapter. Unless otherwise indicated within a specific guideline, these apply to all healthcare settings.

Section II

Section II, Selection of Principal Diagnosis, describes rules for abstracting the main diagnosis for inpatient settings. The guidelines for inpatient settings are different than for outpatient settings. Principal diagnosis applies only to inpatient settings. It is the "condition established after study to be chiefly responsible for occasioning the admission of the patient to the hospital for care," as defined by the **Uniform Hospital Data Discharge Set (UHDDS)**. Refer to the coding manual to review the topics in this section.

Section III

Section III, Reporting **Additional Diagnoses**, describes rules for abstracting **secondary** or extra diagnoses, in addition to the principal diagnosis, for inpatient settings. Refer to the coding manual to review the topics in this section.

Section IV

Section IV, Diagnostic Coding and Reporting Guidelines for Outpatient Services, describes rules for abstracting diagnoses in outpatient settings. Coding guidelines for outpatient diagnoses vary in several ways from those for inpatient diagnoses. The two most notable differences are the following:

- In the outpatient setting, the first-listed diagnosis is the diagnosis, condition, problem, or other reason for the encounter visit shown in the medical record to be chiefly responsible for the services provided. First-listed diagnosis applies only to outpatient settings; principal diagnosis applies only to inpatient settings. Secondary or additional diagnoses apply to all healthcare settings.
- Coding guidelines for inconclusive or uncertain diagnoses (*diagnoses preceded by the words probable, possible, suspected, questionable, rule out, working diagnosis, or similar word*) were developed for inpatient reporting and do not apply to outpatients.

Refer to the coding manual to review the topics in this section.

SUCCESS STEP

The OGCR is updated each year after the coding manual is published. Although the coding manual is updated in October, the OGCR may not be updated until after the physical manual is published. Refer to the websites of the Center for Medicare and Medicaid Services (CMS) at **www.cms.gov** or the Centers for Disease Control and Prevention (CDC) at **www.cdc.gov** to download the most current guidelines.

Conventions

Coders' skills to recognize and interpret the conventions are crucial to interpreting ICD-10-CM instructions and assigning the accurate codes. Many ICD-10-CM conventions are the same as those used by ICD-9-CM. ■ TABLE 4-5 summarizes the conventions that are similar between the two code sets. Conventions that are new in ICD-10-CM are summarized in ■ TABLE 4-6 (page 48). The tables that follow also identify where each convention is discussed in OGCR. Examples and further discussion of the conventions appear later in this chapter as well as in most other chapters in this text.

Several of the most important conventions are discussed next. Refer to the ICD-10-CM manual and look up the examples that follow. The following conventions are discussed in detail:

- Exclusion notes
- Use additional characters
- Extensions and placeholders
- Laterality

Exclusion Notes

ICD-10-CM Tabular List utilizes two exclusion notes: Excludes1 and Excludes2. Exclusion notes may appear at the beginning of a block, category, subcategory, or after a code. Notes at the category or subcategory level apply to all codes that follow, so it is important to check for these notes not only under the code, but also under the preceding block, category, and subcategory headings. For example, refer to category **K55 Vascular disorder of intestine** in the Tabular List and notice the note **Excludes1: necrotizing enterocolitis of newborn (P77.–)**. This note applies to all the subsequent codes, **K55.0** through **K55.9**. If coders read only the notes for one code, such as **K55.1**, they would miss the added instruction at the beginning of the category **K55**.

Table 4-5 ■ **CONVENTIONS THAT ARE THE SAME FOR ICD-9-CM AND ICD-10-CM**

Convention	Meaning/Use	OGCR Reference
( ) **Parentheses**	Tabular and Index: Nonessential modifiers that describe the default variations of a term. These words are not required to appear in the documentation in order to use the code.	I. A. 7
: **Colon**	Tabular: Appears after an incomplete term that requires one or more modifiers following the colon to be classified to that code or category.	I. A. 7
[ ] **Square brackets**	Tabular: Synonyms, alternative wording, explanatory phrases. Index: Indicates sequencing on etiology/manifestation codes or other paired codes. The code in square brackets [ ] should be sequenced second.	I. A. 7
And	Tabular: Means *and/or.*	I. A. 8 I. A. 14
Boldface (heavy type)	Tabular: Code titles. Index: Main terms.	Appears in Conventions, not OGCR
Code Also	Tabular: More than one code may be required to fully describe the condition.	I. A. 13
Code First/Use Additional Code	Tabular: Provides sequencing instructions for conditions that have both an underlying etiology and multiple body system manifestations and certain other codes that have sequencing requirements.	I. A. 13 I. A. 17
Includes notes	Tabular: Begin with the word "Includes" and further define, clarify, or give examples.	I. A. 10
Inclusion terms	Tabular: A list of synonyms or conditions included within a classification.	I. A. 11
Italics (slanted type)	Tabular: Exclusion notes, manifestation codes.	Appears in Conventions, not OGCR
NEC	Tabular and Index: Not Elsewhere Classifiable. The medical record contains additional details about the condition, but there is not a more specific code available to use.	I. A. 6. a & b
NOS	Tabular: Not Otherwise Specified. Information to assign a more specific code is not available in the medical record.	I. A. 6. a & b
See	Index: It is necessary to reference another Main Term or condition to locate the correct code.	I. A. 16
See Also	Index: Coder may refer to an alternative or additional Main Term if the desired entry is not found under the original Main Term.	I. A. 16
With	Tabular: In a code title, means *both* or *together.*	I. A. 15

Table 4-6 ■ **NEW CONVENTIONS IN ICD-10-CM**

Convention	Meaning/Use	Reference
Excludes1	Tabular: Mutually exclusive codes. None of the codes that appear after it should be used with the original code itself.	OGCR I. A. 12. a
Excludes2	Tabular: The condition excluded is not part of the condition represented by the code, but may be reported together if documented.	OGCR I. A. 12. b
4th 5th 6th 7th	Tabular: Some publishers place a symbol in front of a code to indicate that an additional character is needed for the code to be complete. This text uses the symbols shown here.	Conventions
X	Tabular: A placeholder in codes with less than six characters that require a seventh character extension. The X itself has no meaning and is not replaced with an actual number or letter. In some codes, the X is used to reserve room for future expansion.	OGCR I. A. 4 OGCR I. A. 5
- Short dash	Tabular and Index: Additional characters should be assigned in place of the -. The additional characters may be number or letters.	This symbol is used but not explained in OGCR or Conventions.
With/Without	Tabular: Within a set of alternative codes, describe options for final character.	Conventions

Excludes1 indicates that the condition represented by the code and the condition listed as excluded are mutually exclusive and should not be coded together. When an Excludes1 note appears under a code, none of the codes that appear after it should be used with the code where the note appears. For example, the Excludes1 note under **K55** means that **necrotizing enterocolitis of newborn (P77.-)** should not be reported with any of the codes within the **K55** category.

Excludes2 indicates that the condition excluded is not part of the condition represented by the code, but the patient may have both conditions at the same time. These conditions are not mutually exclusive. When an Excludes2 note appears under a code, it is acceptable to use the main code and the excluded code if the patient is documented to have both conditions. For example, refer to the Tabular List entry **K86.0 Alcohol induced chronic pancreatitis** and notice the note **Excludes2: alcohol induced acute pancreatitis (K85.2)**. The second condition, alcohol induced acute pancreatitis, is not included in code **K86.0**, but may be reported together with it, if the documentation states that the patient has both conditions.

Some codes may have both Excludes1 and Excludes2 notes. For example, the block **Diseases of liver (K70-K77)** has an Excludes1 note for **Jaundice NOS (R17)**, meaning that **R17** should not be reported with any of the codes from **K70** through **K77**. The same block also has several Excludes2 notes. The conditions listed under Excludes2 are not included in any of the codes **K70** through **K77**, but may be reported together with them if the patient is documented to have both conditions. **K77** may appear on a different physical page than the block heading, so the coder who fails to review the beginning of the category will not be aware of these important instructions.

If a code does not have any exclusion notes, then it can be used with any other code that is supported by the medical record and the OGCR.

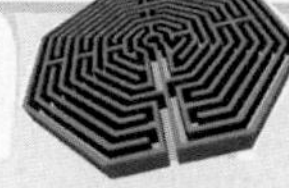

Coding Practice

Now it is your turn to demonstrate your understanding of exclusion notes. Try to answer the questions from memory first, then refer back to the information in this section if you need a little extra help.

Exercise 4.2 Conventions: Exclusion Notes

Instructions: For each pair of codes, indicate if they can be used together based on the exclusion notes. Look up the first code listed in each question. Read the excludes note(s) and determine if the second code can be reported together with the first code. Circle the correct answer.

1. G43.001 and G43.709 OK Do not use together
2. D56.1 and D57.411 OK Do not use together

3. H71.00 and H60.410	OK	Do not use together
4. M21.532 and M21.721	OK	Do not use together
5. O07.0 and O04.84	OK	Do not use together
6. R22.2 and R19.01	OK	Do not use together
7. R29.890 and N63	OK	Do not use together
8. M80.012 and M89.712	OK	Do not use together
9. S83.015A and M23.204	OK	Do not use together
10. T38.0X5D and T49.0X5D	OK	Do not use together

Use Additional Characters

ICD-10-CM alerts coders to use additional characters on a code in two ways:

- a symbol in front of a code
- a short dash (-) at the end of a code number.

When coders see one of these conventions, it means a subcategory needs additional characters and the coder should look down to the next level for more specificity. In ICD-10-CM the additional values for characters 4 through 6 are listed below the subcategory. ■ FIGURE 4-1 illustrates the symbol to use additional characters.

SUCCESS STEP

Many publishing companies print the ICD-10-CM coding manual and each company may use different symbols to alert coders to the need for additional characters. If you do not see the symbols **4th**, **5th**, **6th**, or **7th** in your edition of the coding manual, check the introductory material at the beginning of the manual to learn what symbols the publisher uses.

5th K94.2 Gastrostomy complications

K94.20 Gastrostomy complication, unspecified

K94.21 Gastrostomy hemorrhage

K94.20 Gastrostomy infection

K94.20 Gastrostomy malfunction

Figure 4-1 ■ Example of a Symbol to Use Additional Characters

For example, OGCR C.12.a.2) for Chapter 12, Diseases of Skin and Subcutaneous Tissue (L00-L99), states, **Assignment of the code for Unstageable pressure ulcer (L89.- - 0) should be based on the clinical documentation.** The use of two short dashes (- -) means that this guideline applies to all codes beginning with **L89** and ending in **0**, such as **L89.000**, **L89.010**, **L89.130**, etc. In the earlier example, **Excludes1: necrotizing enterocolitis of newborn (P77.-)**, the designation **P77.-** uses the short dash (-) to indicate all codes beginning with **P77**.

Extensions and Placeholders

Extensions are the seventh character of a code and must appear in that position, regardless of the length of the code. The addition of an extension may be indicated by a symbol, such as **7th**, preceding a code. When a three-, four-, or five-character code requires an extension, the placeholder X must fill any empty positions preceding the seventh character extension. The X itself has no meaning and is not replaced with an actual number or letter. Definitions for the extension character appear preceding the code entry, often at a preceding block, category, or subcategory level.

The extension must appear in the seventh position, regardless of the length of the code itself. The range of codes the extension characters apply to is dictated by where the characters and definitions appear within the organizational hierarchy. Codes that require a seventh-character extension are invalid if the seventh character is omitted; therefore, the claim may be rejected by the payer. ■ FIGURE 4-2 (page 50) illustrates an example entry in the Tabular List that requires both an extension and a placeholder. To assign a code for *unspecified open wound of scalp, initial encounter,* follow these steps in the Tabular List:

- Select code **S01.00**.
- Because the code is only 5 characters in length, the **7th** symbol reminds you to add the placeholder **X**

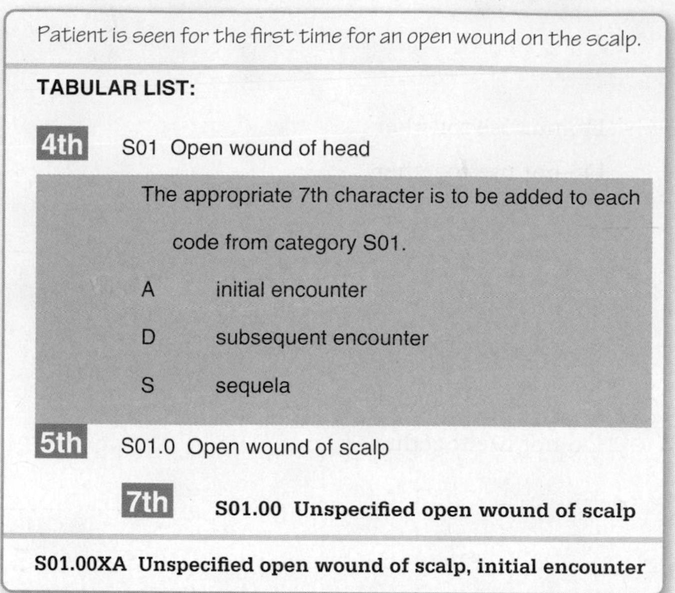

Figure 4-2 ■ Example Use of a Placeholder (X) and an Extension (A)

for the sixth character, before adding the seventh character extension.

- Finally, add the seventh character extension **A** to designate the initial episode of care.
- The final code is **S01.00XA**.

Laterality

ICD-10-CM contains a new OGCR, Section I.B.13, Laterality. For conditions that affect bilateral sites, such as eyes, ears, arms, and legs, the fifth or sixth character indicates whether the condition affects the right or left side. Approximately 28% of ICD-10-CM codes include a designation for laterality. A limited number of these codes also provide an option for bilateral, both sides affected. If there is no designation for bilateral, assign separate codes for the right side and the left side. If laterality is unspecified, assign the code for **unspecified** side. The implementation of laterality is one example of why ICD-10-CM has many times the number of codes as ICD-9-CM does. In ICD-9-CM a condition such as *Marginal corneal ulcer* has one code number, 370.01, whereas ICD-10-CM has four codes plus a subcategory heading (five entries total) for the same condition (■ FIGURE 4-3).

SUCCESS STEP

It is important to notice exactly where a set of extension definitions appears within the organizational hierarchy. When the extension characters and definitions appear at the beginning of a chapter, they are used with all subsequent codes in the chapter; when they appear at the beginning of a block, they are used with all codes in the block; when they appear at the beginning of a category or subcategory, they are used with all codes in the category or subcategory, respectively.

ICD-10-CM code	Description	Level of organization
H16.04	Marginal corneal ulcer	Subcategory
H16.041	Marginal corneal ulcer, right eye	Code
H16.042	Marginal corneal ulcer, left eye	Code
H16.043	Marginal corneal ulcer, bilateral	Code
H16.049	Marginal corneal ulcer, unspecified eye	Code

Figure 4-3 ■ Example of Laterality in ICD-10-CM

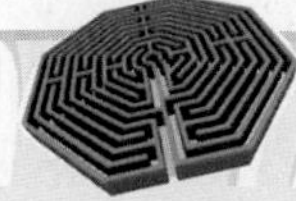

Coding Practice

Now it is your turn to demonstrate your understanding of assigning the correct number of characters in a code. Try to answer the questions from memory first, then refer back to the information in this section if you need a little extra help.

Exercise 4.3 Conventions: Use Additional Characters, Extensions, and Placeholders

Instructions: Look up the following codes in the Tabular list and determine if each is correct, needs additional characters, needs a placeholder, and/or needs an extension. Some codes may need more than one of these items.

If the code is correct, write *Correct* in the space provided. If the code is incorrect, write the correct code for the stated condition in the space provided.

1. E65 Localized adiposity ____________
2. E66 Morbid obesity due to excess calories ________
3. G43.1 Migraine with aura, not intractable, with status migrainosus ____________
4. I48.0 Atrial fibrillation ____________
5. O31.00 Papyraceous fetus, first trimester, fetus 1 ____________
6. O29.8X2 Other complications of anesthesia during pregnancy, second trimester ____________
7. S71.151 Bite, right thigh, sequela ____________
8. S84.22 Injury of cutaneous sensory nerve at lower leg level, left leg, initial encounter ____________
9. S72.02 Displaced fracture of epiphysis, left femur, subsequent encounter for closed fracture with nonunion ____________
10. T59.6X Toxic effect of hydrogen sulfide, accidental, subsequent encounter ____________

HOW TO CODE DIAGNOSES

Diagnosis coding requires three skills of an ace coder:

- Abstract—read the medical record and determine which elements of the encounter require codes.
- Assign—determine codes that accurately describe the patient's condition, reflect the highest level of specificity possible, and contain the correct number of characters for each code.
- Arrange (sequence)—place codes in the order dictated by the OGCR and instructional notes.

Although coders do not need to memorize specific codes, they do need to memorize the skills and steps of the coding process.

When coders begin the process of assigning diagnosis codes, they do not necessarily know how many codes will be required. In some cases, a combination code is available, which describes two or more conditions in a single code. Other times, multiple coding is required, which means that two or more codes are needed to fully describe a condition. Coders learn how many codes are needed by following the guidelines, conventions, and instructional notes in the Index, Tabular List, and OGCR.

Abstracting Diagnoses

The first step in coding is to identify the diagnosis(es) to be coded, based on the documentation. The OGCR provide guidelines for this task in Section I.B., as well as Section IV for outpatient services and Sections II and III for inpatient services. Chapter-specific guidelines in Section I.C. provide more detailed guidance for selected conditions. This section provides an overview of abstracting outpatient and inpatient diagnoses.

Abstracting Outpatient Diagnoses

For outpatient coding, the coder needs to identify the main reason for the services provided, which is the first-listed diagnosis. Recall that this is the diagnosis, condition, problem, or other reason for the encounter visit shown in the medical record to be chiefly responsible for the services provided (OGCR IV.A.). Coding conventions and the general (OGCR I. B.) and chapter-specific (OCGR I.C.) guidelines take precedence over Section IV outpatient guidelines if there is a conflict. Key rules for abstracting outpatient diagnoses follow:

- Do **not** code **signs** or **symptoms** that are an integral part of the disease process when the diagnosis has been established.
- Do **not** code an uncertain diagnosis, which is indicated in the medical record by words such as probable, possible, suspected, questionable, rule out, or working diagnosis.
- **Do** code the presenting signs and symptoms when the diagnosis is uncertain. This guideline for outpatient services is different than the guideline for uncertain diagnoses for inpatient services.
- **Do** code additional conditions and signs or symptoms that are not part of the confirmed disease process, in addition to the first-listed diagnosis, when they are managed during the encounter.
- Do **not** code conditions that are resolved, not treated, or have no bearing on the current encounter.

ICD-10-CM also provides codes for encounters due to reasons other than a disease or injury. These may be routine health screenings, preventive care, diagnostic services only, therapeutic services only, preoperative evaluations, prenatal visits, and similar situations. Codes for most of these situations are classified under Factors Influencing Health Status and Contact with Health services (Z00-Z99). Detailed guidelines appear in OGCR IV and codes are indexed in the Index to Diseases and Injuries.

Abstracting Using the Mini-Medical-Record

This text uses a mini-medical-record format for examples and exercises, which extracts the most essential information from a patient's medical record. Refer to ■ FIGURE 4-4 to become acquainted with this format and to learn how to interpret it.

Guided Example of Abstracting Diagnoses

Refer to the following example, which begins here and continues throughout the chapter, to learn more about abstracting a diagnosis for an outpatient visit. Sherry Whittle, CPC, is a fictitious coder who guides you through this case.

> Date: 4/1/yy Location: Branton Family Practice
>
> Provider: Kristen Conover, MD
>
> Patient: Eric Beardsley Gender: M Age: 24
>
> Chief complaint: Pain and swelling in right ankle. Tripped over rocks while hiking and twisted ankle.
>
> Assessment: X-rays negative for fracture. Right ankle sprain, deltoid ligament
>
> Plan: Ice, compression wrap, crutches. Elevate foot. Keep weight off foot for one week. **OTC** acetaminophen for pain **PRN**. Call office if not better in 2 weeks.

Follow along with coder Sherry Whittle, CPC, as she reads the progress notes from Eric Beardsley's office visit. Check off each step as you complete it.

⇨ First, Sherry reviews the demographic information, then reads Mr. Beardsley's chief complaint.

- ❑ She notes that pain is a subjective symptom experienced by the patient and swelling is an objective sign that Dr. Conover verified.
- ❑ She also notes the cause of the injury.

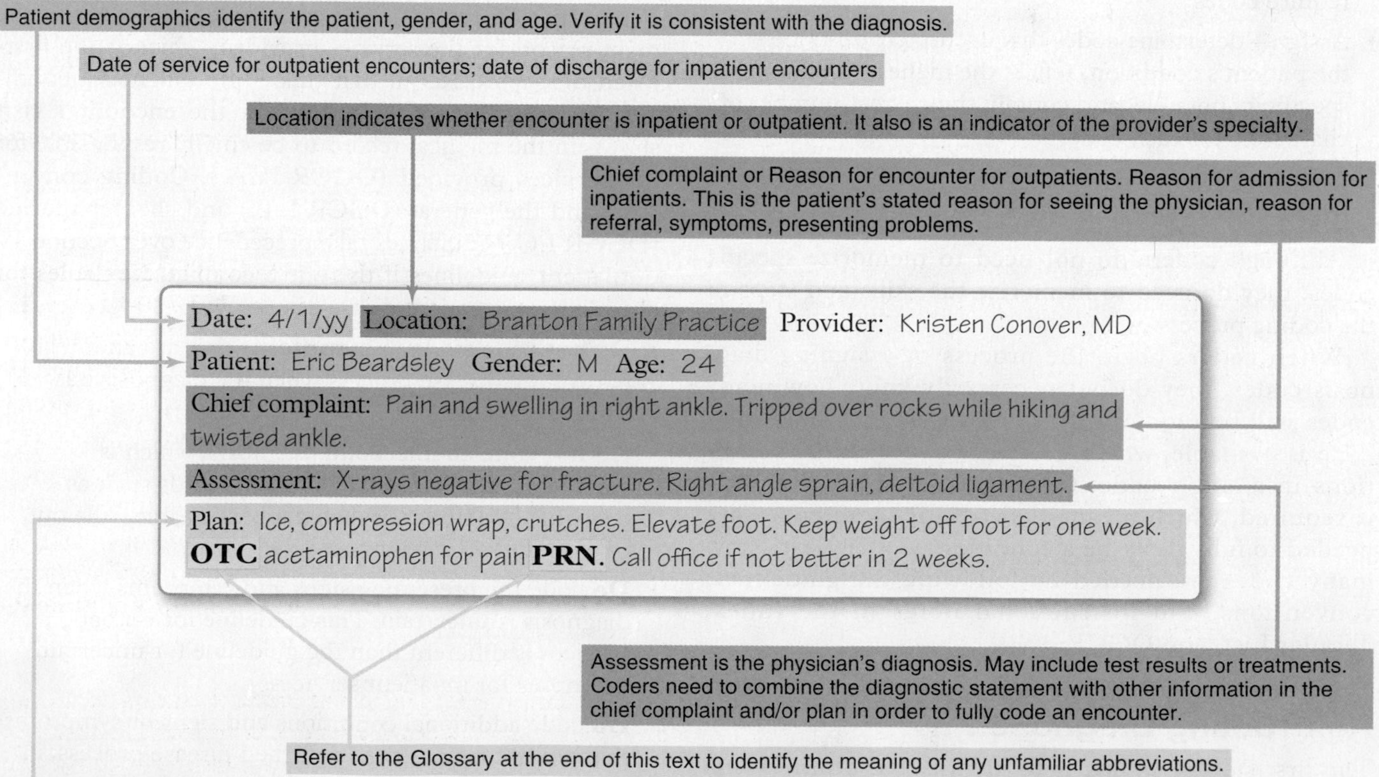

Figure 4-4 ■ Key to Interpreting the Mini-Medical-Record

- She reads the assessment, which is Dr. Conover's diagnosis.
  - She notes that X-rays were taken to determine if there is a fracture, which there is not.
  - Dr. Conover determines that the patient has a sprain of the deltoid ligament in the right ankle.
- She reviews the treatment plan and notes it is consistent with the condition of sprained ankle.
- Sherry compares the signs and symptoms in the chief complaint to the diagnostic statement of a sprained ankle.
  - She confirms that both pain and swelling are integral to a sprained ankle.
  - Because Dr. Conover made a diagnosis of sprained ankle, Sherry does not need to code for the symptoms of pain and swelling.
  - Sherry will code the diagnosis Right ankle sprain, deltoid ligament.

SUCCESS STEP

You do not always know how many codes you will end up with, or even exactly which conditions require a code, at the time of abstracting. You abstract *potential* conditions and elements to be coded. OGCR and instructional notes in the Tabular List provide further direction about how many and what codes are needed in a specific situation.

Abstracting Inpatient Diagnoses

Recall that for inpatient services, the main reason that services were provided is the principal diagnosis. This is "the condition established after study to be chiefly responsible for occasioning the admission of the patient to the hospital for care" (OGCR Section II.). Coding conventions and the general (OGCR I.B) and chapter-specific (OGCR I.C.) guidelines take precedence over Section II and III inpatient guidelines if there is a conflict. Key rules for abstracting inpatient diagnoses follow:

- Do **not** code signs or symptoms that are an integral part of the disease process when the diagnosis has been established.
- **Do** code additional conditions, signs, or symptoms not part of the confirmed disease, in addition to the principal diagnosis, when they are relevant to the current admission. Relevant diagnoses, also called clinically significant conditions, are defined by UHDDS as "all conditions that coexist at the time of admission, that develop subsequently, or that affect the treatment received and/or the length of stay. Diagnoses that relate to an earlier episode which have no bearing on the current hospital stay are to be excluded." (OGCR III.)
- **Do** code for an uncertain diagnosis if a definitive diagnosis is not available at the time of discharge and/or after all test results are reported. This guideline is different for inpatient services than outpatient. For inpatient, code an uncertain diagnosis as if it exists, because it is the reason for the hospital admission and any diagnostic and therapeutic services provided. (OGCR II. H.)

Assigning Diagnosis Codes

After identifying the first-listed diagnosis or principal diagnosis in the medical record, the next step is to assign the most specific code possible that describes the condition. To assign a diagnosis code, first look up the condition in the Index to Diseases and Injuries (Index), then verify the code in the Tabular List.

CODING CAUTION

Coding sounds simple to the casual observer, but as you are about to learn, it is an extended research process that involves many comparisons and cross-checks. Learning the detailed steps of coding will make you a more accurate coder. Unfortunately, there are no shortcuts.

Locate the Main Term in the Index

The first step in assigning the code is to locate the Main Term (*the primary index entry*) in the ICD-10-CM Index to Diseases and Injuries. The Main Term is the name of the condition or reason for the visit, usually presented as a noun. Coders need to be knowledgeable about several details regarding the organization of the Index, which are discussed in the next section.

Anatomical Sites Are Not Indexed. Anatomical sites or organs are rarely indexed as Main Terms, so it is best to look up the condition itself. Main Terms appear in boldface type in the index.

Guided Example of Using the Index. Continue with the example of Eric Beardsley who was treated for an ankle sprain to learn more about using the Index. Follow along in your ICD-10-CM manual as Sherry Whittle, CPC, locates the code for Mr. Beardsley in the Index. Check off each step as you complete it.

➪ Sherry looks up the entry for **Ankle** and observes a cross-reference note that states ***see* condition** (■ FIGURE 4-5).

- ❑ She recalls that this is a cross-reference directing her to look up the term that describes the *condition affecting* the ankle, which in this case is a sprain.
- ❑ She does not look up the word "condition."
- ❑ Sherry will look up the Main Term **Sprain** because that is the condition that affects the ankle.

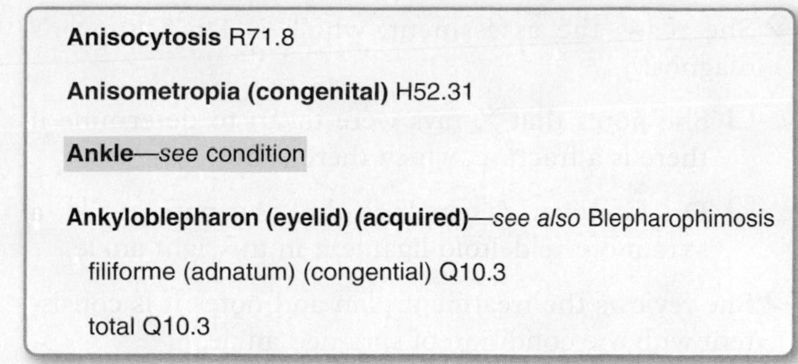

Figure 4-5 ■ Example of a Cross-Reference in Index

Subterms. Subterms are words indented under each Main Term that further describe the Main Term in greater detail, such as anatomical location or other disease variation. Subterms appear in roman type (not boldface) and are indented three spaces under the Main Term. Many subterms have additional subterms indented under them. Each subterm is an expansion of the Main Term or previous subterm it is indented under. In some editions of the coding manual, the ICD-10-CM Index provides light gray guidelines to align the first and third levels of indentation. Refer to ■ FIGURE 4-6 for the layout and compare the figure to the actual coding manual.

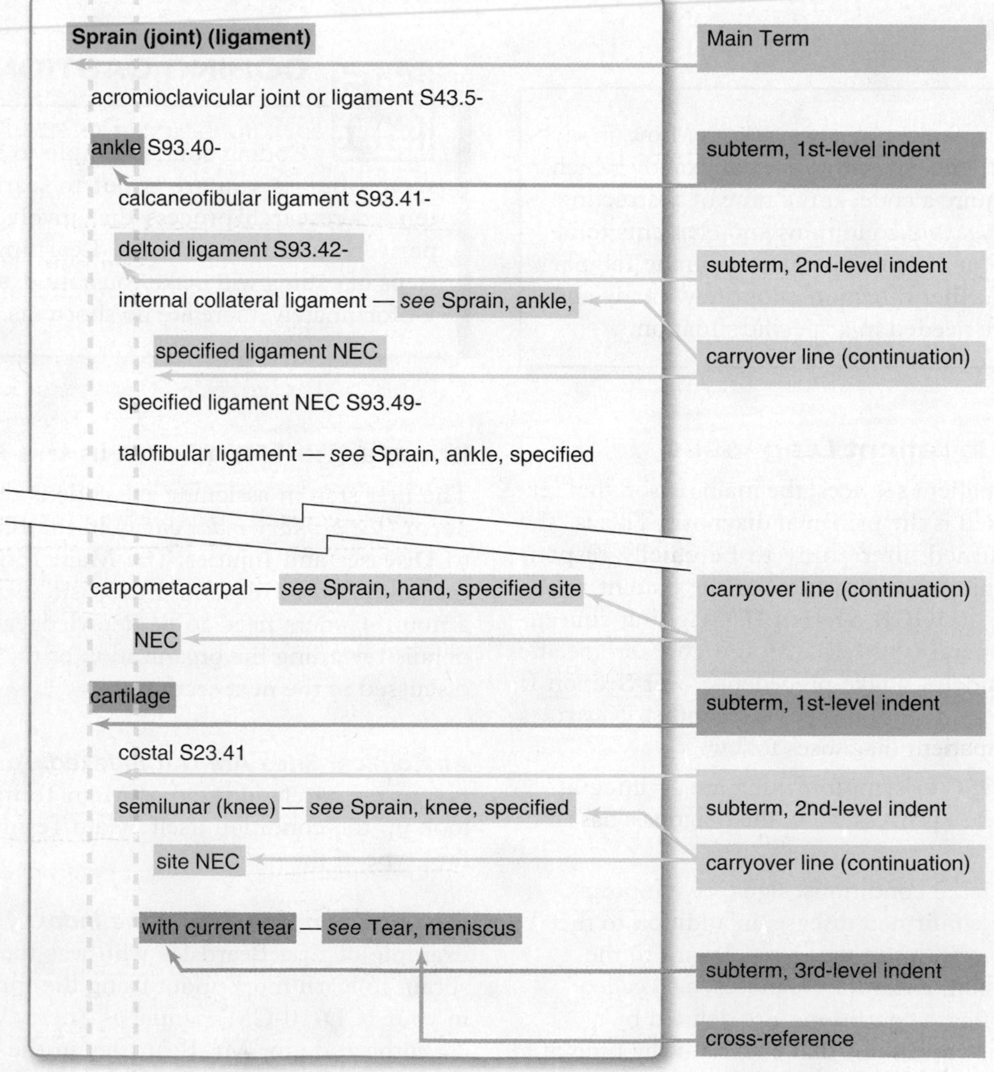

Figure 4-6 ■ Example of Main Term and Subterm Indents in the Index

Guided Example of Locating the Main Term. Continue to follow along in your ICD-10-CM manual as Sherry Whittle, CPC, looks up the Main Term **Sprain** for Mr. Beardsley's case. Check off each step as you complete it.

➩ Sherry locates the Main Term **Sprain** in the Index to Diseases and Injuries.

- ☐ She scans the entire entry for **Sprain** which continues onto the next several columns on the next page. At the top of each column is a heading **Sprain – continued**, telling her which Main Term is being continued.
- ☐ She notices that all the subterms describe anatomical sites of a sprain.
- ☐ She locates the subterm **ankle**, for the anatomical site.
- ☐ She notices that additional subterms further describe the anatomical site within the ankle, such as **calcaneofibular ligament S93.41-** and **deltoid ligament S93.42-**. These subterms are second-level indents. Both of these entries are part of the overall entry for ankle, because they are indented under the subterm **ankle**.
- ☐ Sherry identifies the second-level subterm **deltoid ligament S93.42-** as the best match for Mr. Beardsley's case.
- ☐ The full name of this entry combines the Main Term and each indented subterm: **Sprain + ankle + deltoid ligament** (Figure 4-6).

Also notice in Figure 4-6 that a third-level indent appears further down in the entry for **Sprain**. The subterm **cartilage** is a first-level indent, so it is parallel to the subterm **ankle**. These two subterms are mutually exclusive. Cartilage has second-level indents for the sites **costal** and **semilunar**. Semilunar has a third-level indent, **with current tear**. The full entry for this subterm is **Sprain, cartilage, semilunar, with current tear**.

Cross-References. As previously mentioned, some subterms provide cross-referencing instructions, which begin with the word ***see*** or ***see also***. When the instruction following the word ***see*** or ***see also*** is capitalized, the coder should look under the word listed to find the correct code. For example, under **Sprain, cartilage, semilunar, with current tear**, the subterm **with current tear** provides cross-referencing instructions to ***see*** **Tear, meniscus**. This means the coder should look up the Main Term **Tear** and the subterm **meniscus** in order to locate the code.

Refer to Figure 4-5 for an example of a ***see also*** cross-reference. Notice that the Main Term **Ankyloblepharon** has two subterms. In addition to reviewing these subterms, coders should also cross-reference the Main Term **Blepharophimosis** for additional codes.

SUCCESS STEP

In the beginning, you may experience a process of trial and error while you are learning how to identify and locate Main Terms. Do not let this frustrate you and do not be disturbed by cross-reference notes in the Index. This is ICD-10-CM's way of pointing you in the right direction and is a normal part of coding.

Appendicitis (pneumococcal) (retrocecal) K37

Figure 4-7 ■ Example of Index Entry for a Default Code with Nonessential Modifiers

Default Codes. A code listed next to a Main Term in the ICD-10-CM Index is referred to as a **default code**. The default code may represent the condition most commonly associated with the Main Term, or, it may represent the unspecified code for the condition, which usually ends in 9. Refer to ■ FIGURE 4-7 for an example of a default code. In this example, if appendicitis is documented in the medical record without any additional information, such as acute or chronic, the default code, **K37**, should be assigned because it appears next to the Main Term, **Appendicitis**.

Nonessential Modifiers. The words in parentheses ( ) after a Main Term or subterm are **nonessential modifiers**. Nonessential modifiers are included in the default description of the code and do not need to be present in the medical record in order to use the code. For example, in Figure 4-7, the Main Term **Appendicitis** is followed by the terms **(pneumococcal)** and **(retrocecal)**. These words are nonessential modifiers because they are enclosed in parentheses. This means that pneumococcal and retrocecal appendicitis are automatically included in the default appendicitis code **K37**. However, these words do not need to be present in the medical record in order to assign this code because they are nonessential modifiers. The conditions appendicitis, pneumococcal appendicitis, and retrocecal appendicitis are all classified with the same code, **K37**.

Also notice that in the ICD-10-CM Index, the entry **Appendicitis** has numerous subterms with different codes. Coders must review all the subterms and locate the most specific one before selecting a code to verify. Do not automatically select the default code without reviewing the subterms.

Multiple Coding Paths. Conditions may have multiple **coding paths**, which means they can be indexed under more than one Main Term. For example, chronic rhinopharyngitis (inflammation of the nose and throat) appears under **Rhinopharyngitis, chronic J31.1** and also under

Nasopharyngitis, chronic J31.1. Both Main Terms lead to the same code because the medical terminology combining forms rhin/o and nas/o both mean nose. If coders have difficulty locating a Main Term, they can also look under an eponym (*named after a person*), a synonym, or other alternative term. In addition, coders can reference broad-ranging Main Terms, such as Abnormal, Anomaly, Complication, Disease, Findings, Infection, Injury, or Syndrome. In some cases, coders may need to look in several locations under different Main Terms to identify multiple code options before proceeding. This is a normal part of the coding process.

SUCCESS STEP

There are times when you will not be completely sure of which code to look up based on your research in the Index. That is okay. If you locate two or three possible codes in the Index, make note of all of them. After you verify each one in the Tabular List, you will have more information to help determine which code best describes the patient. You will learn how to verify codes later in this chapter.

Specialized Index Locations. While most conditions and reasons for the encounter are located in the Index to Diseases and Injuries, ICD-10-CM has three additional locations for specialized codes.

- *Neoplasms* are indexed on the Table of Neoplasms, located under "N" in the Index to Diseases and Injuries. This is similar to the ICD-9-CM. Some publishers may locate this table immediately after the Index to Diseases and Injuries.
- *Poisonings, adverse effects, and underdosing caused by drugs and chemicals* are indexed in the ICD-10-CM Table of Drugs and Chemicals, which is located following the Index to Diseases and Injuries. This is similar to the ICD-9-CM.
- *External causes of illness and injury* are located in a separate index, the ICD-10-CM Index to External Causes, which follows the Table of Drugs and Chemicals. This is similar to the E code index in ICD-9-CM. External causes reported under "E codes" in ICD-9-CM are generally reported using codes beginning with the letters V, W, X, and Y in ICD-10-CM and appear within the Tabular List.

SUCCESS STEP

Just as some publishers use different symbols to alert coders to special situations, some may organize the sections of the coding manual in a different order. Refer to the Table of Contents at the beginning of your coding manual to learn how it is organized.

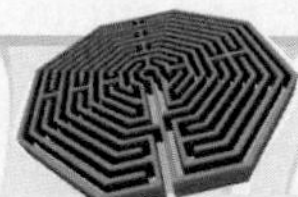

Coding Practice

Now it is your turn to demonstrate your understanding of Main Terms. Try to answer the questions from memory first, then refer back to the information in this section if you need a little extra help.

Exercise 4.4 Locating the Main Term

Instructions: Underline the Main Term in each of these diagnoses. Then look up the Main Term in the Index to confirm that you chose the correct term. If the Index cross-references another entry, write the name of the cross-reference in the space provided. Then look up the cross-referenced entry.

Example: Short arm *Deformity, limb, unequal length*

1. Complicated open wound of left ear, initial encounter ____________________
2. Deprivation of water, subsequent encounter ____________________
3. Urinary tract infection ____________________
4. Chickenpox ____________________
5. Blackwater fever ____________________
6. Gallbladder infection ____________________
7. Quartan malaria ____________________
8. Cerebrovascular disease ____________________
9. Congestive heart failure ____________________
10. Type 1 diabetes ____________________

Verify Codes in the Tabular List

After identifying the potential code(s) in the Index, the next step in assigning a code is to verify it in the Tabular List. This is an essential step because the Index is not designed to provide the full code or full information about how to use the code. Verifying codes requires cross-referencing information at several points.

A short dash (-) at the end of an Index entry indicates that additional characters are required. Even when a dash is not included at the Index entry, it is necessary to refer to the Tabular List to verify that no seventh character is required and to review the instructional notes. Characters for laterality and the seventh position extension can only be assigned in the Tabular List. The Tabular List also includes instructional notes that must be followed, such as those for sequencing, multiple coding, and inclusion and exclusion notes discussed earlier in the chapter.

To verify a code, look up the code number in the Tabular List and follow these steps:

1. Read the code title to confirm that the code accurately describes the intended condition.
2. Read the instructional notes under the code.
3. Check for symbols preceding the entry indicating that additional characters are required.
4. Cross-reference the titles of the subcategory and the three-character category and read any instructional notes under those titles.
5. Cross-reference the titles of the block and the chapter headings and read any instructional notes under those titles.
6. Compare and contrast any other codes being considered for first-listed or principal diagnosis.
7. Assign all required digits and write the code down, taking time to double check for transcription or typographical errors.
8. Repeat this process for each code required.

Guided Example of Verifying Codes in the Tabular List

Continue with the example of Eric Beardsley, who has a right ankle sprain of the deltoid ligament, to learn more about verifying codes in the Tabular List.

Follow along in your ICD-10-CM manual as Sherry Whittle, CPC, verifies the diagnosis code. Check off each step after you complete it.

⇨ Recall that Sherry located the entry **S93.42-** in the Index.

- ❑ Sherry notices the entry ends with a short dash (-). She knows this means that she will need to assign additional digits when she verifies the code in the Tabular List.

⇨ Sherry looks up the entry **S93.42** in the Tabular List.

- ❑ She notices that this is a subcategory, not a code, because additional characters are required. The symbol **6th** in front of the entry tells her that a sixth character is required.
- ❑ She confirms the title of the category **Sprain of deltoid ligament** is consistent with the progress note.

⇨ She reads the code choices listed and notices that the sixth character defines laterality with choices for right ankle, left ankle, and unspecified ankle.

- ❑ She refers back to the progress note to confirm which ankle was affected.
- ❑ She selects code **S93.421** for the right ankle.

⇨ Sherry notices that the symbol **7th** appears in front of the code **S93.421**. This tells her that a seventh character is required to complete the code.

- ❑ The seventh character is not listed under the code, so she knows she needs to review the previous subcategory, category, and block headings to locate the seventh character options. She knows she needs to review these headings anyway in order to locate any possible instructional notes.

⇨ Sherry confirms the subcategory title **S93.4, Sprain of ankle** is the correct anatomic site because other joints, such as the shoulder, also have a **deltoid** muscle or ligament.

- ❑ She reads the note **Excludes2: injury of Achilles tendon (S86.0-)** under the subcategory title and verifies that does not apply to her case because the Achilles tendon was not documented.

⇨ Next she works back up the organizational hierarchy of the Tabular List until she locates the three-character category heading **S93, Dislocation and sprain of joints and ligaments at ankle, foot and toe level** (■ FIGURE 4-8, page 58).

- ❑ Sherry reads the entries for the **Includes** note under the category heading. She observes that one of entries is **sprain of cartilage, joint or ligament of ankle, foot and toe,** which is consistent with the Mr. Beardsley's progress note.
- ❑ Sherry notices the instructional note **Code also any associated open wound** following the Includes list. She understands that if Dr. Conover had documented an open wound in addition to the sprain, she would need an additional code for the wound. Because a wound was not documented, she knows she can bypass this note.
- ❑ Sherry reads the note **Excludes2: strain of muscle and tendon of ankle and foot (S96.-)** and understands that if Dr. Conover had also documented

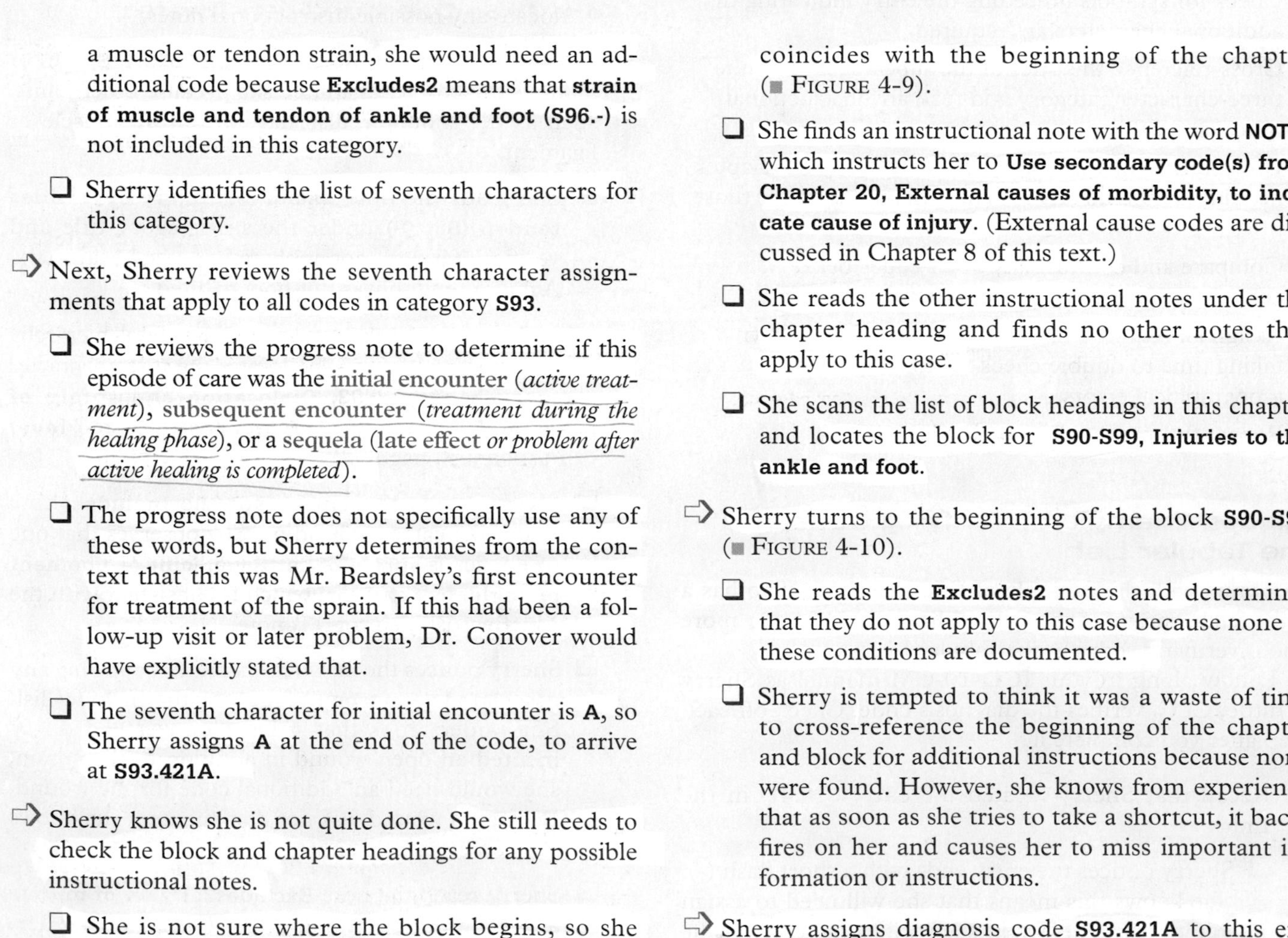

S93 Dislocation and sprain of joints and ligaments at ankle, foot and toe level

Includes:

avulsion of joint or ligament of ankle, foot and toe

laceration of cartilage, joint or ligament of ankle, foot and toe

sprain of cartilage, joint or ligament of ankle, foot and toe

traumatic hemarthrosis of joint or ligament of ankle, foot and toe

traumatic rupture of joint or ligament of ankle, foot and toe

traumatic subluxation of joint or ligament of ankle, foot and toe

traumatic tear of joint or ligament of ankle, foot and toe

Excludes2: strain of muscle and tendon of ankle and foot (S96.-)

Code also any associated open wound

The appropriate 7th character is to be added to each code from category S93

A - initial encounter

D - subsequent encounter

S - sequela

Figure 4-8 ■ Tabular List Entry for Category Heading S93

a muscle or tendon strain, she would need an additional code because **Excludes2** means that **strain of muscle and tendon of ankle and foot (S96.-)** is not included in this category.

❑ Sherry identifies the list of seventh characters for this category.

⇨ Next, Sherry reviews the seventh character assignments that apply to all codes in category **S93**.

❑ She reviews the progress note to determine if this episode of care was the initial encounter (*active treatment*), subsequent encounter (*treatment during the healing phase*), or a sequela (late effect *or problem after active healing is completed*).

❑ The progress note does not specifically use any of these words, but Sherry determines from the context that this was Mr. Beardsley's first encounter for treatment of the sprain. If this had been a follow-up visit or later problem, Dr. Conover would have explicitly stated that.

❑ The seventh character for initial encounter is **A**, so Sherry assigns **A** at the end of the code, to arrive at **S93.421A**.

⇨ Sherry knows she is not quite done. She still needs to check the block and chapter headings for any possible instructional notes.

❑ She is not sure where the block begins, so she refers to the beginning of the entries for codes beginning with **S** in the Tabular List, which coincides with the beginning of the chapter (■ FIGURE 4-9).

❑ She finds an instructional note with the word **NOTE:** which instructs her to **Use secondary code(s) from Chapter 20, External causes of morbidity, to indicate cause of injury**. (External cause codes are discussed in Chapter 8 of this text.)

❑ She reads the other instructional notes under the chapter heading and finds no other notes that apply to this case.

❑ She scans the list of block headings in this chapter and locates the block for **S90-S99, Injuries to the ankle and foot.**

⇨ Sherry turns to the beginning of the block **S90-S99** (■ FIGURE 4-10).

❑ She reads the **Excludes2** notes and determines that they do not apply to this case because none of these conditions are documented.

❑ Sherry is tempted to think it was a waste of time to cross-reference the beginning of the chapter and block for additional instructions because none were found. However, she knows from experience that as soon as she tries to take a shortcut, it backfires on her and causes her to miss important information or instructions.

⇨ Sherry assigns diagnosis code **S93.421A** to this encounter. She will also assign external cause codes for tripping while hiking.

Chapter 19

Injury, poisoning and certain other consequences of external causes (S00-T88)

NOTE: Use secondary code(s) from Chapter 20, External causes of morbidity, to indicate cause of injury. Codes within the T section that include the external cause do not require an additional external cause code.

Use additional code to identify any retained foreign body, if applicable (Z18.-)

Excludes1:

birth trauma (P10-P15)

obstetric trauma (O70-O71)

This chapter contains the following blocks:

S00-09	Injuries to the head
S10-19	Injuries to the neck
S20-29	Injuries to the thorax
S70-79	Injuries to the hip and thigh
S80-89	Injuries to the knee and lower leg
S90-99	Injuries to the ankle and foot
T07	Injuries involving multiple body regions
T14	Injury of unspecified body region
T79	Certain early complications of trauma
T80-88	Complications of surgical and medical care, not elsewhere classified

Figure 4-9 ■ Tabular List Entry for Chapter 19

Injuries to the ankle and foot (S90-S99)

Excludes2:

burns and corrosions (T20-T32)

fracture of ankle and malleolus (S82.-)

frostbite (T33-T34)

insect bite or sting, venomous (T63.4)

Figure 4-10 ■ Tabular List Entry for Block Heading S90-S99

Arranging Diagnosis Codes

The final step in diagnosis coding is to arrange, or sequence, codes in correct order when there is more than one diagnosis code. Coders may need to assign more than one diagnosis code when patients have more than one condition that is being treated or managed during an encounter; there is an etiology/manifestation relationship; multiple coding is required; or instructional notes in the Tabular List direct the coder to additional codes needed. Each of these situations is discussed below. In addition, the OGCR discusses requirements for multiple coding related to specific diseases.

SUCCESS STEP

This text uses the term *arrange* as a learning mnemonic for *sequence* in order to remind you of the coding skills of **A**bstract, **A**ssign, and **A**rrange. In the workplace, most professional coders simply use the term *sequence*.

More Than One Condition Treated

When more than one condition is treated or managed during an encounter, sequence the principal or first-listed diagnosis first. When it is difficult to determine which condition is the principal diagnosis, refer to the following guidelines:

- When two or more interrelated conditions each potentially meet the definition for principal diagnosis, either condition may be sequenced first if the circumstances of admission (*facts, signs, and symptoms that require the admission*), the Index, or the Tabular List provide no further guidance (OGCR II. B.).
- When two or more distinct conditions equally meet the definition for principal diagnosis, either condition may be sequenced first if the circumstances of admission, the Index, or the Tabular List provide no further guidance (OGCR II. C.).

When the principal or first-listed diagnosis is clear, sequence the additional conditions in order of importance to the encounter or in order of severity or risk to the patient's health and well-being.

Etiology/Manifestation

Etiology/manifestation is an ICD-10-CM convention for certain conditions that have both an underlying etiology (*cause*) and manifestations (*signs and symptoms*) in multiple body systems (OGCR I.A.13). Sequence the etiology first and the manifestation second. Coders may not always know in advance if a particular combination of diseases is an etiology/manifestation relationship, so the ICD-10-CM manual alerts coders with sequencing instructions.

CODING CAUTION

Do not apply etiology/manifestation rules if ICD-10-CM does not list instructional notes or other conventions indicating this relationship.

Refer to the following example of dementia in Parkinson's disease, where Parkinson's disease is the etiology and dementia is a manifestation. Common sequencing instructions for etiology/manifestation follow with examples:

- The Index lists both conditions and both codes together. The etiology code is first; the manifestation code is second and appears in [brackets]. Always sequence the code in brackets second (■ FIGURE 4-11).
- In the Tabular List entry for the manifestation code, the manual provides an instructional note **Code first** and lists codes for possible etiologies. The condition listed after this note should be sequenced second (■ FIGURE 4-12).
- The manifestation code title often includes the phrase **in diseases classified elsewhere**. Code titles with this phrase are highlighted in blue in the Tabular List as a reminder that manifestation codes may never be the first-listed or principal diagnosis.

CODING CAUTION

Do not assign a code from the **Use additional code** list for any condition that is not documented in the medical record. If the etiology documented in the medical record does not appear in the list, you should refer to the Index and locate the code for the specific etiology you need.

CODING CAUTION

Notice that Figure 4-13 has an **Excludes1** note for **dementia with Parkinsonism** and cross-references the coder to **G31.83**. When you cross-reference **G31.83**, you see the code title is **Dementia with Lewy bodies**, which is a specific kind of dementia. Since this condition is not documented in the medical record, use the original code **G20**.

- When two codes are listed in the Index, remember to verify both codes in the Tabular List. ■ FIGURE 4-13 shows the Tabular List entry for the etiology code **G20**.
- In some instances, the etiology code in the Tabular List provides the instructional note **Use additional code** and lists common manifestations. Refer to ■ FIGURE 4-14 (page 62) to see how this note is used for **Alzheimer's disease, late onset, and dementia with behavioral disturbance**. Assign and arrange the codes as follows:

  (1) **G30.0 Alzheimer's disease with early onset**

  (2) **F02.81 Dementia with behavioral disturbance**

Use Additional Code

The Tabular List also lists the instructional note **Use additional code** in other situations besides etiology/manifestation. The note may appear under code, subcategory, category, block, or chapter titles, so the coder must always review these headings for instructions. Refer to the ICD-10-CM manual Chapter 10, Diseases of the Respiratory System (J00-J99), and locate the note **Use additional code**

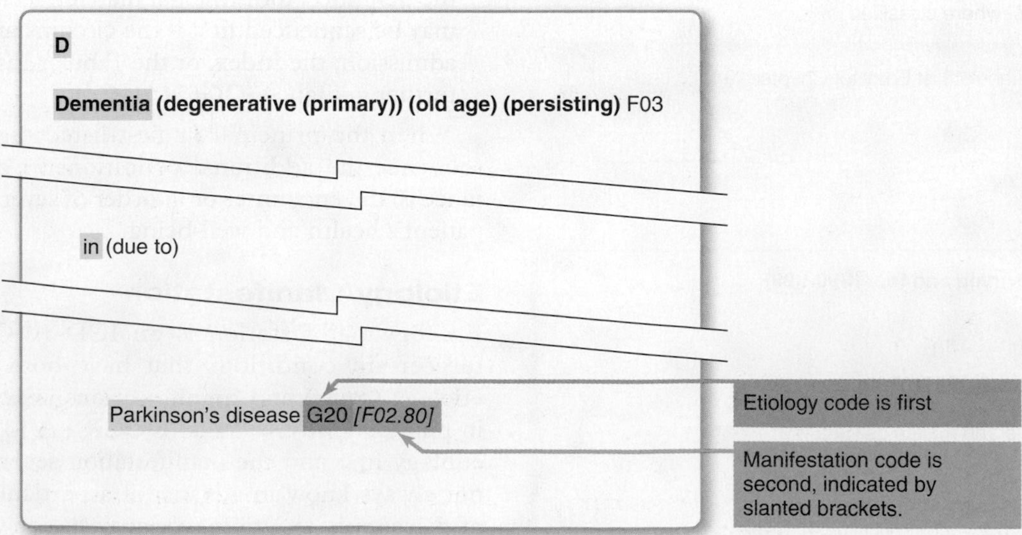

Figure 4-11 ■ Example of Index Entry for Etiology and Manifestation Codes

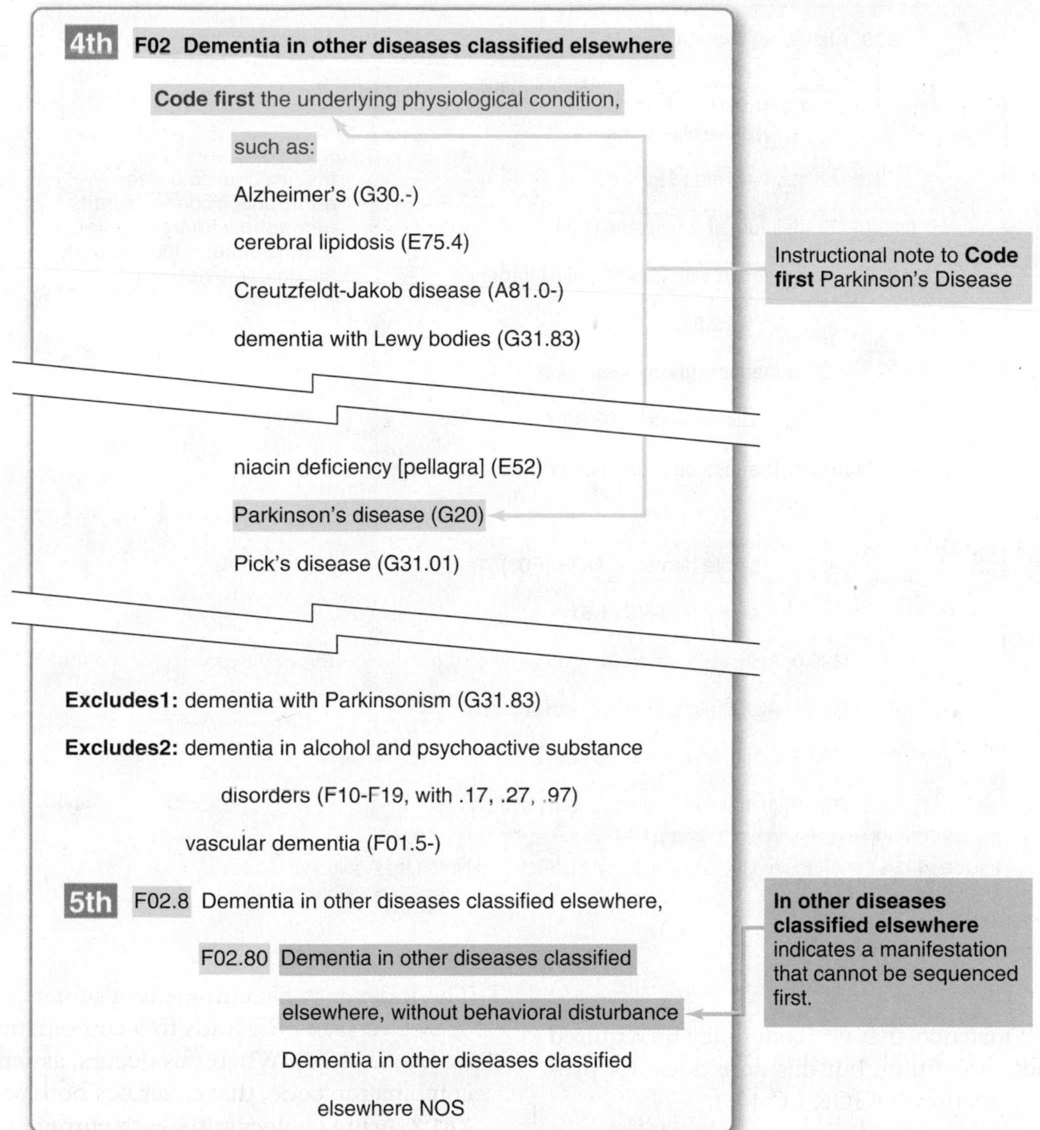

4th **F02 Dementia in other diseases classified elsewhere**

Code first the underlying physiological condition,

such as:

Alzheimer's (G30.-)

cerebral lipidosis (E75.4)

Creutzfeldt-Jakob disease (A81.0-)

dementia with Lewy bodies (G31.83)

niacin deficiency [pellagra] (E52)

Parkinson's disease (G20)

Pick's disease (G31.01)

Excludes1: dementia with Parkinsonism (G31.83)

Excludes2: dementia in alcohol and psychoactive substance disorders (F10-F19, with .17, .27, .97)

vascular dementia (F01.5-)

5th F02.8 Dementia in other diseases classified elsewhere,

F02.80 Dementia in other diseases classified elsewhere, without behavioral disturbance

Dementia in other diseases classified elsewhere NOS

Figure 4-12 ■ Example of Tabular List Entry for Code First Instructions

under the chapter title. This instructional note applies to all codes in the chapter (OGCR I.A.13.).

G20 Parkinson's disease

Hemiparkinsonism

Idiopathic Parkinsonism or Parkinson's disease

Paralysis agitans

Parkinsonism or Parkinson's disease NOS

Primary Parkinsonism or Parkinson's disease

Excludes1: dementia with Parkinsonism (G31.83)

Figure 4-13 ■ Example of Tabular List Entry for an Etiology Code (G20)

Code First

Code first notes also appear under certain codes that are not specifically manifestation codes, but may be due to an underlying cause. When there is a **Code first** note and an underlying condition is present, the underlying condition should be sequenced first (OGCR I.A.13. and I.B.7.).

Code, if Applicable, Any Causal Condition First

Code, if applicable, any causal condition first notes indicate that this code may be assigned as a principal diagnosis when the causal condition is unknown or not applicable. If a causal condition is known, then the code for that condition should be sequenced as the principal or first-listed diagnosis (OGCR I.B.7.).

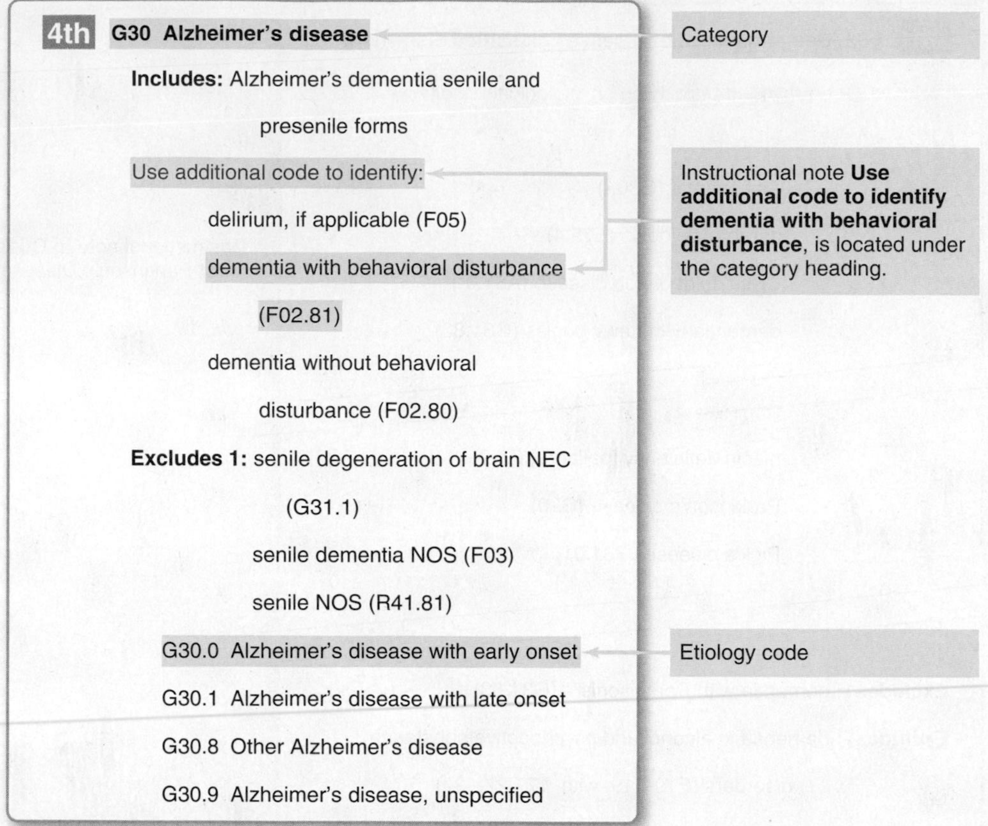

Figure 4-14 ■ Tabular List Entry with the Instructional Note Use Additional Code

Code Also

A **Code also** note instructs that two codes may be required to fully describe a condition, but this note does not provide sequencing direction (OGCR I.C.17.).

CODING CAUTION

Do not automatically assign additional codes when you see an instructional note. The condition must be documented in the medical record in order to assign a code.

Acute and Chronic

Providers may document that a patient has both acute and chronic forms of the same condition, such as bronchitis or cholecystitis. The sequencing is determined by how the Index presents the acute and chronic conditions. The Index lists acute and chronic conditions in one of two ways:

- The Index may list subterms for both acute and chronic at the same level of indentation.

  When this occurs, sequence the code for acute first and the code for chronic second (OGCR I.B.8.) (■ FIGURE 4-15).

- The Index may list **chronic** as a subterm of **acute**, or vice versa, which leads to a combination code (■ FIGURE 4-16). When this occurs, assign one code, the combination code, that describes both conditions:

  K81.2 Acute cholecystitis with chronic cholecystitis

Regardless of how the Index lists the entries, always verify the codes in the Tabular List and follow any instructional notes.

Other Multiple Code Situations

In addition to the general guidelines for sequencing multiple codes, multiple codes may be needed in many specific situations such as obstetrics, injuries, surgical or procedural complications, and late effects. OGCR Section I C., Chapter Specific-Coding Guidelines, defines these rules.

SUCCESS STEP

As you have seen, there is not one simple rule that tells you how to sequence multiple codes. Your knowledge of OGCR and ability to read all instructional notes in the Tabular List guide you in each situation.

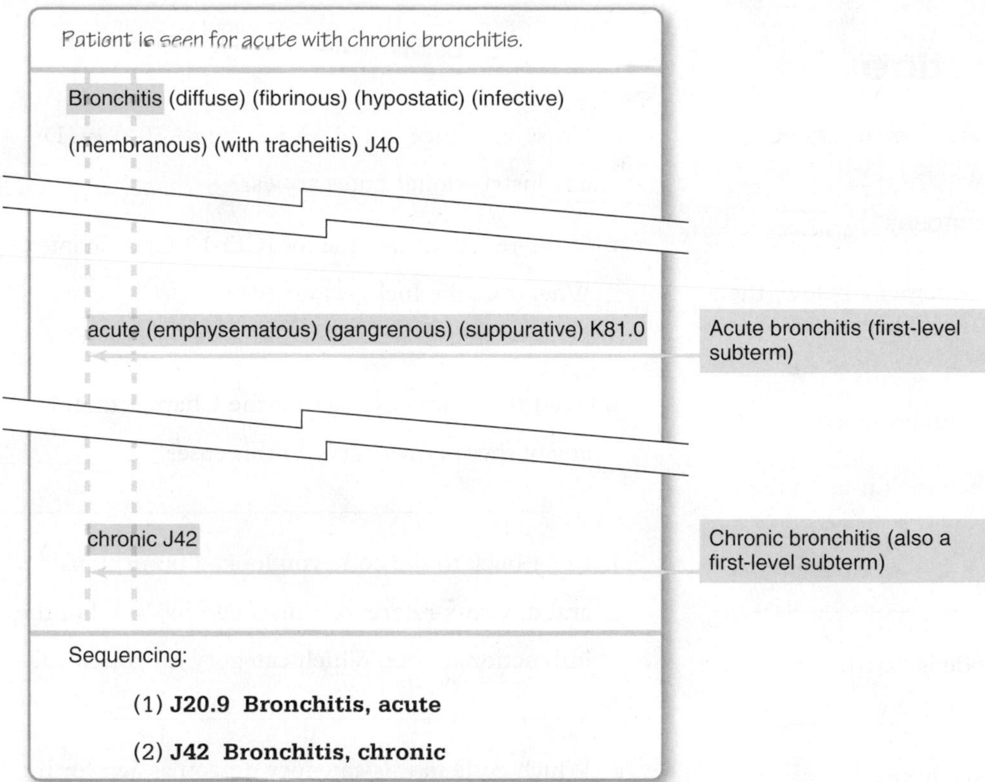

Figure 4-15 ■ Example of Multiple Coding for an Acute and Chronic Condition

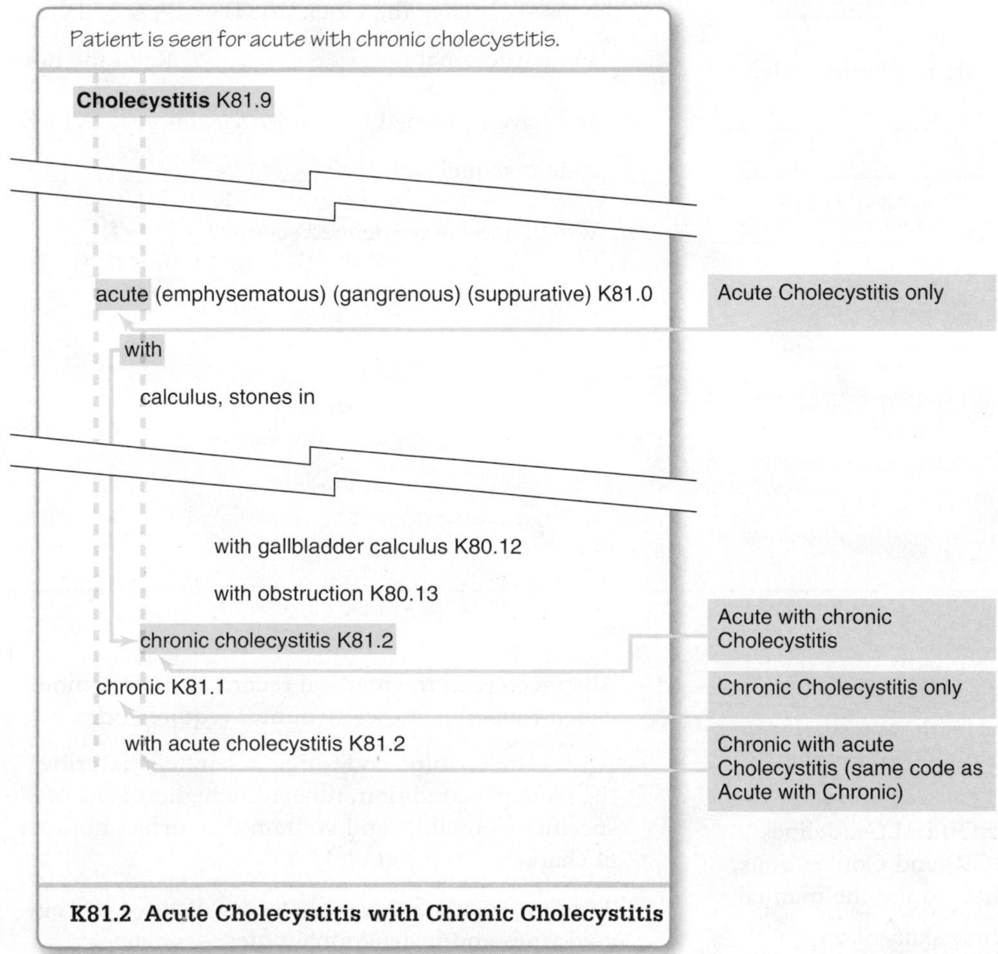

Figure 4-16 ■ Example of a Combination Code for an Acute with Chronic Condition

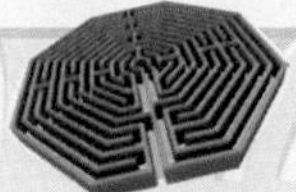

Coding Practice

Now it is your turn to demonstrate how to assign and arrange diagnosis codes.

Exercise 4.5 How to Code Diagnoses

Instructions: Read the diagnostic statement below, then answer the questions that follow to assign the correct codes. Sequence multiple codes in correct order.

1. Toxic shock syndrome due to streptococcus A

   a. Underline the Main Term, then look it up in the Index.

   b. What is the subterm? ______________________

   c. Locate the subterm. What code is listed?

   ____

   d. Locate the code listed in step c in the Tabular List. Is there a symbol indicating that an additional digit is required? ______________________

   e. What instructional note appears under the code?

   ____

   ____

   f. What is the name of the organism? ____________

   ____

   g. Cross-reference the block heading A30-A49. Do any instructional notes appear? ______________

   h. Cross-reference the title for ICD-10-CM Chapter 1. What does the Includes note say?

   ____

   i. Read the other notes under the Chapter title. Do any of these notes apply to this case? __________

   ____

   j. Refer back to the code you looked up in steps c and d. Cross-reference the categories listed in the instructional note. Which category do you need?

   ____

   k. Which code in this category do you assign for the organism? ______________________

   l. Cross-reference the block title B95-B97. Is there an instructional note? __________ Read the note.

   m. You have identified two codes for this case. Which code is sequenced first? ______________

   n. Which code is sequenced second? ____________

   ____

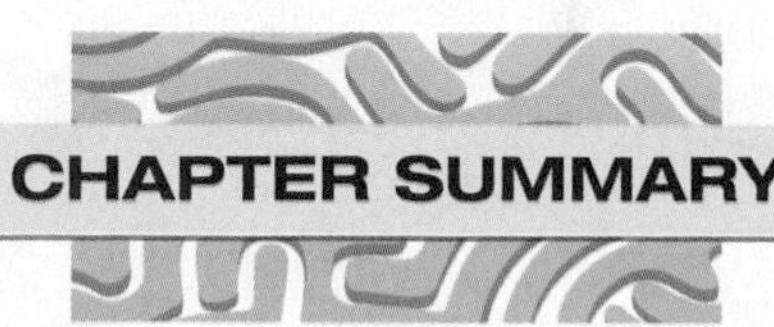

CHAPTER SUMMARY

In this chapter you learned that:

- The ICD-10-CM manual (2012 Draft) is a single volume and is not separated into three volumes as the ICD-9-CM is.
- ICD-10-CM is accompanied by Official Guidelines for Coding and Reporting (OGCR) and Conventions, both of which direct the coder how to use the manual.
- Diagnosis coding involves the three skills of an ace coder:
  - Abstract—read the medical record and determine which elements of the encounter require codes
  - Assign—determine codes that accurately describe the patient's condition, reflect the highest level of specificity possible, and contain the correct number of characters for that code
  - Arrange—place codes in the order dictated by the guidelines and instructional notes (sequence).

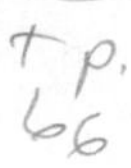

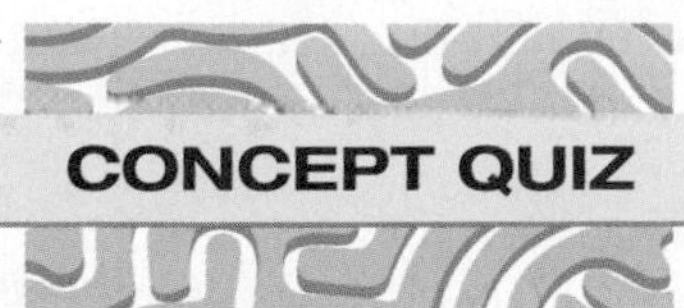

CONCEPT QUIZ

– All the questions.

Take a moment to look back at your trip through diagnosis coding and solidify your new skills. This is your opportunity to pull together everything you have learned.

Completion

Instructions: Write the term that answers each question based on the information you learned in this chapter. Choose from the list below. Some choices may be used more than once and some choices may not be used at all. Refer to the discussion in this chapter and the Glossary at the end of this book if you need a little extra help.

-	Code Also
( )	Code First
4th	Excludes1
5th	Excludes2
6th	Includes
7th	*See*
★	Use Additional Code
:	X
[ ]	

1. The convention _______________ identifies nonessential modifiers that describe the default variations of a term.
2. The convention _______________ identifies mutually exclusive codes that should not be used together.
3. The convention _______________ tells the coder that additional characters should be assigned to a code.
4. A code that appears in _______________ in the Index should be sequenced second.
5. The convention _______________ appears in front of a four-digit code to indicate that a fifth digit is required.
6. The convention _______________ is a placeholder in codes with less than six characters that require a seventh character extension.
7. The convention _______________ indicates that the condition excluded is not part of the condition represented by the code, but the patient may have both conditions at the same time.
8. The convention _______________ instructs the coder to sequence the etiology first.
9. The convention _______________ instructs the coder to sequence the manifestation second.
10. The convention _______________ instructs the coder to reference another Main Term or condition to locate the correct code.

Multiple Choice

Instructions: Circle the letter of the best answer to each question based on the information you learned in this chapter. Refer to the discussion in this chapter and the Glossary at the end of this book if you need a little extra help.

1. _________ are the seventh characters of codes that must appear in that position, regardless of the length of the code.
   A. Extensions
   B. Modifiers
   C. Conventions
   D. Exclusions
2. In the outpatient setting, the _________ diagnosis is the diagnosis, condition, problem, or other reason for the encounter visit shown in the medical record to be chiefly responsible for the services provided.
   A. principal
   B. uncertain
   C. first-listed
   D. Main Term
3. _________ diagnoses are preceded by the words probable, possible, suspected, questionable, rule out, working diagnosis, or similar word.
   A. Principal
   B. Uncertain
   C. First-listed
   D. Main Term
4. In an inpatient setting, the _________ diagnosis is the condition established after study to be chiefly responsible for occasioning the admission of the patient to the hospital for care.
   A. principal
   B. uncertain
   C. first-listed
   D. Main Term
5. _________ are rules that complement the conventions and instructional notes to provide additional information and direction in identifying the diagnoses to be reported.
   A. OGCR
   B. Conventions
   C. Exclusions
   D. Instructional notes

6. ________ are the use of symbols, typeface, and layout features to succinctly convey interpretive information.
   A. OGCR
   B. Conventions
   C. Exclusions
   D. Instructional notes
7. ________ means to read the medical record and determine which elements of the encounter require codes.
   A. Abstracting
   B. Assigning
   C. Arranging
   D. Cross-referencing
8. A ________ is a contiguous range of codes within a chapter in ICD-10-CM.
   A. block
   B. category
   C. section
   D. subcategory
9. ________ is a new OGCR that defines separate codes for the right and left sides of the body.
   A. Bilateral
   B. Multiple coding
   C. Arranging
   D. Laterality
10. Do not code signs or symptoms that are a/an ________ part of the disease process when the diagnosis has been established.
   A. uncertain
   B. nonessential
   C. etiology
   D. integral

CODING CHALLENGE

Instructions: Read the mini-medical-record, then answer the questions that follow to abstract, assign, and arrange (sequence) the correct codes.

> Date: 4/1/yy Location: Branton Family Practice
>
> Provider: Kristen Conover, MD
>
> Patient: Paul Bucci Gender: M Age: 75
>
> Chief complaint: Visit to monitor hypertension and **CHF**. **C/o** increased **SOB**.
>
> Assessment: Chronic combined systolic and diastolic heart failure, due to hypertension. Patient is a current and long-term tobacco user. Change diuretic. Use supplemental $\mathbf{O_2}$ PRN.

Part 1: Abstract

1. Read through the mini-medical-record. Observe the patient demographics. Compare the chief complaint to the final assessment.
   a. What symptom did the patient report in the chief complaint? ________________
   b. What two conditions are stated in the assessment?
   ____
   ____
2. a. Is the symptom integral to one of the conditions stated in the assessment? ________________
   b. Should you code for the symptom? ________________
   c. Why or why not? ________________
   What is the first condition due to? ________________
   ____

Part 2: Assign

3. You can look up the conditions in any order you wish, as long as you sequence them correctly in the end based on the instructional notes you will find during this exercise.

   Today, begin by coding the underlying (due to) condition.

   a. Look up the Main Term **Hypertension** in the Index, then the subterm **with, heart failure**. What code is listed? ________________
   b. Verify this code in the Tabular List. Is there a symbol in front of this code indicating that you need additional characters? ________________

(continued)

4. a. What does the instructional note under the code say? ______

b. Based on this instructional note, should the code for **Hypertension** be sequenced first or second? ______

5. a. Locate the beginning of this block for **Hypertensive diseases**. Read the instructional notes. Now refer back to the mini-medical-record. What lifestyle habit is documented? ______

b. Which instructional note applies to this patient? (Tip: *history* describes a past condition that no longer exists.) ______

You will verify this code later in this exercise.

c. Review the instructional notes at the beginning of ICD-10-CM Chapter 9. Do any of these notes apply to this patient? ______

6. a. Now you will determine the code for heart failure. Look again at the instructional note under the code for **Hypertension**. What code is listed in the instructional note? ______

b. What does the - at the end of the code mean? ______

7. a. Verify the code listed in the instructional note. Review the four-digit subcategories under this heading and locate the one that describes **Combined systolic and diastolic heart failure**. Write down the subcategory code. ______

b. Now review the five-digit codes under this subcategory. What code describes **Chronic combined systolic and diastolic heart failure**? ______

8. Cross-reference the three-digit category heading for **Heart failure**. Read through the instructional notes. What condition should be coded first that applies to this patient? ______

This code should match the one you assigned in step 3.a. The instructional note confirms that you assigned the correct first code or alerts you to the fact that the first code was not correct.

9. Now you need to assign a third code for the lifestyle habit you listed in step 5.a. above. List the code here. ______ Verify the code. (This code is sequenced last.)

Part 3: Arrange

10. You have identified three codes for this case. Review your answers in the previous questions to determine the correct sequencing.

a. What code is sequenced first, based on the instructional notes in steps 4.b. and 8? ______

b. What code is sequenced second? ______

c. What code is sequenced third? ______

KEEP ON CODING

As a coder, you can never have too much experience. Apply everything you have learned in this chapter to code the following diagnostic statements. Use the OGCR and instructional notes in the Tabular List to help determine how many codes are required.

Instructions: Read the diagnostic statement, then use the Index and Tabular List to assign and sequence ICD-10-CM (CM) diagnosis codes. Write the code(s) on the line provided.

1. Acquired flat foot, left: CM Code(s) ______
2. Encounter for immunotherapy: CM Code(s) ______
3. Stage 3 pressure ulcer, left buttock: CM Code(s) ______

4. Alcohol dependence: CM Code(s) ______

5. Fistula, left elbow: CM Code(s) ______

6. Family history of alcohol abuse: CM Code(s) ______

7. Body mass index of 38 in an adult: CM Code(s) ______

8. Benign hypertension: CM Code(s) ______

9. Dysphagia following a cerebral infarction with difficulty swallowing: CM Code(s) ______

10. Severe abdominal pain with abdominal rigidity: CM Code(s) ______

11. Repeated falls: CM Code(s) ______

12. Merkel cell carcinoma of the right eyelid: CM Code(s) ______

13. Pain due to malignant neoplasm: CM Code(s) ______

14. Type 2 diabetes mellitus with moderate diabetic retinopathy with macular edema: CM Code(s) ______

15. Insect bite, left ankle, subsequent encounter: CM Code(s) ______

16. Second and third degree chemical burns, right ankle, initial encounter: CM Code(s) ______

17. Fused toes, bilateral: CM Code(s) ______

18. Chronic cystitis with hematuria: CM Code(s) ______

19. Pneumocystis pneumonia: CM Code(s) ______

20. Anemia: CM Code(s) ______

21. Encounter for blood typing: CM Code(s) ______

22. Ventilator associated pneumonia: CM Code(s) ______

23. Head lice: CM Code(s) ______

24. Polyhydramnios, second trimester, fetus 3: CM Code(s) ______

25. Acute otitis externa, right ear: CM Code(s) ______

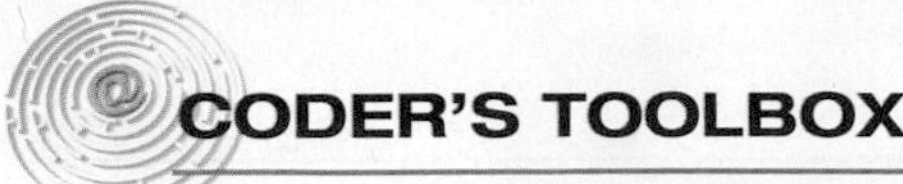

CODER'S TOOLBOX

The following resources are a starting point for learning more about diagnosis coding. The > symbol indicates a menu selection within the website in order to navigate to a specific page.

AAPC > ICD-10 **http://www.aapc.com/ICD-10/index.aspx**

American Health Information Management Association **http://www.ahima.org/icd10/default.aspx**

Centers for Disease Control and Prevention > Coordination and Maintenance Committee **http://www.cdc.gov/nchs/icd/icd9cm_maintenance.htm**

Centers for Medicare and Medicaid/Medicare > ICD-9-CM Coordination and Maintenance Committee **http://www.cms.gov/ICD9ProviderDiagnosticCodes/03_meetings.asp**

Healthcare Financial Management Association **http://www.hfma.org/**

Healthcare Information Management Systems Society **http://www.himss.org/ASP/index.asp**

Reliable information about specific diseases can be located at the following websites:

eMedicineHealth **http://www.emedicinehealth.com**

Mayo Clinic **http://www.mayoclinic.com**

MedicineNet **http://www.medicinenet.com**

MedlinePlus **http://www.nlm.nih.gov/medlineplus**

National Institutes for Health **http://www.ncbi.nlm.nih.gov**

Web MD **http://www.webmd.com**

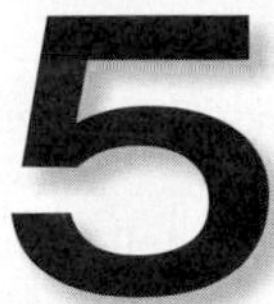

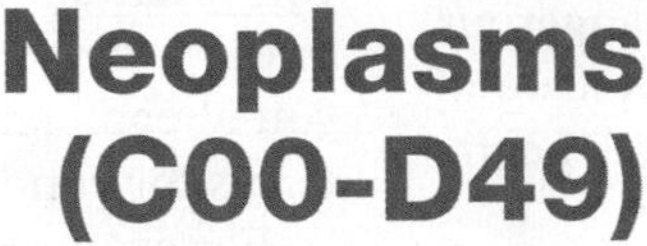

5 Neoplasms (C00-D49)

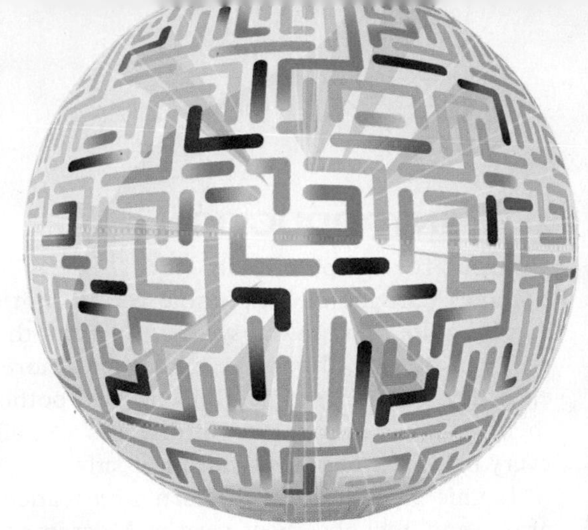

Learning Objectives

After completing this chapter, you should have the skills to:

- Spell and define the key words, medical terms, and abbreviations related to neoplasms.
- Discuss the behavior and common types of neoplasms.
- Identify the main characteristics of coding for neoplasms.
- Abstract diagnostic information from the medical record for coding neoplasms.
- Assign codes for neoplasms and related conditions.
- Arrange codes for neoplasms and related conditions.
- Discuss the Official Guidelines for Coding and Reporting related to neoplasms.

Key Terms and Abbreviations

adenocarcinoma
adjuvant
behavior
benign
CA
CA in situ
cancer
carcinoma
carcinoma of unknown primary (CUP)
cell type
external radiotherapy
family history
histology
internal radiotherapy
leukemia
malignant
metastasize
neoplasm
oncologist
overlapping lesion
personal history
primary
prognosis
secondary
site of origin
staging
topography

In addition to the key terms listed here, students should know the terms defined within tables in this chapter.

Chapter Outline

- **Neoplasm Refresher**
- **Coding Overview of Neoplasms**
- **Abstracting for Neoplasms**
- **Assigning Codes for Neoplasms**
- **Arranging Codes for Neoplasms**

ICD-10-CM codes in this chapter are from the ICD-10-CM 2014 Draft code set from the Department of Health and Human Services, Centers for Disease Control and Prevention.

INTRODUCTION

On your road trip you will inevitably encounter some potholes. Driving into a pothole you do not see coming can be quite a jolt to the system. When potholes are not repaired quickly, they grow bigger and more dangerous each day. The medical field has its own potholes. One of them is cancer, a collection of diseases that affects nearly every person either directly or indirectly.

In this chapter you will learn what cancer is, how it arises, and how physicians treat it. Most importantly, you will practice coding for patient encounters related to neoplasms, a skill that requires you to abstract information from the mini-medical-record, assign correct codes, and arrange (sequence) the codes in the proper order.

An oncologist is a physician who specializes in diagnosing and treating tumors. Medical oncologists specialize in medical treatments such as chemotherapy. Surgical oncologists specialize in surgical treatment, such as the surgical excision of malignant (cancerous) tumors. Radiation oncologists specialize in treating malignant tumors with radiation therapy. Physician specialists of a particular body system may also be involved in treating patients with tumors and cancer affecting that body system.

As you read this chapter, open up your medical terminology book and keep a medical dictionary handy to refresh your memory of any unfamiliar terms. Think of these resources as your travel brochures that tell you more about an area. This way, you have the information you need at your fingertips.

NEOPLASM REFRESHER

Neoplasms are abnormal growth of new tissue, which may be **malignant** (*life threatening*) or **benign** (*not life threatening*). Malignant neoplasms are commonly referred to as cancer. Neoplasms may occur in any body system and at any anatomical site. **Oncologists** are physicians who specialize in the diagnosis and treatment of tumors. In order to code neoplasms, coders need to be familiar with neoplasm related terminology, benign neoplasm behavior, and malignant neoplasm behavior.

Neoplasm Related Terminology

Neoplasms are classified based on the **behavior** (*malignant or benign*), **topography** or **site of origin** (*anatomic site where the growth begins*), **histology** (*type of tissue*), and **cell type** (*characteristics or appearance of the cell*) of the growth. As you learn about different types of neoplasms, remember to put together the root or combining form for body parts you already know with suffixes and prefixes to define new terms for conditions and procedures related to neoplasms.

For example, the suffix -oma means tumor, and gastr/o means stomach, so gastroma refers to a neoplasm in the stomach (gastr/oma). Sarc/o refers to connective tissue, so sarcoma refers to a neoplasm of connective tissue (sarc/oma) and is nearly always malignant.

Terms for neoplasms frequently contain more than one root to fully describe the tumor. For example, **adenocarcinoma** (adeno/carcin/oma) has two roots to describe a cancerous (carcin/o) tumor in a gland (aden/o). Refer to ■ TABLE 5-1 for a refresher on how to build medical terms related to neoplasms.

CODING CAUTION

Be alert for medical word terms that are spelled similarly and have different meanings.

adenoma (*tumor of a gland*) and
adeno<u>carcin</u>oma (*cancerous tumor of a gland*)
<u>diag</u>nosis (*complete knowledge—determining the nature of a disease*) and **<u>prog</u>nosis** (*future knowledge—the expected course of the disease*)

Benign Neoplasm Behavior

A benign neoplasm does not have the ability to invade surrounding tissue or spread to other parts of the body. Types of benign neoplasms are tumors, warts, moles, polyps, and fibroids. In some cases, physicians can determine if a neoplasm is benign or malignant through visual inspection. If they believe the growth could be malignant or are unsure of its behavior, they perform a **biopsy** to obtain a specimen. They send the specimen to the laboratory where a **pathologist** examines it microscopically.

Table 5-1 ■ **EXAMPLE OF CONSTRUCTING MEDICAL TERMS FOR NEOPLASMS**

Prefix/Combining Form	Suffix	Complete Medical Term
neo- (*new*) **sarc/o** (*connective tissue*) **my/o** (*muscle*) **carcin/o** (*cancerous*) **aden/o** (*gland*)	**-plasm** (*growth*)	**neo + plasm** (*new growth*)
	-oma (*tumor*)	**sarc + oma** (*tumor of connective tissue*) **aden + oma** (*tumor of a gland*)
		myo + sarc + oma (*tumor of connective tissue and muscle*) **adeno + carcin + oma** (*cancerous tumor of a gland*)

Many benign neoplasms present no health problems and require no treatment. However, a large benign neoplasm can apply pressure to or interfere with surrounding organs or structures and this can create health problems. For example, a benign brain tumor is not cancerous, but it can compress cranial nerves or apply pressure to areas of the brain and may need to be removed to protect brain function. ■ TABLE 5-2 outlines the differences between benign and malignant neoplasms.

Malignant Neoplasm Behavior

The ability of malignant neoplasms to metastasize (*spread and invade organs*) makes them life threatening. When tumors invade vital organs, they cause organ malfunction, leading to death if not treated. It is important to distinguish between the common term cancer (CA) and the medical terms malignant neoplasm and carcinoma. Refer to the following to review the similarities and differences in these terms:

- Carcinoma is a malignant tumor of epithelial cells, which line body cavities and organs. Not all areas of the body have epithelial cells, so true carcinoma only occurs in structures that contain epithelial cells.
- Carcinoma in situ (CA in situ) refers to cells that have begun to change but are contained within the epithelial layer. When malignant cells break through the epithelial membrane into the organ, they become a primary malignant neoplasm (■ FIGURE 5-1).

Table 5-2 ■ COMPARISON OF BENIGN AND MALIGNANT NEOPLASM CHARACTERISTICS

Characteristic	Benign Neoplasm	Malignant Neoplasm
Rate of growth	Grows slowly	Grows rapidly
Encapsulation	Is encapsulated	Is not encapsulated
Differentiation	Has cells that resemble the normal cells from which they arose (well-differentiated)	Has cells that undergo permanent change, abnormal rapid proliferation (anaplastic and undifferentiated)
Growth pattern	Grows by expansion and causes pressure on surrounding tissue	Has invasive growth and metastasis
Mestastasis	Remains localized (non-metastatic)	Spreads through bloodstream and lymphatic system Causes extensive tissue destruction due to invasiveness
Recurrence	Does not recur when surgically removed	Can recur when surgically removed if invasive growth has occurred
Cachexia	Produces no cachexia (extreme weakness, fatigue, wasting, and malnutrition)	Produces cachexia

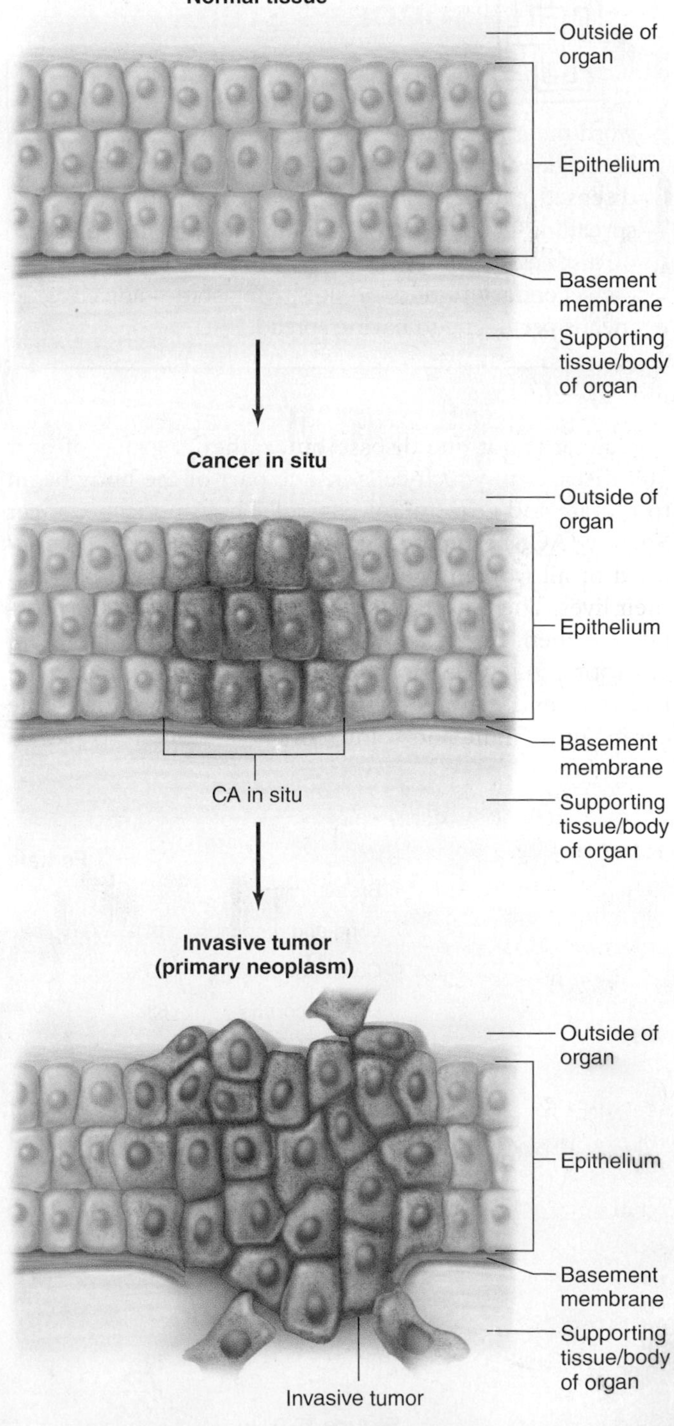

Figure 5-1 ■ Progression of CA in Situ to Primary Neoplasm

- Malignant neoplasm is a life-threatening new growth of any type of tissue. Although malignant neoplasms are cancerous, not all are classified as carcinoma. Malignant neoplasms can also occur in other types of cells such as bone, muscle, and fat.
- Cancer, in its most limited meaning, is synonymous with carcinoma. However, our language uses cancer loosely to refer to many types of malignancies, including ones that are not tumors. For example, cancer is often used to describe leukemia, which is a malignant disease of the blood-forming organs, but does not produce tumors.

SUCCESS STEP

Be aware of different forms of the word metastasize, which literally means *beyond control.* Metastasize (verb) means to transform or spread diseased cells. Metastasis (noun) is the process of spreading or the condition resulting from the spread of diseased cells. Metastases (plural) refer to multiple secondary tumors or sites. Metastatic (adjective) means pertaining to having spread.

Cancer is not one disease but, rather, a group of over 100 diseases in which cells in one part of the body begin to mutate and grow out of control. The American Cancer Society (ACS) estimates that one-half of all men and one-third of all women will develop cancer at some point in their lives. The most common sites of cancer are the prostate for men, breast for women, lung, and colon/rectum (■ FIGURE 5-2). The most common childhood cancers are leukemia and medulloblastoma, a cancer that affects the cerebellum, brain, and spinal cord.

Cells become cancerous due to damaged DNA that is not repaired as it is in normal cells. The damaged cells do not die as they normally should but, rather, replicate and make new damaged cells. Cancer spreads when the damaged cells invade nearby tissues and when damaged cells move into the bloodstream or lymphatic system, which carry them to other areas of the body. The anatomic site where the neoplasm begins is the primary site. The sites it spreads to are the secondary sites or metastases. The most common sites for metastases are the liver, lungs, and bone. Cancer cells that have metastasized retain the characteristics of the organ in which they originated. For example, breast cancer cells that have spread to the lung still look like breast cells under the microscope. Breast cancer that has spread to the lung is called metastatic breast cancer (■ FIGURE 5-3).

Topography is the anatomic site where the neoplasm begins. Many histological and cell types of malignant neoplasms and cancers can affect any given site. For example, types of colorectal cancer include the following histological types, each of which originates from a different type of tissue:

- adenocarcinoma, which originates in the glands
- leiomyosarcoma, which originates in smooth muscle tissue
- lymphoma, which originates in the lymph nodes
- malignant melanoma, which originates in pigment cells of the skin
- neuroendocrine, which originates in hormone-producing cells that are a cross between nerve cells and endocrine cells

Each of these histological types can appear in many different organs. For example, adenocarcinoma may appear in the colon, prostate, lungs, breast, stomach, pancreas, and cervix. Each histological type may have a variety of cell subtypes, which are often named based on their appearance. For example, adenocarcinoma of the colon has a

Female		Male	
Breast	28%	Prostate	28%
Lung and bronchus	14%	Lung and bronchus	15%
Colon and rectum	10%	Colon and rectum	9%
Uterine corpus	6%	Urinary bladder	7%
Thyroid	5%	Melanoma of the skin	5%
Non-Hodgkin's lymphoma	4%	Non-Hodgkin's lymphoma	4%
Melanoma of the skin	4%	Kidney/renal pelvis	4%
Ovary	3%	Oral cavity/pharynx	3%
Kidney and renal pelvis	3%	Leukemia	3%
Leukemia	3%	Pancreas	3%
Other	20%	Other	19%

Figure 5-2 ■ Most Frequent Sites of New Cancer Cases

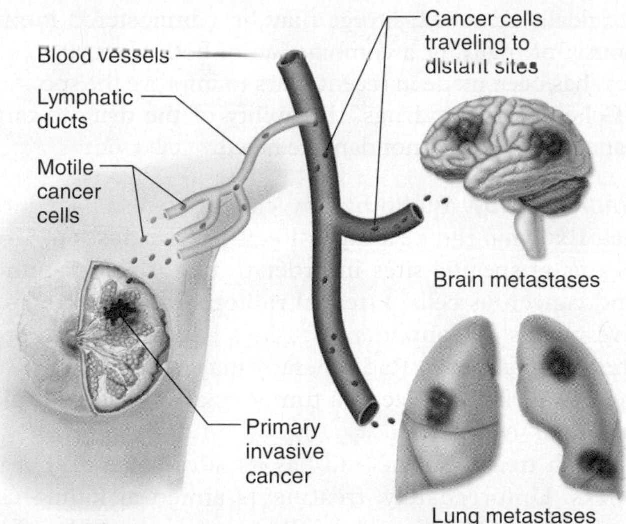

Figure 5-3 ■ Metastasis of Breast Cancer to the Brain and Lung

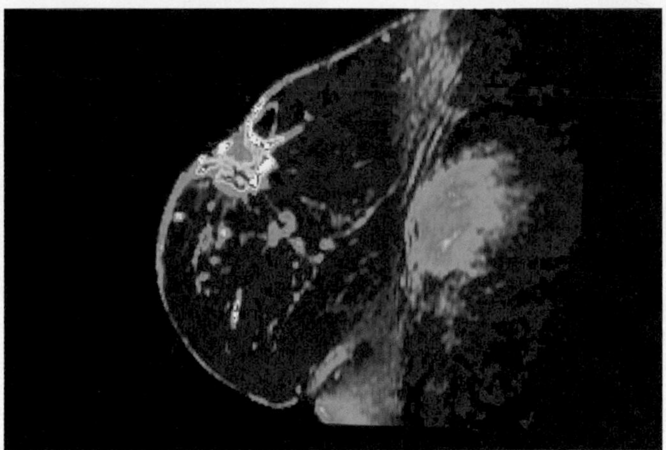

Figure 5-4 ■ MRI Image of the Breast. *Source*: © *Dr. Steven Harmes/National Cancer Institute (NCI).*

mucinous cell subtype (comprised of at least 60% mucus) and a signet ring cell subtype (looks like a ring when viewed microscopically). Physicians must identify the specific subtype of cell in order to determine the behavior, the patient's **prognosis** (*expected outcome*), and treatment plan. Hundreds of different cell subtypes are known for various topographical and histological types of cancer.

Coders need to know how malignant neoplasms and other cancers are diagnosed and treated in order to abstract, assign, and sequence codes.

Diagnosis

Physicians diagnose cancer through **screening** examinations or in response to patient symptoms. Screening examinations detect certain types of cancer at an early stage. Cancer that is detected during an early stage is more likely to respond to treatment. Examples of screening tests include the following:

- colonoscopy—colon cancer
- mammogram—breast cancer
- papanicolaou (PAP) test—cervical cancer
- prostate specific antigen (PSA) blood test—prostate cancer
- digital rectal examination (DRE)—prostate cancer

When patients present with symptoms, physicians may diagnose cancer with blood tests, biopsies, and imaging, such as a CT scan, MRI, or PET scan (■ FIGURE 5-4). After making a diagnosis of cancer, physicians determine the stage and grade of the disease in order to help determine the best course of treatment.

Staging. **Staging** is the process of determining how far the cancer has spread. Several staging systems exist and various systems are used for specific types of cancers. Two common staging systems are TNM and stage grouping. TNM staging assigns numbers to describe how far the primary tumor (T) has grown in its original site; extent of spread to regional (nearby) lymph nodes (N), and whether the cancer has metastasized (M) to other organs of the body. The results of TNM staging are then combined into stage grouping. Stage grouping uses numbers to designate the malignancy from the least advanced (stage 0) to the most advanced (IV). The specific criteria for each stage of TNM and stage grouping are unique to each anatomical site. For example, the definition of stage II colon cancer is different than stage II breast cancer. Physicians state the diagnosis by referencing the stage of cancer at the time it is discovered. However, all cancers will eventually become the highest stage if left untreated. Staging information helps coders confirm if the disease has metastasized.

Grading. Grading describes how closely the cancer cell type looks like a normal cell when viewed microscopically. A pathologist determines the grade through microscopic inspection of a tissue or fluid specimen. The grade is rated from G1, a low grade cell that looks much like normal tissue, to G4, a high grade cell that looks very abnormal. Low grade cancers tend to grow and spread more slowly than high grade cells. Several different grades of cancer cells can affect any given anatomic site, so physicians must determine each patient's exact cell type and its grade. The grade of the cell does not change as the disease progresses.

Physicians use the combination of stage and grade to determine a patient's treatment plan and prognosis. Stage and grade are independent of each other. A patient can have a low stage and high grade, a high stage and a low grade, or any combination in between. For example, a patient with a lymphoma type that is stage IV (widespread) and grade G1 (slow growing), such as follicular cell lymphoma, may have a better outcome than a patient with a type of carcinoma of the uterus that is stage I (localized) but grade G4 (rapidly growing and spreading), such as clear cell carcinoma.

Treatment

Physicians recommend treatment plans based on topography, stage, and grade of cancer as well as the patient's age and health condition. The three primary types of treatment are surgery, chemotherapy, and radiotherapy. They may be used alone or in conjunction with each other. When more than one type of treatment is used, the additional treatments are referred to as **adjuvant** therapies. Some malignancies are more responsive to one type of treatment than another. Which treatments are used, and in what order, is unique to each type of cancer and each patient.

Surgery. Surgery is used to remove the tumor and a portion of the healthy tissue around the tumor to be certain that all the malignancy is removed. It is most successful when a tumor is small and localized. Surgery is also used to treat some complications of cancer, such as blockage or pain due to a tumor.

Chemotherapy. Chemotherapy uses drugs to kill cancer cells. It may be used before surgery, to shrink the size of a large tumor so it is easier to remove, or after surgery, to kill any potentially remaining diseased cells. Chemotherapy is also used to treat widespread metastasis that cannot be surgically removed. Drugs may be administered intravenously or orally, or a combination of both. Immense progress has been made in recent years to improve the specificity of chemotherapy drugs, the ability of the drug to target cancerous cells but not damage healthy cells.

Radiotherapy. Radiotherapy can be external or internal. **External radiotherapy** directs precise doses of X-ray beams at specific sites in order to kill or shrink tumors and cancerous cells. **Internal radiotherapy** uses radioactive pellets or containers within a body cavity to target the malignant area. Radiotherapy may be used before surgery to shrink the size of a tumor or after surgery to slow potential metastasis.

Each treatment method has its advantages and drawbacks. Unfortunately, treatments aimed at killing cancer cells also kill healthy cells, resulting in side effects for patients. Patients, their families, and their physicians make difficult and personal decisions regarding what is best in any given situation.

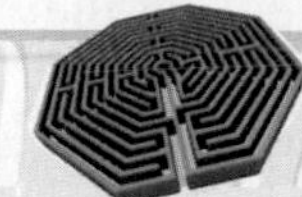

Coding Practice

Refresh your knowledge of neoplasm terminology. Use a medical terminology text or a website such as GlobalRph .com > Medical Terminology **http://www.globalrph .com/medterm.htm** to identify the meaning of word parts that may not be familiar to you.

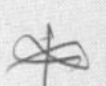

Exercise 5.1 Neoplasm Refresher

Instructions: Use your medical terminology skills and resources to define the following neoplasms. Do not assign codes. Follow these steps:

- Use slash marks "/" to break down each term into its root(s) and suffix.
- Define the meaning of the word, based on the meaning of each word part.

Example: sarcoma sarc/oma Meaning: *neoplasm of connective tissue*

1. osteosarcoma ____________________
2. leiomyoma ____________________
3. lipoma ____________________
4. liposarcoma ____________________
5. adenoma ____________________
6. adenocarcinoma ____________________
7. osteoma ____________________
8. melanoma ____________________
9. neuroblastoma ____________________
10. lymphoma ____________________

CODING OVERVIEW OF NEOPLASMS

ICD-10-CM Chapter 2, Neoplasms (C00-D49), contains 21 blocks or subchapters that are divided by anatomical site. Review the block names and code ranges listed at the beginning of Chapter 2 in the ICD-10-CM manual to become familiar with the content and organization. This chapter classifies all malignant and most benign neoplasms. Some benign neoplasms are classified in the specific body system chapter. For example, adenomas of the prostate are classified in ICD-10-CM Chapter 14, Diseases of the Genitourinary System (N00-N99).

Notice the following characteristics of codes in the neoplasm chapter:

- Codes beginning with C classify malignant neoplasms.
- Codes beginning with D classify neoplasms in situ, benign, and of uncertain or unspecified behavior.
- Some codes contain an alphabetic character in the third position of the code, such as C7A, C7B, D3A.

This ICD-10-CM chapter compares to Chapter 2 in ICD-9-CM and reflects numerous category expansions. Characters have been added to code for laterality and more specific sites. Codes for leukemia contain characters to identify whether the disease is in remission or relapse. OGCR I.C.2.c.1), Anemia associated with malignancy, has been updated.

Instructional notes at the beginning of ICD-10-CM Chapter 2 address functional activity, morphology, overlapping sites, and malignant neoplasm of ectopic tissue.

CODING CAUTION

When diagnosis codes have a letter for other than the first or last character, they can be tricky to locate because they do not appear in a manner consistent with alphanumeric rules. For example, category **C7A** is sequenced after **C75** and before **C76**, but category **D3A** appears after **D36** and before **D37**. Be aware of this inconsistency and know that you may need to take a few moments to locate the code.

ICD-10-CM provides Official Guidelines for Coding and Reporting (OGCR) for neoplasms in OGCR section I.C.2. OGCR provides specific direction for sequencing codes for multiple neoplasms, complications, adjuvant therapies, and other situations. In addition, frequent instructional notes throughout the chapter direct coders to use multiple codes to describe harmful lifestyle habits that contribute to neoplasms.

ABSTRACTING FOR NEOPLASMS

When abstracting patient cases with neoplasms, coders must look for several pieces of information that will help determine the first-listed or principal diagnosis and the sequencing of any additional diagnoses. Refer to OGCR I.C.2. for detailed guidance on abstracting neoplasms. ■ TABLE 5-3 highlights key questions to answer when reviewing the medical record. Coders use answers to these questions when assigning and sequencing codes. Remember that the abstracting questions are a guide and that not every question applies to, or can be answered for, every case. For example, complications of cancer may not be present in every patient.

Abstracting Metastases

An important task in abstracting is determining the sites of the primary and any secondary neoplasms. Coders must give special attention to the specific wording used to describe various neoplasm sites. In particular, take note of the prepositions *from*, *to*, and *in* because they describe the direction in which the neoplasm has spread. Refer to ■ TABLE 5-4 to better understand how metastases are documented.

Table 5-3 ■ KEY CRITERIA FOR ABSTRACTING NEOPLASMS

- ❑ What is the histologic description of the neoplasm or cancer?
- ❑ What is the anatomic site of the neoplasm?
- ❑ Is the neoplasm stated as malignant or benign?
- ❑ If malignant, is the neoplasm primary, secondary, in situ, or of unknown histologic origin?
- ❑ Has the malignant neoplasm metastasized? If so, to what sites?
- ❑ What complications are documented, such as anemia, dehydration, or a surgical complication?
- ❑ If anemia is present, is it due to the malignancy itself or due to a treatment such as chemotherapy, radiotherapy, or immunotherapy?
- ❑ Is the reason for the encounter or admission the malignancy or an unrelated condition?
- ❑ If the reason for the encounter is the malignancy, what is the specific purpose?
  - treatment of the primary site
  - treatment of a metastatic site(s)
  - treatment of a complication
  - chemotherapy
  - radiotherapy
  - immunotherapy
  - pain management
  - determination of the extent of malignancy
  - aftercare
  - follow-up care
- ❑ Is the patient in remission from leukemia, multiple myeloma, or malignant plasma neoplasm?
- ❑ If the primary malignancy was previously excised, is there any remaining evidence of primary malignancy, metastasis, or any related treatment?
- ❑ Does the patient have a personal history or family history of malignant neoplasm?

Table 5-4 ■ ALTERNATIVE DESCRIPTIONS OF METASTASES

Statement	Primary Site	Secondary Site(s)
Colon cancer with metastasis *to* the liver	Colon	Liver
Metastatic liver cancer *from* the colon	Colon	Liver
Metastatic colon cancer	Colon	Unknown
Metastatic cancer *in* lung, liver, and bone	Unknown	Lung, liver, and bone
Liver metastases	Unknown	Liver

Guided Example of Abstracting Neoplasms

Refer to the following example here and throughout the chapter to learn more about coding for neoplasms. Karla Destefano, CPC, is a fictitious certified coder who guides you through the coding process.

> Date: 5/1/yy Location: East Side Oncology
>
> Provider: Richard Blackford, MD
>
> Patient: Anthony Payne Gender: M Age: 68
>
> Reason for encounter: review test results to determine extent of prostate cancer
>
> Assessment: adenocarcinoma of prostate with metastasis to colon
>
> Plan: surgery to be followed with radiotherapy

Follow along in your ICD-10-CM manual as Karla abstracts the diagnosis. Check off each step after you complete it.

⇨ Karla begins by reviewing the medical record to abstract the diagnosis. She refers to the Key Criteria for Abstracting Neoplasms (Table 5-3).

- ❑ *What is the histologic description of the neoplasm or cancer?* adenocarcinoma
- ❑ *What is the anatomic site of the neoplasm?* prostate
- ❑ *Is the neoplasm stated as malignant or benign?* Adenocarcinoma by definition is malignant. In addition, the fact that it has spread indicates it is malignant.
- ❑ *If malignant, is the neoplasm primary, secondary, in situ, or of unknown histologic origin?* The prostate is primary because it is not stated as secondary.
- ❑ *Has the malignant neoplasm metastasized? If so, to what sites?* She notes that the secondary site is the colon.
- ❑ *What complications are documented?* None
- ❑ *Is the reason for the encounter or admission the malignancy or an unrelated condition?* The malignancy
- ❑ *Does the patient have a personal history or family history of malignant neoplasm?* None stated

⇨ Next, Karla will assign the codes.

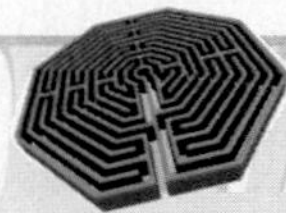

Coding Practice

Now it is your turn to practice abstracting diagnoses for neoplasms. Questions help guide your analysis.

Exercise 5.2 Abstracting Diagnoses for Neoplasms

Instructions: Read the mini-medical-record of each patient's encounter and answer the abstracting questions. Write the answer on the line provided. Do not assign any codes.

> **1.** Date: 5/2/yy Location: East Side Oncology
>
> Provider: Richard Blackford, MD
>
> Patient: Terry Putnam Gender: F Age: 59
>
> Reason for encounter: chemotherapy
>
> Assessment: adenocarcinoma of the right breast, lower outer quadrant, with metastasis to the brain
>
> Plan: return for next treatment in 3 weeks
>
> a. What is the primary site? ____________
>
> *(continued)*

> **1.** (continued)
>
> b. Is metastasis documented? Where? ____________
>
> c. Are any complications documented? ____________
>
> d. What is the specific purpose of the visit? ____________

> **2.** Date: 5/2/yy Location: Branton Medical Center
>
> Provider: Tanya Schmitt, MD
>
> Patient: Roberta Sydnor Gender: F Age: 44
>
> Procedure: embolization of uterine fibroids
>
> Postprocedural diagnosis: intramural (*within the muscle wall*) leiomyoma, uterus
>
> Plan: FU in office in 4 weeks
>
> *(continued)*

2. (continued)

a. What is embolization? ____________________

b. What is a leiomyoma? ____________________

c. What is the anatomic site? ____________________

d. Is the neoplasm malignant or benign? ____________________

3. Date: 5/2/yy Location: East Side Oncology

Provider: Richard Blackford, MD

Patient: Tony Barone Gender: M Age: 43

Reason for encounter: review results of biopsy and CT scan

Assessment: gastric adenocarcinoma, fundus

Plan: surgery to be followed by radiotherapy

a. What is the primary site? ____________________

b. What part of the stomach is the fundus? ____________________

bottom or base of an organ

c. Is metastasis documented? Where? ____________________

d. Are any complications documented? ____________________

e. What is the specific purpose of the visit? ____________________

4. Date: 5/2/yy Location: Branton Medical Center

Provider: Richard Blackford, MD

Patient: Jessica Salcido Gender: F Age: 15

Reason for admission: limb-salvage surgery after chemotherapy to shrink tumor

Procedure description: successfully cut out tumor from left thigh

Postprocedural assessment: osteosarcoma in the left thigh

Plan: discharge in 1–2 days

Limb salvage SX is a procedure designed to remove cancer, usually bone tumors or bone sarcoma, but also soft tissue sarcoma's affecting the body extremities — w/o amputation, while preserving tendons, nerves, & blood vessels

(continued)

4. (continued)

a. What is the primary site? ____________________

b. Is metastasis documented? ____________________

c. Are any complications documented? ____________________

d. What is the specific purpose of the encounter? ____________________

e. What is the medical term for the bone in the thigh? ____________________

5. Date: 5/2/yy Location: Branton Medical Center

Provider: Richard Blackford, MD

Patient: George Rhoden Gender: M Age: 67

Reason for admission: anemia

Assessment: anemia due to classical lymphocyte depleted Hodgkin lymphoma

Plan: administer IV iron supplements

a. What is the primary neoplasm? ____________________

b. Is metastasis documented? ____________________

c. What complication is documented? ____________________

d. What is the reason for the admission? ____________________

6. Date: 5/2/yy Location: Branton Medical Center

Provider: Richard Blackford, MD

Patient: Leonard Morton Gender: M Age: 61

Reason for procedure: brain stem tumor

Procedure description: used Gamma Knife surgery to destroy tumor

Postprocedural diagnosis: squamous cell carcinoma of the lung with brain stem metastases

Plan: FU in office 1 week, evaluate for chemotherapy

(continued)

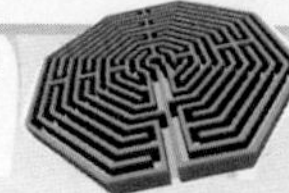

Coding Practice (continued)

6. (continued)

Tip: Look up unfamiliar terms in a medical dictionary or on the Internet.

a. What is the primary neoplasm? ______________________

b. Is metastasis documented? What site? ______________________

(continued)

6. (continued)

c. Which site is the reason for the procedure? ______________________

d. What is Gamma Knife surgery? ______________________

ASSIGNING CODES FOR NEOPLASMS

Assigning codes for neoplasms involves three steps:

1. Search for the histological term in the Index to Diseases and Injuries.
2. Locate the anatomical site and behavior in the Table of Neoplasms.
3. Verify the code(s) in the Tabular List.

Search for the Histological Term in the Index

Coders use both the Index to Diseases and Injuries and the Table of Neoplasms to locate codes for neoplasms. Careful abstracting and attention to the terms in the documentation determine how to locate the code.

When the histological type is documented, search for that term in the Index. The histological term identifies the tissue type of a neoplasm, such as carcinoma, melanoma, sarcoma, or leukemia. When the Index lists a code for the histological type, coders may proceed to the Tabular List to verify the code (■ FIGURE 5-5).

In many cases, the Index lists a cross-reference note to the Table of Neoplasms, such as **specified site - *see* Neoplasm, malignant**. In this situation, coders need to refer to the Table of Neoplasms, locate the column for Malignant Primary, then locate the anatomic site in the left-hand column (■ FIGURE 5-6). Recall that the Table of Neoplasms appears in the Index to Diseases and Injuries under the letter N in most editions of the ICD-10-CM manual.

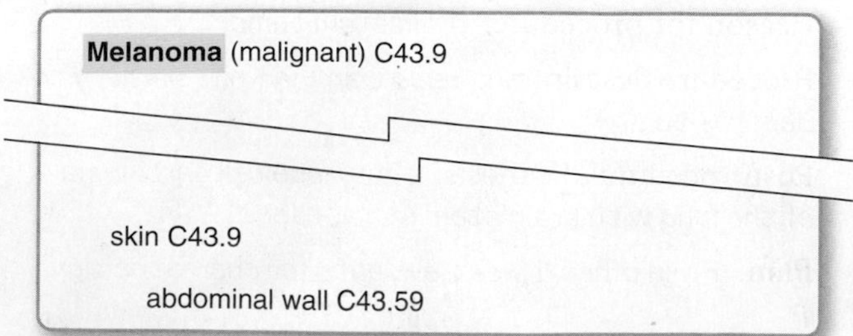

Figure 5-5 ■ Example of Index Entry for a Histological Type of Neoplasm

SUCCESS STEP

To help remember where the Table of Neoplasms is located and to find it quickly, place an adhesive tab along the top edge of the first page of the Table of Neoplasms. By placing it on the top edge, it will not be obscured by other tabs for the Index to Diseases and Injuries and the Tabular List.

Personal or Family History

When physicians document that patients are at risk due to a personal or family history of malignant neoplasm, assign a code for the history. **Personal history** is a condition the patient had in the past, was removed, and is no longer being treated, but has the potential for recurrence, and therefore may require continued monitoring. To locate codes for personal history, search the Index for **History, personal, malignant neoplasm**, then locate the subterm for the anatomic site.

Carcinoma (malignant) — *see also* Neoplasm, by site, malignant
acidophil
specified site — *see* Neoplasm, malignant, by site

Figure 5-6 ■ Example of Cross-Reference to Table of Neoplasms

Family history is a condition that a patient's family member had in the past or currently has that causes the patient to be at higher risk of also contracting the disease. The family member may be alive or deceased. The family member's malignancy may have been removed and/or may still be undergoing treatment. To locate codes for family history, search the Index for **History, family, malignant neoplasm,** then locate the subterm for the body system.

SUCCESS STEP

The significance of personal or family history must be documented by the physician as relevant to the current condition or encounter. Patients must have a blood relationship to the family member, such as a parent or sibling. The history of grandparents, aunts, and uncles may be relevant for certain cancers with proven genetic links, such as breast cancer.

Locate Site and Behavior in the Table of Neoplasms

The Table of Neoplasms lists the codes for neoplasms by anatomical site. Anatomical sites appear in the left column of the table in alphabetical order (■ FIGURE 5-7). Many sites have indented subterms, similar to indentations in the Index to Diseases and Injuries. Subterms in the Table of Neoplasms describe specific locations within a large anatomical site. For example, the anatomic site **abdomen, abdominal** has subterms for **cavity**, **organ**, **viscera**, and **wall. Abdominal wall** has a second-level subterm for **connective tissue**.

The Table of Neoplasms has six columns, one for each anatomic site, that describe the possible behavior of the neoplasm: Malignant Primary, Malignant Secondary, CA in situ, Benign, Uncertain Behavior (*the physician documents that he/she has not determined whether the neoplasm is malignant or benign*), or Unspecified Nature (*the physician does not document whether the neoplasm is malignant or benign*). The description of the neoplasm will often indicate which of the six columns to use. For example, benign fibroadenoma of breast is coded using the Benign column; carcinoma in situ of cervix uteri is coded using the CA in situ column. Some sites do not have codes in all six columns because some behaviors do not occur in certain sites. For example, cancer in situ does not occur in bone, muscle, or connective tissue. Cancer in situ occurs only in epithelial cells and these sites do not have epithelial cells.

SUCCESS STEP

When a malignant neoplasm is not specified as primary, secondary, or in situ, you should code it as primary. Secondary and CA in situ must be stated in the medical record in order to assign codes from those columns.

Unknown Anatomic Site

When the anatomic site of the primary or secondary neoplasm is not known, assign a code from the first line of the Table of Neoplasms, which is labeled **Neoplasm, neoplastic**. The same codes also appear under the subterm **Neoplasm, unknown site or unspecified.** There are two common situations when this may occur:

- Carcinoma of unknown primary (CUP) occurs when the neoplasm is diagnosed at a late stage after it has metastasized and the physician is unable to determine the site of origin.
- The secondary site may not be specified when the neoplasm has metastasized to multiple areas throughout the body and treatment is directed at the overall body rather than one specific site.

	Malignant Primary	Malignant Secondary	Ca in situ	Benign	Uncertain Behavior	Unspecified Behavior
Neoplasm, neoplastic	C80.1	C79.9	D09.9	D36.9	D48.9	D49.9
abdomen, abdominal	C76.2	C79.8-	D09.8	D36.7	D48.7	D49.89
cavity	C76.2	C79.8-	D09.8	D36.7	D48.7	D49.89
organ	C76.2	C79.8-	D09.8	D36.7	D48.7	D49.89
viscera	C76.2	C79.8-	D09.8	D36.7	D48.7	D49.89
wall	C44.59	C79.2-	D04.5	D23.5	D48.5	D49.2
connective tissue	C49.4	C79.8-	-	D21.4	D48.1	D49.2
abdominopelvic	C76.8	C79.8-	-	D36.7	D48.7	D49.89

Figure 5-7 ■ Example of the Table of Neoplasms

	Malignant Primary	Malignant Secondary	Ca in situ	Benign	Uncertain Behavior	Unspecified Behavior
lung	C34.9-	C78.0-	D02.2-	D14.3-	D38.1	D49.1
azygos lobe	C34.1-	C78.0-	D02.2-	D14.3-	D38.1	D49.1
carina	C34.0-	C78.0-	D02.2-	D14.3-	D38.1	D49.1
hilus	C34.0-	C78.0-	D02.2-	D14.3-	D38.1	D49.1
linqula	C34.1-	C78.0-	D02.2-	D14.3-	D38.1	D49.1
lobe NEC	C34.9-	C78.0-	D02.2-	D14.3-	D38.1	D49.1
lower lobe	C34.3-	C78.0-	D02.2-	D14.3-	D38.1	D49.1
main bronchus	C34.0-	C78.0-	D02.2-	D14.3-	D38.1	D49.1
middle lobe	C34.2 -	C78.0-	D02.21	D14.31	D38.1	D49.1
overlapping lesion	C34.8-	-	-	-	-	-
upper lobe	C34.1-	C78.0-	D02.2-	D14.3-	D38.1	D49.1

Figure 5-8 ■ Example of Entry in Table of Neoplasms for an Overlapping Lesion

The subterm for **unknown site** provides codes in all six columns, so coders should select the appropriate column. For example, it is possible for the primary site to be specified, but not the secondary; for the secondary site to be specified, but not the primary; or for neither to be specified. In all cases, coders should query the physician and review all information in the medical record before assigning a code for unspecified site.

Overlapping Lesions

Some anatomic sites provide a listing for **overlapping lesions**. Overlapping lesions are contiguous sites where the tumor continues from one site to the adjacent one without interruption. Refer to ■ FIGURE 5-8 and review the entries for **lung** in the Table of Neoplasms. Separate entries describe distinct sites within the lung with separate codes. Use the entry for overlapping lesion when the physician documents that two contiguous sites within the lung are affected and the lesions have overlapping boundaries.

Patients may also have multiple tumors in contiguous sites that are not overlapping. For example, distinct tumors in two different lobes of the same lung that do not meet or overlap should be assigned two separate codes for primary malignant neoplasm of each lobe. Coders must review the documentation carefully to determine if the sites are overlapping or distinct.

Malignant Neoplasm of the Liver

The liver is a common site for metastasis because it filters the blood, which is a route through which cancer spreads. Primary liver cancer is rare, but does occur as the result of cirrhosis and alcoholism. When abstracting and assigning codes for malignant neoplasms of the liver, coders must take extra care to determine if it is primary or secondary.

Verify Codes in the Tabular List

All codes in the Table of Neoplasms must be verified in the Tabular List. Codes listed with a short dash - at the end require an additional character for laterality, which must be determined from the Tabular List. The Tabular List also provides instructional notes directing coders when additional codes are required and what sequencing is required. The beginning of ICD-10-CM Chapter 2 (C00-D49) provides several instructional notes that apply to all codes in the chapter.

Guided Example of Assigning Neoplasm Codes

Continue with the example from earlier in this chapter of Anthony Payne who saw Dr. Blackford for prostate cancer. Follow along in your ICD-10-CM manual as Karla Destefano, CPC, assigns the codes for the conditions she abstracted. Check off each step after you complete it.

⇨ Karla reviews the conditions she abstracted.

- ☐ *adenocarcinoma of prostate*
- ☐ *metastasis to colon*

➪ Karla locates the Main Term for the primary neoplasm in the Index.

❑ She looks up **A, adenocarcinoma**.

❑ The Main Term entry contains an instructional note **(*see also* Neoplasm, malignant, by site)**.

❑ She searches the subterms for **prostate** but cannot find it (■ FIGURE 5-9).

- Therefore, she knows she needs to refer to the Table of Neoplasms as directed in the instructional note.

❑ Karla searches for **N** in the Index to Diseases and Injuries and locates the Table of Neoplasms.

❑ She searches the left column for the subterm **prostate** and locates the entry.

❑ She checks the medical record to confirm that prostate cancer is primary.

❑ She refers to the first code column of the Table of Neoplasms, **Malignant Primary**, and selects the code **C61**.

➪ Next, Karla proceeds to verify the code in the Tabular List.

❑ Karla locates **C61** in the Tabular List and verifies the code title, **Malignant neoplasm of prostate**.

❑ She reviews the **Excludes1** note under the code and sees that **Malignant neoplasm of seminal vesicles** should not be coded here. She double-checks the medical record to be certain that seminal vesicles are not documented.

❑ Karla confirms that the block title **Malignant neoplasms of male genital organs (C60-C63)** contains no additional instructional notes.

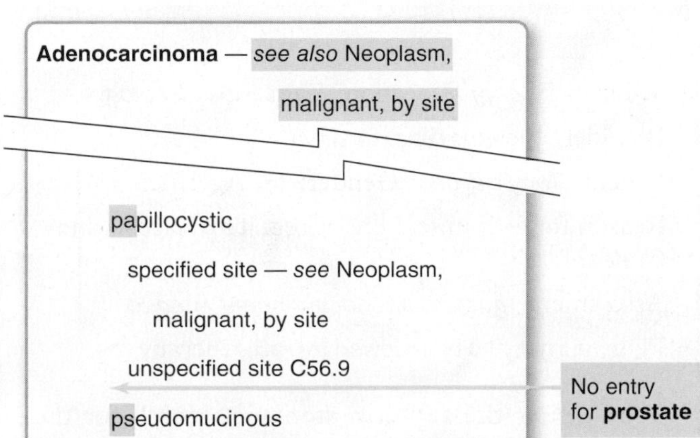

Figure 5-9 ■ Index Entry for Adenocarcinoma, Subterms Beginning with p

❑ Karla reviews the instructional notes at the beginning of **Chapter 2 Neoplasms (C00-D49)**. She determines that they do not apply to this case because she has no functional activity to report (first note); morphology codes are not required for billing (second note); there are no overlapping boundaries (third note); and the neoplasm does not involve ectopic tissue (fourth note).

➪ Karla assigns code **C61, Malignant neoplasm of prostate** for the primary neoplasm.

➪ Karla reviews the medical record and identifies the metastatic site is the colon.

❑ She returns to the Table of Neoplasms and locates the subterm for **intestine**.

❑ Under **intestine** she locates the subterm for **large**, then **colon** (■ FIGURE 5-10, page 82).

❑ She refers to the column **Malignant Secondary** and locates the code **C78.5**.

➪ Karla locates code in the Tabular List and verifies the title, **C78.5, Secondary malignant neoplasm of large intestine and rectum**.

❑ She reviews the category heading **C78, Secondary malignant neoplasm of respiratory and digestive organs** and confirms this case does not include any of the conditions listed under the **Excludes1** note.

CODING CAUTION

Although the Table of Neoplasms provides an entry for **C, colon**, it cross-references you to **C79.89 Secondary malignant neoplasm of other specified sites**, which is less specific than **C78.5**. Therefore, it is best to search for colon under the subterms **intestine, large** in order to locate the most specific code.

❑ She reviews the block heading **Malignant neoplasms of ill-defined, other secondary and unspecified sites (C76-C80)** and notes that there are no instructional notes.

❑ She already checked the notes at the beginning of **Chapter 2** so she does not need to do so again.

➪ Karla double-checks the medical record one last time to be sure she did not overlook anything. She has assigned the codes:

❑ **C61, Malignant neoplasm of prostate** for the primary neoplasm

❑ **C78.5, Secondary malignant neoplasm of large intestine and rectum** for the metastatic site

➪ Next, Karla needs to sequence the codes.

	Malignant Primary	Malignant Secondary	Ca in situ	Benign	Uncertain Behavior	Unspecified Behavior
intestine, intestinal	C26.0	C78.80	D01.40	D13.9	D37.8	D49.0
large	C18.9	C78.5	D01.0	D12.6	D37.4	D49.0
appendix	C18.1	C78.5	D01.0	D12.1	D37.3	D49.0
caput coli	C18.0	C78.5	D01.0	D12.0	D37.4	D49.0
cecum	C18.0	C78.5	D01.0	D12.0	D37.4	D49.0
colon	C18.9	C78.5	D01.0	D12.6	D37.4	D49.0
and rectum	C19	C78.5	D01.1	D12.7	D37.5	D49.0

Figure 5-10 ■ Table of Neoplasms Entry for Large Intestine, Colon

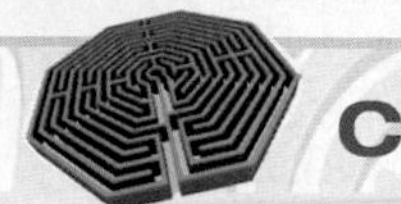

Coding Practice

Now it is your turn to practice assigning codes for neoplasms. Refer to the ***Tip*** at the end of the mini-medical-record if you need a little extra help.

Exercise 5.3 Assigning Codes for Neoplasms

Instructions: Read the mini-medical-record of each patient's encounter, review the information abstracted in Exercise 5.2, and assign ICD-10-CM diagnosis codes (CM) using the Index and Tabular List. Write the code(s) on the line provided.

1. Date: 5/2/yy Location: Branton Medical Center

Provider: Tanya Schmitt, MD

Patient: Roberta Sydnor Gender: F Age: 44

Reason for procedure: uterine fibroids

Procedure description: inserted catheter through femoral artery to uterus and injected polyvinyl alcohol (PVA) to block arteries leading to tumor

Postprocedural diagnosis: intramural (*within the muscle wall*) leiomyoma, uterus

Plan: FU in office in 4 weeks

Tip: The Main Term is the name of the tumor, not its site.

1 CM Code __________

2. Date: 5/2/yy Location: Branton Medical Center

Provider: Richard Blackford, MD

Patient: Jessica Salcido Gender: F Age: 15

Reason for admission: limb-salvage surgery after chemotherapy to shrink tumor

Procedure description: successfully cut out tumor from left thigh

Postprocedural assessment: osteosarcoma in the left thigh

Plan: discharge in 1–2 days

Tip: Remember to identify the medical term for the thigh bone.

1 CM Code __________

3. Date: 5/2/yy Location: East Side Oncology

Provider: Richard Blackford, MD

Patient: Tony Barone Gender: M Age: 43

Reason for encounter: review results of biopsy and CT scan

Assessment: gastric adenocarcinoma, fundus

Plan: surgery to be followed by radiotherapy

Tip: Under the subterm stomach, search for the specific location within the stomach.

1 CM Code __________

ARRANGING CODES FOR NEOPLASMS

Sequencing of neoplasm codes is determined by the circumstances of the encounter or admission. The findings from abstracting (Table 5-3) help coders determine how to sequence multiple codes. In particular, be alert for the following circumstances which call for specific sequencing:

- evaluation or treatment directed at the primary neoplasm
- evaluation or treatment directed at the metastasis
- encounter solely for chemotherapy, radiotherapy, or immunotherapy
- evaluation or treatment for a complication
- personal or family history of malignant neoplasm

Refer to ■ TABLE 5-5 for a summary of sequencing rules for neoplasms, then read the more detailed instructions that follow.

Evaluation or Treatment Directed at the Primary Malignancy

When the reason for the encounter is evaluation or treatment of the malignancy, sequence the primary neoplasm first, followed by codes for metastatic sites, complications, or any other relevant conditions (OGCR I.C.2.a. and OGCR I.C.2.l.1)). Treatment of the malignancy includes surgical removal of the neoplasm, diagnostic testing to determine the location or extent of the malignancy, and therapies such as **paracentesis** or **thoracentesis**.

When *both* the primary and secondary sites are being treated or evaluated, sequence the primary malignancy first, followed by the code(s) for the secondary site(s). Use a code for the primary malignancy as long as the patient is receiving treatment for it, even if the tumor has been surgically removed (OGCR I.C.2.l.1)).

CODING CAUTION

Be careful to understand the difference between primary or secondary malignant neoplasm and principal or first-listed diagnosis. The terms primary and secondary refer to the progression of the malignancy: where it started and where it spread to. Principal and first-listed diagnoses refer to the sequencing of codes. A code for primary neoplasm is not always sequenced first and a code for secondary neoplasm is not always sequenced second.

Table 5-5 ■ **SUMMARY OF COMMONLY USED SEQUENCING RULES FOR NEOPLASMS**

Reason for Encounter	Sequencing
Evaluation or treatment of primary neoplasm or *both* primary and secondary sites	1. Primary neoplasm 2. Secondary neoplasm
Evaluation or treatment of metastasis	1. Secondary neoplasm 2. Primary neoplasm
Evaluation or treatment *only* for complication of neoplasm (except anemia)	1. Complication 2. Primary neoplasm 3. Secondary neoplasm
Evaluation or treatment of anemia due to neoplasm	1. Neoplasm 2. Anemia
Encounter solely for chemotherapy, radiotherapy, or immunotherapy	1. Encounter for chemotherapy, radiotherapy, or immunotherapy 2. Complications during the therapy, if any 3. Primary neoplasm 4. Secondary neoplasm
Treatment, such as surgery, followed by chemotherapy, radiotherapy, or immunotherapy	1. Neoplasm 2. Encounter for chemotherapy, radiotherapy, or immunotherapy
Screening due to family history of malignant neoplasm	1. Screening 2. Family history of malignant neoplasm
Follow-up after completing treatment for a malignant neoplasm that no longer exists	1. Follow-up 2. Personal history of malignant neoplasm
Evaluation or treatment for an unrelated condition	1. Unrelated condition 2. Neoplasm, if documented as relevant

Evaluation or Treatment of the Metastasis

When the reason for the encounter is evaluation or treatment of the secondary malignancy or metastasis *only*, sequence the code for the secondary site as the principal or first-listed diagnosis; sequence the code for the primary malignancy as an additional code (OGCR I.C.2.b. and OGCR I.C.2.l.2)).

When *both* the primary and secondary sites are evaluated or treated, sequence the primary site first.

Encounter Solely for Chemo-, Radio-, or Immunotherapy

When the reason for the encounter or admission is *only* for administration of chemotherapy, radiotherapy, or immunotherapy, assign the principal or first-listed diagnosis for **Encounter for**, followed by the name of the therapy (OGCR I.C.2.e.2)) (■ FIGURE 5-11). To locate the code in the Index, search for the Main Term **Chemotherapy**, **Radiotherapy**, or **Immunotherapy**, respectively. Sequence codes for the primary and/or secondary neoplasms as additional codes.

CODING CAUTION

The codes titled **Encounter for** are diagnosis codes that describe the *reason* for the encounter. They are not procedure codes. You must also assign procedure codes that describe the service(s) provided using ICD-10-PCS codes for inpatient hospitals or CPT codes for physician office and outpatient services.

When the primary malignancy has been surgically removed but the patient is still receiving treatment, assign the code for **Encounter for** the therapy first, followed by the code for malignant neoplasm. Do not assign a code for personal history of malignant neoplasm when the patient is still receiving treatment, even when it has been surgically removed.

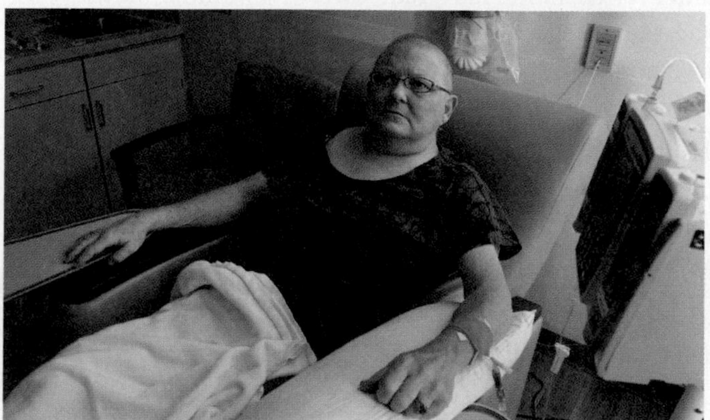

Figure 5-11 ■ A patient receives chemotherapy. *Source*: © *Norma Jean Gargasz/Alamy*.

When an episode of care involves surgical removal of the neoplasm, followed by chemotherapy or radiation therapy during the *same* episode of care, sequence the neoplasm code first, followed by the **Encounter for** therapy code(s) (OGCR I.C.2.e.1)).

Evaluation or Treatment for a Complication

When an encounter is for management of a complication associated with a neoplasm, such as dehydration, and the treatment is *only* for the complication, sequence the complication first, followed by the appropriate code(s) for the neoplasm (OGCR I.C.2.e.4)). However, if treatment is directed at the neoplasm and the complication is *also* treated, sequence the appropriate neoplasm code first, followed by the codes for the complications.

The exception to these sequencing rules is when the complication is anemia. When the encounter is for management of an anemia associated with the malignancy, and the treatment is *only* for anemia, sequence the appropriate code for the *malignancy* as the principal or first-listed diagnosis followed by code **D63.0, Anemia in neoplastic disease** (OGCR e.4)).

SUCCESS STEP

To locate the code for anemia due to cancer in the Index, search for **Anemia**, then the subterm **in**, then the subterm **neoplastic disease**.

CODING CAUTION

Coders familiar with ICD-9-CM should note that the OGCR for sequencing of anemia in neoplastic disease is different in ICD-10-CM.

Personal or Family History of Malignant Neoplasm

When a physician documents that family history of malignant neoplasm contributes to a patient's health risk, sequence the diagnosis code for screening first, followed by the history code. For example, a patient with a history of colonic polyps and a family history of colorectal cancer may need a colonoscopy more frequently than the general population. Sequence the codes as follows:

1. Screening for malignant neoplasm of colon
2. Personal history of colon polyps (benign neoplasm)
3. Family history, malignant neoplasm of digestive organs

When a physician sees a patient for follow-up after cancer treatment has been completed and the disease no longer exists, assign a code for follow-up first, followed by the appropriate personal history code (OGCR I.C.21.c.8)).

SUCCESS STEP

Although it takes a lot of experience to memorize every OGCR for the coding of neoplasms, even new coders can memorize the *fact* that this ICD-10-CM chapter has many guidelines. This serves as a reminder to refer to the OGCR for specific guidance.

The circumstances discussed here are the most common that coders encounter. Refer to the OGCR I.C.2.c. for additional detailed guidance on sequencing related to neoplasms.

Guided Example of Arranging Neoplasm Codes

Continue with the example from earlier in this chapter of Anthony Payne who saw Dr. Blackford for prostate cancer.

Follow along in your ICD-10-CM manual as Karla Destefano, CPC, sequences the codes. Check off each step after you complete it.

⇨ Karla reviews the codes she assigned.

- ❑ **C61, Malignant neoplasm of prostate**
- ❑ **C78.5, Secondary malignant neoplasm of large intestine and rectum**

⇨ She reviews the reason for the encounter in the medical record: review test results to determine extent of prostate cancer

- ❑ Therefore, she sequences the primary neoplasm as the first-listed diagnosis, followed by the metastatic site:

(1) **C61, Malignant neoplasm of prostate**

(2) **C78.5, Secondary malignant neoplasm of large intestine and rectum**

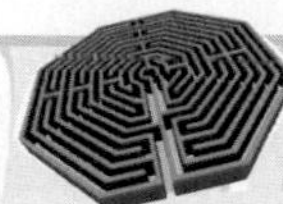

Coding Practice

Now it is your turn to practice coding and sequencing neoplasms. Refer to the ***Tip*** at the end of the mini-medical-record if you need a little extra help.

Exercise 5.4 Arranging Codes for Neoplasms

Instructions: Read the mini-medical-record of each patient's encounter, review the information abstracted in Exercise 5.2, assign ICD-10-CM diagnosis codes (CM) using the Index and Tabular List, and sequence the codes correctly. Write the code(s) on the line provided.

1. Date: 5/2/yy Location: East Side Oncology
Provider: Richard Blackford, MD
Patient: Terry Putnam Gender: F Age: 59
Reason for encounter: chemotherapy
Assessment: adenocarcinoma of the right breast, lower outer quadrant, which metastasized to multiple overlapping sites in the brain
Plan: return for next treatment in 3 weeks

Tip: Refer to OGCR I.C.2.e.2) for a reminder on how to sequence these codes. Remember to verify all codes in the Tabular List.

3 CM Codes ① chemo ② mets ③ breast

2. Date: 5/2/yy Location: Branton Medical Center
Provider: Richard Blackford, MD
Patient: Leonard Morton Gender: M Age: 61
Reason for procedure: brain stem tumor
Procedure description: used Gamma Knife surgery to destroy tumor
Postprocedural diagnosis: squamous cell carcinoma of the lung with brain stem metastases
Plan: FU in office 1 week, evaluate for chemotherapy

Tip: The site that is the reason for surgery should be sequenced first.

2 CM Codes Brainstem mets Sq. cell of the lung

3. Date: 5/2/yy Location: Branton Medical Center
Provider: Richard Blackford, MD
Patient: George Rhoden Gender: M Age: 67
Reason for admission: anemia
Assessment: anemia due to classical lymphocyte depleted Hodgkin lymphoma
Plan: administer IV iron supplements

Tip: Refer to OGCR e.4) for sequencing guidance.

2 CM Codes Lymphoma depleted Hodgkin Anemia

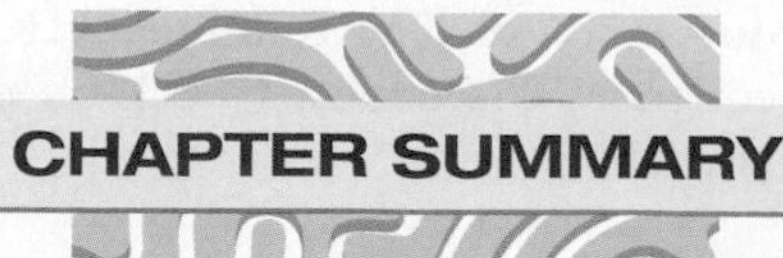

CHAPTER SUMMARY

In this chapter you learned that:

- Neoplasms are abnormal growth of new tissue, which may be malignant or benign.
- ICD-10-CM Chapter 2, Neoplasms (C00-D49), contains 21 blocks or subchapters that are divided by anatomical site.
- When abstracting patient cases with neoplasms, coders must look for several pieces of information that will help determine the first-listed or principal diagnosis and the sequencing of any additional diagnoses.
- Coders use both the Index to Diseases and Injuries and the Table of Neoplasms to locate codes for neoplasms.
- Sequencing of neoplasm codes is determined by the circumstances of the encounter or admission. OGCR provides detailed guidance on sequencing.
- ICD-10-CM provides Official Guidelines for Coding and Reporting (OGCR) for neoplasms in OGCR section I.C.2., which provide specific direction for sequencing codes for multiple neoplasms, complications, adjuvant therapies, and other situations.

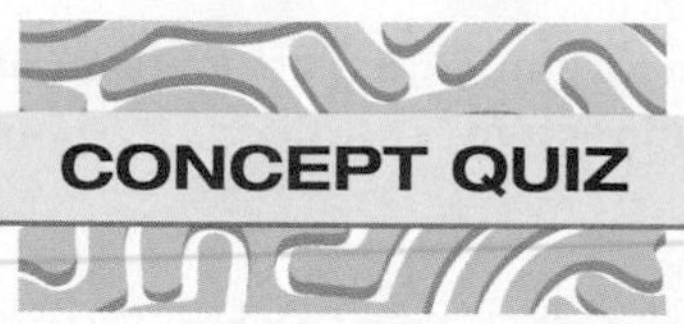

CONCEPT QUIZ

Take a moment to look back at your trip through neoplasms and solidify your skills. This is your opportunity to pull together everything you have learned.

Completion

Instructions: Write the term that answers each question based on the information you learned in this chapter. Choose from the following list. Some choices may be used more than once and some choices may not be used at all. Refer to the discussion in this chapter and the Glossary at the end of this book if you need a little extra help.

adjuvant	malignant
behavior	metastasis
benign	overlapping
CA in situ	primary neoplasm
carcinoma	radiotherapy
chemotherapy	sarcoma
CUP	secondary neoplasm
grading	staging
histology	topography
immunotherapy	

1. _______________ describes the anatomical site where the neoplasm begins.
2. _______________ describes the tissue type.
3. _______________ describes a neoplasm that has spread to other sites.
4. _______________ is the process of determining how far the cancer has spread.
5. Chemotherapy, radiotherapy, and immunotherapy are examples of _______________ therapy.
6. _______________ uses drugs to kill cancer cells.
7. _______________ occurs only in epithelial cells.
8. _______________ tumors are contiguous sites where the neoplasm continues from one site to the adjacent one without interruption.
9. _______________ describes how closely the cancer cell looks like a normal cell when viewed microscopically.
10. _______________ means life threatening.

Multiple Choice

Instructions: Circle the letter of the best answer to each question based on the information you learned in this chapter. Refer to the discussion in this chapter and the Glossary at the end of this book if you need a little extra help.

1. Which of the following is NOT a characteristic of malignant neoplasms?
   A. Are not encapsulated
   B. Have invasive growth and metastasis
   C. Produce no cachexia
   D. Can recur when surgically removed
2. Malignant neoplasms metastasize through
   A. exchange of bodily fluids.
   B. the bloodstream and lymphatic system.
   C. genetic transmission.
   D. bacteria.

3. Personal history of malignant neoplasm is
   A. a condition that a patient's family member had in the past or currently has that causes the patient to be at higher risk of also contracting the disease.
   B. a primary neoplasm that has metastasized.
   C. a condition the patient currently has and is receiving treatment for.
   D. a condition the patient had in the past, was removed, and is no longer being treated, but has the potential for recurrence.
4. Which of the following is NOT a column on the Table of Neoplasms?
   A. Personal History
   B. Malignant Primary
   C. Benign
   D. Uncertain Behavior
5. Which of the following statements about the Table of Neoplasms is TRUE?
   A. Coders always should consult the Table of Neoplasms instead of the Index to Diseases and Injuries.
   B. Codes in the Table of Neoplasms must always be verified in the Tabular List.
   C. The Table of Neoplasms classifies only malignant neoplasms.
   D. The Table of Neoplasms combines the Index and Tabular list into one document.
6. When a patient is seen for evaluation or treatment of metastasis, which code should be sequenced first?
   A. Primary neoplasm
   B. Secondary neoplasm
   C. CA in situ
   D. Complication
7. When a patient is seen for dehydration due to colon cancer that has metastasized to multiple sites, which code should be sequenced first?
   A. Colon cancer
   B. Metastatic site
   C. Dehydration
   D. Encounter for chemotherapy
8. When a patient is admitted for surgery to remove a tumor from the breast, then receives chemotherapy while still in the hospital, which code should be sequenced first?
   A. Breast cancer
   B. Encounter for surgery
   C. Encounter for chemotherapy
   D. Aftercare
9. When a patient receives a colonoscopy more frequently than normal, due to a family history of colon cancer, which code should be sequenced first?
   A. Screening
   B. Family history of malignant neoplasm
   C. Personal history of malignant neoplasm
   D. Colon cancer
10. When a patient who previously had surgery to remove a malignant neoplasm of the lung has an encounter only for radiotherapy, which code(s) should be assigned?
    A. Malignant neoplasm only
    B. Encounter for radiotherapy only
    C. Malignant neoplasm first and encounter for radiotherapy second
    D. Encounter for radiotherapy first and malignant neoplasm second

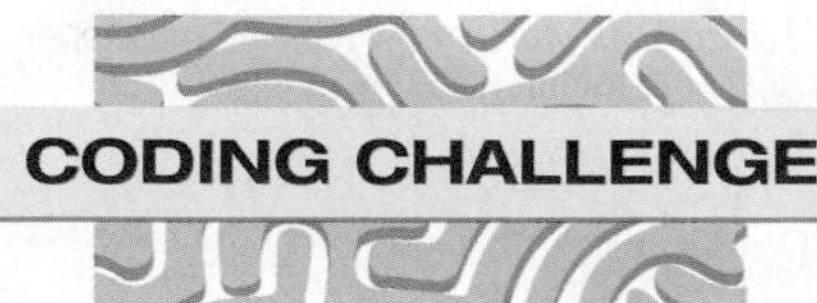

CODING CHALLENGE

Now it is your turn to demonstrate coding all aspects of neoplasms. Refer back to the examples and discussion in this chapter when you need a little extra help. Use your medical dictionary and anatomy references when needed.

Instructions: Read the mini-medical-record of each patient's encounter, then abstract, assign, and sequence ICD-10-CM diagnosis codes (CM) using the Index and Tabular List. Write the code(s) on the line provided.

1. Date: 5/9/yy Location: East Side Oncology

Provider: Richard Blackford, MD

Patient: Alicia Shelby Gender: F Age: 32

Chief complaint: management of multiple myeloma

Assessment: multiple myeloma in remission

Plan: recheck in 6 months

Tip: The fifth character in the code specifies remission.

1 CM Code __________

(continued)

(continued from page 87)

2. Date: 5/9/yy Location: Branton Medical Center Outpatient Procedure Center

Provider: Tanya Schmitt, MD (general surgeon)

Patient: Joseph Twigg Gender: M Age: 67

Reason for procedure: removal of tumor in left cheek

Procedure description: removed one lesion, 0.5 cm

Postprocedural diagnosis: basal cell adenoma left parotid salivary gland

Plan: recheck in 6 months

Tip: The parotid salivary gland is located in the cheek.

1 CM Code __________

3. Date: 5/9/yy Location: East Side Oncology

Provider: Richard Blackford, MD

Patient: Dianne Pedersen Gender: F Age: 57

Chief complaint: review colon biopsy results

Assessment: adenocarcinoma in situ in sigmoid colon

Plan: schedule surgery

Tip: What is another term for the colon? Search for this term to find the code you need.

1 CM Code __________

4. Date: 5/9/yy Location: East Side Oncology

Provider: Richard Blackford, MD

Patient: Adam Montiel Gender: M Age: 27

Chief complaint: evaluate unusual mole on forehead

Assessment: malignant melanoma

Plan: schedule removal next week

Tip: Remember to search for the subterm *skin.*

1 CM Code __________

5. Date: 5/9/yy Location: East Side Oncology

Provider: Richard Blackford, MD

Patient: Louise Fleenor Gender: F Age: 35

Chief complaint: review pathology results of lesion removed from skin of left breast 1 week ago

Assessment: CA in situ, completely removed

(continued)

5. (continued)

Plan: self-check entire skin once a month to watch for any additional lesions. Schedule a re-check appointment with office in 6 months.

1 CM Code __________

6. Date: 5/9/yy Location: East Side Oncology

Provider: Richard Blackford, MD

Patient: Anna Lapointe Gender: F Age: 71

Reason for encounter: radiotherapy to lung

Assessment: metastatic cancer in the right lung, CUP

Plan: 5 treatments per week for 6 weeks

Tip: The site being treated is the first-listed diagnosis.

2 CM Codes __________ __________

7. Date: 5/9/yy Location: Branton Gastroenterology Provider: Stanley Garrett, MD (gastroenterologist)

Patient: Tara Abshire Gender: F Age: 63

Chief complaint: monitoring of benign neoplasm

Assessment: benign Islet cell neoplasm of the pancreas

Plan: return visit if any new problems arise

1 CM Code __________

8. Date: 5/9/yy Location: Branton Medical Center Outpatient Procedure Center Provider: Stanley Garrett, MD (gastroenterologist)

Patient: Patricia Davidson Gender: F Age: 66

Reason for encounter: screening colonoscopy

Assessment: personal history of carcinoma of the colon which was successfully removed five years ago, no new findings today

Plan: colonoscopy in 5 years

Tip: Refer to OGCR I.C.21.c.8) for coding and sequencing guidance.

2 CM Codes __________ __________

9. Date: 5/9/yy Location: Branton Medical Center
Provider: Cynthia Hiatt, MD
Patient: Dennis Kohn Gender: M Age: 48
Reason for admission: Admitted from emergency department where he was seen due to an accident while riding off road recreational vehicle
Assessment: fracture right tibia shaft, notified patient's oncologist who is currently treating him for prostate cancer
Plan: follow up with oncologist and orthopedic surgeon in office

Tip: This is the patient's initial encounter for the fracture.

2 CM Codes __________ __________

10. Date: 5/9/yy Location: Branton Medical Center
Provider: Richard Blackford, MD
Patient: Angela Dash Gender: F Age: 81
Reason for admission: admitted from Emergency Department after collapsing at home, arrived by ambulance
Assessment: dehydration and hyponatremia (*sodium deficiency*) due to chemotherapy for metastatic bilateral ovarian cancer

Tip: The code for the complication is a combination code. Metastatic ovarian cancer means that the ovary is the primary site and the secondary site is unknown. Refer to OGCR I.B.13 to review rules for coding bilateral conditions. Refer to OGCR I.C.2.e.4) for sequencing guidance.

4 CM Codes __________ __________
__________ __________

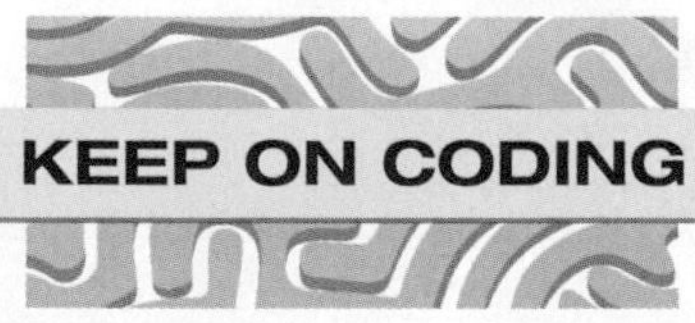

KEEP ON CODING

As a coder, you can never have too much experience. Apply everything you have learned in this chapter to code the following diagnostic statements. Use the OGCR and instructional notes in the Tabular List to help determine how many codes are required.

Instructions: Read the diagnostic statement, then use the Index and Tabular List to assign and sequence ICD-10-CM (CM) diagnosis codes. Write the code(s) on the line provided.

1. Carcinoma in situ of false vocal cord: CM Code(s) __________
2. Benign neoplasm of the mouth: CM Code(s) __________
3. Benign carcinoid tumor of the right kidney: CM Code(s) __________
4. Mesothelioma of lung: CM Code(s) __________
5. Metastatic carcinoma of the parietal lobe of the brain: CM Code(s) __________
6. Benign polyps of colon: CM Code(s) __________
7. Chief cell adenoma: CM Code(s) __________
8. Kaposi's sarcoma with HIV of stomach: CM Code(s) __________
9. Basal cell carcinoma of right hand: CM Code(s) __________
10. Malignant melanoma of skin of abdominal wall: CM Code(s) __________

11. Malignant neoplasm of nipple of the right breast: CM Code(s) ____________

12. Follicular lymphoma, Grade IIIb, inguinal region: CM Code(s) ____________

13. Acute leukemia, in relapse: CM Code(s) ____________

14. Melanoma of left forearm: CM Code(s) ____________

15. Carcinoma in situ, cervical stump: CM Code(s) ____________

16. Family history of breast cancer: CM Code(s) ____________

17. Personal history of brain cancer: CM Code(s) ____________

18. Malignant neoplasm of the right upper and lower lobes of the lung, primary: CM Code(s) ____________

19. Admission for chemotherapy for ovarian cancer: CM Code(s) ____________

20. Malignant primary cancer of the body of the pancreas: CM Code(s) ____________

21. Metastatic cancer to the rib: CM Code(s) ____________

22. Anemia due to left intra-ocular cancer: CM Code(s) ____________

23. Metastatic cancer of the liver, with unknown primary site: CM Code(s) ____________

24. Invasive hydatidiform mole: CM Code(s) ____________

25. Adenocarcinoma of the parotid gland with metastasis to the spine: CM Code(s) ____________

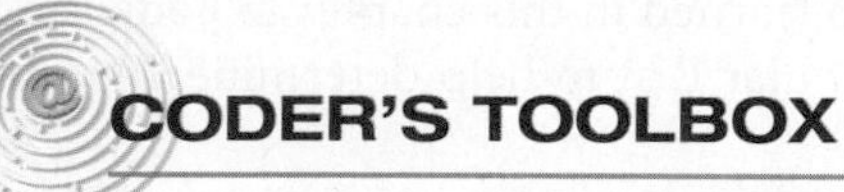

CODER'S TOOLBOX

The following resources are a starting point for learning more about neoplasms.

American Cancer Society (ACS) **http://www.cancer.org/index**

American Society of Clinical Oncology (ASCO) **http://www.cancer.net/**

Cancer Treatment Watch **http://www.cancertreatmentwatch.org/index.html**

Centers for Disease Control and Prevention (CDC)/ Cancer **http://www.cdc.gov/CANCER/**

Colon Cancer Alliance **http://www.ccalliance.org/**

LungCancer.org **http://www.lungcancer.org/**

National Cancer Institute (NCI) **http://www.cancer.gov/**

Prostate Cancer Foundation **http://www.pcf.org/**

Susan G. Komen for the Cure **http://ww5.komen.org/**

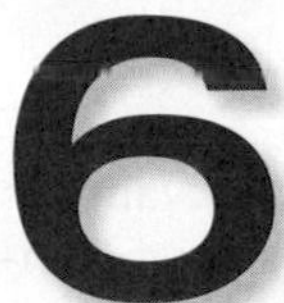

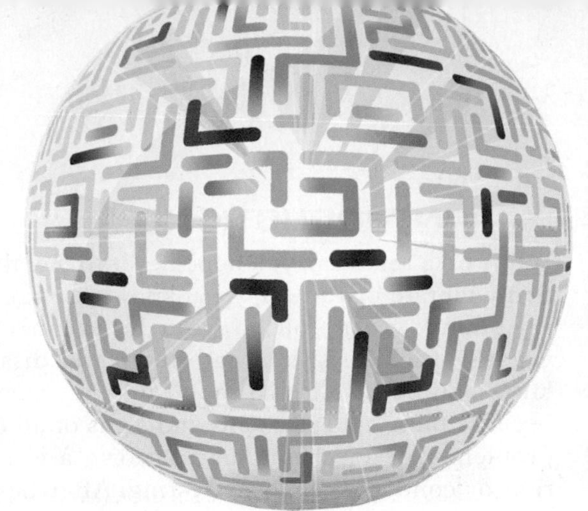

6 Symptoms, Signs, and Abnormal Clinical and Laboratory Findings, Not Elsewhere Classified (R00-R99)

Learning Objectives

After completing this chapter, you should have the skills to:

- Spell and define the key words, medical terms, and abbreviations in this chapter.
- Distinguish between symptoms, signs, abnormal clinical findings and abnormal laboratory findings, and confirmed diagnoses.
- Identify the main characteristics of coding symptoms, signs, and abnormal findings.
- Abstract symptoms, signs, abnormal findings, and confirmed diagnoses from the medical record.
- Assign codes for symptoms, signs, abnormal findings, and confirmed diagnoses.
- Arrange codes for symptoms, signs, abnormal findings, and confirmed diagnoses.
- Discuss the Official Guidelines for Coding and Reporting related to symptoms, signs, and abnormal findings.

Key Terms and Abbreviations

abnormal finding
confirmed
Impression
integral
modifier
qualified
qualifier
related
unrelated

In addition to the key terms listed here, students should know the terms defined within tables in this chapter.

Chapter Outline

- **Symptoms and Signs Refresher**
- **Coding Overview of Symptoms and Signs**
- **Abstracting Symptoms and Signs**
- **Assigning Codes for Symptoms and Signs**
- **Arranging Codes for Symptoms and Signs**

ICD-10-CM codes in this chapter are from the ICD-10-CM 2014 Draft code set from the Department of Health and Human Services, Centers for Disease Control and Prevention.

INTRODUCTION

While on a road trip, you hope never to feel the car suddenly vibrate or to hear an unknown clanging or hissing sound. When you do, your heart sinks and your visions of a few days of carefree travel dissipate. You know you need to get to the nearest mechanic quickly because these are symptoms and signs of an underlying problem. The mechanic may perform a visual inspection or conduct diagnostic testing. After he diagnoses the malfunction, he usually can repair it, so you can get on your way. Occasionally, the breakdown cannot be identified immediately and further tests or investigation are needed. Medical problems work in a similar manner although, unfortunately, some are not easy to diagnose or repair. Just as new drivers may not be familiar with all the sounds and motions a vehicle makes, new coders must learn to distinguish patient symptoms, signs, abnormal findings, and test results from the underlying diagnosis. Physicians of all specialties evaluate symptoms, signs, and abnormal findings.

This chapter helps you learn when to assign codes for symptoms, signs, and abnormal findings. Most importantly, you will practice coding for patient encounters related to symptoms, signs, and abnormal findings, a skill which requires you to abstract information from the mini-medical-record, assign correct codes, and arrange (sequence) the codes in the proper order.

As you read this chapter, open up your medical terminology book and keep a medical dictionary handy to refresh your memory of any unfamiliar terms. Also bookmark reliable Internet sites. These resources are especially important to help you learn what symptoms or signs are common with various conditions. By having the information you need at your fingertips, you will be able to better focus on coding skills.

SYMPTOMS AND SIGNS REFRESHER

To determine a patient's diagnosis, a physician evaluates numerous sources of information: the patient's chief complaint and description of the problem, a visual observation of the patient, a physical examination, and results of laboratory tests, imaging, and other evaluations. The physician's goal is to establish a definitive diagnosis and prescribe a treatment plan to cure the problem and/or alleviate the symptoms. Sometimes a confirmed diagnosis is not possible because the physician needs multiple encounters, extended testing, evaluation by specialists, surgery, or other procedures to arrive at a diagnosis.

Refer to ■ TABLE 6-1 to review the meanings of various types of diagnostic data.

Remember to use medical terminology skills to put together word roots, prefixes, and suffixes you already know to define new terms that describe symptoms, signs, and abnormal findings. Symptoms and signs are often identified with prefixes or suffixes that are applied to word roots from specific body systems. Refer to ■ TABLE 6-2 for a refresher on how to build medical terms related to symptoms, signs, and abnormal findings.

CODING CAUTION

Be aware of easily confused medical terms that have similar spellings and different meanings, such as:

dysphagia (*difficulty swallowing*) and **dysphasia** (*difficulty speaking*)

hem/e (*blood*) and **hemi-** (*half, side*)

hypo- (*low, below*) and **hyper-** (*high, excessive*)

Table 6-1 ■ **DEFINITION AND EXAMPLES OF DIAGNOSTIC DATA SOURCES**

Data	Definition	Example
Symptom	Subjective evidence of a disease or condition, usually reported by the patient	Pain, anxiety, fatigue, nausea
Sign	Objective evidence of a disease or condition that can be observed by the physician	Fever, limp, crying, bleeding, vomiting
Abnormal clinical finding	Evidence of a disease or condition discovered through physical examination or testing	Palpation of a lump or mass, irregular EKG, X-ray showing a fracture
Abnormal laboratory test	Result of a chemistry test, blood test biological culture that is outside of (higher or lower than) the normal numerical range, or microscopic specimen examination that differs from the standard visual features	Elevated or low glucose, high or low complete blood count, microscopic dysplasia

Table 6-2 ■ **EXAMPLE OF CONSTRUCTING MEDICAL TERMS FOR SYMPTOMS, SIGNS, AND ABNORMAL FINDINGS**

Root/Combining Form	Suffix	Complete Medical Term
dys- (*abnormal, painful*)	**-uria** (*condition of urine*) **-ptysis** (*to spit, cough*) **meno + rrhea** (*menstrual flow*)	**dys + uria** (*difficulty urinating*) **dys + phagia** (*difficulty swallowing*) **dys + meno + rrhea** (*difficulty or painful menstrual flow*)
hem/e (*blood*)		**hemat + uria** (*blood in urine*) **hemo + ptysis** (*coughing up blood*)
poly- (*many*)		**poly + uria** (*frequent urination*) **poly + meno + rrhea** (*frequent menstrual flow*)

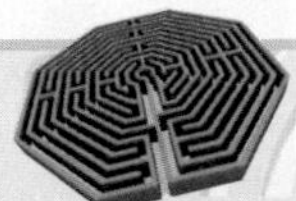

Coding Practice

Refresh your knowledge of terminology related to symptoms, signs, abnormal findings, and confirmed diagnoses. Use a medical terminology text or a website such as GlobalRph .com > Medical Terminology http://www.globalrph.com /medterm.htm to identify the meaning of word parts that may not be familiar to you.

Exercise 6.1 Symptoms and Signs Refresher

Instructions: Define the following symptoms, signs, and abnormal findings, then assign the diagnosis code.

Follow these steps:

- Use slash marks "/" to break down each term into its root(s) and suffix.
- Define the meaning of the word, based on the meaning of each word part.
- Assign the default ICD-10-CM diagnosis code (CM) for the condition using the Index and Tabular List.

Example: dysuria dys/ur/ia Meaning: condition of painful urination CM Code: R30.0

1. dyspnea Meaning difficulty breathing CM Code R06.00
2. nocturia Meaning urination at night CM Code R35.1
3. aphagia Meaning unable to swallow CM Code R13.0
4. epistaxis epi + staxis Meaning bleeding from above (nosebleed) CM Code R04.0
5. lymphadenopathy Meaning abnormal condition of lymph nodes CM Code R59.1
6. hyperemesis Meaning excessive vomiting CM Code R11.10
7. hypoxemia Meaning low oxygen in the blood CM Code R09.02
8. cyanosis cyan + osis Meaning yellow skin CM Code R23.0
9. glycosuria Meaning sugar in urine CM Code R81
10. tachycardia Meaning rapid heartbeat CM Code R00.0

CODING OVERVIEW OF SYMPTOMS AND SIGNS

ICD-10-CM Chapter 18, Symptoms, Signs, and Abnormal Clinical and Laboratory Findings, Not Elsewhere Classified (R00-R99), contains 14 blocks or subchapters that are divided by anatomical site. Review the block names and code ranges listed at the beginning of Chapter 18 in the ICD-10-CM manual to become familiar with the content and organization.

This chapter includes symptoms, signs, and abnormal results of clinical and laboratory procedures. It also includes ill-defined conditions that do not fit anywhere else in ICD-10-CM or that can be indicative of multiple conditions. Signs and symptoms that point to a specific diagnosis appear in other chapters of the classification. For example, fevers of unknown origin or that are drug induced appear in this chapter, but fevers with a known cause, such as a fever due to heat or a specific organism, appear in other chapters. An abnormal blood culture appears in this chapter, but an abnormal white blood cell count is classified to ICD-10-CM Chapter 3, Diseases of the Blood and Blood Forming Organs.

This chapter is comparable to ICD-9-CM Chapter 16 (780-799). Codes have been added, deleted, and expanded for clarity and specificity. Significant expansions have been made to codes in the block **Abnormal findings on examination of other body fluids, substances and tissues, without diagnosis (R83-R89)** in order to further specify the type of finding. Coding for **Coma (R40.2-)** has been expanded from a single code in ICD-9-CM (780.01) to 16 codes, each with one of five extensions to reflect the Glasgow Coma Scale ratings. Review the instructional notes at the beginning of the chapter that discuss how coders should report codes in this chapter. Also review the **Excludes2** note, which lists several conditions not classified to this chapter. Frequent instructional notes throughout the chapter direct coders to use multiple codes to describe related or underlying conditions associated with various symptoms.

ICD-10-CM provides Official Guidelines for Coding and Reporting (OGCR) for symptoms, signs, and abnormal clinical and laboratory findings in OGCR section I.C.18. OGCR provides a detailed discussion of when to report and not report codes from this chapter. OGCR also discusses coding of symptoms and signs related to several specific conditions: repeated falls, coma, **functional quadriplegia, systemic inflammatory response syndrome (SIRS)**, and death not otherwise specified (NOS). Additional OGCR related to symptoms, signs, and abnormal findings appear in OGCR I.B.4, 5, and 6; II.A., II.E.; IV.D., and IV.H.

ABSTRACTING SYMPTOMS AND SIGNS

Abstracting requires coders to be knowledgeable of disease processes and the related symptoms, signs, abnormal clinical findings, and abnormal laboratory test results, so they can distinguish which elements should be coded and which should not. They also must distinguish when a physician makes a confirmed diagnosis, in contrast to when the diagnosis is uncertain, because different coding rules apply to these situations. ■ TABLE 6-3 highlights key questions to answer when reviewing the medical record. Coders use answers to these questions when assigning and sequencing codes. Remember that the abstracting questions are a guide and that not every question applies to, or can be answered for, every case. For example, not all patients have abnormal laboratory findings. Details that will help answer these questions follow in the remainder of this section of the chapter.

Table 6-3 ■ KEY CRITERIA FOR ABSTRACTING SYMPTOMS, SIGNS, ABNORMAL FINDINGS, AND CONFIRMED CONDITIONS

- ❑ What symptoms does the patient report?
- ❑ What signs does the physician document?
- ❑ What abnormal laboratory findings are reviewed?
- ❑ What confirmed diagnoses are documented?
- ❑ What diagnoses are identified as uncertain with words such as possible, probable, rule out, suspected?
- ❑ Which symptoms, signs, and abnormal findings are integral to the condition?
- ❑ Which symptoms, signs, and abnormal findings are related but not integral to the condition?
- ❑ Which symptoms, signs, and abnormal findings are unrelated to the condition?

Integral, Related, and Unrelated Findings

Coders must distinguish between symptoms, signs, and abnormal findings that are an **integral** (*routine*) part of a disease process, those that are **related** but not integral, and those that are **unrelated**. They need a solid understanding of common conditions and their symptoms so they can make these distinctions. Refer to ■ TABLE 6-4 to review symptoms, signs, and abnormal findings for commonly diagnosed conditions.

Integral Symptoms

When a diagnosis is confirmed, assign codes to the named condition, but do *not* assign codes for the symptoms, signs, and abnormal findings that are integral to the condition (OGCR I.B.4. and 5.; I.C.18.a). Integral or routine symptoms are those that most patients with the condition experience. For example:

- The physician documents *Fever and RLQ pain due to acute ruptured appendicitis*. Fever and pain are symptoms integral to a ruptured appendix, so the coder assigns a code only for the appendicitis. Do *not* assign codes for fever and pain.

SUCCESS STEP

Be proactive and keep a reference book on diseases on your desk so you can consult it when you are unsure if a symptom is integral, related, or unrelated. Consider creating "cheat sheets" with notes on conditions commonly coded in your office to guide you through the learning process. If you are unsure about a symptom, consult a colleague or supervisor; do not guess.

Do not code clinical findings that are integral to the condition. For example:

- The physician documents *Three elevated BP readings over the past three months. Hypertension* (■ FIGURE 6-1). The coder assigns a code for hypertension, but not for elevated blood pressure, because a series of elevated blood pressure readings is the definition of hypertension.

Table 6-4 ■ **SYMPTOMS, SIGNS, AND ABNORMAL FINDINGS FOR COMMONLY DIAGNOSED CONDITIONS**

Condition	Symptoms and Signs	Abnormal Findings
Allergic contact dermatitis	Rash, erythema, pruritus, burning	
Anemia	Fatigue, **SOB**, decreased exercise tolerance	Folic acid
Asthma	Dyspnea, difficulty exhaling, wheezing	
Appendicitis	**RLQ** pain, fever, nausea, vomiting	
Benign prostatic hyperplasia (BPH)	Nocturia, polyuria, dysuria, oliguria	
Cerebrovascular accident (CVA)	Headache, muscular weakness, speech disturbance, loss of consciousness	Angiography, CT scan, MRI
Colorectal cancer	Melena, change in bowel habits, lower abdominal pain	Biopsy, colonoscopy
Congestive heart failure (CHF)	SOB, fatigue, edema	EKG, echocardiogram, **BP**, X-ray
Dementia	Language, memory, and mood deficits	
Depression	Prolonged sadness, sleep and appetite changes, feelings of guilt and anxiety	
Diabetes mellitus (DM)	Polyuria, polydipsia	Hyperglycemia, elevated glucose, elevated **HbA1C**
Endometriosis	Pelvic pain, diarrhea, constipation, menorrhagia, fatigue	
Epilepsy	Convulsions, seizures	**EEG**
Gastroenteritis	Nausea, vomiting, diarrhea, abdominal pain	Stool culture
Gout	Joint pain, heat, swelling, redness	
Hiatal hernia	Indigestion, heartburn, acid reflux, esophagitis	
Hypercholesterolemia	**Asymptomatic**	Elevated serum cholesterol
Hypertension (HTN)	Asymptomatic	Elevated blood pressure
Leukemia	Fatigue, weight loss, fever, hemorrhages	Blood tests
Osteoarthritis (OA)	Joint pain and stiffness, muscle weakness, enlarged joints	X-ray
Pneumonia	Chest pain, fluid in lungs, fever, productive cough	X-ray
Rosacea	Flushing, persistent erythema, papules pustules, telangiectasia	
Urinary tract infection (UTI)	Polyuria, dysuria, hematuria	Urinalysis

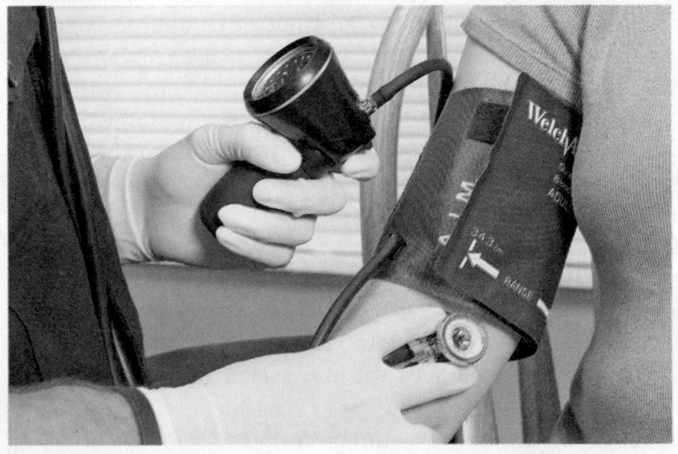

Figure 6-1 ■ Taking Blood Pressure. *Source: Michal Heron/ Pearson Education/PH College.*

Do not code laboratory test results that are integral to the condition. For example:

- The physician documents *Elevated glucose HbA1C results, type 2 diabetes*. The coder assigns a code for type 2 diabetes, but not for elevated glucose or HbA1C because those tests are used to establish the diagnosis.

Do code for the symptoms, signs, abnormal clinical findings, or abnormal test results when a diagnosis is not stated. For example:

- The physician documents *Three elevated BP readings over the past three months*. The coder assigns a code for elevated blood pressure, but not hypertension, because the physician did not document hypertension as a diagnosis.

- The physician documents Elevated glucose HbA1C results. Refer to dietician for meal plan. The coder assigns a code for elevated glucose, but not diabetes, because the physician did not document diabetes as a diagnosis. Coders should not assign a diagnosis that is not documented.

CODING CAUTION

The physician's diagnosis stands on its own. Coders do not assign codes to symptoms to justify *why* the physician arrived at the diagnosis. Assign codes for the symptoms *only* if the diagnosis is not confirmed. When the diagnosis is confirmed, code *only* the diagnosis, not the symptoms.

Related Symptoms

Do code for symptoms that are related to the disease process, but not integral to it (OGCR I.B.6.). Related symptoms are those that patients occasionally experience with the confirmed diagnosis, but are not common or routine. For example:

- The physician documents RLQ pain, fever, vomiting, dehydration due to acute ruptured appendicitis. Administered IV fluids. Dehydration is the result of the fever and vomiting associated with appendicitis, but is not a routine part of the condition. Additional treatment was provided for the dehydration. Therefore, assign a code for dehydration in addition to ruptured appendicitis.

Unrelated Symptoms

Do code for symptoms that are unrelated to the confirmed diagnosis (OGCR I.C.18.b). Unrelated symptoms are those that are not associated with the confirmed diagnosis and may indicate an additional problem or condition. For example:

- The physician documents Fever, difficulty breathing, hemoptysis, X-ray positive for pneumonia, sputum culture for hemoptysis. Fever and difficulty breathing are integral to pneumonia, which the physician confirmed with a chest X-ray. Hemoptysis is not a symptom associated with pneumonia, so it should be coded in addition to pneumonia.

Uncertain Diagnoses

When physicians cannot establish a definite diagnosis, outpatient coders assign codes for the symptoms, signs, and abnormal findings until a diagnosis is established (OGCR IV.H.). Coders must interpret the terms physicians use in documentation in order to understand whether a diagnosis is confirmed or uncertain. An uncertain diagnosis is one that the physician is not completely confident of. Particularly in the outpatient setting, physicians may require multiple visits, consultation with a specialist, and test results in order to determine a diagnosis. Coders assign codes for symptoms until the diagnosis is established. After the diagnosis is established, they no longer code the symptoms that are integral to the condition.

Table 6-5 ■ TERMS INDICATING UNCERTAIN DIAGNOSES

❑ likely	❑ rule out (R/O)
❑ possible	❑ still to be ruled out
❑ probable	❑ suspected
❑ questionable	

By default, interpret any diagnostic statement as **confirmed**, one the physician is confident of, *unless* the physician indicates it is uncertain. A diagnosis may be uncertain when a patient has symptoms and signs that can be attributed to many different conditions or when test results do not provide clear data. An uncertain diagnostic statement contains **qualifiers** or **modifiers** (*word(s) that limit the meaning of another*) before the name of the condition (■ TABLE 6-5).

An uncertain diagnosis is also called a **qualified** diagnosis. The words *qualified* and *qualifier* have two opposite meanings. One common meaning is *meeting a standard or set of criteria*. An alternative meaning is one of *limiting or restricting*. When coders and physicians use the expression, *qualified diagnosis*, they are using the second meaning of the word, a *diagnosis that is limited or uncertain*.

Physicians may use the heading **Impression** in their progress notes for the diagnostic statement. This word also carries multiple meanings, which sometimes causes confusion for new coders. One meaning is *an idea or belief that is vague or unclear*. Physicians use an alternate meaning, *an effect produced on the mind by outside stimuli*. Therefore, use of the word *impression* does not describe an uncertain diagnosis.

In the outpatient setting, do not assign a code to an uncertain diagnosis. Instead, code the symptoms, signs, and abnormal test results documented by the physician (OGCR IV.D. and H.). In the inpatient setting, when the diagnosis documented at the time of discharge is stated as uncertain, code the condition as if it existed (OGCR III.A. and H.). The rationale for this guideline is that the diagnostic workup, arrangements for further workups, and initial treatments provided must relate to the principal diagnosis.

SUCCESS STEP

When you code for an uncertain diagnosis in an inpatient setting, assign the usual code for the condition. You do not assign any additional codes to indicate it is uncertain.

Abnormal Clinical and Laboratory Findings

When coding inpatient services, abstract abnormal (*the readings are not within the normal average range established for that particular test*) clinical and laboratory findings *only* when the provider documents their clinical significance. Do not automatically abstract and code all findings that are outside the normal range. In rare cases, the provider may order additional tests to further evaluate abnormal findings, or prescribe a treatment, but not document their clinical significance. In this situation, coders should query the provider regarding the possible significance of the findings (OGCR III.B.).

Guided Example of Abstracting Symptoms and Signs

Refer to the following example to learn more about abstracting symptoms, signs, and abnormal findings. Sherry Whittle, CPC, is a fictitious coder who guides you through this case.

> Date: 6/1/yy Location: Branton Family Practice
> Provider: Kristen Conover, MD
> Patient: Chad Wang Gender: M Age: 6
> Chief Complaint: nausea, vomiting, and diarrhea
> Assessment: gastroenteritis
> Plan: bed rest and plenty of fluids

Follow along as Sherry Whittle, CPC, reviews the medical record and abstracts the diagnosis. Check off each step after you complete it.

⇨ Sherry begins by referring to Key Criteria for Abstracting Symptoms, Signs, Abnormal Findings, and Confirmed Conditions (Table 6-3).

- ❑ *What symptoms does the patient report?* nausea, vomiting, and diarrhea
- ❑ *What signs does the physician document?* None
- ❑ *What abnormal laboratory findings are reviewed?* None
- ❑ *What confirmed diagnoses are documented?* gastroenteritis
- ❑ *What diagnoses are identified as uncertain with words such as possible, probable, rule out, suspected?* None
- ❑ *Which symptoms, signs, and abnormal findings are integral to the condition?* All
- ❑ *Which symptoms, signs, and abnormal findings are related but not integral to the condition?* None
- ❑ *Which symptoms, signs, and abnormal findings are unrelated to the condition?* None

⇨ Because the symptoms of nausea, vomiting, and diarrhea are all integral to gastroenteritis, Sherry does not abstract these items to code.

- ❑ The only diagnosis code to be assigned is gastroenteritis. (You will learn how to do this when you study the digestive system.)

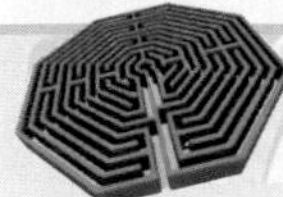

Coding Practice

Now it is your turn to practice abstracting symptoms, signs, abnormal findings, and confirmed diagnoses. Questions help guide your analysis.

Exercise 6.2 Abstracting Symptoms and Signs

Instructions: Read the mini-medical-record of each patient's encounter and answer the abstracting questions. Write the answer on the line provided. Do not assign any codes.

> **1.** Date: 6/2/yy Location: Branton Family Practice
> Provider: Kristen Conover, MD
> Patient: Ernest Watts Gender: M Age: 61
> Reason for encounter: review result of liver function study
> Assessment: abnormal liver function test
> Plan: biopsy
>
> a. Does the physician state a confirmed diagnosis?
> NO
> ______________________________
>
> b. Is this a sign, a symptom, an abnormal clinical finding, or an abnormal laboratory test?
> abnormal laboratory tst
> ______________________________
>
> c. What Main Term will you look up in the Index?
> abnormal
> ______________________________

(*continued*)

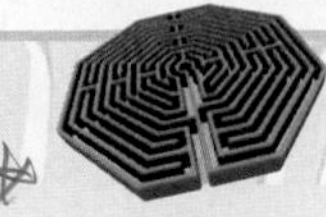

Coding Practice (continued)

2. Date: 6/2/yy Location: Branton Medical Center
Provider: Cynthia Hiatt, MD
Patient: Albert Wexler Gender: M Age: 74
Reason for admission: irregular heartbeat, chest pain, and lightheadedness
Assessment: atrial fibrillation
Plan: cardiologist evaluation

Tip: Do not code symptoms that are integral to a confirmed condition.

a. What symptoms and signs are mentioned? irregular heart beat, chest pain, & light headedness

b. Does the physician state a confirmed diagnosis? yes

c. Are all of the symptoms and signs integral to the diagnosis? yes

d. Which symptoms and signs should be coded? none

e. What condition will you code? a-fib

3. Date: 6/2/yy Location: Branton Medical Center
Provider: Kristen Conover, MD
Patient: Yvonne Macpherson Gender: F Age: 16
Reason for admission: repeated seizures
Assessment: seizures of unknown cause
Plan: continued follow-up with neurologist, medication

a. Does the physician state a confirmed diagnosis? no

b. What symptom should be coded? seizures

c. What is the Main Term? seizures

4. Date: 6/2/yy Location: Branton Family Practice
Provider: Kristen Conover, MD
Patient: Debra Giroux Gender: F Age: 45
Chief complaint: polydipsia, polyuria, and difficulty sleeping, most recent blood test showed hyperglycemia
Assessment: type 2 diabetes, possible sleep apnea
Plan: evaluate for sleep apnea

a. What symptoms and signs are mentioned? polydipsia, polyuria, difficulty sleeping hyperglycemia

b. Does the physician state a confirmed diagnosis? yes What is it? type 2 diabetes

c. Does the physician state an uncertain diagnosis? yes What is it? sleep apnea

d. Should you code an uncertain diagnosis for an outpatient encounter? no What should you code instead? signs & symptoms

e. Which symptoms and signs are integral to the confirmed diagnosis? polydipsia, polyuria, hypergly

f. Which symptoms and signs relate to the unconfirmed diagnosis? difficulty sleeping

g. What two conditions/symptoms will you code? type 2 diabetes, difficulty sleeping

5. Date: 6/2/yy Location: Branton Family Practice
Provider: Kristen Conover, MD
Patient: Mark Greenfield Gender: M Age: 29
Chief complaint: extreme nervousness and irritability
Assessment: R/O hyperthyroidism
Plan: thyroid workup

a. What symptoms and signs are mentioned? extreme nervousness & irritability

b. What does R/O (rule out) mean? uncertain condition that the doctor wants to try and eliminate

c. Does the physician state a confirmed diagnosis? no

d. Does the physician state an uncertain diagnosis? yes What is it? hyperthyroidism

e. What two conditions/symptoms will you code? nervousness, irritability

6. Date: 6/2/yy Location: Branton Medical Center
Provider: Kristen Conover, MD
Patient: Stanley Nicholson Gender: M Age: 52
Reason for admission: abdominal pain
Discharge diagnosis: epigastric pain due to acute pancreatitis or cholangitis (*inflammation of the common bile duct*)
Plan: pain medication, antibiotics as precaution, further imaging

(continued)

6. (continued)

Tip: This is a hospital discharge, so inpatient OGCR apply.

a. What symptoms and signs are mentioned? epigastric pain

b. Does the physician state a confirmed diagnosis? No

c. What alternative or comparative diagnoses does the physician document? acute pancreatitis or cholangitis

ASSIGNING CODES FOR SYMPTOMS AND SIGNS

The most challenging aspect of coding for symptoms, signs, and abnormal findings is distinguishing integral, related, and unrelated symptoms and distinguishing confirmed and uncertain diagnoses. After this is accomplished, assigning codes is relatively straightforward. The Main Term for many symptoms and signs codes is the name of the symptom or sign. Combination codes also exist for definitive diagnoses and certain related symptoms. Coding for abnormal test results can be more challenging and is discussed later in this section.

Codes for Symptoms and Signs

Main Term entries for most symptoms and signs in the Index often are the name of the symptom or sign, such as pain, fever, vomiting, or weakness. Review the subterms carefully for anatomic sites or other descriptions of the condition. If none of the specific subterms apply, use the default code immediately following the Main Term.

Refer to the Main Term **Fever** in the ICD-10-CM Index (■ FIGURE 6-2). The default code is **R50.9**. Over 200 subterms describe specific types or causes of fever. When a subterm applies, verify and assign the code listed with the subterm. When no subterm applies, verify and assign the default code.

Combination Codes

Do use combination codes when available. ICD-10-CM contains combination codes that identify both the definitive diagnosis and certain related symptoms. When using this kind of combination code, do not assign an additional code for the related symptom. For example:

- The physician documents Type 2 diabetes with gastroparesis. ICD-10-CM provides an entry in the Index for **Diabetes, with gastroparesis E11.43**. Use the combination code and do not assign a separate code for gastroparesis.

SUCCESS STEP

ICD-10-CM uses combination codes more frequently than ICD-9-CM did. In ICD-9-CM coders assigned additional codes for manifestations and symptoms of diabetes, but in ICD-10-CM, most of these have been replaced with combination codes.

Fever (inanition) (of unknown origin) (persistent) (with chills) (with rigor) R50.9
- abortus A23.1
- Aden (dengue) A90
- African tick-borne A68.1
- American
  - mountain (tick) A93.2
  - spotted A77.0
- aphthous B08.8
- arbovirus, arboviral A94

Figure 6-2 ■ Example of Index Entry for a Sign (Fever) with Subterms

Codes for Abnormal Findings

Physicians may receive test results from the laboratory that are abnormal, but they are still unable to establish a firm diagnosis. In this situation, coders assign codes for the abnormal test result (■ FIGURE 6-3). To locate the Main Term for abnormal clinical and laboratory findings, identify the word in the diagnostic statement that describes how the result *differs* from normal. Refer to ■ TABLE 6-6 for commonly used Main Terms and examples of subterm entries. Also be alert for instructional notes and cross-references in the Index that may lead to alternative entries.

Guided Example of Assigning Symptoms and Signs Codes

Refer to the following example to learn how to assign codes for symptoms. This case is similar to the earlier example of Chad Wang who was seen for nausea, vomiting, and diarrhea and was diagnosed with gastroenteritis. However, notice how this example should be coded differently based on the wording of the Assessment.

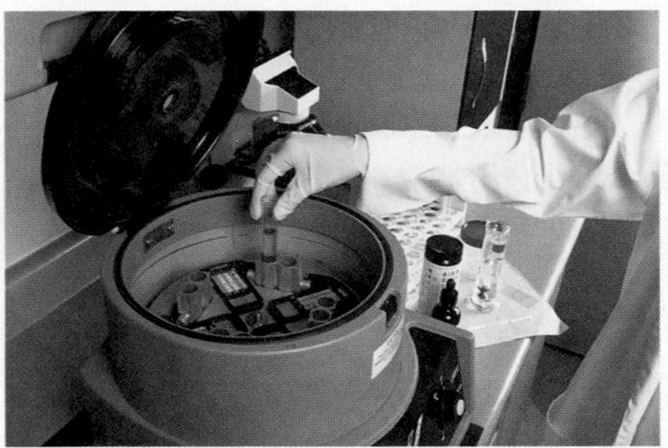

Figure 6-3 ■ Laboratory Technician Performing a Urinalysis Test.
Source: Michal Heron/Pearson Education/PH College.

Date: 6/1/yy Location: Branton Family Practice
Provider: Kristen Conover, MD
Patient: Charlene Winger Gender: F Age: 15
Chief Complaint: nausea, vomiting, and diarrhea
Assessment: suspected gastroenteritis
Plan: stool culture, bed rest, and plenty of fluids

Follow along as Sherry Whittle, CPC, assigns codes for nausea, vomiting, and diarrhea. Check off each step as you complete it.

⇨ First, Sherry abstracts the case.

- ❑ She reads the presenting symptoms nausea, vomiting, and diarrhea.
- ❑ She reads the Assessment suspected gastroenteritis.
- ❑ She notes that "suspected" makes gastroenteritis an uncertain diagnosis.
- ❑ As a result, she identifies the three symptoms—nausea, vomiting, and diarrhea—to code and does not code gastroenteritis.

⇨ Sherry searches the Index for the Main Term **Nausea** (■ FIGURE 6-4).

- ❑ She reads the nonessential modifier **(without vomiting)** which is the default for code R11.0.
- ❑ She locates the subterm **with vomiting, R11.2**, which provides a combination code for two of the symptoms of this patient.

⇨ Sherry verifies code **R11.2** in the Tabular List.

- ❑ She reads the code title for **R11.2, Nausea with vomiting, unspecified** and confirms that this accurately describes the symptoms.

Table 6-6 ■ **COMMONLY USED MAIN TERMS FOR ABNORMAL FINDINGS**

Main Term	Diagnostic Statement Examples	Index Entry Examples
Abnormal	Abnormal liver function test Abnormal hemoglobin in urine	Abnormal, function studies, liver Abnormal, urine, hemoglobin
Anomaly	Heart auricle anomaly Hip anomaly	Anomaly, heart, auricle Anomaly, hip, NEC
Deficiency	Low growth hormone Vitamin D deficiency	Deficiency, hormone, growth Deficiency, vitamin D
Elevated	High fasting glucose Elevated blood pressure	Elevated, fasting glucose Elevated, blood pressure
Findings, abnormal, inconclusive, without diagnosis	Lead in blood Abnormal urine glucose	Findings, in blood, lead Findings, urine, glucose
Loss	Transient loss of consciousness	Loss, consciousness, transient

➩ Sherry checks for instructional notes in the Tabular List.

- ❑ She cross-references the beginning of category **R11** and reads the **Excludes1** instructional note. None of the conditions listed describe the patient, so she may proceed.
- ❑ She cross-references the beginning of the block **R10-R19** and reads the **Excludes1** instructional note. None of the conditions listed describe the patient, so she may proceed.
- ❑ She cross-references the beginning of **Chapter 18 (R00-R99)** and reads the detailed instructional notes. She determines that note **(e) cases in which a more precise diagnosis was not available** describes this case and that she is coding correctly.

➩ Next, Sherry searches the Index for the Main Term **Diarrhea**.

- ❑ She reads through all of the available subterms but finds none that apply. She checks the documentation to confirm that the diarrhea is not stated as either viral or bacterial. It is not and that is likely the reason a stool culture was obtained.
- ❑ She selects the default entry **Diarrhea, diarrheal (disease) (infantile) (inflammatory) R19.7**.

➩ Sherry verifies code **R19.7** in the Tabular List.

- ❑ She reads the code title for **R19.7, Diarrhea, unspecified** and confirms that this accurately describes the symptom because more detailed information is not provided in the medical record.

Figure 6-4 ■ Index Entry for Nausea, with Vomiting

➩ Sherry checks for instructional notes in the Tabular List.

- ❑ She cross-references the beginning of category **R19** and identifies the instructional note **Excludes1: acute abdomen (R10.0)**. This does not describe the patient's symptoms so she knows she can proceed.
- ❑ She cross-references the beginning of the block **R10-R19** and chapter in the previous step and recalls that there are no notes that would change the code she selected.

➩ Sherry reviews the codes she has assigned for this case.

- ❑ **R11.2, Nausea with vomiting, unspecified**
- ❑ **R19.7, Diarrhea, unspecified**

➩ Next, Sherry must determine how to sequence the codes.

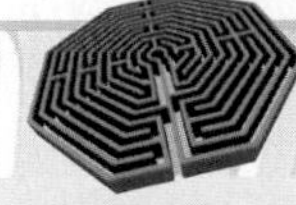

Coding Practice

Now it is your turn to practice assigning codes for symptoms, signs, abnormal findings, and confirmed diagnoses. Refer to the ***Tip*** at the end of the mini-medical-record if you need a little extra help.

Exercise 6.3 Assigning Codes for Symptoms and Signs

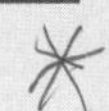

Instructions: Read the mini-medical-record of each patient's encounter, review the information abstracted in Exercise 6.2, and assign ICD-10-CM diagnosis codes (CM) using the Index and Tabular List. Write the code(s) on the line provided.

1. Date: 6/2/yy Location: Branton Family Practice
Provider: Kristen Conover, MD
Patient: Ernest Watts Gender: M Age: 61
Reason for encounter: review result of liver function study

(continued)

1. (continued)
Assessment: abnormal liver function test
Plan: biopsy
1 CM Code R94.5 Index → Abnormal → fxn studies → liver

2. Date: 6/2/yy Location: Branton Medical Center
Provider: Cynthia Hiatt, MD
Patient: Albert Wexler Gender: M Age: 74
Reason for admission: irregular heartbeat, chest pain, and lightheadedness
Assessment: atrial fibrillation

(continued)

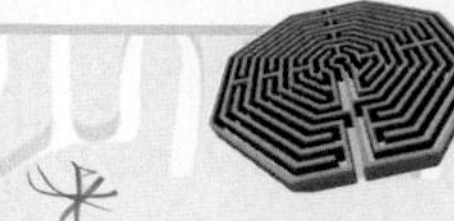

Coding Practice (continued)

2. (continued)
Plan: *cardiologist evaluation*

Tip: Do not code symptoms that are integral to a confirmed condition.

1 CM Code I48.91 (fibrillation atrial)

3. Date: 6/2/yy Location: Branton Medical Center
Provider: Kristen Conover, MD
Patient: Yvonne Macpherson Gender: F Age: 16
Reason for admission: repeated seizures
Assessment: seizures of unknown cause
Plan: continued follow-up with neurologist, medication

1 CM Code R56.9 Seizures

ARRANGING CODES FOR SYMPTOMS AND SIGNS

In general, multiple codes for symptoms, signs, and abnormal findings are sequenced using the same guidelines as any other codes. Special situations include coding for a confirmed diagnosis and related symptoms, coding a confirmed diagnosis and unrelated symptoms, coding symptoms followed by a diagnosis, and coding symptoms with no confirmed diagnosis. These are discussed next.

Confirmed Diagnosis and Related Symptoms

The physician may document a confirmed diagnosis and a symptom, sign, or abnormal finding that is related, but not integral. Sequence the confirmed diagnosis first, followed by the related symptom (■ FIGURE 6-5).

Confirmed Diagnosis and Unrelated Symptoms

The physician may document a confirmed diagnosis and an unrelated symptom, sign, or abnormal finding. Sequence the code chiefly responsible for the services provided first. When both the confirmed diagnosis and the unrelated symptom are equally responsible, sequence either code first (■ FIGURE 6-6).

Symptom Followed by Diagnoses

Occasionally, the physician may document a symptom, sign, or abnormal finding followed by two contrasting or comparative diagnoses. Sequence the symptom code first. Code all the contrasting or comparative diagnoses as additional diagnoses (OGCR II.E.) (■ FIGURE 6-7).

Patient seen for RLQ pain, fever, vomiting, dehydration due to acute ruptured appendicitis. Administered IV fluids.

(1) **K35.2 Acute ruptured appendicitis**

(2) **E86.0 Dehydration**

Figure 6-5 ■ Example of Sequencing for Confirmed Diagnosis and Related Symptom

Patient c/o of fever, difficulty breathing, hemoptysis. X-ray is positive for pneumonia. Sputum culture is ordered for hemoptysis.

(1) **J18.9 Pneumonia**

(2) **R04.2 Hemoptysis**

Figure 6-6 ■ Example of Sequencing for a Confirmed Diagnosis and Unrelated Symptom

Patient is seen for right shoulder pain due to rotator cuff syndrome or loose body in shoulder joint.

(1) **M25.511 Pain in right shoulder**

(2) **M75.11 Incomplete rotator cuff tear or rupture of right shoulder, not specified as traumatic**

(3) **M24.011 Loose body in right shoulder**

Figure 6-7 ■ Example of Sequencing for Symptom Followed by Contrasting or Comparative Diagnoses

Symptoms with No Confirmed Diagnosis

The physician may document only symptoms, signs, and abnormal findings, and no confirmed diagnosis. Assign the main reason for the encounter as the principal or first-listed diagnosis. When more than one symptom is equally responsible for the encounter, sequence either code first.

Guided Example of Arranging Symptoms and Signs Codes

To practice skills for sequencing codes for symptoms and signs, continue with the example from earlier in the chapter about patient Charlene Winger, who was seen for symptoms of nausea, vomiting, and diarrhea, with no confirmed diagnosis.

Follow along in your ICD-10-CM manual as Sherry Whittle, CPC, sequences the codes. Check off each step after you complete it.

⇨ First, Sherry confirms the diagnosis codes she assigned.

- ❑ **R11.2, Nausea with vomiting, unspecified**
- ❑ **R19.7, Diarrhea, unspecified**

⇨ Sherry determines that the physician documented only symptoms but no confirmed diagnosis.

- ❑ The documentation does not state that one symptom was chiefly responsible for the encounter.
- ❑ Therefore, either diagnosis may be sequenced first.

⇨ Sherry finalizes the codes and sequencing for this case:

- ❑ **R11.2, Nausea with vomiting, unspecified**
- ❑ **R19.7, Diarrhea, unspecified**

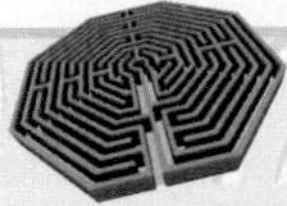

Coding Practice

Now it is your turn to practice arranging codes for symptoms, signs, abnormal findings, and confirmed diagnoses. Refer to the *Tip* at the end of the mini-medical-record if you need a little extra help.

Exercise 6.4 Arranging Codes for Symptoms and Signs

Instructions: Read the mini-medical-record of each patient's encounter, review the information abstracted in Exercise 6.2, assign ICD-10-CM diagnosis codes (CM) using the Index and Tabular List, and arrange the codes in proper sequence. Write the code(s) on the line provided.

1. Date: 6/2/yy Location: Branton Family Practice
Provider: Kristen Conover, MD
Patient: Debra Giroux Gender: F Age: 45
Chief complaint: polydipsia, polyuria, and difficulty sleeping, most recent blood test showed hyperglycemia
Assessment: type 2 diabetes, possible sleep apnea
Plan: evaluate for sleep apnea

Tip: Determine which symptoms are integral to diabetes and which one is unrelated.

2 CM Codes E11.9 DB type 2 G47.9 sleep→disorder

2. Date: 6/2/yy Location: Branton Family Practice
Provider: Kristen Conover, MD
Patient: Mark Greenfield Gender: M Age: 29
Chief complaint: extreme nervousness and irritability
Assessment: R/O hyperthyroidism
Plan: thyroid workup

Tip: A condition described as "rule out" means it is uncertain.

2 CM Codes R45.0 nervousness, R45.4 irritability

3. Date: 6/2/yy Location: Branton Medical Center
Provider: Kristen Conover, MD
Patient: Stanley Nicholson Gender: M Age: 52
Reason for admission: abdominal pain
Discharge diagnosis: epigastric pain due to acute pancreatitis or cholangitis (*inflammation or infection of the common bile duct*)
Plan: pain medication, antibiotics as precaution, further imaging

Tip: Because this is a hospital discharge, follow inpatient OCGR.

3 CM Codes R10.13 pain→epigastric, K85.9 (Pancreatitis acute) K83.0 (cholangitis)

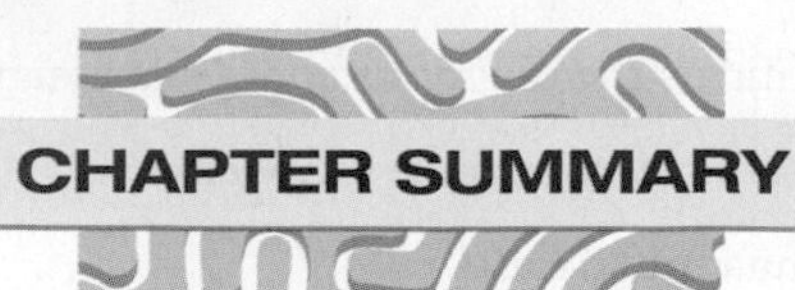

CHAPTER SUMMARY

In this chapter you learned that:

- Sometimes a confirmed diagnosis is not possible because the physician needs multiple encounters, extended testing, evaluation by specialists, surgery, or other procedures to arrive at a diagnosis.
- ICD-10-CM Chapter 18, Symptoms, Signs, and Abnormal Clinical and Laboratory Findings, Not Elsewhere Classified (R00-R99), contains 14 blocks or subchapters that are divided by anatomical site.
- Abstracting requires coders to be knowledgeable of disease processes and the related symptoms, signs, abnormal clinical findings, and abnormal laboratory test results so they can distinguish which elements should be coded and which should not.
- The Main Term for many symptoms and signs codes is the name of the symptom or sign. Coding for abnormal test results can be more challenging.
- In general, multiple codes for symptoms, signs, and abnormal findings are sequenced using the same guidelines as any other codes, but a few special situations exist.
- ICD-10-CM provides Official Guidelines for Coding and Reporting (OGCR) for symptoms, signs, and abnormal clinical and laboratory findings in OGCR section I.C.18.

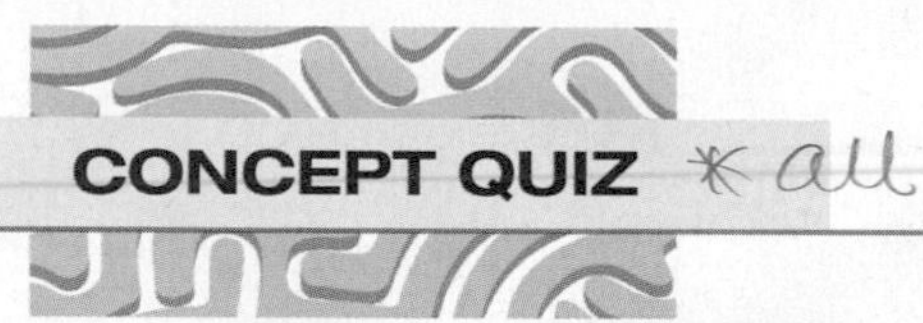

CONCEPT QUIZ

Take a moment to look back at your trip through symptoms, signs, and abnormal findings and solidify your skills. This is your opportunity to pull together everything you have learned.

Completion

Instructions: Write the term that answers each question based on the information you learned in this chapter. Choose from the following list. Some choices may be used more than once and some choices may not be used at all. Refer to the discussion in this chapter and the Glossary at the end of this book if you need a little extra help.

abnormal	outpatient
clinical	related
confirmed	sign
finding	symptom
inpatient	uncertain
integral	unrelated
laboratory	

1. A (an)_______________ is the subjective evidence of a disease or condition, usually reported by the patient.
2. A symptom that is _______________ is a routine part of the disease process.
3. A qualified diagnosis is _______________.
4. An abnormal _______________ finding is evidence of a disease or condition discovered through physical examination.
5. A (an)_______________ is objective evidence of a disease or condition that can be observed by the physician.
6. _______________ symptoms are those which patients occasionally experience with the confirmed diagnosis, but are not common or routine.
7. Rule out, suspected, and likely are words physicians use to describe a (an) _______________ diagnosis.
8. _______________ symptoms are those which are not due to the confirmed diagnosis and may indicate an additional problem or condition.
9. A laboratory test result that is outside of the normal numerical range is _______________.
10. In the _______________ setting, if the diagnosis documented at the time of discharge is uncertain, code the condition as if it existed.

Multiple Choice

Instructions: Circle the letter of the best answer to each question based on the information you learned in this chapter. Refer to the discussion in this chapter and the Glossary at the end of this book if you need a little extra help.

1. Which of the following is an example of a symptom?
   A. Nausea
   B. Vomiting
   C. Bleeding
   D. Fever

2. Which of the following is an example of an abnormal clinical finding?
   A. Elevated glucose
   B. Bleeding
   C. Irregular EKG
   D. Microscopic dysplasia
3. All of the following are integral to a CVA EXCEPT
   A. headache.
   B. muscular weakness.
   C. speech disturbance.
   D. dysuria.
4. Which of the following conditions are asymptomatic?
   A. Osteoarthritis
   B. Hypertension
   C. Gastroenteritis
   D. Anemia
5. ________ symptoms should NOT be coded when the physician provides a confirmed diagnosis.
   A. Integral
   B. Related
   C. Unrelated
   D. All
6. When should an uncertain diagnosis be coded as though it existed?
   A. Inpatient setting
   B. Outpatient setting
   C. Emergency department
   D. Never
7. All of the following Main Terms can be used to locate abnormal findings in the Index EXCEPT
   A. Abnormal.
   B. Deficiency.
   C. Findings.
   D. Uncertain.
8. Physicians may use all of the following terms EXCEPT ________ to indicate an uncertain diagnosis.
   A. possible
   B. integral
   C. suspected
   D. rule out
9. A physician may not be able to document a confirmed diagnosis because
   A. additional testing is necessary.
   B. the code is difficult to locate.
   C. the patient has multiple symptoms.
   D. the OGCR is unclear.
10. Which of the following statements is TRUE?
    A. Coders should assign codes for all symptoms and all conditions documented.
    B. Coders should assign codes for symptoms that are related but not integral to the diagnosis.
    C. Coders should never assign codes for uncertain diagnoses.
    D. Coders should assign a rule out code when coding for uncertain diagnoses.

CODING CHALLENGE

Now it is your turn to demonstrate coding all aspects of symptoms, signs, and abnormal findings. Refer back to the examples and discussion in this chapter when you need a little extra help. Use your medical dictionary and anatomy references when needed.

Instructions: Read the mini-medical-record of each patient's encounter, then abstract, assign, and sequence ICD-10-CM diagnosis codes (CM) using the Index and Tabular List. Write the code(s) on the line provided.

1. Date: 6/9/yy Location: Branton Family Practice
Provider: Kristen Conover, MD
Patient: Tiffany Risinger Gender: F Age: 41
Reason for visit: review abnormal mammogram results
Assessment: microcalcifications in right breast
Plan: mammogram with magnification to r/o ca
1 CM Code R92.8 abnormal mammogram → microcalcification

2. Date: 6/9/yy Location: Branton Family Practice
Provider: Kristen Conover, MD
Patient: Rhonda Straight Gender: F Age: 31
Reason for encounter: review lung X-ray
Assessment: abnormal shadow, right lung, inferior lobe
Plan: refer to pulmonologist

Tip: An X-ray is classified as diagnostic imaging.
1 CM Code R91.8 (Abnormal → diagnostic imaging, lung

3. Date: 6/9/yy Location: Branton Family Practice
Provider: Kristen Conover, MD
Patient: Holly Derosier Gender: F Age: 23

(continued)

(continued from page 105)

3. (continued)

Chief complaint: review results of blood test performed last week because patient was concerned he'd been exposed to HIV

Assessment: Nonconclusive HIV test

Plan: further testing needed

Tip: Search for the Main Term *HIV* or *Test.*

1 CM Code R75 (HIV → lab evidence or test → HIV → nonconclusive)

4. Date: 6/9/yy Location: Branton Family Practice

Provider: Kristen Conover, MD

Patient: Juan Dunlop Gender: M Age: 24

Chief complaint: sneezing, scratchy throat, postnasal drip

Assessment: suspected seasonal allergies

Plan: OTC antihistamine

3 CM Codes R06.7 Sneezing R09.89 Scratchy throat R09.82 Drip → Postnasal

5. Date: 6/9/yy Location: Branton Medical Center

Provider: Kristen Conover, MD

Patient: Phillip Higginbotham Gender: M Age: 27

Reason for admission: lumbar pain, weakness in left leg

Discharge diagnosis: probable herniated intervertebral lumbar disc, sciatica

Plan: refer to physical therapy

Tip: The description of the admission and discharge indicates that this was an inpatient stay so follow the OCGR for inpatient settings.

1 CM Code M51.16 Hernia → intervebral disc → see displacement → intervertebral disc → lumbar region → w/ sciatica

6. Date: 6/9/yy Location: Branton Family Practice

Provider: Kristen Conover, MD

Patient: Christina Claussen Gender: F Age: 24

Reason for encounter: repeat PAP test

Assessment: abnormal cervical PAP test result, cytologic (*cellular*) evidence of malignancy

Plan: possible colposcopy based on repeat test results

1 CM Code R87.614 Abnormal cervix → w/ cytologic evidence of malignancy

7. Date: 6/9/yy Location: Branton Family Practice

Provider: Kristen Conover, MD

Patient: Russell Maze Gender: M Age: 56

Chief complaint: review blood work results

Assessment: glucose reading of 107, insulin resistant

Plan: HbA1c in 3 months to check long-term glucose levels

1 CM Code E88.81 Resistance → insulin

8. Date: 6/9/yy Location: Branton Family Practice

Provider: Kristen Conover, MD

Patient: Geraldine Calton Gender: F Age: 36

Chief complaint: daily headaches

Assessment: likely migraines

Plan: refer to neurologist for further testing and evaluation

1 CM Code R51 Headache → daily chronic

9. Date: 6/9/yy Location: Branton Medical Center

Provider: Kristen Conover, MD

Patient: Ana Dowling Gender: F Age: 62

Reason for admission: shortness of breath

Assessment: increased edema, congestive heart failure

Discharge instructions: begin new diuretic, follow up with cardiologist

1 CM Code I50.9 Failure → heart congestive

10. Date: 6/9/yy Location: Branton Family Practice

Provider: Kristen Conover, MD

Patient: Joanne Spain Gender: F Age: 50

Chief complaint: review recent lab work

Assessment: Everything was normal except for low Vitamin D.

Plan: Rx 50,000 IU of Vitamin D once a week for 8 weeks; recheck in 8 weeks

Tip: A "low" test result is indexed as a deficiency.

1 CM Code E55.9 Deficiency → vit D

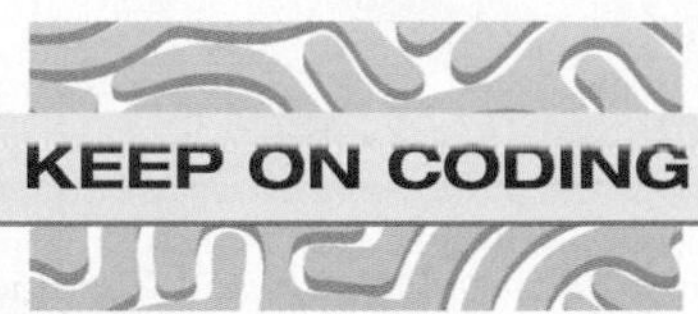

KEEP ON CODING

As a coder, you can never have too much experience. Apply everything you have learned in this chapter to code the following diagnostic statements. Use the OGCR and instructional notes in the Tabular List to help determine how many codes are required.

Instructions: Read the diagnostic statement, then use the Index and Tabular List to assign and sequence ICD-10-CM (CM) diagnosis codes. Write the code(s) on the line provided.

1. Right lower quadrant rebound abdominal tenderness: CM Code(s) ____________
2. Nonvisualization of gallbladder: CM Code(s) ____________
3. Heartburn: CM Code(s) ____________
4. Absent bowel sounds: CM Code(s) ____________
5. Slow heart beat: CM Code(s) ____________
6. Overactivity: CM Code(s) ____________
7. Auditory hallucinations: CM Code(s) ____________
8. Nosebleed: CM Code(s) ____________
9. Shortness of breath: CM Code(s) ____________
10. Severe sepsis with septic shock: CM Code(s) ____________
11. Excessive sweating: CM Code(s) ____________
12. Late walker: CM Code(s) ____________
13. Change in bowel habits: CM Code(s) ____________
14. Heart murmur: CM Code(s) ____________
15. Hiccough: CM Code(s) ____________
16. Finding of cocaine in blood: CM Code(s) ____________
17. Age-related cognitive decline: CM Code(s) ____________
18. Intermittent urinary stream: CM Code(s) ____________
19. Hoarseness: CM Code(s) ____________
20. Abnormal blood-gas level: CM Code(s) ____________
21. Respiratory arrest: CM Code(s) ____________
22. Unsteadiness on feet: CM Code(s) ____________
23. Abnormal liver scan: CM Code(s) ____________
24. Failure to gain weight: CM Code(s) ____________
25. Febrile seizures, simple: CM Code(s) ____________

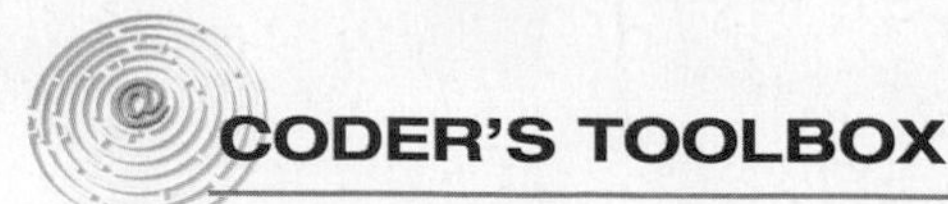

CODER'S TOOLBOX

The following resources are a starting point for learning more about symptoms, signs, and abnormal findings. The > symbol indicates a menu selection within the website in order to navigate to a specific page.

American Cancer Society > Quick Finder > Show All Cancer Types **http://www.cancer.org/Cancer/index#cancerListView**

American Diabetes Association > Diabetes Basics > Symptoms **http://www.diabetes.org/diabetes-basics/symptoms/**

American Heart Association > Conditions > select a condition, then select Symptoms and Diagnosis **http://www.heart.org/HEARTORG/Conditions/Conditions_UCM_001087_SubHomePage.jsp**

Centers for Disease Control and Prevention > Diseases and Conditions **http://www.cdc.gov/DiseasesConditions/**

E-medicine > Medscape **http://emedicine.medscape.com/**

Lab Tests Online **http://labtestsonline.org/**

Mayo Clinic > Diseases and Conditions **http://www.mayoclinic.com/health-information/**

MedicineNet > Symptom Checker **http://www.medicinenet.com/symptoms_and_signs/article.htm**

MedlinePlus **http://www.nlm.nih.gov/medlineplus**

National Institutes for Health **http://www.ncbi.nlm.nih.gov**

WebMD > Symptom Checker **http://symptoms.webmd.com/**

7

Factors Influencing Health Status and Contact with Health Services (Z00-Z99)

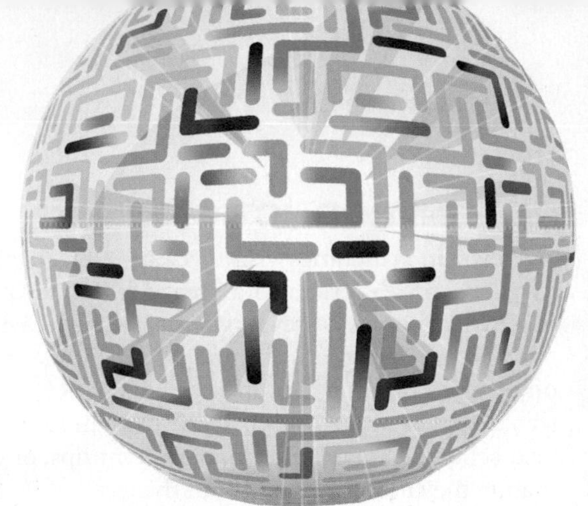

Learning Objectives

After completing this chapter, you should have the skills to:

- Spell and define the key words, medical terms, and abbreviations related to factors influencing health status and contact with health services.
- Describe when to report codes for factors influencing health status and contact with health services.
- Discuss the main characteristics of coding for factors influencing health status and contact with health services.
- Abstract information required for coding factors influencing health status and contact with health services from the medical record.
- Assign codes for factors influencing health status and contact with health services.
- Sequence codes for factors influencing health status and contact with health services and related conditions.
- Discuss the Official Guidelines for Coding and Reporting related to factors influencing health status and contact with health services.

Key Terms and Abbreviations

ostomy

Z codes

In addition to the key terms listed here, students should know the terms defined within tables in this chapter.

Chapter Outline

- **Introduction to Z Codes**
- **Coding Overview of Z Codes**
- **Abstracting Z Codes**
- **Assigning Z Codes**
- **Arranging Z Codes**

ICD-10-CM codes in this chapter are from the ICD-10-CM 2014 Draft code set from the Department of Health and Human Services, Centers for Disease Control and Prevention.

INTRODUCTION

Car owners sometimes visit or call the mechanic although they have not experienced a breakdown. They may seek an oil change, periodic preventive maintenance, winterization, tightening of some loose screws, tire rotation, or a variety of other types of information. Mechanics may apply a windshield sticker or send a postcard to remind owners of the next scheduled maintenance, important tips, or other information they need to know about the car.

In healthcare, patients receive services even though they are not ill or injured. They may seek annual physical examinations, vaccinations, screening examinations, follow-up care, or maternity care. Physicians need to track information about patients' health status, health history, and health risks that do not present current problems but could in the future. In this chapter you will learn how to use ICD-10-CM codes for these purposes. You will practice coding for patient encounters when patients receive healthcare services even though they are not ill or injured, a skill which requires you to abstract information from the mini-medical-record, assign correct codes, and arrange (sequence) the codes in the proper order.

As you read this chapter, open up your medical terminology book and keep a medical dictionary handy to refresh your memory of any unfamiliar terms. Think of these resources as your travel brochures that tell you more about an area. This way, you have the information you need at your fingertips.

INTRODUCTION TO Z CODES

ICD-10-CM Chapter 21 classifies factors influencing health status and contact with health services. For the sake of brevity, this text refers to codes in this chapter as Z codes. Z codes represent reasons for encounters and may be used in any healthcare setting when the reason for the encounter is not a disease, injury, or external cause that is classified in the preceding ICD-10-CM chapters for body systems (A00 to Y99). Z codes are used in two general types of circumstances:

- A person encounters the health services for some specific purpose that, in itself, is not a disease or injury. Examples are to receive limited care or service for a current condition, to donate an organ or tissue, to receive **prophylactic** vaccination, or to discuss a problem.
- A circumstance or problem exists that influences the person's health status, but is not, in itself, a current illness or injury. Examples are being a carrier of a communicable disease, having a family history of certain conditions, wearing a prosthetic device such as a pacemaker or an artificial limb.

Z codes are classified into 15 categories, which are defined in ■ TABLE 7-1. Acquaint yourself with these definitions and examples, as they are the foundation for learning to abstract, assign, and sequence Z codes. Refer to the specific OCGR listed for a full discussion of how to use each category.

SUCCESS STEP

Although you do not need to memorize specific codes, it is helpful to memorize the Z code categories and definitions. By knowing the circumstances in which Z codes are required, you will become more accurate when abstracting.

Table 7-1 ■ **DEFINITIONS AND EXAMPLES OF Z CODE CATEGORIES**

Z Code Category/OGCR	Definition	Example Codes
Contact/Exposure (OGCR I.C.21.c.1))	Patient does not show any sign or symptom of a disease but is suspected to have been exposed to it by close personal contact with an infected individual or are in an area where a disease is epidemic.	Z20.5 Contact with and (suspected) exposure to viral hepatitis Z20.820 Contact with and (suspected) exposure to varicella
Inoculations and vaccinations (OGCR I.C.21.c.2))	Reported for encounters for prophylactic inoculations and vaccinations against a disease.	Z23 Encounter for immunization
Status (OGCR I.C.21.c.3))	A patient is either a carrier of a disease or has the sequela or residual of a past disease or condition.	Z21 Asymptomatic HIV infection status Z67.10 Type A blood, Rh positive Z68.23 Body mass index (BMI) 23.0-23.9, adult Z94.1 Heart transplant status

Table 7-1 ■ (continued)

Z Code Category/OGCR	Definition	Example Codes
History (of) (OGCR I.C.21.c.4))	Personal history codes explain a patient's past medical condition that no longer exists and is not receiving any treatment, but that has the potential for recurrence, and therefore may require continued monitoring. Family history codes are for a patient who has a family member(s) who has had a particular disease, which causes the patient to be at higher risk of also contracting the disease.	Z86.11 Personal history of tuberculosis Z80.3 Family history of malignant neoplasm of breast
Screening (OGCR I.C.21.c.5))	Seemingly well individuals receive testing for disease or disease precursors so that early detection and treatment can be provided for those who test positive for the disease.	Z12.31 Encounter for screening mammogram for malignant neoplasm of breast Z13.1 Encounter for screening for diabetes mellitus
Observation (OGCR I.C.21.c.6))	A person is being observed for a suspected condition that is ruled out. This category is rarely used.	Z03.73 Encounter for suspected fetal anomaly ruled out
Aftercare (OGCR I.C.21.c.7))	The initial treatment of a disease has been performed and the patient requires continued care during the healing or recovery phase, or for the long-term consequences of the disease.	Z44.002 Encounter for fitting and adjustment of unspecified left artificial arm Z51.11 Encounter for antineoplastic chemotherapy
Follow-up (OGCR I.C.21.c.8))	Continuing surveillance following completed treatment of a disease, condition, or injury when the condition has been fully treated and no longer exists.	Z08 Encounter for follow-up examination after completed treatment for malignant neoplasm Z39.2 Encounter for routine postpartum follow-up
Donor (OGCR I.C.21.c.9))	Living individuals are donating blood or other body tissue.	Z52.4 Kidney donor
Counseling (OGCR I.C.21.c.10))	A patient or family member receives assistance in the aftermath of an illness or injury, or when support is required in coping with family or social problems.	Z31.5 Encounter for genetic counseling Z69.010 Encounter for mental health services for victim of parental child abuse
Encounters for Obstetrical and Reproductive Services (OGCR I.C.21.c.11))	A patient receives obstetric or reproductive encounters when none of the problems or complications included in the codes from the obstetrics chapter (ICD-10-CM Chapter 15 (O00-O9A)) exist.	Z34.01 Encounter for supervision of normal first pregnancy, first trimester Z37.0 Single live birth Z3A.17 (Pregnancy, weeks of gestation, 17 weeks)
Newborns and Infants (OGCR I.C.21.c.12))	Reports the health supervision and care of foundling, routine child health examination, and classification of birth status of liveborn infants.	Z00.110 Health examination for newborn under 8 days old
Routine and Administrative Examinations (OGCR I.C.21.c.13))	Used for encounters for routine examinations or administrative purposes.	Z00.00 Encounter for general adult medical examination without abnormal findings Z02.1 Encounter for pre-employment examination Z32.01 Encounter for pregnancy test, result positive
Miscellaneous (OGCR I.C.21.c.14))	Additional codes provide useful information on circumstances that may affect a patient's care and treatment.	Z28.01 Immunization not carried out because of acute illness of patient Z53.09 Procedure and treatment not carried out because of other contraindication Z76.0 Encounter for issue of repeat prescription
Non-specific (OGCR I.C.21.c.15))	Used primarily in inpatient settings when there is no further documentation to permit more precise coding.	Z86.59 Personal history of other mental and behavioral disorders Z92.23 Personal history of estrogen therapy

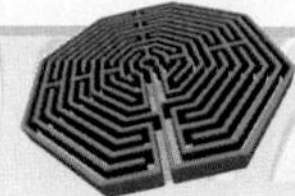

Coding Practice

Now it is your turn to demonstrate your understanding of Z codes. Try to answer the questions from memory first, then refer back to the information in this section if you need a little extra help.

Exercise 7.1 Introduction to Z Codes

Instructions: Write your answer to each question in the space provided.

1. Give three examples of Z codes that describe the main reason for the encounter. aftercare, counseling, follow-up, immunizations, observations obstetrics

2. What is the OGCR location of guidelines for each of the following Z code categories?

   Example: History OGCR I.C.21.4

   a. Contact/Exposure OGCR I.C.21.C.1

   b. Status OGCR I.C.21.C.3

   c. Aftercare OGCR I.C.21.C.7

   d. Routine and Administrative Examinations OGCR I.C.21.C.13

   Tip: Refer to Table 7-1.

3. Identify the Z code category for each of the following codes:

   Example: Z67.10 Type A blood, Rh positive Status

   a. Z12.31 Encounter for screening mammogram for malignant neoplasm of breast Screening

   b. Z52.4 Kidney donor Donor

   c. Z86.59 Personal history of other mental and behavioral disorders Non-Specific

   d. Z86.11 Personal history of tuberculosis History

   Tip: Refer to Table 7-1.

CODING OVERVIEW OF Z CODES

ICD-10-CM Chapter 21, Factors Influencing Health Status and Contact with Health Services (Z00-Z99), contains 14 blocks or subchapters. Review the block names and code ranges listed at the beginning of Chapter 21 in the ICD-10-CM manual to become familiar with the content and organization. This chapter is used to report reasons for encounters that are not due to a current illness or injury or to report health status or risk factors documented as significant by the physician.

ICD-10-CM Z codes are comparable to the ICD-9-CM Supplementary Classification of Factors influencing Health Status and Contract with Health Services (V01-V91). In ICD-10-CM, the codes are part of the regular classification rather than being a supplementary classification.

Some ICD-10-CM Z codes are directly comparable to ICD-9-CM V codes, such as those in the category **Outcome of delivery (Z37)**.

Some ICD-9-CM categories were significantly expanded in ICD-10-CM, including those for examinations (**Z02**), encounters for other specific health care (**Z40-Z53**), health hazards related to socioeconomic and psychosocial circumstances (**Z55 to Z65**), and counseling (**Z70**). For example, ICD-9-CM **V70.3 Other medical examination for administrative purposes**, a single code, is replaced with ICD-10-CM category **Z02 Encounter for administrative examination**, which contains over ten codes.

Some ICD-9-CM V codes were reduced in specificity or eliminated. For example, ICD-9-CM subcategory **V64.4x Closed procedures converted to open procedures** does not have a corresponding category in ICD-10-CM. ICD-9-CM categories V03-V06 for immunizations were reduced to a single ICD-10-CM code, **Z23**.

ICD-10-CM provides Official Guidelines for Coding and Reporting (OGCR) Z codes in OGCR section I.C.21. OGCR contains a detailed discussion of the categories of Z codes, when to report them, and which codes may only be sequenced as the principal or first-listed diagnosis. Additional OGCR related to Z codes appear throughout the guidelines, particularly in OGCR I.B.3., I.C.1.a.(HIV), I.C.2. (neoplasms), I.C.4.(endocrine), I.C.15. (obstetrics), I.C.19. (injuries), I.C.20. (external causes), and IV.B. In the Tabular List, instructional notes throughout all chapters alert coders to many circumstances that require Z codes.

ABSTRACTING FOR Z CODES

Because Z codes are applicable to a wide variety of situations, there is not one concise rule that guides coders when Z codes are needed. Refer to ■ TABLE 7-2 for guidance on how to abstract for the most commonly used Z codes. Locate the patient situation in the left column, then refer to the appropriate Main Term in the right column. Remember that the abstracting questions are a guide and that not every encounter requires a Z code. In addition, some situations not in this table also require Z codes, which are discussed later in this chapter.

Coders receive direction to abstract for Z codes from three sources:

- Z codes describe the reason for the encounter.
- Instructional notes in the Tabular List direct coders to use Z codes.
- Z codes are required by the OGCR.

Reason for the Encounter

When a Z code(s) describes the main reason for the encounter, abstracting is fairly straightforward. Coders identify the main reason for the encounter, then search for the Main Term in the Index to Diseases and Injuries (Index) to locate the Z code. Examples of Z codes describing the main reason for the encounter include the following:

- aftercare
- counseling
- follow up
- immunizations
- observation
- routine pregnancy
- routine or administrative examinations (pre-employment, annual check-up)
- screening examinations (colonoscopy, mammogram)

Instructional Notes

In many circumstances, the Tabular List provides instructional notes directing the coder to assign certain types of Z codes (■ FIGURE 7-1, page 114). Examples of Z codes required by instructional notes include the following:

- birth status of newborn
- long-term use of medication
- occupational risk factors
- outcome of delivery
- tobacco, alcohol, drug use

Coders must distinguish between codes for history and current use. In Figure 7-1, report **history of tobacco use (Z87.891)** when tobacco use occurred in the past, but the patient is not currently using tobacco. Report **tobacco use (Z72.0)** when the patient currently uses tobacco. Report **tobacco dependence (F17.-)** rather than **tobacco use (Z72.0)** when the medical record documents the dependence.

Table 7-2 ■ KEY CRITERIA FOR ABSTRACTING Z CODES

Patient Situation	Main Term
❑ Is the reason for the encounter a routine examination?	Examination
❑ Is the reason for the encounter to receive an inoculation or vaccination against a disease?	Inoculation
❑ Does the physician document a past medical condition that no longer exists and is not receiving any treatment, but that has the potential for recurrence?	History, personal
❑ Does the physician document that patient has a family member(s) who has had a particular disease, which causes the patient to be at higher risk of also contracting the disease?	History, family
❑ Is the reason for the encounter testing for disease or disease precursors in seemingly well individuals so that early detection and treatment can be provided?	Screening
❑ Does the physician document a lifestyle habit that poses a risk factor?	Use
❑ Is the reason for the encounter continued care during the healing or recovery phase after initial treatment has been completed?	Aftercare
❑ Is the reason for the encounter continuing surveillance following completed treatment of a disease, condition, or injury when the condition has been fully treated and no longer exists?	Follow-up
❑ Is the reason for the encounter to receive assistance in the aftermath of an illness or injury, or for support in coping with family or social problems?	Counseling
❑ Did a woman give birth during the encounter?	Outcome of delivery
❑ Is the patient a newborn who was born during the current admission?	Newborn, born

I20 Angina pectoris

Use additional code to identify:

exposure to environmental tobacco smoke (Z77.22)

history of tobacco use (Z87.891)

occupational exposure to environmental tobacco smoke (Z57.31)

tobacco dependence (F17.-)

tobacco use (Z72.0)

Figure 7-1 ■ Example of Instructional Notes in Tabular List Requiring Z Codes (Category I20)

CODING CAUTION

Remember that codes in instructional notes should be reported only when they apply to the patient. For example, do not report **Z87.891 History of nicotine dependence** if the patient does not have a history of tobacco use or dependence.

Official Guidelines

The most challenging situation is when OGCR require Z codes to describe supplemental information related to the encounter, but the Tabular List does not provide instructional notes. The Tabular List cannot anticipate every patient circumstance for every diagnosis in which a Z code is needed. This is when coders' knowledge of OGCR guides them to abstract the information. Examples of Z codes that may be required by the OGCR and rely on coders' knowledge, include the following:

- acquired absence of organ or body part
- artificial opening status
- blood type
- BMI
- carrier
- do not resuscitate (DNR) status
- internal or external prosthetics, functional implements, or enabling devices
- personal or family history
- postprocedural states
- problems related to life circumstances such as education, literacy, employment, unemployment, housing, family situation
- transplant waiting list, recipient, or donor

Guided Example of Abstracting Z Codes

Refer to the following example here and throughout the chapter to learn more about using Z codes. Sherry Whittle, CPC, is a fictitious coder who guides you through coding this case.

Date: 7/1/yy Location: Branton Medical Center Outpatient Procedure Clinic

Provider: Stanley Garrett, MD

Patient: Angela Holmes Gender: F Age: 50

Procedure: screening colonoscopy

Findings: none

Plan: next colonoscopy in 10 years

Follow along as Sherry abstracts the Z code. Check off each step as you complete it.

⇨ Sherry refers to Key Criteria for Abstracting Z Codes (Table 7-2) and looks for questions that may apply to this patient.

- ❑ *Is the reason for the encounter a routine examination?* While this is a routine colonoscopy, a colonoscopy is not considered to be an examination.
- ❑ *Does the physician document a past medical condition that no longer exists and is not receiving any treatment, but that has the potential for recurrence?* No. If the patient were receiving the colonoscopy due to previous colon cancer, then Sherry would answer "yes" and be directed to a different Z code category and a different Main Term.
- ❑ *Does the physician document that the patient has a family member(s) who has had a particular disease, which causes the patient to be at higher risk of also contracting the disease?* No. If the colonoscopy were being done at a more-frequent-than-normal interval due to having family members with colon cancer, Sherry would answer "yes" and would assign a code for family history of colon cancer.
- ❑ *Is the reason for the encounter testing for disease or disease precursors in seemingly well individuals so that early detection and treatment can be provided?* Yes, this is the definition of a screening.

⇨ Next, Sherry will assign the code.

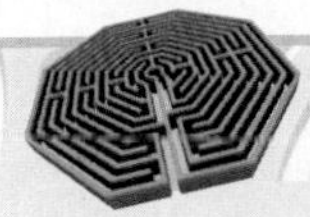

Coding Practice

Now it is your turn to practice abstracting diagnoses for health status and health services. Questions guide your analysis.

Exercise 7.2 Abstracting for Z Codes

Instructions: Read the mini-medical-record of each patient's encounter and answer the abstracting questions. Write the answer on the line provided. Do not assign any codes.

1. Date: 7/3/yy Location: Branton Family Practice Provider: Kristen Conover, MD

Patient: Lawrence Baumgardner Gender: M Age: 52

Reason for encounter: annual medical examination

Assessment: comprehensive metabolic panel test results are normal, no new problems

Plan: **RTO** 1 year

a. What is the reason for the encounter? Annual medical examination

b. Were there any abnormal findings? no

If yes, what are they? ______

2. Date: 7/3/yy Location: New Life Obstetrics

Provider: Kay Pinkney, MD

Patient: Josephine Day Gender: F Age: 24

Reason for encounter: supervision of normal second pregnancy, third trimester, 34 weeks

Assessment: Estimated Date of Delivery (EDD) 8/3/yy

Plan: RTO 1 week

a. What is the reason for the encounter? Supervision of normal second pregnancy, third trimester

b. Were there any abnormal findings? No

If yes, what are they? ______

3. Date: 7/3/yy Location: City Center Cardiology

Provider: Matthew Bunker, MD

Patient: Brandon Woodruff Gender: M Age: 76

Reason for encounter: adjustment of cardiac pacemaker

Assessment: reprogrammed pacemaker, no problems

Plan: RTO 6 months

a. What is the reason for the encounter? adjustment of cardiac pacemaker

b. Were there any abnormal findings? no

If yes, what are they? ______

4. Date: 7/4/yy Location: Branton Medical Center Outpatient Radiology

Provider: Jennifer Kolb, MD (radiologist)

Patient: Monica Heath Gender: F Age: 47

Reason for encounter: screening mammogram

Assessment: normal mammogram, both breasts

Plan: repeat screening 6 months due to personal history of breast cancer

Tip: The National Cancer Institute recommends mammograms every one to two years for women over age 50.

a. What is the reason for the encounter? Normal mammogram, both breasts

b. Were there any abnormal findings? no

If yes, what are they? ______

c. Why is this patient receiving a mammogram more frequently than normal? Personal Hx of breast cancer

(*continued*)

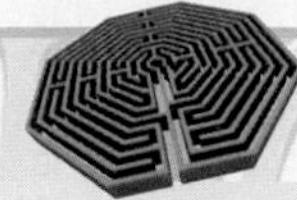

Coding Practice (continued)

5. Date: 7/4/yy Location: East Side Oncology

Provider: Richard Blackford, MD

Patient: Ricardo Ferrari Gender: M Age: 61

Reason for encounter: 6-month follow up after removal of prostate due to malignant neoplasm of prostate

Assessment: no new findings, no recurrence of disease, no current treatment

Plan: next FU 6 months

a. What is the reason for the encounter? 6-month F/u for malignant neoplasm of prostate

b. Were there any abnormal findings? no

If yes, what are they? ______

c. What past condition is documented? malignant neoplasm of prostate

d. A condition that no longer exists but presents potential for recurrence is classified as what? personal history

e. What gland was previously removed? prostate

6. Date: 7/4/yy Location: Branton Medical Center

Provider: Matthew Bunker, MD

Patient: John Binns Gender: M Age: 48

Reason for admission: unresolved angina pectoris, current tobacco use

Assessment: EKG negative for AMI, **ECC** normal, angiogram normal

Discharge Plan: Rx nitroglycerin, follow up in office 1 week

a. What is the reason for the encounter? angina pectoris

b. Were there any abnormal findings? No

If yes, what are they? ______

c. What lifestyle habit is documented? Tobacco use

ASSIGNING Z CODES

When assigning Z codes, coders need to know what Main Terms to search for in the Index, how to distinguish between diagnosis codes and procedure codes, and when to *not* use a Z code.

Locating Main Terms

Coders normally search for the name of a condition or disease in the Index in order to locate codes. Because Z codes are not conditions, new coders may be puzzled about what Main Term to search for. Remember to identify the noun that describes the reason or purpose of the encounter. Refer to ■ Table 7-3 for commonly used Main Terms.

Diagnosis vs. Procedure Codes

When the reason for the encounter is a screening examination or specific health service, the title of the Z code may *look like* a procedure code, but it is a diagnosis code—the reason for the encounter. Coders assign a Z code for the diagnosis and an ICD-10-PCS or CPT code for the procedure. (This chapter discusses only Z codes.) Examples when confusion may occur include the following:

- Persons encountering health services for examinations. For the diagnosis, assign a Z code (**Z00-Z13**) as the reason for the encounter, then assign a procedure code to identify the complexity of the examination.
- Persons encountering health services in circumstances related to reproduction. For the diagnosis, assign

requires Z code

Table 7-3 ■ COMMONLY USED MAIN TERMS FOR Z CODES

❑ Absence, acquired	❑ History, family
❑ Admission (for)	❑ History, personal
❑ Aftercare	❑ Immunization
❑ Contact	❑ Newborn, born
❑ Counseling	❑ Newborn, twin, triplet, quadruplet
❑ Donor	❑ Outcome of delivery
❑ Encounter (for)	❑ Pregnancy
❑ Examination	❑ Status
❑ Exposure	❑ Supervision (of)
❑ Fitting (and adjustment of)	
❑ Follow-up	

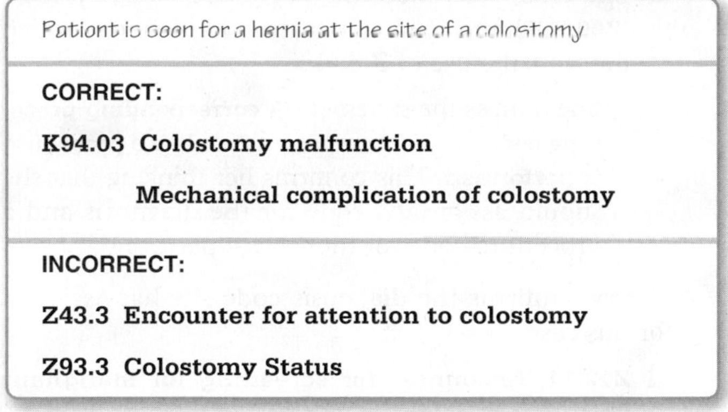

Patient is seen for a hernia at the site of a colostomy

CORRECT:

K94.03 Colostomy malfunction

Mechanical complication of colostomy

INCORRECT:

Z43.3 Encounter for attention to colostomy

Z93.3 Colostomy Status

Figure 7-2 ■ Example of a Diagnosis Code That Overrides the Need for a Z Code

a Z code (**Z30-Z39**) to describe the reason for the encounter, then assign a procedure code to identify the service(s) provided.

- Encounters for other specific health procedures, such as fitting or adjustment of a prosthetic device, prophylactic or cosmetic surgery, or care of an ostomy (*artificial opening between a hollow organ and the skin*). For the diagnosis, assign a Z code (**Z40-Z53**) to describe the reason for the encounter, then assign a procedure code to identify the service(s) provided.

When Not to Use Z Codes

In some cases, diagnosis codes from body system chapters may include information that coders would otherwise report with a status Z code. When this is the case, do not assign a Z code that repeats the same information (OGCR I.C.21.b.3)). In addition, do not assign aftercare codes when the patient has a current condition that is coded from a body system chapter. Aftercare codes are used only after the initial treatment of a disease has been performed and the patient requires continued care during healing or recovery. Refer to ■ FIGURE 7-2 to learn more about body system chapter codes that override the need for Z codes.

In the example in Figure 7-2, because the diagnosis code is specific to a colostomy, do not also assign **Z93.9 Colostomy status**. In addition, because the colostomy malfunction is a current condition, do not assign code **Z43.3 Encounter for attention to colostomy**.

Guided Example of Assigning Z Codes

To learn more about assigning Z codes and procedure codes, continue with the example about Angela Holmes who was seen at Branton Medical Center Outpatient Procedure Clinic for a screening colonoscopy.

Follow along as Sherry Whittle, CPC, assigns the Z code. Check off each step as you complete it.

⇨ Sherry searches the Index for the Main Term **Screening** (■ FIGURE 7-3).

- ❑ She locates the subterm **Colonoscopy, Z12.11**.

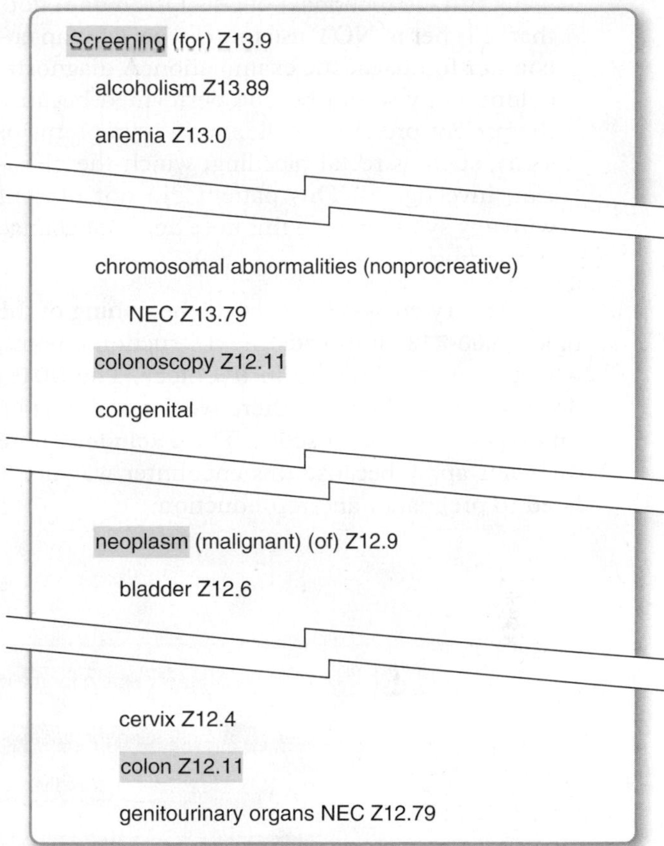

Screening (for) Z13.9
alcoholism Z13.89
anemia Z13.0
chromosomal abnormalities (nonprocreative)
NEC Z13.79
colonoscopy Z12.11
congenital
neoplasm (malignant) (of) Z12.9
bladder Z12.6
cervix Z12.4
colon Z12.11
genitourinary organs NEC Z12.79

Figure 7-3 ■ Index Entry for the Main Term Screening

- ❑ She reviews the rest of the subterms and also locates **neoplasm (malignant)**, which has a second-level subterm **colon Z12.11**.
- ❑ She determines that both entries point to the same code because the purpose of a screening colonoscopy is to identify any benign polyps or sign of malignant neoplasm.

⇨ Next, Sherry verifies code **Z12.11** in the Tabular List.

- ❑ She reads the code title for **Z12.11, Encounter for screening for malignant neoplasm of colon** and confirms that this accurately describes the reason for the encounter.

⇨ Sherry checks for instructional notes in the Tabular List.

- ❑ She cross-references the beginning of category **Z12, Encounter for screening for malignant neoplasms** and reads the instructional notes (■ FIGURE 7-4, page 118).
  - The first instructional note defines what this category is used for. She determines that the patient's encounter meets this definition.
  - The second instructional note states **Use additional code to identify any family history of malignant neoplasm (Z80.-)**. She checks the medical record for documentation of a family history of colon cancer and finds none, so she does not assign a code from **Z80**.

- The third instructional note is an **Excludes1** note that tells her to NOT use this category for an encounter for diagnostic examination. A diagnostic colonoscopy would be one performed because the patient presented with specific symptoms or signs, such as rectal bleeding, which the physician investigates. This patient did not present with any symptoms, so this note does not change the coding.

❑ Next, Sherry cross-references the beginning of the block **(Z00-Z13)** and reads the instructional notes, which apply to all codes in the block. The **NOTE:** does not apply because there were no abnormal findings of the colonoscopy. The **Excludes1** note does not apply because this encounter was unrelated to pregnancy and reproduction.

❑ She cross-references the beginning of **Chapter 21 (Z00-Z99)** and reads the instructional notes, which describe the use of Z codes.

- She notices the statement **A corresponding procedure code must accompany a Z code if a procedure is performed.** This confirms her thinking that she should assign a Z code for the diagnosis and a procedure code for the service performed.

⇨ Sherry confirms the diagnosis code she has assigned for this case.

❑ **Z12.11, Encounter for screening for malignant neoplasm of colon**

⇨ Next, Sherry will assign a CPT code to describe the physician's service of performing the colonoscopy. (CPT coding is not covered in this text.)

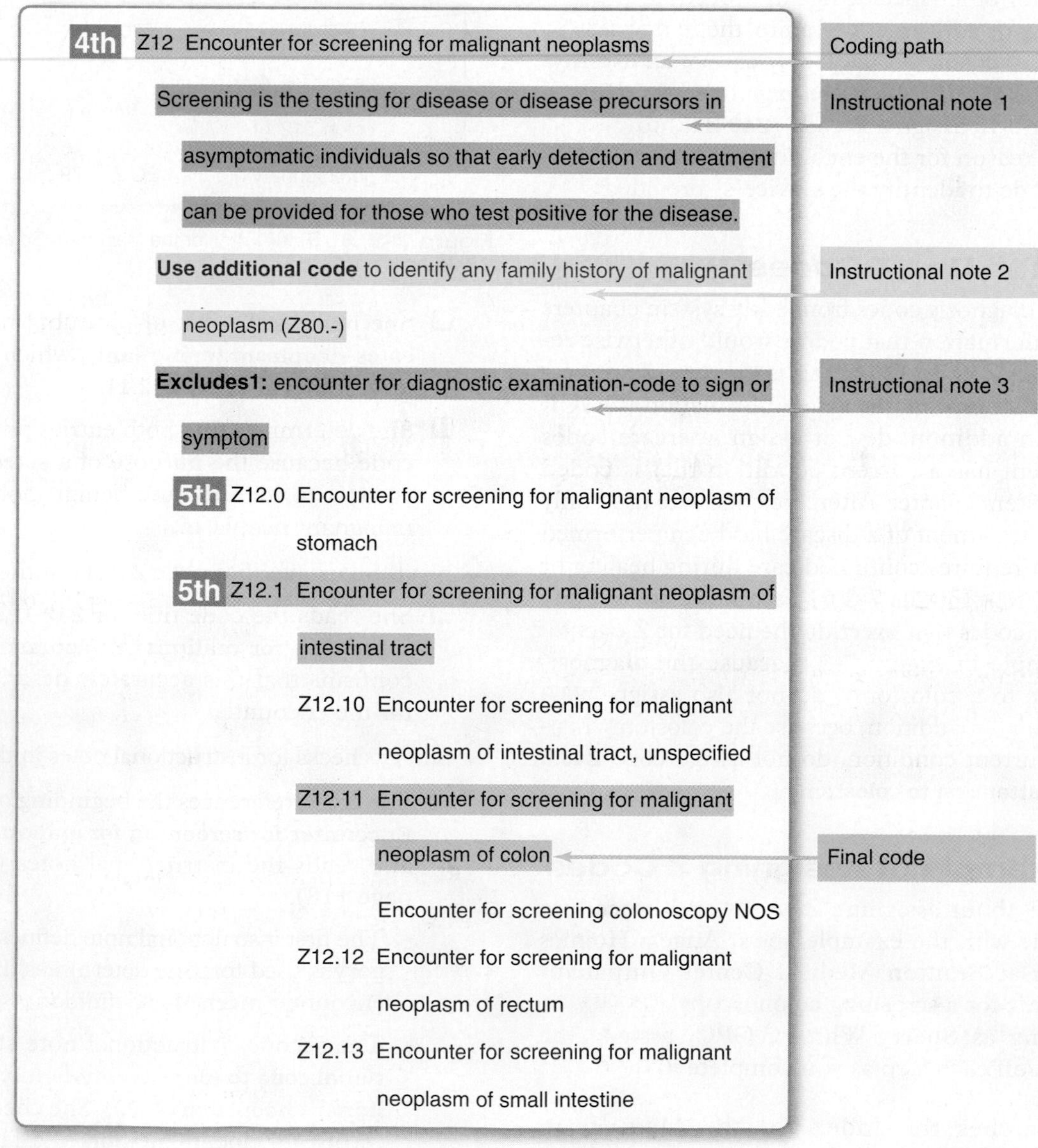

Figure 7-4 ■ Tabular List Entry for Category Z12 and Code Z12.11

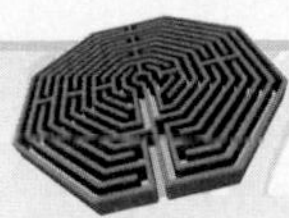

Coding Practice

Now it is your turn to practice assigning codes for health status and health services. Refer to the ***Tip*** at the end of the mini-medical-record if you need a little extra help.

Exercise 7.3 Assigning Z Codes

Instructions: Read the mini-medical-record of each patient's encounter, review the information abstracted in Exercise 7.2, and assign ICD-10-CM diagnosis codes (CM) using the Index and Tabular List. Write the code(s) on the line provided.

1. Date: 7/3/yy Location: Branton Family Practice
Provider: Kristen Conover, MD
Patient: Lawrence Baumgardner Gender: M
Age: 52
Reason for encounter: annual medical examination
Assessment: comprehensive metabolic panel test results are normal, no new problems
Plan: **RTO** 1 year
1 CM Code annual examination Z00.00

2. Date: 7/3/yy Location: New Life Obstetrics
Provider: Kay Pinkney, MD
Patient: Josephine Day Gender: F Age: 24
Reason for encounter: supervision of normal second pregnancy, third trimester, 34 weeks
Assessment: Estimated Date of Delivery (EDD) 8/3/yy
Plan: RTO 1 week

***Tip*:** The subterm for a second pregnancy is classified as "specified NEC." Assign one code for the supervision and a second code for weeks of gestation.

2 CM Codes Z34.83 Z3A.34
pregnancy → supervision → normal → specified NEC → 3rd trimester; pregnancy → weeks of gestation → 34 wks

3. Date: 7/3/yy Location: City Center Cardiology
Provider: Matthew Bunker, MD
Patient: Brandon Woodruff Gender: M Age: 76
Reason for encounter: adjustment of cardiac pacemaker
Assessment: reprogrammed pacemaker, no problems
Plan: RTO 6 months

***Tip*:** The Main Term **Fitting** is defined as **Fitting and adjustment of.**

1 CM Code Z45.018 Fitting & adjustment of → pacemaker

ARRANGING Z CODES

Instructional notes in the Tabular List and the OGCR provide sequencing guidance regarding which Z codes are permitted only as the principal or first-listed diagnosis code and which may be the sole diagnosis code or additional (secondary) diagnosis codes.

Principal or First-Listed Diagnosis

OGCR I.C.21.c.16) lists the Z codes and categories that may *only* be reported as the principal or first-listed diagnosis. The exception is when patients have multiple encounters on the same day and the medical records for the encounters are combined, as may be the case for inpatient records.

Instructional notes in the Tabular List and OGCR from other chapters may also provide direction for Z code sequencing. For example, OGCR I.C.21. c.16) lists the following categories as principal or first-listed diagnosis only:

- **Z51.0 Encounter for antineoplastic radiation therapy**
- **Z51.1- Encounter for antineoplastic chemotherapy and immunotherapy**

However, OGCR I.C.2.e. provides additional guidelines, which state the following:

- When an episode of care involves the surgical removal of a neoplasm, followed by adjunct chemotherapy or radiation therapy during the same episode of care, sequence the *neoplasm* code *first*, then assign the therapy code(s) as additional diagnoses.

When more than one type of antineoplastic therapy is provided during the same encounter, either may be sequenced first.

Therefore, coders must review all the OGCR related to an encounter and apply critical thinking skills to compare and contrast the guidelines.

Sole Diagnosis Code

Any code listed in OGCR I.C.21.c.16) may also be assigned as the only diagnosis code for an encounter. This is often the case when patients seek specific health services, such as routine and administrative medical examinations or supervision of a normal pregnancy, and have no other problems or conditions.

CODING CAUTION

Category **Z38 Liveborn infants according to place of birth and type of delivery** must always be sequenced *first* on *newborn* records that include the birth encounter. However, category **Z37 Outcome of delivery** must always be a *secondary* code on records of *mothers* that include the delivery encounter.

Status codes and history codes are rarely used as the sole diagnosis code because they do not represent the sole reason for an encounter. For example, codes for family history, BMI, blood type, or DNR describe supplemental information and are used in conjunction with other Z codes or codes from the body system chapters.

Additional Diagnosis Codes

Any code not listed in OGCR I.C.21.c.16) may be used as a secondary, or additional, diagnosis code. When no specific OGCR exists for sequencing a Z code, follow OGCR that apply to sequencing all diagnosis codes.

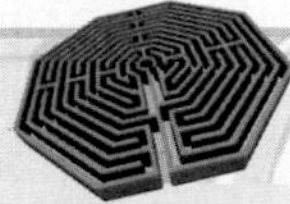

Coding Practice

Now it is your turn to practice arranging codes for health status and health services. Refer to the ***Tip*** the end of the mini-medical-record if you need a little extra help.

Exercise 7.4 Arranging Z Codes

Instructions: Read the mini-medical-record of each patient's encounter, review the information abstracted in Exercise 7.2, assign ICD-10-CM diagnosis codes (CM) using the Index and Tabular List, and sequence them correctly.

1. Date: 7/4/yy Location: Branton Medical Center Outpatient Radiology

Provider: Jennifer Kolb, MD (radiologist)

Patient: Monica Heath Gender: F Age: 47

Reason for encounter: screening mammogram

Assessment: normal mammogram, both breasts

Plan: repeat screening 6 months due to personal history of breast cancer

2 CM Codes Z12.31 Z85.3

(1) Screening → Dz → neoplasm → breast → routine mammogram
(2) Hx → personal → malignant neoplasm → breast

2. Date: 7/4/yy Location: East Side Oncology

Provider: Richard Blackford, MD

Patient: Ricardo Ferrari Gender: M Age: 61

Reason for encounter: 6-month follow up after removal of prostate due to malignant neoplasm of prostate

Assessment: no new findings, no recurrence of disease, no current treatment

Plan: next FU 6 months

Tip: Assign codes for the examination, acquired absence of organ, and history of malignant neoplasm.

3 CM Codes Z08 Z90.79 Z85.46

(1) Examination → F/U → malignant neoplasm (2) Absence → prostate
(3) Hx → personal → malignant neoplasm → prostate

3. Date: 7/4/yy Location: Branton Medical Center

Provider: Matthew Bunker, MD

Patient: John Binns Gender: M Age: 48

Reason for admission: unstable angina pectoris, current tobacco use

Assessment: EKG negative for AMI, **ECC** normal, angiogram normal

Discharge Plan: Rx nitroglycerin, follow up in office 1 week

Tip: Remember to read the instructional notes at the beginning of the three-digit category.

2 CM Codes I20.0 Z72.0

Angina → stable Tobacco → use

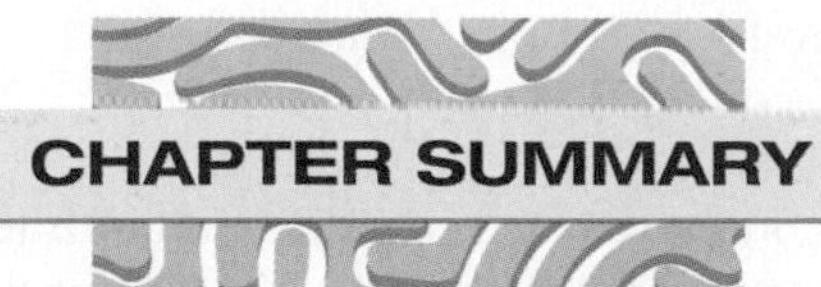

CHAPTER SUMMARY

In this chapter you learned that:

- Z codes represent reasons for encounters and may be used in any healthcare setting when the reason for the encounter is not a disease, injury, or external cause that is classified in the preceding ICD-10-CM chapters for body systems (A00 to Y89).
- ICD-10-CM Chapter 21, Factors Influencing Health Status and Contact with Health Services (Z00-Z99) contains 14 blocks or subchapters.
- Coders abstract information described by Z codes in three different types of circumstances: Z codes describe the reason for the encounter; instructional notes in the Tabular List direct coders to use Z codes; Z codes are required by the OGCR only.
- When assigning Z codes, coders need to know what Main Terms to search for in the Index, how to distinguish between diagnosis codes and procedure codes, and when to not use a Z code.
- Instructional notes in the Tabular List and the OGCR provide sequencing guidance regarding which Z codes are permitted only as the principal or first-listed diagnosis code and which may be the sole diagnosis code or additional (secondary) diagnosis codes.
- ICD-10-CM provides Official Guidelines for Coding and Reporting (OGCR) Z codes in OGCR section I.C.2., which contains a detailed discussion of the categories of Z codes, when to report them, and which codes may only be sequenced as the principal or first-listed diagnosis.

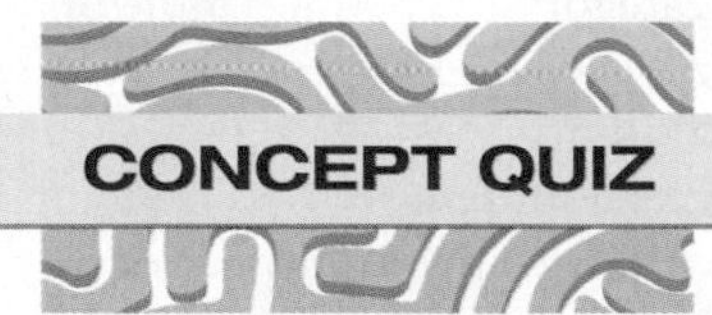

CONCEPT QUIZ

Take a moment to look back at your trip through health status and health services and solidify your skills. This is your opportunity to pull together everything you have learned.

Completion

Instructions: Write the term that answers each question based on the information you learned in this chapter. Choose from the following list. Some choices may be used more than once and some choices may not be used at all. Refer to the discussion in this chapter and the Glossary at the end of this book if you need a little extra help.

aftercare
contact/exposure
counseling
donor
follow-up
personal history
family history
inoculations and vaccinations
newborns and infants
observation
obstetrical and reproductive
routine and administrative examinations
screening
status
miscellaneous

1. ______________________ Z codes describe testing for disease or disease precursors in seemingly well individuals so that early detection and treatment can be provided for those who test positive for the disease.
2. ______________________ Z codes describe a patient's past medical condition that no longer exists and is not receiving any treatment, but that has the potential for recurrence, and therefore may require continued monitoring.
3. ______________________ Z codes describe a person is being observed for a suspected condition that is ruled out.
4. ______________________ Z codes describe when a patient or family member receives assistance in the aftermath of an illness or injury.
5. Z00.00 Encounter for general adult medical examination is an example of the Z code category ______________________.
6. ______________________ Z codes describe when the initial treatment of a disease has been performed and the patient requires continued care during the healing or recovery phase, or for the long-term consequences of the disease.
7. ______________________ Z codes describe a patient who has a family member(s) who has had a particular disease that causes the patient to be at higher risk of also contracting the disease.

8. Z53.09 Procedure and treatment not carried out because of other contraindication is an example of the Z code category for ______________.

9. ______________ Z codes describe continuing surveillance following completed treatment of a disease, condition, or injury when the condition has been fully treated and no longer exists.

10. Z37.0 Single live birth is an example of the Z code category for ______________ services.

Multiple Choice

Instructions: Circle the letter of the best answer to each question based on the information you learned in this chapter. Refer to the discussion in this chapter and the Glossary at the end of this book if you need a little extra help.

1. The formal name for Z codes is
   A. Supplemental Reasons for Health Service Encounters.
   B. Personal and Family History of Certain Diseases.
   C. Factors Influencing Health Status and Health Behavior.
   D. Factors Influencing Health Status and Contact with Health Services.
2. Which of the following is NOT a situation that requires Z codes?
   A. Tobacco, alcohol, drug use
   B. Tobacco dependence
   C. Acquired absence of organ
   D. Transplant waiting list, recipient, or donor
3. A category of Z code that is rarely used is
   A. observation.
   B. history.
   C. outcome of delivery.
   D. screening.
4. All of the following Main Terms lead to Z codes EXCEPT
   A. Absence
   B. Encounter
   C. Abnormal
   D. Follow-up
5. When should you assign a procedure code in addition to a Z code?
   A. Always
   B. When both codes are listed together in the Index
   C. When an instructional note in the Tabular List instructs you to do so
   D. Never
6. Do not assign a Z code when
   A. the initial treatment of a disease has been performed and the patient requires continued care during healing or recovery.
   B. diagnosis codes from body system chapters include the same information.
   C. a CPT code is required.
   D. more than one service is provided during the same encounter.
7. Z codes may be used in what healthcare setting(s)?
   A. Inpatient settings only
   B. Outpatient settings only
   C. Preventive care settings only
   D. Any healthcare setting
8. The code Z23 Encounter for immunization is an example of what category of Z code?
   A. Inoculations and vaccinations
   B. Newborns and infants
   C. Preventive care encounters
   D. Routine and administrative examinations
9. The Z code category Encounters for Obstetrical and Reproductive Services includes which of the following codes?
   A. Z32.01 Encounter for pregnancy test, result positive
   B. Z39.2 Encounter for routine postpartum follow-up
   C. Z38.01 Single liveborn infant, delivered by cesarean
   D. Z34.01 Encounter for supervision of normal first pregnancy, first trimester
10. The Z code category Aftercare includes which of the following codes?
    A. Z03.73 Encounter for suspected fetal anomaly ruled out
    B. Z08 Encounter for follow-up examination after completed treatment for malignant neoplasm
    C. Z44.002 Encounter for fitting and adjustment of unspecified left artificial arm
    D. Z69.010 Encounter for mental health services for victim of parental child abuse

CODING CHALLENGE

Now it is your turn to demonstrate coding all aspects of health status and health services. Refer back to the examples and discussion in this chapter when you need a little extra help. Use your medical dictionary and anatomy references when needed.

Instructions: Read the mini-medical-record of each patient's encounter, then abstract, assign, and sequence ICD-10-CM diagnosis codes (CM) using the Index and Tabular List. Write the code(s) on the line provided.

1. Date: 7/15/yy Location: Branton Medical Center Provider: Kay Pinkney, MD (obstetrician)

Patient: Ralph Newell Gender: M Age: 1 day

Assessment: normal healthy newborn after cesarean delivery here yesterday

Discharge Plan: FU with pediatrician in 2 weeks

***Tip*:** Search under the Main Term, Newborn, and subterm, born.

1 CM Code Z38.01 Newborn→born in hosp→ by cesarean

2. Date: 7/15/yy Location: Branton Medical Center Provider: Richard Blackford, MD

Patient: David Egbert Gender: M Age: 67

Reason for admission: initial antineoplastic chemotherapy, risk of **tumor lysis syndrome** and dehydration

Assessment: small cell carcinoma in both lungs, dehydration due to chemotherapy

Discharge Plan: RTO 1 week

***Tip*:** Refer to OGCR I.C.2.e for guidance on code assignment and sequencing. Remember to code for laterality.

4 CM Codes Z51.0 Chemotherapy, E86.0 Dehydration
C34.91 Table of neoplasms→ lung→Right
C34.92 " " " → lung→Left

3. Date: 7/15/yy Location: Branton Family Practice Provider: Kristen Conover, MD

Patient: Leticia Curry Gender: F Age: 45

Reason for encounter: follow-up exam after completing treatment for surgical removal of uterus due to **endometrial** cancer

Assessment: no new findings

Plan: FU 6 months

***Tip*:** Remember to read all instructional notes in the Tabular List.

3 CM Codes Z08 Examination→F/u→malignant neoplasm
Z90.710 Absence→uterus
Z85.42 history→personal→malignant→neoplasm→uterus

4. Date: 7/15/yy Location: Branton Medical Center Provider: Richard Blackford, MD

Patient: Lynda Liu Gender: F Age: 62

Reason for admission: radical cystectomy followed by inpatient radiotherapy

Assessment: stage III carcinoma of the bladder, invasive into bladder, no metastasis found

Plan: continue radiotherapy as outpatient

2 CM Codes C67.9 Table of neoplasm→bladder→primary
Z51.0 Radiotherapy

5. Date: 7/15/yy Location: Branton Family Practice Provider: Kristen Conover, MD

Patient: Peter Earp Gender: M Age: 15

Reason for encounter: school sports physical

Assessment: cleared for football

Plan: discussed safety precautions and conditioning

1 CM Code Z02.5 examination→physical→sports

(*continued*)

(continued from page 123)

6. Date: 7/15/yy Location: Branton Family Practice Provider: Kristen Conover, MD

Patient: Phillip Rayner Gender: M Age: 12 months

Reason for encounter: Hepatitis B, **MMR**, and **varicella** immunizations

Assessment: child has a heavy cold today, so immunization was not carried out

Plan: reschedule when he is healthy

2 CM Codes Z28.01 Immunization → not done → acute illness of patient ___ J00 Cold → common

7. Date: 7/15/yy Location: Branton Medical Center Provider: Tanya Schmitt, MD

Patient: Daniel Otero Gender: M Age: 29

Reason for admission: Patient is a donor match for brother who has end stage renal disease (ESRD).

Assessment: removal of kidney for transplantation to brother

Plan: FU in office, 4 weeks

1 CM Code Z52.4 Donor → kidney

8. Date: 7/15/yy Location: Branton Family Practice Provider: Kristen Conover, MD

Patient: Candice Chauvin Gender: F Age: 4

Reason for encounter: routine 4-year-old exam

Assessment: no new findings, MMR and varicella immunizations administered

Plan: RTO 1 year, call if any new problems

2 CM Codes Z00.129 Examination → child ___ Z23 Immunization → encounter for

9. Date: 7/15/yy Location: Branton Medical Center Provider: Kay Pinkney, MD

Patient: Gloria Tardiff Gender: F Age: 23

Reason for admission: normal delivery, 39 weeks gestation

Outcome: single liveborn infant

Discharge Plan: FU in office, 2 weeks

Tip: Locate the delivery under the Main Term, Delivery, and subterm, normal. Remember to read the instructional notes in the Tabular List.

3 CM Codes O80 Delivery → normal ___ Z3A.39 pregnancy → week of gestation → 39 wks ___ Z37.0 outcome of delivery → single → liveborn

10. Date: 7/15/yy Location: Branton Family Practice Provider: Kristen Conover, MD

Patient: Angelica Gowan Gender: F Age: 65

Reason for encounter: management of coronary artery disease (CAD)

Assessment: chronic CAD, BP well-controlled

Plan: renew Rx for **anticoagulant** (warfarin) which patient has used successfully for 5 years, discussed eating habits due to borderline cholesterol and the need to quit smoking

Tip: You need one code for the disease. Read the instructional notes at the beginning of the category for the second code. The third code is for long-term drug therapy.

3 CM Codes I25.9 Disease → heart → ischemic ___ Z72.0 Tobacco use ___ Z79.01 Long-term drug therapy → anticoagulants

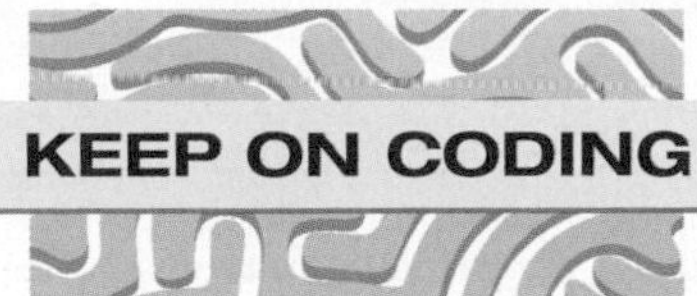

KEEP ON CODING

As a coder, you can never have too much experience. Apply everything you have learned in this chapter to code the following diagnostic statements. Use the OGCR and instructional notes in the Tabular List to help determine how many codes are required.

Instructions: Read the diagnostic statement, then use the Index and Tabular List to assign and sequence ICD-10-CM (CM) diagnosis codes. Write the code(s) on the line provided.

1. Encounter for pregnancy test with a negative result: CM Code(s) Z32.02 Encounter → pregnancy → test → result (-)
2. Blood type AB, Rh positive: CM Code(s) Z67.30 Blood → Type → AB → Rh +
3. Dental examination and cleaning: CM Code(s) Z01.20 Examination → dental
4. Surgical procedure canceled per patient decision: CM Code(s) Z53.20 Canceled procedure → because of → pt's decis
5. Status post heart transplant without complications: CM Code(s) Z94.1 Transplant → heart
6. Renal dialysis status: CM Code(s) Z99.2 status → dialysis
7. Encounter for removal of breast implant: CM Code(s) Z45.81 Encounter → removal → breast implant
8. Status post coronary angioplasty: CM Code(s) Z98.61 Status → angioplasty → coronary artery
9. Family history of diabetes mellitus: CM Code(s) Z83.3 Hx → family → diabetes mellitus
10. History of tobacco use: CM Code(s) Z87.891 Hx → personal → nicotine dependence
11. Encounter for paternity testing: CM Code(s) Z02.81 Encounter → administrative → examination for → paternity testing
12. Encounter for supervision of high risk pregnancy in the twentieth week (second trimester): CM Code(s) ________
13. Liveborn single female, delivered vaginally in the hospital: CM Code(s) ________
14. Lack of physical exercise: CM Code(s) ________
15. Long-term use of non-steroidal anti-inflammatories (NSAID): CM Code(s) ________
16. Allergy to seafood: CM Code(s) ________
17. Presence of a cerebrospinal shunt: CM Code(s) ________
18. Physical restraint status: CM Code(s) ________
19. Do not resuscitate (DNR) status: CM Code(s) ________
20. Homelessness: CM Code(s) ________
21. Pregnant state incidental to encounter: CM Code(s) ________
22. Personal history of kidney stones: CM Code(s) ________
23. Cystic fibrosis carrier: CM Code(s) ________
24. History of adult neglect: CM Code(s) ________
25. Routine well child exam, age six months, with abnormal findings: CM Code(s) ________

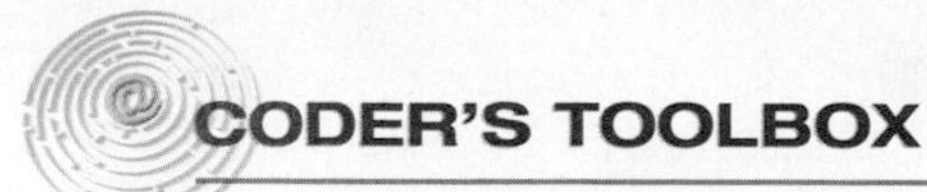

CODER'S TOOLBOX

The following resources are a starting point for learning more about health status and health services. The > symbol indicates a menu selection within the website in order to navigate to a specific page.

American Academy of Family Practice (AAFP) > Geriatric Assessment **http://www.aafp.org/afp/viewRelatedDocumentsByMesh.htm?meshId=D015577**

American Academy of Family Practice (AAFP) > Primary Prevention **http://www.aafp.org/afp/viewRelatedDocumentsByMesh.htm?meshId=D011322**

American Academy of Pediatrics > Children's Health Topics **http://www.aap.org/topics.html**

American Health Information Management Association (AHIMA) > From V Codes to Z Codes: Transitioning to ICD-10 **http://library.ahima.org/xpedio/groups/public/documents/ahima/bok1_022421.hcsp?dDocName=bok1_022421**

Centers for Disease Control and Prevention > Vaccines Home > Immunization Schedules **http://www.cdc.gov/vaccines/recs/schedules/default.htm**

Mayo Clinic Health Solutions > Health Assessment Overview **http://www.mayoclinichealthsolutions.com/products/Health-Assessment.cfm**

Medicare > Preventive Services **https://www.cms.gov/MLNProducts/downloads/MPS_QuickReferenceChart_1.pdf**

Organ Donor.gov **http://organdonor.gov/**

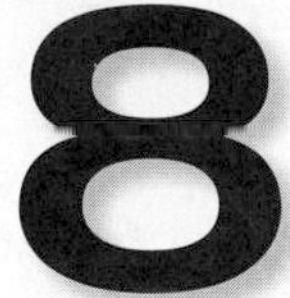

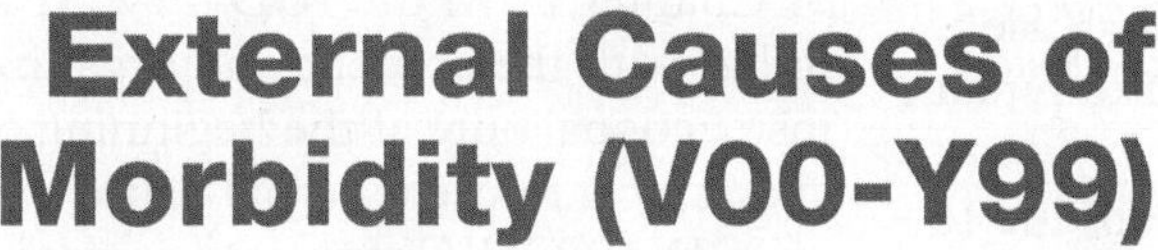

8 External Causes of Morbidity (V00-Y99)

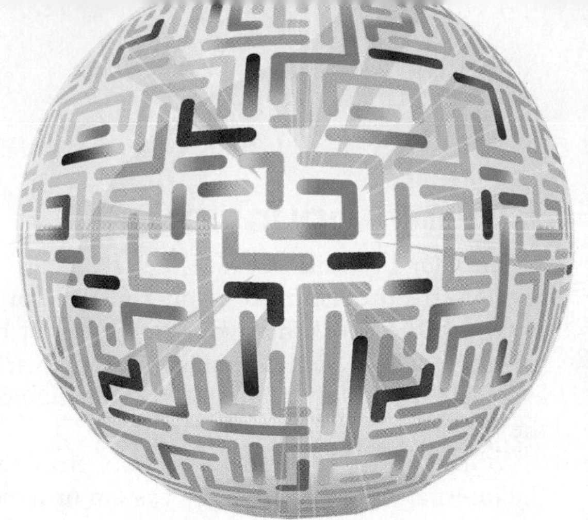

Learning Objectives

After completing this chapter, you should have the skills to:

- Spell and define the key words, medical terms, and abbreviations related to external causes of morbidity.
- Describe the purpose of external cause codes.
- Discuss the main characteristics of coding external causes of morbidity.
- Abstract information required for coding external causes of morbidity and related conditions from the medical record.
- Assign codes for external causes of morbidity and related conditions.
- Arrange codes for external causes of morbidity and related conditions.
- Discuss the Official Guidelines for Coding and Reporting related to external causes of morbidity.

Key Terms and Abbreviations

activity
adverse effect
cause/causal event
complication
external cause
intent
misadventure
place of occurrence
status
terrorism

In addition to the key terms listed here, students should know the terms defined within tables in this chapter.

Chapter Outline

- **Introduction to External Causes**
- **Coding Overview of External Causes**
- **Abstracting for External Causes**
- **Assigning Codes for External Causes**
- **Arranging Codes for External Causes**

ICD-10-CM codes in this chapter are from the ICD-10-CM 2014 Draft code set from the Department of Health and Human Services, Centers for Disease Control and Prevention.

INTRODUCTION

When your tire fails because the treads are worn down or the retread delaminates, you know the problem is inherent to the tire. When your tire goes flat because you pick up a nail or someone slashes your tires, the cause is external to the tire. In either case, you still need to repair the tire.

In healthcare, some medical problems develop due to the internal failure of an organ system or biological function; other medical problems are due to external causes, such as an accident or assault. These special circumstances require you to identify and code for external causes of illness and injuries. In this chapter, you will practice coding for patient encounters related to injury and poisoning, a skill that requires you to abstract information from the mini-medical-record, assign correct codes, and arrange (sequence) the codes in the proper order.

Physicians of any specialty may use external cause codes, but they are often used in the emergency department, family practice, orthopedics, and ophthalmology because these physicians specialize in circumstances or body systems frequently affected by external causes.

As you read this chapter, open up your medical terminology book and keep a medical dictionary handy to refresh your memory of any unfamiliar terms. An anatomy text will also be useful. Think of these resources as your travel brochures that tell you more about an area. This way, you have the information you need at your fingertips.

INTRODUCTION TO EXTERNAL CAUSES

External cause codes describe the event or circumstances that caused an injury or medical problem. Diagnosis codes from the body system chapters describe the actual injury or condition that results. External cause codes may be used in any healthcare setting and with any diagnosis code, but they are secondary codes and should *never* be used as a principal or first-listed diagnosis (OGCR I.C.20.a.1) and 6)).

An **external cause** is an event such as an accident, force of nature, assault, or situation that causes an injury or **adverse effect** (*negative physical reaction*), **complication** (*an abnormal medical reaction that results from a medical or surgical procedure*), or **misadventure** (*an error during a medical or surgical procedure*). Examples of external causes include floods, automobile accidents, falls, prescribed or illegal drugs, and medical or surgical procedures.

Many states require the reporting of external cause codes to track statistics. External cause codes assist third-party payers in tracking the liability (who is at fault) for medical costs and enable health researchers to collect standardized data for injury research and injury prevention strategies.

CODING OVERVIEW OF EXTERNAL CAUSES

ICD-10-CM Chapter 20 External Causes of Morbidity (V00-Y99) contains 33 blocks or subchapters. Review the block names and code ranges listed at the beginning of Chapter 20 in the ICD-10-CM manual to become familiar with the content and organization. Also review the instructional note at the beginning of the chapter that discusses how to use external cause codes.

ICD-10-CM Chapter 20 corresponds with ICD-9-CM Supplementary Classification of External Causes of Injury and Poisoning (E000-E999), commonly referred to as E codes. ICD-10-CM includes external cause codes as part of the main classification rather than as a supplementary classification as ICD-9-CM did. However, ICD-10-CM provides a separate Index to External Causes. Numerous title changes, expansions, and reorganization appear in ICD-10-CM. Nearly all external cause codes require a seventh-character. Many external cause events that were a single code in ICD-9-CM are categories in ICD-10-CM with expansion at the subcategory level in order to add specificity. Transport accidents are reorganized based on the mode of transportation. Codes for complications of medical and surgical care are greatly expanded. Place of occurrence codes have greater specificity, including the type of dwelling and room of the house in which the injury occurred. Late effect of external cause codes are eliminated because late effects are reported with a seventh-character extension in ICD-10-CM.

ICD-10-CM provides Official Guidelines for Coding and Reporting (OGCR) external causes in OGCR section I.C.20. OGCR provides detailed discussion of when to report codes from this chapter and how they are to be used. Additional OGCR for using external cause codes in conjunction with specific conditions appear throughout the OGCR and as instructional notes throughout the Tabular List.

CODING CAUTION

There is no national requirement for mandatory reporting of external cause codes. Providers are encouraged to voluntarily report external cause codes, because they provide valuable data for injury research and evaluation of injury prevention strategies (OGCR I.C.20.).

ABSTRACTING FOR EXTERNAL CAUSES

Whenever patients are treated for injuries, adverse effects, or complications from procedures, coders abstract information related to the external cause of the condition. Multiple external cause codes are required, each

Table 8-1 ■ KEY CRITERIA FOR ABSTRACTING EXTERNAL CAUSES

- ❑ **Diagnosis:** What physical injury(ies) or health condition did the patient sustain?
- ❑ **Intent:** What is the purpose or intent of the injury: accidental, self-harm, assault, legal intervention, military operation, or medical procedure?
- ❑ **Cause/causal event:** How did the injury or health condition happen?
- ❑ **Place:** Where did the event occur?
- ❑ **Activity:** What was the patient doing at the time of the event?
- ❑ **Status:** What was the employment status at the time the event occurred: civilian employment, military, volunteer, or recreational/leisure?

describing a different aspect of the event, if the documentation provides the required information. In addition to the clinical diagnosis, external cause information that must be abstracted appears in ■ TABLE 8-1.

Place of occurrence, Activity, and Status codes are in the block **Supplementary factors related to causes of morbidity classified elsewhere (Y90-Y99)**. An instructional note in the Tabular List instructs coders that these categories may be used to provide supplementary information concerning causes of morbidity. They are not to be used as the only external cause code.

Intent and Cause

Combination codes report both intent and cause. **Intent** describes whether the event was accidental or intentional. **Cause** describes the event or action that resulted in the injury. Code(s) for intent and cause are reported *every* time the patient receives treatment for the injury (OGCR I.C.20.a.2)).

Because intent and cause are described in a combination code, determine the intent first. Doing so helps to locate the Main Term in the Index to External Causes. Options for intent include the following:

- accidental
- self-harm
- assault
- result of legal, military, or terrorist activity
- undetermined

The cause or event code is based on the intent. For example, separate codes exist for an accidental fall, a fall that is a suicide attempt, and a fall that is due to an assault. The vast majority of cause codes are for accidental intent, so accident codes are the most specific. The most common causes of accidents are traffic accidents and falls.

When the intent of the cause of an injury or other condition is unknown or unspecified, code the intent as **accidental**. All transport accident categories assume **accidental** intent (OGCR I.C.20.h.) When the documentation states that the intent cannot be determined, then abstract the intent as **undetermined**.

SUCCESS STEP

Always abstract before you attempt to assign codes. Write down notes with key information to help keep the details organized. When you begin to assign codes, you may need to refer back to the medical record and abstract additional details based on the specificity of information the code requires.

SUCCESS STEP

Coders also need to abstract the episode of care, which describes the phase of treatment. Identifying the episode of care is necessary in order to assign the seventh-character extension of an external cause code. Options for the episode of care are:

- **initial** episode, which identifies that the patient received active treatment for the injury during the encounter;
- **subsequent** episode, which identifies that the patient received routine care during the healing phase at the encounter; and
- **sequela** episode, which identifies an encounter at which the patient was treated for a complication after the healing phase is complete.

CODING CAUTION

The extension for the **initial** episode of care does not refer only to the *first* encounter, but to any encounter during *active treatment*, such as initial stabilization of fracture, initial surgery, and cast application. Use the extension for **subsequent** care during the healing phase, such as for a cast change, X-ray to monitor healing, or surgery to correct malunion.

Place of Occurrence (Y92.-)

The **place of occurrence** code describes where the injury occurred, such as a public street or a single family home. Report only *one* place per injury and *only* at the initial encounter for treatment (OGCR I.C.20.b. and d.). Review the category **Y92.**- to familiarize yourself with the various types of settings. Within each setting, such as single family residence, codes designate the specific room or area where the injury occurred.

Activity (Y93.-)

An activity code describes what the person was doing when the injury occurred, such as running, playing sports, or preparing food. Report *one* activity code per injury when it provides additional information about the event. Report the activity code *only* at the initial encounter for treatment (OGCR I.C.20.c. and d.). Review the category **Y93.**- to familiarize yourself with the various types of activities. Activity codes are not applicable to poisonings, adverse effects, medical misadventures, complications, or late effects.

Be careful to differentiate the activity from the causal event. The causal event, such as a fall, may occur while doing any number of activities, such as running, walking, or working in the yard. When a person is engaged in an activity, such as walking, an injury could occur as a result of a variety of events, such as falling, tripping, or being struck by an object or vehicle. Every injury should be coded with a causal event, but not every injury requires an activity code. Assign an activity code when it provides additional information.

Status (Y99.-)

Status codes describe the person's employment status in relation to the event that caused the injury (OGCR I.C.20.d. and k.). Report *one* status code per injury event and *only* at the initial encounter for treatment. The status code indicates whether the event occurred during military activity or whether a civilian was at work or engaged in a volunteer activity.

Guided Example of Abstracting External Causes

Refer to the following example throughout this chapter in order to practice your abstracting, assigning, and arranging external cause code skills. Marcy Elwood, CCS, is a fictitious coder who guides you through coding this case.

> Date: 8/1/yy Location: Branton Medical Center Emergency Department Provider: Cynthia Hiatt, MD
>
> Patient: Charles Fink Gender: M Age: 24
>
> Reason for encounter: Patient had an accident on his day off. He was painting the outside of his single family home when he fell off a ladder.
>
> Assessment: fractured left tibia
>
> Plan: Applied long leg cast. Use crutches to keep weight off. Follow-up with orthopedic clinic.

Follow along as Marcy abstracts the diagnosis. Check off each step after you complete it.

⇨ Marcy begins by reading the medical record. She refers to the Key Criteria for Abstracting External Causes (Table 8-1) to abstract the diagnosis. She will abstract all the information first, then assign the actual codes later in this chapter.

- ☐ *Diagnosis: What physical injury(ies) or health condition did the patient sustain?* She notes that the diagnosis is fractured left tibia because it describes the injury the patient experienced and writes this down.
- ☐ *Intent: What is the purpose or intent of the injury: accidental, self-harm, assault, legal intervention, military operation, or medical procedure?* She notes that the intent is stated as an accident and writes this down.
- ☐ *Causal event: How did the injury or health condition happen?* She notes that the causal event is a fall. Specifically, the fall was from a ladder. She writes this down.
- ☐ *Place of occurrence: Where did the event occur?* She notes that the fall occurred outside of a single family home. She writes this down.
- ☐ *Activity: What was the patient doing at the time of the event?* Marcy notes that the patient was painting the outside of his house and writes this down.
- ☐ *Status: What was the employment status at the time the event occurred: civilian employment, military, volunteer, or recreational/leisure?* Marcy determines the patient was doing the work for personal purposes on his day off. Even though he is employed, the accident was not related to his employment.

⇨ Marcy reviews all the data she abstracted for this case and verifies it against the medical record.

- ☐ Diagnosis: fractured left tibia, initial encounter
- ☐ Intent and cause: accidental fall from ladder, initial encounter
- ☐ Place: outside of single family home
- ☐ Activity: painting outside of house
- ☐ Status: personal

⇨ Next, Marcy will assign the codes.

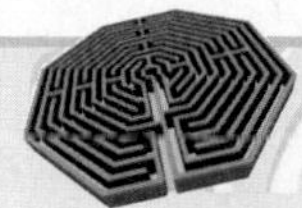

Coding Practice

Now it is your turn to practice abstracting external causes. Questions guide your analysis.

Exercise 8.1 Abstracting for External Causes

Instructions: Read the mini-medical-record of each patient's encounter and answer the abstracting questions. Write the answer on the line provided. Do not assign any codes.

1. Date: 8/2/yy Location: Branton Medical Center Emergency Room Provider: Cynthia Hiatt, MD

Patient: Mildred Stiles Gender: F Age: 85

Chief complaint: Laceration on the forehead. Fell off toilet and hit her head on the sink.

Assessment: 3 cm laceration

Plan: see family physician for suture removal in 10 days

a. What is the diagnosis? ____________________

b. What event caused the injury? ____________________

c. Was this episode of care the initial, subsequent, or sequela? ____________________

2. Date: 8/2/yy Location: Branton Medical Center Emergency Room Provider: Cynthia Hiatt, MD

Patient: Constance Macgregor Gender: F Age: 5

Reason for encounter: burn due to accidentally touching hot stove

Assessment: second degree burn to the right hand

Plan: Dressed wound. Instructed parent on wound care. Follow up with family physician in 2 weeks. Call if any problems develop.

a. What is the diagnosis? ____________________

b. What event caused the injury? ____________________

c. Was this episode of care the initial, subsequent, or sequela? ____________________

3. Date: 8/2/yy Location: Branton Medical Center

Provider: Bruce Prentice, MD

Patient: Frank Bernhardt Gender: M Age: 25

Reason for admission: assault by handgun to leg 6 weeks ago. Patient was treated for fracture to femur caused by a bullet. Bullet was removed but fracture has not healed properly so surgery is needed.

Discharge diagnosis: malunion of non-displaced comminuted (bone broken into fragments) fracture, left femur shaft

Plan: FU in office in 3 weeks

a. What is the diagnosis? ____________________

b. What event caused the injury? ____________________

c. Was this episode of care the initial, subsequent, or sequela? ____________________

4. Date: 8/3/yy Location: Branton Medical Center

Provider: Matthew Bunker, MD

Patient: Anthony Mojica Gender: M Age: 47

Reason for admission: heart attack due to overexertion while shoveling snow in driveway of his single family home.

Discharge diagnosis: AMI

Plan: FU in office in 2 weeks

a. What is the diagnosis? ____________________

b. What event caused the injury? ____________________

c. Was this episode of care the initial, subsequent, or sequela? ____________________

d. Where did the injury occur? ____________________

e. What was the patient doing at the time of the injury? ____________________

f. Was the activity done for civilian work, leisure, volunteer service, or military operations? ____________________

(*continued*)

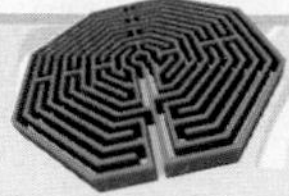

Coding Practice (continued)

5. Date: 8/3/yy Location: Branton Medical Center
Provider: Bruce Prentice, MD (orthopedic surgeon)
Patient: Darlene Thatcher Gender: F Age: 41
Reason for admission: second surgery for fractured scapula, which was the result of a traffic accident. She was driving a van as a volunteer for the swim team and collided with a pickup truck.
Assessment: displaced fracture of body of left scapula

a. What is the diagnosis? ______

b. What event caused the injury? ______

c. Was this episode of care the initial, subsequent, or sequela? ______

d. Where did the injury occur? ______

e. What was the patient doing at the time of the injury? ______

f. What kind of vehicle was the patient in? ______

g. Was she the driver or a passenger? ______

h. What kind of vehicle did she collide with? ______

i. What is the external cause status? ______

6. Date: 8/3/yy Location: Branton Medical Center Emergency Room Provider: Cynthia Hiatt, MD
Patient: Wayne Ramage Gender: M Age: 53
Reason for encounter: Patient was walking on a public sidewalk while making a delivery as part of his job when he was bit on the leg by a German shepherd dog which was running free in the neighborhood.
Assessment: puncture wound, left calf
Plan: follow up with orthopedic physician in 2 weeks

a. What is the diagnosis? ______

b. What event caused the injury? ______

c. Was this episode of care the initial, subsequent, or sequela? ______

d. Where did the injury occur? ______

e. What was the patient doing at the time of the injury? ______

f. Was the activity done for civilian work, leisure, volunteer service, or military operations? ______

ASSIGNING CODES FOR EXTERNAL CAUSES

To assign codes to cases involving external causes, coders use a separate Index to External Causes and verify the codes in the Tabular List.

SUCCESS STEP

Coders familiar with ICD-9-CM will notice that although ICD-10-CM has a separate Index to External Causes, it does *not* have a separate Tabular List as ICD-9-CM did. External cause codes appear in Chapter 20 (V00 to Y99) of the Tabular List.

Index to External Causes

The Index to External Causes is separate from the Index to Diseases and Injuries (Index) and appears immediately before the Tabular List. When coding cases that involve external causes, use both indices, as follows:

- Use the Index to Diseases and Injuries to locate the diagnosis code(s) for the injury or condition.
- Use the Index to External Causes to locate external cause codes for intent and cause, place of occurrence, activity, and employment status.

In order to use the Index to External Causes successfully, coders must locate Main Terms for each type of external cause code. Coders should also learn how to locate codes specifically for traffic accidents, the most commonly used and largest block in the external cause chapter.

SUCCESS STEP

If you have not already done so, apply an adhesive index tab to the first page of the Index to External Causes to help you remember where to find it. This index is not long enough that you need alphabetic tabs for every letter in the index, but it is helpful to insert a few tabs to make it easier to navigate. Good places to mark with tabs are A-B, C-O, and P-Z.

Main Terms

Main Terms for external cause codes for intent and causal event can be located in two ways: search for the intent or search for the event. Regardless of which way coders search for Main Terms, they must be attentive to multiple levels of indented subterms in order to locate the correct code, as follows:

- When searching for intent, the Main Term is the intent, such as **Accident** or **Assault**. Causal events are subterms indented under each Main Term.
- When searching for the causal event, the event is the Main Term, such as **Fall** or **Bite**. Each indent is a subterm under each causal event.

Main Terms for place, activity, and status are located under entries that carry those names: **Place**, **Activity**, and **Status**. Refer to ■ Table 8-2 for a list of commonly used Main Terms in the Index to External Causes. As in the Index to Diseases and Injuries, Main Terms have indented subterms that further define the specifics of entry. Remember to carefully review all available subterms in order to locate the most specific code.

Table 8-2 ■ COMMONLY USED MAIN TERMS IN THE INDEX TO EXTERNAL CAUSES

❑ Accident	❑ Incident
❑ Activity	❑ Jump
❑ Assault	❑ Legal
❑ Bite	❑ Military operations
❑ Burn	❑ Misadventure
❑ Complication	❑ Place
❑ Contact	❑ Radiation
❑ Drowning	❑ Status
❑ Explosion	❑ Striking against
❑ Exposure to	❑ Struck by
❑ Failure	❑ Suicide
❑ Fall	❑ War operations
❑ Forces of nature	

SUCCESS STEP

Three separate status codes exist for Status: (1) **civilian activity done for pay, Y99.0**, (2) **military activity, Y99.1**, and (3) **volunteer activity, Y99.2**. All other status descriptions such as student, hobby, or leisure activity are grouped together under one code, **Other external cause status, Y99.8.**

SUCCESS STEP

When burns are caused by contact with a hot object, such as a stove or iron, search under the Main Term **Burn**. When burns are caused by a fire with flames, such as a campfire or house fire, search under the Main Term **Exposure (to)** and subterm **fire, flames**.

Motor Vehicle Accidents

The Index entry for motor vehicle accidents is several pages long and has numerous levels of subterms (■ Figure 8-1, page 134). The most common types of accidents can be located as follows:

1. Locate the Main Term **Accident**.
2. Locate the subterm **transport**.
3. Locate the next level of subterm for type of vehicle the patient was riding in, such as **bus**, **car**, or **motorcycle**.
4. Locate the next subterm to identify the patient as the **driver** or **passenger**.
5. Locate the next level of subterm that identifies what object the vehicle collided with, such as **animal, car**, or **pedal cycle**.
6. The default code for motor vehicle accidents is for a traffic accident, as indicated by the parentheses for a nonessential modifier, **(traffic)**. When a vehicle accident occurs anywhere except a public highway, use the subterm **nontraffic**. The Tabular List provides definitions for the various types of accidents.
7. When the patient was a pedestrian or bicyclist who was hit by a vehicle, search under **Accident, transport, pedestrian** or **Accident, transport, pedal cyclist**.

Review the extensive instructional notes in the Tabular List at the beginning of the block **V00 to V99, Transport Accidents**. These notes provide definitions of transport vehicles, types of collisions, and vehicle occupants so that all coders use the codes in a consistent manner. A note also instructs coders to **Use additional code to identify** an airbag injury, type of street or road, or use of cellular telephone or electronic device at time of accident.

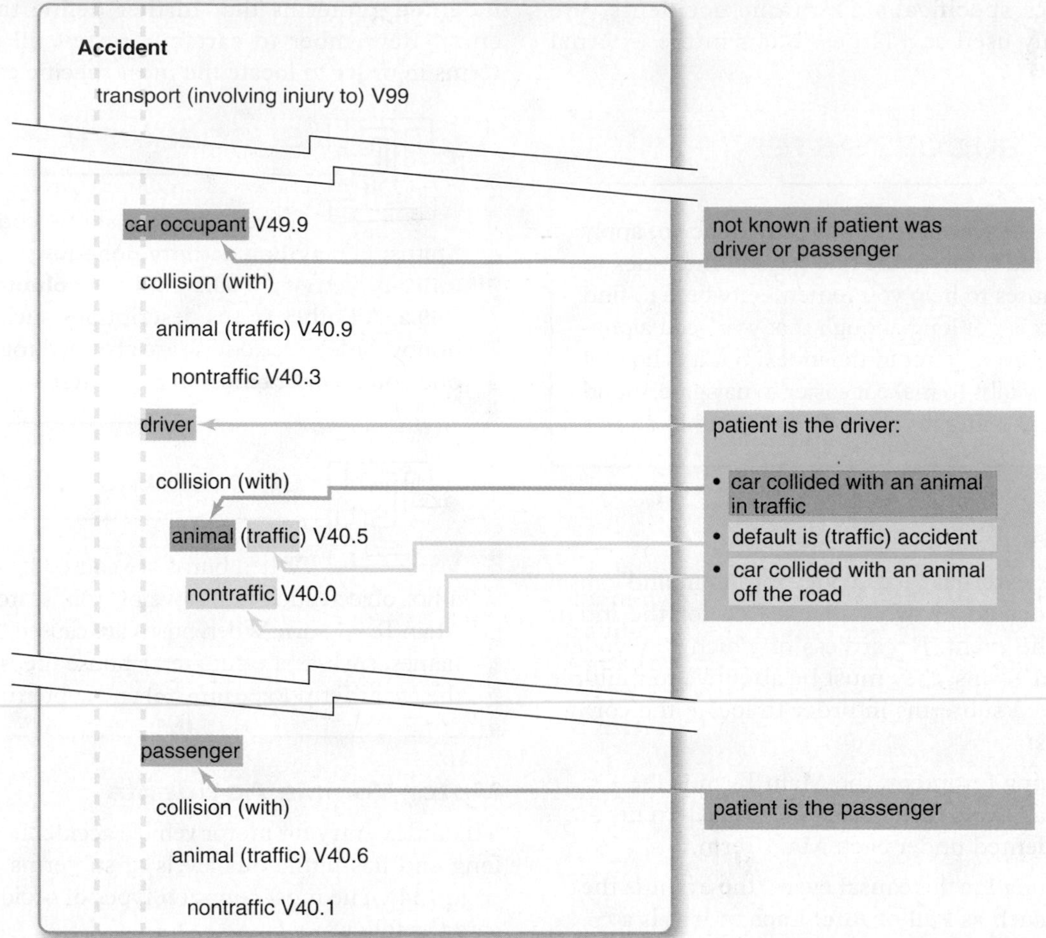

Figure 8-1 ■ Example of Index to External Causes, Main Term and Subterms for an Automobile Accident

Verify in Tabular List

Coders should verify all external cause codes in the Tabular List. Doing so can help catch mistakes that are easily made when navigating multiple levels of indented subterms in the Index to External Causes. In addition, seventh-character extensions can be assigned only from the Tabular List.

Most external cause codes for intent and cause from **V00** to **Y38** require a seventh-character extension to describe the episode of care. Seventh-character extensions for external causes appear under each three-digit category heading in the Tabular List (■ FIGURE 8-2). Refer to ■ TABLE 8-3 to learn when to use each extension (OGCR I.C.19.a.).

CODING CAUTION

External cause codes for place, activity, and status do NOT use seventh-character extensions for the episode of care.

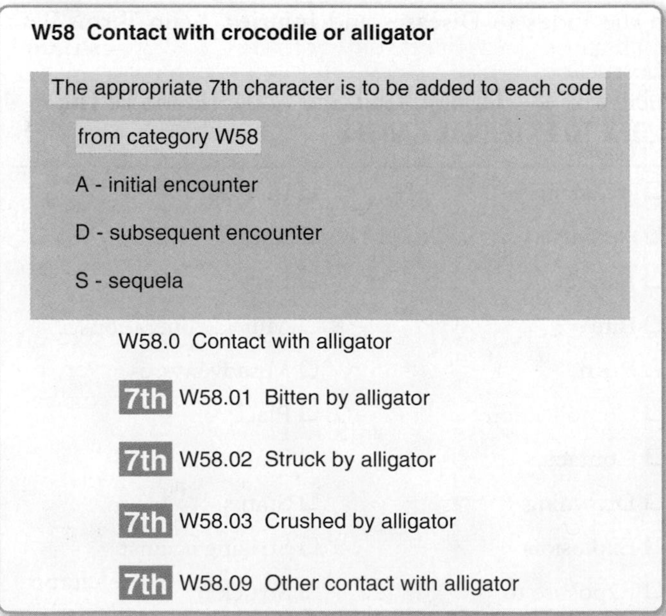

Figure 8-2 ■ Example of the Location of Seventh-Character Extensions Under Category Titles in Index to External Causes

Table 8-3 ■ **SEVENTH-CHARACTER EXTENSION, DEFINITIONS, AND EXAMPLES**

7th-Character Extension	Definition	Example
A Initial Encounter	Use while the patient is receiving active treatment for the injury.	Surgical treatment Emergency department encounter Evaluation and treatment by a new physician
D Subsequent Encounter	Use for encounters after the patient has received active treatment of the injury and is receiving routine care for the injury during the healing or recovery phase.	Cast change or removal Removal of external or internal fixation device Medication adjustment Visits following injury treatment
S Sequela	Use for complications or conditions that arise as a direct result of an injury after the healing phase is complete.	Scar formation after a burn

Recall that the convention 7th means that the extension character must be in the seventh position and coders should assign the placeholder **X** in any unused positions. Because the code **W50.01 Bitten by alligator** is only five characters, add the character **X** in the sixth position, before adding the extension. For example, **Bitten by alligator, initial encounter** is written as **W58.01XA**.

When the external cause and intent are included in a combination code from another chapter, do not report an additional code from Chapter 20 (OGCR I.C.20.a.8)). For example, **Poisoning by penicillin, accidental** is reported with code **T36.0X1-**. Because the diagnosis code describes both cause and intent, an external cause code is not reported. In addition, do not report place, activity, and status codes with poisonings. Poisonings are discussed in detail in Chapter 13 of this text.

Some external cause codes are combination codes that identify two or more related or sequential events that result in an injury, such as a fall that results in striking against an object. Such a code may be used when the injury is due to either the event alone or both at the same time. Assign the combination code that describes the full sequence of events, regardless of whether the most serious injury was from the fall itself or from striking the object (OGCR I.C.20.a.7)).

Assign as many external cause event codes as necessary to fully explain each cause. If only one external cause code can be recorded, assign the code most related to the principal diagnosis (OGCR I.C.20.a.4)). However, assign only one code each for place, activity, and status and report these codes only on the initial encounter.

Guided Example of Assigning External Cause Codes

Continue with the example from earlier in the chapter about patient Charles Fink, who fell off a ladder while painting his house, to learn more about using the Index to External Causes.

Follow along in your ICD-10-CM manual as Marcy Elwood, CCS, assigns codes. Check off each step after you complete it.

⇨ Marcy reviews the information she abstracted:

- ❑ Diagnosis: *fractured left tibia, initial encounter*
- ❑ Intent and cause: *accidental fall from ladder, initial encounter*
- ❑ Place: *outside of single family home*
- ❑ Activity: *painting outside of house*
- ❑ Status: *personal*

⇨ The first code Marcy will assign is the diagnosis code for the injury.

- ❑ She searches the Index to Diseases and Injuries for the diagnosis that she abstracted, *fractured left tibia, initial encounter*.
- ❑ She locates the Main Term **Fracture**, and subterm **tibia S82.20-**.

⇨ Marcy verifies the diagnosis code **S82.20-** in the Tabular List.

- ❑ She locates the subcategory title, **S82.20-, Unspecified fracture of shaft of tibia.**
- ❑ The symbol 6th tells her to assign a sixth character, located below the subcategory title. She assigns the sixth character, **2**, for the left tibia.
- ❑ The symbol 7th tells her to assign a seventh-character extension, located at the beginning of the category **S82**. She assigns the seventh character, **A**, for the initial encounter for closed fracture.
- ❑ The diagnosis code is **S82.202A, Unspecified fracture of shaft of left tibia, initial encounter for closed fracture.**

➩ Marcy turns her attention to the external cause codes. She locates the Index to External Causes, located immediately before the Tabular List. First, she will code the intent and cause.

➩ Marcy searches the Index to External Causes for the intent and cause of the injury, which she abstracted as *accidental fall from ladder*.

- ❑ She locates the Main Term **Fall** and notes that the default intent is **(accidental)**, so she knows she is in the right place.
- ❑ She locates the subterm **from, off, out of**.
- ❑ She locates the second-level subterm, **ladder W11**.

➩ Marcy verifies the first external cause code for **accidental fall off ladder**.

- ❑ She locates the Tabular List entry **W11**. She verifies the external cause code title, **Fall on and from ladder**, which accurately describes the situation.
- ❑ She cross-references the subchapter title **Other External Causes of Accidental Injury (W00-X58)** to verify that the fall code relates to an accidental intent.
- ❑ She notices the symbol **7th** in front of the code, which tells her a seventh character is required.
- ❑ She reviews the seventh character options, which are listed under the code, and identifies that **A** represents **the initial encounter**.
- ❑ She also notices that the **X** in the symbol means that because the code is three digits long, she must use the placeholder holder **X** to fill out the fourth, fifth, and sixth characters of the code.
- ❑ She assigns the code **W11.XXXA** for **Accidental fall from ladder, initial encounter**. Next she will assign the code for Place of occurrence.

➩ Marcy searches the Index to External Causes for the **Place of occurrence** which she abstracted as *outside of single family home*.

- ❑ She locates the Main Term **Place** and the **subterm residence (non-institutional) (private) Y92.00**. She notices there are more subterms for the type of residence, so she does not assign this code.
- ❑ She locates the next level of subterm, **house, single family Y92.019**. She notices there are more subterms for the specific location at the house, so she does not assign this code.
- ❑ She selects the subterm **yard Y92.017** because the accident occurred outside.

➩ Marcy verifies the second external cause code for place of occurrence, **house, single family, yard**.

- ❑ She locates the Tabular List entry for **Y92.017**.
- ❑ She verifies the code title, **Garden or yard in single-family (private) house as the place of occurrence of the external cause**, which accurately describes the situation.
- ❑ She reviews the instructional notes at the beginning of the category **Y92** that instruct her to report this code only at the initial encounter. Next she will assign the code for the Activity.

➩ Marcy searches the Index to External Causes for the **Activity**, which she abstracted as *painting outside of house*.

- ❑ She locates the Main Term **Activity**.
- ❑ She searches for a subterm that describes *painting outside of house*, but cannot find anything that specific.
- ❑ She reviews the subterms again, searching for a broader term that would include *painting outside of house*.
- ❑ She locates the subterm **maintenance**, then the subterm **exterior building NEC Y93.H9**.

➩ Marcy verifies the external cause code for activity, **maintenance, exterior building NEC**.

- ❑ She searches for the Tabular List entry for **Y93.H9**.
- ❑ She locates the category **Y93** and observes that alphabetic characters for the fourth character of the code begin after **Y93.7** and before **Y93.8**.
- ❑ She verifies the code title, **Y93.H9, Activity, other involving exterior property and land maintenance, building and construction**, which accurately describes the situation. Next, Marcy will assign a code for the Status.

➩ Marcy searches the Index to External Causes for the **Status**, which she abstracted as *personal*.

- ❑ She locates the Main Term **Status of external cause** and reviews the subterms.
- ❑ She notices that there is no entry for personal, but there is an entry for **leisure activity Y99.8**.

➩ Marcy verifies the final external cause code for status, **leisure activity**.

- ❑ She locates the Tabular List entry for **Y99.8**.
- ❑ She verifies the code title, **Other external cause status**, which accurately describes the situation

➩ Marcy reviews the information she located in the Index to External Causes.

- ❑ Intent and cause: **accidental fall off ladder W11**
- ❑ Place: **house, single family, yard Y92.017**

- ❑ Activity: **maintenance, exterior building NEC Y93.H9**
- ❑ Status: **leisure activity Y99.8**

⇨ Marcy reviews the diagnosis code, **S82.202A Unspecified fracture of shaft of left tibia, initial encounter.**

⇨ Next, Marcy needs to determine how to sequence the codes.

CODING CAUTION

When place of occurrence, activity, or status are not documented, omit the code. Do not use place of occurrence code **Y92.9** if the place is not stated or is not applicable (OGCR I.C.20.b.). Do not assign **Y93.9 Unspecified activity** if the activity is not stated (OGCR I.C.20.c.) Do not assign code **Y99.9 Unspecified external cause status** if the status is not stated (OGCR I.C.20.k.). Use these codes only when the *documentation specifically states* that the information is not known or available.

Coding Practice

Now it is your turn to practice assigning codes for external causes. Refer to the ***Tip*** at the end of the mini-medical-record if you need a little extra help.

Exercise 8.2 Assigning Codes for External Causes

Instructions: Read the mini-medical-record of each patient's encounter, review the information abstracted in Exercise 8.1, and assign ICD-10-CM diagnosis codes (CM) using the Index to Diseases and Injuries, the Index to External Causes, and the Tabular List. Write the code(s) on the line provided.

1. Date: 8/2/yy Location: Branton Medical Center Emergency Room Provider: Cynthia Hiatt, MD

Patient: Mildred Stiles Gender: F Age: 85

Chief complaint: Laceration on the forehead. Fell off toilet and hit her head on the sink.

Assessment: 3 cm laceration

Plan: see family physician for suture removal in 10 days

***Tip*:** Code the diagnosis and the external cause event. This medical record does not give you information for place, activity, or status codes.

2 CM Codes __________ __________

2. Date: 8/2/yy Location: Branton Medical Center Emergency Room Provider: Cynthia Hiatt, MD

Patient: Constance Macgregor Gender: F Age: 5

Reason for encounter: burn due to accidentally touching hot stove

Assessment: second degree burn to the right hand

Plan: Dressed wound. Instructed parent on wound care. Follow up with family physician in 2 weeks. Call if any problems develop.

***Tip*:** Code the diagnosis and the external cause event. This medical record does not give you information for place, activity, or status codes.

2 CM Codes __________ __________

3. Date: 8/2/yy Location: Branton Medical Center

Provider: Bruce Prentice, MD

Patient: Frank Bernhardt Gender: M Age: 25

Reason for admission: assault by handgun to leg 6 weeks ago. Patient was treated for fracture to femur caused by a bullet. Bullet was removed but fracture has not healed properly so additional surgery is needed.

Discharge diagnosis: malunion of non-displaced comminuted (bone broken into fragments) fracture, left femur shaft

Plan: FU in office in 3 weeks

***Tip*:** Code the diagnosis and the external cause event. This medical record does not give you information for place, activity, or status codes. On the fracture code, assign the seventh character for **subsequent encounter for closed fracture with malunion.**

2 CM Codes __________ __________

ARRANGING CODES FOR EXTERNAL CAUSES

External cause codes are always secondary codes; they can *never* be the principal or first-listed diagnosis. Sequence external cause codes as follows:

1. The principal or first-listed diagnosis.
2. Secondary diagnosis codes from the body system chapters.
3. External cause combination code for the intent and causal event code that most closely supports the principal or first-listed diagnosis. If more than one intent and causal event code applies, sequence them as follows (OGCR I.C.20.b. to f.):
   1) Child and adult abuse
   2) **Terrorism** events (*events designated by the FBI as terrorism*)
   3) Cataclysmic events
   4) Transport accidents
4. Place of occurrence code, if required.
5. Activity code, if required.
6. Status code, if required.

If the reporting format (the claim form or computer screen) limits the number of external cause codes that can be used in reporting clinical data, report the combination code for the intent and causal event most related to the principal diagnosis. If the format permits capture of additional external cause codes, report intent/cause codes of any additional causal events, including misadventures, before reporting the codes for place, activity, or external status (OGCR I.C.20.b. to e.)).

CODING CAUTION

Recall that external cause, place, activity, and status codes are not applicable to poisonings, adverse effects, misadventures, or late effects. When these three types of codes apply, assign them only for the initial encounter.

Guided Example of Arranging External Cause Codes

Continue with the example about Charles Fink, who fell off a ladder while painting his house, in order to practice skills for arranging external cause codes.

➩ Follow along as Marcy Elwood, CCS, sequences the codes she verified earlier. Check off each step after you complete it.

- ❑ Marcy sequences the diagnosis code, **S82.202A, Unspecified fracture of shaft of left tibia, initial encounter** first because it meets the criteria for the first-listed diagnosis.
- ❑ The second code is the external cause code for intent and causal event, **W11.XXXA, Accidental fall from ladder.**
- ❑ The third code is the external cause code for place, **Y92.017, Garden or yard in single-family (private) house as the place of occurrence of the external cause.**
- ❑ The fourth code is the external cause code for activity, **Y93.H9, Activity, other involving exterior property and land maintenance, building and construction.**
- ❑ The fifth code is the external cause code for status, **Y99.8, Other external cause status.**

➩ Finally, Marcy cross-references each code against the medical record to be certain that she did not overlook anything.

➩ The final code assignment and sequencing is

(1) **S82.202A, Unspecified fracture of shaft of left tibia, initial encounter**

(2) **W11.XXXA, Accidental fall from ladder**

(3) **Y92.017, Garden or yard in single-family (private) house as the place of occurrence of the external cause**

(4) **Y93.H9, Activity, other involving exterior property and land maintenance, building and construction**

(5) **Y99.8, Other external cause status**

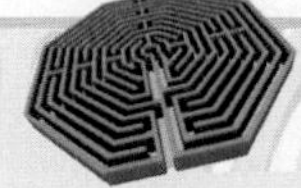

Coding Practice

Now it is your turn to practice sequencing external cause codes. Refer to the ***Tip*** at the end of the mini-medical-record if you need a little extra help.

Exercise 8.3 Arranging Codes for External Causes

Instructions: Read the mini-medical-record of each patient's encounter, review the information abstracted in Exercise 8.1, assign ICD-10-CM diagnosis codes (CM) using the Index to Diseases and Injuries, the Index to External Causes, and the Tabular List, and sequence them correctly.

1. Date: 8/3/yy Location: Branton Medical Center
Provider: Matthew Bunker, MD
Patient: Anthony Mojica Gender: M Age: 47
Reason for admission: heart attack due to overexertion while shoveling snow in driveway of his single family home.
Discharge diagnosis: AMI
Plan: FU in office in 2 weeks

Tip: You need 1 diagnosis code and 4 external cause codes.

5 CM Codes ________ ________ ________ ________ ________

2. Date: 8/3/yy Location: Branton Medical Center
Provider: Bruce Prentice, MD (orthopedic surgeon)
Patient: Darlene Thatcher Gender: F Age: 41
Reason for admission: second surgery for fractured scapula, which was the result of a traffic accident. She was driving a van as a volunteer for the swim team and collided with a pickup truck.
Assessment: displaced fracture of body of left scapula
Plan: follow up in office in 3 weeks

Tip: Report place, activity, and status only for the initial encounter.

2 CM Codes ________ ________

3. Date: 8/3/yy Location: Branton Medical Center Emergency Room Provider: Cynthia Hiatt, MD
Patient: Wayne Ramage Gender: M Age: 53
Reason for encounter: Patient was walking on a public sidewalk while making a delivery as part of his job when he was bit on the leg by a German shepherd dog which was running free in the neighborhood.
Assessment: puncture wound, left calf
Plan: follow up with orthopedic physician in 2 weeks

Tip: This is the initial encounter, so provide the full range of four external cause codes.

5 CM Codes ________ ________ ________ ________ ________

CHAPTER SUMMARY

In this chapter you learned that:

- External cause codes describe the event that created an injury or medical problem.
- ICD-10-CM Chapter 20 External Causes of Morbidity (V00-Y99) contains 33 blocks or subchapters.
- Whenever patients are treated for injuries, adverse effects, or complications from procedures, coders must abstract multiple external cause codes, each describing different aspects of the event.
- Coders use a separate Index to External Causes to locate codes, then verify them in the Tabular List.
- External cause codes are always secondary codes and must be sequenced in a specific order.
- ICD-10-CM provides Official Guidelines for Coding and Reporting (OGCR) in OGCR I.C.20., which discusses when to report codes from this chapter and how they are to be used.

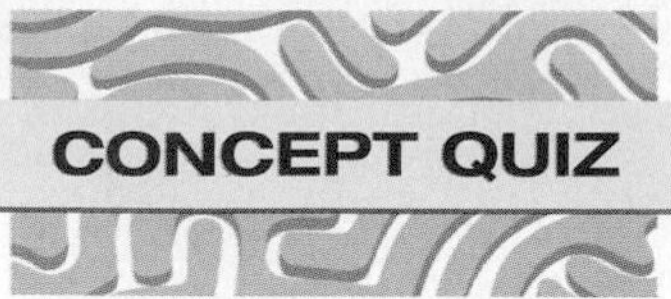

CONCEPT QUIZ

Take a moment to look back at your trip through external causes and solidify your skills. This is your opportunity to pull together everything you have learned.

Completion

Instructions: Write the term that answers each question based on the information you learned in this chapter. Choose from the following list. Some choices may be used more than once and some choices may not be used at all. Refer to the discussion in this chapter and the Glossary at the end of this book if you need a little extra help.

activity	military operations
adverse effect	misadventure
causal event	place
complication	principal
external cause	secondary
falls	status
first-listed	suicide
intent	traffic accident

1. _______________ codes describe the purpose of the injury as accidental or intentional.
2. _______________ is a negative physical reaction.
3. _______________ codes describe what the person was doing at the time of the event.
4. Reporting of _______________ codes allows third-party payers to determine liability for medical costs.
5. _______________ codes describe employment status at the time the event occurred.
6. _______________ and _______________ are reported with a combination code.
7. _______________ is an error during a medical or surgical procedure.
8. External cause codes are always _______________ codes.
9. _______________, _______________, and _______________ codes are NOT applicable to poisonings, adverse effects, misadventures, complications, or late effects.
10. The most commonly used and largest block in the external cause chapter is _______________.

Multiple Choice

Instructions: Circle the letter of the best answer to each question based on the information you learned in this chapter. Refer to the discussion in this chapter and the Glossary at the end of this book if you need a little extra help.

1. What healthcare setting uses external cause codes?
   A. Outpatient setting only
   B. Emergency department only
   C. Inpatient setting only
   D. All healthcare settings
2. Which of the following does NOT describe an intent?
   A. Accidental
   B. Military operation
   C. Assault
   D. Intentional
3. If the intent of the cause of an injury or other condition is unknown or unspecified, code the intent as
   A. undetermined.
   B. accidental.
   C. assault.
   D. external.
4. All transport accident categories assume _______ intent.
   A. assault
   B. accidental
   C. undetermined
   D. external
5. Which of the following is NOT an option for episode of care?
   A. Initial
   B. Subsequent
   C. Final
   D. Sequela
6. Which type of external cause code is reported at every encounter related to the injury?
   A. Intent and cause
   B. Place
   C. Activity
   D. Status
7. Where are external cause codes indexed?
   A. Index to Diseases and Injuries
   B. Index to External Causes
   C. Table of Drugs and Chemicals
   D. Tabular List
8. Which of the following is NOT a Main Term in the Index to External Causes?
   A. Fracture
   B. Failure
   C. Fall
   D. Military operations

9. Which of the following is NOT a status code?
   A. Civilian activity done for pay
   B. Military activity
   C. Volunteer activity
   D. Vacation activity

10. Which code is sequenced first?
   A. Diagnosis code
   B. Causal event code
   C. Place of occurrence code
   D. Status code

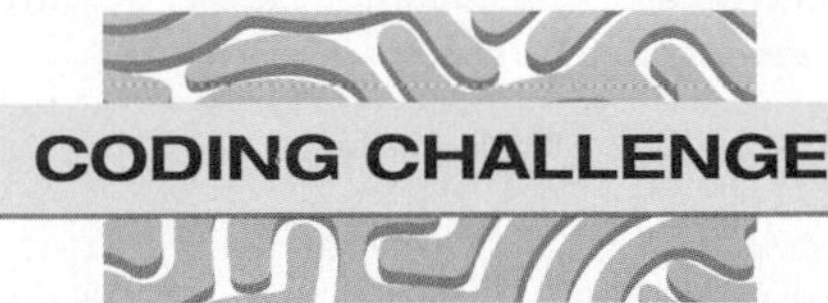

CODING CHALLENGE

Now it is your turn to demonstrate coding all aspects of external causes. Refer back to the examples and discussion in this chapter when you need a little extra help. Use your medical dictionary and anatomy references when needed.

Instructions: Read the mini-medical-record of each patient's encounter and assign diagnosis codes using the Index to Diseases and Injuries, the Index to External Causes, Tabular List, and sequence them correctly. Write the code(s) on the line provided.

1. Date: 8/15/yy Location: Branton Medical Center
Provider: Bruce Prentice, MD
Patient: Olga Mckean Gender: F Age: 20
Reason for admission: Admitted through ED. Patient was on her way home from work and was walking on a local street because there was no sidewalk. It was after dark and a car struck her when the driver did not see her.
Discharge diagnosis: Concussion without loss of consciousness, fracture in the lower end of radius, right arm.
Discharge plan: FU in office 3 weeks. Call if any symptoms such as dizziness or headache.

Tip: Assign a diagnosis code for each injury and assign four external codes. Sequence the concussion as the principal diagnosis.

6 CM Codes __________ __________
__________ __________ __________
____

2. Date: 8/15/yy Location: Branton Medical Center
Provider: Matthew Bunker, MD
Patient: Michael Caruthers Gender: M Age: 19
Reason for admission: Admitted from ED after fall from canoe and submersion in cold water in Branton Lake. He was instructing a class as part of his job.
Discharge diagnosis: bradycardia (*slow heart rate*) due to **hypothermia**, hypoxemia (*oxygen depletion*)
Discharge plan: FU in office, 1 week

Tip: Assign three diagnosis codes and five external cause codes. Instructional notes in the Tabular List for hypothermia direct you to one of the external cause codes.

8 CM Codes __________ __________
__________ __________ __________
__________ __________ __________

3. Date: 8/15/yy Location: Branton Medical Center Provider: Kristen Conover, MD
Patient: Harry Burrus Gender: M Age: 20
Reason for admission: Admitted from ED for dislocated shoulder. He was texting his girlfriend while driving on the freeway and ran his motorcycle into a sign post.
Discharge diagnosis: dislocated right acromioclavicular (shoulder) joint, 100% displacement
Discharge plan: Immobilize joint for 2 weeks. FU in office 2 weeks. Recommended course on motorcycle safety.

Tip: The patient's status is not identified.

4 CM Codes __________ __________
__________ __________

(continued)

(continued from page 141)

4. Date: 8/15/yy Location: Branton Medical Center
Provider: Tanya Schmitt, MD
Patient: Rosa Hayman Gender: F Age: 80
Planned procedure: scheduled for total knee replacement, left knee, due to primary osteoarthritis
Postprocedural diagnosis: procedure performed in error on right knee, which also had degeneration due to osteoarthritis
Discharge plan: Physical therapy and rehab.

***Tip*:** External cause codes for place, activity, and status are not required because this is a misadventure. In the Index to External Causes, under the entry for **Misadventure, performance of inappropriate operation,** you will see a cross-reference to a different Main Term.

2 CM Codes __________ __________

5. Date: 8/15/yy Location: Branton Medical Center Provider: Kristen Conover, MD
Patient: Patrick Bastin Gender: M Age: 21
Reason for admission: knife stab wounds to the chest after a gang fight in a public park
Discharge diagnosis: Intrathoracic wound with laceration of right lung.

***Tip*:** External cause codes for activity and status are not needed.

3 CM Codes __________ __________ __________

6. Date: 8/15/yy Location: Branton Medical Center
Provider: Tanya Schmitt, MD
Patient: Bruce Barnwell Gender: M Age: 22
Reason for admission: Admitted from ED. Patient was riding his bicycle for recreation through a parking lot and was hit by a bus. He impacted the handlebar and appears to have internal injuries.
Assessment: stomach laceration

***Tip*:** The Index to External Causes classifies *bicyclist* using the term **pedal cyclist.**

5 CM Codes __________ __________ __________ __________ __________

7. Date: 8/15/yy Location: Branton Medical Center Emergency Room Provider: Cynthia Hiatt, MD
Patient: Oliver Denison Gender: M Age: 27
Chief complaint: State police officer arrived by ambulance after being struck in the head by a baton while taking down a suspect. Loss of consciousness for 15 minutes.
Assessment: concussion to head

***Tip*:** The causal event is legal intervention. Do not assign an activity code because there is none that adds information to the encounter.

3 CM Codes __________ __________ __________

8. Date: 8/15/yy Location: Branton Medical Center
Provider: Kristen Conover, MD
Patient: Susan Himes Gender: F Age: 18
Reason for admission: stupor, vomiting, muscle cramps, **anhidrosis,** dyspnea, elevated pulse after being outside in the sun all day at the beach where she was working as a lifeguard, body temperature 104 degrees.
Assessment: heat stroke with stupor

***Tip*:** Distinguish integral symptoms of heat stroke from complications that the Tabular List instructional notes direct you to code.

5 CM Codes __________ __________ __________ __________ __________

9. Date: 8/15/yy Location: Branton Family Practice
Provider: Kristen Conover, MD
Patient: Ross Hayman Gender: M Age: 35
Reason for encounter: second visit for sore back after slipping while playing golf
Assessment: MRI negative for disc damage, lumbar sprain
Plan: Refer to physical therapy

2 CM Codes __________ __________

10. Date: 8/15/yy Location: Branton Medical Center Emergency Room Provider: Cynthia Hiatt, MD
Patient: Eugene High Gender: M Age: 28
Chief complaint: put nail through thumb with nail gun while performing his construction job as a carpenter
Assessment: puncture wound, right thumb

4 CM Codes __________ __________ __________ __________

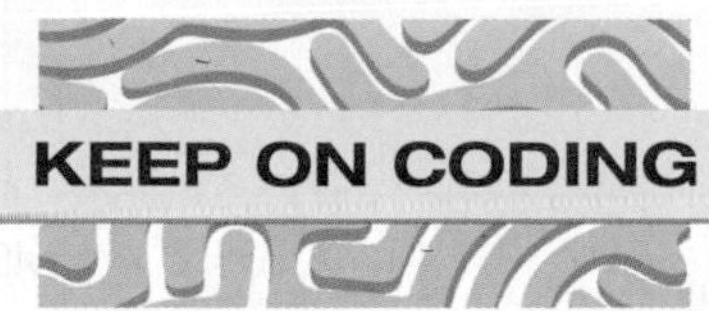

KEEP ON CODING

As a coder, you can never have too much experience. Apply everything you have learned in this chapter to code the following diagnostic statements. Use the OGCR and instructional notes in the Tabular List to help determine how many codes are required.

Instructions: Read the diagnostic statement, then use the Index to External Causes and Tabular List to assign and sequence ICD-10-CM (CM) diagnosis codes. Write the code(s) on the line provided.

1. Burn of the hand while onboard a sailboat, initial encounter: CM Code(s) ________
2. Injury occurred while cheerleading (activity code): CM Code(s) ________
3. Injury while using a chainsaw, subsequent encounter: CM Code(s) ________
4. Late effect of being struck by golf ball: CM Code(s) ________
5. Electrocution by a toaster, suicide attempt, initial encounter: CM Code(s) ________
6. Bitten by a raccoon, initial encounter: CM Code(s) ________
7. Overexposure in a tanning bed, sequela: CM Code(s) ________
8. Incorrect procedure performed on correct patient: CM Code(s) ________
9. Pellet gun injury, intent undetermined, initial encounter: CM Code(s) ________
10. Overexposure to sound waves, subsequent encounter: CM Code(s) ________
11. Burned by a hot toaster, initial encounter: CM Code(s) ________
12. Hunting rifle discharge, unknown intent, initial encounter: CM Code(s) ________
13. Excessive fluid administered during a transfusion: CM Code(s) ________
14. Human bite during an assault, initial encounter: CM Code(s) ________
15. Drowning of undetermined intent after a fall in the swimming pool, initial encounter: CM Code(s) ________
16. Blood alcohol level 65 mg/100 ml: CM Code(s) ________
17. Fall into a well, subsequent encounter: CM Code(s) ________
18. Fall from the steps due to ice, initial encounter: CM Code(s) ________
19. Pecked by a macaw, initial encounter: CM Code(s) ________
20. Fall from a motorcycle, driver, in a nontraffic accident, initial encounter: CM Code(s) ________
21. Fall from scaffolding, initial encounter: CM Code(s) ________
22. Subsequent encounter from being stranded in a snow blizzard: CM Code(s) ________
23. Fall from inline roller skates, subsequent encounter: CM Code(s) ________
24. Injured in the garden of a private house (place of occurrence): CM Code(s) ________
25. Failure of sterile precautions during an injection, initial encounter: CM Code(s) ________

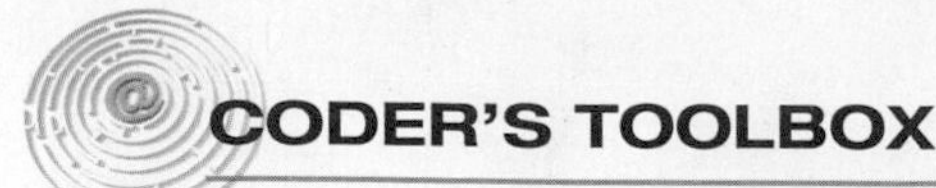

CODER'S TOOLBOX

The following resources are a starting point for learning more about external causes. The > symbol indicates a menu selection within the website in order to navigate to a specific page.

Bureau of Labor Statistics > Injuries, Illnesses, and Fatalities **http://www.bls.gov/iif/**

Centers for Disease Control and Prevention (CDC) > Injury Home **http://www.cdc.gov/HomeandRecreationalSafety/index.html**

Federal Bureau of Investigation (FBI) > Stats & Services > Reports and Publications > Terrorism **http://www.fbi.gov/stats-services/publications**

National Highway Traffic Safety Administration (NHTSA) **http://www.nhtsa.gov/**

National Institute of Mental Health (NIMH) > Health Topics > Publications > Suicide in the US: Statistics and Prevention **http://www.nimh.nih.gov/health/publications/suicide-in-the-us-statistics-and-prevention/index.shtml**

National Institutes of Health > Health Information > Injuries and Wounds **http://health.nih.gov/category/InjuriesandWounds**

Ohio State University Medical Center > Emergency Services > Unintentional Injury Statistics **http://medicalcenter.osu.edu/patientcare/healthcare_services/emergency_services/non_traumatic_emergencies/unintentional_injury_statistics/pages/index.aspx**

Suicide.org > Suicide Statistics **http://www.suicide.org/suicide-statistics.html**

United Stated Department of Labor > Occupational Safety and Health Administration Workplace Injury, Illness and Fatality Statistics **http://www.osha.gov/oshstats/work.html**

US Census Bureau The 2011 Statistical Abstract > Transportation: Motor Vehicle Accidents and Fatalities **http://www.census.gov/compendia/statab/cats/transportation/motor_vehicle_accidents_and_fatalities.html**

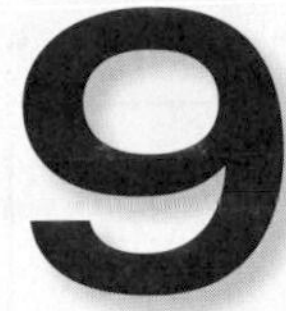

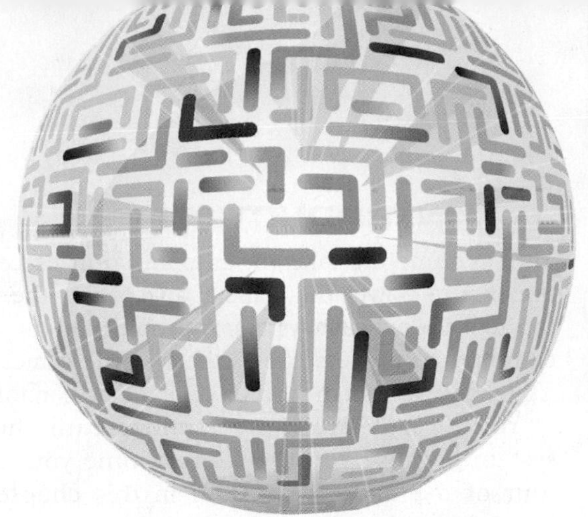

9 Diseases of the Digestive System (K00-K95)

Learning Objectives

After completing this chapter, you should have the skills to:

- Spell and define the key words, medical terms, and abbreviations related to the digestive system.
- Discuss the structure, function, and common conditions of the digestive system.
- Identify the main characteristics of coding for the digestive system.
- Abstract diagnostic information from the medical record for coding diseases of the digestive system.
- Assign codes to patient encounters related to the digestive system.
- Arrange multiple codes for patient encounters related to the digestive system.
- Abstract, assign, and sequence codes for neoplasms of the digestive system.
- Discuss the Official Guidelines for Coding and Reporting for the digestive system.

Key Terms and Abbreviations

accessory organs
alimentary canal
barium enema
comorbidity
digestive system
diverticulosis
diverticula
diverticulitis
endoscopic retrograde cholangiopancreatography (ERCP)
gastrointestinal (GI) system
Helicobacter pylori (H. pylori)
nasogastric

In addition to the key terms listed here, students should know the terms defined within tables in this chapter.

Chapter Outline

- **Digestive System Refresher**
- **Coding Overview of the Digestive System**
- **Abstracting for the Digestive System**
- **Assigning Codes for the Digestive System**
- **Arranging Codes for the Digestive System**
- **Coding Neoplasms of the Digestive System**

ICD-10-CM codes in this chapter are from the ICD-10-CM 2014 Draft code set from the Department of Health and Human Services, Centers for Disease Control and Prevention.

INTRODUCTION

Your automobile takes in gasoline, utilizes certain components to power the vehicle, and expels the byproducts through the exhaust system. A problem at any point in the complicated process affects the way the vehicle functions. The digestive system serves a similar function for your body.

You already are quite familiar with the digestive system because you use it every time you eat. In your tour of the digestive system in this chapter you will learn more about how the digestive system works, why sometimes it does not work as it should, and how physicians treat these conditions. Most importantly, you will practice coding for patient encounters related to digestive diseases and conditions, a skill that requires you to abstract information from the mini-medical-record, assign correct codes, and arrange (sequence) the codes in the proper order.

Gastroenterologists are physicians who specialize in the study, diagnosis, and treatment of digestive system diseases. Dentists specialize in the study, diagnosis, and treatment of disorders of the oral cavity, which is part of the digestive system. Primary care physicians and internal medicine physicians treat many common digestive system disorders. They refer complex cases to a gastroenterologist or dentist.

As you study this chapter, open up your medical terminology and anatomy reference books to the chapters on the digestive system. A medical dictionary (physical or online) will also help you. Just as you take a basic tool kit and first aid kit with you when travelling, your coding resources ensure that you have the information you need at your fingertips.

DIGESTIVE SYSTEM REFRESHER

The function of the **digestive system**, also called the **gastrointestinal (GI) system**, is to receive nutrients, break them down, absorb them into the blood to be used by the body, and eliminate solid waste products. The digestive system consists of the **alimentary canal** and **accessory organs** (■ FIGURE 9-1). The alimentary canal is a continuous tube, approximately 30 feet in length, which begins at the mouth; continues through the esophagus, stomach, small intestine, and large intestine; and exits the body at the rectum and anus. The accessory organs assist in digestion, but are not directly connected to the alimentary canal. They are the salivary glands, liver, gall bladder, and pancreas.

Each structure in the digestive system is labeled with its name as well as its medical terminology root/combining form in Figure 9-1. As you learn about conditions and procedures that affect the digestive system, remember to apply medical terminology skills to combine the root or combining form for the body part with the suffixes you already know to define new terms for conditions and procedures, as shown in ■ TABLE 9-1.

CODING CAUTION

Be alert for medical word roots with similar spellings but different meanings:

chole/o (*bile or gall*), **col/o** (*colon*), and **colp/o** (*vagina*)

cholecyst/o (*gall bladder*) and **cyst/o** (*bladder or sac, often used in reference to the urinary bladder*)

ile/o (*ileum, part of the small intestine*) and **ili/o** (*ilium, the pelvic bone*)

ileum (*small intestine*) and **ileus** (*a paralytic condition of the small intestine*)

Conditions of the Digestive System

The functions of the digestive system are:

- ingestion—taking in food (mouth, esophagus; aided by the salivary glands)
- digestion—breaking down food (stomach, small intestine; aided by the liver, gall bladder, and pancreas)
- absorption—transferring nutrients to the body (small intestine, large intestine)
- elimination—removing solid waste from the body (large intestine, rectum, anus)

SUCCESS STEP

Remember the difference between an organ system and a body region or cavity. Do not confuse the digestive system (an organ system) with the abdomen (a body region or cavity). Digestive system organs are located in the head, neck, thoracic cavity, abdominal cavity, and pelvic cavity.

Digestive system conditions account for approximately 12% of all inpatient procedures and 31% of all ambulatory procedures, according to the National Digestive Diseases Information Clearinghouse (NDDIC). Treating these conditions costs about $98 billion per year. Over 236,000 people die each year from digestive system conditions. Diseases and conditions of the digestive system can be caused by heredity, the type and amount of food consumed, substance abuse, particularly alcohol and tobacco, or mental health conditions. Diseases are diagnosed through a combination of physical examination, medical

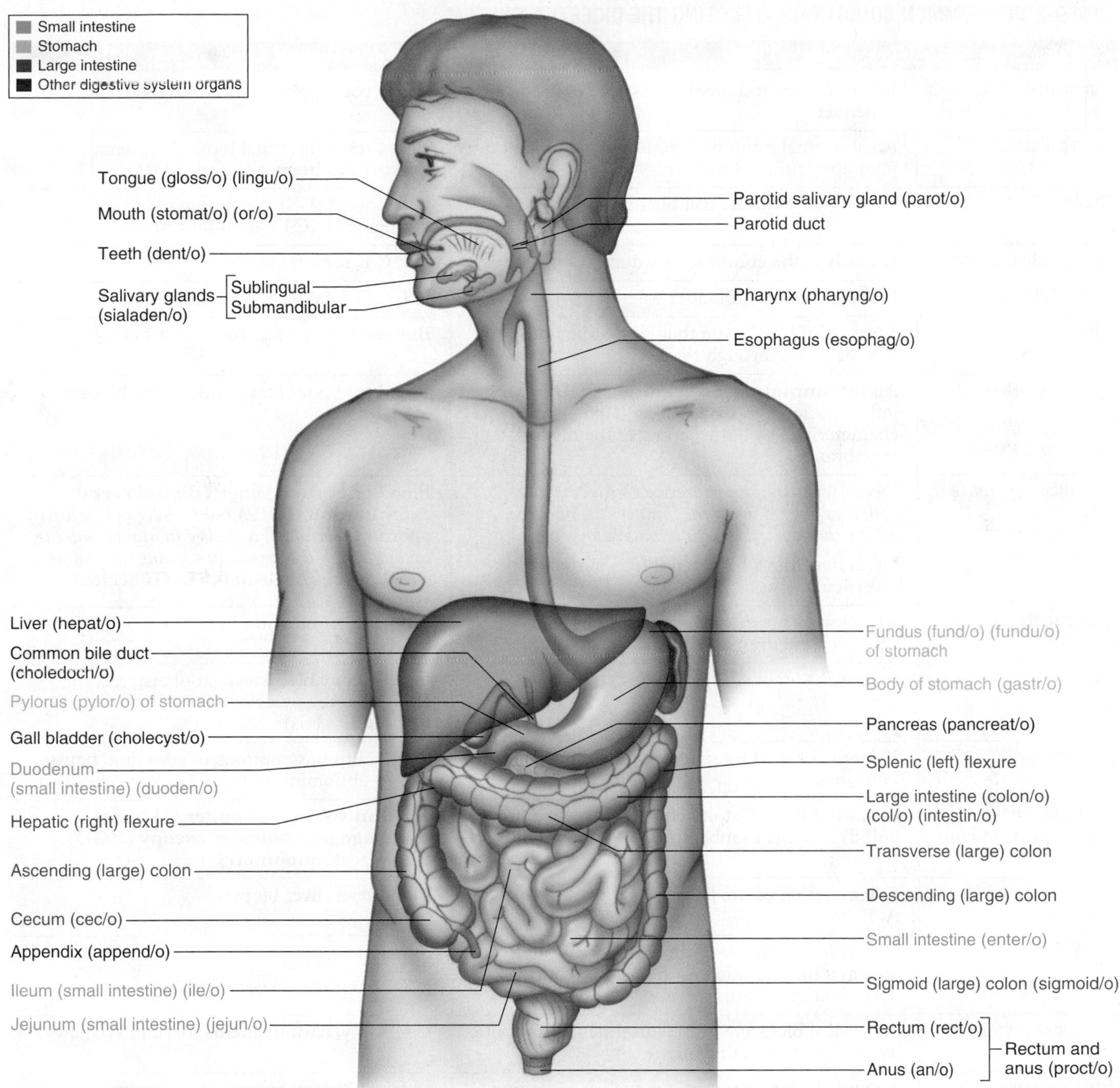

Figure 9-1 ■ The Digestive (Gastrointestinal) System

Table 9-1 ■ EXAMPLE OF CONSTRUCTING MEDICAL TERMS FOR THE DIGESTIVE SYSTEM

Combining Form	Suffix	Complete Medical Term
gastr/o (*stomach*) **enter/o** (*intestines*) **colon/o** (*large intestine*)	**-logy** (*study of*)	**gastro + entero + logy** (*the study of the stomach and intestines*)
	-itis (*inflammation*)	**gastr + itis** (*inflammation of the stomach*) **enter + itis** (*inflammation of the intestines*)
	-scopy (*visual examination*)	**gastro + scopy** (*visual examination of the stomach*) **colono + scopy** (*visual examination of the large intestine*)

Table 9-2 ■ **COMMON CONDITIONS AFFECTING THE DIGESTIVE SYSTEM**

Condition	Description	Diagnostic Methods
Appendicitis	Inflammation and possible rupture of the appendix	Blood count, physical examination
Celiac disease	An abnormal immune reaction to gluten and poor absorption of nutrients	Blood tests, intestinal biopsy, presence of **dermatitis herpetiformis (DH)**
Cholecystitis	Inflammation of the gall bladder	Ultrasound (US), computerized axial tomography (CT), fecal fat test
Choledocholithiasis	**Calculi** in the common bile duct	US, CT, fecal fat test
Cholelithiasis	Calculi in the gall bladder	US, CT, fecal fat test
Cirrhosis	Scarring of liver tissue that blocks the normal flow of blood through the liver	Blood tests, imaging tests, liver biopsy
Crohn's disease	An **inflammatory bowel disease (IBD)** with inflammation and ulcers in the alimentary tract characterized by a thickening of the mucous membrane	Blood tests, stool test, endoscopy, biopsy
Diverticular disease	Diverticulosis: the presence of diverticula (*pouches formed when the lining of the intestine pushes through the intestinal muscle layer*) Diverticulitis: a bacterial infection of diverticula	Blood tests, stool sample, **digital rectal examination (DRE)** colonoscopy, barium enema (*injection of a chalky substance into the colon through the anus and viewing the organs on an X-ray; also called* **lower GI series)**
Esophagitis	Irritation of the esophagus caused by acid reflux and weak **cardiac sphincter**	Physical examination, symptoms of **heartburn**
Gastritis	Inflammation of stomach lining	Gastroscopy blood test, stool test, test for Helicobacter pylori, or H. pylori (*bacteria that causes ulcers*)
Gastroenteritis	Bacterial or viral infection of the stomach and intestines	Stool culture, symptoms of vomiting, nausea, and/or abdominal pain
Gastroesophageal reflux disease (GERD)	Backward flow of stomach contents (food or liquid) into the esophagus	**Barium swallow** or **upper GI series**, **esophagogastroduodenoscopy (EGD)**, esophageal **manometry**
Hepatitis	Inflammation of the liver due to viruses named A, B, or C	Blood tests, liver biopsy
Hernia	Protrusion of an organ through a weakened area in a muscle, such as the diaphragm (hiatal hernia) or groin muscle (inguinal hernia)	X-ray
Intestinal obstruction	A physical blockage of the intestine that prevents waste from passing through	CT, X-ray, barium enema, barium swallow
Irritable Bowel Syndrome (IBS)	A combination of symptoms such as cramping, abdominal pain, bloating, constipation, diarrhea	Medical history, symptoms, examination, rule out other problems
Pancreatitis	Inflammation of the pancreas	US, CT, **endoscopic ultrasound (EUS)**, **magnetic resonance cholangiopancreatography (MRCP)**
Stomatitis	Redness, ulcers, and/or bleeding of the mouth due to bacteria, viruses, or fungi	Physical examination, immunological tests, cultures
Ulcer	A sore on the lining of the stomach (gastric ulcer) or duodenum (peptic ulcer)	Blood test for h. pylori, urea breath test, stool antigen test, endoscopy, barium swallow
Ulcerative colitis	An inflammatory bowel disease (IBD) with inflammation and sores, called ulcers, in the lining of the rectum and colon	Physical examination, medical history, blood tests, stool sample, colonoscopy, sigmoidoscopy
Volvulus	Twisting of a portion of the small or large intestine or stomach into a loop that obstructs the passage of digestive material	CT, X-ray, barium enema, barium swallow, endoscopy blood tests

history, signs and symptoms, blood tests, imaging, endoscopy, and biopsy. Common treatments include dietary changes, alcohol and tobacco abstinence, medication, and/or surgery.

■ TABLE 9-2 highlights common conditions affecting the digestive system and common diagnostic methods. This table provides a general reference to help understand where a particular diagnosis or procedure fits into the overall picture of the digestive system, but it does not list everything you need to know. Use medical terminology skills discussed above to learn the meaning of unfamiliar words. Refer to the resources in the Coder's Toolbox at the end of this chapter to learn more about conditions affecting the digestive system.

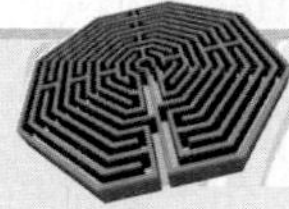

Coding Practice

Refresh your knowledge of digestive system terminology and practice coding simple conditions that affect the digestive system. Use a medical terminology text or a website such as GlobalRph.com > Medical Terminology **http://www.globalrph.com/medterm.htm** to identify the meaning of word parts that may not be familiar to you.

Follow these steps:

- Use slash marks "/" to break down each term into its root(s) and suffix.
- Define the meaning of the word, based on the meaning of each word part.
- Assign the default diagnosis code for the condition using the Index and Tabular List.

Exercise 9.1 Digestive System Refresher

Instructions: Use your medical terminology skills and resources to define the following conditions of the digestive system, then assign the diagnosis code.

Example: gastritis gastr/itis Meaning: *inflammation of the stomach* Code: *K29.70*

1. ileus Meaning ______________ Code ________
2. hematemesis Meaning ______________ Code ________
3. gingivitis Meaning ______________ Code ________
4. volvulus Meaning ______________ Code ________
5. stomatitis Meaning ______________ Code ________
6. hepatoma Meaning ______________ Code ________
7. diverticulitis Meaning ______________ Code ________
8. diverticulosis Meaning ______________ Code ________
9. proctitis Meaning ______________ Code ________
10. cholangitis Meaning ______________ Code ________

CODING OVERVIEW OF THE DIGESTIVE SYSTEM

Chapter 11 of ICD-10-CM, Diseases of the Digestive System (K00-K94), contains 10 blocks or subchapters that are divided by anatomical site. Review the block names and code ranges listed at the beginning of Chapter 11 in the ICD-10-CM manual to become familiar with the content and organization. Review the **Excludes2** note that lists several conditions not classified to this chapter, such as digestive conditions that are perinatal, congenital, pregnancy-related, injuries, symptoms, or neoplasms. Each of these conditions will be discussed in the corresponding chapter of ICD-10-CM, with the exception of neoplasms, which are discussed at the end of this chapter.

ICD-10-CM Chapter 11 corresponds with ICD-9-CM Chapter 9 (520-579). Extensive instructional notes direct coders to assign additional codes to identify certain lifestyle habits involving use or exposure to tobacco and alcohol. Crohn's disease has been expanded from a single code in ICD-9-CM to multiple subcategories and codes, which identify site and complications. Classification of ulcers does not include the presence or absence of an obstruction in ICD-10-CM. Hemorrhoids have been moved from the circulatory system in ICD-9-CM to the digestive system in ICD-10-CM.

ICD-10-CM provides no Official Guidelines for Coding and Reporting (OGCR) for the digestive system. Combination codes that describe complications of digestive system conditions are common. In addition, frequent instructional notes direct coders to use multiple codes to describe the underlying cause or harmful lifestyle habits that contribute to gastrointestinal conditions. Review OGCR section I.B.9. and 7. of the General Coding Guidelines to review the use of combination codes and multiple coding, respectively.

ABSTRACTING FOR THE DIGESTIVE SYSTEM

When abstracting for the digestive system, coders need to look for manifestations, complications, and lifestyle habits associated with digestive system conditions. Key factors to review for coding cases that involve the digestive system appear in ■ TABLE 9-3. Remember that the abstracting questions are a guide and that not every question applies to, or can be answered for, every case. For example, lifestyle habits may not be present for every patient.

Manifestations are symptoms and signs that occur as a result of the underlying condition. Certain digestive system diseases can exist alone or as a manifestation of another condition. For example, liver disorders can be a manifestation of congenital syphilis or congenital **toxoplasmosis**.

Common complications in the digestive system are bleeding, obstruction, and infection. Ulcers, enteritis, colitis, and gastritis may occur with or without bleeding. An obstruction is a blockage of an organ and can be caused by calculi (stones), tumors, organic matter, or volvulus. Gall bladder and intestinal diseases may occur with or without an obstruction. When an infection is present, coders need to abstract the infectious agent, such as *Streptococcus, Escherichia coli*, or *Staphylococcus*.

Lifestyle habits are patient behaviors that cause or contribute to a condition. Lifestyle habits that contribute to many digestive system conditions include use, history of use, dependence, and exposure to tobacco or tobacco smoke and alcohol.

Many digestive system codes are combination codes that include the complication or comorbidity (*two diseases occurring together*). Multiple coding is needed for lifestyle habits and for complications and comorbidities that do not have a combination code. When abstracting, coders do not necessarily know which complications and comorbidities will be assigned a combination code and which will require multiple coding.

Table 9-3 ■ KEY CRITERIA FOR ABSTRACTING DIGESTIVE SYSTEM CONDITIONS

- ❑ What is the condition?
- ❑ What is the anatomic site?
- ❑ What is the laterality, if any?
- ❑ Is bleeding or hemorrhaging documented?
- ❑ What other manifestations or complications are documented?
- ❑ What comorbidities are documented?
- ❑ What lifestyle habits are documented as current or with a history of, such alcohol use or abuse and tobacco exposure, use, or abuse?

Guided Example of Abstracting for the Digestive System

Refer to the following example throughout this chapter to practice skills for abstracting, assigning, and sequencing codes for digestive system conditions. Jill Hynes, CPC, is a fictitious coder who guides you through this case.

Date: 9/1/yy Location: Branton Gastroenterology
Provider: Stanley Garrett, MD
Patient: Gina Addington Gender: F Age: 28
Chief complaint: rectal bleeding, Crohn's disease since age 10
Assessment: Crohn's disease, colon, new complication of rectal bleeding
Plan: liquid diet 1 week, FU if not improved

Follow along as Jill Hynes, CPC, abstracts the diagnosis. Check off each step after you complete it.

⇨ Jill refers to the Key Criteria for Abstracting Digestive System Conditions (Table 9-3).

- ❑ *What is the condition?* Crohn's disease
- ❑ *What is the anatomic site?* colon
- ❑ *Is bleeding or hemorrhaging documented?* Yes, rectal bleeding, which is a new complication.
- ❑ *What other manifestations or complications are documented?* None
- ❑ *What comorbidities are documented?* None
- ❑ *What lifestyle habits are documented as current or with a history of?* None

⇨ Until Jill researches this condition in the ICD-10-CM manual to assign codes, she does not know if Crohn's disease with rectal bleeding will require one or two codes.

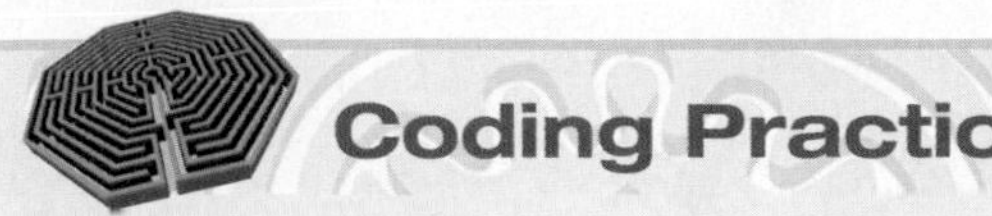

Coding Practice

Now it is your turn to practice abstracting diagnoses for the digestive system. Questions guide your thinking on each scenario. Do not assign any codes.

Exercise 9.2 Abstracting for the Digestive System

Instructions: Read the mini-medical-record of each patient's encounter and answer the abstracting questions. Write the answer on the line provided. Do not assign any codes.

1. Date: 9/3/yy Location: Branton Gastroenterology
Provider: Stanley Garrett, MD
Patient: Mike Dahlberg Gender: M Age: 54
Chief complaint: indigestion
Assessment: chronic perforated peptic ulcer in stomach with bleeding
Plan: change diet, change Rx

a. What symptom is documented? ______

b. Where is the ulcer located? ______

c. What signs or complications are present? ______

d. Is the ulcer acute or chronic? ______

e. Will you code for the symptoms? ______
Why or why not? ______

f. What is the diagnosis to be coded? ______

2. Date: 9/3/yy Location: Valley Hospital Outpatient Surgery Provider: Stanley Garrett, MD
Patient: Natasha Schumacher Gender: F Age: 61
Procedure: repair, right inguinal hernia
Postprocedural diagnosis: recurrent right inguinal hernia
Plan: FU in office

a. Where is an inguinal hernia located? ______

(continued)

2. (continued)

b. Is the hernia unilateral or bilateral? ______

c. Is the hernia documented as recurrent? ______

d. Is an obstruction documented? ______

e. Is gangrene documented? ______

3. Date: 9/3/yy Location: Branton Gastroenterology Provider: Stanley Garrett, MD
Patient: Tony Drennen Gender: M Age: 67
Reason for visit: FU on lower GI series
Assessment: ulcerative colitis with fistula (*an abnormal connection between an organ, vessel, or intestine and another structure*)
Plan: begin liquid diet, Rx antibiotics, FU 2 weeks

a. What test is the follow-up visit for? ______

b. Should you code for the lab test? ______
Why or why not? ______

c. What type of colitis is documented? ______

d. What complication is documented? ______

e. What diagnosis will you code? ______

4. Date: 9/4/yy Location: Branton Gastroenterology Provider: Stanley Garrett, MD
Patient: Jeremy Mcnamara Gender: M Age: 56
Chief complaint: abdominal pain and bloating, fatigue, vomiting
Assessment: alcoholic liver cirrhosis with ascites due to alcohol addiction

(continued)

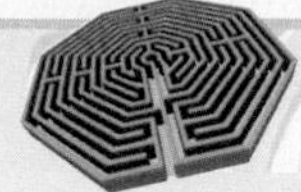

Coding Practice (continued)

4. (continued)

Plan: counseled patient regarding abstinence from alcohol, reduce salt intake

a. What symptoms are documented? ______

b. What is the anatomic site of the cirrhosis? ______

c. What complication is present? ______

d. What is the cause of the cirrhosis? ______

e. What lifestyle habit is documented? ______

f. Will you code the symptoms? ______
Why or why not? ______

g. What diagnosis will you code? ______

5. Date: 9/4/yy Location: Branton Gastroenterology
Provider: Stanley Garrett, MD
Patient: Robin Mitchell Gender: M Age: 59
Chief complaint: hematemesis, history of cirrhosis
Assessment: portal hypertension (*increase in blood pressure in the portal vein*) with portal hypertensive gastropathy
Plan: endoscopic therapy, drug therapy, and dietary changes

a. What symptom(s) are documented? ______

(continued)

5. (continued)

b. Is cirrhosis past or present? ______
Why? ______

c. What is the primary condition diagnosed? ______

d. What is the complication? ______

e. Will you code the symptoms? ______
Why or why not? ______

f. Will you code the cirrhosis? ______
Why? ______

g. What is the first-listed diagnosis? ______

6. Date: 9/4/yy Location: Branton Gastroenterology Provider: Stanley Garrett, MD
Patient: Kenneth Bode Gender: M Age: 33
Chief complaint: redness and tenderness around colostomy site
Assessment: colostomy infection, cellulitis of abdominal wall due to methicillin susceptible staphylococcus aureus (MSSA)

a. What symptom(s) are documented? ______

b. What two conditions are documented? ______

c. What is the infectious agent? ______

d. Will you code the symptoms? ______
Why or why not? ______

ASSIGNING CODES FOR THE DIGESTIVE SYSTEM

Coders frequently assign combination codes to describe common complications or manifestations of digestive system conditions. As a result, the digestive system chapter in ICD-10-CM has more codes and more detail than ICD-9-CM. For example, the category **K50 Crohn's disease** contains over 25 codes, many of which are combination codes that describe common complications of Crohn's disease. This is in contrast to ICD-9-CM, which contained only four codes, to identify the anatomical site, in the category **555 Regional enteritis**. Crohn is an eponym for Burrill Bernard Crohn, a gastroenterologist who identified the condition in 1932. Most codes in category **K50 Crohn's disease** contain six characters:

- Characters 1 to 3 classify Crohn's disease in general.
- Character 4 identifies the site as the small intestine, large intestine, both, or unspecified.
- Character 5 indicates whether a complication is present.
- Character 6 describes the specific complication.

Index entries for conditions with combination codes can be rather long and involved, with many subterms and many levels of indentation, in order to identify all the possible combinations of conditions. Be thorough when searching these entries to be certain to locate the correct item. When verifying the code in the Tabular List, read the description carefully to be sure it matches the combination of conditions in the scenario. Many wrong turns can be caught when verifying.

Guided Example of Assigning Digestive System Codes

Continue with the example from earlier in the chapter about patient Gina Addington, who had Crohn's disease, to practice skills for assigning digestive system codes.

Follow along in your ICD-10-CM manual as Jill Hynes, CPC, assigns codes to the diagnosis. Check off each step after you complete it.

⇨ Jill begins by locating the Main Term in the Index.

- ❑ Jill looks up **C, Crohn's disease**.
- ❑ She reviews the cross-reference note that directs her to **E, Enteritis, regional** (■ Figure 9-2). (With experience, you will learn to go directly to the entry for **Enteritis, regional**.)
- ❑ Under the entry for **E, Enteritis, regional** Jill reviews the subterms that describe the various sites within the intestinal tract.
- ❑ She locates the subterm for **colon**.
- ❑ Jill reviews the instruction to cross-reference the subterm **Enteritis, regional, large intestine**.

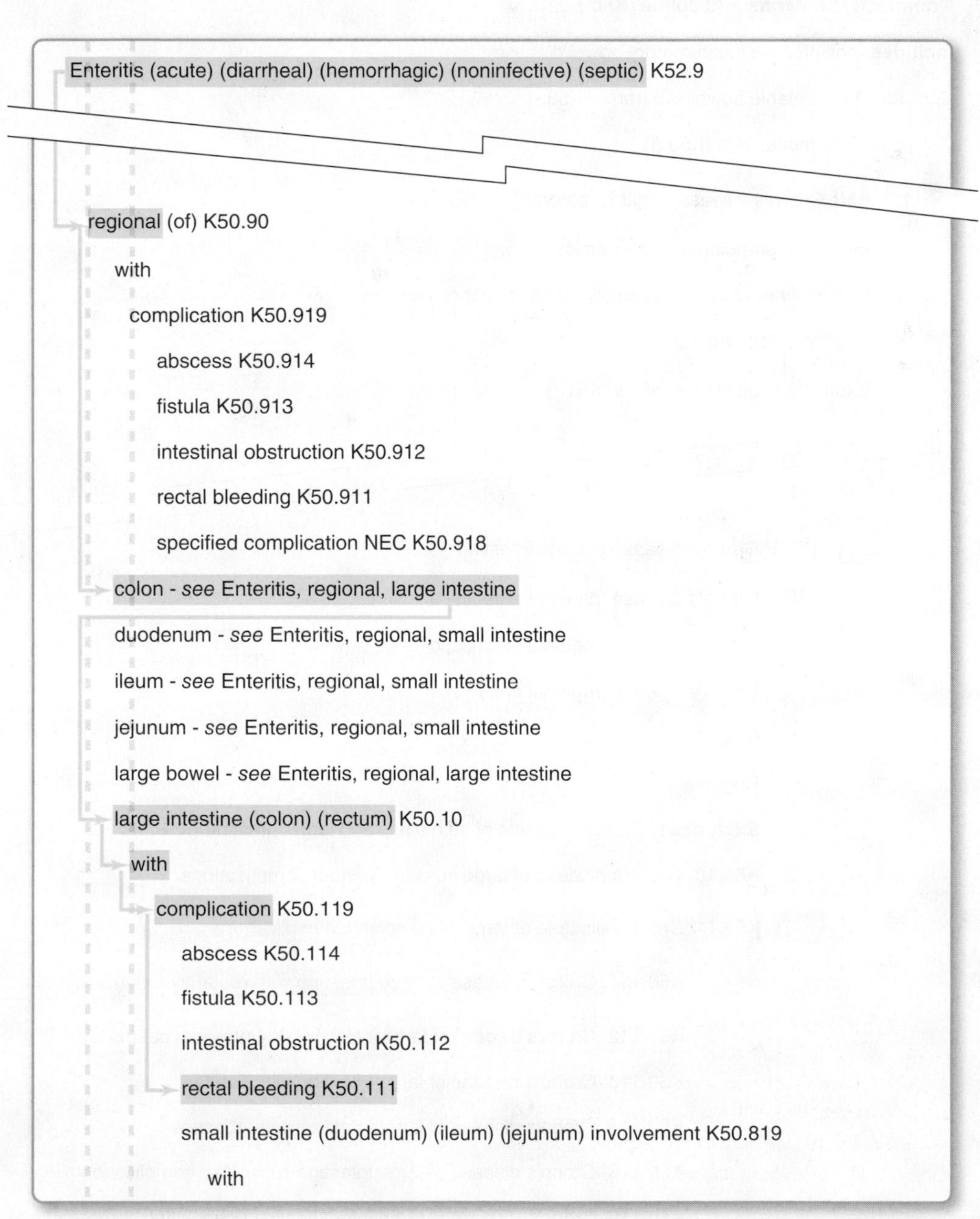

Enteritis (acute) (diarrheal) (hemorrhagic) (noninfective) (septic) K52.9

regional (of) K50.90
  with
    complication K50.919
      abscess K50.914
      fistula K50.913
      intestinal obstruction K50.912
      rectal bleeding K50.911
      specified complication NEC K50.918
  colon - *see* Enteritis, regional, large intestine
  duodenum - *see* Enteritis, regional, small intestine
  ileum - *see* Enteritis, regional, small intestine
  jejunum - *see* Enteritis, regional, small intestine
  large bowel - *see* Enteritis, regional, large intestine
  large intestine (colon) (rectum) K50.10
    with
      complication K50.119
        abscess K50.114
        fistula K50.113
        intestinal obstruction K50.112
        rectal bleeding K50.111
        small intestine (duodenum) (ileum) (jejunum) involvement K50.819
          with

Figure 9-2 ■ Index Entry for Enteritis, Regional

- ❑ Under the subterm for **large intestine,** Jill reviews the additional subterms that describe various associated conditions and complications.
- ❑ She refers back to the medical record and identifies the complication of rectal bleeding.
- ❑ She locates the subentry for **with,** then **rectal bleeding**.
- ❑ Jill confirms that there are no further subentries under **rectal bleeding** and identifies the code **K50.111** that she will verify in the Tabular List.

⇨ Now Jill verifies the code in the Tabular List. She locates the entry for code **K50.111**.

- ❑ Jill confirms that the code description **Crohn's disease of large intestine with rectal bleeding** accurately describes the diagnosis (■ FIGURE 9-3).
- ❑ She notes that a seventh character is not required because there is not a 7th symbol next to it and there are no additional codes under it.
- ❑ Jill reviews the instructional notes at the beginning of the subclassification **K50.1** that state which sites are included. She sees that Crohn's disease of both the colon and rectum are included in this subcategory. The **Excludes1** note reminds her that this entry *excludes* Crohn's disease that affects *both* the large and small intestines and she should

Noninfective enteritis and colitis (K50-K52)

Includes: noninfective inflammatory bowel disease

Excludes1: irritable bowel syndrome (K58.-)

megacolon (K59.3)

4th K50 Crohn's disease [regional enteritis]

Includes: granulomatous enteritis

Use additional code to identify manifestations, such as:

pyoderma gangrenosum (L88)

Excludes1: ulcerative colitis (K51.-)

5th K50.1 Crohn's disease of large intestine

Crohn's disease [regional enteritis] of colon

Crohn's disease [regional enteritis] of large bowel

Crohn's disease [regional enteritis] of rectum

Granulomatous colitis

Regional colitis

Excludes1: Crohn's disease of both small and large intestine (K50.8)

K50.10 Crohn's disease of large intestine without complications

6th K50.11 Crohn's disease of large intestine with complications

K50.111 Crohn's disease of large intestine with rectal bleeding

K50.112 Crohn's disease of large intestine with intestinal obstruction

K50.113 Crohn's disease of large intestine with fistula

K50.114 Crohn's disease of large intestine with abscess

K50.118 Crohn's disease of large intestine with other complication

K50.119 Crohn's disease of large intestine with unspecified complications

Figure 9-3 ■ Tabular List Entry for Crohn's Disease

cross-reference subcategory **K50.8** if that is what she were coding. She makes a mental note of this for future reference.

- ❑ She reviews the instructional notes at the beginning of the category **K50**. She notes there is an instruction to **Use additional code to identify manifestations**. Jill checks the chart note to be certain that it does not mention any manifestations, which it does not. If Dr. Garrett had listed more manifestations, this is how she would know they should be coded in addition to Crohn's disease. She also reads the **Includes** and **Excludes** notes and concludes that she is on the right track.
- ❑ Next, Jill reviews the instructional notes at the beginning of the block **Noninfective enteritis and colitis (K50-K52)**. None of these exclusions apply to the current case.
- ❑ Finally, she checks back to the beginning of ICD-10-CM Chapter 11 and reviews the **Excludes** notes to be sure that none of these exclusions apply to her current case.

SUCCESS STEP

Do not become frustrated by multiple cross-references. When driving, you may see a detour sign that redirects your course. Sometimes part way through the detour the signs seem to stop and you wonder if you are still on the right path or if you missed a sign that directs you to an important turn. When that happens, it can take awhile to get back on the right street. You do not want to let this happen when coding! Cross-references are ICD-10-CM's way of making sure you get to the right place.

⇨ Jill is confident that she completed all verifications and cross-checks, so she assigns code **K50.111, Crohn's disease of large intestine with rectal bleeding**.

SUCCESS STEP

ICD-10-CM uses the term *hemorrhage* when describing a bleeding ulcer, but uses the term *bleeding* when describing bleeding in gastritis, enteritis, duodenitis, and diverticular disease.

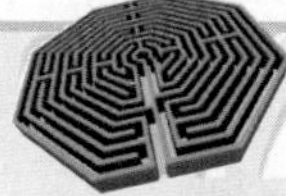

Coding Practice

Now it is your turn to practice combination coding for digestive system conditions. Refer to the ***Tip*** at the end of the mini-medical-record if you need a little extra help.

Exercise 9.3 Assigning Codes for the Digestive System

Instructions: Read the mini-medical-record of each patient's encounter, review the information abstracted in Exercise 9.2 for questions 1, 2, and 3, and assign ICD-10-CM diagnosis codes (CM) using the Index and Tabular List. For questions 4 and 5, abstract the cases on your own, before assigning codes. Write the code(s) on the line provided.

1. Date: 9/3/yy Location: Branton Gastroenterology
Provider: Stanley Garrett, MD
Patient: Mike Dahlberg Gender: M Age: 54
Chief complaint: indigestion
Assessment: chronic perforated peptic ulcer in stomach with bleeding
Plan: change diet, change Rx

Tip: The location of this peptic ulcer is specified, so carefully review all the subterms.

1 CM Code __________

2. Date: 9/3/yy Location: Valley Hospital Outpatient Surgery Provider: Stanley Garrett, MD
Patient: Natasha Schumacher Gender: F Age: 61
Procedure: repair, right inguinal hernia
Postprocedural diagnosis: recurrent right inguinal hernia
Plan: FU in office

Tip: Code for unilateral but not right vs. left side.

1 CM Code __________

3. Date: 9/3/yy Location: Branton Gastroenterology Provider: Stanley Garrett, MD
Patient: Tony Drennen Gender: M Age: 67
Reason for visit: FU on lower GI series
Assessment: ulcerative colitis with fistula
Plan: begin liquid diet, Rx antibiotics, FU 2 weeks

1 CM Code __________

(continued)

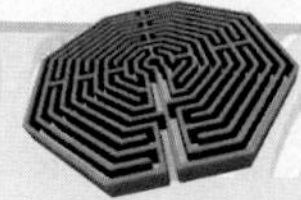

Coding Practice (continued)

4. Date: 9/3/yy Location: Branton Gastroenterology Provider: Stanley Garrett, MD

Patient: Sam Dowdell Gender: M Age: 31

Chief complaint: cramping and diarrhea for 3 days, not helped with OTC antidiarrheals

Assessment: irritable bowel syndrome with diarrhea

Plan: modify diet, Rx antidepressant

Tip: Dr. Stanley prescribed an antidepressant not because the patient was depressed, but because tricyclic antidepressants have proven to be effective in relieving stomach pain in IBS, according to current research (see Coder's Toolbox at the end of the chapter).

1 CM Code __________

5. Date: 9/3/yy Location: Branton Medical Center

Provider: Stanley Garrett, MD

Patient: Penny France Gender: F Age: 47

Reason for admission: rectal bleeding, history of diverticulosis

Assessment: diverticulitis of small and large intestines with bleeding

Plan: IV fluids, monitoring, determine if surgery is needed

Tip: Review the subterms and indentations in the index carefully because you will find several variations of this condition.

1 CM Code __________

ARRANGING CODES FOR THE DIGESTIVE SYSTEM

In order to sequence codes for the digestive system correctly, coders need to follow instructional notes in the Tabular List, which directs coders to assign additional codes for associated conditions, underlying causes, and external causes related to digestive system conditions. Instructional notes direct coders whether the cross-referenced codes should be sequenced as additional codes or whether they should be coded first. ■ TABLE 9-4 highlights the most common instructional notes in the digestive system chapter and the categories where they appear. Notice that multiple coding is often required to describe lifestyle habits, such as alcohol abuse or tobacco abuse, which may contribute to digestive system conditions.

Instructional notes may appear at the beginning of the chapter, the beginning of a block or subchapter, the beginning of a three-character category, the beginning of a subcategory, or under the final code. Therefore, it is important to search for information not only directly under the code, but also at the previous levels of the classification hierarchy.

Guided Example of Arranging Digestive System Codes

Refer to the following new example to practice skills for sequencing codes for the digestive system. Jill Hynes, CPC, is a fictitious coder who guides you through this case. Assume that the abstracting identified an abscess of the submandibular salivary gland and current heavy tobacco use.

Date: 9/2/yy Location: Branton Gastroenterology

Provider: Stanley Garrett, MD

Patient: Gary Spates Gender: M Age: 52

Chief complaint: "lump and tenderness in my jaw"

Assessment: abscess, submandibular salivary gland, heavy current tobacco use

Plan: drain abscess, Rx antibiotics

Follow along in your ICD-10-CM manual as Jill Hynes, CPC, assigns and sequences codes for this case. Check off each step after you complete it.

⇨ Jill begins by locating the Main Term in the Index.

- ❑ Jill looks up **A, Abscess**.
- ❑ She locates the subterm for **salivary (duct) (gland)**.
- ❑ Jill confirms that there are no further subentries under **salivary** and identifies the code **K11.3** that she will verify in the Tabular List.

⇨ Jill locates code **K11.3** in the Tabular List.

- ❑ She confirms that the code description **Abscess of salivary gland** accurately describes the diagnosis. She notes that there are no further breakdowns for the specific salivary gland affected.
- ❑ She reviews the instructional note at the beginning of the category **K11** (■ FIGURE 9-4), which states to **Use additional code**. As she reads the items listed, she observes that they relate to certain lifestyle

Table 9-4 ■ **COMMON INSTRUCTIONAL NOTES FOR THE DIGESTIVE SYSTEM**

Use Additional Code to Identify:	Location of Note
Alcohol abuse and dependence (F10.-)	K20 Esophagitis K25 Gastric ulcer K26 Duodenal ulcer K27 Peptic ulcer K28 Gastrojejunal ulcer K29.0 Acute gastritis K29.2 Alcoholic gastritis K70 Alcoholic liver disease K86.0 Alcohol-induced chronic pancreatitis
Alcohol abuse and dependence (F10.-) Exposure to environmental tobacco smoke (Z77.22) Exposure to tobacco smoke in the perinatal period (P96.81) History of tobacco use (Z87.891) Occupational exposure to environmental tobacco smoke (Z57.31) Tobacco dependence (F17.-) Tobacco use (Z72.0)	K11 Diseases of salivary glands K05 Gingivitis and periodontal diseases K12 Stomatitis and related lesions K13 Other diseases of lip and oral mucosa K14 Diseases of tongue
Specify type of infection	K94.02 Colostomy infection K94.12 Enterostomy infection K94.22 Gastrostomy infection K94.32 Esophagostomy infection

habits. She knows that an instructional note at the beginning of a category applies to all of the codes in that category, so this instructional note applies to all codes from **K11.0** to **K11.9**. The fact that the tobacco use is to be an *additional* code tells her that the abscess should be sequenced first and the tobacco use should be sequenced second.

➩ Next, Jill codes for heavy current tobacco use.

❑ She notices several possible code options in the instructional note:

- **history of tobacco use (Z87.891)**
- **tobacco dependence (F17.-)**
- **tobacco use (Z72.0)**

Jill recalls that even though tobacco use is part of Mr. Spates' medical history, OGCR I.C.21.c.4) states she should use **history (of)** codes only to

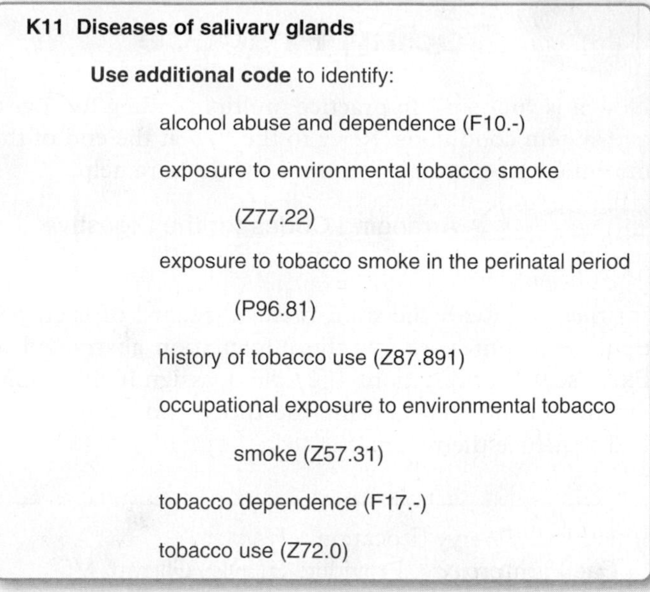

K11 Diseases of salivary glands

Use additional code to identify:

alcohol abuse and dependence (F10.-)

exposure to environmental tobacco smoke (Z77.22)

exposure to tobacco smoke in the perinatal period (P96.81)

history of tobacco use (Z87.891)

occupational exposure to environmental tobacco smoke (Z57.31)

tobacco dependence (F17.-)

tobacco use (Z72.0)

Figure 9-4 ■ Instructional Notes for Category K11 Diseases of the Salivary Glands

describe a past medical condition that no longer exists. Because Mr. Spates' tobacco use is documented as current, she eliminates code **Z87.891, History of tobacco use.**

❑ She checks the medical record to see if Dr. Garrett stated tobacco dependence. He did not, so she eliminates code **F17.- tobacco dependence**. She knows she cannot interpret the word heavy to mean dependence.

❑ She identifies **Z72.0, Tobacco use** as the most appropriate code.

❑ She verifies **Z72.0** in the Tabular List and notes there are no further codes. She reviews the **Excludes1** conditions and verifies that she is on the right path because none of the conditions listed in the note were documented by Dr. Garrett.

❑ Next, Jill goes back to the original code and checks for instructional notes at the beginning of the block **Diseases of the oral cavity and salivary glands (K00-K14)**. This block has no further notes.

❑ Finally, she checks back to the beginning of ICD-10-CM Chapter 11 and reviews the **Excludes** notes to be sure that none of these exclusions apply to her current case.

➩ Jill is confident that she completed all verifications and cross-checks. She sequences **Z72.0** second because the instructional note described it as an additional code.

➩ Jill finalizes the code assignment and sequencing for this case.

(1) **K11.3, Abscess of salivary gland**

(2) **Z72.0, Tobacco use**

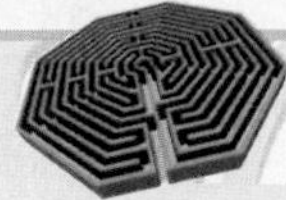

Coding Practice

Now it is your turn to practice multiple coding for digestive system conditions. Refer to the ***Tip*** at the end of the mini-medical-record if you need a little extra help.

Exercise 9.4 Arranging Codes for the Digestive System

Instructions: Read the mini-medical-record of each patient's encounter, review the information abstracted in Exercise 9.2 for questions 1, 2, and 3, assign ICD-10-CM diagnosis codes (CM) using the Index and Tabular List, and sequence them correctly.

1. Date: 9/4/yy Location: Branton Gastroenterology Provider: Stanley Garrett, MD

Patient: Jeremy Mcnamara Gender: M Age: 56

Chief complaint: abdominal pain and bloating, fatigue, vomiting

Assessment: alcoholic liver cirrhosis with ascites due to alcohol addiction

Plan: counseled patient regarding abstinence from alcohol, reduce salt intake

Tip: Read the instructional note at the beginning of the category to use an additional code.

2 CM Codes __________ __________

2. Date: 9/4/yy Location: Branton Gastroenterology Provider: Stanley Garrett, MD

Patient: Robin Mitchell Gender: M Age: 59

Chief complaint: hematemesis, history of cirrhosis

Assessment: portal hypertension *(increase in blood pressure in the portal vein)* with portal hypertensive gastropathy

Plan: endoscopic therapy, drug therapy, and dietary changes

Tip: Code portal hypertension first, then follow the instructional notes to code gastropathy.

3 CM Codes __________ __________ __________

3. Date: 9/4/yy Location: Branton Gastroenterology

Provider: Stanley Garrett, MD

Patient: Kenneth Bode Gender: M Age: 33

Chief complaint: redness and tenderness around colostomy site

Assessment: colostomy infection, cellulitis of abdominal wall due to methicillin susceptible staphylococcus aureus (MSSA)

Plan: Rx antibiotics

Tip: Sometimes coding is like a treasure hunt. You never know where it will take you. Read the instructional notes under the code for colostomy infection to identify the second code. Read the instructional notes under the block heading for cellulitis to identify the third code.

3 CM Codes __________ __________ __________

4. Date: 9/4/yy Location: Branton Gastroenterology

Provider: Stanley Garrett, MD

Patient: Earl Meehan Gender: M Age: 38

Chief complaint: fecal incontinence which has not improved

Assessment: nontraumatic anal sphincter tear

Plan: sphincteroplasty

Tip: Read the instructional notes under the code for nontraumatic anal sphincter tear to identify the second code.

2 CM Codes __________ __________

5. Date: 9/4/yy Location: Buchanan Dentistry

Provider: Alice Buchanan, DDS

Patient: Phillip Nugent Gender: M Age: 14

Procedure: 2 dental fillings

Postprocedural diagnosis: caries *(cavities)*, tooth 2 pit and fissure surface, enamel only; tooth 3 pit and fissure surface, penetrating dentin

Plan: 6 month check-up

Tip: Assign separate codes for each tooth because the depth of the cary was different on each one. Dentists identify each tooth with a number, beginning at the right rear molar on the top of the mouth.

2 CM Codes __________ __________

CODING NEOPLASMS OF THE DIGESTIVE SYSTEM

Neoplasms of the digestive system do not appear in ICD-10-CM Chapter 11 (K00-K94); they appear in Chapter 02 (C00-D49). Codes for neoplasms of the digestive system appear in two different blocks within the neoplasm chapter:

- Malignant neoplasm of lip, oral cavity and pharynx (C00-C14)
- Malignant neoplasm of digestive organs (C15-C26)

Review these two blocks in the ICD-10-CM manual to become familiar with the content.

According to the Centers for Disease Control and Prevention, the most common sites for cancer in the digestive system are the colon and rectum; cancer of these sites is referred to as colorectal cancer. Colorectal cancer is the third most common cancer in the United States and, in most cases, develops slowly over many years. The number of colorectal cancer deaths has declined over the past 15 years, due largely to fewer cases being diagnosed. Colorectal cancer, which most often begins as a polyp, can be detected early through a colonoscopy. Cancer that is detected early is more easily treated. Colorectal cancer can be prevented through removal of polyps during a colonoscopy, before they have time to turn into cancer. When coding for colon cancer, determine if the disease affects only the colon or both the colon and rectum because there are different codes as shown in ■ FIGURE 9-5.

The liver is also a common site of cancer in the digestive system because many types of cancer metastasize to the liver. The liver filters the blood, which is one of the main ways that cancer cells move throughout the body. Most cancer found in the liver is metastatic. Primary liver cancer occurs most often in patients with cirrhosis and alcoholic liver disease. When coding for cancer in the liver, verify if it is primary or is a metastasis.

Malignant neoplasms of the esophagus, stomach, and pancreas have low survival rates because they have few symptoms and are usually not diagnosed until a late stage when they have already metastasized. Cancer of the gall bladder and small intestine are relatively rare.

SUCCESS STEP

Refer to the entry **intestine, large** in the Table of Neoplasms to identify more codes for colon cancer.

	Malignant Primary	Malignant Secondary	Ca in situ	Benign	Uncertain Behavior	Unspecified Behavior
colon	C18.9	C78.5	-	-	-	-
- with rectum	C19	C78.5	D01.1	D12.7	D37.5	D49.0

Figure 9-5 ■ Table of Neoplasms Entry for Colon

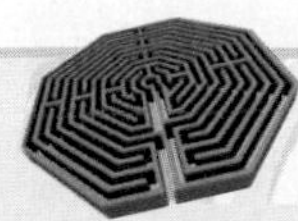

Coding Practice

Now it is your turn to practice coding neoplasms of the digestive system. Refer to the ***Tip*** at the end of the mini-medical-record if you need a little extra help.

Exercise 9.5 Coding Neoplasms of the Digestive System

Instructions: Read the mini-medical-record of each patient's encounter, then abstract, assign, and sequence ICD-10-CM diagnosis codes (CM) using the Index and Tabular List. Write the code(s) on the line provided.

1. Date: 9/5/yy Location: Branton Medical Center Outpatient Procedure Center

Provider: Stanley Garrett, MD

Patient: Agnes Harker Gender: F Age: 57

Procedure: screening colonoscopy due to finding of polyps 5 years ago and family history of colon cancer

Finding: 3 new adenomatous polyps were found at the sigmoid flexure and removed

Plan: 5 year follow up

(continued)

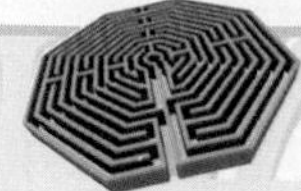

Coding Practice (continued)

1. (continued)

Tip: Identify where the sigmoid flexure is located. Code the patient's personal history as well as the family history because both present risk factors for the patient.

3 CM Codes __________ __________ __________

2. Date: 9/5/yy Location: Branton Gastroenterology Provider: Stanley Garrett, MD

Patient: Renee Dawson Gender: F Age: 61

Reason for visit: FU on CT scan

Assessment: adenocarcinoma of overlapping sites (rectum and sigmoid) of the large intestine

Plan: refer to oncologist

Tip: A tumor in two sites immediately next to each other is considered to be overlapping.

1 CM Code __________

3. Date: 9/5/yy Location: Branton Gastroenterology Provider: Stanley Garrett, MD

Patient: Ross Dasilva Gender: M Age: 54

Reason for visit: FU on liver biopsy

Assessment: hepatocellular cancer due to alcohol dependence and chronic Hepatitis C

Plan: refer to oncologist for evaluation of treatment options

Tip: Read the instructional notes in the Tabular List under the first code to identify the additional conditions that need to be coded.

3 CM Codes __________ __________ __________

4. Date: 9/5/yy Location: Branton Gastroenterology Provider: Stanley Garrett, MD

Patient: Alma Lui Gender: F Age: 70

Reason for visit: FU on colonoscopy results

Assessment: cancer in situ, rectum

Plan: schedule surgery, refer to oncologist for adjuvant therapy

1 CM Code __________

5. Date: 9/5/yy Location: Branton Gastroenterology Provider: Stanley Garrett, MD

Patient: Matthew Bond Gender: M Age: 68

Reason for visit: FU on biopsy and imaging

Assessment: adenocarcinoma of the pancreas with liver and lymph gland metastases

Plan: chemotherapy, palliative care

Tip: Code for the primary cancer and both metastatic sites.

3 CM Codes __________ __________ __________

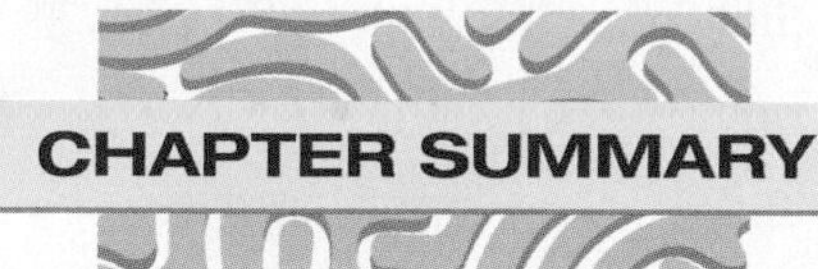

CHAPTER SUMMARY

In this chapter you learned that:

- The digestive system consists of the alimentary canal and accessory organs, which provide for ingestion, digestion, absorption, and elimination of food.
- Chapter 11 of ICD-10-CM, Diseases of the Digestive System (K00-K94), contains 10 blocks or subchapters that are divided by anatomical site.
- When abstracting for the digestive system, coders need to look for manifestations, complications, and lifestyle habits associated with digestive system conditions.
- Coders frequently assign combination codes to describe complications of digestive system conditions.
- In order to sequence codes for the digestive system, follow instructional notes in the Tabular List, which direct coders to assign additional codes for associated conditions, underlying causes, and external causes related to digestive system conditions.
- Colorectal cancer is the third most common cancer in the United States; the liver is a common site of metastases.
- There are no OGCR for the digestive system, but there are many instructional notes in the Tabular List.

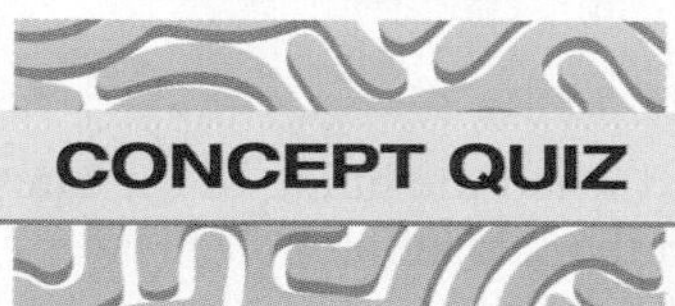

CONCEPT QUIZ

Take a moment to look back at your trip through the digestive system and solidify your skills. This is your opportunity to pull together everything you have learned.

Completion

Instructions: Write the term that answers each question based on the information you learned in this chapter. Choose from the following list. Some choices may be used more than once and some choices may not be used at all. Refer to the discussion in this chapter and the Glossary at the end of this book if you need a little extra help.

calculi	liver
colon	multiple coding
combination coding	pancreas
gall bladder	small intestine
instructional notes	stomach
large intestine	

1. Col/o is the combining form for _______________ or _______________.
2. Cholecyst/o is the combining form for _______________.
3. Hepat/o is the combining form for _______________.
4. Enter/o and ile/o are combining forms for _______________.
5. Fund/o is the combining form for the top portion of the _______________.
6. _______________ describes more than one aspect of a condition, or multiple conditions, in a single code.
7. _______________ requires that more than one code be assigned in order to fully describe the patient's condition.
8. _______________ may appear at the beginning of the chapter, the beginning of a block or subchapter, the beginning of a three-character category, the beginning of a subcategory, or under the final code.
9. Most cancer found in the _______________ is metastatic.
10. _______________ is often required to describe lifestyle habits, such as alcohol abuse or tobacco, which may contribute to digestive system conditions.

Multiple Choice

Instructions: Circle the letter of the best answer to each question based on the information you learned in this chapter. Refer to the discussion in this chapter and the Glossary at the end of this book if you need a little extra help.

1. All of the following are functions of the digestive system EXCEPT
   A. ingestion.
   B. absorption.
   C. circulation.
   D. elimination.
2. The ________ assist in digestion but are not directly connected to the alimentary canal.
   A. large and small intestines
   B. accessory organs
   C. rectum and anus
   D. teeth
3. ________ is an abnormal immune reaction to gluten and poor absorption of nutrients.
   A. Celiac disease
   B. Crohn's disease
   C. Diverticular disease
   D. Gastroesophageal reflux disease
4. What is a barium enema?
   A. Swallowing a chalky substance and viewing it on an X-ray
   B. A group of disorders in which the intestines become red and swollen
   C. Endoscopic examination of the esophagus, stomach, and duodenum
   D. Injecting a chalky substance into the colon through the anus and viewing the organs on an X-ray
5. The Index entry for Crohn's disease cross-references the coder to
   A. Colonitis, large
   B. Diverticulitis
   C. Intestinal obstruction
   D. Enteritis, regional
6. The word root chole/o means
   A. colon.
   B. gall bladder.
   C. bile.
   D. vagina.
7. Category K11 provides instructional notes to code which of the following?
   A. History of tobacco use
   B. Specific type of allergy
   C. Any associated fecal incontinence
   D. Viral hepatitis
8. MRCP refers to a (an)
   A. endoscopic ultrasound.
   B. magnetic resonance cholangiopancreatography.
   C. esophagogastroduodenoscopy.
   D. magnetic resonance imaging of colon and pancreas.
9. Which condition is not a classified as a disease of the digestive system?
   A. Ileus
   B. Obesity
   C. Stomatitis
   D. Hematemesis
10. Diverticulitis is
    A. pouches formed when the lining of the intestine pushes through the intestinal muscle layer.
    B. the presence of diverticula.
    C. diversion of the colon.
    D. a bacterial infection of diverticula.

CODING CHALLENGE

Now it is your turn to demonstrate coding all aspects of digestive system conditions. Refer back to the examples and discussion in this chapter when you need a little extra help. Use your medical dictionary and anatomy references when needed.

Instructions: Read the mini-medical-record of each patient's encounter, then abstract, assign, and sequence ICD-10-CM diagnosis codes (CM) using the Index and Tabular List. Write the code(s) on the line provided.

1. Date: 9/14/yy Location: Branton Medical Center Emergency Department (ED)

Provider: Stanley Garrett, MD

Patient: Greg Allen Gender: M Age: 15

Chief complaint: vomiting, acute abdominal pain, RLQ tenderness, T 101 degrees

Assessment: acute appendicitis with rupture

Plan: laparoscopic appendectomy

1 CM Code ________

2. Date: 9/15/yy Location: Buchannan Dentistry
Provider: Alice Buchanan, DDS
Patient: Yukari Asada Gender: F Age: 41
Reason for visit: referred by her oncologist for mouth ulcers due to chemotherapy for metastatic colon cancer (primary colon cancer that has spread)
Assessment: oral mucositis, side effect from chemotherapy for metastatic colon cancer
Plan: oral debridement, pain relief

Tip: First, code for the condition being treated by Dr. Buchanan. For the second code, read the instructional note in the Tabular List after you verify the first code. Then, code the colon cancer to identify the reason for the chemotherapy. Finally, note that the metastatic sites are unspecified.

4 CM Codes __________ __________ __________ __________

3. Date: 9/15/yy Location: Branton Gastroenterology Provider: Stanley Garrett, MD
Patient: Keith Beeman Gender: M Age: 43
Chief complaint: "My hiatal hernia seems worse than usual"
Assessment: strangulated hiatal hernia
Plan: schedule hernia repair

Tip: Strangulation is classified as an obstruction.

1 CM Code __________

4. Date: 9/15/yy Location: Branton Gastroenterology Provider: Stanley Garrett, MD
Patient: Keith Lewis Gender: M Age: 36
Chief complaint: "I've been having problems with my GERD"
Assessment: GERD
Plan: adjust Rx, call if problems continue
1 CM Code __________

5. Date: 9/15/yy Location: Branton Medical Center Provider: Stanley Garrett, MD
Patient: Megan Brandt Gender: F Age: 52
Reason for admission: pain RUQ, T 102 degrees, vomiting
Procedure: laparoscopic cholecystectomy
Discharge diagnosis: acute cholecystitis with calculi in the common bile duct causing obstruction

Tip: When you search for the Main Term cholecystitis, follow the cross-reference listed in the Index.

1 CM Code __________

6. Date: 9/15/yy Location: Branton Medical Center Outpatient Procedure Center
Provider: Stanley Garrett, MD
Patient: Carl Harville Gender: M Age: 56
Chief complaint: nausea, vomiting, constipation
Assessment: inflammatory colon polyps, intestinal obstruction
Plan: high fiber diet and increased liquids, Rx corticosteroid to reduce inflammation, FU 2 weeks

Tip: Main Term is polyps. Thoroughly review all available subterms to locate the correct combination code.

1 CM Code __________

7. Date: 9/15/yy Location: Buchannan Dentistry
Provider: Alice Buchanan, DDS
Patient: Victor Nolasco Gender: M Age: 26
Chief complaint: yellow teeth
Assessment: amelogenesis imperfecta (*a tooth development disorder in which the teeth are covered with thin, abnormally formed enamel and are easily damaged*)
Plan: apply crowns
1 CM Code __________

(*continued*)

(continued from page 163)

8. Date: 9/15/yy Location: Branton Medical Center ED Provider: Stanley Garrett, MD

Patient: Victor Nolasco Gender: M Age: 12

Chief complaint: "My son forgot that he isn't supposed to eat eggs and ate a hardboiled egg at his friend's house. He has had diarrhea and vomiting for 4 hours and I'm getting worried."

Assessment: allergic gastroenteritis due to eggs

Plan: Rx antiemetic, antidiarrheal

2 CM Codes __________ __________

9. Date: 9/15/yy Location: Branton Medical Center Provider: Stanley Garrett, MD

Patient: Tiffany Cho Gender: F Age: 30

Reason for admission: LUQ pain and swelling increasing over the past 3 days, indigestion

Treatment: IV fluids, pain control, nasogastric suctioning

Discharge diagnosis: acute pancreatitis due to opioid dependence and intoxication

2 CM Codes __________ __________

10. Date: 9/15/yy Location: Branton Medical Center Provider: Stanley Garrett, MD

Patient: Vivian Goss Gender: F Age: 41

Reason for admission: admitted from ED with severe and steady abdominal pain, fever, excessive perspiration, T 101 degrees

Treatment: IV antibiotics, fluids, colectomy

Discharge diagnosis: generalized peritonitis due to e. coli, irritable bowel syndrome

3 CM Codes __________ __________ __________

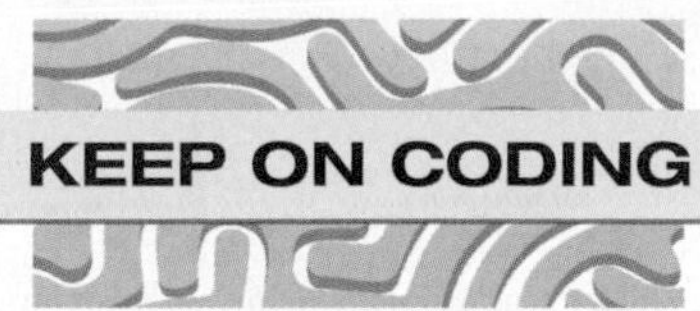

KEEP ON CODING

As a coder, you can never have too much experience. Apply everything you have learned in this chapter to code the following diagnostic statements. Use the OGCR and instructional notes in the Tabular List to help determine how many codes are required.

Instructions: Read the diagnostic statement, then use the Index and Tabular List to assign and sequence ICD-10-CM (CM) diagnosis codes. Write the code(s) on the line provided.

1. Carcinoma of the buccal mucosa: CM Code(s) ______
2. Erosion of teeth due to diet: CM Code(s) ______
3. Enterostomy hemorrhage: CM Code(s) ______
4. Cyst of pancreas: CM Code(s) ______
5. Mucous retention cyst of salivary gland: CM Code(s) ______
6. Cardiospasm: CM Code(s) ______
7. Malignant neoplasm of tongue with a history of tobacco use: CM Code(s) ______
8. Hydrops of the gall bladder: CM Code(s) ______
9. Acute gingivitis, plaque induced: CM Code(s) ______
10. Eosinophilic esophagitis: CM Code(s) ______
11. Hairy leukoplakia: CM Code(s) ______
12. Incisional hernia without obstruction or gangrene: CM Code(s) ______
13. Acute appendicitis with localized peritonitis: CM Code(s) ______
14. Ulcerative pancolitis and abscess: CM Code(s) ______
15. Stage 3 hemorrhoids: CM Code(s) ______
16. Slow transit constipation: CM Code(s) ______
17. Chronic cholecystitis with cholelithiasis without obstruction: CM Code(s) ______
18. Postprocedural liver failure: CM Code(s) ______
19. Cheilosis: CM Code(s) ______
20. Esophageal ulcer with bleeding: CM Code(s) ______
21. Retained dental root: CM Code(s) ______
22. Glossodynia: CM Code(s) ______
23. Alcoholic cirrhosis of liver with ascites: CM Code(s) ______
24. Malignant neoplasm of overlapping sections of the esophagus: CM Code(s) ______
25. Hemoperitoneum: CM Code(s) ______

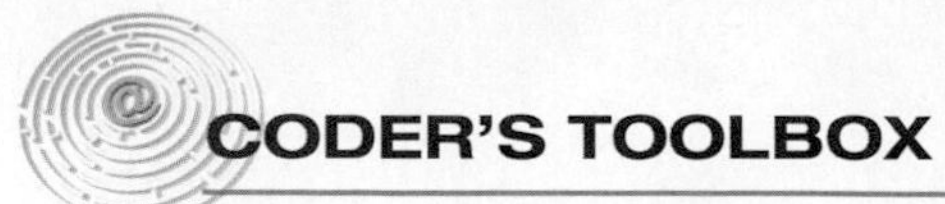

CODER'S TOOLBOX

The following resources are a starting point for learning more about the digestive system.

American Academy of Family Physicians (AAFP) **http://www.aafp.org/online/en/home.html**

American Academy of Periodontology (AAP) **http://www.perio.org/**

American Association for the Study of Liver Diseases (AASLD) **http://www.aasld.org/Pages/Default.aspx**

American Dental Association (ADA) **http://www.ada.org/**

American Gastroenterological Association (AGA) **http://www.gastro.org/**

Celiac Disease Foundation (CDF) **http://www.celiac.org/**

Children's Digestive Health and Nutrition Foundation (CDHNF) **http://www.cdhnf.org/wmspage.cfm?parm1=14**

Clouse, R E. Antidepressants for irritable bowel syndrome, Gut. 2003 April; 52(4): 598–599. Accessed at **http://www.ncbi.nlm.nih.gov/pmc/articles/PMC1773590/**

Crohn's and Colitis Foundation of America (CCFA) **http://www.ccfa.org/info/about/crohns**

International Foundation for Functional Gastrointestinal Disorders (IFFGD) **http://www.iffgd.org/**

National Digestive Diseases Information Clearinghouse (NDDIC) **http://digestive.niddk.nih.gov/index.htm**

National Pancreas Foundation (NPF) **http://pancreasfoundation.org/**

10

Endocrine, Nutritional, and Metabolic Diseases (E00-E89)

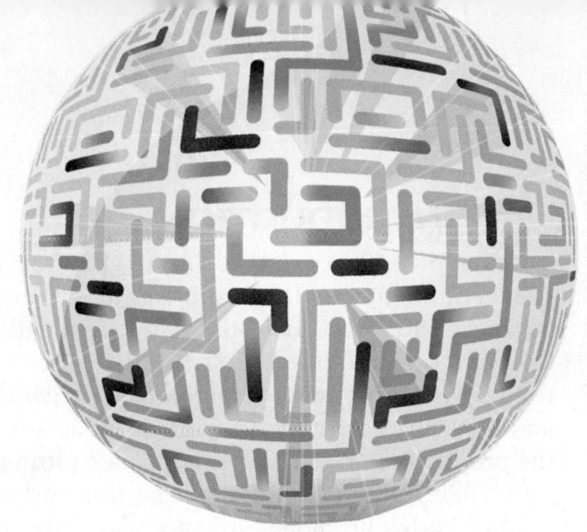

Learning Objectives

After completing this chapter, you should have the skills to:

- Spell and define the key words, medical terms, and abbreviations related to endocrine, nutritional, and metabolic diseases.
- Discuss the structure, function, and common conditions of the endocrine system.
- Identify the main characteristics of coding for endocrine, nutritional, and metabolic diseases.
- Abstract diagnostic information from the medical record for coding endocrine, nutritional, and metabolic diseases.
- Assign codes for endocrine, nutritional, and metabolic diseases and related conditions.
- Arrange codes for endocrine, nutritional, and metabolic diseases and related conditions.
- Code neoplasms of the endocrine system.
- Discuss the Official Guidelines for Coding and Reporting related to endocrine, nutritional, and metabolic diseases.

Key Terms and Abbreviations

causal relationship
diabetes mellitus (DM)
diabetic ketoacidosis (DKA)
endocrine system
HbA1c
hormones
hyperglycemia
hyperosmolarity hyperglycemic nonketotic syndrome (HHNS)
hypoglycemia
metabolism
serum assay
target organ
trachea

In addition to the key terms listed here, students should know the terms defined within tables in this chapter.

Chapter Outline

- **Endocrine System Refresher**
- **Coding Overview of the Endocrine System**
- **Abstracting for the Endocrine System**
- **Assigning Codes for the Endocrine System**
- **Arranging Codes for the Endocrine System**
- **Coding Neoplasms of the Endocrine System**

ICD-10-CM codes in this chapter are from the ICD-10-CM 2014 Draft code set from the Department of Health and Human Services, Centers for Disease Control and Prevention.

INTRODUCTION

When your vehicle gets a little sluggish, you may decide to use oil or fuel additive to boost its performance. The variety of additives available is mind boggling, ranging from friction modifiers that improve fuel economy by reducing friction between parts, to detergents that clean and neutralize impurities, to anti-foam agents that inhibit the production of air bubble that create pitting and corrosion where entrapped air contacts metal surfaces.

Your body's hormones are, in a sense, like fuel additives for your car. They perform a variety of tasks that keep other organ systems and structures working smoothly. It is the endocrine system's job to produce, store, and release hormones.

In your tour of the endocrine system in this chapter you will learn more about how the endocrine system works, why sometimes it does not work as it should, and how physicians treat these conditions. Most importantly, you will practice coding for patient encounters related to endocrine system diseases and conditions, a skill which requires you to abstract information from the mini-medical-record, assign correct codes, and arrange (sequence) the codes in the proper order.

An endocrinologist is a physician who specializes in endocrine, nutritional, and metabolic diseases. When primary care physicians (PCP) are unable to diagnose or manage a complex endocrine, nutritional, or metabolic condition, they refer the patient to an endocrinologist.

As you read this chapter, open up your medical terminology book and keep a medical dictionary handy to refresh your memory of any unfamiliar terms. Resources can be especially helpful to distinguish symptoms that are integral to endocrine system disorders from those that are related, but not integral. This way, you have the information that you need at your fingertips.

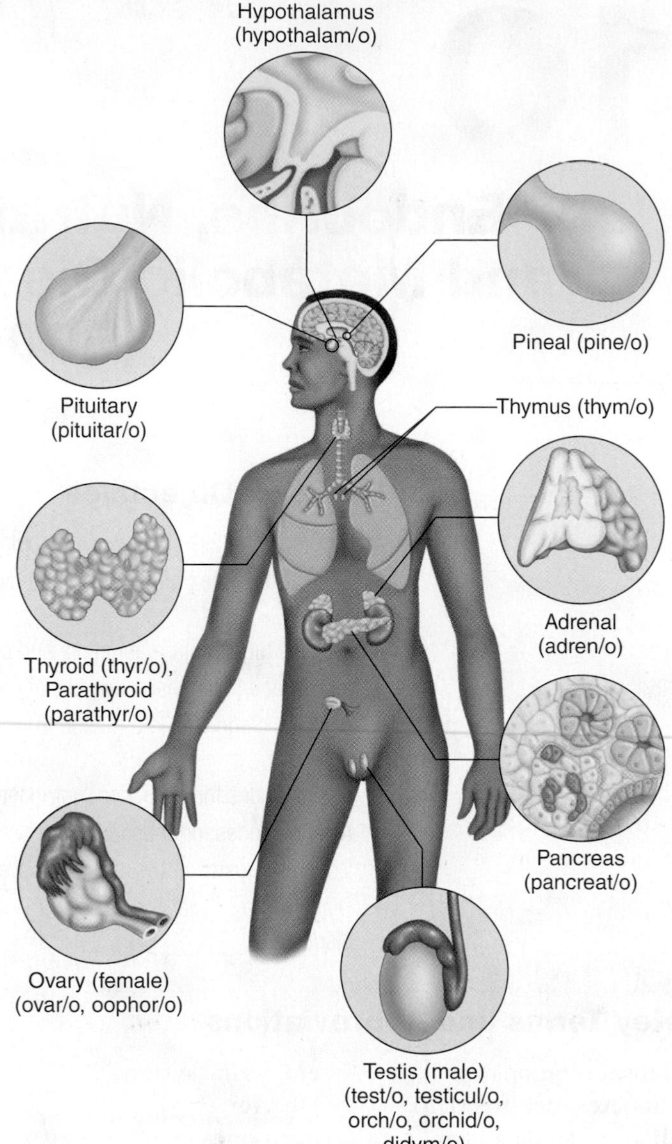

Figure 10-1 ■ The Endocrine System

ENDOCRINE SYSTEM REFRESHER

The function of the endocrine system is to produce, store, and release hormones, which are chemical messengers. Hormones regulate many body functions including growth, development, metabolism (*the processes of digestion, elimination, breathing, blood circulation, and maintaining body temperature*), sexual function, reproduction, and mood. The endocrine system consists of several ductless glands that are not directly connected to each other (■ Figure 10-1). The function of each gland is summarized in ■ Table 10-1. The ovaries and testes function as part of the reproductive system in addition to their endocrine function; the pancreas has an **exocrine** function in the digestive system in addition to its endocrine function.

In Figure 10-1, each structure in the endocrine system is labeled with its name, as well as its medical terminology root/combining form. As you learn about conditions and procedures that affect the endocrine system, remember to use medical terminology skills to combine word roots, prefixes, and suffixes that you already know in order to define new terms related to the endocrine system. Refer to ■ Table 10-2 for a refresher on how to build medical terms related to the endocrine system.

CODING CAUTION

Be alert for medical terms that are spelled similarly and have different meanings.

nephropathy (*kidney disease*) and **neuropathy** (*nerve disease*)

hypothyroidism (*state of low thyroid*) and **hyperthyroidism** (*state of high thyroid*)

thyr/o (*thyroid*), **thym/o** (*thymus gland*), and **thalam/o** (*thalamus, a portion of the brain*)

Table 10-1 ■ **FUNCTION OF ENDOCRINE GLANDS**

Gland	Endocrine Function
Pituitary	Controls most activity in the endocrine system
Hypothalamus	Controls pituitary gland
Pineal	Regulates waking/sleeping functions
Thymus	Produces T-cells used by the immune system
Thyroid	Regulates metabolism
Parathyroid	Regulates the level of circulating calcium
Pancreas (Islets of Langerhans)	Synthesis, storage, and release of **glucagon** and **insulin**
Adrenal	Secretes steroid hormones
Ovaries/Testes (gonads)	Secrete estrogen and testosterone

Conditions of the Endocrine System

Endocrine, nutritional, and metabolic disorders tend to have gradual onsets and generalized symptoms such as fatigue, weakness, weight change, hair loss, muscle weakness, nervousness, appetite change, and irritability, making them difficult to diagnose. When a structure in the endocrine system malfunctions, the result is either hypofunction or hyperfunction of a gland, a hormone, or a target organ (*the organ receiving hormones*).

Endocrine disorders are best diagnosed through serum assays (*lab tests that measure the presence and quantity of a substance in the blood*). Common treatments include injection of hormones, surgical removal of all or part of a gland, and surgical removal of a tumor that is causing the problem.

The most common diseases of the endocrine system are diabetes mellitus (DM) and thyroid disorders. These conditions present concepts and terminology that coders must be familiar with.

Diabetes Mellitus

Diabetes mellitus is a condition resulting in elevated glucose levels over an extended period of time and excess excretion of urine, usually due to malfunction of the pancreas. Coders need to be familiar with several types of diabetes, which are highlighted in ■ TABLE 10-3 (page 170). According to the National Diabetes Association, diabetes affects over 8% of the population or nearly 26 million people, and an additional 79 million people are estimated to have **prediabetes**.

SUCCESS STEP

Diabetes mellitus literally means *sweet urine disease*. The word *diabetes* is based on the Greek word meaning *siphon*. Aretus the Cappadocian, a second-century physician, described patients as having polyuria and passing water like a siphon. In 1675, Thomas Willis, the father of modern neuroscience, added *mellitus* because *mel* is the Latin word for *honey* or *sweetness*.

Diabetes causes both acute and chronic complications. Acute complications consist of the following:

- Hyperglycemia is the condition of severely elevated blood sugar levels, usually occurring in type 1diabetics, due to a lack or deficiency of insulin. Hyperglycemia can cause diabetic ketoacidosis (DKA) in which a high level of ketones (a chemical) accumulate in the blood, turning it acidic. Symptoms include nausea, vomiting, abdominal pain, shock, coma, and death, if not treated immediately.
- Hyperosmolarity hyperglycemic nonketotic syndrome (HHNS) is elevated glucose without ketoacidosis, usually occurring in elderly type 2 diabetics with other conditions, and can result in hyperosmolar coma and death.

Table 10-2 ■ **EXAMPLE OF CONSTRUCTING MEDICAL TERMS FOR THE ENDOCRINE SYSTEM**

Prefix	Root/Combining Form	Suffix	Complete Medical Term
hypo- (*below, low*) **hyper-** (*above, high*)	**glyc/o** (*sugar*)	**-emia** (*condition of the blood*) **-uria** (*condition of the urine*) **-ism** (*state of*)	**hypo + glyc + emia** (*low sugar in the blood*) **hyper + glyc + emia** (*excessive sugar in the blood*) **glyco + uria** (*sugar in the urine*)
	thyr/o- (*thyroid*)		**hypo + thyroid + ism** (*state of low thyroid*) **hyper + thyroid + ism** (*state of high thyroid*)
	protein/o (*protein*)		**protein + emia** (*protein in the blood*) **protein + uria** (*protein in the urine*)

Table 10-3 ■ **OVERVIEW OF DIABETES MELLITUS**

Type of Diabetes	Description	Treatment	Frequency
Type 1 Diabetes (previously called insulin-dependent diabetes mellitus [IDDM] or juvenile-onset diabetes)	Body's immune system attacks pancreatic beta cells so that the pancreas does not produce insulin.	No prevention or cure known. Patients *must* receive insulin, delivered through injection or pump, to survive.	5% of all diagnosed cases of diabetes
Type 2 Diabetes (previously called non–insulin-dependent diabetes mellitus [NIDDM] or adult-onset diabetes)	Pancreas produces insulin, but the body does not use it properly. In some cases, insulin production is decreased also.	Prevent, delay, or reverse the onset of type 2 diabetes with weight loss, increased physical activity, and the medication metformin. Some people *may* need insulin.	90 to 95% of all diagnosed cases of diabetes
Secondary Diabetes	Elevated glucose is caused by an external factor, such as medication, surgery, pancreatic disease, or other illness.	Treat underlying cause if possible. Manage with diet, exercise, medication, and insulin, as needed.	1 to 5% of all diagnosed cases of diabetes
Gestational Diabetes (GDM) (Note: Gestational diabetes is coded under the reproductive system, not the endocrine system.)	Elevated glucose is diagnosed during pregnancy in women with no prior history of diabetes.	Must control the condition quickly to prevent adverse effects on baby. Manage with diet, exercise, and sometimes insulin.	2 to 10% of pregnant women. Using recently updated diagnostic criteria, the rate is expected to increase to 18% of pregnancies.

Table 10-4 ■ **COMMON THYROID DISORDERS**

Condition	Description	Treatment
Hyperthyroidism	Inappropriately elevated thyroid function.	Antithyroid medications (methimazole and propylthiouracil [PTU])
Graves disease (diffuse toxic goiter)	Overproduction by the thyroid gland due to an **autoimmune** condition in which autoantibodies are directed against the thyroid-stimulating hormone (TSH) receptor.	Disable thyroid gland's ability to produce hormones through radioactive iodine and/or antithyroid drugs, beta blockers, thyroidectomy.
Thyrotoxicosis (thyroid storm)	Excessive quantities of circulating thyroid hormone due to overproduction by the thyroid gland, overproduction originating outside the thyroid, or loss of storage function and leakage from the gland.	Cardiac monitor, supplemental oxygen, aggressive hydration, cooling measures, electrolyte replacement, antithyroid medications.
Hypothyroidism	Deficiency of thyroid hormone, usually due to lack of production of the hormone by the thyroid or inadequate secretion of hormones by the pituitary gland or hypothalamus.	Administer supplemental TSH and T4 hormones.
Non-toxic goiter	Enlargement of the thyroid that is not associated with overproduction of thyroid hormone or malignancy.	Supplemental thyroid hormone, thyroidectomy.

- **Hypoglycemia** is abnormally low blood sugar, often due to excessive use of insulin or other glucose-lowering medications. Symptoms are dizziness, confusion, weakness, tremors, seizures, coma, and brain death.

Chronic complications of diabetes can affect nearly every organ system, with the most frequent organ systems affected being the following:

- eye (cataracts, blindness)
- urinary (**nephropathy**, kidney failure)
- nervous (**neuropathy**)
- circulatory (**gangrene**, stroke, hypertension, **peripheral artery disease [PAD]**).

Thyroid Disorders

The thyroid is a butterfly-shaped gland in front of the **trachea** (*windpipe*) that produces two hormones, triiodothyronine (T3) and thyroxine (T4), that regulate how the body breaks down food and uses or stores energy. ■ TABLE 10-4 summarizes the most common thyroid disorders with which coders need to be familiar.

This section provides a general reference to help understand the most common diagnoses of the endocrine system, but does not list everything that you need to know. Remember to keep standard reference books handy in case you get stuck. Refer to the resources in the Coder's Toolbox at the end of this chapter to learn more about conditions affecting the endocrine system.

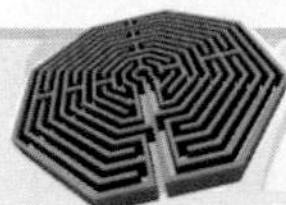

Coding Practice

Refresh your knowledge of terminology related to the endocrine system. Use a medical terminology text or a website such as GlobalRph.com > Medical Terminology **http://www.globalrph.com/medterm.htm** to identify the meaning of word parts that may not be familiar to you.

Exercise 10.1 Endocrine System Refresher

Instructions: Use your medical terminology skills and resources to define the following terms related to the endocrine system, then assign the diagnosis code.

Follow these steps:

- Use slash marks "/" to break down each term into its root(s) and suffix.
- Define the meaning of the word, based on the meaning of each word part.
- Assign the default ICD-10-CM diagnosis code (CM) for the condition using the Index and Tabular List.

Example: hyperthyroidism hyper/thyroid/ism Meaning: pertaining to excessive thyroid CM Code: E05.90

1. thyrotoxicosis Meaning ________ CM Code ________
2. adrenalitis Meaning ________ CM Code ________
3. thyromegaly Meaning ________ CM Code ________
4. thyroiditis Meaning ________ CM Code ________
5. hyperglycemia Meaning ________ CM Code ________
6. hyperlipidemia Meaning ________ CM Code ________
7. panhypopituitarism Meaning ________ CM Code ________
8. parathyroid tetany Meaning ________ CM Code ________
9. hypoparathyroidism Meaning ________ CM Code ________
10. acromegaly Meaning ________ CM Code ________

CODING OVERVIEW OF THE ENDOCRINE SYSTEM

ICD-10-CM Chapter 4, Endocrine, Nutritional, and Metabolic Diseases (E00-E89) contains ten blocks or subchapters that are divided by anatomical site and type of disorder. Review the block names and code ranges listed at the beginning of Chapter 4 in the ICD-10-CM manual to become familiar with the content and organization.

ICD-10-CM Chapter 4 corresponds with ICD-9-CM Chapter 3 (240-279). Diabetes mellitus occupies five categories, divided by etiology, including a new category for drug-induced diabetes. In ICD-10-CM, combination codes identify the type of diabetes and manifestations, reducing the need for multiple coding of this common condition, as required in ICD-9-CM.

In addition to the most common conditions of diabetes and thyroid disorders, this ICD-10-CM chapter also classifies other endocrine system conditions, including the following:

- dysfunction of other endocrine glands, such as adrenal, pituitary, and parathyroid
- endocrine-related disorders of glands that serve multiple systems, such as the pancreas, ovaries, and testes
- nutritional disorders, such as malnutrition and deficiencies of specific vitamins and nutrients
- obesity
- disorders of metabolism, such as electrolyte imbalances and the body's inability to utilize sugar, fat, or copper, properly

ICD-10-CM provides Official Guidelines for Coding and Reporting (OGCR) for endocrine, nutritional, and metabolic diseases in OGCR section I.C.4. OGCR provides detailed guidance regarding assigning and sequencing codes for diabetes mellitus and secondary diabetes mellitus.

SUCCESS STEP

ICD-9-CM classified gout and osteomalacia with diseases of the endocrine system. However, medical science now considers them to be musculoskeletal diseases, so codes for gout and osteomalacia now appear in ICD-10-CM Chapter 13, Diseases of the Musculoskeletal System.

ABSTRACTING FOR THE ENDOCRINE SYSTEM

In order to abstract diagnoses for endocrine system conditions, coders must distinguish between integral symptoms and signs, as opposed to the conditions, complications, and manifestations. It is common for coders to not know all the details of every disease, so when in doubt as to whether a symptom or sign is integral to a disease process, consult a reference book on diseases.

Keep in mind that any diagnosis must be documented by the physician; do not assign a diagnosis based only on test results. Physicians consider a variety of factors, in addition to test results, to establish a diagnosis. They may evaluate a trend of test results over a period of time, order other tests or imaging, or receive an evaluation from a specialist. For example, a patient may have a test result of hyperglycemia, but not be diagnosed as diabetic until the result recurs several times over a period of months and additional tests, such as **HbA1c** (*a blood test that measures glucose attached to hemoglobin*) or a **glucose tolerance test (GTT)**, are evaluated.

Abstracting for Diabetes Mellitus

When coders learn how to accurately abstract for diabetes mellitus, they learn detailed skills that serve them well when abstracting many other conditions as well. In addition, diabetes is a commonly coded condition because patients with diabetes tend to have complications necessitating frequent medical care. Remember that abstracting questions are a general guide and that not all questions apply to every case. For example, not every patient has both acute and chronic complications. ■ TABLE 10-5 lists key criteria for abstracting diabetes.

Do not assume that all conditions documented are complications of diabetes. The specific word choices the physician uses in documentation indicate whether there is a **causal relationship** (*one disease being caused by another*). For example, cataracts may be a complication of diabetes or they may be unrelated. When physicians document diabetic cataracts, where diabetic is a modifier of cataract, they mean that the cataracts are *caused by* diabetes. When they document age-related cataracts, the cataracts are a result of aging and should not be identified as a complication of diabetes, even if the patient also has diabetes.

Similarly, physicians document a condition with the use of **secondary to, due to, with,** or **in**, when they are indicating causality. When physicians document a condition with the use of **and**, the conditions are unrelated. When a physician's documentation is unclear, it is important to query the physician for clarification.

These distinctions are critical when assigning codes. Conditions that arise due to diabetes usually are assigned a

Table 10-5 ■ KEY CRITERIA FOR ABSTRACTING DIABETES MELLITUS

- ❑ What type of diabetes is documented?
- ❑ Are coexisting conditions documented as related to diabetes?
- ❑ What acute complications are documented?
- ❑ What chronic complications are documented?
- ❑ If secondary DM is documented, what is the cause?
- ❑ If either type 2 or secondary DM is documented, is insulin used on a long-term basis?
- ❑ Is a family history of DM documented?
- ❑ Which problem or complication is the reason for the encounter?

Table 10-6 ■ **EXAMPLES OF DOCUMENTATION AND CODING FOR RELATED AND UNRELATED CONDITIONS**

Related Conditions	Unrelated Conditions
Diabetes type 1 with cataracts. E10.36 Type 1 diabetes mellitus with diabetic cataract	Age-related cataracts. Diabetes type 1. H25.9 Unspecified age-related cataract E10.9 Type 1 diabetes mellitus without complications
Diabetic peripheral neuropathy. E11.40 Type 2 diabetes mellitus with diabetic neuropathy, unspecified	Diabetes type 2. Peripheral neuropathy. E11.9 Type 2 diabetes mellitus without complications G62.9 Polyneuropathy, unspecified
Secondary diabetes due to gastroparesis. K31.84 Gastroparesis E08.43 Diabetes mellitus due to underlying condition with diabetic autonomic (poly)neuropathy	Diabetes type 2 and gastroparesis. E11.9 Type 2 diabetes mellitus without complications K31.84 Gastroparesis

combination code describing both conditions. Conditions that are unrelated are assigned separate codes. Refer to ■ TABLE 10-6 for examples of how physicians document related and unrelated conditions and how they are coded differently.

CODING CAUTION

Remember that *type 2* diabetes and *secondary* diabetes are different conditions. In type 2 diabetes, elevated glucose is due to the body's inability to store or release insulin. In secondary diabetes, elevated glucose is caused by an underlying condition or medication. Type 2 and secondary diabetes are identified with different codes.

Abstracting for Thyroid Disorders

When abstracting for thyroid disorders, coders must identify the cause of the condition and whether **goiter** or thyrotoxicosis is documented (■ FIGURE 10-2). The presence of these complications will affect code assignment later. Some thyroid conditions are **congenital**, so this information should also be noted. ■ TABLE 10-7 lists key criteria for abstracting thyroid disorders.

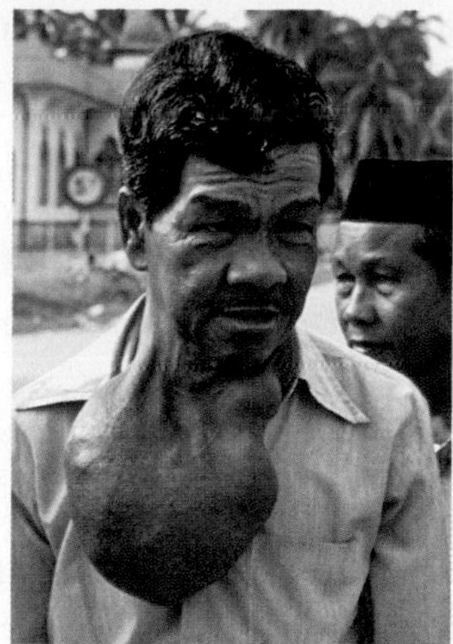

Figure 10-2 ■ Patients with a thyroid condition may also have a goiter. *Source: Eugene Gordon, Pearson Education/PH College.*

Table 10-7 ■ **KEY CRITERIA FOR ABSTRACTING THYROID DISORDERS**

- ❑ Is the condition hyperthyroidism or hypothyroidism?
- ❑ What is the cause of the condition?
- ❑ Is the condition congenital?
- ❑ Is goiter documented?
- ❑ Is thyrotoxicosis crisis documented?

Guided Example of Abstracting for the Endocrine System

Refer to the following example throughout the chapter to practice skills for abstracting and assigning codes for the endocrine system. Tamara Brownlee, CCS-P, is a fictitious coder who guides you through the coding process.

Date: 10/1/yy Location: Branton Medical Center

Provider: Ann Trull, MD

Patient: Justin Kraft Gender: M Age: 12

Reason for admission: hyperglycemia, ketoacidosis, glycosuria, family history (mother and grandmother) of type 1 diabetes

Tests: glucose tolerance test (GTT) positive for diabetes. Abdominal x-ray and CT of pancreas are normal.

Discharge diagnosis: new onset type 1 diabetes

Discharge plan: insulin injections bid (twice a day), FU office 2 weeks

Follow along in your ICD-10-CM manual as Tamara Brownlee, CCS-P, abstracts the diagnosis. Check off each step after you complete it.

⇨ Tamara reads the entire medical record and refers to Key Criteria for Abstracting Diabetes Mellitus (Table 10-5).

- ❑ *What type of diabetes is documented?* new onset type 1 diabetes
- ❑ *Are coexisting conditions documented as related to diabetes?* Tamara notes the symptoms documented under Reason for admission.
  - She identifies that hyperglycemia and glycosuria are integral to type 1 diabetes and should not be coded in addition to the disease (OGCR II.A).
- ❑ *What acute complications are documented?* She identifies that ketoacidosis is an acute complication that should be coded in addition to type 1 diabetes.
- ❑ *Is a family history of DM documented?* She identifies that family history of type 1 diabetes is significant because it poses a risk factor for the patient (OGCR I.C.21.c.4)).
- ❑ *Which problem or complication is the reason for the encounter?* She identifies that type 1 diabetes is the principal diagnosis, the "condition established after study to be chiefly responsible for occasioning the admission of the patient to the hospital for care." (OGCR II.)

⇨ Next, Tamara needs to assign codes.

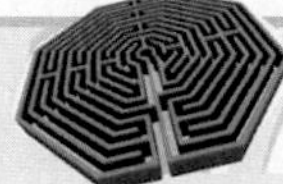

Coding Practice

Now it is your turn to practice abstracting diagnoses for the endocrine system. Questions guide your analysis of each scenario.

Exercise 10.2 Abstracting Diagnoses for the Endocrine System

Instructions: Read the mini-medical-record of each patient's encounter and answer the abstracting questions. Write the answer on the line provided. Do not assign any codes.

1. Date: 10/4/yy Location: North Side Endocrinology Clinic Provider: Ann Trull, MD

Patient: Randy Olney Gender: M Age: 56

Reason for encounter: monitoring of diabetes

Assessment: type 2 diabetes

Plan: HbA1c level is a little high. Discussed further diet management and exercise to better manage glucose

a. What is the reason for the encounter? ______________

b. What type of diabetes does the patient have? ______________

c. What complications are documented? ______________

d. What other conditions exist? ______________

2. Date: 10/3/yy Location: North Side Endocrinology Clinic Provider: Ann Trull, MD

Patient: Roger Ovalle Gender: M Age: 62

Chief complaint: open sore on right heel

Assessment: Patient has developed a foot ulcer with skin breakdown due to type 2 diabetes.

Plan: Refer to wound care.

a. What is the reason for the encounter? open sore on right heel L89.610

b. What type of diabetes does the patient have? Type 2

c. What complications are documented? foot ulcer w/ skin breakdown due to DB2

d. Where is the ulcer located? R heel L89.610

e. What is the extent of damage due to the ulcer? not staged.

3. Date: 10/3/yy Location: Branton Medical Center Provider: Ann Trull, MD

Patient: Alma Hatfield Gender: F Age: 58

Reason for admission: Admitted from emergency department due to weakness, shortness of breath, and severe abdominal pain with vomiting. Patient forgot to take insulin before going out to dinner.

(continued)

3. (continued)

Assessment: DKA, type 1 DM

a. What is the reason for the encounter? ______

b. What type of diabetes does the patient have? ______

c. What complications are documented? ______

d. What symptoms did the patient present with? ______

e. Should the symptoms be coded? ______
Why or why not? ______

f. Should long-term use of insulin be coded? Why or why not? ______

4. Date: 10/4/yy Location: Branton Medical Center Provider: Ann Trull, MD

Patient: Charlotte Strickland Gender: F Age: 36

Reason for admission: insulin-induced hypoglycemia

Assessment: *Patient has chronic pancreatitis for 2 years with secondary diabetes. Patient has struggled to monitor and self-administer insulin correctly.*

Plan: *Prescribe insulin pump. FU in office.*

a. What is the reason for the encounter? insulin – induced hyposlycemia

b. What type of diabetes does the patient have? secondary diabetes

c. What complications are documented? insulin-induced hyposly

d. What other conditions exist? chronic pancreatitis

e. Should long-term use of insulin be coded? Why or why not? ______

f. What Main Term should you look under in the Index to locate long-term use of insulin? Long term Drug therapy

g. What is the principal diagnosis? Insulin-induce
Why? hypoglycemia

5. Date: 10/4/yy Location: Neurology Associates

Provider: Lorene Garman, MD

Patient: Marcia Boggess Gender: F Age: 65

Reason for encounter: management of longstanding neuropathy

Assessment: *peripheral autonomic neuropathy, type 2 diabetes*

Plan: FU 6 months.

a. What is the reason for the encounter? ______

b. What type of diabetes does the patient have? ______

c. Is the neuropathy related to the diabetes? ______
Why or why not? ______

d. What is the first-listed diagnosis? ______

e. What is the additional diagnosis? ______

6. Date: 10/4/yy Location: North Side Endocrinology Clinic Provider: Ann Trull, MD

Patient: James Friday Gender: M Age: 25

Reason for encounter: *follow up on test results after evaluation of proximal muscle weakness, easy bruising, weight gain*

Assessment: *endogenous Cushing's syndrome due to pituitary adenoma*

Plan: *evaluate for surgery to remove tumor*

a. What is the reason for the encounter? follow up on test results after eval of proximal muscle weakness

b. What are the symptoms? easy bruising, muscle weakness, wt gain

c. Should the symptoms be coded? ______
Why or why not? NO b/c related

d. Is the adenoma malignant or benign? benign
Why? ______

e. What is the first-listed diagnosis? Cushing's syndrome

f. What is the cause of the first-listed diagnosis? Due to pituitary adenoma

g. What is the additional diagnosis? pituitary adenoma

ASSIGNING CODES FOR THE ENDOCRINE SYSTEM

When assigning codes for the endocrine system, carefully review the information abstracted from the medical record and determine if the condition is the primary condition or the result of a disease or condition in another body system. This information will affect what codes to assign and how to sequence them. Special attention to the Index is required. Diabetes is used as an example of assigning codes to endocrine system disorders.

Because diabetes has many variations and complications, coders must be especially careful to follow indented subterms in the Index. The Main Term **Diabetes** has only a few first-level subterm entries, each of which have second- and third-level indented subterms that are used as follows:

- First-level subterms identify the type of diabetes.
- Second-level subterms identify that complications are present through the word **with**.
- Third-level subterms identify the specific complication(s) with each type of diabetes.

The exception is when the type of diabetes is not specified. In this case, the complications are listed directly under the Main Term entry, following the indented subterm **with**. Notice that these are the same codes as **Diabetes, type 2** because OGCR directs coders to assign **type 2 diabetes** when the specific type is not documented in the medical record (OGCR I.C.4.a.2)). When the type of diabetes is specified, search for the corresponding first-level subterm before locating the complication.

CODING CAUTION

Selecting the correct *first-level subterm* is critical in order to arrive at the correct code because each type of diabetes can have similar complications. Consequently, the same second- and third-level indented terms appear under each different type of diabetes, but with different codes, which are determined by the first-level subterm.

Refer to ■ FIGURE 10-3 for an abbreviated view of the Index entry **Diabetes**. Selected subterms are shown. Review the first-level subterms and notice that each identifies a different type of diabetes, such as **due to drug or chemical** or **due to underlying condition**. All first-level subterms have the same second- and third-level subterms, **amyotrophy** and **arthropathy**. Each instance of **amyotrophy** and **arthropathy** has a different code because it is a combination code of the manifestation *and* the type of diabetes it is indented under.

SUCCESS STEP

Coders familiar with ICD-9-CM will notice some differences in diabetes coding in ICD-10-CM. Complications are reported with a combination code, reducing the need for multiple coding of complications. In addition, you do not need a fifth digit for *uncontrolled* or *not stated as uncontrolled,* which is no longer a criterion for assigning diabetes codes.

Guided Example of Assigning Endocrine System Codes

Continue with the example from earlier in the chapter about patient Justin Kraft, who was admitted to Branton Medical Center due to new onset of type 1 diabetes, to practice skills for assigning codes.

Follow along in your ICD-10-CM manual as Tamara Brownlee, CCS-P, assigns codes. Check off each step after you complete it.

➩ First, Tamara confirms that type 1 diabetes is the principal diagnosis. Diabetic ketoacidosis (DKA) and family history of diabetes are additional diagnoses.

➩ Tamara searches the Index for the Main Term **Diabetes**.

- ❑ She locates the subterm **type 1**.
- ❑ She reviews the subterms and locates **ketoacidosis**. She determines that the complication of DKA is a combination code with **type 1 diabetes** and she will not need an additional code for ketoacidosis.
- ❑ She notes that **ketoacidosis** has a further subterm for **with coma**, and verifies in the medical record that coma is NOT documented.
- ❑ She makes a note of the code to verify, **E10.10**.

➩ Tamara verifies code **E10.10** in the Tabular List.

- ❑ She reads the code title for **E10.10, Type 1 diabetes mellitus with ketoacidosis without coma** and confirms that this accurately describes the principal diagnosis.

➩ Tamara checks for instructional notes in the Tabular List.

- ❑ Tamara cross-references the beginning of category **E10** and verifies that there are no instructional notes.
- ❑ She cross-references the beginning of the block **Diabetes mellitus (E08-E13)** and verifies that there are no instructional notes that apply to all codes in the block. The instructional notes under **E08** apply only to codes in that category.
- ❑ She cross-references the beginning of **Chapter 4 (E00-E89)** and reviews the **NOTE:**. She determines that it does not apply to this case because the patient's diabetes is not related to another condition.

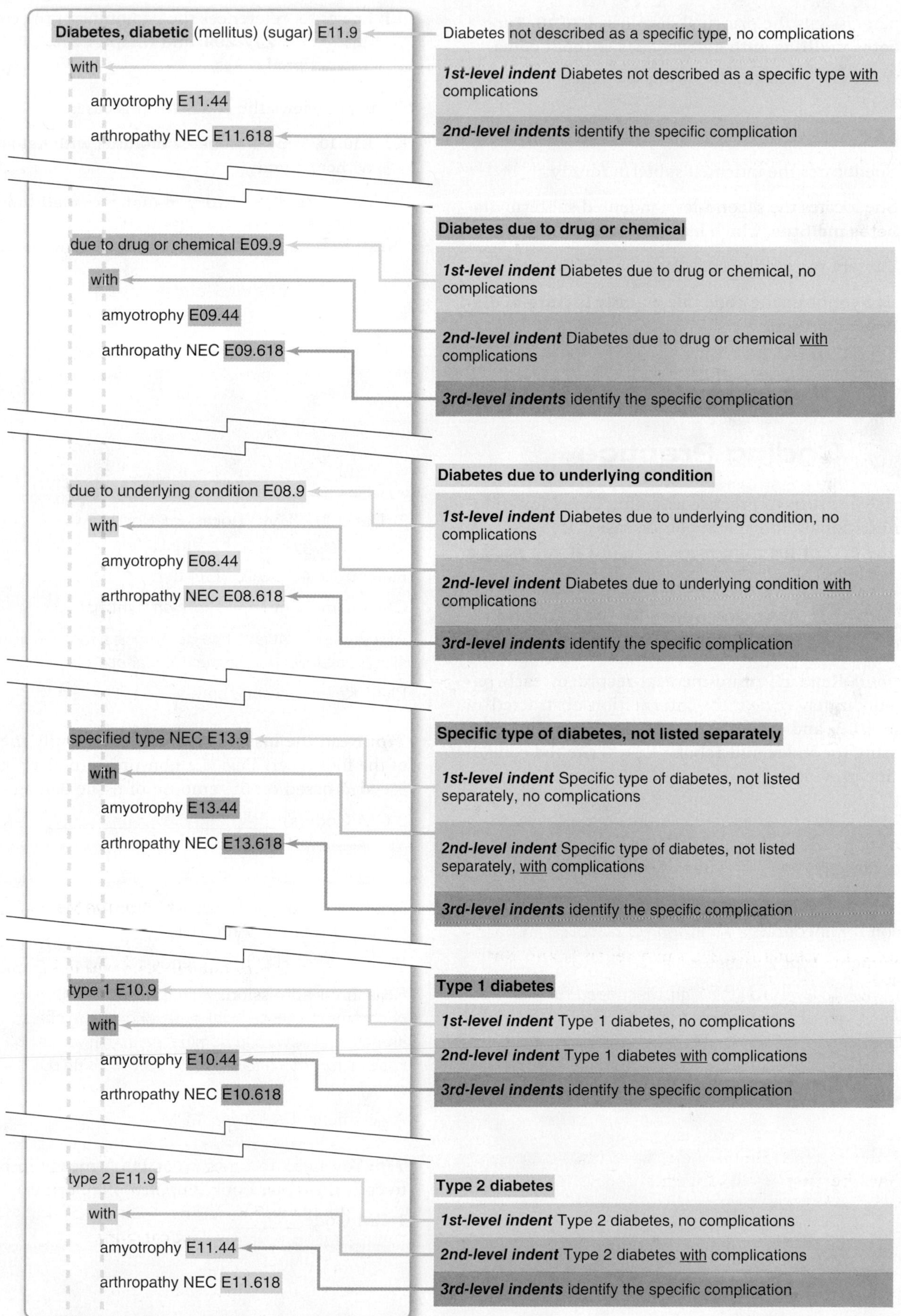

Figure 10-3 ■ Index Entry for Diabetes Showing Structure of Subterms

- Tamara assigns the principal diagnosis **E10.10, Type 1 diabetes mellitus with ketoacidosis without coma.**
- Next, Tamara assigns the code for family history of diabetes.
  - ❑ She locates the Main Term **History** in the Index.
  - ❑ She locates the indented subterm **family**.
  - ❑ She locates the second-level indented subterm **diabetes mellitus,** which has the code **Z83.3**.
  - ❑ Tamara verifies the code **Z83.3** in the Tabular List.
  - ❑ She confirms the code title, **Family history of diabetes mellitus.**
  - ❑ She cross-references the beginning of the category, **Z83**; block, **Z77-Z99**; and **Chapter 21 (Z00-Z99)** for instructional notes.
- Tamara reviews the codes for this case:
  - ❑ **E10.10, Type 1 diabetes mellitus with ketoacidosis without coma**
  - ❑ **Z83.3, Family history of diabetes mellitus**
- Next, Tamara will arrange (sequence) the codes.

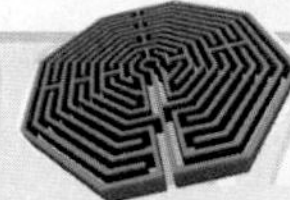

Coding Practice

Now it is your turn to practice assigning codes for endocrine, nutritional, and metabolic diseases. Refer to the ***Tip*** at the end of the mini-medical-record if you need a little extra help.

Exercise 10.3 Assigning Codes for the Endocrine System

Instructions: Read the mini-medical-record of each patient's encounter, review the information abstracted in Exercise 10.2, and assign ICD-10-CM diagnosis codes (CM) using the Index and Tabular List. Write the code(s) on the line provided.

1. Date: 10/4/yy Location: North Side Endocrinology Clinic Provider: Ann Trull, MD

Patient: Randy Olney Gender: M Age: 56

Reason for encounter: monitoring of diabetes

Assessment: type 2 diabetes

Plan: HbA1c level is a little high. Discussed further diet management and exercise to better manage glucose.

1 CM Code __________

2. Date: 10/3/yy Location: North Side Endocrinology Clinic Provider: Ann Trull, MD

Patient: Roger Ovalle Gender: M Age: 62

Chief complaint: open sore on right heel

Assessment: Patient has developed a foot ulcer with skin breakdown due to type 2 diabetes.

Plan: Refer to wound care.

***Tip*:** Read the instructional note to identify the site of the foot ulcer. This is a non-pressure ulcer and it is coded based on the amount of tissue damage.

2 CM Code(s) __________ __________

3. Date: 10/3/yy Location: Branton Medical Center Provider: Ann Trull, MD

Patient: Alma Hatfield Gender: F Age: 58

Reason for admission: Admitted from emergency department due to weakness, shortness of breath, and severe abdominal pain with vomiting. Patient forgot to take insulin before going out to dinner.

Assessment: DKA, type 1 DM

***Tip*:** You need to know what DKA means in order to code this case. Look it up if you are unsure.

1 CM Code __________

ARRANGING CODES FOR THE ENDOCRINE SYSTEM

Multiple coding is required throughout the endocrine system as directed by instructional notes in the Tabular List and conventions in the Index to Diseases and Injuries. When multiple coding is required, there is not one simple rule that dictates sequencing. Refer to OGCR and instructional notes in the Tabular List to determine proper sequencing. Diabetes is used for several examples of multiple coding rules due to its complexity, but the guidelines apply to all conditions. Other examples of multiple coding and sequencing are also provided.

Multiple Coding for Diabetes

Multiple coding is required for diabetes in the following circumstances:

- patients have unrelated conditions in addition to diabetes
- patients have more than one diabetic complication
- to provide additional details about a complication
- to report long-term use of insulin
- to report complications due to the malfunction of an **insulin pump**
- any combination of these situations

Examples of coding and sequencing for each of these situations follow.

Multiple Codes Due to Unrelated Conditions

When patients have coexisting conditions that are not related to or caused by diabetes, multiple codes are required, as shown previously in Table 10-6. Sequence the codes according to the documented reason for the encounter. When the encounter is for treatment or management of diabetes, sequence the diabetes code first (■ FIGURE 10-4). When the encounter is for treatment or management of an unrelated condition, sequence that code first (■ FIGURE 10-5).

Multiple Codes from a Single Diabetes Category

Patients often have more than one complication related to diabetes. Assign as many codes from an ICD-10-CM Chapter 4 category as necessary to describe all documented complications (OGCR I.C.4.a.). Sequence the codes according to the reason for the encounter (■ FIGURE 10-6).

Multiple Codes for Complications

Although all diabetic complications are assigned combination codes from the block **Diabetes mellitus (E00-E13)**, some complications also require codes from other body system chapters to provide additional details. Instructional notes at the beginning of the three-digit category direct the coder and include the following:

- Code first the underlying condition for secondary diabetes.
- Code first the drug or chemical causing secondary diabetes.
- Use an additional code to identify the stage of chronic kidney disease.
- Use an additional code to identify the site of skin ulcer.
- Use an additional code to identify a complication not listed.

For secondary diabetes, sequence the underlying cause first, such as the underlying condition or the drug causing the diabetic reaction. Sequence the code for secondary diabetes as an additional code (OGCR I.C.4.a.6)(b)). The instructional note in the Tabular List indicates this with the words **Code first underlying condition** or **Code first drug or chemical** (■ FIGURE 10-7, page 180).

When assigning multiple codes to describe additional details about a complication, sequence the code for diabetes first and the additional codes for the details about the complication second. The instructional note in the Tabular List indicates this with the words **Use additional code to identify** (■ FIGURE 10-8, page 180).

Patient with type 2 diabetes and peripheral neuropathy sees an endocrinologist for management of diabetes.

(1) **E11.9 Type 2 diabetes mellitus** without complications

(2) **G62.9 Polyneuropathy, unspecified**

Figure 10-4 ■ Example of Sequencing When Diabetes Is the Reason for the Encounter

Patient with type 2 diabetes sees a neurologist for management of peripheral neuropathy.

(1) **G62.9 Polyneuropathy, unspecified**

(2) **E11.9 Type 2 diabetes mellitus without complications**

Figure 10-5 ■ Example of Sequencing When an Unrelated Condition Is the Reason for the Encounter

Patient sees an ophthalmologist for diabetic cataracts and also has neuropathic arthropathy.

(1) **E11.36 Type 2 diabetes mellitus with diabetic cataract**

(2) **E11.40 Type 2 diabetes mellitus with diabetic neuropathy, unspecified**

Figure 10-6 ■ Example of Sequencing Multiple Codes from a Single Diabetes Category

Patient sees an endocrinologist for management of secondary diabetes due to chronic pancreatitis.

Code first the underlying condition

(1) **K86.1 Other chronic pancreatitis**

(2) **E08.9 Diabetes mellitus due to underlying condition without complications**

Figure 10-7 ■ Example of Sequencing the Underlying Condition

Patient with type 1 diabetes sees wound care for a diabetic foot ulcer with muscle necrosis on the heel of the left foot.

(1) **E10.621 Type 1 diabetes mellitus with foot ulcer**

Use additional code to identify site of ulcer (L97.4-, L97.5-)

(2) **L97.423 Non-pressure chronic ulcer of left heel and midfoot with necrosis of muscle**

Figure 10-8 ■ Example of Sequencing Details of a Complication

Multiple Codes for Long-term Use of Insulin

Multiple coding is required to identify long-term insulin use by type 2 diabetics and patients with secondary diabetes. According to the American Diabetic Association, approximately 20% to 25% of type 2 and secondary diabetics require insulin on a continuing basis. Instructional notes in the Tabular List direct coders to use **Z79.4 Long term (current) use of insulin** to identify long-term insulin use by these patients. Do not assign this code if insulin is given temporarily to bring a type 2 patient's blood sugar under control during an encounter (OGCR I.C.4.a.3) and 6)(a)). Sequence the diabetes code first and the **Z** code second (■ FIGURE 10-9).

SUCCESS STEP

Because all type 1 diabetics must use insulin, **Z79.4** is not required and should not be reported with a diagnosis of type 1 diabetes.

Multiple Coding for Complications Due to Insulin Pump Malfunction

Diabetic patients may wear an insulin pump (■ FIGURE 10-10) to regulate insulin evenly and avoid self-administering injections. Underdosing or overdosing of insulin due to insulin pump failure is reported with two codes from ICD-10-CM Chapter 19 Injury, Poisoning and Certain Other Consequences of External Causes (S00-T88) to describe the pump failure and the resulting problem (OGCR I.C.4.a.5)). Also assign codes for the type of diabetes and any related complications (■ FIGURE 10-11).

Patient with type 2 diabetes and diabetic nephropathy sees a nephrologist for management of kidney disease. Patient uses insulin to manage the diabetes.

Use additional code to identify any insulin use (Z79.4)

(1) **E11.21 Type 2 diabetes mellitus with diabetic nephropathy**

(2) **Z79.4 Long term (current) use of insulin**

Figure 10-9 ■ Example of Sequencing Long-Term Use of Insulin

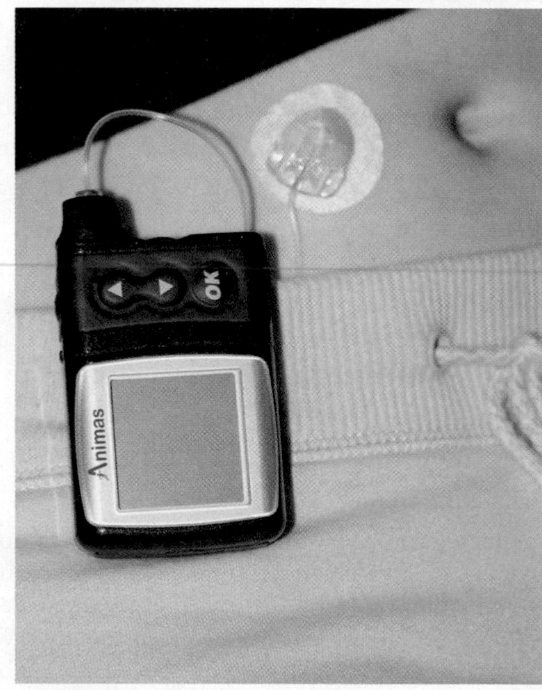

Figure 10-10 ■ An insulin pump detects when a patient needs insulin and dispenses it automatically. *Source: © Scott Camazine/Alamy.*

Multiple Conditions with Multiple Codes

Because diabetes is such a complicated disease, it is not uncommon for coders to encounter cases where several multiple coding situations must be addressed at the same time (■ FIGURE 10-12).

Multiple Coding for Other Endocrine System Conditions

Coders must always be alert for instructional notes in the Tabular List that direct them to assign more than one

Patient is seen in the emergency department for ketoacidosis due to the failure of her insulin pump and underdosing. She has type 1 diabetes and moderate nonproliferative diabetic retinopathy.

(1) **T85.614A Breakdown (mechanical) of insulin pump, initial encounter**

(2) **T38.3X6A, Underdosing of insulin and oral hypoglycemic [antidiabetic] drugs, initial encounter**

(3) **E10.10 Type 1 diabetes mellitus with ketoacidosis without coma**

(4) **E10.33 Type 1 diabetes mellitus with moderate nonproliferative diabetic retinopathy**

Figure 10-11 ■ Example of Sequencing Complications from Insulin Pump Failure

Patient has diabetes due to pituitary-dependent Cushing's disease and uses insulin to manage her diabetes. Patient is seen today for foot ulcer on right great toe with skin breakdown.

(1) **E24.0 Pituitary-dependent Cushing's disease**

(2) **E08.621 Secondary diabetes mellitus with foot ulcer**

(3) **L97.511 Non-pressure chronic ulcer of other part of right foot limited to breakdown of skin**

(4) **Z79.4 Long term (current) use of insulin**

Figure 10-12 ■ Example of Sequencing Multiple Conditions with Multiple Codes

code. Remember to refer to the beginning of the category and block for instructions when assigning codes from the endocrine system. Common situations in this chapter include the following examples and instructional notes:

1. Assign applicable codes from ICD-10-CM Chapter 4 for complications related to neoplasms or other conditions. Example:

   See NOTE: at beginning of Chapter 4.

2. Sequence codes from this chapter as additional codes when they are a manifestation of a disease in a different body system. Example:

   (1) **B90.8 Tuberculous calcification of adrenal gland**

   (2) **E35 Disorders of endocrine glands in diseases classified elsewhere**

3. Assign an additional code to identify the infectious agent in acute infections. Example:

   E06.0 Acute thyroiditis

   Use additional code (B95-B97) to identify infectious agent.

4. Assign an additional code to identify intellectual disabilities associated with congenital conditions. Example:

   E00 Congenital iodine-deficiency syndrome

   Use additional code (F70-F79) to identify associated intellectual disabilities.

5. Assign a code for body mass index (BMI), if known, with codes for obesity. Example:

   E66 Overweight and obesity

   Use additional code to identify body mass index (BMI), if known (Z68.-).

6. Sequence first any drug causing an endocrine condition. Example:

   E06.4 Drug-induced thyroiditis

   Code first (T36-T50) to identify drug.

Guided Example of Arranging Endocrine System Codes

To learn more about sequencing codes for the endocrine system, continue with the example about patient Justin Kraft, who was admitted to Branton Medical Center due to new onset of type 1 diabetes. Follow along as Tamara Brownlee, CCS-P, sequences the codes.

➪ Tamara reviews the codes for this case:

- ❑ **E10.10, Type 1 diabetes mellitus with ketoacidosis without coma**
- ❑ **Z83.3, Family history of diabetes mellitus**

➪ She identifies that type 1 diabetes is the principal diagnosis, the "condition established after study to be chiefly responsible for occasioning the admission of the patient to the hospital for care." (OGCR II).

- ❑ A code for family history of a disease is rarely a principal diagnosis.

➪ Tamara finalizes the codes and sequencing for this case.

- ❑ **E10.10, Type 1 diabetes mellitus with ketoacidosis without coma**
- ❑ **Z83.3, Family history of diabetes mellitus**

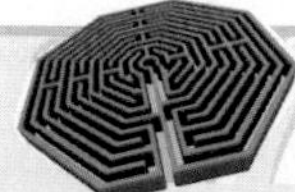

Coding Practice

Now it is your turn to practice sequencing codes for endocrine, nutritional, and metabolic diseases. Refer to the ***Tip*** at the end of the mini-medical-record if you need a little extra help.

Exercise 10.4 Arranging Codes for the Endocrine System

Instructions: Read the mini-medical-record of each patient's encounter, review the information abstracted in Exercise 10.2, assign ICD-10-CM diagnosis codes (CM) using the Index and Tabular List, and sequence them correctly.

1. Date: 10/4/yy Location: Branton Medical Center Provider: Ann Trull, MD

Patient: Charlotte Strickland Gender: F Age: 36

Reason for admission: insulin-induced hypoglycemia

Assessment: Patient has chronic pancreatitis for 2 years and associated diabetes. Patient has struggled to monitor and self-administer insulin correctly.

Plan: Prescribe insulin pump. FU in office.

Tip: Refer to OGCR for secondary diabetes.

3 CM Codes __________ __________ __________

2. Date: 10/4/yy Location: Neurology Associates

Provider: Lorene Garman, MD

Patient: Marcia Boggess Gender: F Age: 65

Reason for encounter: management longstanding neuropathy

Assessment: peripheral autonomic neuropathy, type 2 diabetes

Plan: FU 6 months.

Tip: The neuropathy is not stated as "due to" or "in" the diabetes.

2 CM Codes __________ __________

3. Date: 10/4/yy Location: North Side Endocrinology Clinic Provider: Ann Trull, MD

Patient: James Friday Gender: M Age: 25

Reason for encounter: follow up on test results after evaluation of proximal muscle weakness, easy bruising, weight gain

Assessment: endogenous Cushing's syndrome due to pituitary adenoma

Plan: evaluate for surgery to remove tumor.

Tip: An adenoma is benign, an adenocarcinoma is malignant.

2 CM Codes __________ __________

CODING NEOPLASMS OF THE ENDOCRINE SYSTEM

Neoplasms of the endocrine system do not appear in ICD-10-CM Chapter 4 Endocrine, Nutritional, and Metabolic Diseases (E00-E89); they appear in Chapter 2 (C00-D49). Codes for neoplasms of the endocrine system appear in the following blocks within the neoplasm chapter:

- C73-C75 Malignant neoplasm of thyroid and other endocrine glands
- C7A Malignant neuroendocrine tumors

- C7B Secondary neuroendocrine tumors
- D3A Benign neuroendocrine tumors

Review these blocks in the ICD-10-CM manual to become familiar with the content.

The most common sites for cancer in the endocrine system are the thyroid and pancreas. Thyroid cancer is the fifth most common cancer in women and accounts for 5% of new cancer cases, according to the American Cancer Society (ACS). Most types of thyroid cancer are treatable and most patients are cured and have a normal life expectancy. The American Society of Clinical Oncologists (ASCO) reports that the incidence rates of thyroid cancer in both women and men have been increasing in recent years and researchers are working to learn the reasons. Pancreatic cancer accounts for 3% of new cancer cases but has a poor survival rate because it is usually not diagnosed until after it has metastasized widely and, therefore, is difficult to treat.

Neoplasms of the ovaries and testes appear with neoplasms of other reproductive organs.

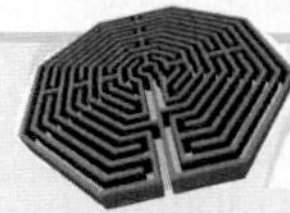

Coding Practice

Now it is your turn to practice coding neoplasms of the endocrine system. Refer to the ***Tip*** at the end of the mini-medical-record if you need a little extra help.

Exercise 10.5 Coding Neoplasms of the Endocrine System

Instructions: Read the mini-medical-record of each patient's encounter, then abstract, assign, and sequence ICD-10-CM diagnosis codes (CM) using the Index and Tabular List. Write the code(s) on the line provided.

1. Date: 10/5/yy Location: Branton Medical Center Provider: Ann Trull, MD

Patient: Sophie Darrah Gender: F Age: 35

Reason for encounter: thyroidectomy

Assessment: serous papillary carcinoma of the thyroid

Plan: thyroid hormone replacement

1 CM Code __________

2. Date: 10/5/yy Location: North Side Endocrinology Clinic Provider: Ann Trull, MD

Patient: Oscar Lampman Gender: M Age: 7

Reason for encounter: follow up on a solitary nodule discovered during a routine check-up 10 days ago

Assessment: Follicular adenoma of the thyroid

Plan: partial thyroidectomy

1 CM Code __________

3. Date: 10/5/yy Location: Branton Medical Center Outpatient Procedure Center

Provider: Ann Trull, MD

Patient: Jay Dames Gender: M Age: 5

(continued)

3. (continued)

Chief complaint: review X-ray and CT performed for dyspnea and cough

Assessment: thymoma

***Tip*:** According to Medscape, the most common location for mediastinal tumors in children is near the trachea, resulting in respiratory symptoms.

1 CM Code __________

4. Date: 10/5/yy Location: Branton Medical Center Provider: Stanley Garrett, MD

Patient: Tom Porcaro Gender: M Age: 51

Reason for Admission: surgical removal of carcinoid tumor

Diagnosis: malignant carcinoid tumor of small intestine with **carcinoid syndrome**

Plan: FU in office.

***Tip*:** Look up **carcinoid** tumor, not cancer or carcinoma.

2 CM Codes __________ __________

5. Date: 10/5/yy Location: Branton Medical Center Provider: Ann Trull, MD

Patient: Elvira McCreight Gender: F Age: 45

Reason for encounter: chemotherapy

Assessment: adenocarcinoma of pancreas with metastases to liver, lung, and colon

***Tip*:** Review OGCR I.C.2.e.2) for coding and sequencing reminders.

3 CM Codes __________ __________ __________

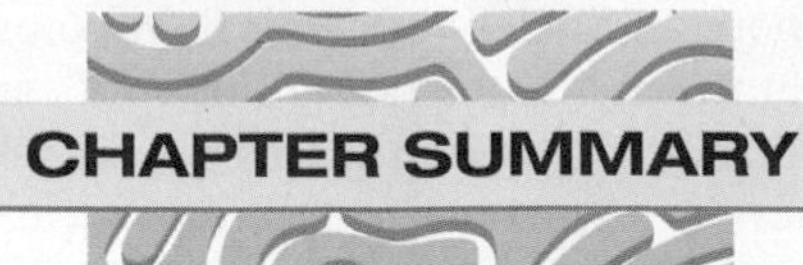

CHAPTER SUMMARY

In this chapter you learned the following:

- The function of the endocrine system is to produce, store, and release hormones, which are chemical messengers that regulate body functions including growth, development, metabolism, sexual function, reproduction, and mood.
- ICD-10-CM Chapter 4, Endocrine, Nutritional, and Metabolic Diseases (E00-E89) contains ten blocks or subchapters that are divided by anatomical site and type of disorder.
- In order to abstract endocrine system conditions, coders must distinguish between integral symptoms and signs as opposed to the conditions, complications, and manifestations.
- When assigning codes for the endocrine system, carefully review the information abstracted from the medical record and determine if the condition is the primary condition or the result of a disease or condition in another body system.
- Multiple coding is required throughout the endocrine system as directed by instructional notes in the Tabular List and conventions in the Index to Diseases and Injuries.
- The most common sites for cancer in the endocrine system are the thyroid and pancreas.

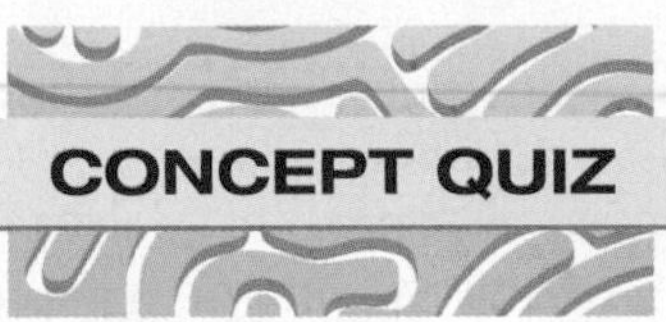

CONCEPT QUIZ

Take a moment to look back at your trip through endocrine, nutritional, and metabolic diseases and solidify your skills. This is your opportunity to pull together everything you have learned.

Completion

Instructions: Write the term that answers each question based on the information you learned in this chapter. Choose from the following list. Some choices may be used more than once and some choices may not be used at all. Refer to the discussion in this chapter and the Glossary at the end of this book if you need a little extra help.

body mass index (BMI)
diabetic ketoacidosis (DKA)
Graves disease
hyperglycemia
hyperosmolarity hyperglycemic nonketotic syndrome (HHNS)
hyperthyroidism
hypoglycemia
hypothalamus
hypothyroidism
metabolism
ovaries
pancreas
pituitary
testes
thyroid
thyrotoxicosis

1. The ______________ gland controls most activity in the endocrine system.
2. The ______________ and ______________ support both the endocrine system and reproductive system.
3. ______________ includes the processes of digestion, elimination, breathing, blood circulation, and maintaining body temperature.
4. ______________ is elevated glucose without ketoacidosis, usually occurring in elderly type 2 diabetics with other conditions.
5. The ______________ is a butterfly-shaped gland in front of the trachea that produces two hormones, tri-iodothyronine (T3) and thyroxine (T4).
6. ______________ is excessive quantities of circulating thyroid hormone due to overproduction by the thyroid gland, overproduction originating outside the thyroid, or loss of storage function and leakage from the gland.
7. ______________ is a deficiency of thyroid hormone, usually due to lack of production of the hormone by the thyroid or inadequate secretion of hormones.
8. Assign a code for ______________, if known, with codes for obesity.
9. ______________ is overproduction by the thyroid gland due to an autoimmune condition.
10. Cancer of the ______________ accounts for three percent of new cancer cases but has a poor survival rate because it is usually not diagnosed until after it has metastasized widely.

Multiple Choice

Instructions: Circle the letter of the best answer to each question based on the information you learned in this chapter. Refer to the discussion in this chapter and the Glossary at the end of this book if you need a little extra help.

1. The type of diabetes in which the body's immune system attacks pancreatic beta cells so that the pancreas does not produce insulin is
   A. type 1 diabetes.
   B. type 2 diabetes.
   C. secondary diabetes.
   D. ketoacidosis.
2. The type of diabetes in which elevated glucose is caused by an external factor, such as medication, surgery, pancreatic disease, or other illness, is
   A. type 1 diabetes.
   B. type 2 diabetes.
   C. secondary diabetes.
   D. ketoacidosis.
3. _________ accounts for 90 to 95% of all diagnosed cases of diabetes.
   A. Type 1 diabetes
   B. Type 2 diabetes
   C. Secondary diabetes
   D. Gestational diabetes
4. In _________ a high level of ketones accumulate in the blood, turning it acidic, and it can be life threatening if not treated immediately.
   A. hyperglycemia
   B. diabetic ketoacidosis
   C. hyperosmolarity hyperglycemic nonketotic syndrome
   D. hypoglycemia
5. Which of the following disorders is not classified in ICD-10-CM Chapter 4, Endocrine, Nutritional, and Metabolic Diseases (E00-E89)?
   A. DKA
   B. HHNS
   C. DM
   D. GDM
6. Which of the following word choices does NOT establish a causal relationship in physician documentation?
   A. due to
   B. in
   C. with
   D. and
7. Which of the following is NOT a key criterion for abstracting thyroid disorders?
   A. Is the condition congenital?
   B. Is goiter documented?
   C. Is insulin used on a long-term basis?
   D. Is thyrotoxicosis crisis documented?
8. Multiple coding may be required in all of the following situations EXCEPT:
   A. A patient has an unrelated condition in addition to diabetes.
   B. A patient has a diabetic complication.
   C. A type 2 diabetic uses insulin on a long-term basis.
   D. A patient experiences complications due to the malfunction of an insulin pump.
9. Under the Main Term Diabetes in the Index, first-level subterms identify
   A. the type of diabetes.
   B. that complications are present.
   C. the specific complication(s) with each type.
   D. long-term use of insulin.
10. The most frequent sites of cancer in the endocrine system are the
    A. thyroid and lung.
    B. thyroid and pancreas.
    C. ovaries and pancreas.
    D. thyroid and parathyroid.

CODING CHALLENGE

Now it is your turn to demonstrate coding all aspects of endocrine, nutritional, and metabolic diseases. Refer back to the examples and discussion in this chapter when you need a little extra help. Use your medical dictionary and anatomy references when needed.

Instructions: Read the mini-medical-record of each patient's encounter, then abstract, assign, and sequence ICD-10-CM diagnosis codes (CM) using the Index and Tabular List. Write the code(s) on the line provided.

1. Date: 10/15/yy Location: Branton Medical Center Provider: Ann Trull, MD

Patient: Lynda Rayburn Gender: F Age: 35

Reason for admission: T 102 F, tachycardia, extreme anxiety, nausea, diarrhea

Assessment: thyrotoxicosis with goiter and thyroid storm

Plan: Rx PTU (Prophylthiouracil) for thyroid and beta blocker Inderal to control heart rate

1 CM Code E05.01

2. Date: 10/15/yy Location: Branton Medical Center Provider: Ann Trull, MD

Patient: Adam Macklin Gender: M Age: 42

Reason for admission: Patient found non-responsive. Family reports patient being on a fast.

Assessment: non-diabetic hypoglycemic coma

Plan: instructed on diet and glucometer, FU 1 week

1 CM Code E15

3. Date: 10/15/yy Location: North Side Endocrinology Clinic Provider: Ann Trull, MD

Patient: Elisa Dewoody Gender: F Age: 25

Chief complaint: weight loss, appetite, sexual drive, and increased sensitivity to cold

Assessment: hypopituitarism

Plan: hormone replacement therapy, FU 4 wk

1 CM Code E23.0

4. Date: 10/15/yy Location: North Side Endocrinology Clinic Provider: Ann Trull, MD

Patient: Jack Edmiston Gender: M Age: 40

Reason for encounter: FU on lab test results of 24-hour aldosterone excretion rate 18 mcg; 24-h urine sodium above 400 mEq (*milliequivalent*) after presenting with severe hypokalemia, fatigue, muscle weakness, cramping, and hypertension

Assessment: primary hyperaldosteronism (Conn's syndrome) with secondary hypertension

Plan: medication to normalize BP, Na (sodium), electrolytes, and aldosterone

2 CM Codes E26.01 I15.2

5. Date: 10/15/yy Location: North Side Endocrinology Clinic Provider: Ann Trull, MD

Patient: Henrietta Whitmire Gender: F Age: 32

Chief complaint: irregular and infrequent menstrual periods, recent weight gain, noticeable loss of body hair under arms and pubic area

Assessment: polycystic ovarian syndrome

Plan: Rx hormones, FU 1 month

1 CM Code E28.2

6. Date: 10/15/yy Location: North Side Endocrinology Clinic Provider: Ann Trull, MD

Patient: Tonya Castanon Gender: F Age: 51

Reason for encounter: Annual check-up

Assessment: Test results show abnormally low vitamin D level. Patient is obese due to excess calories and has a BMI of 30.5.

Plan: Rx megadose vitamin D for 8 weeks, then recheck.

***Tip*:** Remember that you need a Z code for the annual check-up.

4 CM Codes Z00.01 E55.9 E66.09 Z68.30

7. **Date:** 10/15/yy **Location:** North Side Endocrinology Clinic **Provider:** Ann Trull, MD

Patient: Jeffery Swafford **Gender:** M **Age:** 48

Chief complaint: insomnia, hand tremor, hyperactivity, excessive sweating, weight loss

Assessment: Grave's disease with uninodular goiter

Hyperthyroidism goiter

Plan: radioiodine therapy

1 CM Code E05.10

8. **Date:** 10/15/yy **Location:** Branton Medical Center **Provider:** Ann Trull, MD

Patient: Thomas Haworth **Gender:** M **Age:** 57

Reason for admission: cold clammy skin and pallor, rapid breathing & heart rate

Assessment: hypovolemia

Plan: FU 1 wk

1 CM Code E86.1

9. **Date:** 10/15/yy **Location:** North Side Endocrinology Clinic **Provider:** Ann Trull, MD

Patient: Marguerite Silvas **Gender:** M **Age:** 68

Chief complaint: morbid obesity with shortness of breath

Assessment: hyperlipidemia group b

Plan: referred to nutritionist

1 CM Code E78.1

10. **Date:** 10/15/yy **Location:** Branton Medical Center **Provider:** Ann Trull, MD

Patient: Philip Knox **Gender:** F **Age:** 71

Reason for admission: palpitations and muscle weakness

Assessment: hyperkalemia, hyperosmolality

Plan: low potassium diet, referred to nutritionist, FU 1 month

2 CM Codes E87.5 E87.0

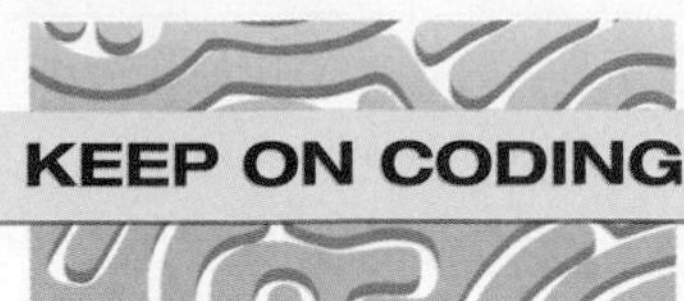

KEEP ON CODING

As a coder, you can never have too much experience. Apply everything you have learned in this chapter to code the following diagnostic statements. Use the OGCR and instructional notes in the Tabular List to help determine how many codes are required.

Instructions: Read the diagnostic statement, then use the Index and Tabular List to assign and sequence ICD-10-CM (CM) diagnosis codes. Write the code(s) on the line provided.

1. Type 1 diabetes mellitus with diabetic cataract, right eye: CM Code(s) ____________
2. Myxedema coma: CM Code(s) ____________
3. Postprocedural hypoparathyroidism: CM Code(s) ____________
4. Malignant neoplasm of the thymus gland: CM Code(s) ____________
5. Argininemia: CM Code(s) ____________
6. Diabetes insipidus: CM Code(s) ____________
7. Postinfectious hypothyroidism: CM Code(s) ____________
8. Drug-induced diabetes mellitus with diabetic neuralgia: CM Code(s) ____________
9. Pickwickian syndrome: CM Code(s) ____________
10. Type V glycogen storage disease: CM Code(s) ____________
11. Thyrotoxicosis factitia without thyrotoxic crisis: CM Code(s) ____________
12. Mixed hyperlipidemia: CM Code(s) ____________
13. Type 2 diabetes mellitus with diabetic gangrene: CM Code(s) ____________
14. Neonatal adrenoleukodystrophy: CM Code(s) ____________
15. Cushing's syndrome: CM Code(s) ____________
16. Constitutional gigantism: CM Code(s) ____________
17. Long chain/very long chain acyl CoA dehydrogenase deficiency: CM Code(s) ____________
18. Infantile osteomalacia: CM Code(s) ____________
19. Accidental puncture of thyroid during parathyroidectomy procedure: CM Code(s) ____________
20. Classical phenylketonuria: CM Code(s) ____________
21. Meconium ileus in cystic fibrosis: CM Code(s) ____________
22. Hypervitaminosis A: CM Code(s) ____________
23. Hypomagnesemia: CM Code(s) ____________
24. Infarction of the thyroid gland: CM Code(s) ____________
25. Estrogen excess: CM Code(s) ____________

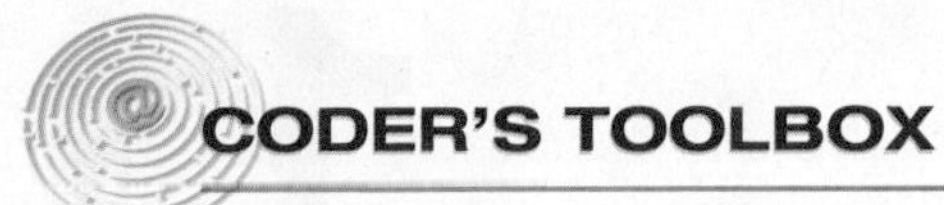

CODER'S TOOLBOX

The following resources are a starting point for learning more about endocrine, nutritional, and metabolic diseases. The > symbol indicates a menu selection within the website in order to navigate to a specific page.

American Association of Clinical Endocrinologists **https://www.aace.com/**

American Diabetes Association **http://www.diabetes.org/**

American Thyroid Association **http://www.thyroid.org/**

Cushing's Support and Research Foundation, Inc. **http://csrf.net/**

Health Indicators > Endocrine and Metabolic Disorders **http://mchb.hrsa.gov/whusa09/hstat/hi/pages/217emd.html**

Health Resources and Services Administration, Women's Health USA > Health Status > KidsHealth > Parents > General Health > Body Basics > Endocrine System **http://kidshealth.org/parent/general/body_basics/endocrine.html**

Lab Tests Online > Endocrine System and Syndromes **http://labtestsonline.org/understanding/conditions/endocrine**

National Adrenal Diseases Foundation **http://www.nadf.us/index.htm**

National Diabetes Information Clearinghouse (NDIC) **http://diabetes.niddk.nih.gov/**

National Endocrine and Metabolic Diseases Information Service **http://endocrine.niddk.nih.gov/index.aspx**

Nature Reviews Neuroscience **http://www.nature.com/nrn/journal/v5/n4/full/nrn1369.html**

Power of Prevention (American Association of Clinical Endocrinologists) **http://www.powerofprevention.com/index.php**

The Hormone Foundation **http://www.hormone.org/endo101/**

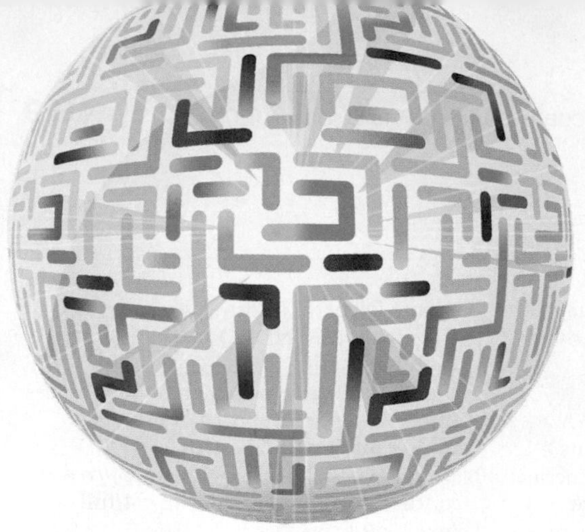

11

Diseases of the Skin and Subcutaneous Tissue (L00-L99)

Learning Objectives

After completing this chapter, you should have the skills to:

- Spell and define the key words, medical terms, and abbreviations related to the diseases of the skin and subcutaneous tissue.
- Discuss the structure, function, and common conditions of diseases of the skin and subcutaneous tissue.
- Identify the main characteristics of coding for diseases of the skin and subcutaneous tissue.
- Abstract diagnostic information from the medical record for coding diseases of the skin and subcutaneous tissue.
- Assign codes for diseases of the skin and subcutaneous tissue.
- Arrange codes for diseases of the skin and subcutaneous tissue.
- Code neoplasms of the integumentary system.
- Discuss the Official Guidelines for Coding and Reporting related to diseases of the skin and subcutaneous tissue.

Key Terms and Abbreviations

actinic keratosis
alopecia
allograft
autograft
basal cell carcinoma (BCC)
biopsy
cellulitis
culture
erythema multiforme
exfoliation
folliculitis
integumentary
keratosis
lichen
melanoma
patch testing
pemphigus
pityriasis
protection
psoriasis
regulation
sebaceous
secretion
sensation
squamous cell carcinoma (SCC)
stage 1 pressure ulcer
stage 2 pressure ulcer
stage 3 pressure ulcer
stage 4 pressure ulcer
subcutaneous
sudoriferous
synthetic
unstageable pressure ulcer
urticaria
vitiligo
xenograft

In addition to the key terms listed here, students should know the terms defined within tables in this chapter.

Chapter Outline

- **Integumentary System Refresher**
- **Coding Overview of the Skin and Subcutaneous Tissue**
- **Abstracting for the Integumentary System**
- **Assigning Codes for the Integumentary System**
- **Arranging Codes for the Integumentary System**
- **Coding Neoplasms of the Integumentary System**

ICD-10-CM codes in this chapter are from the ICD-10-CM 2014 Draft code set from the Department of Health and Human Services, Centers for Disease Control and Prevention.

INTRODUCTION

How does a car's exterior change from being new and polished to old and rusty? A new car's finish consists of a primer layer that helps the paint adhere to the structure of the car, several layers of paint, and a clear coat on top that serves as a protective finish. You dread the day that a new car sustains its first dent or scratch, but that day will inevitably come. How easily the dent or scratch can be repaired depends on how many layers it penetrates. A scratch in the clear coat can easily be buffed out, but a scratch through to the underlying metal can be costly to restore to new condition.

Your skin is the protective covering for your body and also consists of several layers, each with its own function. Repairing damage to the skin can be easy or difficult, depending on how far the damage penetrates. In your tour of the integumentary system in this chapter you will learn more about how the integumentary system works, why sometimes it does not work as it should, and how physicians treat these conditions. Most importantly, you will practice coding for patient encounters related to integumentary system diseases and conditions, a skill that requires you to abstract information from the mini-medical-record, assign correct codes, and arrange the codes in the proper order.

A dermatologist is a physician who specializes in diagnosing and treating conditions of the skin and subcutaneous tissues. Primary care physicians treat uncomplicated conditions of the skin and subcutaneous tissues. They refer patients with more complex conditions to dermatologists.

As you read this chapter, open up your medical terminology book to the chapter on the integumentary system and keep a medical dictionary handy. You will save time and be more accurate by taking a moment to look up unfamiliar terms or conditions.

INTEGUMENTARY SYSTEM REFRESHER

The **integumentary** (*pertaining to a covering*) system consists of the skin and accessory structures: hair, nails, **sebaceous** (*pertaining to oil*) glands, and **sudoriferous** (*pertaining to sweat*) glands (■ FIGURE 11-1). It is the largest organ in the body, weighing approximately six pounds and covering approximately 20 square feet, which is the size of a four-foot by five-foot rug. The integumentary system has four primary functions:

- **protection**—helps prevent invasion by pathogens, mechanical harm, and loss of fluids and electrolytes.

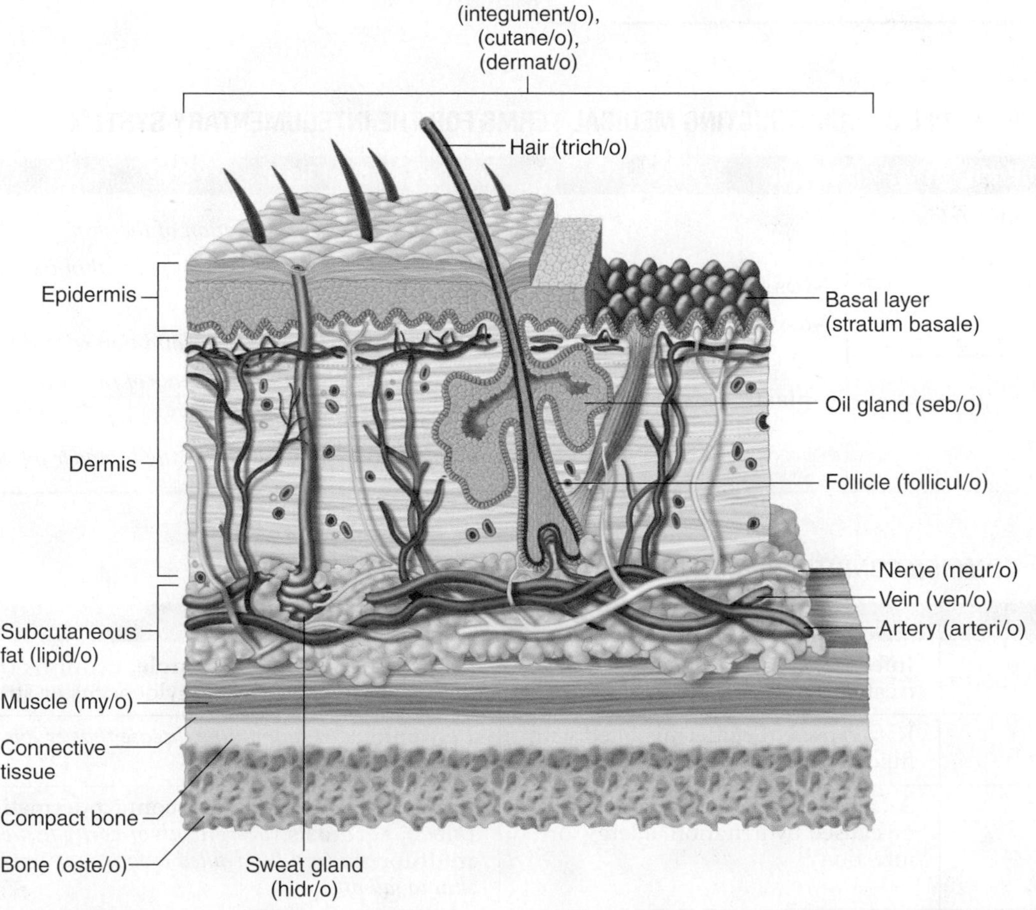

Figure 11-1 ■ The Integumentary System

- **regulation**—raises and lowers body temperature through constriction and dilation of blood vessels and sweat glands.
- **sensation**—contains sensory receptors for pain, touch, heat, cold, and pressure.
- **secretion**—gives off perspiration (water and salt) for temperature control and sebum (oil) to protect from dehydration and penetration by harmful substances.

In Figure 11-1, each structure in the integumentary system is labeled with its name as well as its medical terminology root/combining form. As you learn about conditions and procedures that affect the skin and **subcutaneous** (*under the skin*) structures, remember to apply medical terminology skills to combine word roots, prefixes, and suffixes you already know to define new terms. Refer to ■ TABLE 11-1 for a refresher on how to build medical terms related to the integumentary system.

CODING CAUTION

Be alert for medical terms that are spelled similarly and have different meanings.

myc/o (*fungus*) and **my/o** (*muscle*)

urticaria (*hives*) and **-uresis** (*urinataion*)

onych/o (*nail*) and **onc/o** (*tumor*)

Conditions of the Integumentary System

Common conditions of the integumentary system are summarized in ■ TABLE 11-2. Physicians diagnose problems through visual inspection, **patch testing** (*applying an allergen to the skin to observe the reaction*), **biopsy** (*scraping, punching, or cutting a piece of skin and examining it under a microscope*), and **culture** (*performing a test to identify the microorganism that is causing an infection*). Treatments include the following:

- medication to treat the underlying condition
- incision and drainage of fluid
- surgical removal of the lesion or damaged skin
- applying replacement tissue using an **autograft** (*tissue from the patient*), **allograft** (*tissue from another person*), **xenograft** (*tissue from an animal*), or a **synthetic** (*manmade tissue*) substitute.

This section provides a general reference to help understand the most common diagnoses of the integumentary system but does not list everything you need to know. Use medical terminology skills discussed to learn the meaning of unfamiliar words. Remember to keep standard reference books handy in case you get stuck. Refer to the resources in the Coder's Toolbox at the end of this chapter to learn more about conditions affecting the integumentary system.

Table 11-1 ■ **EXAMPLE OF CONSTRUCTING MEDICAL TERMS FOR THE INTEGUMENTARY SYSTEM**

Combining Form/Prefix	Suffix	Complete Medical Term
derm/o, dermat/o (*skin*) **cutane/o** (*skin*) **myc/o** (*fungus*) **erythr/o** (*redness*) **pachy-** (*thick*) **intra-** (*within*) **sub-** (*below*)	**-itis** (*inflammation*) **-osis** (*condition*) **-al** (*pertaining to*) **-plasty** (*surgical repair*)	**dermat + itis** (*inflammation of the skin*) **intra + derm + al** (*pertaining to within the skin*) **erythro + derma** (*red skin*) **dermo + myc + osis** (*skin condition related to fungus*) **dermo + plasty** (*surgical repair of the skin*) **sub + derm + al** (*pertaining to under the skin*) **sub + cutane + ous** (*pertaining to under the skin*)

Table 11-2 ■ **COMMON CONDITIONS OF THE INTEGUMENTARY SYSTEM**

Condition	Description	Examples
Bacterial infection	Infection caused by bacteria and treatable with antibiotics	Abscess, **furuncle, carbuncle, cellulitis** (*inflammation under the skin*) due to staphylococcus or streptococcus
Bulla (blister)	Raised area of epidermis filled with fluid	**Pemphigus** (*autoimmune disease that erupts in blisters*)
Dermatitis	A flat or raised eruption that can be caused by irritation, allergy, or infection	Eczema, atopic dermatitis, contact dermatitis, **urticaria** (*hives*), **keratosis** (*overgrowth of horny tissue*), **erythema multiforme** (*red fluid-filled lesions that can cause layers of skin to fall off*)

Table 11-2 ■ (continued)

Condition	Description	Examples
Papulosquamous disorders	Papules (*firm bumps*) and scales	**Psoriasis** (*round red patches covered with white scales*), **pityriasis** (*rough, dry scales*), **lichen** (*eruption of flat papules*)
Radiation disorders	Damage to the skin resulting from exposure to radiation	Sunburn, **actinic keratosis** (*a precancerous lesion*), radiodermatitis
Skin appendages	Nails, hair, sweat glands	Ingrowing nail, misshaped nails, **alopecia** (*baldness*), **folliculitis** (*inflammation of space around the hair root*), acne, sweat disorders
Non-pressure ulcers	Breakdown of skin that is not the result of prolonged pressure	Diabetic ulcer, ulcers due to poor circulation or clots (post-phlebitic, post-thrombotic, venostasis)
Decubitus ulcer (pressure ulcer, bed sore)	Breakdown of the skin, usually over bony parts of body, caused by continuous pressure, friction, moistness, and heat	Stage 1—redness that does not go away Stage 2—damage to epidermis that extends into the dermis Stage 3—damage through the full thickness of the dermis and into the subcutaneous tissue (fat) Stage 4—damage extending into the muscle, tendon, or bone Unstageable—ulcers covered with dead cells, **eschar**, or wound exudate that cannot be visually assessed
Pigmentation disorder	Damage to or unhealthy melanin cells that give color to the skin	Age spots, freckles, **vitiligo** (*loss of pigmentation*)

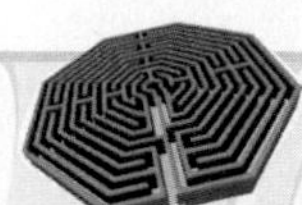

Coding Practice

Refresh your knowledge of terminology related to the integumentary system. Use a medical terminology text or a website such as GlobalRph.com > Medical Terminology http://www.globalrph.com/medterm.htm to identify the meaning of word parts that may not be familiar to you.

Exercise 11.1 Integumentary System Refresher

Instructions: Use your medical terminology skills and resources to define the following terms related to the integumentary system, then assign the diagnosis code.

Follow these steps:

- Use slash marks "/" to break down each term into its root(s) and suffix.
- Define the meaning of the word, based on the meaning of each word part.
- Assign the default ICD-10-CM diagnosis code (CM) for the condition using the Index and Tabular List.

Example: dermatitis dermat/itis Meaning: inflammation of the skin CM Code: L30.9

1. pachyderma Meaning ________ CM Code ________
2. hypertrichosis Meaning ________ CM Code ________
3. perifolliculitis Meaning ________ CM Code ________
4. cellulitis Meaning ________ CM Code ________
5. erythroderma Meaning ________ CM Code ________
6. pyoderma Meaning ________ CM Code ________
7. onychocryptosis Meaning ________ CM Code ________
8. hyperkeratosis Meaning ________ CM Code ________
9. hidraenitis Meaning ________ CM Code ________
10. onychodystrophy Meaning ________ CM Code ________

CODING OVERVIEW OF THE SKIN AND SUBCUTANEOUS TISSUE

ICD-10-CM Chapter 12, Diseases of the Skin and Subcutaneous Tissue (L00-L99), contains nine blocks or subchapters that are divided by anatomical site and type of condition. This chapter includes skin disorders that are not caused by infectious agents, injury, or neoplasms. Review the block names and code ranges listed at the beginning of Chapter 12 in the ICD-10-CM manual to become familiar with the content and organization.

ICD-10-CM Chapter 12 corresponds with ICD-9-CM Chapter 12 (680–709). Many categories have been expanded to reflect the greater specificity available in ICD-10-CM, such as pemphigus, pemphigoid, alopecia areata, carbuncle and furuncle of the trunk, impetigo, and psoriasis. Pressure ulcer codes are combination codes that identify the stage, site, and laterality in a single code, unlike ICD-9-CM which required multiple codes

Take note of the **Excludes2** note which lists skin conditions not classified in this chapter. The following types of skin disorders are classified in other ICD-10-CM chapters:

- Burns (Chapter 19, Injury and Poisoning)
- Neoplasms (Chapter 2, Neoplasms)
- Viral, bacterial, and fungal infections (Chapter 1, Certain Infectious and Parasitic Diseases)
- Parasites (Chapter 1, Certain Infectious and Parasitic Diseases)

ICD-10-CM provides Official Guidelines for Coding and Reporting (OGCR) Diseases of the Skin and Subcutaneous Tissue in OGCR section I.C.12. OGCR provides detailed discussion of assigning codes for pressure ulcer stages. Additional guidelines related to skin infections appears in OGCR I.C.1.b. Guidelines related to burns and other skin injuries appear in OGCR I.C.19.d. Instructional notes throughout the chapter provide information on multiple coding and sequencing.

ABSTRACTING FOR THE INTEGUMENTARY SYSTEM

When abstracting for diseases of the integumentary system, coders need to be familiar with the various types of lesions and complications, as well as the systems used to describe the extent of damage to the skin (■ TABLE 11-3). Remember that the abstracting questions are a guide and that not every question applies to, or can be answered for, every case. For example, not every case has an infectious agent.

Depth of damage is described based on documentation of what layers of tissue are affected. The description varies based on the condition, such as the following:

- Conditions confined to the epidermis by definition, such as contact dermatitis or superficial lesions, do not require depth descriptions.
- Sunburns are classified by the degree of the burn (■ TABLE 11-4).
- Pressure ulcers are assigned a numerical stage from 1 to 4, based on depth (■ FIGURE 11-2).
- Non-pressure ulcers are classified as follows:
  - limited to breakdown of skin
  - fat layer exposed
  - necrosis of muscle
  - necrosis of bone

Table 11-3 ■ KEY CRITERIA FOR ABSTRACTING CONDITIONS OF THE INTEGUMENTARY SYSTEM

- ❑ What is the type of lesion (carbuncle, abscess, urticaria, mole, corn)?
- ❑ What is the anatomic site (face, back, hand)?
- ❑ What is the laterality (right or left side)?
- ❑ Is there an underlying cause (another condition, exposure to a drug, or environmental substance)?
- ❑ What is the infectious agent, if any?
- ❑ Are there complications or manifestations (gangrene)?
- ❑ What is the depth or extent of damage?

Table 11-4 ■ CLASSIFICATION OF BURNS

Degree	Name	Description
1st	Superficial	Damage to the epidermis
2nd	Partial thickness	Damage to the epidermis and part of the dermis
3rd	Full thickness	Damage to the entire depth of the dermis

CODING CAUTION

ICD-10-CM uses Arabic numerals 1, 2, 3, and 4 to identify pressure ulcer stages. The National Pressure Ulcer Advisory Panel, and many physicians, use Roman numerals I, II, III, and IV. Coders need to be familiar with both ways of writing and reading numbers.

Stage 1: Skin discolored, but intact

Epidermis
Dermis
Subcutaneous fat
Muscle
Bone

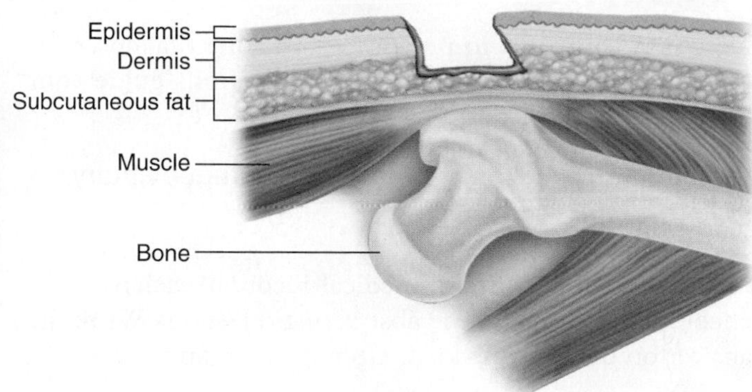

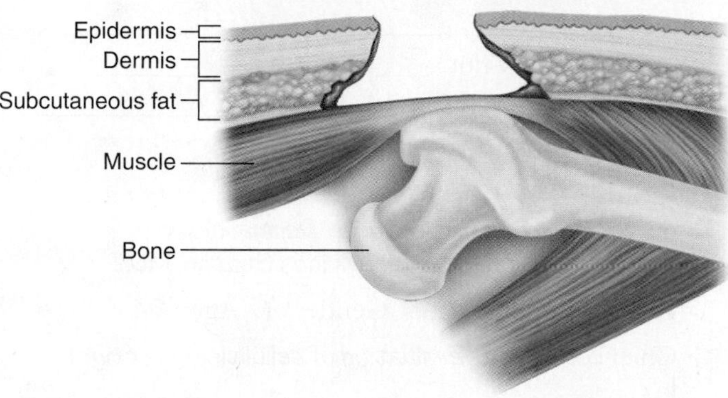

Stage 4: Exposed bone, muscle or tendon

Epidermis
Dermis
Subcutaneous fat
Muscle
Bone

Figure 11-2 ■ Classification of Pressure Ulcer Stages

Guided Example of Abstracting for the Integumentary System

Refer to the following example throughout this chapter to practice skills for abstracting and assigning codes for the integumentary system. Joshua Grider, CPC, is a fictitious coder who guides you through this case.

> Date: 11/1/yy Location: Dermatology Associates
>
> Provider: Lawrence Staton, MD
>
> Patient: Naomi Vargas Gender: F Age: 84
>
> Reason for encounter: debride and change dressing on pressure ulcer per referral from home health care nurse
>
> Assessment: damage through the full thickness of the dermis and into the **subQ** tissue; stage 3 pressure ulcer, right buttock
>
> Plan: FU visits from home health care

Follow along as Joshua Grider, CPC, abstracts the diagnosis. Check off each step after you complete it.

⇨ Joshua reads through the entire record, with special attention to the reason for the encounter and the final assessment.

- ❑ He notes that the procedure of debriding the wound is consistent with a stage 3 ulcer. He refers to Key Criteria for Abstracting Conditions of the Integumentary System (Table 11-3).
- ❑ *What is the type of lesion?* pressure ulcer
- ❑ *What is the anatomic site?* buttock
- ❑ *What is the laterality?* right
- ❑ *Is there an underlying cause?* No
- ❑ *What is the infectious agent, if any?* None
- ❑ *Are there complications or manifestations?* No
- ❑ *What is the depth or extent of damage?* stage 3
- ❑ He refers to the definition of pressure ulcer stages and confirms that the description damage through the full thickness of the dermis and into the subQ tissue is consistent with a stage 3 ulcer.

⇨ Next, Joshua needs to assign the codes.

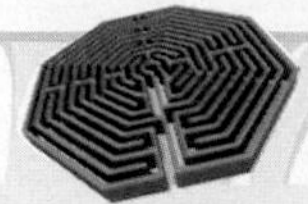

Coding Practice

Now it is your turn to practice abstracting diagnoses for the skin and subcutaneous tissue. Questions guide your analysis of each scenario.

Exercise 11.2 Abstracting for the Integumentary System

Instructions: Read the mini-medical-record of each patient's encounter and answer the abstracting questions. Write the answer on the line provided. Do not assign any codes.

1. Date: 11/3/yy Location: Branton Family Practice Provider: Kristen Conover, MD

Patient: Ethel McCown Gender: F Age: 5

Chief complaint: was at the beach all day and did not have sunscreen applied

Assessment: a severe second degree sunburn

a. What is the chief complaint? ______________________

b. What is the source of the sunburn? ______________________

c. What degree is the sunburn? ______________________

d. What is the definition of a second degree sunburn? ______________________

2. Date: 11/3/yy Location: Branton Family Practice Provider: Kristen Conover, MD

Patient: Thelma Nathan Gender: F Age: 17

Chief complaint: red itchy patches after hiking

Assessment: contact dermatitis due to poison ivy

a. What is the chief complaint? ______________________

b. Should you code for the red itchy patches? ______________________

Why or why not? ______________________

c. What is the diagnosis? ______________________

d. What is the Main Term? ______________________

3. Date: 11/3/yy Location: Dermatology Associates Provider: Lawrence Staton, MD

Patient: Jeremy Laney Gender: M Age: 15

Chief complaint: red and tender area on the left great toe

Assessment: ingrown nail

a. What is the reason for the visit? ______________________

b. What condition does the physician diagnose? ______________________

c. Should you code the redness and tenderness? ______________________

Why or why not? ______________________

4. Date: 11/4/yy Location: Dermatology Associates Provider: Lawrence Staton, MD

Patient: Candice Doss Gender: F Age: 64

Chief complaint: evaluation of cellulitis on her right leg

Assessment: lab results show the cellulitis to be due to streptococcus A

Plan: Rx oral antibiotics. If it does not improve within 3 days or gets worse, she will need to be admitted for IV antibiotics.

a. What condition is being evaluated? ______________________

b. What is the anatomic site? ______________________

c. What is the laterality? ______________________

d. What is the infectious agent? ______________________

5. Date: 11/4/yy Location: Dermatology Associates Provider: Lawrence Staton, MD

Patient: Jonas Wills Gender: M Age: 25

Reason for encounter: follow-up on erythema multiforme minor with stomatitis due to herpes simplex virus

Assessment: Stomatitis showing improvement. 15% of his skin is exfoliated.

a. What condition is being treated? ______________________

b. What is the manifestation? ______________________

c. What virus caused the condition? ______________________

d. What does exfoliation mean? ______________________

e. What is the percentage of exfoliation? ______________________

6. Date: 11/4/yy Location: Dermatology Associates Provider: Lawrence Staton, MD

Patient: Robert Maines Gender: M Age: 73

Reason for encounter: debride and dress chronic ulcer on right calf

Assessment: chronic ulcer due to postphlebitic syndrome. Healing is progressing. At last visit some muscle necrosis was visible. Today only the fat layer is exposed.

a. What condition is being treated? ______________________

b. What is the anatomic site? ______________________

c. What is the laterality? ______________________

d. Is this a pressure ulcer or a non-pressure ulcer? ______________________

e. What is the underlying condition? ______________________

ASSIGNING CODES FOR THE INTEGUMENTARY SYSTEM

When assigning codes for the integumentary system, coders need to be alert for easily confused index entries and must use the information abstracted regarding the depth or extent of skin damage, when applicable.

Skin ulcers are classified into separate categories based on whether they are decubitus (pressure) ulcers or non-pressure ulcers. Pressure ulcers are caused by prolonged pressure on an area, usually a bony prominence, such as the heel, elbow, or hip. Pressure ulcers are indexed under the Main Term **Ulcer**, then the subterm **pressure**, then a second-level subterm for the anatomic site. The most common causes of non-pressure ulcers are diabetes and circulatory problems. Non-pressure skin ulcers are indexed under the Main Term **Ulcer** and a subterm for the anatomic site.

The stage or depth of a pressure ulcer changes as the wound heals or worsens. Assign a code based on the stage documented during the encounter. For an ulcer that worsens during the course of an inpatient admission, assign a code for the highest stage (OGCR I.C.12.a.6). When patients have more than one pressure ulcer, assign separate codes for each ulcer (OGCR I.C.12.a.1).

Some skin conditions cause exfoliation (*falling off in scales or layers*) of the skin. These codes provide the instructional note **Use additional code to identify percentage of skin exfoliation (L49-).**

Guided Example of Assigning Integumentary System Codes

To practice skills for assigning codes for conditions of the integumentary system, continue with the example from earlier in the chapter about patient Naomi Vargas, who was seen by Dr. Stanton due to a stage 3 pressure ulcer on the right buttock.

Follow along in your ICD-10-CM manual as Joshua Grider, CPC, assigns codes. Check off each step after you complete it.

⇨ First, Joshua confirms the diagnosis stage 3 pressure ulcer on the right buttock.

➩ Joshua searches the Index for the Main Term **Ulcer**.

- ❑ He reviews the subterms and notes that many types of ulcers are indexed here, including ulcers in internal organs.
- ❑ He locates a subterm for **buttock**.
- ❑ He locates the second-level subterm for **exposed fat layer L98.412**.

➩ Joshua verifies the code in the Tabular List.

- ❑ He reads the code title **L98.412, Non-pressure chronic ulcer of buttock with fat layer exposed**.
- ❑ Joshua notices that this code is for a *non-pressure* ulcer, which is *not* the diagnosis for this patient.

CODING CAUTION

Remember to distinguish the *cause* of the skin ulcer. A pressure ulcer is due to continuous pressure on an area, often found in patients with limited mobility. A non-pressure ulcer is due to another cause, such as venous insufficiency or diabetes, not due to pressure.

➩ Joshua realizes he selected an incorrect subterm in the Index, so ***he returns to the Index*** entry for the Main Term **Ulcer** to search for a different subterm.

- ❑ He locates the subterm **pressure**.
- ❑ He locates the second-level subterm **buttock L89.3**.

➩ Joshua returns to the Tabular List to verify code **L89.3**.

- ❑ He reads the category title **L89.3, Pressure ulcer of buttock**.
- ❑ He notices the convention **5th** instructing him to assign a fifth character.
- ❑ He reads the titles of the fifth character categories and notes that they indicate laterality.
- ❑ He locates **L89.31, Pressure ulcer of right buttock**.
- ❑ He notices the convention **6th** instructing him to assign a sixth character.
- ❑ He reads the titles of the sixth character codes and notes that they indicate stage.
- ❑ He locates **L89.313, Pressure ulcer of right buttock, stage 3**.
- ❑ He confirms that this accurately describes the diagnosis in the medical record.

➩ Joshua checks for instructional notes in the Tabular List.

- ❑ He cross-references the beginning of category **L89** and reads the instructional notes.
  - The inclusion notes confirm that this category classifies pressure or decubitis ulcers. The **Excludes2** note confirms that other types of ulcers are not coded here.
  - He reads the note to **Code first any associated gangrene (I96)**.
  - He cross-references the medical record to confirm that gangrene is not documented. Because it is not documented, he does *not* assign a code for gangrene.
- ❑ Next, Joshua cross-references the beginning of the block Other disorders of the Skin and Subcutaneous Tissue (L80-L99) and verifies that there are no instructional notes.
- ❑ Finally, he cross-references the beginning of Chapter 12 Diseases of the Skin and Subcutaneous Tissue (L00-L99) and reviews the instructional notes.
  - The only instructional notes are an **Excludes2** note indicating what conditions are not classified in this chapter.
  - He determines that the **Excludes2** does not apply to this case because the patient's condition does not fit the description of any of the listed conditions.

➩ Joshua cross-references the medical record and finalizes the code for this case:

- ❑ **L89.313, Pressure ulcer of right buttock, stage 3.**

Coding Practice

Now it is your turn to practice assigning codes for diseases of the skin and subcutaneous tissue. Refer to the ***Tip*** at the end of the mini-medical-record if you need a little extra help.

Exercise 11.3 Assigning Codes for the Integumentary System

Instructions: Read the mini-medical-record of each patient's encounter, review the information abstracted in Exercise 11.2, and assign ICD-10-CM diagnosis codes (CM) using the Index and Tabular List. Write the code(s) on the line provided.

1. Date: 11/3/yy Location: Branton Family Practice Provider: Kristen Conover, MD

Patient: Ethel McCown Gender: F Age: 5

Chief complaint: was at the beach all day and did not have sunscreen applied

Assessment: a severe second degree sunburn

1 CM Code __________

2. Date: 11/3/yy Location: Branton Family Practice Provider: Kristen Conover, MD

Patient: Thelma Nathan Gender: F Age: 17

Chief complaint: red itchy patches after hiking

(continued)

2. (continued)

Assessment: contact dermatitis due to poison ivy

Tip: Recall that external cause codes for activity are not applicable to poisonings, so you do not need any additional codes.

1 CM Code __________

3. Date: 11/3/yy Location: Branton Family Practice Provider: Kristen Conover, MD

Patient: Jeremy Laney Gender: M Age: 15

Chief complaint: red and tender area on the left great toe

Assessment: ingrown nail

1 CM Code __________

ARRANGING CODES FOR THE INTEGUMENTARY SYSTEM

Sequencing of codes for the integumentary system follows the general coding guidelines OGCR III and IV as well as instructional notes in the Tabular List. In some cases, coders must apply multiple instructional notes for one code. A single category may include notes for **Code first** instructions as well as one or more **Use additional code** instructions. **Code first** means that the code listed should be sequenced before the code from the category in which it appears. **Use additional code** means that the code listed should be sequenced after the code from the category in which it appears.

Guided Example of Arranging Integumentary System Codes

Refer to the following new example of a patient with Stevens-Johnson syndrome to learn how to arrange codes when there are multiple instructional notes. Joshua Grider, CPC, guides you through this case. Review the following mini-medical-record to learn what information Joshua abstracted for each code.

Date: 11/2/yy Location: Branton Medical Center Provider: Lawrence Staton, MD

Patient: Ralph Wray Gender: M Age: 2

Reason for admission: Sudden outbreak of lesions on face, bilaterally on arms and legs, groin after taking a prescribed sulfonamide. Fever. Mouth sores.

Assessment: Stevens-Johnson syndrome, 64% exfoliation

(1) L51.1 Stevens-Johnson syndrome

(2) T37.0X5A Adverse effect of sulfonamides, initial encounter

(3) K12.32 Oral mucositis (ulcerative) due to other drugs

(4) L49.6 Exfoliation due to erythematous condition involving 60-69 percent of body surface

Follow along in your ICD-10-CM manual as Joshua Grider, CPC, assigns and arranges codes. Check off each step after you complete it.

➪ Joshua first assigns the code for Stevens-Johnson syndrome. He locates the Main Term **Stevens-Johnson syndrome L51.1** in the Index, then refers to the Tabular List to verify the code.

- ❑ He reads through the instructional notes at the beginning of category **L51** in the Tabular List (■ FIGURE 11-3).

➪ Joshua reads the first instructional note, which states **Use additional code to identify drug, (T36-T50 with fifth or sixth character 5)**.

- ❑ The documentation states that the condition is the result of taking a *prescribed sulfonamide*.
- ❑ Joshua sequences code **T37.0X5A, Adverse effect of sulfonamides, initial encounter** as the second code because the instructional note states **Use additional code**, which means the drug code should appear *after* the code from this category **(L51)** for the condition.

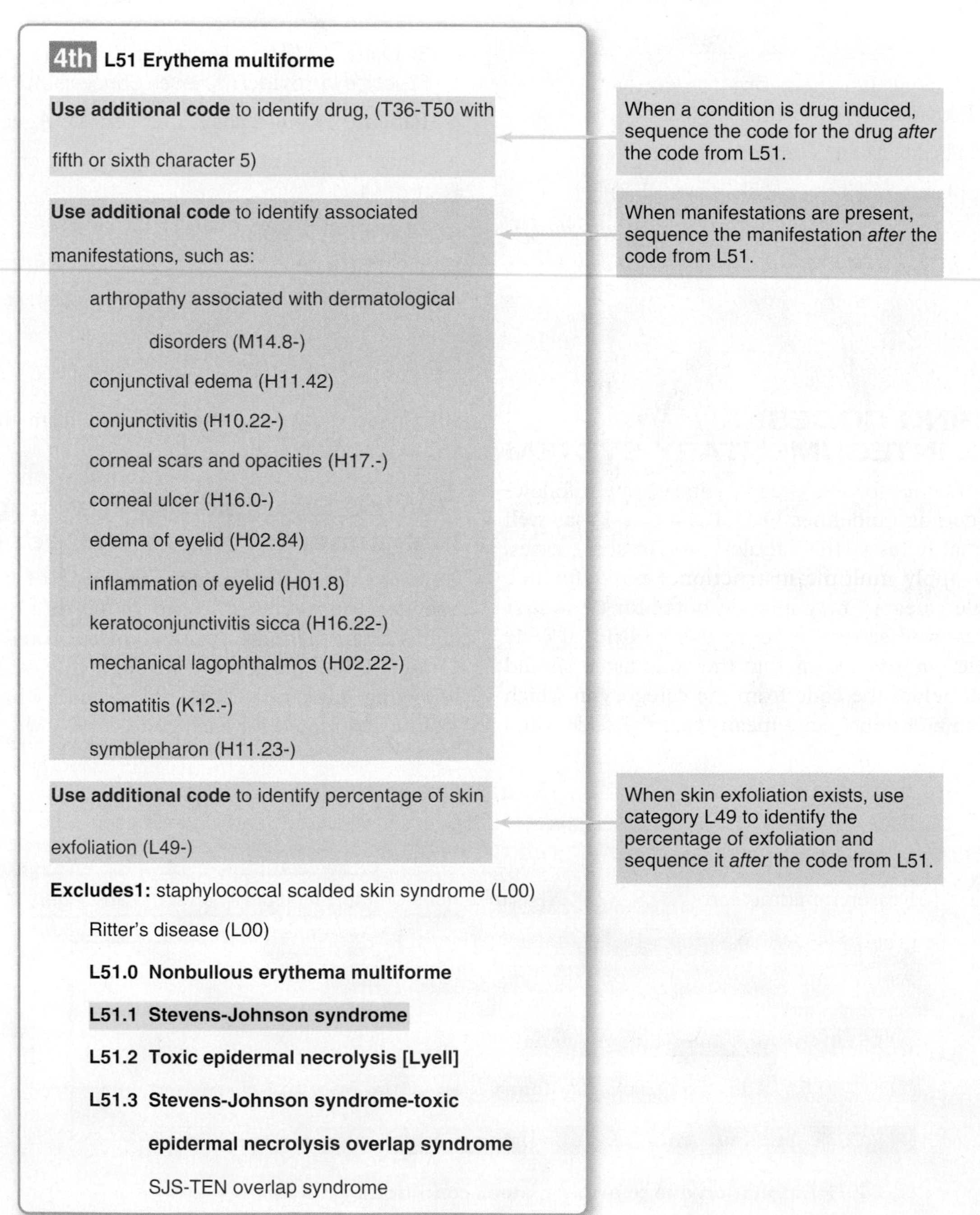

Figure 11-3 ■ Multiple Coding and Sequencing Instructions for All Codes within a Category

⇨ Joshua sequences the condition code first, **L51.1, Stevens-Johnson syndrome**.

⇨ Joshua reads the second instructional note, which states **Use additional code to identify associated manifestations: stomatitis (K12.-)**.

- ❑ He refers to the documentation and confirms the manifestation, **Mouth sores**.
- ❑ He sequences the third code as **K12.32, Oral mucositis (ulcerative) due to other drugs** because the instructional note **Use additional code** means the manifestation code should be sequenced *after* the code from this category **(L51)** for the condition.

⇨ Joshua reads the third instructional note, which states **Use additional code to identify percentage of skin exfoliation (L49-)**.

- ❑ He refers to the documentation and confirms 64% exfoliation.
- ❑ He sequences the fourth code as **L49.6, Exfoliation due to erythematous condition involving 60-69 percent of body surface** because this is also stated to be an *additional* code.

Coding Practice

Now it is your turn to practice arranging codes for diseases of the skin and subcutaneous tissue. Refer to the ***Tip*** at the end of the mini-medical-record if you need a little extra help.

Exercise 11.4 Arranging Codes for the Integumentary System

Instructions: Read the mini-medical-record of each patient's encounter, review the information abstracted in Exercise 11.2, assign ICD-10-CM diagnosis codes (CM) using the Index and Tabular List, and arrange them correctly.

1. Date: 11/4/yy Location: Dermatology Associates Provider: Lawrence Staton, MD

Patient: Candice Doss Gender: F Age: 64

Chief complaint: evaluation of cellulitis on her right leg

Assessment: lab results show the cellulitis to be due to streptococcus A

Plan: Rx oral antibiotics. If it does not improve within 3 days or gets worse, she will need to be admitted for IV antibiotics.

Tip: Read the instructional notes at the beginning of the three-character category to learn if the code for the infectious organism should be sequenced first or additional.

2 CM Codes __________ __________

2. Date: 11/4/yy Location: Dermatology Associates Provider: Lawrence Staton, MD

Patient: Jonas Wills Gender: M Age: 25

Reason for encounter: follow-up on erythema multiforme and stomatitis minor due to herpes simplex virus

Assessment: Stomatitis showing improvement. 15% of his skin is exfoliated.

Tip: Sequence the condition first, the manifestation second, and the exfoliation third.

3 CM Codes __________ __________ __________

3. Date: 11/4/yy Location: Dermatology Associates Provider: Lawrence Staton, MD

Patient: Robert Maines Gender: M Age: 73

Reason for encounter: debride and dress chronic ulcer on right calf

Assessment: chronic ulcer due to postphlebitic syndrome. Healing is progressing. At last visit some muscle necrosis was visible. Today only the fat layer is exposed.

Tip: Sequencing is indicated in the instructional notes.

2 CM Codes __________ __________

CODING NEOPLASMS OF THE INTEGUMENTARY SYSTEM

Neoplasms of the integumentary system do not appear in ICD-10-CM Chapter 12, Diseases of the Skin and Subcutaneous Tissue (L00-L99). Codes for neoplasms of the integumentary system appear in block C43-C44 in the neoplasm chapter.

Skin cancers are named after the type of cell in which they start. The most common cancer in the integumentary system is **basal cell** (*lowest layer of the epidermis*) **carcinoma (BCC)**, which accounts for 75% of new skin cancer cases, according to the American Cancer Society. **Squamous cell carcinoma (SCC)**, named after the flat squamous cells in which it begins, is also common. BCC and SCC, while malignant, tend to spread slowly and are usually treated with a high degree of success.

The most serious neoplasm of the integumentary system is malignant **melanoma**, a tumor of melanocytes, which causes 75% of skin cancer deaths. If found early, melanoma is treatable, but it can metastasize to other areas of the body, in which case it is difficult to treat and usually fatal.

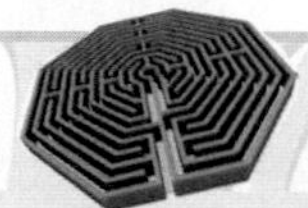

Coding Practice

Now it is your turn to practice coding neoplasms of the integumentary system. Refer to the ***Tip*** at the end of the mini-medical-record if you need a little extra help.

Exercise 11.5 Coding Neoplasms of the Integumentary System

Instructions: Read the mini-medical-record of each patient's encounter, then abstract, assign, and arrange ICD-10-CM diagnosis codes (CM) using the Index and Tabular List. Write the code(s) on the line provided.

1. Date: 11/5/yy Location: Dermatology Associates Provider: Lawrence Staton, MD

Patient: Estelle Pleasants Gender: F Age: 45

Reason for encounter: removal of lesions from eyebrow, chin, and lip

Assessment: removed three lesions, basal cell carcinoma

Plan: instructed patient to perform skin check monthly

Tip: Remember that you should not report the same diagnosis code twice for the same encounter (OGCR I.B.12).

2 CM Codes __________ __________

2. Date: 11/5/yy Location: Dermatology Associates Provider: Lawrence Staton, MD

Patient: Alexander Wilcox Gender: M Age: 42

Reason for encounter: unusual mole on nose

Assessment: melanoma in situ

(continued)

2. (continued)

Plan: schedule outpatient surgery to remove

Tip: Remember to look up melanoma before deciding if you should go to the Table of Neoplasms.

1 CM Code __________

3. Date: 11/5/yy Location: Branton Medical Center Provider: Richard Blackford, MD (oncologist)

Patient: Mindy Drost Gender: F Age: 51

Reason for admission: immunotherapy

Assessment: metastatic melanoma which started on the back

3 CM Codes __________ __________ __________

4. Date: 11/5/yy Location: Dermatology Associates Provider: Lawrence Staton, MD

Patient: Kari Lock Gender: F Age: 36

Reason for encounter: suspicious mole between nose and lip

Assessment: nevus nasolabial groove

Plan: no treatment necessary

1 CM Code __________

5. Date: 11/5/yy Location: Dermatology Associates Provider: Lawrence Staton, MD

Patient: Don Sterling Gender: M Age: 68

Reason for encounter: referred by family physician for areas on left arm where skin is breaking down

Assessment: Merkel cell carcinoma in kidney transplant recipient

(continued)

5. (continued)

Plan: schedule removal in one week

***Tip*:** Chronic immune suppression is a risk factor for the rare Merkel cell carcinoma. Therefore, code the patient's organ transplant status.

2 CM Codes __________ __________

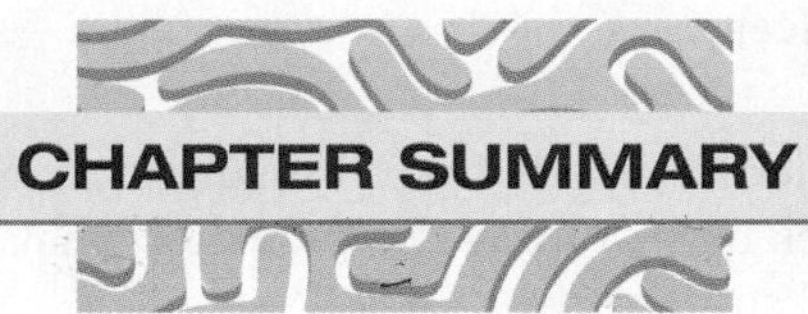

CHAPTER SUMMARY

In this chapter you learned that:

- The integumentary system consists of the skin and accessory structures: hair, nails, sebaceous glands, and sudoriferous glands.
- ICD-10-CM Chapter 12, Diseases of the Skin and Subcutaneous Tissue (L00-L99), contains nine blocks or subchapters that are divided by anatomical site and type of condition.
- When abstracting for diseases of the integumentary system, coders need to be familiar with the various types of lesions and complications, as well as the systems used to describe the extent of damage to the skin.
- When assigning codes for the integumentary system, coders need to be alert for easily confused index entries and must use the information abstracted regarding the depth or extent of skin damage for certain conditions.
- Sequencing of codes for the integumentary system follows the general coding guidelines OGCR III and IV as well as instructional notes in the Tabular List.
- Skin cancers are named after the type of cell in which they start, with the most common being basal cell carcinoma (BCC).

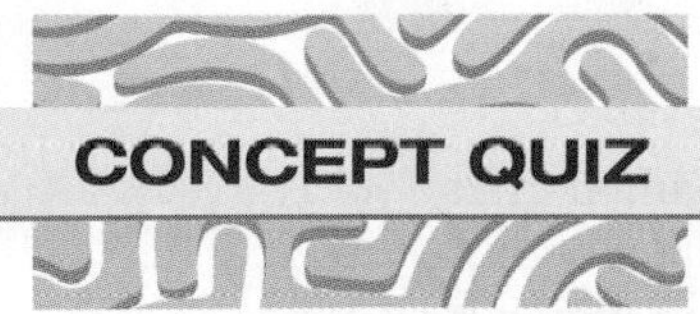

CONCEPT QUIZ

Take a moment to look back at your trip through diseases of the skin and subcutaneous tissue and solidify your skills. This is your opportunity to pull together everything you have learned.

Completion

Instructions: Write the term that answers each question based on the information you learned in this chapter. Choose from the following list. Some choices may be used more than once and some choices may not be used at all. Refer to the discussion in this chapter and the Glossary at the end of this book if you need a little extra help.

allograft
autograft
BCC
cellulitis
decubitus
erythema multiforme
exfoliation
folliculitis
hair
melanoma
nails
protection
regulation
SCC
secretion
sensation
skin
stage 1
stage 2
stage 3
stage 4
urticaria
xenograft

1. The skin's __________ function raises and lowers body temperature through constriction and dilation of blood vessels and sweat glands.

2. __________________ is an inflammation of space around the hair root.

3. __________________ is an inflammation under the skin.

4. A __________________ ulcer is a breakdown of the skin, usually over bony parts of body, caused by continuous pressure, friction, moistness, and heat.

5. __________________ is the medical term for hives.

6. __________________ is the most common cancer in the integumentary system and accounts for 75% of new skin cancer cases.

7. __________________ occurs when skin falls off in layers.

8. Trich/o is the combining form for __________________.

9. Replacement skin tissue from another person is a/an __________________.

10. The skin's __________________ function helps prevent invasion by pathogens, mechanical harm, and loss of fluids and electrolytes.

Multiple Choice

Instructions: Circle the letter of the best answer to each question based on the information you learned in this chapter. Refer to the discussion in this chapter and the Glossary at the end of this book if you need a little extra help.

1. Which of the following is NOT a common method used to diagnose skin conditions?
   A. Patch testing
   B. Biopsy
   C. X-ray
   D. Visual inspection

2. Psoriasis, pityriasis, and lichen are examples of ________ disorders.
   A. papulosquamous
   B. decubitus
   C. pigmentation
   D. dermatitis

3. Pressure ulcers are classified into ________ stages.
   A. two
   B. three
   C. four
   D. five

4. An unstagable pressure ulcer is one that
   A. extends into the muscle, tendon, or bone.
   B. has metastasized to other areas of the body.
   C. is not documented by a physician.
   D. cannot be visually assessed due to dead cells, eschar, or exudate.

5. Which of the following disorders is classified in ICD-10-CM Chapter 12?
   A. Burns
   B. Viral infections
   C. Parasites
   D. Radiation exposure

6. All of the following are non-pressure ulcers of the skin EXCEPT
   A. diabetic ulcer.
   B. peptic ulcer.
   C. venostasis ulcer
   D. post-phlebitic ulcer.

7. Coders should locate a code for a pressure ulcer on the right buttock by searching the Index for what Main Term and subterm?
   A. Pressure, buttock
   B. Buttock, ulcer
   C. Ulcer, buttock
   D. Ulcer, pressure

8. For an ulcer that worsens during the course of an inpatient admission, assign a code for
   A. the highest stage.
   B. the lowest stage.
   C. the stage at admission.
   D. each stage that occurred during the hospital stay.

9. If skin exfoliation exists, use category L49 to identify the percentage of
   A. healthy skin.
   B. lesions.
   C. exfoliation.
   D. dermatitis.

10. Skin cancers are named after
    A. the anatomic site where they start.
    B. the type of cell in which they start.
    C. the rate at which they spread.
    D. the site they metastasize to.

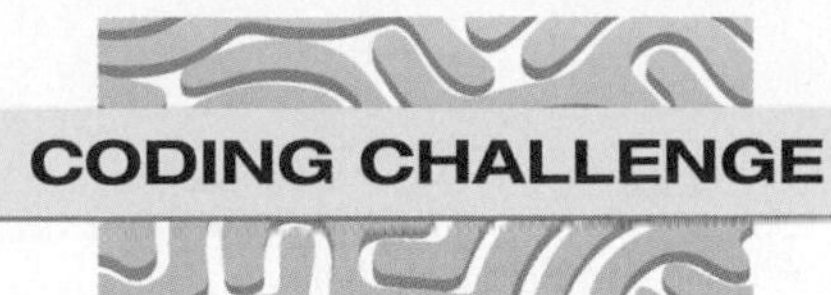

CODING CHALLENGE

Now it is your turn to demonstrate coding all aspects of diseases of the skin and subcutaneous tissue. Refer back to the examples and discussion in this chapter when you need a little extra help. Use your medical dictionary and anatomy references when needed.

Instructions: Read the mini-medical-record of each patient's encounter, then abstract, assign, and sequence ICD-10-CM diagnosis codes (CM) using the Index and Tabular List. Write the code(s) on the line provided.

1. Date: 11/15/yy Location: Dermatology Associates Provider: Lawrence Staton, MD

Patient: Rosie Eskridge Gender: F Age: 27

Reason for encounter: localized pain in the tail bone area

Assessment: abscessed pilonidal cyst

Plan: use depilatory cream and antibiotic, call office if symptoms do not subside

1 CM Code ____________

2. Date: 11/15/yy Location: Branton Medical Center Provider: Lawrence Staton, MD

Patient: Beatrice Boles Gender: F Age: 33

Reason for admission: body covered with blisters, child appears to be in pain

Assessment: Ritters disease, involving 68 percent of body surface

Plan: Rx pain medication, return to burn center for skin debridement

2 CM Codes ____________ ____________

3. Date: 11/15/yy Location: Branton Medical Center Provider: Lawrence Staton, MD

Patient: Elaine Medlin Gender: F Age: 24

Reason for admission: painful blisters on the skin and mucous membrane of the mouth

Assessment: pemphigus vulgaris

Plan: Rx steroids, FU PCP 2 wk

1 CM Code ____________

4. Date: 11/15/yy Location: Dermatology Associates Provider: Lawrence Staton, MD

Patient: Sean Aleman Gender: M Age: 47

Reason for encounter: referred by PCP for red, sore, skin lesion

Assessment: inflamed seborrheic keratosis

Plan: local anesthetic provided and lesion removed, call office if any redness occurs

1 CM Code ____________

5. Date: 11/15/yy Location: Dermatology Associates Provider: Lawrence Staton, MD

Patient: Glenn Martinson Gender: M Age: 89

Reason for encounter: Red open skin area in sacral region

Assessment: pressure ulcer, stage 3, sacral region

Plan: Debrided wound and applied dressing. Refer to wound care clinic for FU.

1 CM Code ____________

6. Date: 11/15/yy Location: Dermatology Associates Provider: Lawrence Staton, MD

Patient: Vera Kauffman Gender: F Age: 52

Reason for encounter: redness on the central face across the cheeks, nose, and forehead

Assessment: rosacea

Plan: Rx oral Antibiotics. FU 6 weeks. Advised on diet and lifestyle changes to minimize symptoms.

1 CM Code ____________

7. Date: 11/15/yy Location: Branton Medical Center Outpatient Procedure Center

Provider: Lawrence Staton, MD

Patient: Earl Pirtle Gender: M Age: 44

Reason for encounter: repair of scar

Assessment: keloid scar

Plan: repaired scar, monitor for infection

1 CM Code ____________

(continued)

(continued from page 205)

8. Date: 11/15/yy Location: Dermatology Associates Provider: Lawrence Staton, MD

Patient: Ryan Borrego Gender: M Age: 41

Reason for encounter: swollen lump under skin in armpit for 2 weeks, fever

Assessment: carbuncle due to methicillin susceptible staphylococcus aureus (MSSA)

Plan: antibiotic, call if no improvement within 1 week

2 CM Codes L02.431 B95.61

9. Date: 11/15/yy Location: Branton Medical Center Provider: Lawrence Staton, MD

Patient: Melody Choe Gender: F Age: 70

Reason for admission: swelling in left leg with apparent infection

Assessment: cellulitis, left leg, streptococcus A

Plan: Rx antibiotics, topical medication, call office if symptoms worsen

2 CM Codes L03.116 B95.0

10. Date: 11/15/yy Location: Branton Family Practice Provider: Kristen Conover, MD

Patient: Chad Vieira Gender: M Age: 6 months

Reason for encounter: Mother is concerned about severe rash and blistering in child's perinanal area, hips, and buttocks that seems to be getting worse.

Assessment: diaper dermatitis

Plan: Reviewed diaper hygiene. Rx ointment.

1 CM Code L22.

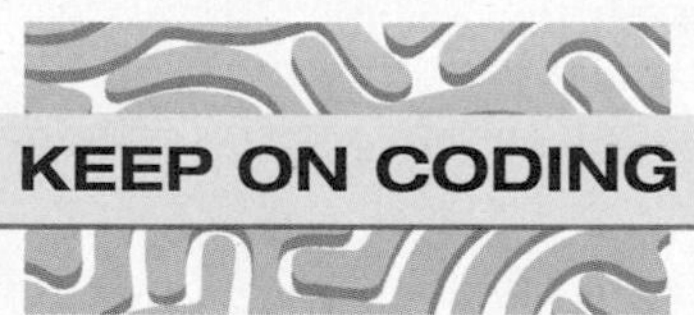

KEEP ON CODING

As a coder, you can never have too much experience. Apply everything you have learned in this chapter to code the following diagnostic statements. Use the OGCR and instructional notes in the Tabular List to help determine how many codes are required.

Instructions: Read the diagnostic statement, then use the Index and Tabular List to assign and sequence ICD-10-CM (CM) diagnosis codes. Write the code(s) on the line provided.

1. Infantile eczema: CM Code(s) L20.83
2. Retiform parapsoriasis: CM Code(s) ________
3. Café au lait spots: CM Code(s) ________
4. Discoid lupus erythematosus: CM Code(s) ________
5. Eosinophilic cellulitis: CM Code(s) ________
6. Stage 3 decubitus ulcer of the right lower back: CM Code(s) ________
7. Trichorrhexis nodusa: CM Code(s) ________
8. Allergic urticaria: CM Code(s) ________
9. Carbuncle of the face: CM Code(s) ________

10. Basal cell carcinoma of skin of right calf: CM Code(s) ______________________

11. Allergic contact dermatitis due to cosmetics: CM Code(s) ______________________

12. Solar urticaria: CM Code(s) ______________________

13. Acne keloid: CM Code(s) ______________________

14. Non-pressure ulcer of the back with necrosis of the bone: CM Code(s) ______________________

15. Neurodermatitis: CM Code(s) ______________________

16. Bockhart's impetigo: CM Code(s) ______________________

17. Anetoderma of Jadassohn-Pellizzari: CM Code(s) ______________________

18. Nonbullous erythema multiforme with 45% skin exfoliation: CM Code(s) ______________________

19. Infantile acne: CM Code(s) ______________________

20. Vitiligo: CM Code(s) ______________________

21. Alopecia mucinosa: CM Code(s) ______________________

22. Onychogryphosis: CM Code(s) ______________________

23. Malignant melanoma in situ of the right eyelid: CM Code(s) ______________________

24. Postprocedural hemorrhage of skin following dermatologic procedure: CM Code(s) ______________________

25. Omphalitis of an adult: CM Code(s) ______________________

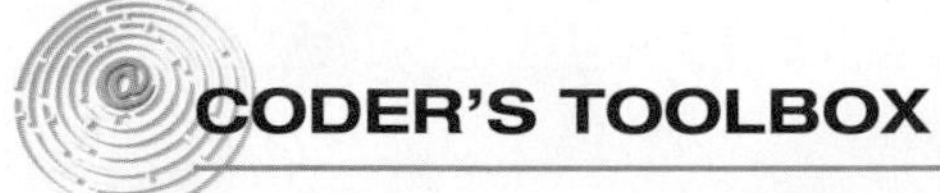

CODER'S TOOLBOX

The following resources are a starting point for learning more about diseases of the skin and subcutaneous tissue.

American Academy of Dermatology (AAD) **http://www.aad.org/**

Merkel Cell Carcinoma **http://www.merkelcell.org/**

National Institute of Arthritis and Musculoskeletal and Skin Diseases (NIAMS) **http://www.niams.nih.gov/**

National Pressure Ulcer Advisory Panel (NPUAP) **http://www.npuap.org/index.html**

National Psoriasis Foundation **http://www.psoriasis.org/**

National Rosacea Society **http://www.rosacea.org/**

National Vitiligo Foundation **http://www.vitiligofoundation.org/**

Poison Ivy, Oak, and Sumac Information Center **http://poisonivy.aesir.com/view**

Skin Cancer Foundation **http://www.skincancer.org/**

Stevens-Johnson Foundation **http://www.sjsupport.org/**

Sturge-Weber Foundation **http://www.sturge-weber.org/**

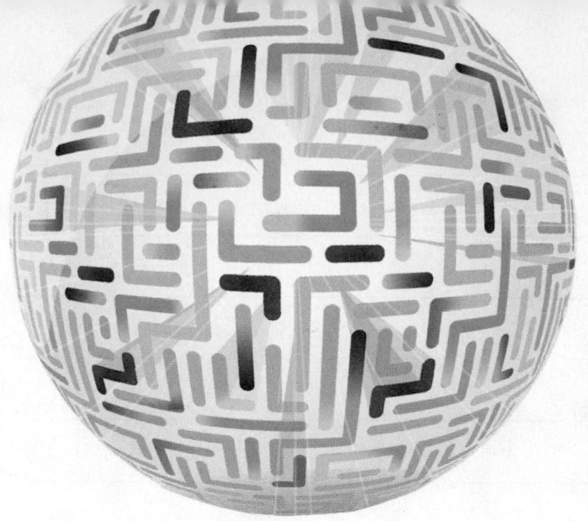

12

Diseases of the Musculoskeletal System and Connective Tissue (M00-M99)

Learning Objectives

After completing this chapter, you should have the skills to:

- Spell and define the key words, medical terms, and abbreviations related to diseases of the musculoskeletal system and connective tissue.
- Discuss the structure, function, and common conditions of the musculoskeletal system.
- Identify the main characteristics of coding for diseases of the musculoskeletal system and connective tissue.
- Abstract information from the medical record required for coding diseases of the musculoskeletal system and connective tissue.
- Assign codes for diseases of the musculoskeletal system and connective tissue.
- Arrange codes for diseases of the musculoskeletal system and connective tissue.
- Code neoplasms of the musculoskeletal system.
- Discuss the Official Guidelines for Coding and Reporting related to diseases of the musculoskeletal system and connective tissue.

Key Terms and Abbreviations

appendicular skeleton
axial skeleton
body
cartilage
delayed
diaphysis
distal epiphysis
fascia
fatigue fracture
femur
fragility fracture
insertion
involuntary
joint
ligament
malunion
march fracture
metastatic bone disease (MBD)
muscular system
musculoskeletal (MS) system
neck
nonunion
origin
osseous
pathologic fracture
proximal epiphysis
shaft
skeletal system
tendon
traumatic
vertebra
voluntary

In addition to the key terms listed here, students should know the terms defined within tables in this chapter.

Chapter Outline

- **Musculoskeletal System Refresher**
- **Coding Overview of the Musculoskeletal System**
- **Abstracting for the Musculoskeletal System**
- **Assigning Codes for the Musculoskeletal System**
- **Arranging Codes for the Musculoskeletal System**
- **Coding Neoplasms of the Musculoskeletal System**

ICD-10-CM codes in this chapter are from the ICD-10-CM 2014 Draft code set from the Department of Health and Human Services, Centers for Disease Control and Prevention.

INTRODUCTION

When you are driving down the road on your trip, the last thing you think about is the framework of your vehicle. If it is working properly, you should *not* think about it. Automotive engineers spend thousands of hours to design an amazing chassis that supports and protects you and also allows you to drive in comfort. In the human body, the musculoskeletal is the chassis that everything else is built on.

In your tour of the musculoskeletal system in this chapter you will learn more about how the musculoskeletal system works, why sometimes it does not work as it should, and how physicians treat conditions of the musculoskeletal system. Most importantly, you will practice coding for patient encounters related to musculoskeletal diseases and conditions, a skill that requires you to abstract information from the mini-medical-record, assign correct codes, and arrange (sequence) the codes in the proper order.

Orthopedic physicians specialize in diagnosing and treating conditions of the musculoskeletal system. Orthopedic surgeons may be subspecialists in a particular anatomic site, such as the spine or the knee. Rheumatologists specialize in diagnosing and treating arthritis and other diseases of the joints, muscles, and bones. Physical therapists, or physiotherapists, are non-physician practitioners who hold a master's or doctorate degree and use various physical treatments and exercises to help patients with musculoskeletal conditions or injuries restore function, improve mobility, and reduce pain. Primary care physicians treat uncomplicated conditions of the musculoskeletal system. They refer patients in need of rehabilitation to physical therapists and refer patients with more complex conditions to orthopedic specialists.

As you read this chapter, open up your medical terminology book to the musculoskeletal system and keep a medical dictionary handy to refresh your memory of any unfamiliar terms. The musculoskeletal system has hundreds of structures with scientific names and no one can remember all of them. Resources ensure that you have the information you need at your fingertips.

MUSCULOSKELETAL SYSTEM REFRESHER

The musculoskeletal (MS) system consists of the skeletal system and the muscular system. The function of the skeletal system is to support the body, protect internal organs, produce blood cells, store minerals, and serve as a point of attachment for the skeletal muscles. The function of the muscular system is to provide for movement of the body as well as the operation of individual organs, maintain body posture, and help produce heat.

Skeletal System

The skeletal system consists of 206 bones, as well as cartilage (*fibrous tissue found at the ends of bones*), ligaments (*fibrous tissue that connects bones to bones*), tendons (*fibrous tissue that connects bones to muscles*), and fascia (*fibrous tissue that connects muscle to muscle*). Joints are where two or more bones meet (■ Figure 12-1). The skeleton has two divisions: the axial skeleton and the appendicular skeleton. The axial skeleton contains 80 bones that are basically stationary and make up the skull, sternum, ribs, and vertebrae (*bony segments of the spine*). The appendicular skeleton contains 126 bones and consists of the arms, shoulders, wrists, hands, legs, hips, ankles, and feet.

Bones are also described by their shapes: long, short, flat, and irregular. Long bones comprise the arms and

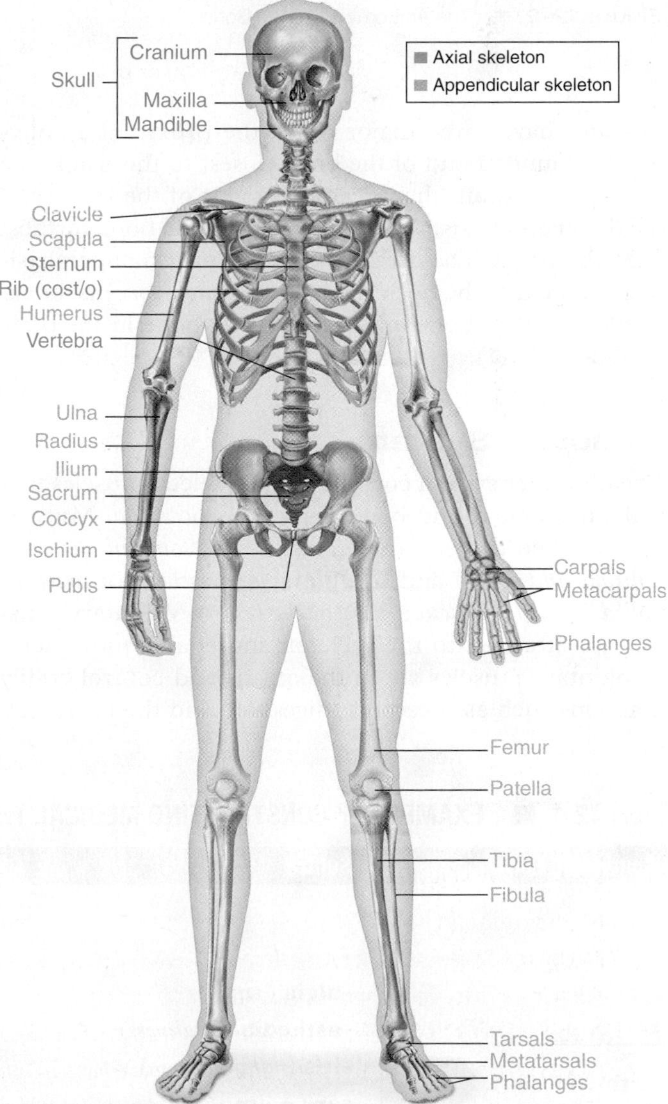

Figure 12-1 ■ The Skeletal System

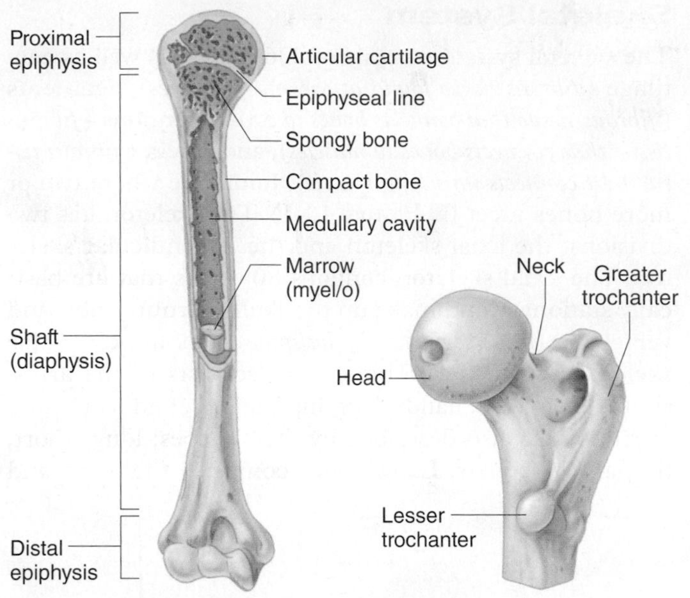

Figure 12-2 ■ The Anatomy of a Long Bone

legs and have three major parts: the **proximal epiphysis**, the rounded end of the bone closest to the trunk; the **diaphysis** or **shaft**, the long narrow part of the bone; and the **distal epiphysis**, the rounded end of the bone furthest from the trunk. The area between the proximal epiphysis and the shaft is the **neck**. The **femur** (*thigh bone*) is an example of a long bone and is the largest bone in the body (■ FIGURE 12-2).

Muscular System

The muscular system consists of 600 skeletal muscles that make movement and bodily processes possible. Muscles are classified as **voluntary** (*muscles a person can choose to contract and relax*) and **involuntary** (*muscles that are controlled by a subconscious part of the brain*). Voluntary muscles are attached to the skeleton and enable movement. Involuntary muscles are in the organs and control bodily functions such as breathing, digestion, and the heartbeat.

Muscles are named based on their location and function. Muscles have three distinct parts: the **origin**, where the muscle is fixed; the **body**, or main portion of the muscle; and the **insertion**, where the muscle attaches to a bone that moves.

Remember to apply medical terminology skills to combine word roots, prefixes, and suffixes you already know to define new terms related to the musculoskeletal system. Refer to ■ TABLE 12-1 for a refresher on how to build medical terms related to the musculoskeletal system.

CODING CAUTION

Remember to distinguish between medical terms with similar spellings, but different meanings:

cost/o (*rib*) and **chondr/o** (*cartilage*)

il<u>i</u>um (*pelvic bone*) and **il<u>e</u>um** (*small intestine*)

my/o (*muscle*) and **my<u>el</u>/o** (*bone marrow*)

sa<u>cr</u>/o (*sacrum, lowest part of back*) and **sa<u>rc</u>/o** (*flesh, connective tissue*)

Conditions of the Musculoskeletal System

Coders use medical resources, such as a reference book on diseases, to understand conditions of the musculoskeletal system, diagnostic methods, and common treatments. Common conditions of the musculoskeletal system are highlighted in ■ TABLE 12-2. Conditions are diagnosed through physical examination, imaging, biopsy, and lab tests. X-rays are used to evaluate conditions of the bone because they clearly show the difference between hard tissue and soft tissue. Computerized tomography (CT) and magnetic resonance imaging (MRI) are used to evaluate muscle and other soft tissue disorders because they show more contrast between different types of soft tissue. Blood tests are used for conditions such as

Table 12-1 ■ **EXAMPLE OF CONSTRUCTING MEDICAL TERMS FOR THE MUSCULOSKELETAL SYSTEM**

Combining Form	Suffix	Complete Medical Term
my/o (*muscle*)	**-algia** (*pain*) **-asthenia** (*weakness*) **-itis** (*inflammation*) **sarc + oma** (*malignant tumor*)	**myo + sitis** (*muscle inflammation*) **my + asthenia** (*muscle weakness*) **my + algia** (*muscle pain*) **myo + sarc + oma** (*malignant tumor in the muscle*)
arthr/o (*joint*)		**arthr + itis** (*inflammation of a joint*) **arthr + algia** (*pain in a joint*)
oste/o (*bone*)		**osteo + arthr + itis** (*inflammation of a bone and joint*) **osteo + sarc + oma** (*malignant tumor in the bone*)

Table 12-2 ■ **COMMON CONDITIONS OF THE MUSCULOSKELETAL SYSTEM**

Condition	Description
Arthritis	Damage or inflammation of the joints
Bursitis	Inflammation of fluid around a joint
Degeneration	Breakdown of bone or tissue
Dislocation	Two bones out of place at the joint
Fracture	Broken bone
Infection	Muscle or bone inflammation due to an infectious agent
Osteoporosis	Thinning of bone tissue and loss of bone density
Sprain	Overstretching, bruise, or tear of a ligament
Strain	Overstretching, bruise, or tear of a bone or tendon
Subluxation	Partial dislocation of bones in a joint
Tendonitis	Inflammation of a tendon, often due to overuse

rheumatoid arthritis, which is detected by the presence of Rh factor, and infections, which elevate the white blood cell count. Noninvasive treatments are pain medication, antibiotics for infections, and physical therapy to improve or restore function. Surgery may be performed to reshape a structure, remove an abnormal growth, or repair and stabilize by inserting orthopedic hardware, such as rods, pins, or screws.

SUCCESS STEP

The shoulder is the most frequently dislocated joint in the body because its shallow socket allows it to move in many directions. As a result, it can slip out of place when force is applied. You may have seen an athlete dislocate a shoulder during a sporting event, "pop" it back into place, and continue participating in the event.

This information provides a starting point to understand the MS system. Use medical terminology skills discussed earlier in this chapter to learn the meaning of unfamiliar words. Remember to keep standard reference books handy. Refer to the resources in the Coder's Toolbox at the end of this chapter to learn more about conditions affecting the musculoskeletal system.

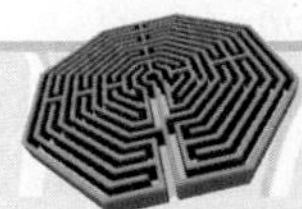

Coding Practice

Refresh your knowledge of terminology related to the musculoskeletal system. Use a medical terminology text or a website such as GlobalRph.com > Medical Terminology **http://www.globalrph.com/medterm.htm** to identify the meaning of word parts that may not be familiar to you.

Exercise 12.1 Musculoskeletal System Refresher

Instructions: Use your medical terminology skills and resources to define the following conditions related to the musculoskeletal system, then assign the diagnosis code.

Follow these steps:

- Use slash marks "/" to break down each term into its root(s) and suffix.
- Define the meaning of the word, based on the meaning of each word part.
- Assign the default ICD-10-CM diagnosis code (CM) for the condition using the Index and Tabular List.

Example: arthritis arthr/itis Meaning: *inflammation of a joint* CM Code: *M19.90*

1. arthropathy Meaning ____________ CM Code ________
2. osteomyelitis Meaning ____________ CM Code ________
3. fibromyalgia Meaning ____________ CM Code ________
4. lordosis Meaning ____________ CM Code ________
5. chondrocalcinosis Meaning ____________ CM Code ________
6. spondylolisthesis Meaning ____________ CM Code ________
7. chondromalacia Meaning ____________ CM Code ________
8. osteolysis Meaning ____________ CM Code ________
9. tenosynovitis Meaning ____________ CM Code ________
10. fascitis Meaning ____________ CM Code ________

CODING OVERVIEW OF THE MUSCULOSKELETAL SYSTEM

ICD-10-CM Chapter 13, Diseases of the Musculoskeletal System and Connective Tissue (M00-M99), contains 18 blocks or subchapters that are divided by type of tissue, such as bone, joint, spine, vertebrae, cartilage, and tendon. Review the block names and code ranges listed at the beginning of Chapter 13 in the ICD-10-CM manual to become familiar with the content and organization.

ICD-10-CM Chapter 13 corresponds with ICD-9-CM Chapter 13 (710-739). ICD-10-CM has expanded a majority of codes in this chapter including laterality, specificity of site, and/or episode of care. Expanded instructional notes in the ICD-10-CM Tabular List direct coders to assign additional codes for underlying and associated conditions. New codes appear for osteoporosis with and without a current pathological fracture, as well as for osteoarthritis and rheumatoid arthritis.

This chapter includes chronic or recurrent conditions of the joint, bone, and soft tissue, including those of the jaw. It does not include codes for **traumatic** (*acute current injury that results from an accident*) fractures, injuries, congenital and perinatal conditions, neoplasms, or symptoms and signs, which are classified in other ICD-10-CM chapters. Review the Excludes2 note at the beginning of the chapter to cross-reference the locations of these codes.

ICD-10-CM provides Official Guidelines for Coding and Reporting (OGCR) for the musculoskeletal system in OGCR section I.C.13. OGCR discusses coding for site and laterality, pathologic fractures, and osteoporosis. Additional OGCR related to conditions of the musculoskeletal system appear in OGCR I.C.19 and 20.

ABSTRACTING FOR THE MUSCULOSKELETAL SYSTEM

The keys to abstracting diagnoses for the MS system are familiarity with the anatomy, knowledge of medical terms, and careful attention to the details of the documented condition. ■ TABLE 12-3 highlights key questions to ask when abstracting MS conditions. Pathologic fractures require additional abstracting, shown in ■ TABLE 12-4. Remember that abstracting questions are a general guide and all questions may not apply to every patient. For example, not all conditions have laterality. When there is a traumatic injury, also abstract the external cause.

Table 12-3 ■ KEY CRITERIA FOR ABSTRACTING MUSCULOSKELETAL CONDITIONS

- ❑ What type of condition is documented: fracture, dislocation, subluxation, sprain, infection, inflammation, or degeneration?
- ❑ What type of tissue or structure is affected: bone, joint, cartilage, muscle, tendon, or ligament?
- ❑ What is the specific subtype of condition (e.g. osteo- vs. rheumatoid arthritis)?

(continued)

Table 12-3 ■ (continued)

- ❑ What is the anatomic site?
- ❑ What is the laterality?
- ❑ For a patient with osteoporosis, does the patient have a pathologic fracture? Does the patient have a history of healed pathologic fractures?
- ❑ Is the condition acute, chronic, or a late effect?
- ❑ Is the encounter for active treatment?
- ❑ Is the encounter for aftercare during the healing phase?
- ❑ Is the encounter for follow-up after active healing is complete?

Table 12-4 ■ KEY CRITERIA FOR ABSTRACTING PATHOLOGIC FRACTURES

- ❑ Is the fracture traumatic or pathologic?
- ❑ What type of pathologic fracture is it?
- ❑ What is the underlying disease?
- ❑ What bone is fractured?
- ❑ What is the laterality?
- ❑ Is the fracture open or closed?
- ❑ Is the fracture displaced or non-displaced?
- ❑ Were any additional bones fractured?
- ❑ Is the healing routine, **delayed** (*patient waited to seek care*), **nonunion** (*failure of the ends of the fractured bone segments to reunite*), or **malunion** (*ends of fractured bone segments did not heal with proper alignment*)?
- ❑ Is the encounter for active treatment?
- ❑ Is the encounter for aftercare during the healing phase?
- ❑ Is the encounter for follow-up after active healing is complete?

Guided Example of Abstracting for the Musculoskeletal System

Refer to the following example throughout this chapter to learn skills for abstracting and assigning codes for conditions affecting the musculoskeletal system. Jacob Bates, CCS, is a fictitious coder who guides you through this case.

Date: 3/1/yy Location: Valley Hospital

Provider: Bruce Prentice, MD

Patient: Nadine Tubbs Gender: F Age: 80

Reason for admission: admitted from physician office where she was seen for hip pain. X-rays showed fracture.

Procedure performed: repair of fracture with a metal rod

Discharge plan: pathologic fracture of right femoral neck due to osteoporosis. Referred to rehab for 6 weeks.

Follow along as Jacob Bates, CCS, abstracts the diagnosis. Check off each step after you complete it.

➡ Jacob reads through the entire record, with special attention to the reason for the admission and the discharge plan. He refers to the Key Criteria for Abstracting Pathologic Fractures (Table 12-4).

- ❑ *Is the fracture traumatic or pathologic?* pathologic
- ❑ *What is the underlying disease?* osteoporosis
- ❑ *What bone is fractured?* femur
- ❑ *What site on the bone is fractured?* neck
- ❑ *What is the laterality?* right
- ❑ *Is the fracture open or closed?* The fracture is not stated as open or closed, so he will use the default of closed.
- ❑ *Is the fracture displaced or non-displaced?* The fracture is not stated as displaced or non-displaced, so he will use the default of displaced.
- ❑ *Is the encounter for active treatment?* Yes, the episode of care is the initial encounter because the fracture was repaired and there is no mention of previous treatment for it.
- ❑ He will not abstract pain, because pain is a symptom integral to the condition.

➡ Jacob has completed abstracting. Next, he will assign the codes.

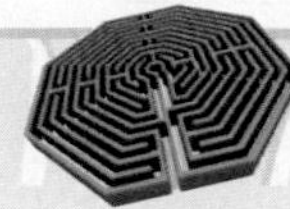

Coding Practice

Now it is your turn to practice abstracting diagnoses for the musculoskeletal system and connective tissue. Questions guide your analysis of each scenario.

Exercise 12.2 Abstracting for the Musculoskeletal System

Instructions: Read the mini-medical-record of each patient's encounter and answer the abstracting questions. Write the answer on the line provided. Do not assign any codes.

1. Date: 12/3/yy Location: Northwest Orthopedics and Rheumatology

Provider: Mark Stollings, MD

Patient: Minnie John Gender: F Age: 48

Chief complaint: Patient came in for management of fibromyalgia which was diagnosed last year. C/o increased pain in lower back and hips.

Assessment: fibromyalgia

Plan: Refer to physical therapy for modified exercise program and pain relief. Adjusted medication.

a. What are the presenting symptoms? ____________

____

b. What is the underlying condition? ____________

____

c. Should you code the symptoms? ____________
Why or why not? ____________

____

d. Should you code an encounter for physical therapy? ____________ Why or why not? ____________

____

2. Date: 12/3/yy Location: Northwest Orthopedics and Rheumatology

Provider: Bruce Prentice, MD

Patient: Elsie Rousseau Gender: F Age: 66

Reason for encounter: management and monitoring osteoarthritis

Assessment: degenerative osteoarthritis of the right knee

a. What type of arthritis does the patient have?

____

b. What is the anatomic site? ____________

____

c. What is the laterality? ____________

____

d. Is the arthritis described as generalized?

____

e. Is the arthritis post-traumatic? ____________

____

3. Date: 12/3/yy Location: Northwest Orthopedics and Rheumatology Provider: Bruce Prentice, MD

Patient: Walter Studer Gender: M Age: 72

Chief complaint: acute hip pain

Assessment: X-rays show a fracture of the ilium due to age-related osteoporosis

a. What is the presenting symptom? ____________

____

(continued)

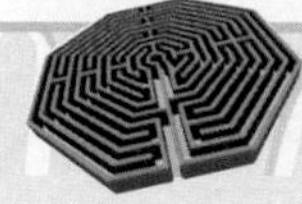

Coding Practice (continued)

3. (continued)

b. What is the diagnosis of the cause of the pain? ______

c. What is the underlying condition? ______

d. What type of fracture is this? ______

e. Should the symptom be coded? ______
Why or why not? ______

4. Date: 12/4/yy Location: Valley Hospital
Provider: Bruce Prentice, MD
Patient: Jeremiah Rayburn Gender: M Age: 56
Reason for encounter: vertebroplasty (*injection of acrylic cement a fractured vertebra to stabilize it*) to correct compression fracture
Assessment: collapsed vertebrae L3 and L4 due to bone metastasis from prostate cancer

a. What procedure was performed? ______

b. What is the reason for the procedure? ______

c. What is the anatomic site? ______

d. What type of fracture is this? ______

e. What additional diagnoses exist? ______

f. What is the principal diagnosis? ______

g. What is the second diagnosis? ______

h. What is the third diagnosis? ______

5. Date: 12/4/yy Location: Northwest Orthopedics and Rheumatology
Provider: Bruce Prentice, MD
Patient: Jesse Saito Gender: M Age: 36
Reason for encounter: left knee pain
Assessment: chronic knee derangement due to an old injury of the anterior horn of the medial meniscus. Injury was sustained during a tackle in a college football game 15 years ago.

a. What is the symptom? ______

b. Should you code the symptom? ______
Why or why not? ______

c. What is the episode of care? ______

d. What is the site within the knee where the original injury occurred? ______

e. What is the laterality? ______

f. What external cause event caused the injury?
______

g. Should you code for the activity? ______
Why or why not? ______

6. Date: 12/4/yy Location: Northwest Orthopedics and Rheumatology

Provider: Bruce Prentice, MD

Patient: Dawn Rife Gender: F Age: 70

Reason for encounter: follow up on test results after complaints of hand pain

Assessment: elevated WBC, calcification evident on X-rays. Arthritis in crystal arthropathy (*presence of calcification within soft tissues*) of the right hand due to dicalcium phosphate crystals. Patient previously diagnosed with primary hyperparathyroidism which is associated with this condition.

Plan: corticosteroid injection, RTO 4 wk

a. What condition is newly diagnosed? ___________

____

(continued)

6. (continued)

b. What is the cause of the condition? ___________

____

c. What is the anatomic site? ___________

____

d. What is the laterality? ___________

____

e. What is the previously existing condition?

____

f. Should the previously existing condition be coded? ___________ Why or why not? ___________

____

ASSIGNING CODES FOR THE MUSCULOSKELETAL SYSTEM

Assigning codes for MS disorders may require coders to cross-reference the medical record multiple times in order to accurately capture the details of the disorder. This serves as a cross-check for abstracting because it is easy to overlook one or more details. Coders may not know exactly what information is required until they assign the code, review the subterms in the Index, and read the instructional notes in the Tabular List. In addition, careful attention to the spelling of medical terms is necessary in order to locate the correct term in the Index. Conventions in the Index and Tabular List indicate when multiple coding is required for infections, underlying conditions, and complications. The Tabular List conventions also notify coders when a seventh-character extension is required and what the seventh-character choices are for any given code.

SUCCESS STEP

Because there are 206 bones and 600 muscles, it is common to encounter terms you may be unfamiliar with when coding the MS system. Just as you keep a map or global positioning navigator handy when driving in unfamiliar areas, a quick check in a medical terminology or anatomy book will help smooth out the bumps in the road.

Most of the codes within Chapter 13 have site and laterality designations. The site represents the bone, joint, or muscle involved. For some conditions where more than one bone, joint, or muscle is usually involved in the same type of injury, the Index provides a combination for multiple sites available (OGCR I.C.13.a.) (■ FIGURE 12-3).

For some conditions, such as **avascular necrosis of bone** and osteoporosis, the bone may be affected at the upper or lower end. Although the portion of the bone

Patient has osteochondropathy of ankles, knees, and hip.

Osteochondropathy M93.90

- ankle M93.97-
- elbow M93.92-
- foot M93.97-
- hand M93.94-
- hip M93.95-
- Kienböck's disease of adults M93.1
- knee M93.96-
- multiple joints M93.99

Figure 12-3 ■ Example of a Combination Code for Multiple Sites

Patient has avascular necrosis at the proximal epiphysis of the left radius.

Index:

Necrosis, bone *see also* Osteonecrosis

Osteonecrosis, idiopathic, radius M87.03-

Tabular List:

M87.032 Idiopathic aseptic necrosis of left radius

Figure 12-4 ■ Example of Coding the Site as Bone, Not Joint 1

affected may be at the joint, code the site as the bone, not the joint (OGCR I.C.13.a.1.). (■ FIGURE 12-4). Code the joint when the joint capsule itself is affected, as in arthritis.

Guided Example of Assigning Musculoskeletal System Codes

Continue with the example from earlier in the chapter about patient Nadine Tubbs, who was admitted to Valley Hospital due to a pathologic fracture, to practice skills for assigning codes for the MS system.

Follow along in your ICD-10-CM manual as Jacob Bates, CCS, assigns codes. Check off each step after you complete it.

⇨ First, Jacob confirms that the diagnosis is pathologic fracture of the right femoral neck due to osteoporosis.

- ❑ Jacob searches the Index for the Main Term **Fracture, pathological**. He notes that this is a separate Main Term from **Fracture, traumatic.**
- ❑ He locates the subterm **due to.**
- ❑ He locates the second-level subterm **osteoporosis M80.00.**
- ❑ He notes that there are no further subterms for anatomic site.
- ❑ However, he does notice a cross-reference for **postmenopausal *see* Osteoporosis, postmenopausal, with pathological fracture.**
- ❑ He cross-references the Main Term **Osteoporosis** and the subterm **postmenopausal.**
- ❑ Now he sees a second-level subterm **with pathological fracture**
- ❑ Under this entry he notices no entry for femur, but does see an additional subterms for **ilium, ischium, and pelvis,** all of which point to **M80.05.** He decides to research this option because these bones are adjacent to the femoral joint and he knows that the ICD-10-CM often classifies them together.

CODING CAUTION

If Jacob does not follow the cross-reference, **Osteoporosis, postmenopausal, with pathological fracture,** he will verify **M80.00 Age-related osteoporosis with current pathological fracture, unspecified site.** The words **unspecified site** should be a red flag and cause him to either return to the Index, or review the Tabular List to locate a more specific code for the **femur.**

⇨ Jacob verifies code **pelvis M80.05** in the Tabular List.

- ❑ He reads the code title for **M80.05, Age-related osteoporosis with current pathological fracture, femur** and confirms that this accurately describes the principal diagnosis and identifies the anatomic site of the femur.
- ❑ Jacob looks for any conventions or instructional notes with the code.
- ❑ He notices the convention 6th that directs him to use a sixth character with **M80.05** for laterality.
- ❑ He double-checks the medical record to verify the laterality as **right.**
- ❑ The code for right femur is **M80.051.**
- ❑ He notices the convention 7th that tells him a seventh-character extension is required with **M80.051.**
- ❑ He refers to the beginning of category **M80** to locate the seventh-character extension.
- ❑ He selects the extension **A, initial encounter** because the episode of care is for active treatment. Even though the patient was previously seen in the physician's office, there was no treatment, so extension **D, subsequent encounter for fracture with routine healing** is not appropriate.
- ❑ Jacob verifies that the complete code is **M80.051A.**

⇨ Jacob checks for any additional instructional notes in the Tabular List.

- ❑ Since he is already at the beginning of the three-digit category, he reviews the notes that appear, including the definition of a fragility fracture.

- ❑ He reviews the note **Use additional code to identify major osseous defect, if applicable** and double-checks the medical record to be certain no defects are documented.
- ❑ He also double-checks the medical record to see if there is a personal history of (healed) osteoporosis fracture, which there is not. If there were, he would need to assign code **Z87.310** for the history.
- ❑ He cross-references the beginning of the block **M80-M94** and verifies that there are no instructional notes.
- ❑ He cross-references the beginning of **Chapter 12 (M00-M99)** and reviews the instructional notes. He determines he does not need to assign an external cause code because the patient's fracture was not due to an external cause, but was due to a disease.

⇨ Jacob finalizes the code for this case:

- ❑ **M80.051A, Age-related osteoporosis with current pathological fracture, right femur, initial encounter.**

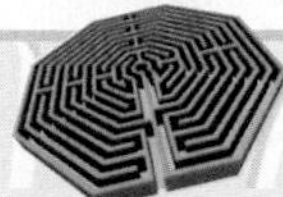

Coding Practice

Now it is your turn to practice abstracting diagnoses for the musculoskeletal system and connective tissue. Refer to the ***Tip*** at the end of the mini-medical-record if you need a little extra help.

Exercise 12.3 Assigning Codes for the Musculoskeletal System

Instructions: Read the mini-medical-record of each patient's encounter, review the information abstracted in Exercise 12.2, and assign ICD-10-CM diagnosis codes (CM) using the Index and Tabular List. Write the code(s) on the line provided.

1. Date: 12/3/yy Location: Northwest Orthopedics and Rheumatology Provider: Mark Stollings, MD

Patient: Minnie John Gender: F Age: 48

Chief complaint: Patient came in for management of fibromyalgia which was diagnosed last year. C/o increased pain in lower back and hips.

Assessment: fibromyalgia

Plan: Refer to physical therapy for modified exercise program and pain relief. Adjusted medication.

1 CM Code __________

2. Date: 12/3/yy Location: Northwest Orthopedics Provider: Bruce Prentice, MD

Patient: Elsie Rousseau Gender: F Age: 66

Reason for encounter: management and monitoring osteoarthritis

Assessment: degenerative osteoarthritis of the right knee

1 CM Code __________

3. Date: 12/3/yy Location: Northwest Orthopedics and Rheumatology Provider: Bruce Prentice, MD

Patient: Walter Studer Gender: M Age: 72

Chief complaint: acute hip pain

Assessment: X-rays show a fracture of the ilium due to age-related osteoporosis

Tip: The ilium is classified with the femur in the Tabular List, so do not be confused when you read the code title.

1 CM Code __________

ARRANGING CODES FOR THE MUSCULOSKELETAL SYSTEM

When MS disorders require multiple coding, coders must be attentive to the sequencing indicated in the instructional notes. Because there is a wide variety of code sequencing situations, this section provides several short examples rather than a single guided example of arranging codes. Examples of the most commonly encountered situations follow, including pathologic fracture, infections conditions, osseous defects, and external causes.

Pathologic Fractures

Pathologic fractures, also called **fragility fractures**, are fractures caused by disease rather than trauma. OGCR I.C.12.d.2). The instructional **NOTE:** at the beginning of block **M80-M85** defines a pathological fracture as

Table 12-5 ■ **DEFINITIONS AND SEQUENCING INSTRUCTIONS FOR PATHOLOGIC FRACTURES**

Type of Fracture	Definition	Instructional Note
Osteoporosis	A fragility fracture in person with osteoporosis.	Use additional code to identify major **osseous** (*bone*) defect, if applicable (M89.7-). Use additional code to identify personal history of (healed) osteoporosis fracture, if applicable (Z87.310).
Neoplastic	A fragility fracture due to neoplastic disease.	Code also underlying neoplasm.
Stress	Fracture of a bone that has been subjected to repeated use or impact. Also called a **march fracture** or **fatigue fracture**.	Use additional external cause code(s) to identify the cause of the stress fracture.
Other	A fragility fracture due to a disease other than osteoporosis or neoplasm. Any other type of pathological fracture.	Code also underlying condition.

"a fracture sustained with trauma no more than a fall from a standing height or less that occurs under circumstances that would not cause a fracture in a normal healthy bone." ICD-10-CM classifies four types of pathologic fractures and provides instructional notes for sequencing codes (■ TABLE 12-5).

Infectious Conditions

Infectious conditions, such as **pyogenic arthritis** and myositis, require coders to use an additional code for the infectious agent (■ FIGURE 12-5).

Osseous Defects

Pathologic fractures, osteomyelitis, and osteonecrosis require coders to use an additional code to describe any major bone defects. Pathologic fractures also require an additional code for a history of healed pathologic fractures (■ FIGURE 12-6).

External Cause

Stress fractures and soft tissue disorders, which are due to overuse or pressure, require coders to assign and sequence an external cause code as a secondary code. In many cases, the only external cause code will be an activity code because there is not an applicable event code. This is an exception to the general rule that requires that activity codes be assigned only in conjunction with external cause event codes (■ FIGURE 12-7).

Multiple Sites

Earlier in the chapter, Figure 12-3 demonstrated how to assign a combination code for multiple sites, rather than coding each site separately, when more than one bone, joint, or muscle is involved. However, not all categories provide a combination code for multiple sites. When the Index does not provide a code for multiple sites, assign separate codes to indicate each of the sites involved, as shown in (■ FIGURE 12-8) (OGCR I.C.13.a)). When each site is equally responsible for the encounter, sequence any of the codes first (OGCR II.C. and IV.).

Patient is seen for pyogenic arthritis in the right elbow due to methicillin susceptible Staphylococcus aureus.

(1) M00.021 Staphylococcal arthritis, right elbow

(2) B95.61 Methicillin susceptible staphylococcus aureus as the cause of diseases classified elsewhere

Figure 12-5 ■ Sequencing for an Infectious Condition

Patient is seen for chronic osteomyelitis of left scapula due to methicillin susceptible Staphylococcus aureus with major osseous defect.

(1) M86.612 Other chronic osteomyelitis, left shoulder

(2) B95.61 Methicillin susceptible staphylococcus aureus as the cause of diseases classified elsewhere

(3) M89.712 Major osseous defect, left shoulder region

Figure 12-6 ■ Example of Sequencing for Osseous Defects

Patient is seen for tendonitis of the left forearm due to overuse in baseball.

Index Entry for Main Term, Tendonitis:

Tendinitis, tendonitis — *see also* Enthesopathy

Achilles M76.6-

due to use, overuse, pressure — *see also* Disorder, soft tissue, due to use

specified NEC — *see* Disorder, soft tissue, due to use, specified NEC

Index Entry for Cross-referenced Main Term, Disorder:

Disorder

soft tissue M79.9

ankle M79.9

due to use, overuse and pressure M70.90

ankle M70.97-

bursitis — *see* Bursitis

foot M70.97-

forearm M70.93-

hand M70.94-

lower leg M70.96-

Tabular List for Category M70:

Other soft tissue disorders (M70-M79)

M70 Soft tissue disorders related to use, overuse and pressure

Includes: soft tissue disorders of occupational origin

Use additional external cause code to identify activity causing disorder (Y93.-)

Final Code Assignment and Sequencing:

(1) **M70.932 Unspecified soft tissue disorder related to use, overuse and pressure, left forearm**

(2) **Y93.64 Activity, baseball**

Figure 12-7 ■ Example of Sequencing of External Causes

Patient is seen for ruptured synovium in the right shoulder and right elbow.

Index:

Rupture

abscess (spontaneous) - code by site under Abscess

aneurysm — *see* Aneurysm

synovium (cyst) M66.10

ankle M66.17-

elbow M66.12-

finger M66.14-

foot M66.17-

forearm M66.13-

hand M66.14-

pelvic region M66.15-

shoulder region M66.11-

specified site NEC M66.18

thigh M66.15-

toe M66.17-

upper arm M66.12-

wrist M66.13-

The Index does not provide a subterm for **synovium, multiple sites.**

Tabular List:

(1) **M66.111 Rupture of synovium, right shoulder**

(2) **M66.121 Rupture of synovium, right elbow**

Figure 12-8 ■ Example of Assigning Separate Codes for Multiple Sites

CODING CAUTION

When the Index does not provide a subterm for **multiple sites**, it is helpful to also review the Tabular List entries to be certain that no code for multiple sites exists. In some cases, a multiple site code exists even though it is not listed as a subterm in the Index. The code for **multiple sites** usually appears at the end of a category and ends in the number **8**.

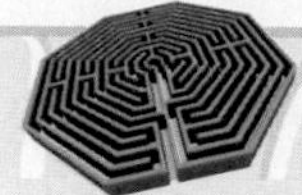

Coding Practice

Now it is your turn to practice sequencing codes for diseases of the musculoskeletal system and connective tissue. Refer to the ***Tip*** at the end of the mini-medical-record if you need a little extra help.

Exercise 12.4 Arranging Codes for the Musculoskeletal System

Instructions: Read the mini-medical-record of each patient's encounter, review the information abstracted in Exercise 12.2, assign ICD-10-CM diagnosis codes (CM) using the Index and Tabular List, and sequence them correctly.

1. Date: 12/4/yy Location: Valley Hospital
Provider: Bruce Prentice, MD
Patient: Jeremiah Rayburn Gender: M Age: 56
Reason for encounter: vertebroplasty (*injection of acrylic cement a fractured vertebra to stabilize it*) to correct compression fracture
Assessment: collapsed vertebrae L3 and L4 due to bone metastasis from prostate cancer

Tip: The reason for the vertebroplasty is the principal diagnosis. Sequence metastasis second because it caused the compression fracture. Sequence the primary neoplasm third.

3 CM Codes __________ __________ __________

2. Date: 12/4/yy Location: Northwest Orthopedics and Rheumatology Provider: Bruce Prentice, MD
Patient: Jesse Saito Gender: M Age: 36
Reason for encounter: left knee pain
Assessment: chronic knee derangement due to an old injury of the anterior horn of the medial meniscus. Injury was sustained during a tackle in a college football game 15 years ago.

Tip: The fact that this is due to an "old injury" makes it a sequela. Remember to use the Index of External Causes to locate the external cause (event) code.

2 CM Codes __________ __________

3. Date: 12/4/yy Location: Northwest Orthopedics and Rheumatology Provider: Bruce Prentice, MD
Patient: Dawn Rife Gender: F Age: 70
Reason for encounter: follow up on test results after complaints of hand pain
Assessment: elevated WBC, calcification evident on X-rays. Impression: arthritis in crystal arthropathy (*presence of crystal-like deposits in the joints*) of the right hand due to dicalcium phosphate crystals. Patient previously diagnosed with primary hyperparathyroidism which is associated with this condition.
Plan: corticosteroid injection, RTO 4 wk

Tip: You may start with the Main Term arthritis or arthropathy.

2 CM Codes __________ __________

CODING NEOPLASMS OF THE MUSCULOSKELETAL SYSTEM

Neoplasms of the musculoskeletal system do not appear in ICD-10-CM Chapter 12 Diseases of the Musculoskeletal System and Connective Tissue (M00-M99). Codes for neoplasms of the musculoskeletal system appear in the block C40-C41 within the neoplasm chapter. Codes for leukemia, which originates in the bone marrow, appear in categories C90 to C96.

The most common cancer in the musculoskeletal system is **metastatic bone disease (MBD)** because the bone is a frequent site of metastasis from primary neoplasms in other organs, including the breast, lung, prostate, kidney, and thyroid. According to the American Academy of Orthopaedic Surgeons, approximately 50% of tumors can metastasize to the bone.

Cancer that begins in the bone is called primary bone cancer, or sarcoma, and is named after the specific type of tissue in which it originates, such as osteosarcoma (sarcoma of bone) or chondrosarcoma (sarcoma of cartilage). Ewing's sarcoma forms in the shaft of long bones, the hip, and ribs. Children and young people are more likely than adults to have bone cancers. Soft-tissue sarcomas are relatively rare, but are quite aggressive and dangerous, particularly when they occur in adults.

Leukemia is a cancer that starts in the bone marrow and affects the cells that form new blood cells. About one-third of childhood cancers are leukemias, the most common of which is acute lymphoblastic leukemia.

All malignant neoplasms in the musculoskeletal system are either primary or secondary. CA in situ does not exist because bone and connective tissue do not have the epithelial cells that give rise to CA in situ.

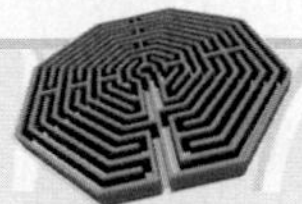

Coding Practice

Now it is your turn to practice coding neoplasms of the musculoskeletal system. Refer to the ***Tip*** at the end of the mini-medical-record if you need a little extra help.

Exercise 12.5 Coding Neoplasms of the Musculoskeletal System

Instructions: Read the mini-medical-record of each patient's encounter, then abstract, assign, and sequence ICD-10-CM diagnosis codes (CM) using the Index and Tabular List. Write the code(s) on the line provided.

1. Date: 12/5/yy Location: Valley Hospital
Provider: Bruce Prentice, MD
Patient: Jimmy Scarbrough Gender: M Age: 14
Reason for admission: surgical removal of tumor
Assessment: osteosarcoma in the right tibia
1 CM Code ________

2. Date: 12/5/yy Location: Valley Hospital
Provider: Bruce Prentice, MD
Patient: Rhonda Culver Gender: F Age: 48
Reason for encounter: pain management for MBD
Assessment: left breast cancer with metastasis to bone

Tip: The code for neoplasm related pain may be assigned as the principal or first-listed code when the stated reason for the admission/encounter is documented as pain control/pain management. The underlying neoplasm should be reported as an additional diagnosis. OGCR I.C.6.b.5).

3 CM Codes ________ ________ ________

3. Date: 12/5/yy Location: Valley Hospital
Provider: Bruce Prentice, MD
Patient: Sharon Alderete Gender: F Age: 13
Reason for admission: induction chemotherapy with a goal of remission
Assessment: acute lymphoblastic leukemia
2 CM Codes ________ ________

4. Date: 12/5/yy Location: Northwest Orthopedics and Rheumatology
Provider: Bruce Prentice, MD
Patient: Cynthia Doe Gender: F Age: 63
Reason for encounter: pain and lump on diaphysis of humerus
Assessment: possible chondrosarcoma
Plan: CT, MRI

Tip: Remember the guidelines about coding uncertain conditions (OGCR II.H., IV.D., and IV.H.). You need to determine if this is an inpatient or outpatient encounter based on the location stated. You also need to identify where the humerus is.

2 CM Codes ________ ________

5. Date: 12/5/yy Location: Valley Hospital
Provider: Bruce Prentice, MD
Patient: Eugene Pickard Gender: M Age: 16
Reason for admission: surgical removal of tumor, followed by chemotherapy
Assessment: Ewings sarcoma, left femur

Tip: Refer to OGCR I.C.2.a. and e.1). for sequencing guidance.

2 CM Codes ________ ________

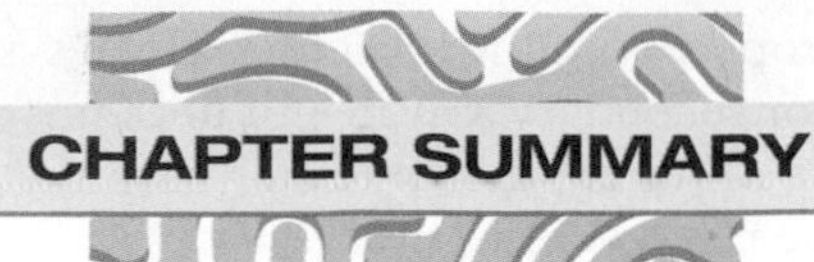

CHAPTER SUMMARY

In this chapter you learned that:

- The musculoskeletal (MS) system consists of the skeletal system, which supports the body, protects internal organs, produces blood cells, stores minerals, and serves as a point of attachment for the skeletal muscles; and the muscular system, which provides for movement of the body, operates individual organs, maintains body posture, and helps produce heat.
- ICD-10-CM Chapter 13, Diseases of the Musculoskeletal System and Connective Tissue (M00-M99) contains 18 blocks or subchapters that are divided by type of tissue, such as bone, joint, spine, vertebrae, cartilage, and tendon.
- The keys to abstracting for the MS system are familiarity with the anatomy, knowledge of medical terms, and careful attention to the details of the documented condition.
- Assigning codes for MS disorders may require coders to cross-reference the medical record multiple times in order to accurately capture the details of the disorder.
- When codes for MS disorders require multiple coding, coders must be attentive to the sequencing indicated in the instructional notes.
- The most common cancer in the musculoskeletal system is metastatic bone disease (MBD) because the bone is a frequent site of metastasis from primary neoplasms in other organs, including the breast, lung, prostate, kidney, and thyroid.
- ICD-10-CM provides Official Guidelines for Coding and Reporting (OGCR) for the musculoskeletal system in OGCR section I.C.13. OGCR discusses coding for site and laterality, pathologic fractures, and osteoporosis.

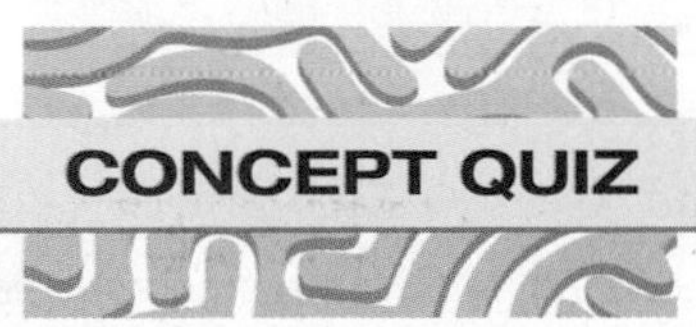

CONCEPT QUIZ

Take a moment to look back at your trip through diseases of the musculoskeletal system and connective tissue and solidify your skills. This is your opportunity to pull together everything you have learned.

Completion

Instructions: Write the term that answers each question based on the information you learned in this chapter. Choose from the following list. Some choices may be used more than once and some choices may not be used at all. Refer to the discussion in this chapter and the Glossary at the end of this book if you need a little extra help.

appendicular
axial
cartilage
delayed
diaphysis
distal epiphysis
involuntary
joints
ligaments
malunion
nonunion
osteoporosis
pathologic
proximal epiphysis
stress
tendons
traumatic
voluntary

1. A ________________ fracture is an acute current injury that results from an accident.
2. A ________________ fracture is a fracture of a bone that has been subjected to repeated use or impact.
3. ________________ are fibrous tissue that join muscles to bones.
4. ________________ healing occurs when a patient waits to seek care for a fracture.
5. ________________ is when the ends of fractured bone segments do not heal with proper alignment.
6. The ________________ is the shaft, or long narrow portion of a long bone.
7. The ________________ is the rounded end of the bone closest to the trunk.
8. The ________________ consists of the arms, shoulders, wrists, hands, legs, hips, ankles and feet.
9. ________________ are fibrous tissue that connect bones to bones.
10. ________________ muscles are controlled by a subconscious part of the brain and control bodily functions such as breathing and digestion.

Multiple Choice

Instructions: Circle the letter of the best answer to each question based on the information you learned in this chapter. Refer to the discussion in this chapter and the Glossary at the end of this book if you need a little extra help.

1. A fracture that occurs as the result of a disease process is a _________ fracture.
   A. neoplastic
   B. traumatic
   C. pathologic
   D. stress
2. All of the following are key criteria for abstracting pathologic fractures EXCEPT
   A. What is the underlying disease?
   B. Is the fracture open or closed?
   C. What is the laterality?
   D. Is the encounter for aftercare during the healing phase?
3. When more than one bone, joint, or muscle has the same condition, how should the coder assign codes?
   A. Assign individual codes for each site.
   B. Assign a code for the most serious injury only.
   C. Assign a seventh-character extension that indicates the number of sites.
   D. Assign a code for multiple sites.
4. When a bone is affected by osteoporosis at the end near the joint, coders should
   A. assign a code for the bone.
   B. assign a code for the joint.
   C. assign a combination code for both the bone and the joint.
   D. assign a not elsewhere classified (NEC) code.
5. Arthritis that occurs due to another disease requires coders to
   A. sequence the underlying condition first and the arthritis second.
   B. sequence the arthritis first and the underlying condition second.
   C. sequence either first, based on the main reason for the encounter.
   D. None of the above.
6. X-rays are used to evaluate conditions of the _________ because they clearly show the difference between hard tissue and soft tissue.
   A. tendons
   B. ligaments
   C. muscles
   D. bones
7. The presence of Rh factor in the blood allows physicians to use blood tests to diagnose
   A. infections.
   B. rheumatoid arthritis.
   C. osteoarthritis.
   D. fractures.
8. _________ is the failure of the ends of fractured bone segments to reunite.
   A. Delayed healing
   B. Malunion
   C. Nonunion
   D. Pathologic fracture
9. A frequent site for metastatic cancer is
   A. muscle.
   B. joints.
   C. tendons.
   D. bone.
10. Leukemia starts in
    A. blood.
    B. joints.
    C. bone marrow.
    D. tendons.

CODING CHALLENGE

Now it is your turn to demonstrate coding all aspects of Diseases of the Musculoskeletal System and Connective Tissue. Refer back to the examples and discussion in this chapter when you need a little extra help. Use your medical dictionary and anatomy references when needed.

Instructions: Read the mini-medical-record of each patient's encounter, then abstract, assign, and sequence ICD-10-CM diagnosis codes (CM) using the Index to Diseases and Injuries, the Index to External Causes, and the Tabular List. Write the code(s) on the line provided.

1. Date: 12/15/yy Location: Northwest Orthopedics and Rheumatology
Provider: Bruce Prentice, MD
Patient: Phyllis Tunnell Gender: F Age: 61
Reason for encounter: pain, redness and swelling in left knee
Assessment: abscess of bursa, left knee, due to streptococcus A
Plan: Reapply dressing as directed. Take antibiotic as instructed.
2 CM Codes __________ __________

2. Date: 12/15/yy Location: Valley Hospital
Provider: Bruce Prentice, MD
Patient: Karen Rand Gender: F Age: 32
Reason for admission: repair of C5 and C6 disc
Assessment: acute and chronic pain due to herniated cervical disc at C5-C6
Plan: FU with rehab, FU up with surgeon 1 wk.
1 CM Code __________

3. Date: 12/15/yy Location: Valley Hospital
Provider: Bruce Prentice, MD
Patient: Victoria Money Gender: F Age: 28
Reason for admission: admitted for lumbar spinal fusion. She was previously diagnosed with spinal stenosis in her lumbar region. I told her that if the pain could not be controlled, she could opt for surgery. After ongoing efforts to manage the pain unsuccessfully, she decided to have surgery.
Assessment: osseous stenosis at L3-L4-L5
Plan: FU 1 wk
1 CM Code __________

4. Date: 12/15/yy Location: Northwest Orthopedics and Rheumatology
Provider: Bruce Prentice, MD
Patient: Stephen Sansom Gender: M Age: 15
Reason for encounter: Swollen glands and high fever with pain in right shoulder, right elbow and right hand. Abdominal spasmodic pain and diarrhea
Assessment: juvenile arthritis with systemic onset (Still's disease), shoulder, elbow, hand and ulcerative colitis
Plan: Rx anti-inflammatory. RTO 3 wk
2 CM Codes __________ __________

5. Date: 12/15/yy Location: Valley Hospital
Provider: Bruce Prentice, MD
Patient: Yvonne Kinser Gender: F Age: 21
Reason for admission: continuing pain in right shoulder after ineffective physical therapy (PT)
Assessment: frozen right shoulder
Plan: Manipulation under anesthesia for shoulder. Return to PT. FU office 1 wk.
1 CM Code __________

6. Date: 12/15/yy Location: Valley Podiatry
Provider: Michael Glick, DPM (podiatrist)
Patient: Anita Nunez Gender: F Age: 57
Reason for encounter: pain on left big toe area when walking
Assessment: hallux valgus, left
Plan: Referred to orthopedic surgeon following unsuccessful treatment with orthotics
1 CM Code ___________

7. Date: 12/15/yy Location: Northwest Orthopedics and Rheumatology
Provider: Bruce Prentice, MD
Patient: Randall Gearhart Gender: M Age: 47
Reason for encounter: weakness in the right forefoot
Assessment: drop foot
Plan: Refer to PT for fitting of lightweight orthoses
1 CM Code ___________

8. Date: 12/15/yy Location: Valley Hospital
Provider: Bruce Prentice, MD
Patient: Thelma Giffin Gender: F Age: 23
Reason for admission: rotator cuff repair
Assessment: recurrent rotator cuff syndrome
Plan: PT, RTO 1 wk
1 CM Code ___________

9. Date: 12/15/yy Location: Valley Hospital
Provider: Bruce Prentice, MD
Patient: Richard Langham Gender: M Age: 1 year
Reason for encounter: Repair of club foot
Assessment: acquired right talipes equinovarus (clubfoot)
Plan: PT, RTO 1 wk
1 CM Code ___________

10. Date: 12/15/yy Location: Valley Hospital
Provider: Bruce Prentice, MD
Patient: Ernest Ingham Gender: M Age: 45
Reason for admission: sudden onset of pain and swelling in left hip, fever
Testing: arthrocentisis (*removing fluid from a joint with a needle*), blood culture, X-ray
Assessment: bacterial pyogenic arthritis due to pseudomonas aeruginosa, likely due to patient's intravenous drug abuse
3 CM Codes ___________ ___________ ___________

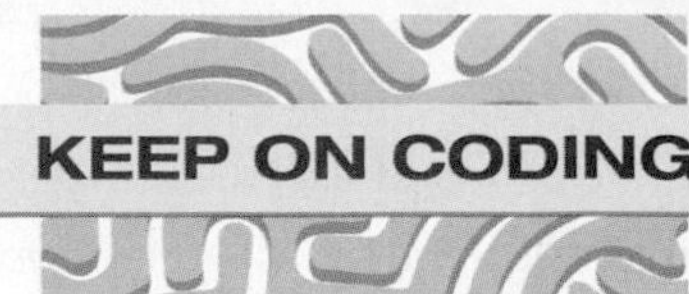

KEEP ON CODING

As a coder, you can never have too much experience. Apply everything you have learned in this chapter to code the following diagnostic statements. Use the OGCR and instructional notes in the Tabular List to help determine how many codes are required.

Instructions: Read the diagnostic statement, then use the Index and Tabular List to assign and sequence ICD-10-CM (CM) diagnosis codes. Write the code(s) on the line provided.

1. Pneumococcal arthritis of left ankle: CM Code(s) ____________________
2. Felty's syndrome, left hip: CM Code(s) ____________________
3. Dysplastic osteoarthritis of right hip: CM Code(s) ____________________
4. Lead-induced chronic gout, vertebrae: CM Code(s) ____________________
5. Panarteritis nodosa: CM Code(s) ____________________
6. Low back pain: CM Code(s) ____________________
7. Rheumatoid nodule, right wrist: CM Code(s) ____________________
8. Stress fracture, right foot, initial encounter: CM Code(s) ____________________
9. Plica syndrome, left knee: CM Code(s) ____________________
10. Psoas tendinitis, right hip: CM Code(s) ____________________
11. Subacute osteomyelitis, right humerus: CM Code(s) ____________________
12. Sicca syndrome with myopathy: CM Code(s) ____________________
13. Rhabdomyosarcoma of the hip, left: CM Code(s) ____________________
14. Relapsing polychondritis: CM Code(s) ____________________
15. Spondylolysis, lumbar region: CM Code(s) ____________________
16. Postsurgical lordosis: CM Code(s) ____________________
17. Arthralgia of temporomandibular joint: CM Code(s) ____________________
18. Rheumatoid bursitis, left hand: CM Code(s) ____________________
19. Age-related osteoporosis with current pathologic fracture of the right ankle, initial encounter:
    CM Code(s) ____________________
20. Achilles tendinitis, right leg: CM Code(s) ____________________
21. Spinal stenosis, cervical region: CM Code(s) ____________________
22. Diastasis of muscle of the left shoulder: CM Code(s) ____________________

23. Spontaneous rupture of the flexor tendon, lower leg: CM Code(s) ____________________

24. Fibromyalgia: CM Code(s) ____________________

25. Osteitis deformans of skull: CM Code(s) ____________________

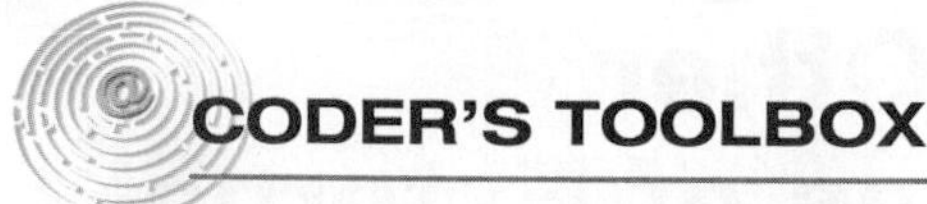

CODER'S TOOLBOX

The following resources are a starting point for learning more about diseases of the musculoskeletal system and connective tissue. The > symbol indicates a menu selection within the website in order to navigate to a specific page.

American Association of Hip & Knee Surgeons (AAHKS) http://www.aahks.org
American Academy of Orthopaedic Surgeons (AAOS) http://www.aaos.org/
American College of Rheumatology http://www.rheumatology.org/
Arthritis Foundation www.arthritis.org/
Association of Bone and Joint Surgeons http://www.abjs.org/
Clinical Orthopaedics and Related Research http://www.clinorthop.org/index.html
Healthline Body Maps > Body Menu http://www.healthline.com/human-body-maps/
Musculoskeletal Infection Society http://msis-na.org/
Musculoskeletal Tumor Society http://msts.org/
National Fibromyalgia Association www.fmaware.org
National Osteoporosis Foundation www.nof.org
NIH Consensus Statement on Hip Replacement > Previous Conferences > Older > 1994 > Total Hip Replacement http://consensus.nih.gov/1994/1994Hipreplacement098html.htm
Orthopaedia Collaborative Orthopaedic Knowledgebase http://www.orthopaedia.com/display/Main/Home
The Hip Society http://www.hipsoc.org/web/index.html
The Knee Society http://www.kneesociety.org/web/index.html
United States Bone and Joint Decade, NFP (USBJD) http://www.usbjd.org/

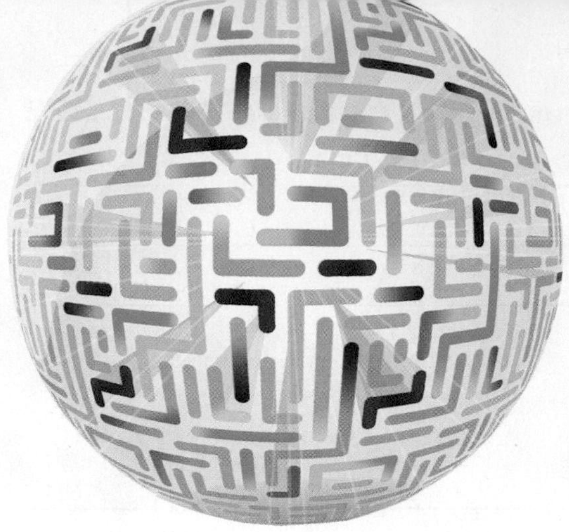

13

Injury, Poisoning, and Certain Other Consequences of External Causes (S00-T88)

Learning Objectives

After completing this chapter, you should have the skills to:

- Spell and define the key words, medical terms, and abbreviations related to injury, poisoning, and certain other consequences of external causes.
- Discuss the common forms of injury and poisoning.
- Identify the main characteristics of coding for injury, poisoning, and certain other consequences of external causes.
- Abstract information from the medical record required for coding injury, poisoning, and certain other consequences of external causes.
- Assign codes for injury, poisoning, and certain other consequences of external causes.
- Arrange codes for injury, poisoning, and certain other consequences of external causes.
- Discuss the Official Guidelines for Coding and Reporting related to injury, poisoning, and certain other consequences of external causes.

Key Terms and Abbreviations

abuse
burn
circumstances of admission
clavicle
closed
complications of care
contusion
corrosion
degree
displaced
foreign body
Gustilo classification system
laceration
nondisplaced
open
open wound
penetrating wound
puncture wound
perforation
Salter-Harris classification
physis
Rule of Nines
superficial injury
total body surface area (TBSA)
traumatic amputation
wound

In addition to the key terms listed here, students should know the terms defined within tables in this chapter.

Chapter Outline

- **Injury and Poisoning Refresher**
- **Coding Overview of Injury and Poisoning**
- **Abstracting for Injury and Poisoning**
- **Assigning Codes for Injury and Poisoning**
- **Arranging Codes for Injury and Poisoning**

ICD-10-CM codes in this chapter are from the ICD-10-CM 2014 Draft code set from the Department of Health and Human Services, Centers for Disease Control and Prevention.

INTRODUCTION

As you are driving down the road, you occasionally need to pull over to let an ambulance pass. Your heart may pause for a moment as you wonder, "Is the ambulance coming or going? What happened? Who is in it? Who are their loved ones?" You never learn the answers, but you always send a prayer and good energy their way. Unfortunately, accidents and injuries are part of the trip of life, and coders follow special requirements to code these situations.

In your tour of injury and poisoning in this chapter you will learn about different types of injuries and poisonings and how physicians treat these conditions. Most importantly, you will practice coding for patient encounters related to injury and poisoning, a skill that requires you to abstract information from the mini-medical-record, assign correct codes, and arrange (sequence) the codes in the proper order.

Any physician may treat injuries and poisonings because they can affect any body system. Physician specialties that most commonly treat these conditions are emergency medicine, primary care, orthopedics, and dermatology.

As you read this chapter, refer to anatomic resources on the integumentary system and musculoskeletal systems, both of which are frequently affected by injuries. Think of these resources as your travel brochures that tell you more about an area. This way, you have the information you need at your fingertips.

INJURY AND POISONING REFRESHER

Injury and poisoning can encompass a wide variety of conditions and a range of definitions, so it is critical that coders understand how ICD-10-CM defines terms, rather than rely on how they might use the words in everyday conversation. Coders use medical resources, such as a reference book on diseases, to understand injuries, diagnostic methods, and common treatments. In particular, coders must be familiar with specific terminology related to burns, traumatic fractures, and poisoning and adverse effects, which are reviewed in detail. Other types of injuries are summarized in ■ TABLE 13-1. Also refer to Table 12-2, Common Conditions of the Musculoskeletal System, for a refresher on dislocations, subluxations, sprains, and strains.

Burns

Burns are damage to skin by heat, electricity, or radiation. In ICD-10-CM, **corrosions** are damage to skin due to chemicals. Both burns and corrosions are described by the **degree** (*depth*) of the burn (■ FIGURE 13-1, page 230). Burns of the eye and internal organs are *not* assigned degrees (OGCR I.C.19.d.).

Table 13-1 ■ **TYPES OF INJURIES**

Injury	Description
Abuse	Physical, emotional, or sexual mistreatment by one person towards another
Complications of care	Unanticipated results of a medical or surgical procedure
Foreign body	An object that does not belong in the body
Laceration	A torn or jagged wound
Open wound	A wound in which underlying tissue is exposed to the air
Penetrating wound puncture wound	A wound caused by a sharp pointed object passing through the skin into the underlying tissues
Perforation	Cutting or puncturing the wall or membrane of an internal organ or structure
Superficial injury	An injury to the surface of the skin, such as abrasion, blister, **contusion** (*bruise*), constriction, insect bite, superficial foreign body
Traumatic amputation	Severing a body part accidentally
Wound	A cut or opening in the skin or mucous membrane

Traumatic Fractures

Traumatic fractures result from an accident rather than a disease. The most frequently broken bone in the body is the **clavicle** (*collar bone*), often caused by a direct blow to the shoulder, such as during a fall, as the result of an automobile collision, or by an outstretched arm that is attempting to break a fall. In babies, clavicle fractures can occur during a difficult delivery. Traumatic fractures are described based on combinations of several criteria:

- body region
- specific bone
- site on the bone
- line of break (■ FIGURE 13-2, page 230)
- **open** (*the bone breaks through the skin*) or **closed** (*the bone does not break the skin*)
- **displaced** (*the fragments of bone move out of alignment*) or **nondisplaced** (*the fragments of bone remain properly aligned*)

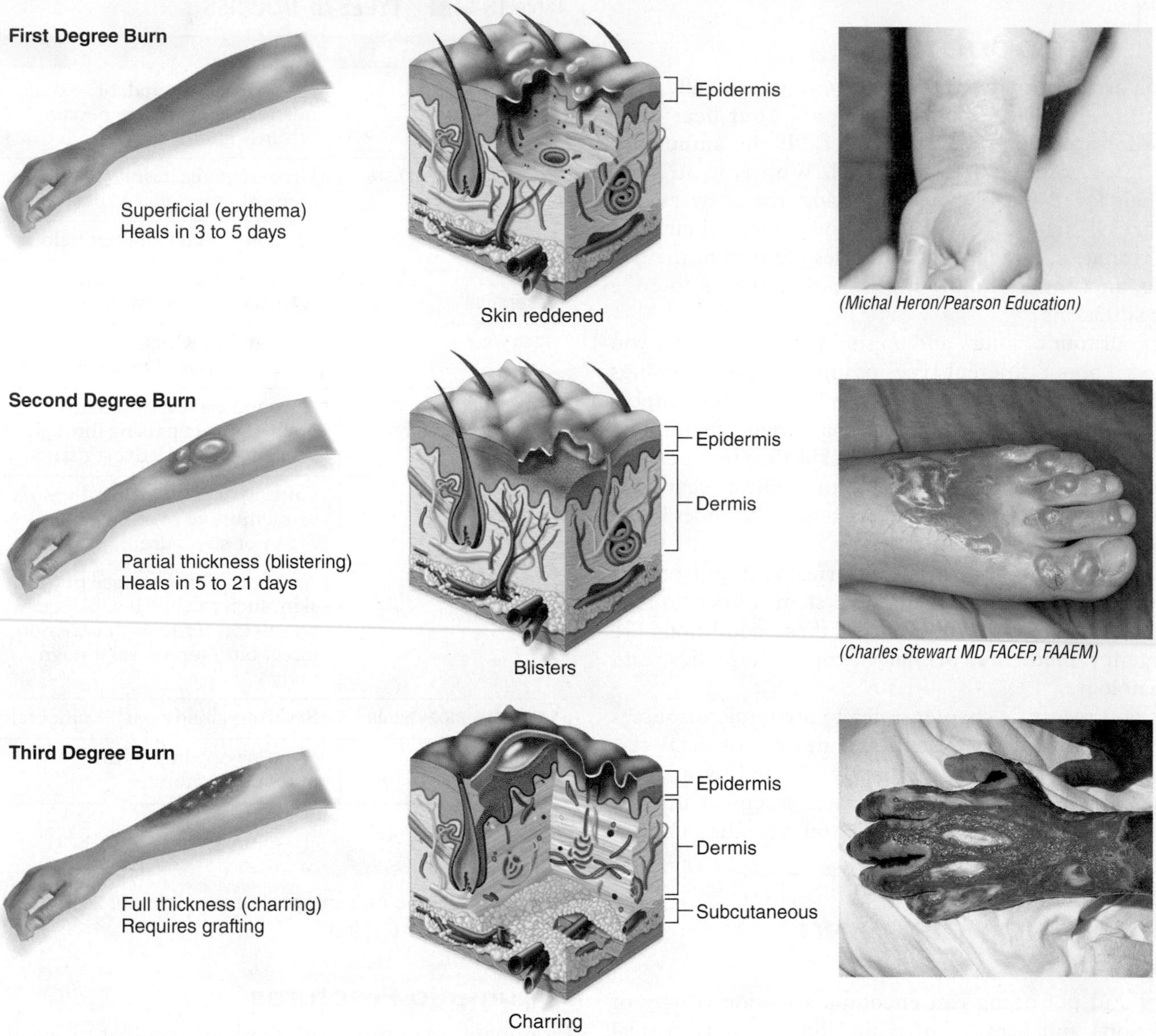

First Degree Burn
Superficial (erythema)
Heals in 3 to 5 days
Epidermis
Skin reddened
(Michal Heron/Pearson Education)
Second Degree Burn
Partial thickness (blistering)
Heals in 5 to 21 days
Epidermis
Dermis
Blisters
(Charles Stewart MD FACEP, FAAEM)
Third Degree Burn
Full thickness (charring)
Requires grafting
Epidermis
Dermis
Subcutaneous
Charring

Figure 13-1 ■ Comparison of Burn Depth. *Source: Pearson Education/PH College.*

Proximal
Midshaft
Distal
Normal bone
Transverse
Oblique
Spiral
Comminuted
Segmental
Greenstick
Impacted

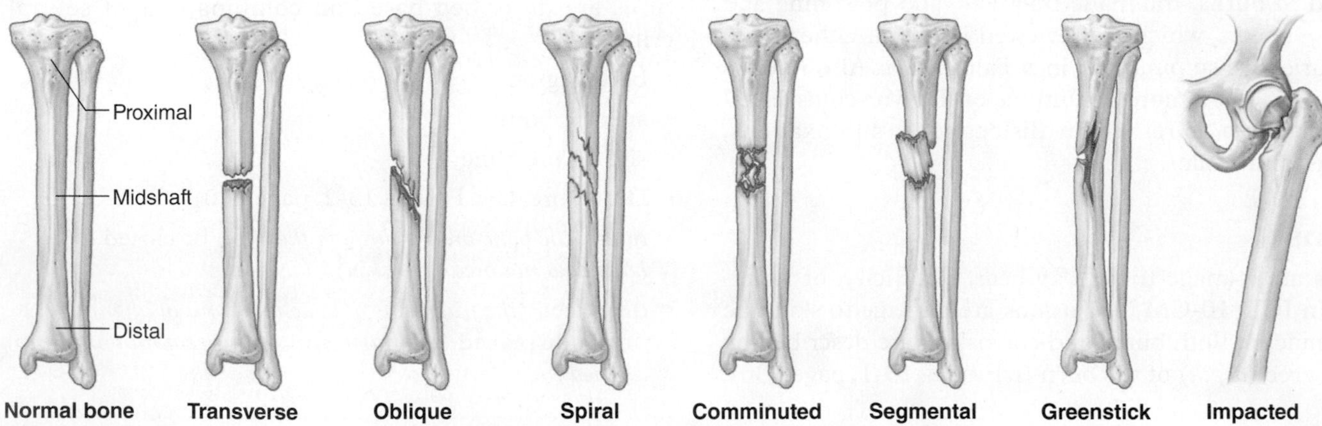

Figure 13-2 ■ Common Lines of Fracture Breaks

SUCCESS STEP

The classification of fractures as displaced or nondisplaced is a new concept in ICD-10-CM that did not exist in ICD-9-CM.

Physicians further classify fractures using specially-developed classification systems, based on the type of fracture. Two such systems that are incorporated into ICD-10-CM are the Gustilo system for open fractures and the Salter-Harris system for epiphysis fractures. Coders must refer to the documentation to determine how the fracture is classified, then assign the corresponding diagnosis code.

Gustilo Open Fracture Classification

Open fractures are classified using the **Gustilo classification system** (■ TABLE 13-2), which organizes open fractures into three major types depending on the method of injury, soft tissue damage, and degree of skeletal involvement. Progression from type I to IIIC describes a higher degree of force involved in the injury, increased soft tissue and bone damage, and greater potential for complications.

Table 13-2 ■ GUSTILO CLASSIFICATION OF OPEN FRACTURES

Type		Description
I		Wound less than 1 cm with minimal soft tissue injury and clean wound bed. Fracture is usually a simple transverse, short oblique fracture, with minimal comminution (fragmentation).
II		Wound greater than 1 cm with moderate soft tissue damage, without flaps, avulsions. Fracture is usually a simple transverse, short oblique fracture, with minimal comminution.
III		Fractures that involve extensive damage to the soft tissues, including muscle, skin, and neurovascular structures. The injury is often accompanied by a high velocity injury or a severe crushing component.
SUBTYPE	IIIA	Adequate soft tissue coverage despite soft tissue laceration regardless of the size of the wound. This includes segmental fractures or severely comminuted fractures.
	IIIB	Extensive soft tissue lost and bony exposure. This is usually associated with massive contamination.
	IIIC	Fracture in which there is a major arterial injury requiring repair for limb salvage.

Salter-Harris Epiphysis Fracture Classification

Epiphysis fractures are classified using the **Salter-Harris classification**, in order to identify the involvement of the growth plate (■ FIGURE 13-3). Fracture of the growth plate is an injury unique to childhood and usually heals without permanent deformity. A small percentage, however, are complicated by growth arrest and subsequent deformity. The Salter-Harris classification aids in estimating both the prognosis and the potential for growth disturbance (■ TABLE 13-3).

Poisoning, Adverse Effects, and Underdosing

ICD-10-CM provides specific definitions for injuries from drugs, chemicals, and biological substances (■ TABLE 13-4, page 232). Coders need to learn how ICD-10-CM uses these terms and not rely on the common language

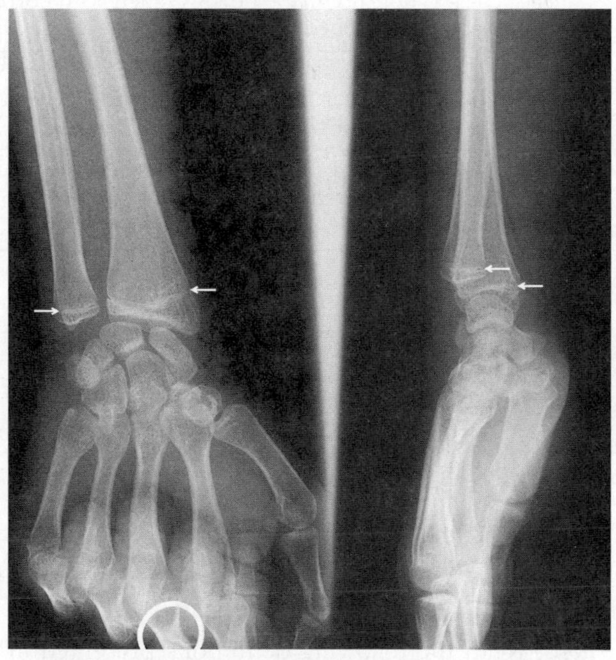

Figure 13-3 ■ X-ray Showing the Epiphysis (Growth Plate).
Source: Courtesy of Teresa Resch.

Table 13-3 ■ SALTER-HARRIS CLASSIFICATION OF EPIPHYSIS FRACTURES

Type	Description
I	A transverse fracture through the growth plate (also referred to as the **physis**).
II	A fracture through the growth plate and the metaphysis, sparing the epiphysis.
III	A fracture through growth plate and epiphysis, sparing the metaphysis.
IV	A fracture through all three elements of the bone, the growth plate, metaphysis, and epiphysis.
V	A crush or compression fracture of the growth plate.

definition. The use of these definitions when assigning codes is discussed later in this chapter.

Over 50% of all exposures to poisoning occur in children age five and younger, but this age group accounts for less than 2% of fatalities. Nearly 40% of fatalities occur in persons age 40 to 59. Intentional poisonings account for nearly 14% of all exposures (American Association of Poison Control Centers).

Table 13-4 ■ **DEFINITIONS FOR INJURIES FROM DRUGS, CHEMICALS, AND BIOLOGICAL SUBSTANCES**

Injury	Definition	Example
Adverse effect	A medication that was correctly prescribed and properly administered causes an undesired physical response.	Allergic reaction to an initial dose of penicillin Interaction between prescribed lithium and Diuril, both taken correctly
Poisoning	The improper use of a medication that causes an undesired physical response: • overdose of any drug, whether intentional or accidental • error made in prescription, wrong drug given or taken in error • interaction of drugs and alcohol • non-prescribed drugs taken with correctly prescribed and administered drug	Administering penicillin to someone known to be allergic Nausea, vomiting, and tachycardia from drinking alcohol while taking metformin
Underdosing	Taking less of a medication than is prescribed by a provider or a manufacturer's instruction causes an undesired physical response.	Diabetic ketoacidosis due to taking too little insulin
Toxic effect	A harmful substance is ingested, or comes in contact with a person, and causes an undesired physical response.	Swallowing bleach Rash from wearing latex gloves

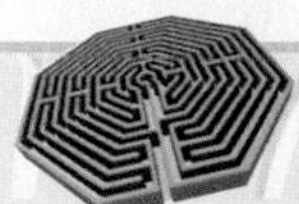

Coding Practice

Refresh your knowledge of terminology related to injury and poisoning.

Exercise 13.1 Injury and Poisoning Refresher

Part A

Instructions: Read the following definitions presented in this section. Write the term being defined in the space provided.

1. ______________________ the fragments of bone move out of alignment.

2. ______________________ unanticipated results of a medical or surgical procedure.

3. ______________________ cutting or puncturing the wall or membrane of an internal organ or structure.

4. ______________________ skin damage due to chemicals.

5. ______________________ a classification system used for open fractures.

Part B

Instructions: Read each of the following patient situations and determine if it is an **adverse effect**, **poisoning**, **underdosing**, or **toxic effect**. Write the answer in the space provided.

6. ______________________ A patient sees her doctor when she breaks out in hives and has shortness of breath after taking prescribed sulfa for an infection. She has never taken sulfa or had this reaction to any medication before.

7. ______________________ A diabetic patient who takes prescribed metformin drinks alcohol at a party. He experiences severe nausea, vomiting, and tachycardia and is taken to the emergency department.

8. ______________________ A two-year-old gets into rubbing alcohol while his mother's back is turned. She does not think he drank any of it, but he did rub it in his eyes and is screaming. She calls Poison Control, then rushes him to the emergency department.

9. ________________________ An elderly woman is seen in the emergency department for an electrolyte imbalance after having taken a newly prescribed diuretic with lithium, which had been prescribed for her last year.

10. ________________________ A type 1 diabetic is seen in the emergency department for ketoacidosis after getting confused and taking too little insulin.

CODING OVERVIEW OF INJURY AND POISONING

ICD-10-CM Chapter 19, Injury, Poisoning, and Certain Other Consequences of External Causes (S00-T88), contains 20 blocks or subchapters that are divided by anatomical site and type of injury. Review the block names and code ranges listed at the beginning of Chapter 19 in the ICD-10-CM manual to become familiar with the content and organization.

ICD-10-CM Chapter 19 compares to ICD-9-CM Chapter 17 (800-999). The ICD-10-CM chapter is reorganized, grouping together all types of injuries for each anatomic region. Codes have been expanded due to additional details and laterality. Most codes also required seventh-character extensions to identify the episode of care. The Table of Drugs and Chemicals has also been reorganized and expanded.

This ICD-10-CM chapter includes traumatic injuries to all body systems. The **S** section classifies injuries related to single body regions, such as head, neck, and hip/thigh. The **T** section classifies injuries to unspecified body regions, effects of foreign bodies, burns, frostbite, poisonings, and other complications and consequences of external causes.

This chapter does not include obstetric trauma, which is classified in categories **O70** and **O71**, or birth trauma, which is classified in categories **P10** through **P15**. It also does not include conditions that arise from a disease process, even though the resulting condition may be similar to a traumatic injury. For example, a pathologic fracture is classified in ICD-10-CM Chapter 13, Diseases of the Musculoskeletal System and Connective Tissue (M00-M99), but a traumatic fracture is classified in ICD-10-CM Chapter 19, Injury, Poisoning, and Certain Other Consequences of External Causes (S00-T88).

ICD-10-CM Official Guidelines for Coding and Reporting (OGCR) for injury and poisoning appear in section I.C.19, which is divided into the following topics:

a. Code Extensions
b. Coding of Injuries
c. Coding of Traumatic Fractures
d. Coding of Burns and Corrosions
e. Adverse Effects, Poisoning, Underdosing and Toxic Effects
f. Adult and child abuse, neglect and other maltreatment
g. Complications of care

Instructional notes at the beginning of ICD-10-CM Chapter 19 direct coders to use secondary codes ICD-10-CM from Chapter 20, External Causes of Morbidity, to indicate the cause of injury. Many codes within section **T** already include the external cause, so those codes do not require an additional external cause code. When a retained foreign body is involved, use an additional code from category **Z18 Retained foreign body fragments** to identify the object.

ABSTRACTING FOR INJURY AND POISONING

Each type of injury has unique criteria for abstracting. Most conditions in ICD-10-CM Chapter 19 also require information on the external cause. Refer to Table 8-1, Key Criteria for Abstracting External Causes, as a refresher on how to abstract data for external causes, and remember to abstract for external causes in addition to the injury. Key criteria for abstracting burns, traumatic fractures, and poisoning and adverse effect follow.

Abstracting Burns

Because burns often involve multiple body areas, specific anatomic sites may not be documented. When that is the case, report the percentage of the **total body surface area (TBSA)** affected by second- and third-degree burns. In addition, when a death occurs or more than 20% of the body is affected by third-degree burns, OGCR recommends, but does not require, reporting the percentage of TBSA involved (OGCR I.C.19.d.6)). Physicians calculate the percentage of TBSA using the **Rule of Nines**, which divides the body into areas, each of which comprises 9% of the total body surface area (■ FIGURE 13-4, page 234). The percentages vary slightly among adults, children, infants, obese patients, and pregnant women. Key criteria for abstracting burns appear in ■ TABLE 13-5 (page 234).

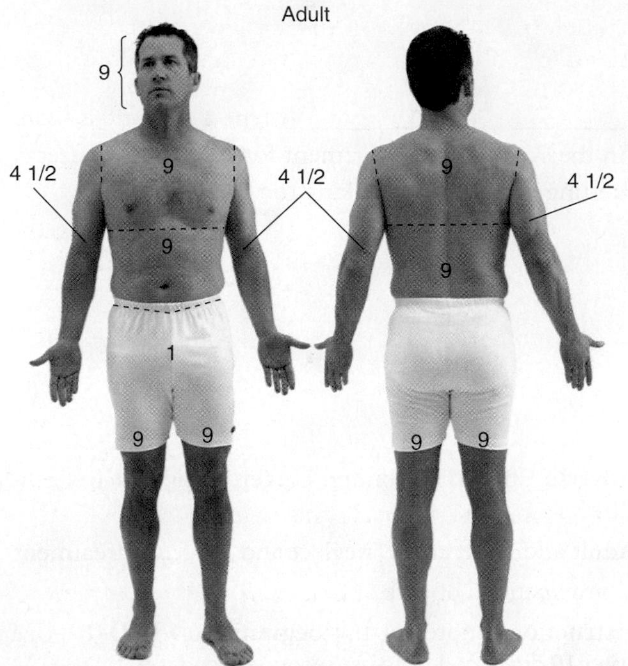

Figure 13-4 ■ Rule of Nines for Reporting Burns (All numbers are percent of total body surface area.). *Source: Michal Heron/Pearson Education*.

Table 13-5 ■ **KEY CRITERIA FOR ABSTRACTING BURNS**

- ❑ Is the burn due to heat or a chemical (corrosion)?
- ❑ What is the anatomic site?
- ❑ What is the laterality?
- ❑ What is the greatest depth (degree) of burn on each site?
- ❑ Are any burns non-healing?
- ❑ Are any burns infected?
- ❑ What is the episode of care?
- ❑ What percent of the body surface involves third-degree burns?

Abstracting Traumatic Fractures

Criteria for abstracting traumatic fractures are more detailed than criteria for pathologic fractures. Knowledge of the anatomy of the skeletal system is essential because fractures are identified by their anatomic location. Knowledge of different types of fracture lines is also critical (Figure 13-2). Key criteria for abstracting traumatic fractures appear in ■ TABLE 13-6.

Abstracting Poisoning

When abstracting poisoning, adverse effects, and underdosing, coders must identify the name of the drug or substance involved. Careful attention to spelling is required because drug names may have similar spelling but belong to a different class of drugs (■ FIGURE 13-5). Key criteria for abstracting poisoning and adverse effects appear in ■ TABLE 13-7.

Table 13-6 ■ **KEY CRITERIA FOR ABSTRACTING TRAUMATIC FRACTURES**

- ❑ Is the fracture traumatic or pathologic?
- ❑ Does the patient have osteoporosis?
- ❑ What bone is fractured?
- ❑ What is the laterality?
- ❑ Were any additional bones fractured?
- ❑ Where on the bone is the fracture located?
- ❑ What type of fracture occurred?
- ❑ Is the fracture displaced or nondisplaced? (*Default is displaced.*)
- ❑ Is the fracture open or closed? (*Default is closed.*)
- ❑ For open fractures, what is the Gustilo classification type?
- ❑ For epiphysis fractures, what is the Salter-Harris classification type?
- ❑ What is the episode of care?
- ❑ Is the healing routine, delayed, nonunion, or malunion?
- ❑ Is the encounter for follow-up after active healing is complete?

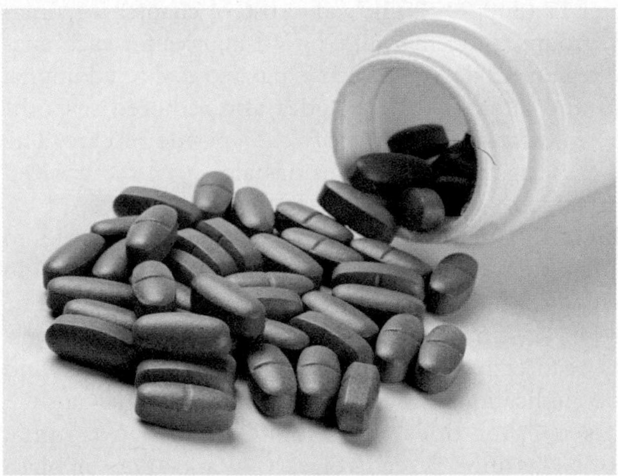

Figure 13-5 ■ According to the American Association of Poison Control Centers, analgesics are the leading cause of accidental poisonings. *Source: © Petr Malyshev/Dreamstime.com*.

Table 13-7 ■ **KEY CRITERIA FOR ABSTRACTING POISONING, ADVERSE EFFECTS, AND UNDERDOSING**

- ❑ What substance is involved?
- ❑ Is a diagnosis of abuse or dependence on the substance documented?
- ❑ Is the injury a poisoning, adverse effect, or underdosing?
- ❑ Is the injury documented as accidental, intentional self-harm, an assault, or of undetermined intent? (*Default is accidental.*)
- ❑ What conditions (manifestations) resulted from the injury?
- ❑ What is the episode of care?

Guided Example of Abstracting for Injury and Poisoning

Refer to the following example throughout this chapter to practice skills for abstracting, assigning, and sequencing injury and poisoning codes. Chelsea Kutcher, CPC-H, is a fictitious coder who guides you through this case.

> Date: 03/1/yy Location: Branton Medical Center Emergency Department Provider: Cynthia Hiatt, MD
>
> Patient: Gwen Beene Gender: F Age: 23
>
> Reason for encounter: hives and has shortness of breath
>
> Assessment: Patient has allergic reaction to Trimethoprim-Sulfamethoxazole prescribed two days ago by her family physician, Dr. Conover, for a urinary tract infection (UTI). She has never taken sulfa or had this reaction to any medication before.
>
> Plan: d/c Trimethoprim-Sulfamethoxazole, notify PCP

Follow along as Chelsea Kutcher, CPC-H, abstracts the diagnosis. Check off each step after you complete it.

⇨ Chelsea reads through the entire record, with special attention to the reason for the encounter and the final assessment. She notes that the patient has a new allergic reaction to a medication, so she refers to the Key Criteria for Abstracting Poisoning, Adverse Effects, and Underdosing (Table 13-7).

- ☐ *What substance is involved?* She notes that the substance is Trimethoprim-Sulfamethoxazole, which is a sulfa-based anti-infective.
- ☐ *Is a diagnosis of abuse or dependence on the substance documented?* No.
- ☐ *Is the injury a poisoning, adverse effect, or underdosing?* She determines that this is an adverse effect because the medication was taken as prescribed and the patient has not had this reaction before.
- ☐ *Is the injury documented as accidental, intentional self-harm, an assault, or of undetermined intent?* Accidental.
- ☐ *What conditions (manifestations) resulted from the injury?* Hives and shortness of breath.
- ☐ *What is the episode of care?* It is the initial encounter because it is a new problem.

⇨ Next, Chelsea needs to assign the codes.

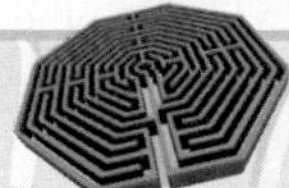

Coding Practice

Now it is your turn to practice abstracting diagnoses for injury and poisoning. Questions guide your analysis of each scenario.

Exercise 13.2 Abstracting for Injury and Poisoning

Instructions: Read the mini-medical-record of each patient's encounter and answer the abstracting questions. Write the answer on the line provided. Do not assign any codes.

> **1.** Date: 3/3/yy Location: Branton Medical Center Emergency Department Provider: Cynthia Hiatt, MD
>
> Patient: Willie Munoz Gender: M Age: 8
>
> Chief complaint: pain, tenderness, swelling, and distortion on right knee after being tackled while playing football at school
>
> Assessment: X-ray shows type III fracture of growth plate at the upper end of the tibia
>
> Plan: surgery and internal fixation to ensure proper alignment of the growth plate and the joint surface
>
> a. What bone is fractured? Tibia, plate & upper ______
>
> What is the laterality? Right knee ______
>
> *(continued)*

> **1.** (continued)
>
> b. What site on the bone is injured? upper end & Growth plate of tibia ______
>
> c. How are fractures to the growth plate classified? Salter Harris ______
>
> d. What is the type (classification system level) of this fracture? type III ______
>
> e. What are the symptoms? pain, tenderness, swelling & distortion on (R) knee ______
>
> f. Should the symptoms be coded? NO ______
>
> Why or why not? b/c its integral to DX ______
>
> g. What is the episode of care? initial ______
>
> h. What is the causal event? tackle in sports ______
>
> i. What is the intent? accidental ______
>
> j. What is the location? School ______
>
> k. What is the external cause status? recreational while playing football ______
>
> l. What activity was he engaged in? Playing foot ball @ school ______

(continued)

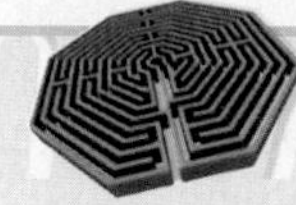

Coding Practice (continued)

2. Date: 3/3/yy Location: Branton Medical Center

Provider: Cynthia Hiatt, MD

Patient: Earl Dews Gender: M Age: 23

Reason for admission: patient arrived by ambulance after a barn fire that occurred on his own farm which is his job

Assessment: third degree burns to left forearm, second degree burns to left upper arm and shoulder, smoke inhalation

a. Is the burn due to a controlled flame or an uncontrolled fire? uncontrolled fire

b. What is the degree, site, and laterality of the most serious burn? third degree burns to Ⓛ forearm

c. What is the degree, site, and laterality of other burns? Second degree burns to Ⓛ upper arm & shoulder.

d. What does OGCR I.C.19.d.2) instruct regarding burns of the same local site (three-digit category)? assign one code for highest degree of burn

e. What other problems does the patient have? Smoke inhalation

f. What is the episode of care? initial

g. What is the causal event? exposed to fire & smoke

h. What is the intent? accidental

i. What is the location? Barn

j. What is the external cause status? Farm Job

k. What activity was he engaged in? Info. not available

3. Date: 3/4/yy Location: Branton Family Practice

Provider: Kristen Conover, MD

Patient: Florence Collard Gender: F Age: 35

Reason for encounter: suture removal from wound to right index finger, sustained when she accidentally cut her finger with a butcher knife while preparing dinner

Assessment: Wound is healed. Removed sutures.

a. What is the injury? wound, *laceration

b. What is the anatomic site and laterality? Index finger Ⓡ

(continued)

3. (continued)

c. What is the reason for the encounter? Suture removal from wound

d. What is the episode of care? Subsequent

e. What is the causal event? Cut finger c̄ knife

f. Should you assign an aftercare code for removal of sutures? NO

Why or why not? Not documented

4. Date: 3/4/yy Location: Branton Medical Center Emergency Department

Provider: Cynthia Hiatt, MD

Patient: Jose Erickson Gender: M Age: 67

Chief complaint: irregular pulse, palpitations, confusion

Assessment: Cumulative intoxication effect (*a build-up in the body*) from digitalis which had been taken as prescribed for atrial fibrillation. Patient also has stage 2 chronic kidney disease which put him at risk for intoxication.

a. What are the symptoms? irregular pulse, Palpitations, confusion

Should they be coded? NO

Why or why not? Because they are integral to cumulative intoxication

b. Is this an adverse effect or accidental poisoning? Adverse effect

Please give the reason for your answer. the med was taken as prescribed

c. What is the substance Digitalis ~~for A-fib~~

d. What condition was the medication prescribed for? A-fibrillation

e. What condition raised the patient's risk for intoxication? stage 2 CKD

f. What is the episode of care? initial

5. Date: 3/4/yy Location: Branton Medical Center Emergency Department Provider: Cynthia Hiatt, MD

Patient: Stefanie Frechette Gender: F Age: 19

Chief complaint: examination after alleged date rape by her boyfriend

(continued)

5. (continued)

Assessment: Conducted physical examination and urine test. Flunitrazepam was found in a urine test. The injury was determined to be sexual assault.

a. What is the substance? Flunitrazepam

b. What is the intent? Assault

c. What is the reason for the encounter? Physical Examination of alleged date rape

d. What event occurred? alleged date rape

e. What is the episode of care? initial

f. Who is the perpetrator? Boyfriend

g. Should you assign a code to identify the perpetrator? Yes
Why or why not? to identify the person who raped

6. Date: 3/3/yy Location: Branton Family Practice Provider: Kristen Conover, MD

Patient: Luke Kershaw Gender: M Age: 31

Chief complaint: accident in which automobile battery exploded and something got in his eyes while he was working on his car in the driveway at his single family home

(continued)

6. (continued)

Assessment: sulfuric acid burn on both eyelids and right cornea, second degree sulfuric acid burn to forehead and right cheek

a. Is the burn due to heat or a chemical? Chemical

b. What is the coding term for this type of burn? Corrosion

c. What is the substance? Sulfuric acid

d. What is the anatomic site? eyelids, cornea, forehead & cheek

e. What is the laterality? eyelids are bilateral, (R) cornea (R) cheek

f. What is the greatest depth (degree) of burn on each site? Second degree

g. What is the episode of care? initial

h. What is the causal event? automobile battery explosion

i. What is the intent? accidental

j. What is the location? Driveway at a single family home

k. What is the external cause status? working on his car/fixing the car

l. What is the activity? Automobile repair

ASSIGNING CODES FOR INJURY AND POISONING

Each type of injury has unique coding guidelines, so coders need to become familiar with a variety of situations. Because the most severe injuries are often accompanied by less serious injuries, the OGCR instruct coders *not* to assign codes for superficial injuries, such as abrasions or contusions, when more severe injuries, such as an open wound or fracture of the *same* site, are present. Assign codes for the more severe injuries (OGCR I.C.19.b.1)).

Most codes in ICD-10-CM Chapter 19 require a seventh-character extension for the episode of care. Refer to Table 8-3 to review the three most common extensions, **A**, **D**, and **S**.

This section of the chapter demonstrates how to assign codes for the three major types of injuries—burns, traumatic fractures, and poisoning—then also discusses two special topics—child or adult abuse and complications of care.

CODING CAUTION

Use extension **S Sequela** for all follow-up and aftercare of injuries. Do not report aftercare **Z** codes with injuries (OGCR I.C.21.c.7) and 19.a)).

Assigning Codes for Burns

Burns are classified by anatomic site, depth (degree), extent, and causal event or agent (source). Burns of the eye and internal organs are classified by site and causal event or agent, but not by degree. Event and agent codes are external cause codes that are located in the Index to External Causes. The following information summarizes key guidelines to keep in mind when assigning codes for burns (■ FIGURE 13-6, page 238):

- Assign separate codes for each burn site (OGCR I.C.19.d.5)). Search the Index for the Main Term **Burn** and a subterm for the anatomic site.

Patient is treated for multiple third degree burns to her left arm, multiple second degree burns to her left leg, and first degree burns to both feet. She sustained the burns in a house fire of a single family home where she was trapped in a bedroom.

(1) Code the 3rd degree burns

(2) Code the 2nd degree burns

(3) Code the 1st degree burns, left foot

(4) Code the 1st degree burns, right foot because there is no code for bilateral

(5) Code for percent of TBSA burned based on the body areas identified

(6) External cause code for causal event

(7) External cause code for place of occurrence

(1) Index to Diseases: **Burn, upper limb, multiple sites, left, third degree**

Tabular List: **T22.392A Burn of third degree of multiple sites of left shoulder and upper limb, except wrist and hand, initial encounter**

(2) Index to Diseases: **Burn, lower limb, multiple sites, left, second degree**

Tabular List: **T24.292A Burn of second degree of multiple sites of right lower limb, except ankle and foot, initial encounter**

(3) Index to Diseases: **Burn, foot, left, first degree**

Tabular List: **T25.122A Burn of first degree of left foot, initial encounter**

(4) Index to Diseases: Burn, foot, right, first degree

Tabular List: **T25.121A Burn of first degree of right foot, initial encounter**

(5) Index to Diseases: **Burn, extent, 20–29 percent of body surface, 0–9 percent with third degree**

Tabular List: **T31.20 Burns involving 20–29% of body surface with 0% to 9% third degree burns, initial encounter**

(6) External Cause Index: **Exposure, fire, uncontrolled, in building or structure**

Tabular List: **X00.0XXA Exposure to flames in uncontrolled fire in building or structure, initial encounter**

(7) External Cause Index: **Place of occurrence, residence, house, single family, bedroom**

Tabular List: **Y92.013 Bedroom of single-family (private) house as the place of occurrence of the external cause**

Figure 13-6 ■ Example of Assigning Codes for Burns

- When the same local site (three-character category level, **T20-T28**) has multiple burns of different degrees, assign a code only for highest degree recorded in the diagnosis (OGCR I.C.19.d.2)).
- Assign additional codes for any infection of the burn site (OGCR I.C.19.d.4)) and for other related conditions, such as smoke inhalation or respiratory failure (OGCR I.C.19.d.1)c)).
- Assign a code for the percentage of TBSA involved from categories **T31 Burns classified according to extent of body surface involved** or **T32 Corrosions classified according to extent of body surface involved** in the following situations (OGCR I.C.19.d.6)):
  - when the site of the burn is not specified
  - when there is a need for additional data, such as that required by the state health department
  - to provide data for evaluating burn mortality, such as that needed by burn units
  - when a third-degree burn involves 20% or more of TBSA

SUCCESS STEP

Non-healing burns and necrosis of burned skin are coded in the same way as an acute burn (OGCR I.C.19.d.3)).

Assigning Codes for Traumatic Fractures

In addition to the seventh-character extensions **A**, **D**, and **S** used for most injury and poisoning codes, traumatic fracture codes use several additional extensions that describe combinations of the following criteria:

- open or closed
- Gustilo type for open fractures (■ FIGURE 13-7)
- routine or delayed healing
- normal union, malunion, or nonunion

Seventh character options appear at the beginning of each three-digit category and are summarized in ■ TABLE 13-8.

The details of code selection vary with the type of fracture. For example, some categories provide separate codes for displaced and nondisplaced fractures. Categories **S49**, **S59**, **S79**, and **S89** classify epiphysis fractures using the Salter-Harris system.

OGCR I.C.19.c. provides guidance on the default coding of fractures when certain details are not documented, as follows:

- When a fracture is not documented as open or closed, assign a code for closed.
- When a fracture is not documented as displaced or not displaced, assign a code for displaced.

Patient is seen for follow-up on an open fracture or the right tibia plateau. The fracture occurred at the lateral condyle. The physician classifies the fracture as Type II using the Gustilo scale. X-rays show that the fracture is healing well.

Index: **Fracture, tibia, plateau, *see* upper end, bicondylar**

Tabular List:

S82.14 Bicondylar fracture of tibia

1 sixth digit for **right tibia, displaced**

E seventh character extension for **subsequent encounter for open fracture type I or II with routine healing**

Final code: **S82.141E Displaced bicondylar fracture of right tibia, subsequent encounter for open fracture type I or II with routine healing**

Figure 13-7 ■ Example of Coding a Gustilo Fracture

Table 13-8 ■ **MATRIX OF SEVENTH-CHARACTER EXTENSIONS FOR TRAUMATIC FRACTURES**

Treatment Phase	Closed	Open Type I or II	Open Type IIIA, B, or C
Initial	A	B	C
Routine healing	D	E	F
Delayed healing	G	H	J
Nonunion healing	K	M	N
Malunion healing	P	Q	R
Sequela	S	S	S

SUCCESS STEP

When a patient with known osteoporosis suffers a fracture, remember to assign a code from category **M80 Osteoporosis with current pathological fracture**, NOT a traumatic fracture code. Do this even when the patient has a minor fall or trauma. If the fall or trauma would not usually break a normal, healthy bone, you should assign a code for pathologic fracture due to osteoporosis (OGCR I.C.19.c.1).

Assigning Codes for Poisoning

To assign codes for poisoning, adverse effects, toxic effects, and underdosing, use the Table of Drugs and Chemicals (■ FIGURE 13-8). Assign as many codes as necessary to describe completely all drugs or medicinal or biological substances (OGCR I.C.19.e.2)). When two or more drugs or medicinal or biological substances are reported, code each individually unless a combination code is listed in the Table of Drugs and Chemicals (OGCR I.C.19.f.4)). Do not assign an additional external cause code because the external cause is included in the injury code.

SUCCESS STEP

The Table of Drugs and Chemicals is located at the end of the Index to Diseases and before the Index to External Causes. If you haven't already done so, place a red self-adhesive tab along the top edge of the page to make it easier to find.

To use the Table of Drugs and Chemicals follow these steps:

1. Locate the name of the substance in the left-hand column. Some substances have subterms indented below them on the next line.
2. Select the substance code in the column that corresponds to the intent determined during abstracting. When the intent is not stated, code it as accidental. When the intent is underdosing, assign codes as follows:
    a. If underdosing exacerbates the condition for which the medication was prescribed, assign a code for the condition.
    b. Assign a code for noncompliance or complication of care to further indicate intent, if known.
3. Verify the code in the Tabular List. Do not code directly from the Table of Drugs and Chemicals.
4. Confirm that the code title reflects the intent.
5. Assign the seventh-character extension for the episode of care.
6. When more than one substance is involved, repeat the steps for the each substance.
7. Assign additional codes to identify the condition(s) or manifestation(s) that resulted.

SUCCESS STEP

ICD-10-CM introduces some changes to the Table of Drugs and Chemicals. Underdosing is a new concept not present in ICD-9-CM and has a separate column on the table. Poisonings are reported with a combination code that describes both the substance and intent. A separate external cause code for intent is no longer required. The Therapeutic Use column from ICD-9-CM is renamed Adverse Effect and appears as the fifth column.

Substance	Poisoning, Accidental (unintentional)	Poisoning, Intentional self-harm	Poisoning, Assault	Poisoning, Undetermined	Adverse effect	Underdosing
Trimethobenzamide	T45.0X1	T45.0X2	T45.0X3	T45.0X4	T45.0X5	T45.0X6
Trimethoprim	T37.8X1	T37.8X2	T37.8X3	T37.8X4	T37.8X5	T37.8X6
with sulfamethoxazole	T36.8X1	T36.8X2	T36.8X3	T36.8X4	T36.8X5	T36.8X6
Trimethylcarbinol	T51.3X1	T51.3X2	T51.3X3	T51.3X4	-	-
Trimethylpsoralen	T49.3X1	T49.3X2	T49.3X3	T49.3X4	T49.3X5	T49.3X6
Trimeton	T45.0X1	T45.0X2	T45.0X3	T45.0X4	T45.0X5	T45.0X6
Trimetrexate	T45.1X1	T45.1X2	T45.1X3	T45.1X4	T45.1X5	T45.1X6

Figure 13-8 ■ Table of Drugs and Chemicals

Guided Example of Assigning Injury and Poisoning Codes

To practice skills for using the Table of Drugs and Chemicals, continue with the example from earlier in the chapter about patient Gwen Beene, who was seen in the Branton Medical Center Emergency Department due to an allergic reaction to Trimethoprim-Sulfamethoxazole.

Follow along in your ICD-10-CM manual as Chelsea assigns codes. Check off each step after you complete it.

⇨ First, Chelsea confirms the diagnosis of hives and shortness of breath due to adverse effect of Trimethoprim-Sulfamethoxazole.

⇨ Chelsea locates the Table of Drugs and Chemicals at the end of the Index to Diseases.

- ❑ She searches for the Main Term **Trimethoprim** in the left-hand column of the table (Figure 13-8).
- ❑ She locates the subterm **with Sulfamethoxazole** on the next line.
- ❑ She locates the column for **Adverse Effects.**
- ❑ She locates code where the column for **Adverse Effects** crosses the row for **with Sulfamethoxazole.**
- ❑ She identifies the code **T36.8X5.**

⇨ Chelsea verifies code **T36.8X5** in the Tabular List.

- ❑ She reads the code title for **T36.8X5, Adverse effect of other systemic antibiotics** and confirms that this accurately describes the diagnosis.
- ❑ She notes the convention **7th** that directs her to assign a seventh-character extension.
- ❑ She refers to the beginning of category **T36** to review the available seventh-character extensions for episode of care.
- ❑ The episode of care is **A, initial encounter** because this is the first encounter for the problem.
- ❑ She assigns code **T36.8X5A.**

⇨ Chelsea checks for instructional notes in the Tabular List.

- ❑ She cross-references the beginning of the block **Poisoning by, adverse effects of and underdosing of drugs, medicaments and biological substances (T36-T50)** and sees several instructional notes.
- ❑ She reviews the **Includes** notes that give the definition of poisoning and adverse effect and concludes that she chose the correct category of adverse effect because the medication was properly administered.
- ❑ She reads another instructional note that says **Code first for adverse effects, the nature of the adverse effect.** Therefore, she knows that she should code for hives and shortness of breath.
- ❑ She cross-references the beginning of **Chapter 19 (S00-T88)** and reviews the instructional notes. She reads the note that says **Use secondary code(s) from Chapter 20, External causes of morbidity, to indicate cause of injury. Codes within the T section that include the external cause do not require an additional external cause code.** She determines she does not need an additional code for external cause because the code from section **T** includes the cause, which is an adverse effect to a medication.

⇨ Chelsea assigns the codes for the manifestations.

- ❑ She searches the Index for the Main Term **Hives,** which cross-references her to **Urticaria.**
  - She searches for the Main Term **Urticaria** and the subterm **due to drug,** which directs her to code **L50.0.**
  - She verifies the code in the Tabular List and confirms the code title **L50.0, Allergic urticaria.**
  - She cross-references the beginning of the category, block, and chapter for any applicable instructional notes.
- ❑ She searches the Index for the Main Term **Shortness** and subterm **breath,** which directs her to code **R06.02.**
  - She verifies the code in the Tabular List and confirms the code title **R06.02, Shortness of breath.**
  - After cross-referencing the beginning of the category, block, and chapter for any applicable instructional notes, she returns to the Index to locate the code for hives.

⇨ Chelsea identifies the codes for this case:

- ❑ **T36.8X5A, Adverse effect of other systemic antibiotics, initial encounter**
- ❑ **L50.0, Allergic urticaria**
- ❑ **R06.02, Shortness of breath**

CODING CAUTION

Use the Table of Drugs and Chemicals only for poisoning, adverse effects, and underdosing. Do *not* use this table to report the fact that a patient is taking, or has been prescribed, a medication when no injury is involved.

Special Topics

OGCR provide guidelines for adult and child abuse and complications of care. Coding for these topics is summarized next.

Adult and Child Abuse, Neglect, and Other Maltreatment

Coding of adult and child abuse or neglect is based on whether the medical record documents the abuse as confirmed or suspected (OGCR I.C.19.f)). To learn how to code for abuse, neglect, and other maltreatment, review the following guidelines:

- When the medical record documents abuse or neglect, assign a code for confirmed maltreatment from category **T74.-**.
  1. Search the Index for the Main Term **Maltreatment**.
     - Select a subterm that identifies the victim as **adult** or **child**.
     - Select a second-level subterm for **confirmed**.
  2. Assign an external cause code from the assault section **(X92-Y08)** to identify the cause of any physical injuries.
     - Search the External Cause Index for the Main Term **Assault**, then select the applicable subterm to identify the method of assault.
  3. Assign a perpetrator code **(Y07)** when the perpetrator of the abuse is known.
     - Search the External Cause Index for the Main Term **Perpetrator**, then select the applicable subterm to identify the relationship of the perpetrator to the victim.
- When the medical record documents suspected abuse, assign a code for suspected maltreatment from category **T76.-**.
  1. Search the Index for the Main Term **Maltreatment**.
     - Select a second level subterm for **suspected**.
  2. For suspected cases of abuse or neglect, *do not* report external cause or perpetrator code.

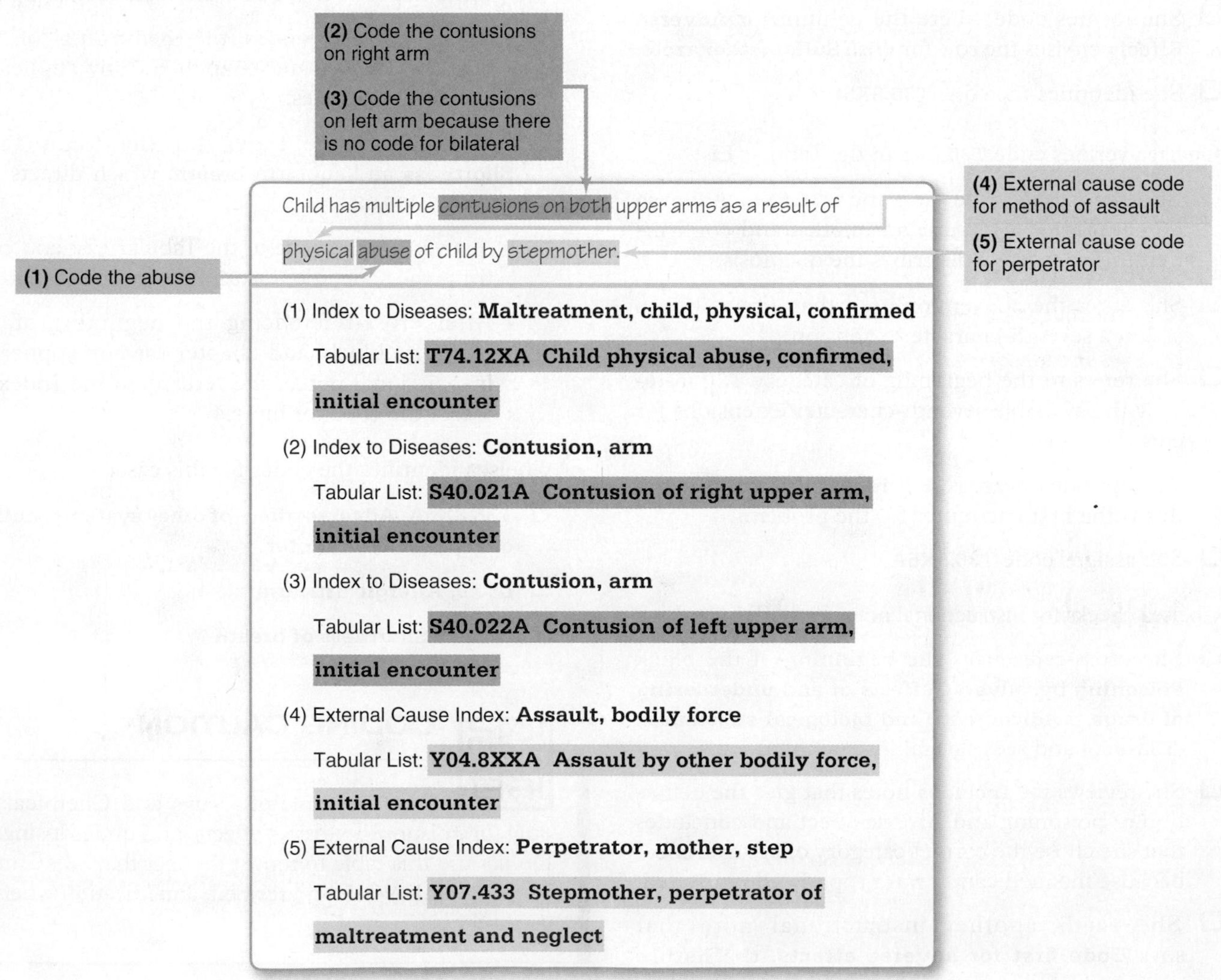

Figure 13-9 ■ Example of Code Assignment and Sequencing for Child Abuse

3. If a suspected case of abuse, neglect, or mistreatment is ruled out during an encounter, assign code **Z04.71, Encounter for examination and observation following alleged adult physical abuse**, or code **Z04.72, Encounter for examination and observation following alleged child physical abuse**, *not* a code from **T76**. The inclusion notes under **Z04.71** and **Z04.72** state **Suspected . . . physical and sexual abuse, ruled out.**

- Sequence the codes as follows (■ FIGURE 13-9):
  1. The code from category **T74.-** or **T76.-** to identify confirmed or suspected abuse, neglect and other maltreatment.
  2. Additional codes to identify any associated mental health condition or injury (OGCR I.C.19.f).
  3. An external cause code to identify the method of assault.
  4. An external cause code to identify the perpetrator (for confirmed abuse only).

Complications of Care

When providers document that a medical or surgical procedure is the cause of a condition, assign a code for the event of a complication (OGCR I.C.19.g.1)(a)) as well as the resulting condition(s) or manifestation(s), as follows:

- Search the Index for the Main Term **Complication**.
  - Locate the first-level subterm that describes the event or procedure that *caused* the problem (■ FIGURE 13-10).
  - Locate the second-level subterm that describes the condition that *resulted*.
  - Locate the third-level subterm that identifies the anatomic site.
- Some complications of care codes are combination codes that describe the nature of the complication as well as the type of procedure that caused the complication.
  - When the external cause is included in a combination code, do not assign an additional external cause code.
- When a complication code is available from a body system chapter, sequence the body system code first, followed by code(s) for the specific complication condition or manifestation, if applicable (OGCR I.C.19.g.5)).

Complications of care include a broad range of conditions that may be due to external causes or may be physical reactions. Complications due to external causes include performing an incorrect procedure, operating on an incorrect site, leaving foreign objects in a patient, perforating a nearby organ or structure during a procedure, malfunction of prosthetic devices, and certain infections. Complications that are physical reactions include cardiac arrest, respiratory failure, hemorrhaging, or **ileus**.

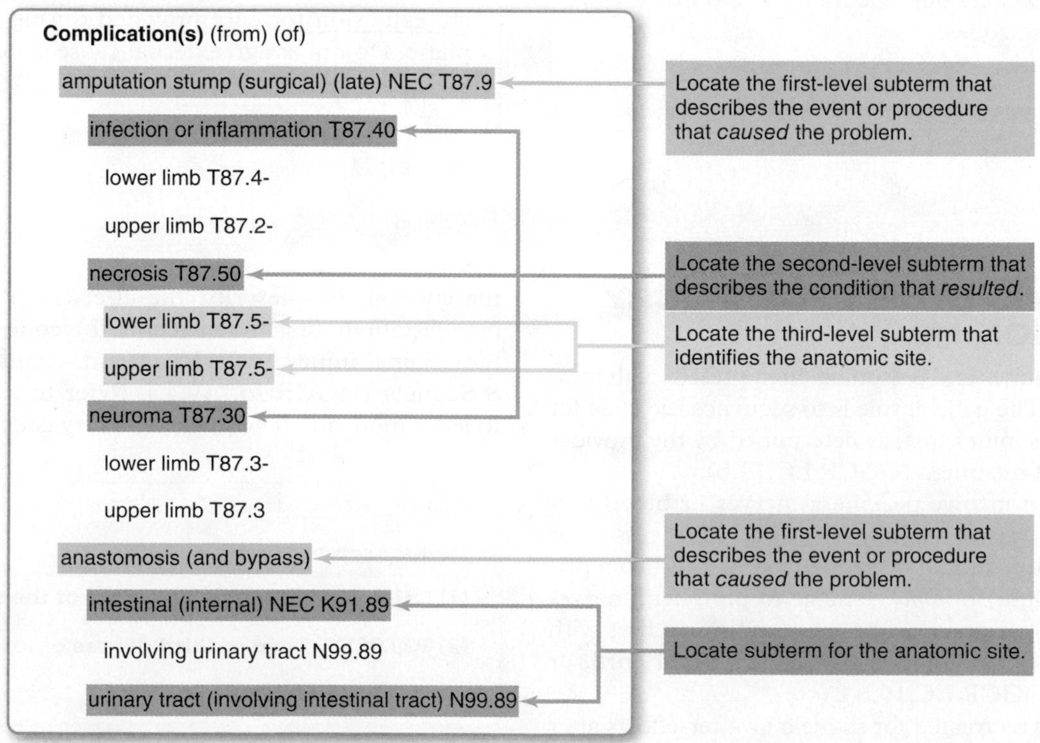

Figure 13-10 ■ Example of Index Entry for the Main Term Complication

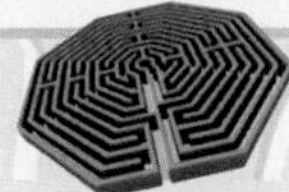

Coding Practice

Now it is your turn to practice assigning codes for injury and poisoning. Refer to the ***Tip*** at the end of the mini-medical-record if you need extra help.

Exercise 13.3 Assigning Codes for Injury and Poisoning

Instructions: Read the mini-medical-record of each patient's encounter, review the information abstracted in Exercise 13.2, and assign ICD-10-CM diagnosis codes (CM) using the Index to Diseases, Table of Drugs and Chemicals, and Tabular List. Assign codes for the injuries only. Do NOT assign external cause codes in this exercise. Write the code(s) on the line provided.

1. Date: 3/3/yy Location: Branton Medical Center Emergency Department Provider: Cynthia Hiatt, MD

Patient: Willie Munoz Gender: M Age: 8

Chief complaint: pain, tenderness, swelling, and distortion on right knee after being tackled while playing football at school

Assessment: X-ray shows type III fracture of growth plate at the upper end of the tibia

Plan: surgery and internal fixation to ensure proper alignment of the growth plate and the joint surface

Tip: Physis (physeal) is the medical term for the growth plate. Code only the fracture. Do not assign external cause codes.

1 CM Code __________

2. Date: 3/3/yy Location: Branton Medical Center Provider: Cynthia Hiatt, MD

Patient: Earl Dews Gender: M Age: 23

Reason for admission: patient arrived by ambulance after a barn fire that occurred on his own farm which is his job

Assessment: third degree burns to left forearm, second degree burns to left upper arm and shoulder, smoke inhalation

Tip: Assign a code for the burns and a code for the smoke. Do not code activity, status, or location external cause codes.

2 CM Codes __________ __________

3. Date: 3/4/yy Location: Branton Family Practice

Provider: Kristen Conover, MD

Patient: Florence Collard Gender: F Age: 35

Reason for encounter: suture removal from wound to right index finger, sustained when she accidentally cut her finger with a butcher knife while preparing dinner

Assessment: Wound is healed. Removed sutures.

Tip: Assign a code for the injury with the appropriate extension for care provided during the healing phase. Do not assign external cause codes.

1 CM Code __________

ARRANGING CODES FOR INJURY AND POISONING

Patients with injuries and poisoning often present with multiple problems. The general rule is to sequence the code for the most serious injury first, as determined by the provider and the focus of treatment (OGCR I.C.19.b).

Injuries often involve peripheral nerves or blood vessels. When the *primary* injury is to the blood vessels or nerves, that injury should be sequenced first. When a primary injury results in *minor* damage to peripheral nerves or blood vessels, sequence the primary injury first with additional codes for injuries to nerves, spinal cord, or blood vessels (OGCR I.C.19.b.2)).

Patients may be treated for sequela or after-effects after the primary injury has healed, such as scars. Sequence the code(s) that describe the after-effect conditions or manifestations first. Then report the code that identifies the original injury, with the seventh-character extension S Sequela (OGCR I.C.19.a.). Refer to ■ Figure 13-11 to learn more about sequencing injury codes and sequela.

A patient is treated for a keloid scar that forms following a third degree burn on the right cheek.

(1) **L91.0 Hypertrophic disorders of the skin**

(2) **T20.36XS Burn of third degree of forehead and cheek, sequela**

Figure 13-11 ■ Example of Coding the Sequela of an Injury

CODING CAUTION

Remember to assign the extension to the injury code only. Do not assign an extension to the code for the condition that resulted unless directed to do so by instructional notes in the Tabular List, as occurs with traumatic fractures.

Arranging Codes for Burns

When more than one burn is present, the first code should reflect the highest degree of burn (OGCR I.C.19.d.1)). The size of the damaged area is *not* a factor in sequencing burn codes.

The OGCR state that circumstances of admission govern the selection of the principal diagnosis or first-listed diagnosis in certain situations. This means that sequencing is based on the specific reason for admission and which injuries are most serious. The circumstances of admission apply when a patient has both internal and external burns (OGCR I.C.19.d.1)(b)) or has other related conditions, such as smoke inhalation and or respiratory failure (OGCR I.C.19.d.1)(c)).

For example, consider a patient with second degree burns and life-threatening respiratory failure due to smoke inhalation. Sequence respiratory failure first because it is more serious than second degree burns.

Arranging Codes for Traumatic Fractures

Sequence multiple fractures based on the severity of the fracture (OGCR I.C.19.c.2)). The severity may be determined by either the location of the fracture or the type of fracture. Review the following examples to learn more about sequencing multiple fractures:

- A fracture to the skull is more serious than a fracture to a finger.
- An open fracture is more serious than a closed fracture.
- A fracture that causes damage to another organ, such as a fractured rib that punctures a lung, is more serious than one that does not, such as a fractured arm.

If coders cannot determine the relative severity of multiple fractures based on the documentation, they should consult with the supervisor or query the physician.

Arranging Codes for Poisoning

The OGCR are different for sequencing poisonings, adverse effects, and underdosings (OGCRI.C.19.e). When coding poisonings, the first code should be from categories **T36** through **T65** to identify the type and intent of injury. Next, report the codes that identify all resulting conditions or manifestations.

When coding for adverse effects,sequence first the code(s) for the manifestations or resulting conditions first. Then, sequence the **T** code for the drug and the intent of adverse effect.

Sequence codes for underdosing encounters as follows:

1. The principal or first-listed diagnosis should be the resulting condition or manifestation.
2. Sequence the underdosing **T** code as an additional code.
3. Sequence a code for complication of care or a **Z** code for noncompliance, as applicable.

Guided Example of Arranging Injury and Poisoning Codes

To practice skills for sequencing codes for adverse effects, continue with the example from earlier in the chapter about patient Gwen Beene, who was seen at Branton Medical Center Emergency Department due to an allergic reaction to Trimethoprim-Sulfamethoxazole.

Follow along in your ICD-10-CM manual as Chelsea sequences the codes. Check off each step after you complete it.

➪ First, Chelsea confirms the three diagnoses:

- ☐ **T36.8X5A, Adverse effect of other systemic antibiotics, initial encounter**
- ☐ **R06.02, Shortness of breath**
- ☐ **L50.0, Allergic urticaria**

➪ Chelsea reviews the instructional notes she found earlier at the beginning of the block **T36-T50** that said **Code first for adverse effects, the nature of the adverse effect.**

- ☐ The words **Code first** mean that the manifestations should be sequenced before the **T** code for the drug that causedadverse effect.

➪ Chelsea also reviews OGCR I.C.19.5)(a) that states **When coding an adverse effect of a drug that has been correctly prescribed and properly administered, assign the appropriate code for the nature of the adverse effect followed by the appropriate code for the adverse effect of the drug (T36-T50).**

- ☐ This confirms that the manifestation codes should be sequenced first, followed by the **T** code.
- ☐ She sequences **R06.02, Shortness of breath** first because it is a more serious condition than hives.

➪ Chelsea finalizes the sequencing for this case:

(1) **R06.02, Shortness of breath**

(2) **L50.0, Allergic urticaria**

(3) **T36.8X5A, Adverse effect of other systemic antibiotics, initial encounter**

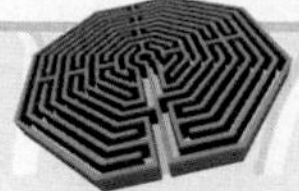

Coding Practice

Now it is your turn to practice sequencing codes for injury and poisoning. Refer to the ***Tip*** at the end of mini-medical-record if you need extra help.

Exercise 13.4 Arranging Codes for Injury and Poisoning

Instructions: Read the mini-medical-record of each patient's encounter, review the information abstracted in Exercise 13.2, assign ICD-10-CM diagnosis codes (CM) using the Index to Diseases, the Index to External Causes, the Table of Drugs and Chemicals, and the Tabular List, and sequence them correctly. DO assign external cause codes in this exercise.

1. Date: 3/4/yy Location: Branton Medical Center Emergency Department Provider: Cynthia Hiatt, MD

Patient: Jose Erickson Gender: M Age: 67

Chief complaint: irregular pulse, palpitations, confusion

Assessment: Cumulative intoxication effect (*a build-up in the body*) from digitalis which had been taken as prescribed for atrial fibrillation. Patient also has stage 2 chronic kidney disease which put him at risk for intoxication.

***Tip*:** Sequence codes as follows: 1) the condition that described the adverse effect, 2) the drug that caused the adverse effect, 3) reason he was at risk.

3 CM Codes __________ __________ __________

2. Date: 3/4/yy Location: Branton Medical Center Emergency Department Provider: Cynthia Hiatt, MD

Patient: Stefanie Frechette Gender: F Age: 19

Chief complaint: examination after alleged date rape by her boyfriend

Assessment: Conducted physical examination and urine test. Flunitrazepam was found in a urine test. The injury was determined to be sexual assault.

(continued)

2. (continued)

***Tip*:** Assign a code from the Table of Drugs and Chemicals, a code for the examination as the reason for the encounter, and two external causes codes for the type of assault and the perpetrator.

4 CM Codes (1) T42.4X3A = Table of Drugs & chemicals for Flunitrazepam, assault (2) Z04.41 examination, following alleged rape (3) T74.21XA (rape, adult, initial encounter) (4) Y07.03 perpetrator, boyfriend.

3. Date: 3/3/yy Location: Branton Family Practice

Provider: Kristen Conover, MD

Patient: Luke Kershaw Gender: M Age: 31

Chief complaint: accident in which automobile battery exploded and something got in his eyes while he was working on his car in the driveway at his single family home

Assessment: sulfuric acid burn on both eyelids and right cornea, second degree sulfuric acid burn to forehead and right cheek

***Tip*:** Assign a code from the Table of Drugs and Chemicals, four codes for the injuries, and two external cause codes for place and status. Read the instructional notes in the Tabular List for help on sequencing. Recall that burns to the eye are not rated by degree. The burn to the cornea is the most serious and the burns to the cheek and forehead are the least serious.

7 CM Codes __________ __________ __________ __________ __________ __________ __________

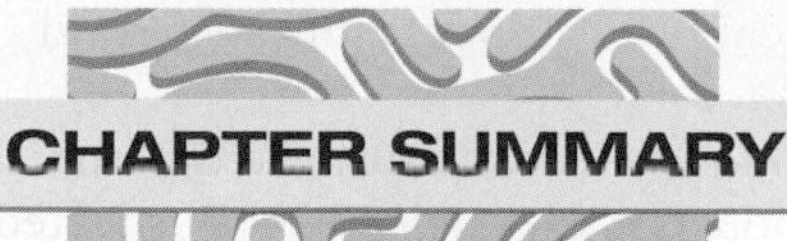

CHAPTER SUMMARY

In this chapter you learned that:

- Injury and poisoning can encompass a wide variety of conditions and a range of definitions, so it is critical that coders understand how ICD-10-CM defines terms.
- ICD-10-CM Chapter 19, Injury, Poisoning, and Certain Other Consequences of External Causes (S00-T88), contains 20 blocks or subchapters that are divided by anatomical site and type of injury.
- The most common injuries are burns, fractures, and poisonings, each of which has unique criteria for abstracting.
- Each type of injury has unique coding guidelines, so coders need to become familiar with a variety of situations.
- In general, sequence the code for the most serious injury first, as determined by the provider and the focus of treatment.
- ICD-10-CM Official Guidelines for Coding and Reporting (OGCR) for injury and poisoning appear in section I.C.19, which is divided into sections based on the type of injury.

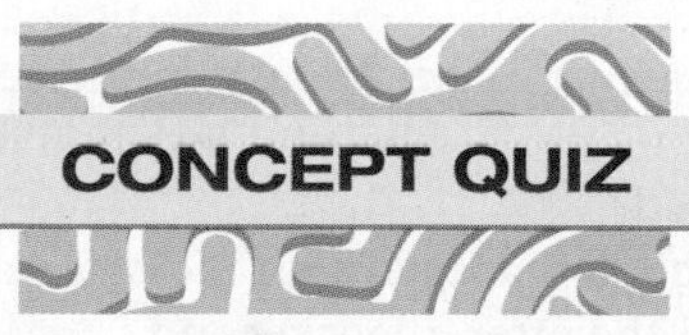

CONCEPT QUIZ

Take a moment to look back at your trip through injury and poisoning and solidify your skills. This is your opportunity to pull together everything you have learned.

Completion

Instructions: Refer to category **S72 Fracture of femur** in the ICD-10-CM manual. Read the descriptions of the seventh-character extensions. Write the letter that matches each definition in the space provided. Some choices may be used more than once and some choices may not be used at all. Refer to the discussion in this chapter and the Glossary at the end of this book if you need a little extra help.

A	J
B	K
C	M
D	N
E	P
F	Q
G	R
H	S

1. The extension _____ describes subsequent encounter for closed fracture with malunion.
2. The extension _____ describes subsequent encounter for open fracture type IIIA, IIIB, or IIIC with routine healing.
3. The extension _____ describes subsequent encounter for closed fracture with nonunion.
4. The extension _____ describes initial encounter for closed fracture.
5. The extension _____ describes initial encounter for open fracture type IIIA, IIIB, or IIIC.
6. The extension _____ describes subsequent encounter for open fracture type I or II with delayed healing.
7. The extension _____ describes sequela.
8. The extension _____ describes initial encounter for open fracture type I or II.
9. The extension _____ describes subsequent encounter for closed fracture with routine healing.
10. The extension _____ describes subsequent encounter for open fracture type I or II with routine healing.

Multiple Choice

Instructions: Circle the letter of the best answer to each question based on the information you learned in this chapter. Refer to the discussion in this chapter and the Glossary at the end of this book if you need a little extra help.

1. Which is NOT a criteria used in assigning codes for burns?
   A. Depth
   B. Anatomic site
   C. Open or closed
   D. Extent
2. Traumatic fracture codes have seventh-character extensions for all of the following EXCEPT
   A. displaced or nondisplaced.
   B. open or closed.
   C. routine or delayed healing.
   D. sequela.
3. When a patient with osteoporosis has a minor fall, coders should assign
   A. a code for a traumatic fracture only.
   B. a code for osteoporosis fracture only.
   C. a code for a traumatic fracture AND a code for osteoporosis fracture.
   D. a code for external cause only.
4. Which of the following is NOT true regarding the Table of Drugs and Chemicals?
   A. Locate the name of the substance in the left-hand column.
   B. Select the substance code in the column that corresponds to the intent.
   C. Assign codes directly from the table without verifying in the Tabular List.
   D. Assign additional codes to identify the condition(s) or manifestation(s) that resulted.
5. To assign a code for adult or child abuse, search the Index for the Main Term
   A. Abuse.
   B. Maltreatment.
   C. Child.
   D. Confirmed.
6. When the medical record documents suspected abuse,
   A. assign a code to identify the suspected perpetrator.
   B. search the Index for the Main Term Suspected.
   C. assign a code only for the injuries, but not the abuse.
   D. search the Index for the Main Term Maltreatment and subterm suspected.
7. Assign a complications of care code when
   A. patients have more than one condition.
   B. providers document that a medical or surgical procedure is the cause of a condition.
   C. providers perform complicated procedures.
   D. you are unclear what the physician documented.
8. When a patient has multiple injuries, how should codes be sequenced?
   A. Sequence the codes in numerical order.
   B. Sequence conditions in the order the physician mentions them in the medical record.
   C. Sequence burns first, fractures second, and wounds third.
   D. Sequence the code for the most serious injury first.
9. When patients are treated for sequela or after-effects after the primary injury has healed, how should codes be sequenced?
   A. Sequence the code that identifies the original injury first and the after-effect second.
   B. Sequence the after-effect condition first and the primary injury second.
   C. Assign codes for the after-effect but not the original injury.
   D. Sequence according to the circumstances of admission.
10. When coding poisoning and adverse effects, how should codes be sequenced?
    A. Sequence according to the circumstances of admission.
    B. Sequence the external cause code first.
    C. Sequence the code for the resulting condition or manifestation first.
    D. Sequence the code for type and intent of injury first.

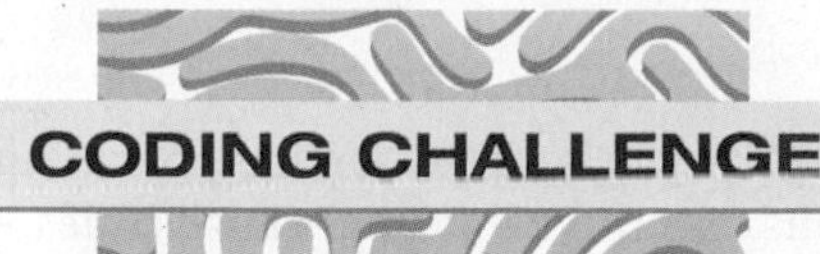

CODING CHALLENGE

Now it is your turn to demonstrate coding all aspects of injury and poisoning. Refer back to the examples and discussion in this chapter when you need a little extra help. Use your medical dictionary and anatomy references when needed.

Instructions: Read the mini-medical-record of each patient's encounter, then abstract, assign, and sequence ICD-10-CM diagnosis codes (CM) using the Index to Diseases, the Index to External Causes, and the Tabular List. Write the code(s) on the line provided.

1. Date: 3/15/yy Location: Branton Family Practice Provider: Kristen Conover, MD

Patient: Claire Lennon Gender: F Age: 71

Chief complaint: swollen and painful right wrist and large bruises on right calf after she tripped and fell in the living room of her apartment yesterday.

Assessment: Colles' fracture. Extensive hematoma on the calf is due to her long term Coumadin (*anticoagulant/blood thinner*) therapy. Patient was previously diagnosed with age-related osteoporosis.

Plan: Arm casted, **INR** (*international normalized ratio blood clotting test*) performed, RTO to access healing of fracture and cast removal

Tip: Assign three diagnosis codes and two external cause codes.

5 CM Codes __________ __________

__________ __________ __________

2. Date: 3/15/yy Location: Northwest Orthopedics Provider: Bruce Prentice, MD

Patient: Peter Rice Gender: M Age: 21

Reason for encounter: follow-up on shoulder dislocation sustained when the motorcycle he was driving collided with an automobile three weeks ago.

Current status: Patient continues to have persistent pain and is unable to work

Assessment: dislocated right shoulder, acromioclavicular joint, 150% displacement

Plan: Outpatient surgery scheduled for reducing dislocation. This will be performed under IV sedation. Preop instructions provided to the patient.

(continued)

2. (continued)

Tip: Assign a code for the injury and an external cause code for the accident.

2 CM Codes __________ __________

3. Date: 3/15/yy Location: Branton Medical Center Emergency Department

Provider: Cynthia Hiatt, MD

Patient: Geraldine Downes Gender: F Age: 19

Reason for encounter: infected wound where she stepped on nail last week

Assessment: puncture wound left foot

Plan: Continue antibiotic ointment, begin 10 day regime of antibiotics, review status of tetanus immunization. Redress wound. RTO in 3 days

Tip: Assign a code for the injury and an external cause code.

2 CM Codes __________ __________

4. Date: 3/15/yy Location: Branton Medical Center Provider: Cynthia Hiatt, MD

Patient: Howard Toole Gender: M Age: 45

Reason for admission: Admitted from emergency department due to skull fracture. He was unconscious for 90 minutes, but returned to his normal state of consciousness.

Assessment: open occipital condylar fracture (Type I) of base of skull with subarachnoid hemorrhage.

Plan: Craniotomy performed based on CT results which showed bleeding. Vessel occlusion performed. Patient in ICU following surg. RTO 4 days post discharge and weekly thereafter for two weeks.

Tip: A combination code describes the injury and the loss of consciousness. The external cause is not documented. Do not assign external cause codes.

2 CM Codes __________ __________

(continued)

(continued from page 249)

5. Date: 3/15/yy Location: Branton Medical Center Emergency Department

Provider: Cynthia Hiatt, MD

Patient: George Lutes Gender: M Age: 37

Reason for encounter: ketoacidosis with coma. Admit for observation. Stat blood chemistry and insulin administration.

Assessment: Type 1 diabetic forgot to take insulin. He is here on vacation and got confused due to the time zone change and an erratic schedule.

Plan: FU with endocrinologist when returns home. 1 week.

Tip: Follow the guidelines for underdosing. OGCR I.C. 19.e.5.(c)

3 CM Codes __________ __________ __________

6. Date: 3/15/yy Location: Northwest Orthopedics Provider: Bruce Prentice, MD

Patient: Dennis Albertson Gender: M Age: 34

Reason for encounter: removal of cast

Assessment: X-rays show full healing of oblique fracture of left radius shaft. Cast removed.

Tip: Do not assign aftercare Z codes with injury codes. OGCR I.C.19.a.

1 CM Code __________

7. Date: 3/15/yy Location: Branton Medical Center Emergency Department

Provider: Cynthia Hiatt, MD

Patient: Faith Ulrich Gender: F Age: 28

Chief complaint: Patient was brought in by her neighbor. She was at home stripping wood furniture inside on a rainy day. She got a severe headache and nausea due to the fumes and began vomiting.

Assessment: acetone toxicity

Plan: OTC medication for headache, restore fluids orally, postpone furniture finishing until it is possible to have better ventilation

(continued)

7. (continued)

Tip: Assign three diagnosis codes for the poisoning and manifestations and three external cause codes.

6 CM Codes __________ __________ __________ __________ __________ __________

8. Date: 3/15/yy Location: Northwest Orthopedics Provider: Bruce Prentice, MD

Patient: Arlene Borkowski Gender: F Age: 25

Reason for admission: surgery to right clavicle, 4 weeks following an accident while riding as a passenger in an off-road vehicle

Assessment: Malunion of displaced right clavicle, acromonial end

Plan: RTO 2 weeks, immobilization sling

Tip: Assign an injury code and an external cause code.

2 CM Codes __________ __________

9. Date: 3/15/yy Location: Branton Medical Center

Provider: Kristen Conover, MD

Patient: Greg Waites Gender: M Age: 18 months

Reason for admission: Child got into some open whiskey and was found unconscious. He had been left alone by his stepfather who ran out to the corner store. Admit for overnight observation.

Assessment: Child neglect and abandonment. Alcohol toxicity. Blood alcohol level (BAC) of .360 (360 mg per 100 ml of blood)

Plan: Stabilized with oxygen and IV fluids. Social service evaluation of home, mandatory report to dept of human services

Tip: Assign three diagnosis codes and three external cause codes for BAC, perpetrator, and place of occurrence. (Do not assign codes for the coma scale.)

6 CM Codes __________ __________ __________ __________ __________ __________

10. Date: 3/15/yy Location: Branton Medical Center

Provider: Kristen Conover, MD

Patient: Antoinette Brashear Gender: F Age: 22

Chief complaint: admitted from physician's office after complaining of fast heart beat

Assessment: supraventricular tachycardia that is a late effect of a heroin overdose during a suicide attempt 3 months ago

(continued)

10. (continued)

Plan: Stabilized rhythm with vagal maneuvers. Discharged on regime of antiarrhythmic med. Referral for substance addiction.

Tip: Assign codes for the injury and the current manifestation.

2 CM Codes __________ __________

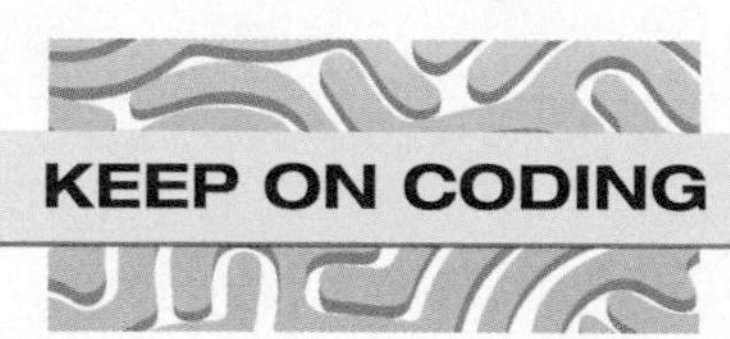

KEEP ON CODING

As a coder, you can never have too much experience. Apply everything you have learned in this chapter to code the following diagnostic statements. Use the OGCR and instructional notes in the Tabular List to help determine how many codes are required.

Instructions: Read the diagnostic statement, then use the Index and Tabular List to assign and sequence ICD-10-CM (CM) diagnosis codes. Write the code(s) on the line provided.

1. Abrasion of the scalp, initial encounter: CM Code(s) ____________________
2. Fracture of the mandible, subsequent encounter: CM Code(s) ____________________
3. Laceration of the left carotid artery, initial encounter: CM Code(s) ____________________
4. Muscle strain of the lower back, initial encounter: CM Code(s) ____________________
5. Accidental ingestion of toxic mushrooms, initial encounter: CM Code(s) ____________________
6. Bone marrow transplant failure: CM Code(s) ____________________
7. Crushing injury of the left upper arm, initial encounter: CM Code(s) ____________________
8. Heat collapse, initial encounter: CM Code(s) ____________________
9. Fracture of the left sacrum, type 3, subsequent encounter: CM Code(s) ____________________
10. Complete amputation of right breast, traumatic injury, late effect: CM Code(s) ____________________
11. Late effect of a moderate laceration of the spleen: CM Code(s) ____________________
12. Nonunion of fracture of femoral neck, right: CM Code(s) ____________________
13. Acute transfusion reaction due to Rh incompatibility, initial encounter: CM Code(s) ____________________
14. Traumatic compartment syndrome of the left hip, initial encounter: CM Code(s) ____________________

15. Partial traumatic amputation, left leg, subsequent encounter: CM Code(s) ____________

16. Blast injury of right ear, initial encounter: CM Code(s) ____________

17. Traumatic hemopneumothorax, subsequent encounter: CM Code(s) ____________

18. Foreign body in nostril, initial encounter: CM Code(s) ____________

19. Late effect of a third degree burn of the left ankle: CM Code(s) ____________

20. Displaced avulsion fracture of the right ischium, initial encounter: CM Code(s) ____________

21. Major contusion of left kidney, traumatic, initial encounter: CM Code(s) ____________

22. Displaced longitudinal fracture of right patella, initial encounter: CM Code(s) ____________

23. Open bite of the right buttock, subsequent encounter: CM Code(s) ____________

24. Sprain of right ankle, initial encounter: CM Code(s) ____________

25. Adverse effect of overuse of laxatives, subsequent encounter: CM Code(s) ____________

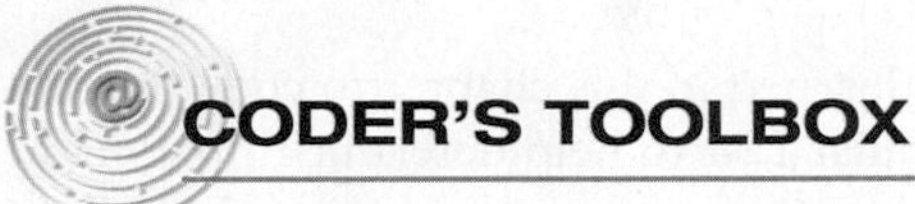

CODER'S TOOLBOX

The following resources are a starting point for learning more about injury and poisoning. The > symbol indicates a menu selection within the website in order to navigate to a specific page.

American Association of Poison Control Centers **http://www.aapcc.org/dnn/default.aspx**

American Burn Association **http://www.ameriburn.org/index.php**

Burn Resource Center **http://www.burnsurvivor.com/**

Centers for Disease Control and Prevention > NCHS Home > FastStats Home **http://www.cdc.gov/nchs/fastats/ervisits.htm**

Centers for Disease Control > Injury Prevention & Control > Data & Statistics (WISQARSTM) **http://www.cdc.gov/injury/wisqars/index.html**

National Safety Council > News & Resources > Injury & Death Statistics **http://www.nsc.org/NEWS_RESOURCES/INJURY_AND_DEATH_STATISTICS/Pages/InjuryDeathStatistics.aspx**

Ohio State University Medical Center > Healthcare Services > Emergency Services > Non-Traumatic Injuries > Unintentional Injury Statistics **http://medicalcenter.osu.edu/patientcare/healthcare_services/emergency_services/non_traumatic_emergencies/unintentional_injury_statistics/pages/index.aspx**

14

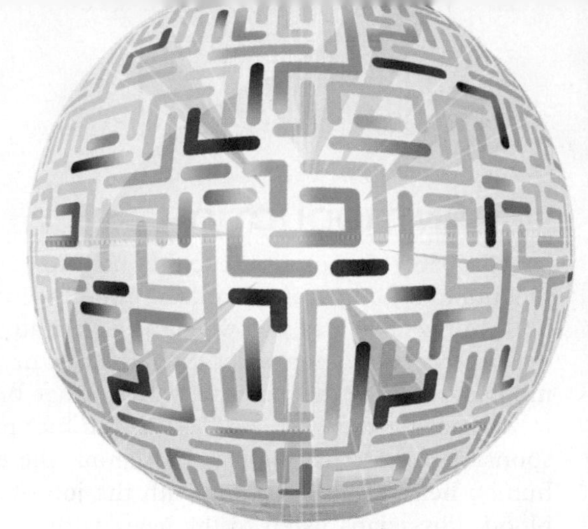

Diseases of the Circulatory System (I00-I99)

Learning Objectives

After completing this chapter, you should have the skills to:

- Spell and define the key words, medical terms, and abbreviations related to diseases of the circulatory system.
- Discuss the structure, function, and common conditions of the circulatory system.
- Identify the main characteristics of coding for diseases of the circulatory system.
- Abstract diagnostic information from the medical record for coding diseases of the circulatory system.
- Assign codes for diseases of the circulatory system.
- Arrange codes for diseases of the circulatory system.
- Discuss the Official Guidelines for Coding and Reporting related to diseases of the circulatory system.

Key Terms and Abbreviations

acute myocardial infarction (AMI)
angiography
angioplasty
aorta
aortic valve
arrhythmia
artery
arteriole
atrioventricular bundle (bundle of His)
atrioventricular (AV) node
atrioventricular (AV) valves
atrium/atria
autologous
Barlow's syndrome
bundle branch
bypass graft
capillary
cardiac catheterization
cardiac function test
cardiac scan
cardiovascular (CV) system
cerebral
circulatory system
click murmur syndrome
coronary artery bypass graft (CABG)
coronary circulation
current MI
diastole
Doppler ultrasonography
echocardiography
electrocardiography (ECG, EKG)
embolectomy
endarterectomy
endocardium
epicardium
Holter monitor
inferior vena cava
internal mammary artery (IMA)
left atrium
left ventricle
mitral valve
mitral valve prolapse (MVP)
mitral valve stenosis
myocardial infarction (MI)
myocardium
native
nonautologous
nonbiological
non-ST elevation MI (NSTEMI)
nontransmural
occlusion
old (healed) MI
pacemaker
parietal pericardium
pericardium
plaque
precerebral
pulmonary circulation
pulmonary valve
Purkinje fibers
regurgitation
right atrium
right ventricle
sinoatrial (SA) node
ST elevation MI (STEMI)
stent insertion
stress testing
subendocardial
subsequent MI
superior vena cava
systemic circulation
systole
transmural MI
tricuspid valve
valve repair
valve replacement
vein
venography
ventricle
venule
visceral pericardium

In addition to the key terms listed here, students should know the terms defined within tables in this chapter.

Chapter Outline

- **Circulatory System Refresher**
- **Conditions of the Circulatory System**
- **Coding Overview of the Circulatory System**
- **Abstracting for the Circulatory System**
- **Assigning Codes for the Circulatory System**
- **Arranging Codes for the Circulatory System**

ICD-10-CM codes in this chapter are from the ICD-10-CM 2014 Draft code set from the Department of Health and Human Services, Centers for Disease Control and Prevention.

INTRODUCTION

You probably do not give much thought to your vehicle's fuel pump as long as it is working properly. But when it is not, your vehicle may stall when the accelerator is pressed or not start at all. Mechanics listen to hear the pump running and test the fuel pressure with a gauge on their way to diagnosing the problem. Just as the fuel pump is responsible for circulating gas throughout the engine, the human heart is also a pump with the job of circulating blood. Physicians listen to the heart with a stethoscope and measure blood pressure as part of their diagnostic methods.

In your tour of the circulatory system in this chapter you will learn more about how the circulatory system works, why sometimes it does not work as it should, and how physicians treat these conditions. Most importantly, you will practice coding for patient encounters related to circulatory diseases and conditions, a skill that requires you to abstract information from the mini-medical-record, assign correct codes, and arrange (sequence) the codes in the proper order.

Cardiologists are physicians who specialize in diagnosing and treating diseases of the circulatory system. Subspecialities in cardiology include pediatric cardiology and cardiothoracic surgery. Primary care physicians diagnose and treat common conditions of the circulatory systems and refer complex cases to cardiologists.

As you read this chapter, open up your medical terminology book and an anatomy reference to the chapters on the cardiovascular system. Coding for the circulatory system requires detailed knowledge of anatomy. You will save time when you have the information you need at your fingertips.

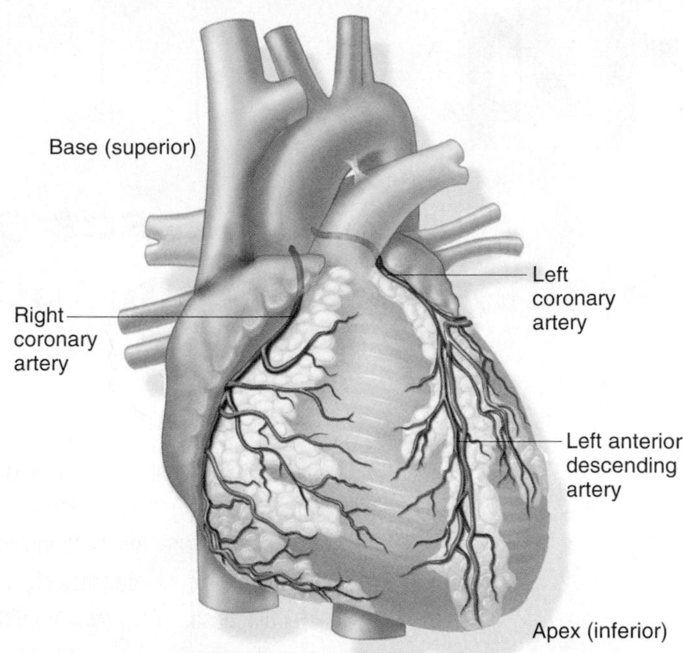

Figure 14-1 ■ The Major Arteries and Vessels of Coronary Circulation

CIRCULATORY SYSTEM REFRESHER

The function of the **circulatory system**, also called the **cardiovascular (CV) system**, is to distribute blood throughout the body. It consists of the heart, which is the pump, and blood vessels, which are the tubes that carry blood. The distribution or transportation task provides three functions:

- carries oxygen and nutrients to the body tissues for metabolism
- carries waste products of metabolism to the kidneys and other excretory organs
- circulates electrolytes and hormones needed to regulate body functions

The circulatory system consists of pulmonary circulation, systemic circulation, and coronary circulation. **Pulmonary circulation**, which occurs between the heart and the lungs, carries deoxygenated blood from the heart to the lungs, where it is replenished with oxygen, then back to the heart. **Systemic circulation**, which occurs between the heart and the rest of the body, carries oxygenated blood away from the heart to the tissues and cells of the body, then carries oxygen-depleted blood back to the heart. **Coronary circulation**, which occurs within the heart, carries blood from the aorta to the tissues of the heart in order to maintain the function of the heart itself (■ FIGURE 14-1).

According to the Centers for Disease Control and Prevention, heart disease is the leading cause of death in the United States for both men and women, accounting for over 25% of all deaths each year. Every year about 785,000 people have a first heart attack and another 470,000, who previously had a heart attack, have another one. Heart disease costs the United States over $315 billion per year for healthcare services, medication, and lost productivity.

To understand disorders of the circulatory system, coders need to understand the structure and operation of the heart muscle, the conduction system, and the blood vessels.

The Heart Muscle

The heart is a muscular organ that contains four chambers: two **atria**, which receive blood from the body (**right atrium**) and the lungs (**left atrium**), and two **ventricles**, which eject blood to the lungs (**right ventricle**) and the body (**left ventricle**) (■ FIGURE 14-2). Four valves control the one-way flow of blood into, through, and out of the heart: the **tricuspid** (*right atrium to right ventricle*), **mitral** (*left atrium to left ventricle*), **pulmonary** (*right ventricle to pulmonary artery*), and **aortic** (*left ventricle to aorta*) **valves**. The mitral and tricuspid valves are **atrioventricular (AV)**

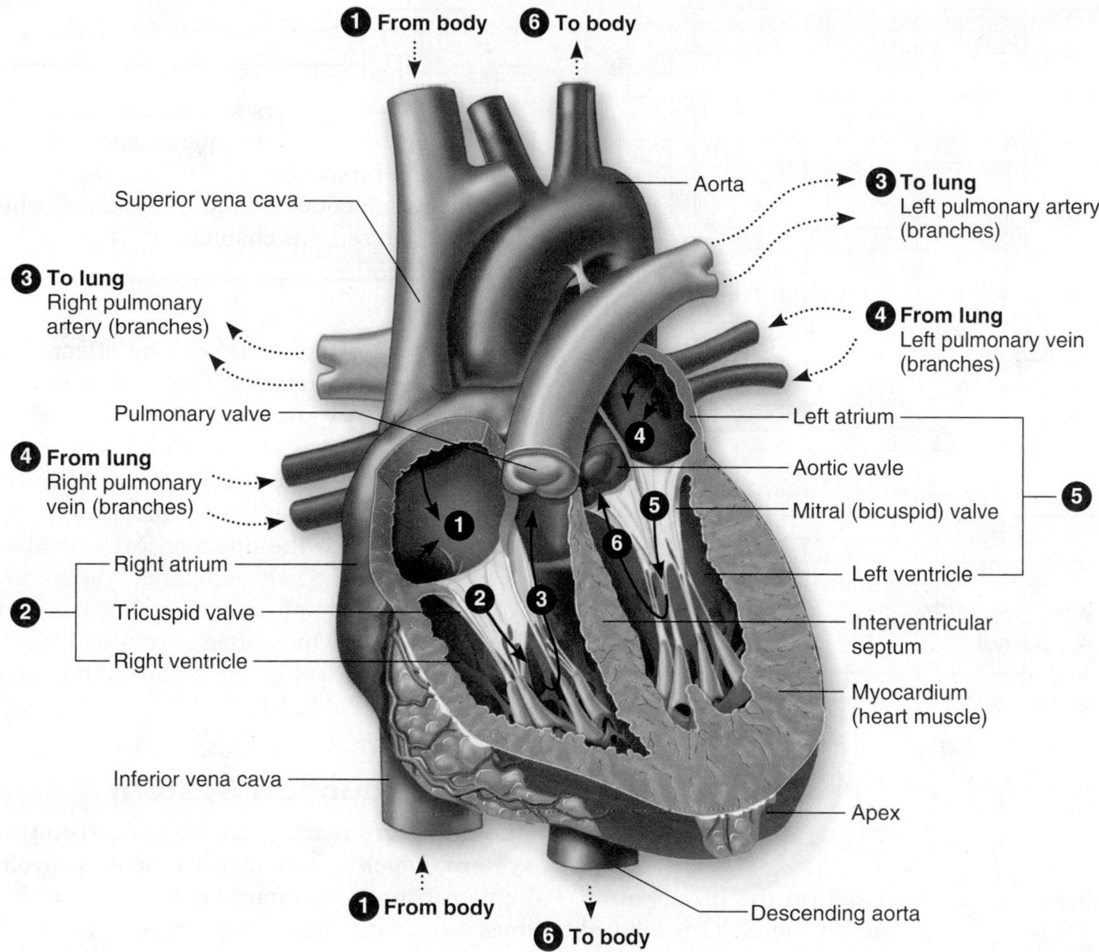

Figure 14-2 ■ The Path of Blood Flow Through the Heart

valves because they control the flow of blood from atria to ventricles. During every heart cycle, each chamber relaxes as it fills with blood during diastole and contracts as it ejects blood during systole.

The heart wall is a thick muscle consisting of three layers:

- the endocardium, the smooth inner layer that reduces the friction as the blood flows through the heart;
- the myocardium, the thick muscular inner layers that contract to pump blood; and
- the pericardium, a double-walled sac filled with fluid, which is the outer layer.

The pericardium consists of the epicardium or visceral pericardium (*inner layer*), the parietal pericardium (*outer layer*).

Disorders of the Heart Muscle

Myocardial infarction (MI), commonly known as a heart attack, is the death of heart tissue caused by an interruption to the blood supply. The most common cause of MI is occlusion (blockage) of a coronary artery by plaque. MIs are described by the heart wall that is affected: anterior, posterior, or inferior. A transmural MI extends through the entire thickness of the heart muscle. A subendocardial or nontransmural infarction affects only a small portion of the heart wall, usually due to a decreased, but not totally occluded, blood supply.

An MI that has occurred within the past four weeks is an acute myocardial infarction (AMI), also referred to as a current MI. An MI that occurs within four weeks of a previous AMI is also clinically acute, but is referred to as a subsequent MI in order to distinguish it from the original MI. An MI more than four weeks old is an old (healed) MI.

CODING CAUTION

If you are familiar with ICD-9-CM, it is important to note that the timeframe for acute MI has changed. Under ICD-9-CM, an acute MI was eight weeks, but in ICD-10-CM, an acute MI is only four weeks.

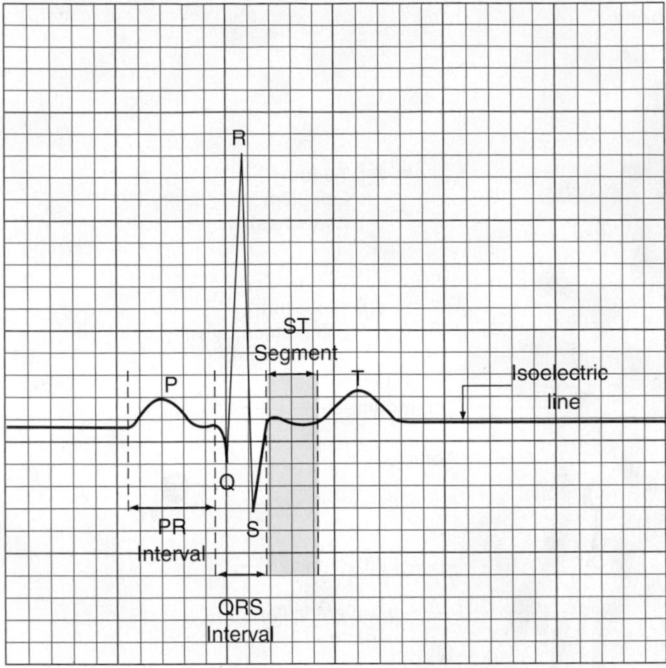

Figure 14-3 ■ Example of an ECG Report Showing the ST Segment

MIs are further described based on the results of an ECG (■ FIGURE 14-3). Each part of the ECG is labeled with a letter denoting a specific phase of the heart's electrical activity. The ST segment is elevated in an MI that completely occludes a vessel, known as ST elevation MI (STEMI). When the vessel is partially blocked, the ST segment is not elevated, resulting in a non-ST elevation MI (NSTEMI).

> **SUCCESS STEP**
>
> Coders should memorize the definitions of current, subsequent, and old MI, as well as STEMI and NSTEMI. These distinctions determine which codes should be assigned, which is discussed later in this chapter.

The valves of the heart can be affected by prolapse, regurgitation, or stenosis. The most common **valvular** disorder is mitral valve prolapse (MVP), also called click murmur syndrome and Barlow's syndrome. The two leaflets that comprise the valve fall backward into the left atrium, which results in regurgitation, blood leaking backward through the opening. Mitral valve stenosis is a narrowing of the valve opening, which may be caused by calcification, as often occurs with the aortic valve, or rheumatic fever, which often occurs with the mitral valve. Additional disorders of the heart are highlighted later in this chapter in Table 14-2.

The Conduction System

The heart rate is regulated by the **autonomic nervous system**, which means that it functions involuntarily and humans cannot voluntarily control it. Specialized neuromuscular tissue within the heart conducts an electrical impulse that stimulates each chamber to contract in the proper order. The electrical impulses begin in the sinoatrial (SA) node, which is the pacemaker of the heart, through the atrioventricular (AV) node to the atrioventricular bundle (bundle of His), then to bundle branches to the Purkinje fibers in the ventricular myocardium (■ FIGURE 14-4).

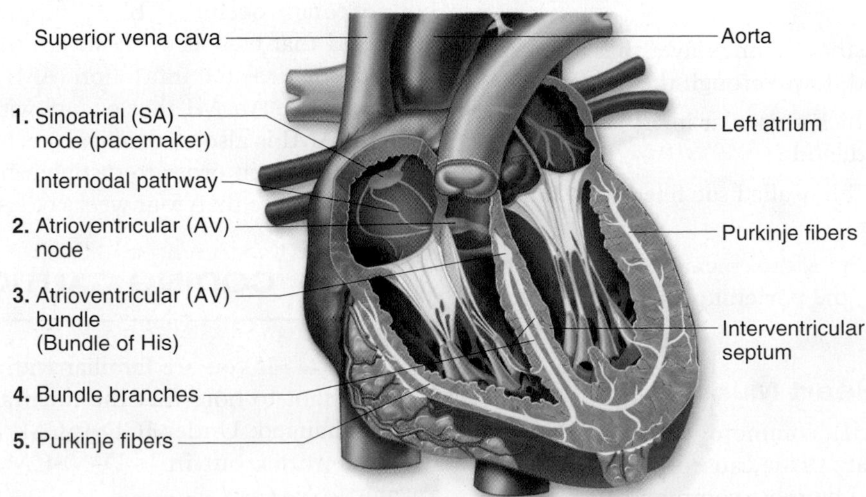

Figure 14-4 ■ The Conduction System of the Heart

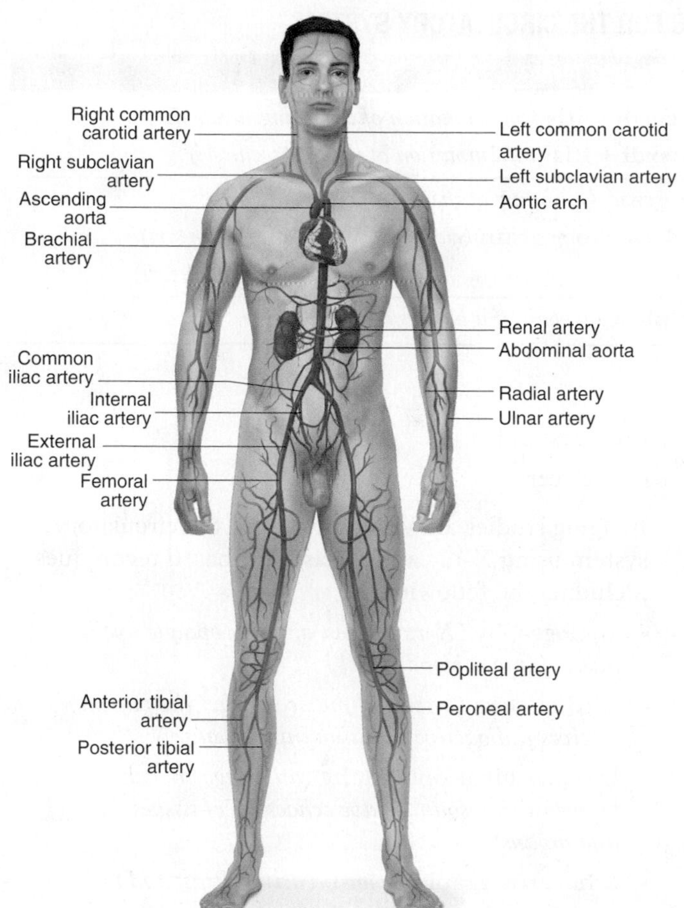

Figure 14-5 ■ The Major Arteries of Systemic Circulation

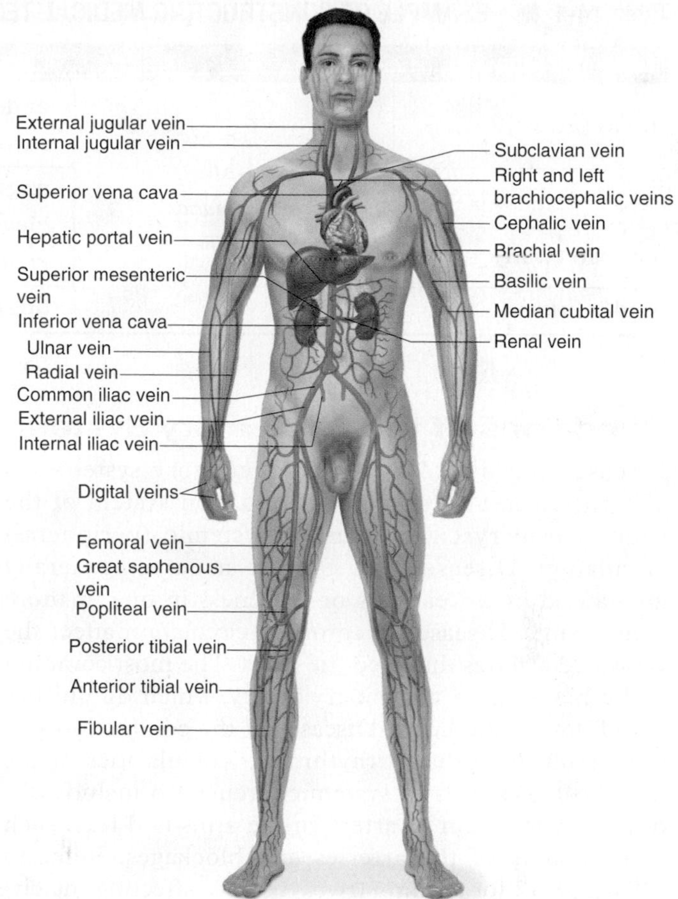

Figure 14-6 ■ The Major Veins of Systemic Circulation

Faulty electrical signaling in the heart causes arrhythmia (*an abnormal heartbeat*). A pacemaker is a small electronic device that is implanted in the chest to correct arrhythmia by speeding up, slowing down, smoothing out, or coordinating the heartbeat. Additional disorders of the conduction system are highlighted later in this chapter in Table 14-2.

The Blood Vessels

Blood vessels are the pipes that carry the blood through the body. Arteries are large, thick-walled vessels that carry blood away from the heart. The aorta is the first artery leading out of the heart to the body, which then repeatedly subdivides into smaller arteries that lead to each body region and anatomic site (■ Figure 14-5). Capillaries are very thin-walled membranes at the end of arterioles (*small arteries*) that allow blood to diffuse into body tissues and receive waste products from the tissues to send back into the bloodstream. Veins and venules (*small veins*) carry blood from the capillaries back to the heart in successively larger veins leading the superior vena cava and inferior vena cava, the largest veins that carry deoxygenated blood back to the right ventricle (■ Figure 14-6). Disorders of the blood vessels are highlighted later in this chapter in Table 14-2.

In the preceding figures, each structure in the circulatory system is labeled with its name as well as its medical terminology root/combining form, where applicable. Arteries and veins generally are named after the anatomic site where they are located. For example, the artery in the thigh (femur) is the femoral artery and the vein in the upper leg is the femoral vein. As you learn about conditions and procedures that affect the circulatory system, remember to apply medical terminology skills to combine word roots, prefixes, and suffixes you already know to define new terms related to the circulatory system. Refer to ■ Table 14-1 (page 258) for a refresher on how to build medical terms related to the circulatory system.

CODING CAUTION

Be alert for medical terms that are spelled similarly and have different meanings.

hemorrhoid (*resembling blood*) and **hemorrhage** (*flow of blood*)

ather/o (*plaque*) and **arteri/o** (*artery*) and **arthr/o** (*joint*)

pericardium (*sack around the heart*) and **perineum** (*the area between the external genitalia and the anus*)

Table 14-1 ■ **EXAMPLE OF CONSTRUCTING MEDICAL TERMS FOR THE CIRCULATORY SYSTEM**

<table>
<tr><th>Combining Form</th><th>Suffix</th><th>Complete Medical Term</th></tr>
<tr><td>my/o (muscle)</td><td rowspan="4">-gram (recording)
-itis (inflammation)
-plasty (repair)</td><td>endo + cardi + itis (inflammation of the lining inside the heart)
myo + cardi + itis (inflammation of the heart muscle)</td></tr>
<tr><td>angi/o (vessel)</td><td rowspan="2">angio + gram (recording of the vessels)
electro + cardio + gram (electrical recording of the heart)
echo + cardio + gram (recording of the sound of the heart)</td></tr>
<tr><td>cardi/o (heart)</td></tr>
<tr><td>end/o (within)</td><td>angio + plasty (repair of a blood vessel)</td></tr>
</table>

Conditions of the Circulatory System

Diseases and disorders of the circulatory system can affect the heart muscle, the conduction system of the heart, coronary circulation, or systemic (peripheral) circulation. Diseases of the heart structure generally are caused by a weakness or looseness in one or more components. Diseases of coronary circulation affect the veins and arteries that feed the heart. The most common is the blockage of a coronary artery, which diminishes blood flow to the heart. Diseases of the conduction system result in cardiac arrhythmias, irregularities of the heartbeat. Diseases of systemic circulation include abnormality in a vein or artery in the arms and legs, such as hardening of the arteries and blockages. Refer to ■ Table 14-2 for a summary of diseases affecting the circulatory system.

This section provides a general reference to help understand the most common diagnoses of the circulatory system, but does not list everything you need to know. Use medical terminology skills discussed earlier in this chapter to learn the meaning of unfamiliar words. Remember to keep standard reference books handy in case you get stuck. Refer to the resources in the Coder's Toolbox at the end of this chapter to learn more about conditions affecting the circulatory system.

Neoplasms of the Circulatory System

Neoplasms of the cardiovascular system are rare, and when they do occur, most are benign. Secondary or metastatic neoplasms of the heart occur in 1% of the population; primary neoplasms are even more infrequent.

Diagnostic Methods

Diseases of the circulatory system are diagnosed with laboratory tests, imaging studies, and cardiac function studies, which are described as follows:

- Laboratory tests measure the levels of substances in the blood, such as the following:
  - cardiac enzymes
    - creatine phosphokinase (CPK)
    - lactate dehydrogenase (LDH)
    - glutamic oxaloacetic transaminase (GOT)
  - cholesterol
  - triglycerides
- Imaging studies are visualizations of the circulatory system using X-ray and ultrasound-based techniques, including the following:
  - angiography (*X-ray taken after an opaque dye is injected into a blood vessel*)
  - cardiac scan (*a scan of the heart after the patient receives radioactive thallium intravenously*)
  - Doppler ultrasonography (*an image created by measuring sound-wave echoes off of tissues and organs*)
  - echocardiography (*non-invasive ultrasound to visualize internal cardiac structures*)
  - venography (*X-ray of the veins by tracing the venous pulse*)
- Cardiac function tests measure the capacity of the heart in real time, including the following:
  - cardiac catheterization (*passage of a thin tube through a blood vessel to the heart to visualize the structure, collect blood samples, and determine the blood pressure of the heart*)
  - electrocardiography (ECG, EKG) (*a graphical recording of the electrical activity of the heart*)
  - Holter monitor (*a portable ECG worn by the patient for an extended period of hours or days to measure heart activity in a variety of situations*)
  - stress testing (*measuring ECG and oxygen levels as a patient performs an increasing level of exercises on a treadmill or stationary bicycle*)

Treatment Methods

Heart disease is treated with a wide range of medications that regulate circulatory system functions, medical procedures such as a pacemaker or **implantable cardioverter-defibrillator** to regulate heart activity, and surgery to repair defects. Common procedures include the following:

- angioplasty (*insertion of an inflatable catheter in a blood vessel that expands to compress plaque against the walls of the vessel*)

Table 14-2 ■ **COMMON DISEASES OF THE CIRCULATORY SYSTEM**

Condition	Definition
Aneurysm	A bulge in the wall of an artery due to weakening, most commonly occurring in the abdominal aorta and cerebral arteries
Angina	Intense pain and spasms
Arrhythmia	Irregularity of the heartbeat
Arteriosclerotic heart disease (ASHD)	Atherosclerosis occurring in the coronary arteries; also called ischemic heart disease or coronary heart disease
Atherosclerosis	The formation of plaque on the inner walls of arteries in the heart
Atrial fibrillation (A-fib)	Irregular heartbeat in the atria characterized by an abnormal quivering of heart fibers
Bundle branch block (BBB)	The blockage of the conduction of electrical impulse through the branches of the atrioventricular bundle
Cerebrovascular accident (CVA)	A sudden drop in blood supply to the brain; also called stroke
Congestive heart failure (CHF)	The inability of the heart to maintain circulation, often resulting in water retention and edema
Coronary artery disease (CAD)	Insufficient blood supply to the heart due to an obstruction of one or more coronary arteries
Coronary heart disease (CHD)	Also called ischemic heart disease or arteriosclerotic heart disease
Deep vein thrombosis (DVT)	The formation of a thrombus within a deep vein, usually in the leg or pelvis
Embolus	An abnormal particle circulating in the blood, such as an air bubble or thrombus that has broken loose from its point of origin
Endocarditis	Inflammation of the lining of the heart or valves, due to bacteria or another disease
Hypertension (HTN)	High blood pressure readings exceeding 140/90, documented repeatedly over an extended period of time
Ischemia	Deficient blood supply to a local area due to obstruction of the arterial blood flow, usually due to narrowing of the arteries; also called coronary heart disease or arteriosclerotic heart disease when it affects the heart
Mitral valve prolapse (MVP)	Weakness in the flaps of the mitral valve, which allows blood to flow backward from the right ventricle into the right atrium
Myocardial infarction (MI)	The death of heart tissue due to a blockage of the blood supply
Pericarditis	Inflammation of the pericardial sac that surrounds the heart
Peripheral artery disease (PAD)	Damage to arteries outside the heart resulting in decreased blood flow
Stenosis	A narrowing of a valve or vessel
Thrombus	A clot of blood formed within a blood vessel that remains attached to its point of origin
Transient ischemic attack (TIA)	A brief episode of cerebral ischemia
Ventricular fibrillation (V-fib)	Irregular heartbeat in the ventricles, characterized by an abnormal quivering of heart fibers, which can result in cardiac arrest

- **bypass graft** (*creation of a new route around a blockage in a blood vessel using a vessel from another part of the body, another person, or a synthetic substitute*)
- **coronary artery bypass graft (CABG)** (*open heart surgery to create a bypass around a blocked coronary artery, usually using the* **internal mammary artery** *[IMA] or a vein from the leg*)
- **embolectomy** (*removal of a clot from a blood vessel*)
- **endarterectomy** (*removal of the diseased or damaged inner lining of an artery*)
- **stent insertion** (*placement of a mesh tube in a blood vessel to keep it open, due to atherosclerosis*)
- **valve repair** (*correction of a physical defect*)
- **valve replacement** (*replacement of a heart valve with an synthetic or porcine [pig] valve*)

Heart transplants, first done in 1967, are the third most common organ transplant in the United States and are performed in extreme cases of heart failure when other treatments have failed. According to the American Heart Association, approximately 2,100 heart transplants are performed each year in the United States. However, the need is far greater than that, but cannot be met, due to a shortage of available donor organs.

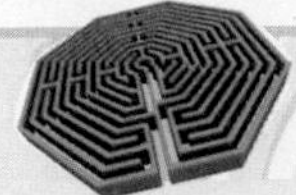

Coding Practice

Refresh your knowledge of terminology related to the circulatory system. Use a medical terminology text or a website such as GlobalRph.com > Medical Terminology **http://www.globalrph.com/medterm.htm** to identify the meaning of word parts that may not be familiar.

Exercise 14.1 Circulatory System Refresher

Instructions: Use your medical terminology skills and resources to define the following conditions related to the circulatory system, then assign the diagnosis code.

Follow these steps:

- Use slash marks "/" to break down each term into its root(s) and suffix.
- Define the meaning of the word, based on the meaning of each word part.
- Assign the default ICD-10-CM diagnosis code (CM) for the condition using the Index and Tabular List.

Example: endocarditis endo/card/itis Meaning: *inflammation of the lining of the heart* CM Code: I38

1. hypertension Meaning ______________________ CM Code __________
2. myocarditis Meaning ______________________ CM Code __________
3. cardiomyopathy Meaning ______________________ CM Code __________
4. atheroma Meaning ______________________ CM Code __________
5. arteriosclerosis Meaning ______________________ CM Code __________
6. arrhythmia Meaning ______________________ CM Code __________
7. lymphocele Meaning ______________________ CM Code __________
8. thrombophlebitis Meaning ______________________ CM Code __________
9. thromboangiitis Meaning ______________________ CM Code __________
10. pyopneumopericardium Meaning ______________________ CM Code __________

CODING OVERVIEW OF THE CIRCULATORY SYSTEM

ICD-10-CM Chapter 9, Diseases of the Circulatory System (I00-I99), contains 11 blocks or subchapters that are divided by the type of disease. Review the block names and code ranges listed at the beginning of Chapter 9 in the ICD-10-CM manual to become familiar with the content and organization.

ICD-10-CM Chapter 9 corresponds with ICD-9-CM Chapter 7 (390-459). Many codes have been expanded to identify specific anatomic sites and laterality. Terminology has been updated for angina pectoris, myocardial infarction, atherosclerosis, pulmonary embolism, cardiac arrest, and nontraumatic subarachnoid hemorrhage in order to be consistent with current clinical practice. ICD-9-CM category 438, Late effects of cerebrovascular disease, has been significantly expanded in ICD-10-CM category I69, Sequelae of cerebrovascular disease. OGCR for myocardial infarction and hypertensive heart disease have also been updated.

This chapter includes disorders that affect the heart and the pulmonary, systemic, and coronary circulatory systems. Conditions may consist of acquired physical dysfunctions or infections.

This chapter does not include congenital diseases of the circulatory system, which are classified in ICD-10-CM Chapter 17, Congenital Malformations, Deformations, and Chromosomal Abnormalities (Q00-Q99) or diseases of the blood, which are classified in ICD-10-CM Chapter 3, Diseases of the Blood and Blood-Forming Organs and Certain Disorders Involving the Immune Mechanism (D50-D89).

ICD-10-CM provides Official Guidelines for Coding and Reporting (OGCR) for the circulatory system in OGCR section I.C.9. OGCR provides detailed discussion regarding hypertension, atherosclerotic coronary artery disease and angina, cerebrovascular accident and disease, and acute myocardial infarction. The Tabular List contains no instructional notes at the beginning of the chapter, but does provide many instructional notes throughout the chapter regarding additional codes that are required to identify related conditions and lifestyle habits related to tobacco use.

ABSTRACTING FOR THE CIRCULATORY SYSTEM

Coders need to pay close attention to detail when abstracting for the CV system because codes must be specific to anatomic site, nature of the disease, and comorbidities. Coders rely on their knowledge of anatomy in order to identify the exact site of the disorder and their knowledge of diseases in order to identify the specific form of the disease and co-existing conditions. They also must identify circumstances that require Z codes. Key factors to review when coding cases that involve the circulatory system appear in ■ TABLE 14-3. Remember that the abstracting questions are a guide and that not every question applies to, or can be answered for, every case. For example, the questions about myocardial infarction do not apply to patients who have not had this condition.

Table 14-3 ■ KEY CRITERIA FOR ABSTRACTING CONDITIONS OF THE CIRCULATORY SYSTEM

- ❑ What part of the circulatory system is affected?
- ❑ What is the specific anatomic site?
- ❑ What type of disorder is present?
- ❑ Is the condition further specified as complete, partial, current, or old?
- ❑ What is the underlying cause?
- ❑ What symptoms are documented that are not integral to the condition?
- ❑ Is the condition acquired or congenital?
- ❑ Is the condition related to pregnancy?
- ❑ Does the patient have a current, subsequent, or old MI?
- ❑ Has the patient had more than one AMI in the past four weeks?
- ❑ What other CV conditions coexist?
- ❑ What conditions exist in other organ systems?
- ❑ Which conditions are documented as being related to the CV condition?
- ❑ What is the patient's exposure to or use of tobacco?
- ❑ Does the patient use anticoagulants or antithrombotics on a long-term basis?
- ❑ Does the patient have a family history of CV disease?
- ❑ Does the patient wear a pacemaker?
- ❑ Has the patient had a CABG?
- ❑ If a vessel is blocked or diseased, is it an artery or vein? Is it **native** (*the patient's original vessel*) or a graft?
- ❑ If a grafted vessel is blocked, is the grafted vessel **autologous** (*from the patient*), biological **nonautologous** (*from a source other than the patient, such as a cadaver or animal*), or **nonbiological** (*synthetic*)?
- ❑ Is the patient waiting for or a recipient of a heart transplant?

Guided Example of Abstracting for the Circulatory System

Refer to the following example throughout this chapter to learn skills for abstracting, assigning, and sequencing circulatory system codes. Tanisha Riemann, CCS-P, is a fictitious coder who guides you through the coding process.

> Date: 4/1/yy Location: Branton Medical Center
>
> Provider: Matthew Bunker, MD
>
> Patient: Gordon Rothe Gender: M Age: 76
>
> Reason for admission: admitted from emergency department due to unstable angina, patient has been on warfarin since a CABG of the left anterior descending coronary artery (LAD) 11 years ago using the left saphenous vein, continues to use tobacco although he states that his usage has decreased
>
> Assessment: atherosclerosis of grafted vessel
>
> Plan: balloon angioplasty to clear the partially blocked graft, Rx atorvastatin to address lipid rich plaque

Follow along as Tanisha Riemann, CCS-P, abstracts the diagnosis. Check off each step after you complete it.

⇨ Tanisha reads through the entire record, with special attention to the reason for the encounter and the final assessment. She refers to the Key Criteria for Abstracting Conditions of the Circulatory System (Table 14-3) to guide her review.

- ❑ She notes the presenting symptom of unstable angina.
- ❑ *What part of the circulatory system is affected?* grafted vessel
- ❑ *What is the specific anatomic site?* The heart, near the left anterior descending coronary artery
- ❑ *What type of disorder is present?* blocked graft and atherosclerosis
- ❑ Is the condition further specified as complete, partial, current, or old? partially blocked
- ❑ *Does the patient have a current, subsequent, or old MI?* No
- ❑ *What other CV conditions coexist?* lipid rich plaque
- ❑ *What is the patient's exposure to or use of tobacco?* The patient continues to use tobacco although he states that his usage has decreased.
- ❑ Does the patient use anticoagulants or antithrombotics on a long-term basis? Yes, the patient has been on warfarin since a CABG 11 years ago.
- ❑ *Has the patient had a CABG?* Yes, 11 years ago

- ❑ *If a vessel is blocked or diseased, is it an artery or vein?* vein *Is it native or a graft?* graft
- ❑ *If a grafted vessel is blocked, is the grafted vessel autologous, biological nonautologous, or nonbiological?* The graft used the left saphenous vein, so it is autologous.

➩ At this point, Tanisha is not sure of how many codes she will need. She knows that she needs to search the Index and cross-reference any instructional notes in the Tabular List before she knows what her final codes will be.

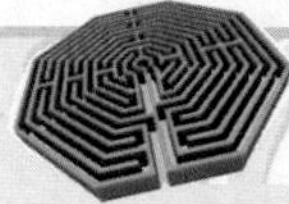

Coding Practice

Now it is your turn to practice abstracting diagnoses for the circulatory system. Questions guide your analysis of each scenario. Refer to the content of this chapter and to your outside resources, when needed, to answer the questions.

Exercise 14.2 Abstracting for the Circulatory System

Instructions: Read the mini-medical-record of each patient's encounter and answer the abstracting questions. Write the answer on the line provided. Do not assign any codes.

1. Date: 4/3/yy Location: Branton Medical Center
Provider: Matthew Bunker, MD
Patient: Susana Lampton Gender: F Age: 42
Reason for admission: admitted from emergency department with subendocardial infarction
Assessment: nontransmural myocardial infarction
Plan: This is her first event so we will treat it with medication and diet.

a. What is a subendocardial infarction? ____________

____

b. What is a nontransmural infarction? ____________

____

c. What is the Main Term? ____________

____

2. Date: 4/3/yy Location: City Center Cardiology
Provider: Matthew Bunker, MD
Patient: Isabelle Mcloud Gender: F Age: 68
Reason for encounter: Patient has been taking her BP at home and is concerned about readings that have been increasing over the past 3 months. She claims to be taking the diuretic and beta blocker as directed. Lab results show slightly low potassium.

(continued)

2. (continued)
Assessment: hypertensive cardiomegaly
Plan: Add spironolactone to the medication regime.

a. What is the cause of the patient's cardiomegaly?

____

b. Should you code for low potassium? ____________

____

c. What is the Main Term? ____________

____

3. Date: 4/3/yy Location: Branton Medical Center
Provider: Matthew Bunker, MD
Patient: Derrick Grunwald Gender: M Age: 68
Reason for admission: mitral porcine valvoplasty
Assessment: mitral valve regurgitation due to prolapse

a. Where is the mitral valve located? ____________

____

b. In your own words, explain what procedure was done. ____________

____

c. In your own words, explain why the procedure was done. ____________

____

4. Date: 4/4/yy Location: Branton Medical Center
Provider: Matthew Bunker, MD
Patient: Keisha Wier Gender: F Age: 71
Reason for admission: Admitted from emergency department with angina. Patient has history of MI 2 years ago, as well as history of TIAs, although the TIAs did not leave any residual deficits.

(continued)

4. (continued)

Assessment: STEMI involving 90% occlusion of the right coronary artery

Procedure: CABG

a. Should you code for angina? ________

Why or why not? ________

b. What is TIA? ________

c. What is STEMI? ________

d. What is the site of the STEMI? ________

____

e. Should you code for the old MI? ________

____

f. In your own words, describe the procedure that was done. ________

____

5. Date: 4/4/yy Location: City Center Cardiology

Provider: Matthew Bunker, MD

Patient: Dustin Napper Gender: M Age: 65

Chief complaint: increased edema and SOB since last visit

Assessment: HTN and decompensated CHF, A-fib

Plan: We will start by adjusting the diuretic, then evaluate the need for other adjustments based on response after 4 weeks. Continue long term warfarin and clopidrogel (*an antiplatelet medication*).

a. Define the abbreviations in this scenario. ________

____

b. Which condition are the edema and SOB most related to? ________

c. What is the causal relationship between HTN and CHF? ________

d. Which condition is the first listed diagnosis?

________ Why? ________

e. What type of medication is warfarin? ________

____

f. What type of medication is clopidrogel? ________

____

6. Date: 4/4/yy Location: Branton Medical Center

Provider: Matthew Bunker, MD

Patient: Dennis Lehto Gender: M Age: 57

Reason for admission: transferred from Valley hospital where patient was admitted for cerebral infarct 20 hours ago and received tPA (tissue plasminogen activator), but now it is evident that a mechanical or surgical embolectomy is needed

Assessment: cerebral infarction d/t embolus in right middle cerebral artery, cerebral atherosclerosis, HTN, history of tobacco use

Procedure: surgical embolectomy

a. What is the common term for cerebral infarction?

____

b. What is the cause of the cerebral infarction?

____

c. What is an embolus? ________

____

d. Is the middle cerebral artery **cerebral** (*located within the brain*) or **precerebral** (*outside of the brain*)? ________

e. What other medical conditions exist? ________

____

f. What lifestyle habit is documented?

____

g. In your own words, describe the procedure that was performed. ________

____

ASSIGNING CODES FOR THE CIRCULATORY SYSTEM

Diseases of the circulatory system frequently occur with multiple comorbidities from within the cardiovascular system and/or from other systems. The choice of codes is dependent on the precise wording physicians use in the documentation. The coding of hypertension, a common circulatory system condition, is an example of how documentation affects code choices. Hypertension may occur by itself, in conjunction with chronic kidney disease, heart disease, both kidney and heart disease, or many other conditions. Refer to the following examples to better understand how to interpret physician documentation when assigning codes.

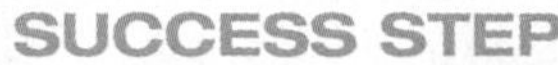

SUCCESS STEP

ICD-10-CM does not have a separate Hypertension Table as ICD-9-CM did. Locate the Main Term **Hypertension** in the Index, then locate the appropriate subterm(s) for the condition being coded. In addition, ICD-10-CM does not distinguish between essential, benign, and malignant hypertension as ICD-9-CM did.

Hypertension

Physicians diagnose hypertension when patients have elevated blood pressure over an extended period of time. Assign a code for hypertension only when the physician has documented for this condition. Do not assign a code for hypertension simply because a patient has a random high blood pressure reading, referred to as an incidental high blood pressure reading (■ FIGURE 14-7).

When the diagnosis of hypertension is documented, search for the Main Term **Hypertension** in the Index. Assign the default code, **I10 Essential (primary) hypertension**, for hypertension described with the following terms:

- accelerated
- benign
- essential

High
altitude effects T70.20
blood pressure — *see also* Hypertension
reading (incidental) (isolated) (nonspecific), without diagnosis
of hypertension R03.0

Figure 14-7 ■ Index Entry for Incidental High Blood Pressure Reading

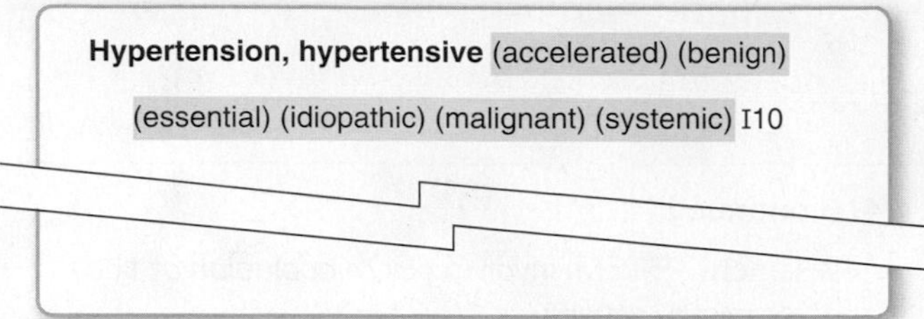

Hypertension, hypertensive (accelerated) (benign) (essential) (idiopathic) (malignant) (systemic) I10

Figure 14-8 ■ Index Entry for Main Term Hypertension with Nonessential Modifiers

- idiopathic
- malignant
- systemic

Refer to the Index entry in the ICD-10-CM manual, which identifies these terms as nonessential modifiers by the use of parentheses (■ FIGURE 14-8). Subterms identify codes for use when hypertension occurs with or due to another condition, which is discussed later in this chapter.

In the Tabular List, an instructional note, **Excludes1**, reminds coders that hypertension complicating pregnancy, childbirth, and the puerperium is not coded here. Another instructional note, **Excludes2**, directs coders to look elsewhere for hypertension involving vessels of the brain and eye.

Hypertension and Chronic Kidney Disease

ICD-10-CM presumes a causal relationship between hypertension and **chronic kidney disease (CKD)** because hypertension is known to cause CKD and CKD is known to cause hypertension.

OGCR I.C.9.a. provides guidelines on coding these conditions when they occur together. Assign codes as follows (■ FIGURE 14-9):

1. Assign a code from category **I12 Hypertensive chronic kidney disease** based on the stage of CKD documented. Refer to category **I12** in the ICD-10-CM manual to review the available codes and locate the instructional notes.
2. Assign a code from category **N18 Chronic kidney disease** as an additional code to identify the stage of CKD, as stated in the instructional note (OGCR I.C.9.a.2)).

Patient is seen for stage 4 CKD and HTN.

(1) **I12.9 Hypertensive chronic kidney disease with stage 1 through stage 4 chronic kidney disease, or unspecified chronic kidney disease**

(2) **N18.4 Chronic kidney disease, stage 4 (severe)**

Figure 14-9 ■ Example of Assigning Codes for Hypertension and Chronic Kidney Disease

Hypertension and Heart Disease

Although hypertension is a major cause of heart failure, ICD-10-CM does *not* presume a causal relationship between hypertension and heart disease. A causal relationship must be stated or implied in order to assign a code for *hypertensive* heart disease. A causal relationship is stated definitively by documentation such as heart disease due to hypertension or hypertension with heart involvement. A causal relationship is implied by documentation such as hypertensive heart disease.

SUCCESS STEP

Hypertensive heart disease is the leading cause of illness and death due to hypertension.

No Causal Relationship

When no causal relationship is documented, assign separate codes for the heart condition and hypertension. Do not assign a code for *hypertensive* heart disease (■ FIGURE 14-10).

Causal Relationship Stated or Implied

When a causal relationship exists between heart failure and hypertension, assign codes as follows:

1. Assign a code from category **I11 Hypertensive heart disease**. This category includes any condition in **I51.4** to **I51.9** that is due to hypertension (■ FIGURE 14-11).
2. Also assign a code from category **I50 Heart failure** to identify the type of heart failure as left ventricular, systolic, diastolic, combined, or unspecified. Sequence the code for hypertensive heart disease first and the code for heart failure second (■ FIGURE 14-12).

SUCCESS STEP

To locate CHF in the Index, search for the Main Term **Failure,** and the subterm **heart.**

Patient is seen for myocarditis, chronic combined congestive heart failure, and hypertension.

(1) **I51.4 Myocarditis, unspecified**

(2) **I50.42 Chronic combined systolic (congestive) and diastolic (congestive) heartfailure**

(3) **I10 Essential (primary) hypertension**

Figure 14-10 ■ Example of Assigning Codes for Hypertension and Heart Disease When a Causal Relationship Is NOT Documented

I51.4 Myocarditis, unspecified
Chronic (interstitial) myocarditis
Myocardial fibrosis
Myocarditis NOS
Excludes1: acute or subacute myocarditis (I40.-)

I51.5 Myocardial degeneration
Fatty degeneration of heart or myocardium
Myocardial disease
Senile degeneration of heart or myocardium

I51.7 Cardiomegaly
Cardiac dilatation
Cardiac hypertrophy
Ventricular dilatation

I51.8 Other ill-defined heart diseases

I51.81 Takotsubo syndrome
Reversible left ventricular dysfunction following sudden emotional stress
Stress induced cardiomyopathy
Takotsubo cardiomyopathy
Transient left ventricular apical ballooning syndrome

I51.89 Other ill-defined heart diseases
Carditis (acute)(chronic)
Pancarditis (acute)(chronic)

I51.9 Heart disease, unspecified

Figure 14-11 ■ Tabular List Entry for I51.4 to I51.9

Patient is seen for hypertensive myocarditis with chronic combined congestive heart failure.

(1) **I11.0 Hypertensive heart disease with heart failure**

(2) **I50.42 Chronic combined systolic (congestive) and diastolic (congestive) heart failure**

Figure 14-12 ■ Example of Assigning Codes for Heart Disease and Hypertension When a Causal Relationship IS Documented

Hypertensive Kidney Disease and Hypertensive Heart Disease

The documentation may state that both hypertensive kidney disease and *hypertensive* heart disease exist. The causal relationship between hypertension and heart disease must be stated or implied, but a causal relationship between hypertension and CKD should be assumed. Assign codes as follows (■ FIGURE 14-13):

1. Assign a code from category **I13 Hypertensive heart and chronic kidney disease.**
2. Also assign a code from category **I50** when heart failure is present.
3. Assign a code from category **N18** to identify the stage of CKD.

Hypertension and Other Conditions

Whenever hypertension exists with another condition, searching Main Terms for both conditions helps ensure that nothing is omitted. Carefully review all available subterms under **Hypertension** to locate any applicable code for the comorbidity. Also locate the Index Main Term entry for the comorbid condition and search for a subterm of hypertension. Refer to OGCR I.C.9.a. for additional guidelines on coding hypertension with cerebrovascular disease and retinopathy, as well as secondary, transient, controlled, and uncontrolled hypertension.

Guided Example of Assigning Circulatory System Codes

To practice skills for assigning codes for the circulatory system, continue with the example from earlier in the chapter about patient Gordon Rothe, who was admitted to Branton Medical Center due to unstable angina.

Follow along in your ICD-10-CM manual as Tanisha assigns codes. Check off each step after you complete it.

Patient is seen for hypertensive myocarditis with chronic combined CHF and stage 4 CKD.

(1) **I13.0 Hypertensive heart and chronic kidney disease with heart failure and stage 1 through stage 4 chronic kidney disease, or unspecified chronic kidney disease**

(2) **N18.4 Chronic kidney disease, stage 4 (severe)**

(3) **I50.42 Chronic combined systolic (congestive) and diastolic (congestive) heart failure**

Figure 14-13 ■ Example of Assigning Codes for Hypertensive Heart Disease and Hypertensive Chronic Kidney Disease

➩ First, Tanisha confirms the information she abstracted from the medical record:

- ❑ Unstable angina.
- ❑ ASHD with occlusion in grafted vein.
- ❑ Lipid rich plaque.
- ❑ Anti-coagulant use for 11 years.
- ❑ Tobacco use.

➩ Tanisha searches the Index for the Main Term **Angina**.

- ❑ She locates the subterm **unstable I20.0**.

➩ Tanisha verifies code **I20.0** in the Tabular List.

- ❑ She reads the code title for **I20.0, Unstable angina** and confirms that this accurately describes the medical record documentation.

➩ Tanisha checks for instructional notes in the Tabular List.

- ❑ Tamara cross-references the beginning of category **I20** and reads the **Excludes1** note that states **atherosclerosis of coronary artery bypass graft(s) and coronary artery of transplanted heart with angina pectoris (I25.7-).**
- ❑ The note tells her that **I20.0** cannot be used with a code from **I25.7-** because **Excludes1** means the codes are mutually exclusive.
- ❑ She decides to research the rest of her codes before deciding if she should include **I20.0**.

➩ Next, Tanisha searches the Index for the Main Term **Atherosclerosis** (■ FIGURE 14-14).

- ❑ She locates the instructional note to cross-reference the Main Term **Arteriosclerosis**.
- ❑ She follows the indented subterms for **coronary (artery), bypass graft, autologous vein, with, angina pectoris, unstable I25.710**.
- ❑ She identifies that she will have a combination code for ASHD and unstable angina.

SUCCESS STEP

Arteriosclerosis (hardening of an artery) is usually caused by atherosclerosis (hardening of a vessel due to plaque), so ICD-10-CM indexes both conditions to the Main Term **Arteriosclerosis**. When you remember this, you can go directly to **Arteriosclerosis** in the Index, then locate the needed subterm, rather than searching **Atherosclerosis** first.

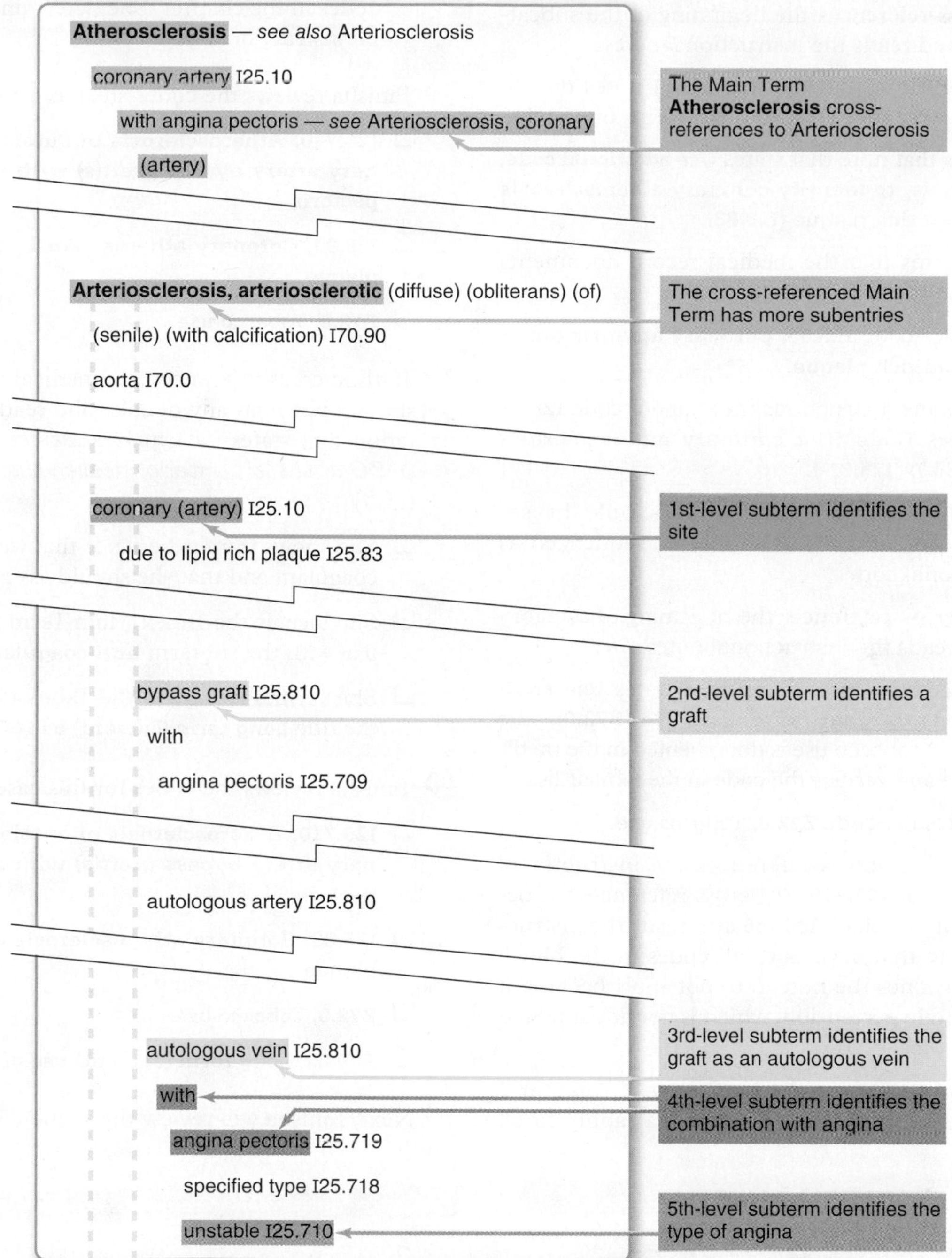

Figure 14-14 ■ Index Entry for Arteriosclerosis of a Grafted Autologous Vein with Unstable Angina

➩ Tanisha verifies code **I25.710** in the Tabular List.

- ❑ She locates the code title **Atherosclerosis of autologous vein coronary artery bypass graft(s) with unstable angina pectoris** and confirms that all components of the code description are consistent with the documentation.
- ❑ She also refers to OGCR I.C.9.b. which states:
  - ICD-10-CM has combination codes for atherosclerotic heart disease with angina pectoris. When using one of these combination codes it is not necessary to use an additional code for angina pectoris. A causal relationship can be assumed in a patient with both atherosclerosis and angina pectoris, unless the documentation indicates the angina is due to something other than the atherosclerosis.
- ❑ She determines that because this is a combination code, she should *not* also assign **I20.0, Unstable angina.**

⇨ Tanisha cross-references the beginning of the subcategory **I25.7** and reads the instructional notes.

- ❑ She determines that the **Excludes1** notes do not apply because they refer to other forms of ASHD.
- ❑ She reads that note that states **Use additional code, if applicable, to identify coronary atherosclerosis due to lipid rich plaque (I25.83).**
- ❑ She confirms that the medical record documents lipid rich plaque.
- ❑ She verifies code **I25.83, Coronary atherosclerosis due to lipid rich plaque**.
- ❑ She reads the instructional note under code **I25.83** that states **Code first coronary atherosclerosis (I25.1-, I25.7-, I25.81-).**
- ❑ The note confirms that **I25.710** should be sequenced first and **I25.83** should be sequenced as an additional code.
- ❑ Tanisha cross-references the beginning of category I25 and reads the instructional notes.
- ❑ She notices the instruction that states **Use additional code to identify: tobacco use (Z72.0)**. She verifies that tobacco use is documented in the medical record and verifies the code in the tabular list.
- ❑ She locates the code **Z72.0, Tobacco use**.
- ❑ Next, Tanisha cross-references the instructional notes for code **I25.710**. She cross-references the beginning of the block **I20-I25** and reads the instructional note that applies to all codes in the block. She determines the note does not apply because it pertains to hypertension, which is not documented in the medical record.
- ❑ She cross-references the beginning of **Chapter 9 (I00-I99)** for instructional notes that apply to all codes in the chapter. She determines that there are no instructional notes.

⇨ Tanisha reviews the codes she has assigned so far:

- ❑ **I25.710, Atherosclerosis of autologous vein coronary artery bypass graft(s) with unstable angina pectoris**
- ❑ **I25.83, Coronary atherosclerosis due to lipid rich plaque**
- ❑ **Z72.0, Tobacco use**

⇨ Tanisha cross-references the medical record to ensure she did not miss any details. She reads the documentation that states patient has been on warfarin since a CABG of the left anterior descending coronary artery (LAD) 11 years ago.

- ❑ She knows from experience that warfarin is an anticoagulant and that she should assign a code for it.
- ❑ She locates the Index Main Term **Long term drug use** with the subterm **anti-coagulant Z79.01**.
- ❑ She verifies **Z79.01** in the Tabular List and locates the title **Long term (current) use of anticoagulants**.

⇨ Tanisha reviews the codes for this case:

- ❑ **I25.710, Atherosclerosis of autologous vein coronary artery bypass graft(s) with unstable angina pectoris**
- ❑ **I25.83, Coronary atherosclerosis due to lipid rich plaque**
- ❑ **Z72.0, Tobacco use**
- ❑ **Z79.01, Long term (current) use of anticoagulants**

⇨ Next, Tanisha will review the sequencing of the codes.

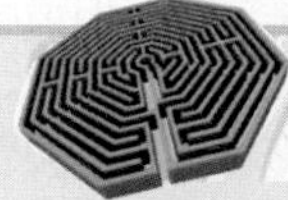

Coding Practice

Now it is your turn to practice assigning codes for diseases of the circulatory system. Refer to the ***Tip*** at the end of the mini-medical-record if you need a little extra help.

Exercise 14.3 Assigning Codes for the Circulatory System

Instructions: Read the mini-medical-record of each patient's encounter, review the information abstracted in Exercise 14.2 for questions 1 to 3. For questions 4 and 5, do the abstracting on your own. Assign ICD-10-CM diagnosis codes (CM) using the Index and Tabular List. Write the code(s) on the line provided.

1. Date: 4/3/yy Location: Branton Medical Center

Provider: Matthew Bunker, MD

Patient: Susana Lampton Gender: F Age: 42

Reason for admission: admitted from emergency department with subendocardial infarction

Assessment: nontransmural myocardial infarction

Plan: this is her first event so we will treat it with medication and diet

1 CM Code ___________

2. Date: 4/3/yy Location: City Center Cardiology

Provider: Matthew Bunker, MD

Patient: Isabelle Mcloud Gender: F Age: 68

Reason for encounter: Patient has been taking her BP at home and is concerned about readings that have been increasing over the past 3 months. She claims to be taking the diuretic and beta blocker as directed. Lab results show slightly low potassium.

Assessment: hypertensive cardiomegaly

Plan: Add spironolactone to the medication regime.

1 CM Code __________

3. Date: 4/3/yy Location: Branton Medical Center

Provider: Matthew Bunker, MD

Patient: Derrick Grunwald Gender: M Age: 68

Reason for admission: mitral porcine valvoplasty

Assessment: mitral valve regurgitation

Tip: Remember to follow the cross-references in the Index.

1 CM Code __________

4. Date: 4/13/yy Location: Branton Medical Center Emergency Department

Provider: Matthew Bunker, MD

Patient: Maurice Rybicki Gender: M Age: 53

Chief complaint: tachycardia

Assessment: ventricular flutter

Plan: CPR, external electric shock

Tip: You did not practice abstracting this case earlier, so see how you do on your own.

1 CM Code __________

5. Date: 4/13/yy Location: City Center Cardiology

Provider: Matthew Bunker, MD

Patient: Cecilia Widener Gender: F Age: 38

Chief complaint: referred by primary care physician for pain in right leg due to varicose veins that have not improved with compression stockings

Assessment: varicose veins right calf

Plan: ultrasound to evaluate for thrombus or valve problems. Consider for sclerotherapy.

Tip: You did not practice abstracting this case earlier, so see how you do on your own.

1 CM Code __________

ARRANGING CODES FOR THE CIRCULATORY SYSTEM

The circumstances of admission, OGCR, and instructional notes in the Tabular List always determine the selection of the principal or first-listed diagnosis and the sequencing of codes. In some cases sequencing is fairly straightforward and in other cases it can be challenging to sort through multiple sets of instructions. This holds true for patients who have AMI, and especially for patients who have had multiple MIs. Refer to the following examples to better understand how to sequence codes for MI.

SUCCESS STEP

To locate MI in the Index, use the Main Term **Infarct** and the subterm **myocardium.**

Myocardial Infarction and Coronary Artery Disease

When a patient with CAD is admitted for an AMI, sequence codes as follows (OGCR I.C.9.b.):

1. Sequence the AMI first.
2. Sequence the CAD as an additional code (■ FIGURE 14-15, page 270).

SUCCESS STEP

To locate CAD in the Index, search for the Main Term **Disease**, the first-level subterm **heart**, and the second-level subterm **ischemic**. As an alternative, you can also use the Main Term **Ischemia**.

Patient was admitted for inferior wall STEMI and also has atherosclerotic heart disease.

(1) **I21.19 ST elevation (STEMI) myocardial infarction involving other coronary artery of inferior wall**
(2) **I25.10 Atherosclerotic heart disease of native coronary artery without angina pectoris**

Figure 14-15 ■ Example of Sequencing AMI and ASHD

Acute and Subsequent Myocardial Infarction

ICD-10-CM classifies an MI as acute or current for four weeks after the event. Patients may have two or more MI events within the four week timeframe. When this occurs, assign the first MI a code from category **I21.- ST elevation (STEMI) and non-ST elevation (NSTEMI) myocardial infarction** and assign the second event a code for a subsequent AMI from category **I22.- Subsequent ST elevation (STEMI) and non-ST elevation (NSTEMI) myocardial infarction**. Sequencing is determined by the AMI that is *chiefly responsible* for the encounter, as shown in the following examples (OGCR I.C.9.e.). Refer to the examples that follow to better understand sequencing rules.

SUCCESS STEP

During the course of an admission, STEMI may evolve to NSTEMI and NSTEMI may evolve to STEMI. In both cases, assign the STEMI code (OGCR I.C.9.e.1)).

Sequencing in an Admission for AMI Followed by a Subsequent MI

When a patient is admitted for an AMI and has a second AMI during the stay, sequence the codes as follows:

1. Assign a code from category **I21.-** for the original AMI and sequence this condition first because it is the condition chiefly responsible for the admission and services provided.
2. Assign a code from category **I22.-** for subsequent AMI to the second event and sequence it second, as shown in ■ FIGURE 14-16.

SUCCESS STEP

Read the instructional notes at the beginning of categories I21, I22, and I23 for definitions and sequencing guidance on MI.

Patient was admitted for STEMI of the anterolateral wall. Two days later, the patient had a separate NSTEMI.

(1) **I21.09 ST elevation (STEMI) myocardial infarction involving other coronary artery of anterior wall**
(2) **I22.2 Subsequent non-ST elevation (NSTEMI) myocardial infarction**

Figure 14-16 ■ Example of Sequencing in an Admission for AMI Followed by a Subsequent MI

Sequencing in an Admission for a Subsequent MI

When a non-hospitalized patient is admitted for a second AMI within four weeks of a previous AMI, assign and sequence codes as follows (■ FIGURE 14-17):

1. Assign a code from category **I22.-** for subsequent MI to the second event. Sequence the subsequent event as the principal diagnosis because it is the reason for the admission and services provided.
2. Assign a code from category **I21.-** for acute MI to the first event. Sequence this code second because it was not the reason for admission.

Sequencing a Current AMI and an Old MI

When more than four weeks elapse between MI events, the first MI is classified as an old or healed MI and only the new AMI is coded as acute. When a non-hospitalized patient is admitted for a second AMI that occurs more than four weeks after a previous AMI, assign and sequence codes as follows (■ FIGURE 14-18):

1. Assign a code for a current AMI from category **I21.-** for the new AMI. Sequence the new event as the principal diagnosis because it is the reason for the admission and services provided.
2. Assign the code **I25.2 Old myocardial infarction** to the first event. Sequence this condition as an additional code because it was not the reason for admission.

Patient was admitted for a STEMI involving the inferior wall. Three weeks ago, the patient had a transmural MI to the inferoposterior wall.

(1) **I22.1 Subsequent ST elevation (STEMI) myocardial infarction of inferior wall**
(2) **I21.11 ST elevation (STEMI) myocardial infarction involving right coronary artery**

Figure 14-17 ■ Example of Sequencing in an Admission for a Subsequent AMI

Patient was admitted for AMI involving the LAD coronary artery.

Three months ago, the patient had a MI to the anterior wall.

(1) **I21.02 ST elevation (STEMI) myocardial infarction involving left anterior descending coronary artery**

(2) **I25.2 Old myocardial infarction**

Figure 14-18 ■ Example of Sequencing a Current AMI and an Old MI

SUCCESS STEP

After four weeks, an MI is no longer considered acute, but is defined as an old MI.

Guided Example of Arranging Circulatory System Codes

In order to practice skills for sequencing codes for the circulatory system, continue with the example from earlier in the chapter about patient Gordon Rothe, who was admitted to Branton Medical Center due to unstable angina.

Follow along in your ICD-10-CM manual as Tanisha sequences the codes. Check off each step after you complete it.

⇨ Tanisha reviews the codes she identified for this case:

- ❑ **I25.710, Atherosclerosis of autologous vein coronary artery bypass graft(s) with unstable angina pectoris**
- ❑ **I25.83, Coronary atherosclerosis due to lipid rich plaque**
- ❑ **Z72.0, Tobacco use**
- ❑ **Z79.01, Long term (current) use of anticoagulants**

⇨ Tanisha determines the principal diagnosis.

- ❑ She reviews the medical record for the reason for admission, which is documented as unstable angina.
- ❑ She reviews the reason that balloon angioplasty was performed, which is documented as atherosclerosis of grafted vessel.
- ❑ She confirms that **I25.710, Atherosclerosis of autologous vein coronary artery bypass graft(s) with unstable angina pectoris** meets the definition of principal diagnosis, which is "that condition established after study to be chiefly responsible for occasioning the admission of the patient to the hospital for care" (OGCR II).
- ❑ She double-checks the instructional note under code **I25.710** in the Tabular List that directs her to use **I25.83, Coronary atherosclerosis due to lipid rich plaque** as an *additional* code, meaning **I25.83** should *not* be the principal diagnosis.
- ❑ She double-checks the instructional note under code **I25.83** in the Tabular List that directs her to *Code first* a code from **I25.7-**, meaning that **I25.7.-** should be sequenced *before* **I25.83.**
- ❑ She also refers to OGCR I.C.9.b. which states:
  - If a patient with coronary artery disease is admitted due to an acute myocardial infarction (AMI), the AMI should be sequenced before the coronary artery disease.
- ❑ She determines that the guideline does not affect the sequencing because the patient did not have an AMI.
- ❑ Therefore, she is confident that **I25.710** is the principal diagnosis and **I25.83** is sequenced second.
- ❑ She sequences **Z72.0, Tobacco use** third because it was specified in an instructional note.
- ❑ She sequences **Z79.01, Long term (current) use of anticoagulants** as the final code.

⇨ Tanisha finalizes the codes and the sequencing for this case:

(1) **I25.710, Atherosclerosis of autologous vein coronary artery bypass graft(s) with unstable angina pectoris**

(2) **I25.83, Coronary atherosclerosis due to lipid rich plaque**

(3) **Z72.0, Tobacco use**

(4) **Z79.01, Long term (current) use of anticoagulants**

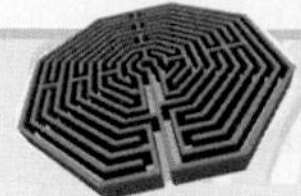

Coding Practice

Now it is your turn to practice sequencing codes for diseases of the circulatory system. Refer to the ***Tip:*** at the end of the mini-medical-record if you need a little extra help.

Exercise 14.4 Arranging Codes for the Circulatory System

Instructions: Read the mini-medical-record of each patient's encounter, review the information abstracted in Exercise 14.2 for questions 1 to 3. For questions 4 and 5, do the abstracting on your own. Assign ICD-10-CM diagnosis codes (CM) using the Index and Tabular List, and sequence them correctly.

1. Date: 4/4/yy Location: Branton Medical Center
Provider: Matthew Bunker, MD
Patient: Keisha Wier Gender: F Age: 71
Reason for admission: Admitted from emergency department with angina. Patient has history of MI 2 years ago, as well as history of TIAs, although the TIAs did not leave any residual deficits
Assessment: STEMI involving 90% occlusion of the right coronary artery
Procedure: CABG

Tip: Assign a Z code for history of TIA.

3 CM Codes __________ __________

____

2. Date: 4/4/yy Location: City Center Cardiology
Provider: Matthew Bunker, MD
Patient: Dustin Napper Gender: M Age: 65
Chief complaint: increased edema and SOB since last visit
Assessment: HTN and decompensated CHF, A-fib
Plan: We will start by adjusting the diuretic, then evaluate the need for other adjustments based on response after 4 weeks. Continue long term warfarin and clopidrogel (an antiplatelet medication).

Tip: Remember to assign Z codes for the long term use of the medications.

5 CM Codes __________ __________

__________ __________ __________

3. Date: 4/4/yy Location: Branton Medical Center Provider: Matthew Bunker, MD
Patient: Dennis Lehto Gender: M Age: 57
Reason for admission: transferred from Valley hospital where patient was admitted for cerebral infarct 20 hours ago and received tPA (tissue plasminogen activator), but now it is evident that a mechanical or surgical embolectomy is needed
Assessment: cerebral infarction d/t embolus in right middle cerebral artery, cerebral atherosclerosis, HTN, history of tobacco use
Procedure: surgical embolectomy

Tip: Remember to read the instructional notes at the beginning of the category and the beginning of the block in order to identify what you need Z codes for.

5 CM Codes __________ __________

__________ __________ __________

4. Date: 4/14/yy Location: City Center Cardiology Provider: Matthew Bunker, MD
Patient: Glenna Shirah Gender: F Age: 55
Reason for encounter: management of CHF and A-fib
Assessment: A-fib, chronic diastolic CHF
Plan: Refer to wound clinic for a stage 1 venous stasis ulcer on left thigh

Tip: You did not practice abstracting this case earlier, so see how you do on your own.

Use your resources if you need assistance in defining any terms or conditions.

3 CM Codes __________ __________

____

5. Date: 4/14/yy Location: Branton Medical Center Provider: Matthew Bunker, MD
Patient: Lewis Hubbs Gender: M Age: 45
Reason for admission: Admitted from emergency department with angina, SOB, tachycardia, hemoptysis. Undergoing treatment for DVT and
Assessment: pulmonary embolism, chronic DVT of left femoral vein

Tip: You did not practice abstracting this case earlier, so see how you do on your own.

2 CM Codes __________ __________

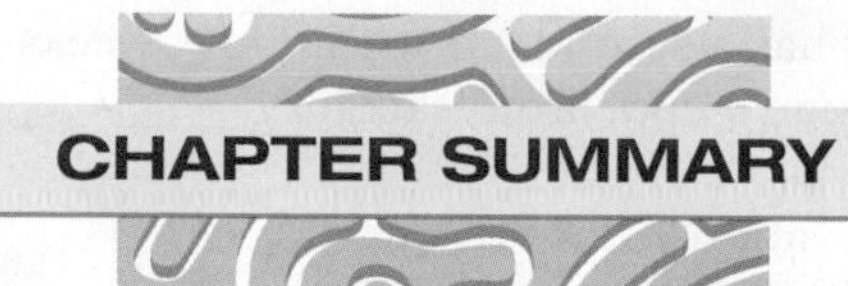

CHAPTER SUMMARY

In this chapter you learned that:

- The function of the circulatory system, also called the cardiovascular (CV) system, is to distribute blood throughout the body.
- ICD-10-CM Chapter 9, Diseases of the Circulatory System (I00-I99) contains 11 blocks or subchapters that are divided by the type of disease.
- Coders need to pay close attention to detail when abstracting for the CV system because they assign codes that are very specific to anatomic sites, nature of the disease, and comorbidities.
- Diseases of the circulatory system frequently occur with multiple comorbidities from within the cardiovascular system and/or from other systems; consequently, the choice of codes is dependent on the precise wording physicians use in the documentation.
- Sequencing of codes for multiples MIs depends on the circumstances of admission.
- ICD-10-CM provides Official Guidelines for Coding and Reporting (OGCR) for the circulatory system in OGCR section I.C.9. and provides detailed discussion regarding hypertension, atherosclerotic coronary artery disease and angina, cerebrovascular accident and disease, and acute myocardial infarction.

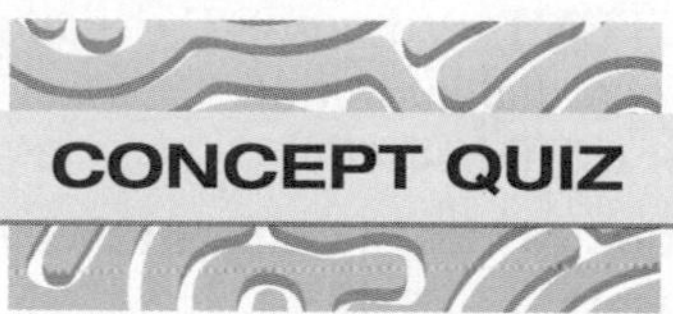

CONCEPT QUIZ

Take a moment to look back at your trip through the circulatory system and solidify your skills. This is your opportunity to pull together everything you have learned.

Completion

Instructions: Write the term that answers each question based on the information you learned in this chapter. Choose from the list below. Some choices may be used more than once and some choices may not be used at all. Refer to the discussion in this chapter and the Glossary at the end of this book if you need a little extra help.

angioplasty
arrhythmia
atherosclerosis
bypass graft
cardiac catheterization
cerebrovascular accident (CVA)
congestive heart failure (CHF)
days
deep vein thrombosis (DVT)
electrocardiography
embolectomy
embolus
endarterectomy
endocarditis
Holter monitor
ischemia
months
NSTEMI
STEMI
stenosis
weeks

1. Another term for arteriosclerotic heart disease (ASHD) is ______________.
2. The medical term for stroke is ______________.
3. A thrombus that has broken loose from its point of origin and circulates through the bloodstream is a/an ______________.
4. The inability of the heart to maintain circulation, often resulting in water retention and edema, is ______________.
5. The formation of a thrombus within a deep vein, usually in the leg or pelvis, is ______________.
6. Taking a vessel from another part of the body to create a new route around a blockage in a blood vessel is a/an ______________.
7. A myocardial infarction is classified as current or acute for four ______________.
8. A myocardial infarction that completely occludes a vessel is called ______________.
9. Removal of the diseased or damaged inner lining of an artery is a/an ______________.
10. A portable ECG worn by the patient for an extended period of hours or days to measure heart activity in a variety of situations is a/an ______________.

Multiple Choice

Instructions: Circle the letter of the best answer to each question based on the information you learned in this chapter. Refer to the discussion in this chapter and the Glossary at the end of this book if you need a little extra help.

1. Which of the following diagnostic statements states or implies a causal relationship?
   A. Chronic kidney disease and congestive heart failure
   B. Hypertensive heart disease
   C. Hypertension and heart disease
   D. STEMI and HTN
2. To locate acute myocardial infarction in the Index, you should search under the Main Term
   A. heart.
   B. acute.
   C. myocardial.
   D. infarction.
3. OGCR instructs coders to presume a causal relationship between hypertension and
   A. chronic kidney disease.
   B. acute myocardial infarction.
   C. congestive heart failure.
   D. chronic heart disease.
4. Assign a Z code for any of the following when they are present EXCEPT
   A. history of myocardial infarction.
   B. status post CABG.
   C. history of tobacco use.
   D. long term use of anticoagulant.
5. To locate congestive heart failure in the Index, you should search under the Main Term
   A. congestive.
   B. heart.
   C. failure.
   D. myocardial.
6. Which of the following is NOT a key criterion for abstracting circulatory system disorders?
   A. Is the condition acquired or congenital?
   B. What is the patient's alcohol use?
   C. Has the patient had more than one AMI in the past four weeks?
   D. Which conditions are documented as being related to the CV condition?
7. When a patient has a second MI within four weeks of another MI, assign a code from category ________ to the FIRST MI.
   A. I21.- ST elevation (STEMI) and non-ST elevation (NSTEMI) myocardial infarction
   B. I22.- Subsequent ST elevation (STEMI) and non-ST elevation (NSTEMI) myocardial infarction
   C. I23 Certain current complications following ST elevation (STEMI) and non-ST elevation (NSTEMI) myocardial infarction
   D. I25.2 Old myocardial infarction
8. When a patient has a second MI within four weeks of another MI, assign a code from category ________ to the SECOND MI.
   A. I21.- ST elevation (STEMI) and non-ST elevation (NSTEMI) myocardial infarction
   B. I22.- Subsequent ST elevation (STEMI) and non-ST elevation (NSTEMI) myocardial infarction
   C. I23 Certain current complications following ST elevation (STEMI) and non-ST elevation (NSTEMI) myocardial infarction
   D. I25.2 Old myocardial infarction
9. ________ circulation carries blood from the aorta to the tissues of the heart.
   A. Coronary
   B. Endocardial
   C. Pulmonary
   D. Systemic
10. Mitral, tricuspid, aortic, and pulmonary are
    A. coronary arteries.
    B. chambers of the heart.
    C. valves of the heart.
    D. types of myocardial infarction.

CODING CHALLENGE

Now it is your turn to demonstrate coding all aspects of diseases of the circulatory system. Refer back to the examples and discussion in this chapter when you need a little extra help. Use your medical dictionary and anatomy references when needed.

Instructions: Read the mini-medical-record of each patient's encounter, then abstract, assign, and sequence ICD-10-CM diagnosis codes (CM) using the Index and Tabular List. Write the code(s) on the line provided.

1. Date: 4/15/yy Location: Branton Medical Center

Provider: Matthew Bunker, MD

Patient: Wesley Orris Gender: M Age: 91

Reason for admission: arrived by ambulance to emergency department for severe abdominal pain

Assessment: ruptured abdominal aortic aneurysm

Discharge status: deceased

1 CM Code ___________

2. Date: 4/15/yy Location: Branton Medical Center Provider: Matthew Bunker, MD

Patient: Pedro Poulter Gender: M Age: 71

Reason for admission: admitted from emergency department for inferolateral STEMI.

Assessment: On the third day after admission, patient had a second STEMI in the same location.

Procedure: CABG x3

Tip: A CABG was performed to bypass three coronary arteries.

2 CM Codes ___________ ___________

3. Date: 4/15/yy Location: Branton Medical Center

Provider: Matthew Bunker, MD

Patient: Jolene Moorefield Gender: F Age: 59

Reason for admission: spells of dizziness, slow heart rate, and near fainting. Admitted for cardiac work up.

(continued)

3. (continued)

Assessment: EKG showed abnormal waves. Left anterior bundle branch block.

Plan: patient discharged with FU with cardiologist in 3 weeks

1 CM Code ___________

4. Date: 4/15/yy Location: Branton Medical Center Provider: Matthew Bunker, MD

Patient: Sam Necaise Gender: M Age: 42

Reason for admission: shortness of breath, generalized weakness, agitation, elevated BP, fever, rapid pulse, history of hyperthyroidism

Assessment: cardiomyopathy due to thyrotoxicosis with thyroid storm

Plan: Inhibit thyroid hormone synthesis with Methimazole. Beta blockers, body cooling, FU with cardiologist for cardiomyopathy management

2 CM Codes ___________ ___________

5. Date: 4/15/yy Location: Branton Medical Center

Provider: Matthew Bunker, MD

Patient: Leola Patt Gender: F Age: 26

Reason for admission: feet and ankle edema, chest pain, shortness of breath, fever

Assessment: pericarditis due to Staphylococcus aureus

Plan: Drain fluid from pericardial space, sensitivity testing for suitable antibiotic shows response to methicillin. FU 3 days after discharge

2 CM Codes ___________ ___________

(continued)

(continued from page 275)

6. Date: 4/15/yy Location: Branton Medical Center
Provider: Matthew Bunker, MD
Patient: Debora Gatling Gender: F Age: 66
Reason for admission: painful sore on left calf area, nausea, vomiting
Assessment: atherosclerosis of nonautologous biological bypass graft with ulceration of left calf with muscle necrosis
Plan: intravenous fluids, CBC, surgical debridement and re bypass graft, wound care. Visiting nurse scheduled daily upon discharge
2 CM Codes __________ __________

7. Date: 4/15/yy Location: Branton Medical Center
Provider: Matthew Bunker, MD
Patient: Roberto Salo Gender: M Age: 75
Reason for admission: angina pectoris with documented spasm
Assessment: CAD of grafted autologous artery following CABG 8 years ago, hypertensive chronic systolic with diastolic CHF
Plan: Oxygen, vasodilators, beta and calcium channel blockers, angioplasty with stent
3 CM Codes __________ __________ __________

8. Date: 4/15/yy Location: City Center Cardiology
Provider: Matthew Bunker, MD
Patient: Polly Racette Gender: F Age: 52
Chief complaint: dizziness upon sudden standing, temporary visual dimming, numbness and tingling in arms and hands
Assessment: orthostatic hypotension
Plan: BP to be checked daily and follow instructions related to life style changes (i.e. improve diet and exercise)
1 CM Code __________

9. Date: 4/15/yy Location: Branton Medical Center
Provider: Matthew Bunker, MD
Patient: Derrick Tacey Gender: M Age: 82
Reason for admission: left sided paralysis, inability to walk, inability to formulate words
Assessment: cerebral infarction due to embolism in right common carotid artery with pharyngeal dysphagia and left non-dominant hemiplegia
Plan: Rehab for mobility and speech, medication to address blood pressure issues. FU with primary care physician

Tip: The carotid artery is located in the neck.
4 CM Codes __________ __________ __________ __________

10. Date: 4/15/yy Location: Branton Medical Center Provider: Matthew Bunker, MD
Patient: Hector Barrie Gender: M Age: 47
Reason for admission: chest pain
Assessment: post-infarctional angina following LAD STEMI 2 weeks ago
Plan: FU 1 week
2 CM Codes __________ __________

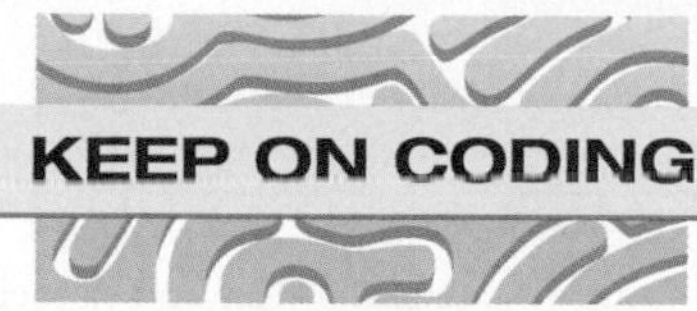

KEEP ON CODING

As a coder, you can never have too much experience. Apply everything you have learned in this chapter to code the following diagnostic statements. Use the OGCR and instructional notes in the Tabular List to help determine how many codes are required.

Instructions: Read the diagnostic statement, then use the Index and Tabular List to assign and sequence ICD-10-CM (CM) diagnosis codes. Write the code(s) on the line provided.

1. Rheumatic myocarditis: CM Code(s) ______
2. Acute cor pulmonale: CM Code(s) ______
3. Floppy nonrheumatic mitral valve syndrome: CM Code(s) ______
4. Non-ruptured cerebral aneurysm: CM Code(s) ______
5. Dissection of the iliac artery: CM Code(s) ______
6. Rupture of brachial artery: CM Code(s) ______
7. Postthrombotic syndrome, both legs with inflammation: CM Code(s) ______
8. Intraoperative cardiac arrest during cardiac surgery: CM Code(s) ______
9. Hypertensive heart and stage 3 chronic kidney disease without heart failure: CM Code(s) ______
10. Acute cerebral infarction, due to embolism of the posterior cerebral artery, left with tPA administered prior to admission: CM Code(s) ______
11. Variant angina with tobacco use: CM Code(s) ______
12. Intra-dialytic hypotension: CM Code(s) ______
13. Phlebitis of the right iliac vein: CM Code(s) ______
14. Acute mesenteric lymphadenitis: CM Code(s) ______
15. Portal vein obstruction: CM Code(s) ______
16. Esophageal varices with bleeding: CM Code(s) ______
17. Asymptomatic varicose veins of both legs: CM Code(s) ______
18. Malignant neoplasm of the abdominal aorta: CM Code(s) ______
19. ST elevation myocardial infarction involving the anterior wall: CM Code(s) ______
20. Alcoholic cardiomyopathy with alcohol abuse: CM Code(s) ______
21. Myocardial infarction (STEMI) of left anterior descending coronary artery with old myocardial infarction involving left main coronary artery: CM Code(s) ______
22. Second degree atrioventricular block, type I: CM Code(s) ______
23. Stuttering following a cerebral infarction, non-traumatic: CM Code(s) ______
24. Premature atrial beats: CM Code(s) ______
25. Chronic venous hypertension, both legs with inflammation: CM Code(s) ______

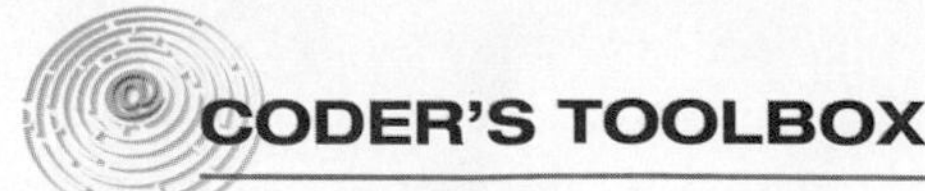

CODER'S TOOLBOX

The following resources are a starting point for learning more about the circulatory system. The > symbol indicates a menu selection within the website in order to navigate to a specific page.

American Heart Association http://www.heart.org/HEARTORG/

American Stroke Association http://www.strokeassociation.org/STROKEORG/

Cardio Source: American College of Cardiology (ACC) http://www.cardiosource.org/

Cardiology.org http://www.cardiology.org/

CardioSmart (American College of Cardiology) http://www.cardiosmart.org/default.aspx

Cardiovascular Physiology Concepts http://www.cvphysiology.com/index.html

Mayo Clinic > Diseases and Conditions > Heart disease http://www.mayoclinic.com/health/heart-disease/DS01120

Mayo Clinic > Tests and Procedures > Heart transplant http://www.mayoclinic.com/health/heart-transplant/MY00361

Multimedia Manual of Cardio Thoracic Surgery http://mmcts.ctsnetjournals.org/

New York University Cardiac and Vascular Institute > Video library http://cvi.med.nyu.edu/news/video-library

The Cardiothoracic Surgery Network http://www.ctsnet.org/

The Heart Surgery Forum http://www.hsforum.com/

The Society of Thoracic Surgeons http://www.sts.org/

15

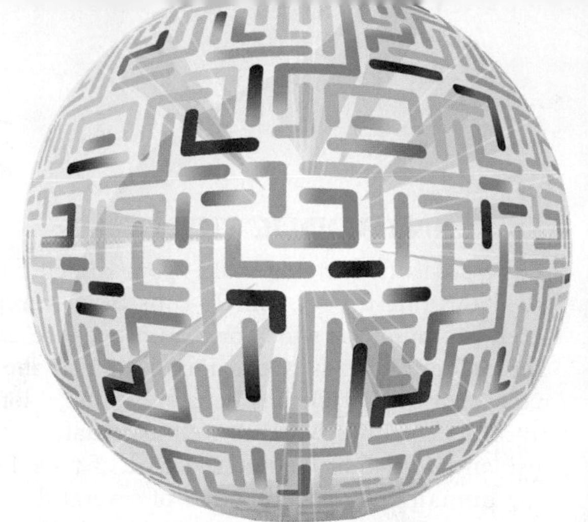

Diseases of the Blood and Blood-Forming Organs and Certain Disorders Involving the Immune Mechanism (D50-D89)

Learning Objectives

After completing this chapter, you should have the skills to:

- Spell and define the key words, medical terms, and abbreviations related to diseases of the blood and blood-forming organs.
- Discuss the structure, function, and common conditions of the blood and blood-forming organs.
- Identify the main characteristics of coding for diseases of the blood and blood-forming organs.
- Abstract diagnostic information from the medical record for coding diseases of the blood and blood-forming organs.
- Assign codes for diseases of the blood and blood-forming organs.
- Arrange codes for diseases of the blood and blood-forming organs.
- Code malignancies of the blood and blood-forming organs.
- Discuss the Official Guidelines for Coding and Reporting related to diseases of the blood and blood-forming organs.

Key Terms and Abbreviations

anemia
aplastic anemia
blood
bone marrow
erythrocytes
formed element
hemic system
hemoglobin (Hb)
hemolytic anemia
hemostasis
leukocytes
nutritional anemia
plasma
relapse
remission
thrombocytes
vasoocclusive crisis
white blood cell disorders

In addition to the key terms listed here, students should know the terms defined within tables in this chapter.

Chapter Outline

- **Blood Refresher**
- **Coding Overview of the Blood**
- **Abstracting for the Blood**
- **Assigning Codes for the Blood**
- **Arranging Codes for the Blood**
- **Coding Malignancies of the Blood**

ICD-10-CM codes in this chapter are from the ICD-10-CM 2014 Draft code set from the Department of Health and Human Services, Centers for Disease Control and Prevention.

INTRODUCTION

Gasoline is the fuel that makes your vehicle run. You need to determine if your vehicle runs best on regular grade fuel, premium, or super premium because each has different components. Occasionally, when the weather is cold or if the vehicle has been sitting for a long time, the gasoline may not work as well as usual, so you need to use an additive or change the type of fuel. The blood in the human body is comprised of several distinct components and, sometimes, they become out of balance and require medical attention.

In your tour of the blood and blood-forming organs in this chapter you will learn more about how the blood and blood-forming organs work, why sometimes they do not work as they should, and how physicians treat these conditions. Most importantly, you will practice coding for patient encounters related to diseases and conditions of the blood and blood-forming organs, a skill that requires you to abstract information from the mini-medical-record, assign correct codes, and arrange (sequence) the codes in the proper order.

A hematologist specializes in diagnosing and treating conditions of the blood and blood-forming organs. Hematologists may specialize in oncology and treat malignancies of the blood. Primary care physicians treat uncomplicated conditions of the blood and refer complex cases to a hematologist.

As you read this chapter, open up your medical terminology book to the chapter on the blood and keep a medical dictionary handy to refresh your memory of any unfamiliar terms. Think of these resources as travel brochures that tell you more about an area. This way, you have needed information at your fingertips, which will assist you in accurate code assignment.

BLOOD REFRESHER

The function of the **blood**, also called the **hemic system**, is to transport and pass nutrients, oxygen, carbon dioxide, water, proteins, and hormones to cells and to transport waste products to excretory organs. Blood consists of **plasma** (*clear fluid*) and **formed elements**, or blood cells. There are three types of blood cells, which are created in the **bone marrow** (*connective tissue in the cavities of bones*): **erythrocytes** (*red blood cells, RBC*), **leukocytes** (*white blood cells, WBC*), and **thrombocytes** (*platelets*) (■ FIGURE 15-1). Blood cells are named based on their appearance and ability to accept **stain** during lab testing (■ FIGURE 15-2). **Hemoglobin (Hb)** is the oxygen-carrying component of erythrocytes. The spleen destroys old erythrocytes, filters microorganisms from the blood, and serves as a reservoir for blood.

SUCCESS STEP

The spleen functions as part of both the hemic and digestive systems.

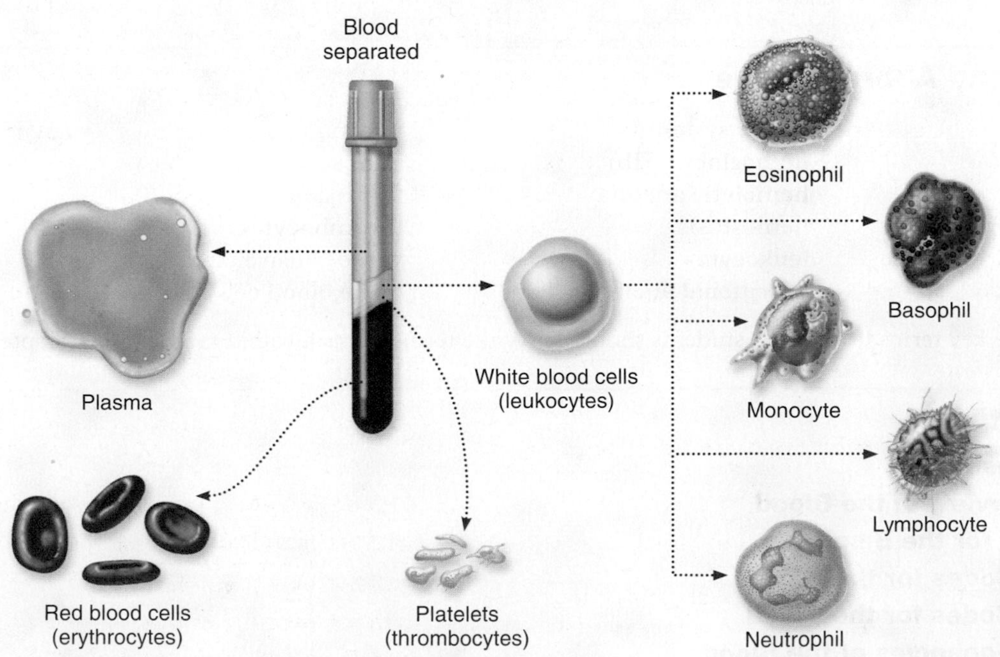

Figure 15-1 ■ Formed Elements of the Blood (Hemic System)

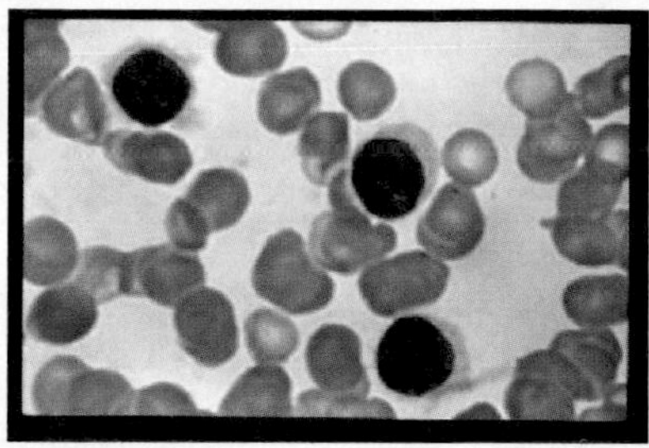

Figure 15-2 ■ Microscopic Image of a Stained Blood Cell.
Source: © National Institutes of Health.

In Figure 15-1, each component of blood is labeled with its name, which is based on the medical terminology root. As you learn about conditions and procedures that affect the hemic system, remember to apply medical terminology skills to combine word roots, prefixes, and suffixes you already know to define new terms. Refer to ■ TABLE 15-1 for a refresher on how to build medical terms related to the blood and lymphatic systems.

CODING CAUTION

Be alert for medical terms that are spelled similarly and have different meanings.

-emia (*blood condition*) and **-penia** (*lack of*)

hemostatis (*stoppage of bleeding*) and **homeostasis** (*the maintenance of a stable internal physical state*)

Conditions of the Blood

Diseases and disorders of the blood include anemias, hemostasis disorders, and white blood cell disorders. Coders use medical resources, such as a reference book on diseases, to understand conditions of the blood, diagnostic methods, and common treatments.

Anemia is a blood disorder characterized by a reduction in the number of red blood cells, which results in less oxygen reaching the tissues. Although there are over 400 different types of anemia, they are classified into the following three types:

- nutritional anemia—anemia due to malabsorption or poor dietary intake
- hemolytic anemia—anemia due to excessive loss of erythrocytes
- aplastic anemia—anemia due to loss of red bone marrow

Anemia can result as a complication of other diseases and treatments, including chronic kidney disease (CKD), malignant neoplasms, and antineoplastic therapy such as chemotherapy, radiotherapy, and immunotherapy.

Hemostasis disorders include a range of medical problems that lead to poor clotting and continuous bleeding. Causes include platelet dysfunction, vitamin K deficiency, and clotting factor deficiencies.

White blood cell disorders diminish the body's immune response and increase the risk of infection.

Common blood conditions are summarized in ■ TABLE 15-2 (page 282). Physicians diagnose blood disorders through blood tests, microscopic examination of blood cells, and bone marrow biopsy. Treatments include correction of nutritional deficiencies and other lifestyle changes, medication to correct the symptom or underlying problem, and transfusion of whole blood or a particular component of the blood.

This section provides a general reference to help understand the most common diagnoses of the blood, but does not list everything you need to know. Use medical terminology skills discussed earlier in this chapter to learn the meaning of unfamiliar words. Remember to keep standard reference books handy and refer to the resources in the Coder's Toolbox at the end of this chapter to learn more about conditions affecting the blood and blood-forming organs.

Table 15-1 ■ EXAMPLE OF CONSTRUCTING MEDICAL TERMS FOR THE HEMIC SYSTEM

Combining Form	Suffix	Complete Medical Term
hem/e, hemat/o (*blood*)	**-emia** (*blood condition*) **-penia** (*lack of*) **-cyte** (*cell*) **-phil** (*attraction*) **-poiesis** (*formation*)	**hemato + poiesis** (*formation of blood*) **an + emia** (*lack of blood condition*)
erythr/o- (*red*)		**erythro + cyte** (*red blood cell*) **erythro + cyto + penia** (*lack of red blood cells*) **erythro + poiesis** (*formation of red blood cells*)
leuk/o (*white*)		**leuko + cyte** (*white blood cell*) **leuko + penia** (*lack of white blood cells*) **leuk + emia** (*condition of white blood cells*)

Table 15-2 ■ **COMMON BLOOD CONDITIONS**

Condition	Description
Folic acid deficiency anemia	Anemia due to lack of **folic acid**
Hemophilia	A genetic disorder in which blood takes too long to clot
Hypogammaglobulinemia	A deficiency of gamma globulins (protein fraction) and antibodies in the blood
Iron deficiency anemia	Anemia due to insufficient iron to manufacture hemoglobin
Neutropenia	A decrease in neutrophils
Pancytopenia	An abnormal reduction in the number of all (medical prefix pan-) types of blood cells: red, white, and platelets
Pernicious anemia	Anemia due to insufficient absorption of Vitamin B12, which is necessary for erythrocyte production
Polycythemia	An abnormal increase in the number of circulating red blood cells
Purpura	Small hemorrhages in the skin
Sarcoidosis	Formation of nodules in the lymph nodes, lungs, bone, and skin
Sickle cell anemia	A genetic disorder in which red blood cells take on a sickle (curved) shape and lead to hemolytic anemia; also called sickle cell disease (SCD)
Thalessemia	A genetic disorder that results in defective formation of hemoglobin
Thrombophilia	A tendency to create blood clots (thrombi)
Von Willebrand's disease	A genetic disorder marked by bleeding of the mucosa

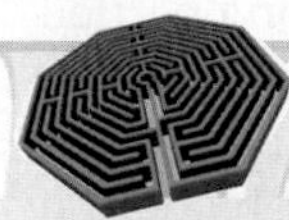

Coding Practice

Refresh your knowledge of terminology related to the blood and blood-forming organs. Use a medical terminology text or a website such as GlobalRph.com > Medical Terminology **http://www.globalrph.com/medterm.htm** to identify the meaning of word parts that may not be familiar.

Exercise 15.1 Refresher on the Blood

Instructions: Use your medical terminology skills and resources to define the following conditions related to the blood and blood-forming organs, then assign the diagnosis code. Follow these steps:

- Use slash marks "/" to break down each term into its root(s) and suffix.
- Define the meaning of the word, based on the meaning of each word part.
- Assign the default ICD-10-CM diagnosis code (CM) for the condition using the Index and Tabular List.

Example: leukemia leuk/emia Meaning: *disorder of white blood cells* CM Code: *C95.90*

1. hemophilia Meaning ____________ CM Code ________
2. neutropenia Meaning ____________ CM Code ________
3. thrombocytopenia Meaning ____________ CM Code ________
4. leukocytosis Meaning ____________ CM Code ________
5. eosinophilia Meaning ____________ CM Code ________
6. hemoglobinemia Meaning ____________ CM Code ________
7. panhematopenia Meaning ____________ CM Code ________
8. hemolymphangioma Meaning ____________ CM Code ________
9. erythroblastophthisis Meaning ____________ CM Code ________
10. leukoerythroblastosis Meaning ____________ CM Code ________

CODING OVERVIEW OF THE BLOOD

ICD-10-CM Chapter 3, Diseases of the Blood and Blood-Forming Organs and Certain Disorders Involving the Immune Mechanism (D50-D89), contains seven blocks or subchapters that are divided by type of condition. This chapter begins at D50, in the middle, rather than at the beginning, of a letter division. Review the block names and code ranges listed at the beginning of Chapter 3 in the ICD-10-CM manual to become familiar with the content and organization.

ICD-10-CM Chapter 3 is comparable to ICD-9-CM Chapter 4 (280-289) but also includes codes that were in ICD-9-CM Chapter 3, Endocrine, Nutritional and Metabolic Disorders, as well as some codes from ICD-9-CM Chapter 1, Infectious and Parasitic Diseases.

Many categories have been expanded to increase specificity. For example, ICD-9-CM had one code for thalassemia and ICD-10-CM has seven codes for specific types of thalassemia.

This ICD-10-CM chapter includes anemia due to nutritional deficiencies, hemolytic anemia, aplastic anemia, coagulation disorders, and disorders of blood-forming organs. It does not include infectious diseases, most diseases of the lymphatic system, or disorders of the circulatory system, all of which are classified in other ICD-10-CM chapters.

ICD-10-CM does not provide Official Guidelines for Coding and Reporting (OGCR) for this chapter. OGCR I.C.2.c.1) and 2) in the ICD-10-CM Chapter 2, Neoplasms, discuss the coding of anemia associated with malignancy, chemotherapy, radiotherapy, and immunotherapy. The Tabular List contains frequent instructional notes to use an additional code for associated conditions and to code first underlying diseases.

ABSTRACTING FOR THE BLOOD

Many of the conditions in this ICD-10-CM chapter can have multiple underlying causes and multiple manifestations. Therefore, coders should thoroughly abstract the symptoms, manifestations, and underlying causes documented in the medical record.

Some of these situations use combination codes, some require multiple coding, and others do not need to be coded because they are integral to the condition. For example, approximately 75 ICD-10-CM codes classify the different types of anemia. Closely related anemias are classified to the same code. Refer to ■ TABLE 15-3 for guidance on how to abstract conditions of the blood and blood-forming organs, then work through the detailed example that follows. Remember that the abstracting questions are a guide and that not every question applies to, or can be answered for, every case.

■ Table 15-3 KEY CRITERIA FOR ABSTRACTING CONDITIONS OF THE BLOOD

- ❑ What is the condition?
- ❑ What part of the hemic system does the condition involve?
- ❑ Is the condition acquired or congenital?
- ❑ Does the condition have an underlying cause?
- ❑ If anemia exists, is it due to a neoplasm or chronic disease?
- ❑ If sickle cell disease exists, what is the specific type?
- ❑ If sickle cell disease exists, is the patient in crisis?
- ❑ If sickle cell disease exists, does the patient have a fever?
- ❑ What symptoms are integral to the condition?
- ❑ What manifestations require an additional code?
- ❑ Is the condition drug-induced?

Guided Example of Abstracting for the Blood

Refer to the following example throughout this chapter to learn skills for abstracting, assigning, and sequencing codes for disorders of the blood and blood-forming organs. Scott Hood, CPC, is a fictitious coder who guides you through the coding process.

> Date: 05/11/yy Location: Branton Medical Center Emergency Department Provider: Robyn Akin, MD
>
> Patient: Douglas Ketron Gender: M Age: 10 months
>
> Reason for encounter: fever, cough, SOB, bilateral dactylitis (*painful and swollen hands and/or feet*)
>
> Assessment: vasoocclusive crisis and acute chest syndrome due to HbSS sickle cell disease (SCD)
>
> Plan: administer oxygen and IV antibiotics, then admit as inpatient

Follow along as Scott Hood, CPC, abstracts the diagnosis. Check off each step after you complete it.

⇨ Scott reads through the entire record, with special attention to the reason for the encounter and the final assessment. Scott reviews all the medical terms in the documentation to be sure he understands the case.

- ❑ He knows from his experience at East Side Hematology that **vasoocclusive crisis** is a form of **sickle cell crisis** in which the patient experiences severe pain due to infarctions, and that the pain may occur in nearly any location (■ FIGURE 15-3, page 284).

Hemoglobin S and Red Blood Cell Sickling

Sickle cell anemia is caused by an inherited autosomal recessive defect in Hb synthesis. Sickle cell hemoglobin (HbS) differs from normal hemoglobin only in the substitution of the amino acid valine for glutamine in both beta chains of the hemoglobin molecule.

When HbS is oxygenated, it has the same globular shape as normal hemoglobin. However, when HbS loses its oxygen, it becomes insoluble in intracellular fluid and crystallizes into rodlike structures. Clusters of rods form polymers (long chains) that bend the erythrocyte into the characteristic crescent shape of the sickle cell.

Incorrect amino acids

β chains

Hemoglobin S molecule

α chains

Polymerized deoxyhemoglobin S

Oxyhemoglobin S

O_2

Deoxyhemoglobin S

Oxygenated erythrocyte

Deoxygenated erythrocyte

Sickled erythrocyte

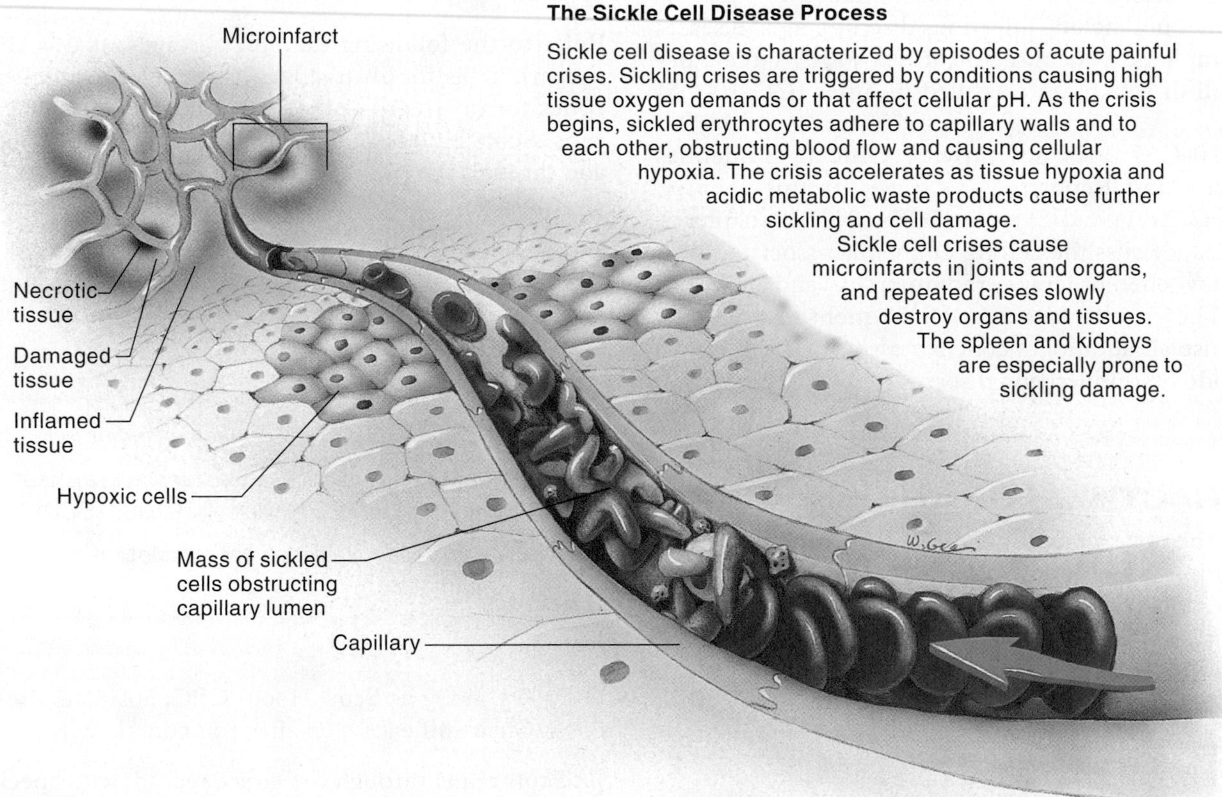

Figure 15-3 ■ How Sickle Cell Disease Affects the Patient. *Source: Pearson Education/PH College.*

❑ He is also aware that acute chest syndrome (ACS) is a group of symptoms, often due to a bacterial infection or lung infarction, seen in patients with SCD and can bring on a vasoocclusive crisis.

❑ He notes the presenting symptoms of fever, cough, SOB, and bilateral dactylitis

⇨ Scott refers to the Key Criteria for Abstracting Conditions of the Blood (Table 15-3).

❑ *What is the condition?* vasoocclusive crisis and acute chest syndrome

❑ *What part of the hemic system does the condition involve?* circulation

- ❑ *Is the condition acquired or congenital?* Sickle cell is congenital.
- ❑ Does the condition have an underlying cause? sickle cell disease
- ❑ *If anemia exists, is it due to a neoplasm or chronic disease?* Not applicable.
- ❑ *If sickle cell disease exists, what is the specific type?* HbSS
- ❑ *If sickle cell disease exists, is the patient in crisis?* Yes, vasoocclusive crisis.
- ❑ *If sickle cell disease exists, does the patient have a fever?* Yes.
- ❑ *What symptoms are integral to the condition?* fever, cough, SOB are symptoms of ACS, dactylitis is a manifestation of SCD.
- ❑ *What manifestations require an additional code?* fever
- ❑ *Is the condition drug-induced?* No.

SUCCESS STEP

At the time of initial abstracting, it may not be clear that a separate code for fever is required, but it will become clear later when assigning codes in the Tabular List. That is the reason the abstracting questions specifically ask about fever with sickle cell crisis.

⇨ Scott double-checks the medical record to be certain that he has identified all of the symptoms, conditions, and manifestations.

⇨ At this point, Scott has abstracted the information he needs, but he is still unsure of how many codes he will need for this case. He knows that he will need to research the Index and Tabular List to learn what combination codes are available for this case.

Coding Practice

Now it is your turn to practice abstracting diagnoses for diseases of the blood and blood-forming organs. Questions guide your analysis of each scenario.

Exercise 15.2 Abstracting for the Blood

Instructions: Read the mini-medical-record of each patient's encounter and answer the abstracting questions. Write the answer on the line provided. Do not assign any codes.

1. Date: 5/13/yy Location: East Side Hematology
Provider: Robyn Akin, MD
Patient: Alan Swafford Gender: M Age: 81
Chief complaint: referred by family physician for reduction in lymphocyte count which appeared on lab results for annual physical
Assessment: lymphocytopenia
Plan: further testing to determine underlying cause

a. What is the reason for referral? ________________

____

b. What is the diagnosis? ________________

____

c. Should you code the abnormal lab results? __________ Why or why not? ________________

____

2. Date: 5/13/yy Location: Branton Family Practice Provider: Kristen Conover, MD
Patient: Juanita Calzada Gender: F Age: 35
Reason for encounter: numbness in extremities, nausea and vomiting
Assessment: pernicious anemia
Plan: vitamin B-12 injections, refer to hematologist

a. What are the symptoms and signs? ________________

____

b. What is the diagnosis? ________________

____

c. Are the symptoms and signs integral to the diagnosis? ________________

____

d. Should you code for the symptoms? ________________

3. Date: 5/13/yy Location: East Side Hematology
Provider: Robyn Akin, MD
Patient: Eugene Albert Gender: M Age: 52
Reason for encounter: referred by family physician for pain and swelling in LUQ
Assessment: splenomegaly due to splenitis
Plan: schedule splenectomy ASAP

(continued)

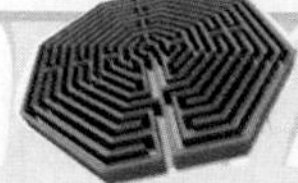

Coding Practice (continued)

3. (continued)

a. What are the symptoms? ______

b. What is splenomegaly? ______

c. What is splenitis? ______

d. What is a splenectomy? ______

e. Where is the spleen located? ______

f. What condition should you code for? ______

4. Date: 5/14/yy Location: Branton Medical Center Provider: Robyn Akin, MD

Patient: Sheri Chapin Gender: F Age: 59

Reason for admission: weakness, fatigue, confusion

Assessment: anemia due to chemotherapy for metastatic colon cancer

a. What are the symptoms? ______

b. Are the symptoms integral to anemia? ______

c. What is the cause of the anemia? ______

d. What is the primary cancer site? ______

e. What is metastatic cancer? ______

f. What condition should be sequenced first? ______

g. What condition should be sequenced second? ______

h. What condition should be sequenced third? ______

5. Date: 5/14/yy Location: Branton Medical Center Provider: Robyn Akin, MD

Patient: Edward Reid Gender: M Age: 61

(continued)

5. (continued)

Reason for admission: tachycardia, headaches, fatigue

Assessment: anemia in due to stage 3 chronic kidney disease

Plan: erythropoiesis stimulating agents (ESAs), supplemental iron

a. What are the symptoms? ______

b. What is the diagnosis? ______

c. Are the symptoms integral to the diagnosis? ______

d. What is the underlying condition? ______

e. Which condition is the principal diagnosis? ______

f. What is the additional diagnosis? ______

6. Date: 5/14/yy Location: Branton Family Practice Provider: Kristen Conover, MD

Patient: Michelle Harper Gender: F Age: 50

Reason for encounter: follow up on glucose tolerance test (GTT) and complete chemistry analysis

Assessment: hyperglycemia due to pre-diabetes, lab result also indicate iron (Fe)-deficiency anemia

Plan: manage pre-diabetes with 1,500 calorie diabetic diet, Rx Fe supplements

a. What is hyperglycemia? ______

b. Should both hyperglylcemia and pre-diabetes be coded? ______

Why or why not? ______

c. Should anemia be coded? ______

Why or why not? ______

d. What type of anemia is present? ______

e. What should be the first-listed diagnosis? ______

f. What is the additional diagnosis? ______

ASSIGNING CODES FOR THE BLOOD

When an ICD-10-CM chapter does not have any OGCR, as is the case with diseases of the blood and blood-forming organs, coders apply the general OGCR (I.A, I.B, II, and III) and follow instructional notes in the Tabular List. When coders conduct thorough abstracting, they are poised to assign codes correctly.

Most types of anemia are indexed under the Main Term **Anemia,** followed by subterms that identify the specific type. Because the Index contains over 350 subterms for **Anemia,** remember to search them carefully to locate the most specific code. Refer to ■ FIGURE 15-4 for a sample Index entry showing how to locate aplastic anemia due to drugs.

SUCCESS STEP

Anemia of newborns and anemia related to pregnancy are not classified in this chapter. ICD-10-CM has separate chapters for conditions of the newborn and pregnancy-related conditions. To locate the codes for anemia of the newborn, search the Main Term **Anemia,** and subterm **newborn.** To locate codes for anemia in pregnancy, search the Main Term, **Pregnancy** and subterm **complicated by anemia.**

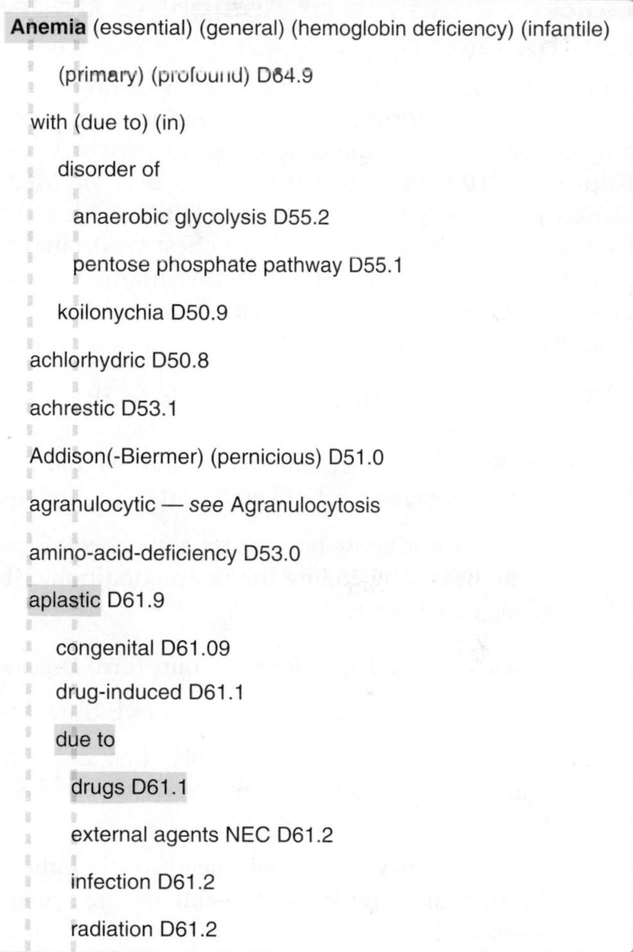

Anemia (essential) (general) (hemoglobin deficiency) (infantile)
(primary) (profound) D64.9
with (due to) (in)
disorder of
anaerobic glycolysis D55.2
pentose phosphate pathway D55.1
koilonychia D50.9
achlorhydric D50.8
achrestic D53.1
Addison(-Biermer) (pernicious) D51.0
agranulocytic — *see* Agranulocytosis
amino-acid-deficiency D53.0
aplastic D61.9
congenital D61.09
drug-induced D61.1
due to
drugs D61.1
external agents NEC D61.2
infection D61.2
radiation D61.2

Figure 15-4 ■ Index Entry for Aplastic Anemia Due to Drugs

Anemia is often associated with cancer and may be caused by the disease itself or by adjunct therapy such as chemotherapy, radiotherapy, or immunotherapy. Review the documentation carefully to clearly identify the cause. Chemotherapy may cause anemia or aplastic anemia, which is a result of bone marrow not producing erythrocytes, and each has separate codes (■ TABLE 15-4). Information about multiple coding for anemia in cancer patients is discussed later in this chapter.

Anemia may be caused by other drugs, in addition to chemotherapy. Drugs such as nonsteriodal anti-inflammatory drugs (NSAIDs) can cause bleeding which, in turn, causes anemia. Drugs that suppress the immune system can cause anemia because the hemapoetic function of the bone marrow is suppressed. Other drugs, such as certain antibiotics, **antihypertensives,** and **antiarrythmics,** can occasionally destroy erythrocytes prematurely, causing hemolytic anemia. When anemia is drug-induced, the Tabular List instructs coders to assign an external cause code for the substance. Use the Table of Drugs and Chemicals to locate the substance and intent.

Anemia may also be caused by CKD, in which case an additional code to identify the stage of kidney disease is required.

Table 15-4 ■ **ANEMIA CODES FOR CANCER PATIENTS**

Cause of Anemia	Code Assignment
Anemia due to the cancer itself	D63.0 Anemia in neoplastic disease
Aplastic anemia due to chemotherapy	D61.1 Drug-induced aplastic anemia
Other anemia due to chemotherapy	D64.81 Anemia due to antineoplastic chemotherapy

SUCCESS STEP

Refer to OGCR I.C.19.e. to review the definitions of each intent column in the Table of Drugs and Poisonings.

Guided Example of Assigning Codes for the Blood

To practice skills for assigning codes for disorders of the blood and blood-forming organs, continue with the example from earlier in the chapter about patient Douglas Ketron, age 10 months, who was seen in Branton Medical Center Emergency Department with HbSS sickle cell disease, vasoocclusive crisis, and acute chest syndrome.

Follow along in your ICD-10-CM manual as Scott Hood, CPC, assigns codes. Check off each step after you complete it.

⇨ First, Scott confirms the diagnosis in the medical record: *HbSS sickle cell with vasoocclusive crisis* and *acute chest syndrome*; and the symptoms and manifestations: *fever*, *cough*, *SOB*, and *bilateral dactylitis*.

- ❑ He does not know how many codes he will need, so he begins by coding the main condition, HbSS sickle cell disease.

⇨ Scott searches the Index for the Main Term **Disease**.

- ❑ He locates the subterm **sickle-cell** (■ FIGURE 15-5).
- ❑ He reviews the second-level subterms and notices that there are subterms for several types of SCD, but not HbSS.
- ❑ He determines that he will need to use either the default entry under **sickle-cell** or the entry for **specified NEC**, but he will not know for sure until he gets to the Tabular List.
- ❑ Scott reviews the subterms under **sickle-cell** and locates a third-level subterm **with crisis (vasoocclusive pain)**.
- ❑ He locates an additional fourth-level subterm **with** that provides a combination code for **acute chest syndrome D57.01**.

⇨ Scott verifies code **D57.01** in the Tabular List.

- ❑ He verifies the code title **D57.01, Hb-SS disease with acute chest syndrome**, and confirms that this accurately describes the diagnosis.

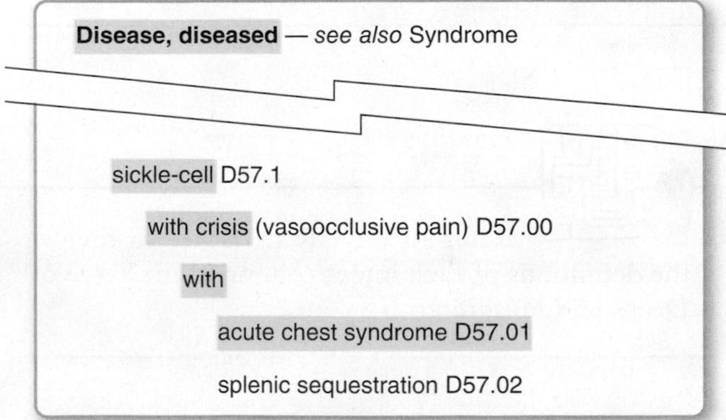

Figure 15-5 ■ Index Entry Showing a Combination Code for Sickle Cell Disease with Crisis and Acute Chest Syndrome

- ❑ He notes that the Tabular List specifies the **D57.0-** category includes HbSS, so he is in the right place and does not need to locate the code for **Other specified sickle cell, NEC** that he had considered in the Index.
- ❑ He also verifies that this is a combination code for SCD, vasoocclusive crisis, and acute chest syndrome, so he does not need to assign additional codes for vasoocclusive crisis or ACS.

⇨ Scott checks for instructional notes in the Tabular List.

- ❑ He cross-references the beginning of category **D57** and reads the instructional note that states **Use additional code for any associated fever (R50.81)** (■ FIGURE 15-6).
- ❑ Before looking up the code for fever, Scott completes the verification of **D57.01**. He cross-references the beginning of the block **Hemolytic anemias (D55-D59)** and verifies that there are no instructional notes.
- ❑ He then cross-references the beginning of **Chapter 3 (D50-D89)** and verifies that there are no instructional notes.

⇨ Now Scott verifies the code for fever contained in the first instructional note, **R50.81.**

- ❑ He verifies the code title **R50.81, Fever presenting with conditions classified elsewhere**, and confirms that this accurately describes the fever.
- ❑ He recognizes that the code is from ICD-10-CM Chapter 18, Symptoms, Signs and Abnormal Clinical and Laboratory Findings, Not Elsewhere Classified (R00-R99). He normally would hesitate to assign a code for a sign with a confirmed diagnosis that includes the three main conditions. However, because the instructional note directs him to assign a code for fever, if present, he knows he should assign it. He knows that fever is a sign of infection and that infection is a life-threatening event for a patient with SCD.

⇨ Scott is unsure if he needs to assign a code for bilateral dactylitis, so he researches this condition in the Index and Tabular List.

- ❑ He locates the Index Main Term for **Dactylitis.**
- ❑ The subterms **sickle cell**, then **HbSS** lead him to **D57.00.**
- ❑ He instantly recognizes that **D57.00** is from the same category as his previous code, **D57.01.**
- ❑ He verifies **D57.00** in the Tabular List and reads the code title **Hb-SS disease with crisis, unspecified.**

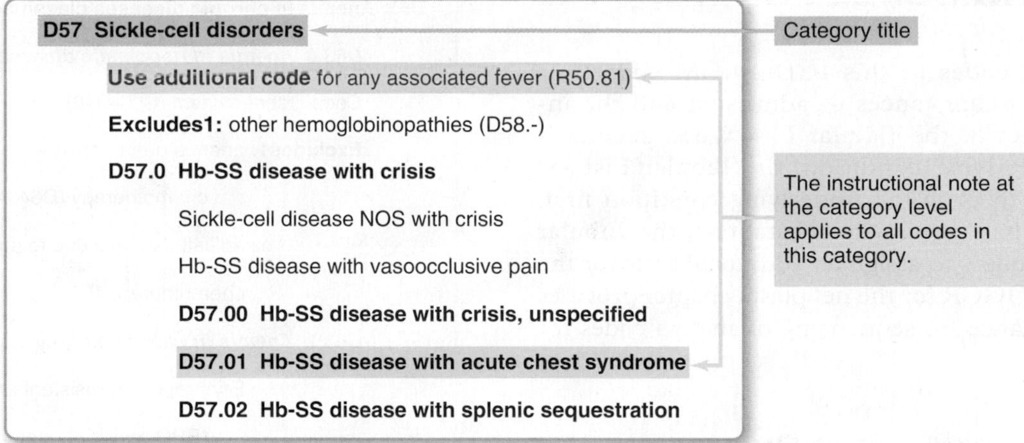

Figure 15-6 ■ Instructional Note at the Category Level in the Tabular List to Use Additional Code

- ❑ This confirms his thinking that dactylitis is a manifestation of SCD crisis. Because he has already identified **D57.01**, which is a *more specific code* for SCD crisis, he does not also assign **D57.00**. **D57.00** is a code with unspecified manifestations, so it adds no further information (OGCR I.A.9.b).

➩ Scott reviews the codes he has assigned for this case:

- ❑ **R50.81, Fever presenting with conditions classified elsewhere**
- ❑ **D57.01, Hb-SS disease with acute chest syndrome**

➩ Next, Scott needs to confirm the sequencing.

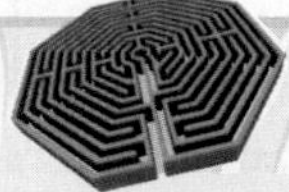

Coding Practice

Now it is your turn to practice assigning codes for diseases of the blood and blood-forming organs. Refer to the ***Tip*** at the end of the mini-medical-record if you need a little extra help.

Exercise 15.3 Assigning Codes for the Blood

Instructions: Read the mini-medical-record of each patient's encounter, review the information abstracted in Exercise 15.2, and assign ICD-10-CM diagnosis codes (CM) using the Index and Tabular List. Write the code(s) on the line provided.

1. Date: 5/13/yy Location: East Side Hematology
Provider: Robyn Akin, MD
Patient: Alan Swafford Gender: M Age: 81
Chief complaint: referred by family physician for reduction in lymphocyte count which appeared on lab results for annual physical
Assessment: lymphocytopenia
Plan: further testing to determine underlying cause

Tip: The name of the condition is the Main Term.
1 CM Code ___________

2. Date: 5/13/yy Location: Branton Family Practice Provider: Kristen Conover, MD
Patient: Juanita Calzada Gender: F Age: 35
Reason for encounter: numbness in extremities, nausea and vomiting
Assessment: pernicious anemia
Plan: vitamin B-12 injections, refer to hematologist

Tip: Look for the Main Term anemia, then look for the subterm that identifies the type of anemia.
1 CM Code ___________

3. Date: 5/13/yy Location: East Side Hematology
Provider: Robyn Akin, MD
Patient: Eugene Albert Gender: M Age: 52
Reason for encounter: referred by family physician for pain and swelling in LUQ
Assessment: splenomegaly due to splenitis
Plan: schedule splenectomy ASAP
1 CM Code ___________

ARRANGING CODES FOR THE BLOOD

Sequencing of codes in this ICD-10-CM chapter is based on the circumstances of admission and the instructional notes in the Tabular List. When anemia is due to an underlying condition, the Tabular List instructs coders to code the underlying condition first. When anemia has certain manifestations, the Tabular List instructs coders to assign an additional code for the manifestation. OGCR for the neoplasm chapter provides additional guidance for sequencing of anemia codes for cancer patients.

Admission for Anemia Due to Neoplastic Disease

Patients with a malignancy and anemia may be admitted in order to treat the neoplasm or in order to treat the anemia. Assign and sequence codes in the same way for both situations. Assign and sequence codes as follows (OGCR I.C.2.c.1)):

1. Assign a code for the neoplasm.
2. Assign code **D63.0 Anemia in neoplastic disease** for the anemia.

Notice that the Tabular List entry for **D63.0 Anemia in neoplastic disease** is highlighted in blue with an italic typeface. The key at the bottom of the page indicates that codes highlighted in blue are manifestation codes, which are never to be sequenced as the first-listed or principal diagnosis (OGCR I.A.13) (■ FIGURE 15-7).

D63 Anemia in chronic diseases classified elsewhere

D63.0 Anemia in neoplastic disease

Code first neoplasm (C00-D49)

Excludes1: anemia due to antineoplastic chemotherapy (D64.81)

aplastic anemia due to antineoplastic chemotherapy (D61.1)

D63.1 Anemia in chronic kidney disease

Erythropoietin resistant anemia (EPO resistant anemia)

Code first underlying chronic kidney disease (CKD) (N18.-)

Manifestation Code

Figure 15-7 ■ Tabular List Convention for a Manifestation Code

CODING CAUTION

Sequencing guidelines for anemia in neoplastic disease are different in ICD-10-CM than they were in ICD-9-CM. In ICD-10-CM, always sequence the anemia *after* the neoplasm code, even when the reason for the encounter is treatment of the anemia.

Admission for Anemia Due to Chemotherapy or Immunotherapy

When the admission or encounter is for management of an anemia associated with an adverse effect of chemotherapy or immunotherapy and the *only* treatment is for the anemia, assign and sequence codes as follows (OGCR I.C.2.c.2)):

1. Assign a code for the anemia.
2. Assign a code for the neoplasm.
3. Assign a code for the adverse effect from the Table of Drugs and Chemicals.

SUCCESS STEP

Although code **D64.81 Anemia due to antineoplastic chemotherapy** may appear to be a combination code that includes the external cause, it is not. You must assign an external cause code from the Table of Drugs and Chemicals when using this code.

Admission for Anemia Due to Radiotherapy

When the admission or encounter is for management of an anemia associated with an adverse effect of radiotherapy, assign and sequence codes as follows (OGCR I.C.2.c.2)):

1. Assign a code for the anemia.
2. Assign a code for the neoplasm.
3. Assign an external cause code for the complication, **Y84.2 Radiological procedure and radiotherapy as the cause of abnormal reaction of the patient, or of later complication, without mention of misadventure at the time of the procedure.**

CODING CAUTION

Notice that when the admission or encounter is for management of an anemia associated with an adverse effect of radiotherapy, anemia is sequenced first. This sequencing is different than when anemia is due to the neoplasm itself.

Admission for Adjunct Therapy

When the admission or encounter is for the purpose of administering adjunct therapy and the patient develops anemia *during* the encounter, assign and sequence codes as follows (OGCR I.C.2.e.3)):

1. Assign the appropriate Z code for the therapy encounter:
   a. **Z51.11 Encounter for antineoplastic chemotherapy**
   b. **Z51.12 Encounter for antineoplastic immunotherapy**
   c. **Z51.0 Antineoplastic radiation therapy**
2. When the encounter is for chemotherapy or immunotherapy, assign a code for the adverse effect from the Table of Drugs and Chemicals.
3. Assign a code for the anemia (See Table 15-4).
4. Assign a code for the neoplasm.
5. If the encounter was for radiotherapy, assign code **Y84.2.**

Guided Example of Arranging Codes for the Blood

To practice skills for sequencing codes for disorders of the blood and blood-forming organs, continue with the example from earlier in the chapter about patient Douglas Ketron, age 10 months, who was seen in Branton Medical Center Emergency Department with HbSS sickle cell disease, vasoocclusive crisis, and acute chest syndrome.

Follow along in your ICD-10-CM manual as Scott sequences the codes. Check off each step after you complete it.

⇨ First, Scott confirms the diagnosis codes he believes should be assigned:

- ❑ **R50.81, Fever presenting with conditions classified elsewhere**
- ❑ **D57.01, Hb-SS disease with acute chest syndrome**

⇨ Scott needs to cross-reference back to the Tabular List to read the sequencing instructions.

- ❑ Scott reads the instructional note that appears in the Tabular List under code **R50.81.** The note states **Code first underlying condition when associated fever is present, such as with: sickle cell disease (D57.-)** (■ FIGURE 15-8).
  - This instruction tells him that SCD should be sequenced first.
- ❑ Scott double-checks the Tabular List entry for code **D57.01.**
  - He is reminded of the instructional note at the beginning of category **D57,** which states **Use additional code for any associated fever (R50.81).**
  - This note confirms that the code for the fever should be sequenced as an additional, or second, code after the code for SCD.

⇨ Scott finalizes the codes and sequencing for this case:

(1) **D57.01, Hb-SS disease with acute chest syndrome**

(2) **R50.81, Fever presenting with conditions classified elsewhere**

R50.8 Other specified fever

R50.81 Fever presenting with conditions classified

elsewhere

Code first underlying condition when associated

fever is present, such as with:

leukemia (C91-C95)

neutropenia (D70.-)

sickle cell disease (D57.-)

Figure 15-8 ■ Instructional Note in the Tabular List to Code First

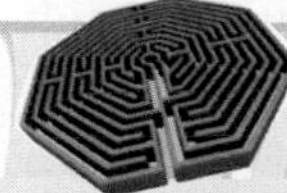

Coding Practice

Now it is your turn to practice sequencing codes for diseases of the blood and blood-forming organs. Refer to the ***Tip*** at the end of the mini-medical-record if you need a little extra help.

Exercise 15.4 Arranging Codes for the Blood

Instructions: Read the mini-medical-record of each patient's encounter, review the information abstracted in Exercise 15.2, assign ICD-10-CM diagnosis codes (CM) using the Index and Tabular List, and sequence them correctly.

1. Date: 5/14/yy Location: Branton Medical Center Provider: Robyn Akin, MD

Patient: Sheri Chapin Gender: F Age: 59

Reason for admission: *weakness, fatigue, confusion*

Assessment: *new anemia due to chemotherapy for metastatic colon cancer*

(continued)

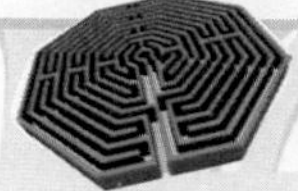

Coding Practice (continued)

1. (continued)

Tip: Read the instructional notes in the Tabular List and refer to OGCR I.C.2c.1) to identify all codes needed and the sequencing.

3 CM Codes __________ __________ __________

2. Date: 5/14/yy Location: Branton Medical Center Provider: Robyn Akin, MD

Patient: Edward Reid Gender: M Age: 61

Reason for admission: tachycardia, headaches, fatigue

Assessment: anemia in due to stage 3 chronic kidney disease

Plan: erythropoiesis stimulating agents (ESAs), supplemental iron

(continued)

2. (continued)

Tip: Read the instructional notes in the Tabular List for sequencing guidance.

2 CM Codes __________ __________

3. Date: 5/14/yy Location: Branton Family Practice Provider: Kristen Conover, MD

Patient: Michelle Harper Gender: F Age: 50

Reason for encounter: follow up on glucose tolerance test (GTT) and complete chemistry analysis

Assessment: hyperglycemia due to pre-diabetes, lab result also indicate iron (Fe)-deficiency anemia

Plan: manage pre-diabetes with 1,500 calorie diabetic diet, Rx Fe supplements

Tip: The main focus of the visit is pre-diabetes.

2 CM Codes __________ __________

CODING MALIGNANCIES OF THE BLOOD

Malignancies of the blood and blood-forming organs do not appear in ICD-10-CM Chapter 3, Diseases of the Blood and Blood-Forming Organs and Certain Disorders Involving the Immune Mechanism (D50-D89). Codes for malignancies of the blood and blood-forming organs appear in block C81 to C96 within the neoplasm chapter.

Neoplasms, which are solid tumors, do not form in the blood, so there is no entry for blood in the Table of Neoplasms. However, hematological malignancies do affect blood, bone marrow, and lymph nodes. Leukemia and myeloma, which begin in the bone marrow, and lymphoma, which begins in the lymphatic system, are the most common types of blood cancer. The blood is also one of the primary vehicles for metastasis of malignant neoplasms in any organ because it circulates through all organs and body tissues.

Lymphomas, leukemias, and myelomas are named based on the type of cell affected and whether the disease begins in mature or immature cells, so coders must be attentive to the exact name of the malignancy. Examples include the following:

- anaplastic large cell lymphoma
- ALK-negative or acute myeloid leukemia with 11q23-abnormality
- multiple myeloma

Acute myeloid leukemia (AML) and chronic lymphocytic leukemia (CML) are the most common leukemias, according to the Leukemia and Lymphoma Society, and increase significantly in adults over age 55. Leukemia is the most common type of cancer in children, accounting for over 27% of childhood cancer. Acute lymphoblastic leukemia (ALL) accounts for 65% of acute leukemias in children, according to the Children's Cancer Research Fund.

To locate codes, search the Index for the Main Term that describes the condition, such as **Lymphoma**, **Leukemia**, or **Myeloma**. Then search for subterms that describe the type and location. Do not search the Table of Neoplasms unless the Index directs you to do so.

Each type of leukemia has three separate codes based on the status of the disease, as follows (OGCR I.C.2.n):

- not having achieved **remission** (*the blood counts return to normal and bone marrow samples show no sign of disease*), final digit of **0**
- in remission, final digit of **1**
- in **relapse** (*the return of the disease after remission*), final digit of **2**

When the medical record does not specifically document the status of the disease, assign a code for **not having achieved remission** because the Tabular List classifies

leukemia NOS under the codes for **leukemia, not having achieved remission** (■ FIGURE 15-9). Also assign a code for **not having achieved remission** when leukemia is documented as *failed remission*.

CODING CAUTION

Remember to distinguish between remission and a personal history of the disease. Personal history defines a condition that no longer exists and is not receiving treatment, but has the potential for recurrence, and therefore may require continued monitoring (OGCR I.C.21.c.4)). If the documentation is unclear whether the patient is in remission, query the provider (OGCR I.C.2.n).

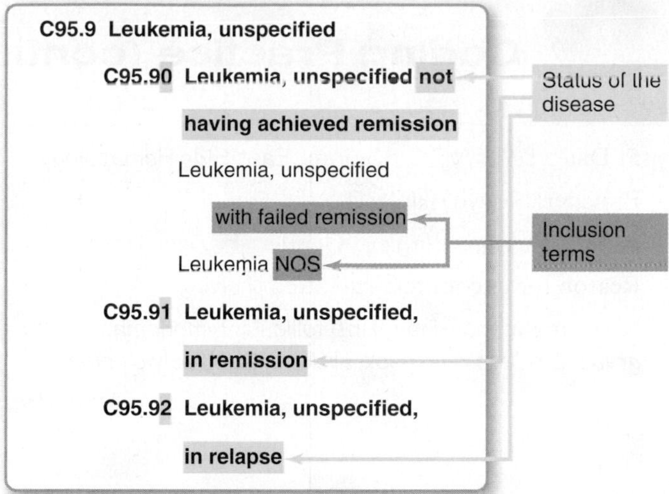

Figure 15-9 ■ Tabular List Entry for Leukemia Showing Separate Codes for the Status of the Disease

Coding Practice

Now it is your turn to practice coding malignancies of the blood and blood-forming organs. Refer to the ***Tip*** at the end of the mini-medical-record if you need a little extra help.

Exercise 15.5 Coding Malignancies of the Blood

Instructions: Read the mini-medical-record of each patient's encounter, then abstract, assign, and sequence ICD-10-CM diagnosis codes (CM) using the Index and Tabular List. Write the code(s) on the line provided.

1. Date: 5/15/yy Location: Branton Medical Center Provider: Robyn Akin, MD

Patient: Derek Micheals Gender: M Age: 78

Reason for admission: induction chemotherapy

Assessment: acute myeloid leukemia M7

Tip: Acute myeloid leukemia has eight subtypes. The goal of induction chemotherapy is to achieve remission.

2 CM Codes __________ __________

2. Date: 5/15/yy Location: Branton Medical Center Provider: Robyn Akin, MD

Patient: Laurel Fargo Gender: F Age: 65

Reason for admission: chemotherapy

(continued)

2. (continued)

Assessment: early stage chronic lymphocytic leukemia, B-cell type

Plan: FU in office 1 week. Repeat treatment 3 weeks.

Tip: Refer to OGCR I.C.2.e.

2 CM Codes __________ __________

3. Date: 5/15/yy Location: East Side Hematology

Provider: Robyn Akin, MD

Patient: Nell Cremer Gender: M Age: 9

Reason for encounter: monitoring of acute lymphoblastic leukemia (ALL)

Assessment: ALL, in remission

Plan: RTO 3 months

1 CM Code __________

4. Date: 5/15/yy Location: East Side Hematology

Provider: Robyn Akin, MD

Patient: Rebekah Thorton Gender: F Age: 22

Reason for encounter: follow up biopsy of lump in neck

Assessment: classical Hodgkin's lymphoma with mixed cellularity

Plan: radiation therapy to neck

1 CM Code __________

(continued)

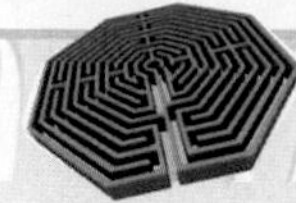

Coding Practice (continued)

5. Date: 5/15/yy Location: East Side Hematology
Provider: Robyn Akin, MD
Patient: Adriana Wrigley Gender: F Age: 36
Reason for encounter: radiation therapy
Assessment: non-Hodgkin's follicular lymphoma, grade 2, stage 3, in neck, abdomen, and pelvic nodes

(continued)

5. (continued)
Plan: treatment 5x/week for 6 weeks

Tip: Remember to distinguish between grade (how aggressive it is) and stage (how far it has spread).

2 CM Codes __________ __________

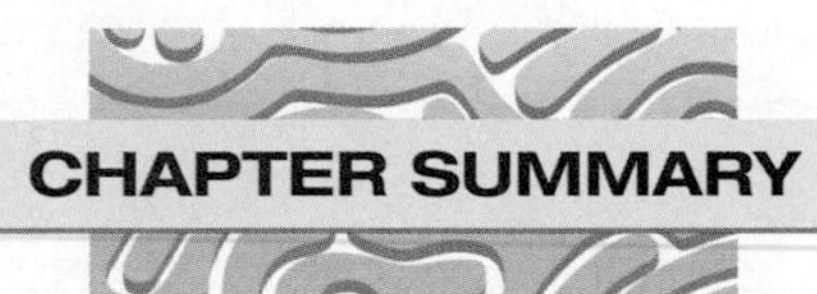

CHAPTER SUMMARY

In this chapter you learned that:

- The function of the blood, also called the hemic system, is to transport and pass nutrients, oxygen, carbon dioxide, water, proteins, and hormones to cells and to transport waste products to excretory organs.
- ICD-10-CM Chapter 3, Diseases of the Blood and Blood-Forming Organs and Certain Disorders Involving the Immune Mechanism (D50-D89), contains seven blocks or subchapters that are divided by type of condition.
- Many of the conditions in this ICD-10-CM chapter can have multiple underlying causes and multiple manifestations, so coders should thoroughly abstract the symptoms, manifestations, and underlying causes documented in the medical record.
- When an ICD-10-CM chapter does not have any OGCR, as is the case with diseases of the blood and blood-forming organs, coders apply the general OGCR (I.A, I.B, II, and III) and follow instructional notes in the Tabular List.
- Sequencing of codes in this ICD-10-CM chapter is based on the circumstances of admission and the instructional notes in the Tabular List.
- Neoplasms, which are solid tumors, do not form in the blood, but leukemia and myeloma, which begin in the bone marrow, and lymphoma, which begins in the lymphatic system, are the most common types of blood cancer.
- ICD-10-CM does not provide Official Guidelines for Coding and Reporting (OGCR) for this chapter, but the Tabular List contains frequent instructional notes to use an additional code for associated conditions and to code first underlying diseases.

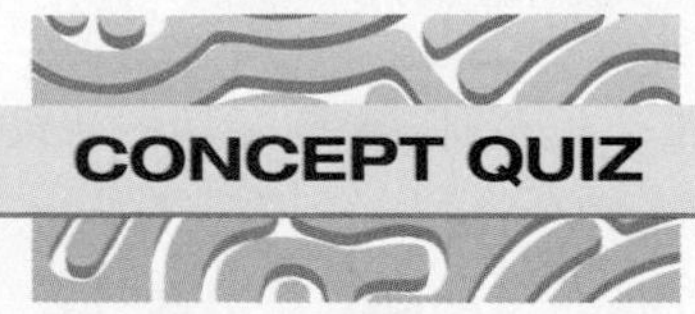

CONCEPT QUIZ

Take a moment to look back at your trip through diseases of the blood and blood-forming organs and solidify your skills. This is your opportunity to pull together everything you have learned.

Completion

Instructions: Write the term that answers each question based on the information you learned in this chapter. Choose from the list below. Some choices may be used more than once and some choices may not be used at all.

Refer to the discussion in this chapter and the Glossary at the end of this book if you need a little extra help.

aplastic	nutritional
bone marrow	plasma
erythrocytes	polycythemia
formed elements	sarcoidosis
hemic	sickle cell disease
hemoglobin	spleen
hemolytic	thrombocytes
leukocytes	thrombophilia

1. Hb, an abbreviation for ______________, is the oxygen-carrying component of erythrocytes.
2. Blood cells are created in the ______________.
3. ______________ anemia is due to excessive loss of erythrocytes.
4. ______________ are white blood cells.
5. The blood is referred to as the ______________ system.
6. ______________ is the formation of nodules in the lymph nodes, lungs, bone, and skin.
7. Erythrocytes, leukocytes, and thrombocytes are blood cells or the ______________ of the blood.
8. The spleen destroys old ______________ and filters the blood.
9. ______________ is an abnormal increase in the number of circulating red blood cells.
10. HbSS is a type of ______________.

Multiple Choice

Instructions: Circle the letter of the best answer to each question based on the information you learned in this chapter. Refer to the discussion in this chapter and the Glossary at the end of this book if you need a little extra help.

1. Which of the following disorders is NOT classified in ICD-10-CM Chapter 3, Diseases of the Blood and Blood-Forming Organs?
   A. Aplastic anemia
   B. Congestive heart failure
   C. Coagulation disorders
   D. Hemophilia
2. Which medical term means "formation of blood"?
   A. Hematapoiesis
   B. Hematologist
   C. Hemoglobin
   D. Hemophilia
3. Code D63.0, Anemia in neoplastic disease, describes what type of anemia?
   A. Aplastic anemia due to chemotherapy
   B. Anemia due to radiotherapy
   C. Anemia due to the cancer itself
   D. Anemia due to antineoplastic chemotherapy
4. ________ disorders include a range of medical problems that lead to poor clotting and continuous bleeding.
   A. Hemostasis
   B. Hemoglobin
   C. Anemia
   D. Purpura
5. When an ICD-10-CM chapter does not have OGCR, how does the coder know how to assign and sequence codes?
   A. Use common sense.
   B. Assign the default code listed in the Index.
   C. Ask the supervisor.
   D. Follow instructional notes in the Tabular List.
6. When anemia is due to an underlying condition, the Tabular List instructs coders to code which condition first?
   A. Anemia
   B. The underlying condition
   C. Either condition may be sequenced first.
   D. Sequencing is determined by the circumstances of admission.
7. When anemia is drug-induced, the Tabular List instructs coders to assign an external cause code for
   A. the neoplasm.
   B. the injury.
   C. the substance.
   D. the anemia.
8. All of the following are key criteria for abstracting conditions of the blood EXCEPT
   A. What part of the hemic system does the condition involve?
   B. Is heart failure involved?
   C. Is the condition drug-induced?
   D. Is the condition acquired or congenital?
9. All of the following are options when coding leukemia EXCEPT
   A. whether leukemia is in remission.
   B. whether leukemia has metastasized.
   C. whether leukemia has relapsed.
   D. whether leukemia has not achieved remission.
10. When the admission or encounter is for management of an anemia associated with an adverse effect of radiotherapy, the first sequenced code is
    A. anemia.
    B. neoplasm.
    C. an external cause code.
    D. Z code for the therapy encounter.

CODING CHALLENGE

Now it is your turn to demonstrate coding all aspects of the blood and blood-forming organs. Refer back to the examples and discussion in this chapter when you need a little extra help. Use your medical dictionary and anatomy references when needed.

Instructions: Read the mini-medical-record of each patient's encounter, then abstract, assign, and sequence ICD-10-CM diagnosis codes (CM) using the Index and Tabular List. Write the code(s) on the line provided.

1. Date: 5/19/yy Location: East Side Hematology
Provider: Robyn Akin, MD
Patient: Darrell Tanksley Gender: M Age: 61
Reason for encounter: bruising and petechiae, SOB, rapid heart rate, pelvic pain
Assessment: aplastic anemia due to chemotherapy for prostate cancer with metastasis to the pelvic bones
Plan: Admitted and started on immunosuppressant drugs, receive blood transfusion, and pain management. Referral to interventional radiologist to deliver targeted ablation (RFA) to bone metastasis. Pain management at weaker opioid level, RTO weekly for CBC

Tip: Refer to OGCR I.C.2.c.1) for sequencing rules.

4 CM Codes __________ __________ __________ __________

2. Date: 5/19/yy Location: Branton Medical Center Provider: Robyn Akin, MD
Patient: Trent Faria Gender: M Age: 47
Reason for admission: severe anemia
Assessment: anemia due to lung cancer in right lower lobe with metastasis to the bone.
Plan: He received blood transfusions and was discharged home.

Tip: Refer to OGCR I.C.2.c.1) for sequencing rules.

3 CM Codes __________ __________ __________

3. Date: 5/19/yy Location: East Side Hematology
Provider: Robyn Akin, MD
Patient: Janette Vreeland Gender: F Age: 12
Reason for encounter: management and monitoring of thrombophilia
Assessment: congenital antithrombin III deficiency
Plan: INR protocol, anticoagulation medication

1 CM Code __________

4. Date: 5/19/yy Location: Branton Medical Center Emergency Department
Provider: Robyn Akin, MD
Patient: Iva Liverman Gender: F Age: 53
Chief complaint: Patient states she ran out of the anticoagulant warafin 5 days ago and now "feels funny."
Assessment: lupus anticoagulant syndrome, systemic lupus erythematosus
Plan: restart warfarin, FU in office

Tip: Remember to assign an external cause code for the medication.

3 CM Codes __________ __________ __________

5. Date: 5/19/yy Location: Branton Medical Center Provider: Robyn Akin, MD
Patient: Greg Glasscock Gender: M Age: 74
Reason for admission: bruising, petechiae, hemorrhages, nosebleeds, bleeding gums, extreme fatigue
Assessment: leukemia, anemia, and thrombocytopenia
Plan: Pt received platelet transfusion. Schedule, chemotherapy, Rx anemia support medications

Tip: Pancytopenia is deficiency of WBC, RBC, and platelets.

1 CM Code __________

6. Date: 5/19/yy Location: East Side Hematology
Provider: Robyn Akin, MD
Patient: Rosetta Paiz Gender: F Age: 32
Reason for encounter: FU on lab results from daily renal dialysis showing Hb in urine
Assessment: hemoglobinuria due to dialysis, end-stage renal failure
Plan: erythropoietin protocol, place on kidney replacement list, investigate possibility of family kidney donor. FU for test results in five days

***Tip*:** Remember to assign an external cause code for complication from dialysis.

3 CM Codes __________ __________ __________

7. Date: 5/19/yy Location: Branton Medical Center Provider: Robyn Akin, MD
Patient: Corey Ebersole Gender: M Age: 64
Reason for admission: Fever, oral cavity lesions. CBC shows absolute neutrophil count (ANC) Is below 500/ microliter
Assessment: neutropenia with fever
Plan: At discharge patient provided guidelines to avoid infections, including use of saline mouth rinses. antibiotic and/or antifungal meds as directed. RTO weekly for CBC.

***Tip*:** Remember to read the instructional notes in the Tabular List.

2 CM Codes __________ __________

8. Date: 5/19/yy Location: Branton Medical Center Provider: Robyn Akin, MD
Patient: Cassie Purdom Gender: F Age: 28
Reason for Admission: Palpitations, rapid heartbeat, long bone pain, enlarged, painful spleen. Admit patient for transfusion, IV therapy, pain management, and splenectomy.
Assessment: Sickle cell crisis with splenic sequestration
Plan: RTO in one week for CBC and post operative check

1 CM Code __________

9. Date: 5/19/yy Location: Branton Medical Center Provider: Robyn Akin, MD
Patient: Jenifer Quayle Gender: F Age: 45
Reason for Admission: bone marrow transplant
Assessment: secondary myelofibrosis due to right breast cancer

***Tip*:** Remember that "due to" means secondary.

2 CM Codes __________ __________

10. Date: 5/19/yy Location: Branton Medical Center Provider: Robyn Akin, MD
Patient: William Pepin Gender: M Age: 36
Chief complaint: unexplained loss of weight, fever, weakness, night sweats, itching, tingling in legs, SOB, elevated red cell count
Assessment: Leukocytosis with polycythemia vera
Plan: FU with clinic one week

2 CM Codes __________ __________

KEEP ON CODING

As a coder, you can never have too much experience. Apply everything you have learned in this chapter to code the following diagnostic statements. Use the OGCR and instructional notes in the Tabular List to help determine how many codes are required.

Instructions: Read the diagnostic statement, then use the Index and Tabular List to assign and sequence ICD-10-CM (CM) diagnosis codes. Write the code(s) on the line provided.

1. Sideropenic dysphagia: CM Code(s) ______________________________
2. Alpha thalassemia: CM Code(s) ______________________________

3. Sickle cell disease without crisis: CM Code(s) ____________________
4. Hereditary factor IX deficiency: CM Code(s) ____________________
5. Bandemia: CM Code(s) ____________________
6. Cyst of the spleen: CM Code(s) ____________________
7. Diffuse large B-cell lymphoma, of axilla: CM Code(s) ____________________
8. Megaloblastic anemia: CM Code(s) ____________________
9. Pancytopenia due to chemotherapy for metastatic pancreatic cancer: CM Code(s) ____________________
10. Encounter for chemotherapy for acute monocytic leukemia: CM Code(s) ____________________
11. Sarcoid arthropathy: CM Code(s) ____________________
12. Postprocedural hematoma of the spleen following gastric surgery: CM Code(s) ____________________
13. Cyclic neutropenia: CM Code(s) ____________________
14. Histiocytic sarcoma: CM Code(s) ____________________
15. Pyruvate-kinase (PK) deficiency anemia: CM Code(s) ____________________
16. Hemolytic-uremic syndrome: CM Code(s) ____________________
17. Infantile pseudoleukemia: CM Code(s) ____________________
18. Heparin induced thrombocytopenia: CM Code(s) ____________________
19. Leukopenia: CM Code(s) ____________________
20. Di George's syndrome: CM Code(s) ____________________
21. Essential cryoglobulinemia: CM Code(s) ____________________
22. Protein deficiency anemia: CM Code(s) ____________________
23. Evans syndrome: CM Code(s) ____________________
24. Acquired pure red cell aplasia: CM Code(s) ____________________
25. Polycythemia due to stress: CM Code(s) ____________________

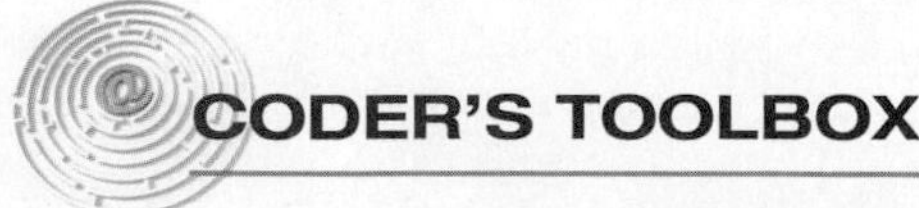

CODER'S TOOLBOX

The following resources are a starting point for learning more about the blood and blood-forming organs. The > symbol indicates a menu selection within the website in order to navigate to a specific page.

American Sickle Cell Anemia Association (ASCAA) http://www.ascaa.org/

American Society of Hematology > Patients http://www.hematology.org/Patients/Blood-Basics/5222.aspx

Cooley's Anemia Foundation http://www.thalassemia.org/

Iron Disorders Institute http://www.irondisorders.org/

Iron Disorders Institute, Hemochromatosis Information Center http://www.hemochromatosis.org/

Leukemia and Lymphoma Society http://www.lls.org/diseaseinformation/leukemia/

National Hemophilia Foundation http://www.hemophilia.org/

Polycythemia Vera Website http://www.polycythemia.org/

16

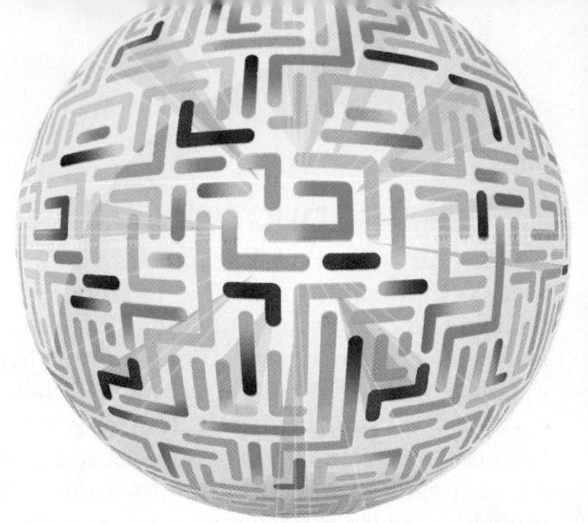

Diseases of the Respiratory System (J00-J99)

Learning Objectives

After completing this chapter, you should have the skills to:

- Spell and define the key words, medical terms, and abbreviations related to the respiratory system.
- Discuss the structure, function, and common conditions of the respiratory system.
- Identify the main characteristics of coding for the respiratory system.
- Abstract diagnostic information from the medical record for coding diseases of the respiratory system.
- Assign codes for diseases of the respiratory system.
- Arrange codes for diseases of the respiratory system.
- Code neoplasms of the respiratory system.
- Discuss the Official Guidelines for Coding and Reporting related to the respiratory system.

Key Terms and Abbreviations

acute exacerbation
acute rhinitis
aerosol therapy
airway obstruction
allergic rhinitis
alveoli
atopic
bronchodilator
bronchogenic
bronchi
bronchial tree
bronchioles
chronic bronchitis
chronic obstructive pulmonary disease (COPD)
culture and sensitivity
emphysema
endotracheal intubation
exchange
extrinsic
hospital acquired condition (HAC)
hypercapnia
hypoxemia
laryngitis
larynx
lobes
lower respiratory tract
lungs
intrinsic
non-atopic
pharyngitis
pharynx
productive cough
pulmonary function test
respiratory system
sinusitis
status asthmaticus
thoracentesis
trachea
tracheal cartilage
tracheostomy tube
upper respiratory tract
ventilation-perfusion scan
ventilator associated pneumonia (VAP)
ventilator

In addition to the key terms listed here, students should know the terms defined within tables in this chapter.

Chapter Outline

- **Respiratory System Refresher**
- **Coding Overview of the Respiratory System**
- **Abstracting for the Respiratory System**
- **Assigning Codes for the Respiratory System**
- **Arranging Codes for the Respiratory System**
- **Coding Neoplasms of the Respiratory System**

ICD-10-CM codes in this chapter are from the ICD-10-CM 2014 Draft code set from the Department of Health and Human Services, Centers for Disease Control and Prevention.

INTRODUCTION

When your road trip takes you through a mountainous area, you probably notice the difference in the air surprisingly quickly. Even at 4,000 or 5,000 feet of elevation above sea level, breathing becomes more difficult for many people. The higher you go, the more difficult breathing becomes, not because there is less oxygen in the air, but because a decrease in air pressure causes us to inhale less air with each breath. Breathing is a body function you probably take for granted until it becomes difficult.

In your tour of the respiratory system in this chapter you will learn more about how the respiratory system works, why sometimes it does not work as it should, and how physicians treat these conditions. Most importantly, you will practice coding for patient encounters related to respiratory diseases and conditions, a skill that requires you to abstract information from the mini-medical-record, assign correct codes, and arrange (sequence) the codes in the proper order.

A pulmonologist specializes in diagnosing and treating conditions of the lungs and lower respiratory system. An otolaryngologist specializes in diagnosing and treating conditions of the upper respiratory system. Primary care physicians treat uncomplicated conditions of the respiratory system and refer more complicated cases to specialists.

As you read this chapter, keep your medical resources handy to help you understand unfamiliar conditions. An anatomical reference on the respiratory system will help you identify the structures needed to code accurately.

RESPIRATORY SYSTEM REFRESHER

The function of the **respiratory system** is to obtain oxygen (O_2) from the air and deliver it to the lungs and blood for distribution to tissue cells and to remove the gaseous waste product carbon dioxide (CO_2) from the blood and lungs and expel it. This process is called **exchange.** The respiratory system also makes it possible to cough, sneeze, and talk.

The respiratory system is divided into the **upper respiratory tract**, which consists of the nose, **pharynx** (*throat*), and **larynx** (*voice box*); and the **lower respiratory tract**, which consists of the **trachea** (*windpipe*), bronchi, and **lungs** (■ Figure 16-1). As air enters the nasal cavity or oral cavity, it is warmed and moistened, then passes through the pharynx, larynx, and trachea. The trachea divides into two **bronchi** (*bronchial tubes*) that lead to the two lungs.

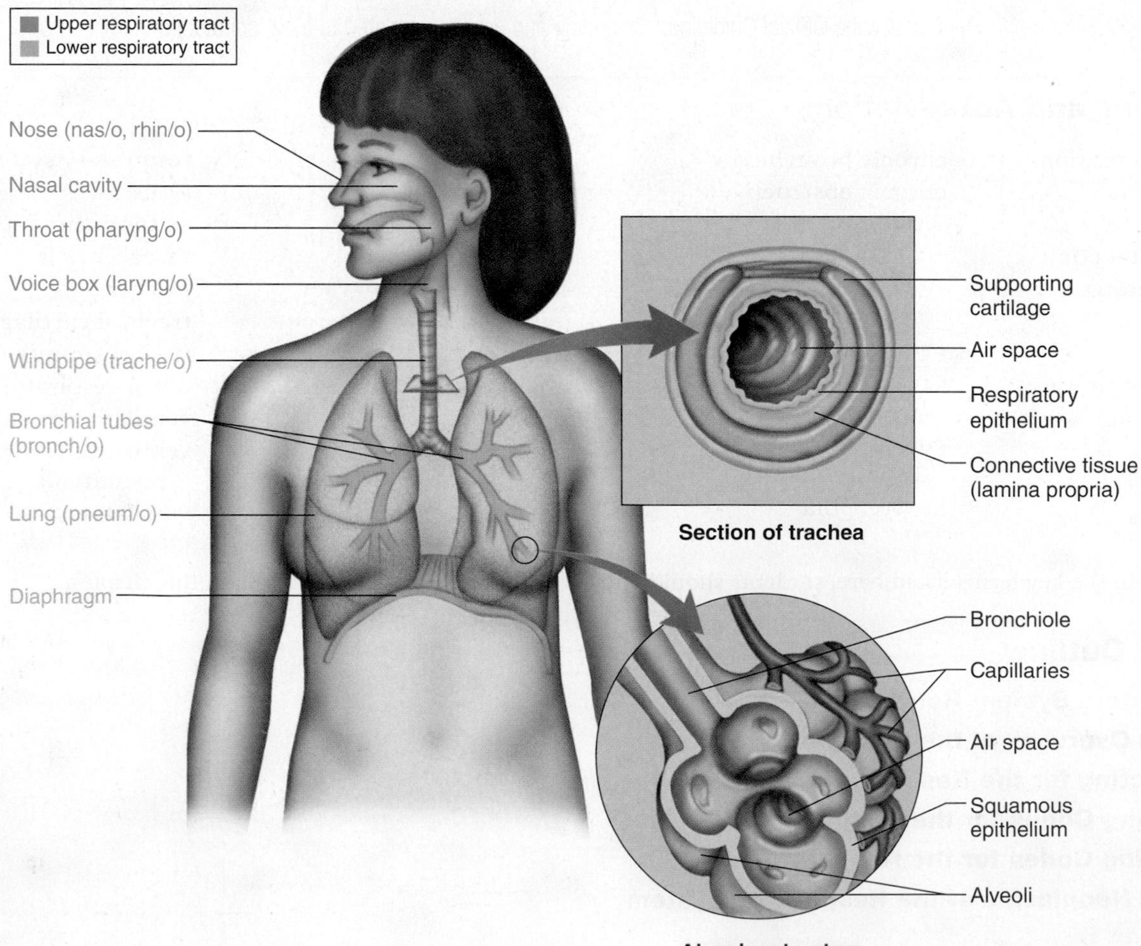

Figure 16-1 ■ The Respiratory System

Table 16-1 ■ **EXAMPLE OF CONSTRUCTING MEDICAL TERMS FOR THE RESPIRATORY SYSTEM**

Prefix/Combining Form	Suffix	Complete Medical Term
dys- (*abnormal, painful*)	**-scope** (*instrument to view the inside*) **-ectasis** (*dilation*) **-pnea** (*breathing*) **-phonia** (*voice*)	**dys + phonia** (*difficulty speaking*) **dys + pnea** (*difficulty breathing*)
bronch/o (*bronchus*)		**broncho + scope** (*instrument to view the bronchus*) **bronchi + ectasis** (*dilated bronchus*)

Rings of tracheal cartilage keep the trachea and bronchi open. In the bronchial tree, the bronchi subdivide into smaller and smaller branches, with the smallest being the bronchioles, which do not contain rings of cartilage. Bronchioles end in small air sacs in the lungs, alveoli.

The lungs consist of spongy tissue with interlacing networks of bronchioles, alveoli, alveolar sacs, blood vessels, and capillaries. The lungs are divided into lobes (*segments*). The right lung has three lobes: the superior, middle, and inferior. The left lung has two lobes: the superior and inferior. The lungs receive deoxygenated blood from the heart through the pulmonary artery, reoxygenate it, and send it back to the heart through the pulmonary vein, so the heart can pump the blood out to the rest of the body.

In Figure 16-1, each structure in the respiratory system is labeled with its name as well as its medical terminology root/combining form, where applicable. As you learn about conditions and procedures that affect the respiratory system, remember to apply medical terminology skills to combine word roots, prefixes, and suffixes you already know to define new terms related to the respiratory system. Refer to ■ TABLE 16-1 for a refresher on how to build medical terms related to the respiratory system.

SUCCESS STEP

Remember to drop the last one or two letters of a medical term and substitute new letters that create the plural form of the word. For example, one bronch**us** becomes two bronch**i**.

CODING CAUTION

Be alert for medical terms that are spelled similarly and have different meanings.

bronchitis (*inflammation of the bronchus*) and **bronchiolitis** (*inflammation of the bronchiole*)

pyothorax (*pus in the chest*) and **pneumothorax** (*air in the chest*)

emphysema (*abnormal accumulation of air in body tissue*) and **empyema** (*pus in a body cavity*)

Conditions of the Respiratory System

Respiratory conditions are divided based on whether they affect the upper or lower respiratory tract. Conditions affecting the upper respiratory tract, frequently caused by viruses, include acute rhinitis (*common cold*), allergic rhinitis (*hay fever*), sinusitis (*sinus infection*), pharyngitis (*sore throat*), and laryngitis (*irritated vocal cords*). Conditions affecting the lower respiratory tract include obstructive diseases (narrowing of the air passages), infection and inflammatory diseases (viral and bacterial infections), and mechanical damage (nontraumatic structural damage to the lung). Refer to ■ TABLE 16-2 (page 302) a summary of respiratory system conditions.

Coders should have an understanding of asthma, COPD, and ventilator associated pneumonia because they pose special coding challenges. These are discussed next, followed by an overview of diagnostic and treatment methods.

Asthma

Asthma is a chronic lung disease that affects the bronchi and is characterized by inflammation and narrowing of the airway. A common symptom is wheezing due to **bronchospasms**. Asthma may be extrinsic or atopic (*due to allergens*), or intrinsic or non-atopic (*not due to allergens*). According to the American College of Allergy, Asthma, and Immunology (ACAAI), approximately 34.1 million people in the United States are diagnosed with asthma, resulting in 500,000 hospitalizations and over 10 million office visits per year.

Physicians diagnose asthma based on the frequency and type of symptoms, forced expiratory volume (FEV), and peak expiratory flow (PEF), which are measurements of lung function. Based on this information, patients' asthma is rated as intermittent or persistent and is classified into one of four severity levels:

1. Mild intermittent
2. Mild persistent
3. Moderate persistent
4. Severe persistent

An acute exacerbation, commonly called an asthma attack, is a sudden increase in the intensity or type of symptoms, such as shortness of breath, wheezing, and chest tightness. Status asthmaticus is an acute exacerbation that does not respond to the standard medical treatments of bronchodilators and **steroids**.

Table 16-2 ■ **CONDITIONS OF THE RESPIRATORY SYSTEM**

Condition	Definition
Acute respiratory distress syndrome (ARDS)	Acute respiratory failure that result for widespread injury to the endothelium in the lung, caused by sepsis, massive blood transfusion, **aspiration** of gastric contents, or pneumonia
Acute respiratory failure (ARF)	Insufficient oxygen passing from the lungs to the blood, due to **hypercapnia** (*high carbon dioxide level*), **hypoxemia** (*low oxygen level*), or both
Asthma	A chronic lung disease that affects the bronchi and is characterized by inflammation of the airway, a reversible obstruction, and reshaping of the airway
Atelectasis	Collapse of a lung, preventing the exchange of oxygen and carbon dioxide
Chronic bronchitis	Inflammation of the bronchi with a productive cough for three months, in two consecutive years
Chronic obstructive pulmonary disease (COPD)	The combination of chronic bronchitis and emphysema as comorbidities
Emphysema	An enlargement and rupture of alveolar sacs at the end of the bronchioles, causing an abnormal accumulation of air in the tissue
Influenza	An acute respiratory infection with sudden onset caused by a virus and characterized by fever, chills, headache, muscle aches, cough, and sore throat
laryngitis	Inflammation of the larynx, resulting in hoarseness
lobar pneumonia	Bacterial pneumonia that primarily affects one lobe of the lung
lobular pneumonia	Pneumonia that primarily affects the bronchi and lobules (clusters of alveoli that surround each bronchial branch); also called bronchopneumonia
Pharyngitis	Inflammation of the throat
Pleurisy	Inflammation of the lining of the lungs and thoracic cavity with oozing of fluid or fibrinous material into the pleural cavity
Pneumonconiosis	Abnormal condition of the lung caused by inhalation of dust particles, such as coal dust (anthracosis), asbestos (asbestosis), iron dust (siderosis), or quartz (silicosis)
Pneumonia	Inflammatory condition of the lung in which the alveoli and air spaces fill with fluid; caused by bacterial, virus, fungi, or chemical irritants (■ FIGURE 16-2)
Pneumothorax	A collection of air between the chest wall and lungs, which may cause the lung to collapse
Pulmonary edema	An abnormal accumulation of fluid in the lungs, especially the alveoli, resulting in dyspnea
Tonsillitis	Inflammation of the tonsils

Chronic Obstructive Pulmonary Disease

Chronic obstructive pulmonary disease (COPD), one of the most common lung diseases, is the combination of **chronic bronchitis** and **emphysema** as comorbidities. An **airway obstruction** is a reduction in the amount of inhaled air in each breath, most commonly caused by a reduction in the diameter of the bronchioles due to inflammation.

According to the Centers for Disease Control and Prevention, approximately 13% of nursing home residents have COPD and over 6% of non-institutionalized adults suffer from either chronic bronchitis or emphysema. COPD accounts for over 17 million physician office visits per year.

Physicians diagnose chronic bronchitis when patients present with a **productive cough** (*cough with sputum*) on most days for three months, in two consecutive years. The most common cause is long term inhalation of irritants. Emphysema is an enlargement and rupture of alveolar sacs at the end of the bronchioles, causing an abnormal accumulation of air in the tissue. The damage it causes is irreversible, unlike asthma, in which the obstruction is reversible.

Ventilator Associated Pneumonia

Ventilator associated pneumonia (VAP) is pneumonia that develops 48 hours or more after mechanical ventilation is given using an endotracheal tube or **tracheostomy tube** (*a surgical opening in the neck leading to the trachea*). Intubation allows microorganisms from oral and gastric secretions to invade the tissues of the lower respiratory tract and lung. VAP is more serious than other types of pneumonia because patients who acquire it are in poorer health than the average person. In addition, the types of germs present in a hospital are often more dangerous and more resistant to treatment than those found in the community at large.

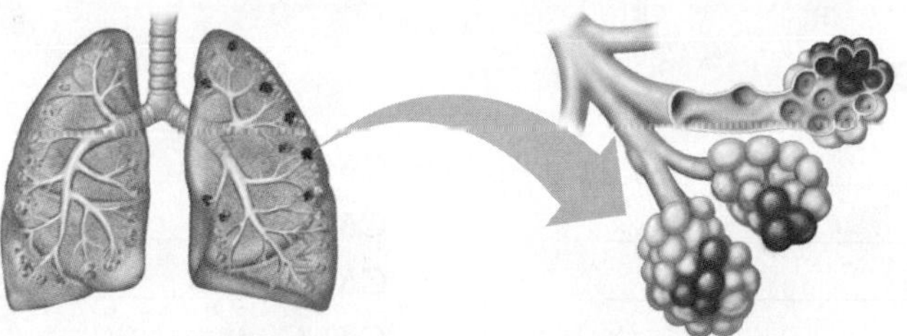
A. Lobular or bronchopneumonia

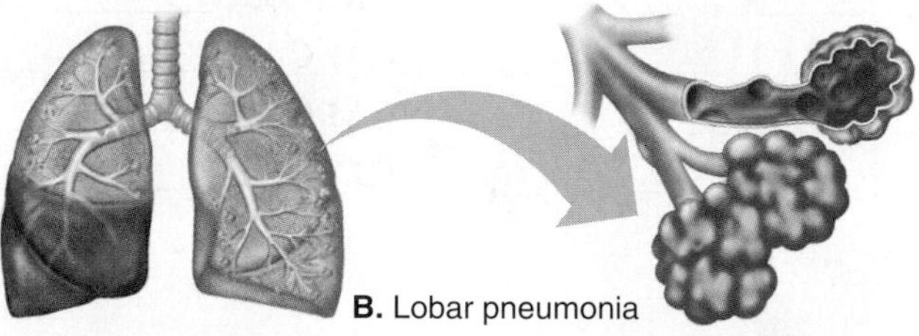
B. Lobar pneumonia

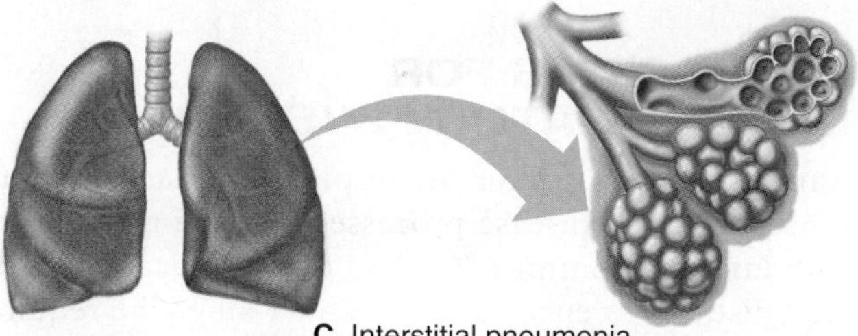
C. Interstitial pneumonia

Figure 16-2 ■ (**A**) Lobular or Bronchopneumonia with Localized Pattern (**B**) Lobar Pneumonia with a Diffuse Pattern within a Lung Lobe (**C**) Interstitial Pneumonia Is Typically Diffuse and Bilateral

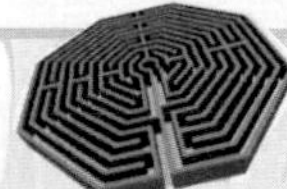

SUCCESS STEP

VAP is an example of a **hospital acquired condition (HAC)**, a serious condition that develops after admission. Medicare does not pay hospitals for the costs incurred to care for HACs and hospitals cannot bill patients for them.

Diagnosis and Treatment of Respiratory Conditions

Diseases of the respiratory system are diagnosed with a wide variety of techniques, including the following:

- arterial blood gasses to determine O_2 and CO_2 levels
- biopsy
- chest X-ray
- computed tomography scan
- **culture and sensitivity**—a lab test of secretions, such as sputum, to observe bacterial growth and determine antibiotic effectiveness
- endoscopy (laryngoscopy, bronchoscopy)
- **pulmonary function tests**—diagnostic tests that measure air flow in and out of the lungs, lung volumes, and gas exchange between the lungs and blood
- ultrasound scanning
- **ventilation-perfusion scan**—a nuclear medicine test useful in identifying pulmonary emboli by showing if blood is flowing to all parts of the lung

Respiratory diseases are treated by medications, surgery, and respiratory therapy, including the following:

- **aerosol therapy**—medication suspended in a mist that is inhaled
- **bronchodilator**—a medication that relaxes muscle spasms in bronchial tubes
- **endotracheal intubation**—placement of a tube through the mouth and glottis into the trachea to create a viable airway
- pulmonectomy or lobectomy
- **thoracentesis**—surgical puncture of the chest wall to remove fluids
- tracheostomy

Coding Practice

Refresh your knowledge of terminology related to the respiratory system. Use a medical terminology text or a website such as GlobalRph.com > Medical Terminology **http://www.globalrph.com/medterm.htm** to identify the meaning of word parts that may not be familiar.

Exercise 16.1 Respiratory System Refresher

Instructions: Use your medical terminology skills and resources to define the following conditions related to the respiratory system, then assign the diagnosis code. Follow these steps:

- Use slash marks "/" to break down each term into its root(s) and suffix.
- Define the meaning of the word, based on the meaning of each word part.
- Assign the default ICD-10-CM diagnosis code (CM) for the condition using the Index and Tabular List.

Example: tonsillitis tonsil/itis Meaning: *inflammation of the tonsils* CM Code: *J03.90*

1. pneumatocele Meaning ________________ CM Code __________
2. bronchiolitis Meaning ________________ CM Code __________

(continued)

Coding Practice (continued)

3. pneumohemothorax Meaning ______________________ CM Code __________
4. rhinorrhea Meaning ______________________ CM Code __________
5. nasopharyngitis Meaning ______________________ CM Code __________
6. bronchoalveolitis Meaning ______________________ CM Code __________
7. laryngoplegia Meaning ______________________ CM Code __________
8. pyothorax Meaning ______________________ CM Code __________
9. tracheostenosis Meaning ______________________ CM Code __________
10. hydropneumothorax Meaning ______________________ CM Code __________

CODING OVERVIEW OF THE RESPIRATORY SYSTEM

ICD-10-CM Chapter 10, Diseases of the Respiratory System (J00-J99), contains 11 blocks or subchapters that are divided by type of disorder and anatomic site. Review the block names and code ranges listed at the beginning of Chapter 10 in the ICD-10-CM manual to become familiar with the content and organization.

ICD-10-CM Chapter 10 compares to ICD-9-CM Chapter 8 (460-519). ICD-10-CM includes more codes than ICD-9-CM did to report manifestations, infectious organisms, and comorbidities. It also introduces new terminology for certain conditions, such as asthma.

This chapter includes infections of the upper and lower respiratory tracts, acute and chronic obstructive diseases, lung diseases due to external agents, and respiratory failure. It does not include infectious diseases, toxic effects of smoke, symptoms and signs, perinatal conditions, or obstetric-related conditions. These conditions are classified in other ICD-10-CM chapters.

ICD-10-CM provides Official Guidelines for Coding and Reporting (OGCR) for the respiratory system in OGCR section I.C.10. OGCR provides a detailed discussion of chronic obstructive pulmonary disease and asthma, acute respiratory failure, influenza, and ventilator associated pneumonia.

An instructional note at the beginning of the ICD-10-CM Chapter 10 in the Tabular List directs coders when they should use an additional code to identify circumstances and lifestyle habits related to tobacco use and tobacco smoke exposure. An additional instructional note directs coders how to assign codes when more than one site in the respiratory system is affected. Instructional notes appear throughout the Tabular List directing coders when additional codes are required for certain categories.

ABSTRACTING FOR THE RESPIRATORY SYSTEM

Abstracting diagnoses for the respiratory system requires knowledge of the disease processes because multiple comorbidities are common. Coders need to distinguish between diseases to ensure they abstract all of the required details. In addition to identifying the conditions, coders must also identify the infectious organism and lifestyle habits related to tobacco. ■ TABLE 16-3 lists important questions to ask when abstracting respiratory system conditions.

Guided Example of Abstracting for the Respiratory System

Refer to the following example throughout this chapter to practice skills for abstracting, assigning, and sequencing respiratory system codes. Leanne Riehl, CCS, is a fictional coder who guides you through the coding process.

> Date: 6/16/yy Location: Branton Medical Center
>
> Provider: Gilbert Stagg, MD
>
> Patient: Jared Hershman Gender: M Age: 73
>
> Reason for admission: dehydration, started IV fluids
>
> Assessment: Patient who previously smoked cigarettes for 50 years (nicotine dependence) was placed on ventilator due to COPD exacerbation. Patient acquired ventilator associated pneumonia (VAP) due to Pseudomonas. Hospital stay was prolonged due to the VAP.
>
> Plan: discharged home after 10 days, continue antibiotics, start supplemental O_2

Table 16-3 KEY CRITERIA FOR ABSTRACTING CONDITIONS OF THE RESPIRATORY SYSTEM

- ❑ What is the specific type of condition?
- ❑ Does the record document any of the following:
  - exposure to environmental tobacco smoke
  - exposure to tobacco smoke in the perinatal period
  - history of tobacco use
  - occupational exposure to environmental tobacco smoke
  - tobacco dependence or tobacco use
- ❑ What is the lowest anatomic site affected by a respiratory infection?
- ❑ Is the condition acute or chronic?
- ❑ Does a lung abscess exist?
- ❑ What is the infectious organism? Is it a virus or bacteria?
- ❑ What are all of the respiratory-related comorbidities?
- ❑ Does influenza or asthma coexist with another respiratory condition?
- ❑ Is the condition in acute exacerbation?
- ❑ If asthma is documented, what is the level of severity?
- ❑ Is asthma in acute exacerbation or status asthmaticus?
- ❑ Is the condition the result of an external cause or procedural complication?
- ❑ If influenza is documented, what manifestations exist?
- ❑ Is the condition recurrent?
- ❑ Does the patient use supplemental oxygen or a ventilator (*a machine that assists in breathing*)?

Follow along as Leanne Riehl, CCS, abstracts the diagnosis. Check off each step after you complete it.

⇨ Leanne reads through the entire record, with special attention to the reason for the encounter and the final assessment.

- ❑ She sees that there are quite a few things going on with this patient, so she needs to break it down step by step. She refers to the Key Criteria for Abstracting Conditions of the Respiratory System (Table 16-3). Because there are several coexisting conditions, she must review all the abstracting questions for each condition.
- ❑ *What is the specific type of condition?* The reason for the admission is dehydration. She notes that this condition was treated with IV fluids.
- ❑ *What are all of the respiratory-related comorbidities?* After he was admitted, the patient experienced an acute exacerbation of the COPD. Patient also developed VAP.
- ❑ *Does the patient use supplemental oxygen or a ventilator?* Yes, patient was placed on ventilator.
- ❑ *What is the infectious organism?* Pseudomonas. *Is it a virus or bacteria?* Bacteria
- ❑ *Is the condition the result of an external cause or procedural complication?* Yes, the pneumonia is ventilator associated.
- ❑ *Does the record document any current or past tobacco use?* Previously smoked cigarettes for 50 years (nicotine dependence).

⇨ Leanne reviews all the information she has gathered about this case.

- ❑ The patient was admitted for dehydration.
- ❑ He has COPD.
- ❑ He experienced an acute exacerbation of COPD.
- ❑ He has a history of cigarette smoking.
- ❑ He acquired VAP due to Pseudomonas.

⇨ At this time, Leanne does not know which of these conditions may need to be coded, nor how many codes she will end up with. She will learn about this when she moves on to assigning codes.

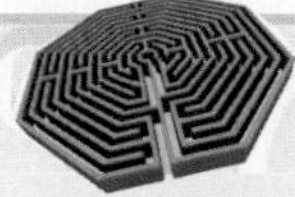

Coding Practice

Now it is your turn to practice abstracting for diseases of the respiratory system. Questions guide your analysis of each scenario. Do not assign any codes.

Exercise 16.2 Abstracting for the Respiratory System

Instructions: Read the mini-medical-record of each patient's encounter and answer the abstracting questions. Write the answer on the line provided. Do not assign any codes.

1. Date: 6/13/yy Location: Branton Family Practice Provider: Kristen Conover, MD

Patient: Allan Westra Gender: M Age: 31

Reason for encounter: patient with previously diagnosed extrinsic asthma presents with increased symptoms of coughing, wheezing, and SOB

(continued)

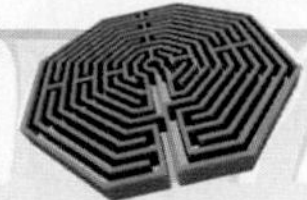

Coding Practice (continued)

1. (continued)

Assessment: Symptoms are due to acute exacerbation of mild intermittent asthma.

Plan: oral steroids and quick relief bronchodilator inhaler

a. What condition was previously diagnosed? ____________

b. What are the presenting symptoms? ____________

c. What is the cause of the symptoms? ____________

d. Which symptoms should you code? ____________

e. What is the severity of the patient's asthma? ____________

2. Date: 6/13/yy Location: North Side Pulmonology Provider: Gilbert Stagg, MD

Patient: Noreen Ewers Gender: F Age: 69

Reason for encounter: productive cough and fever, patient is concerned that she may need medication for COPD which she has not needed for several years

Assessment: viral pneumonia unrelated to patient's past history of COPD

Plan: Rx cough medicine with expectorant, take aspirin for fever, drink plenty of fluids to prevent dehydration

a. What are the patient's symptoms? ____________

b. Why was the patient concerned about the symptoms? ____________

c. What condition did the physician diagnose? ____________

d. What is the difference between viral pneumonia and bacterial pneumonia? ____________

e. Is the pneumonia related to the past COPD? ____________

f. Should you code the symptoms? ____________
Why or why not? ____________

g. Should you code the COPD? ____________
Why or why not? ____________

(continued)

2. (continued)

Tip: If you are unsure about this, refer to OGCR IV.J.

h. Should you code the pneumonia? ____________
Why or why not? ____________

3. Date: 6/13/yy Location: Branton Medical Center

Provider: Gilbert Stagg, MD

Patient: Ted Atteberry Gender: M Age: 72

Reason for encounter: management of chronic obstructive pulmonary disease, recent self-administered spirometry results have been declining, increased SOB

Assessment: COPD with chronic bronchitis and emphysema

Plan: nebulizer treatment to administer bronchodilators

a. What chronic disease was previously diagnosed? ____________

b. What symptoms does the patient report at this encounter? ____________

c. Do these symptoms lead to a new diagnosis? ____________

d. Should you code the symptoms? ____________
Why or why not? ____________

e. Should you code the COPD? ____________
Why or why not? ____________

f. Should you code chronic bronchitis and/or emphysema? ____________
Why or why not? ____________

4. Date: 6/14/yy Location: Branton Medical Center Provider: Gilbert Stagg, MD

Patient: Darren Kaup Gender: M Age: 80

Reason for admission: patient with congestive heart failure admitted from physician's office after presenting with low fever, chills, cough. CHF increases patient risk for complications.

Assessment: lobular pneumonia and acute bronchitis, both due to Mycoplasma pneumoniae

(continued)

4. (continued)

a. What are the symptoms? ______________

b. Should the symptoms be coded? ______________
Why or why not? ______________

c. What is the role of CHF in this case?
____

d. What two conditions were diagnosed? ______________
____

e. Is the bronchitis acute or chronic? ______________
____

f. What is the infectious organism? ______________
____

g. Does the patient have COPD? ______________
____

h. What is the principal diagnosis? ______________
____

Tip: Refer to OGCR II.B.

i. What is the second diagnosis? ______________
____

j. What is the third diagnosis? ______________
____

k. What ongoing medical treatment does the patient use? ______________

5. Date: 6/14/yy Location: Branton Medical Center
Provider: Gilbert Stagg, MD
Patient: Penelope Amor Gender: F Age: 76
Reason for admission: acute bronchitis
Assessment: COPD with acute bronchitis exacerbation and chronic bronchitis
Plan: begin oxygen therapy, patient must cease cigarette smoking as it continues to impact her respiratory conditions, counseled her regarding treatment options for tobacco dependence

a. What is the reason for admission? ______________
____

b. What other conditions are documented?
____

(continued)

5. (continued)

c. What is the relationship between COPD and the acute bronchitis? ______________

d. Should the acute bronchitis be coded? ______________
Why or why not? ______________

e. Should chronic bronchitis be coded? ______________
Why or why not? ______________

f. What lifestyle habit should be coded? ______________
____

Tip: You will learn the sequencing when you begin assigning the codes in Exercise 16.4.

6. Date: 6/14/yy Location: Branton Medical Center Provider: Gilbert Stagg, MD
Patient: Jeanie Emig Gender: F Age: 78
Reason for admission: asbestosis which is thought to be due to exposure to asbestos particles brought home by her late husband who worked in the fireproofing industry for many years and died of mesothelioma
Assessment: asbestosis, clubbing of fingers due to the asbestosis, mild persistent asthma
Plan: O_2, thoracentesis, medication, respiratory therapy

a. What is the reason for admission? ______________
____

b. What is clubbing of the fingers due to? ______________
____

c. Should clubbing of the fingers be coded?
____
Why or why not? ______________

d. What other diagnosis exists? ______________
____

e. What is the severity of the asthma? ______________
____

f. Should asthma be coded? ______________
Why or why not? ______________

g. What is the principal diagnosis? ______________
____

ASSIGNING CODES FOR THE RESPIRATORY SYSTEM

Coders must be attentive to the details of the case, instructional notes in the Tabular List, and the OGCR in order to accurately assign codes for respiratory system conditions. They should become familiar with chapter-wide coding considerations as well as information specifically for asthma, COPD, and influenza.

Chapter-Wide Coding

ICD-10-CM Chapter 10, Diseases of the Respiratory System (J00-J99) begins with two instructional notes that apply to all codes in the chapter. One instruction pertains to assigning additional codes for lifestyle habits; the other instruction describes how to code when multiple sites within the respiratory system are affected. Coders should also assign status **Z** codes when needed.

Lifestyle Habits

ICD-10-CM Chapter 10 provides an instructional note at the beginning of the chapter that instructs coders to use an additional code, when applicable, to identify various situations related to tobacco use, dependence, and exposure to tobacco smoke (■ Figure 16-3). Exposure may include environmental tobacco smoke, occupational exposure to tobacco smoke, and exposure to tobacco smoke during the perinatal period (before birth through the first 28 days after birth).

SUCCESS STEP

ICD-9-CM provided a chapter-wide note to assign an additional code to identify the infectious organism. Because ICD-10-CM has many combination codes that describe the condition and the organism, this chapter-wide note was eliminated. However, you still see a similar note in certain categories that do not provide a combination code.

Use additional code, where applicable, to identify:

exposure to environmental tobacco smoke (Z77.22)

exposure to tobacco smoke in the perinatal period (P96.81)

history of tobacco use (Z87.891)

occupational exposure to environmental tobacco smoke (Z57.31)

tobacco dependence (F17.-)

tobacco use (Z72.0)

Figure 16-3 ■ Tabular List Instructional Notes That Apply to All Codes in Chapter 10

Multiple Sites Affected

Respiratory conditions may affect more than one site within the respiratory system, such as the tonsils and adenoids, trachea and bronchi, or bronchi and lung. When the site is not specifically indexed, assign a code for the lowest anatomical site. This requires coders to follow conventions in the Index carefully and to have knowledge of respiratory system anatomy.

For example, consider a patient seen for tracheobronchitis, an inflammation (-itis) of the trachea (trache/o) and bronchi (bronch/o). The Index entry for the Main Term **Tracheobronchitis** cross-references coders to the Main Term **Bronchitis** because the bronchi are located lower than the trachea. The Index entry for the Main Term **Bronchitis** lists a nonessential modifier for **(tracheobronchitis)** and directs coders to **J40** (■ Figure 16-4). In the Tabular List, **Tracheobronchitis** appears as an inclusion term under the code **J40 Bronchitis, not specified as acute or chronic.**

Z Codes

Certain treatments for respiratory conditions require status **Z** codes. The most common are the existence of a tracheostomy, an encounter for tracheostomy care, long term use of oxygen, and or ventilator assistance in breathing. If there are complications from any of these devices, code the complication and do not assign a **Z** code.

Locate codes for tracheostomy status and tracheostomy care under the Main Term **Tracheostomy** in the Index. Locate the **Z** codes for oxygen and ventilator use under the Main Term **Dependence** in the Index (■ Figure 16-5).

Assigning Codes for Asthma

Assigning codes for asthma has new requirements in ICD-10-CM. To assign codes for asthma, coders need to identify how the physician has documented the severity of the patient's condition. Be attentive when navigating the Main Term for **Asthma** in the Index because the second-level subterms **with exacerbation** and **with status asthmaticus** appear under multiple first-level subterms, and it is easy to become confused.

By searching the Index for the Main Term **Asthma**, then locating a subterm for either **intermittent** or **persistent**, coders can locate most of the codes they need. The

J40 Bronchitis, not specified as acute or chronic

Bronchitis NOS

Bronchitis with tracheitis NOS

Catarrhal bronchitis

Tracheobronchitis NOS

Figure 16-4 ■ Tabular List Entry for Bronchitis with Tracheobronchitis as an Inclusion Term

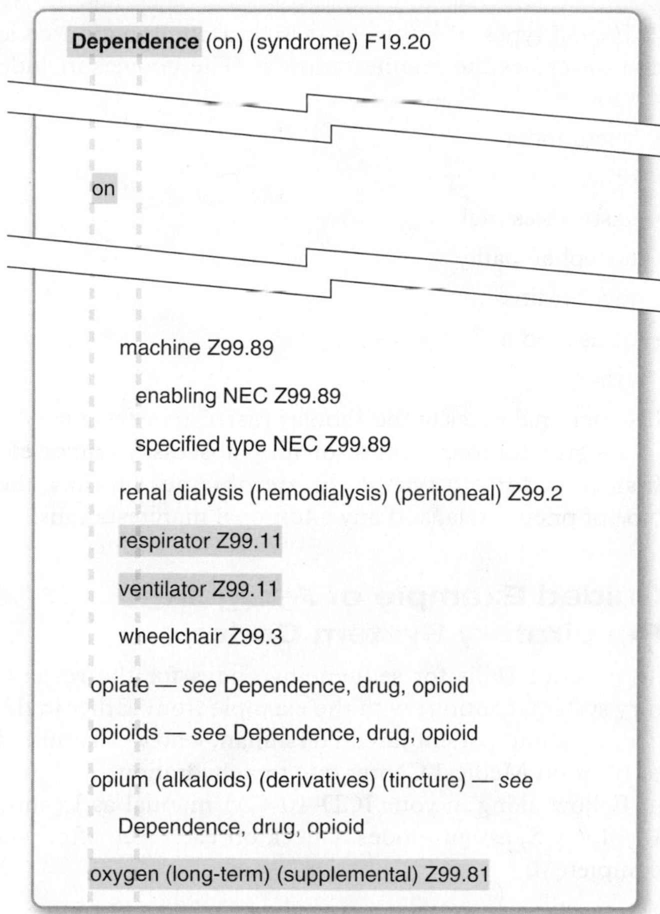

Figure 16-5 ■ Index Entries for Dependence on Ventilator or Oxygen

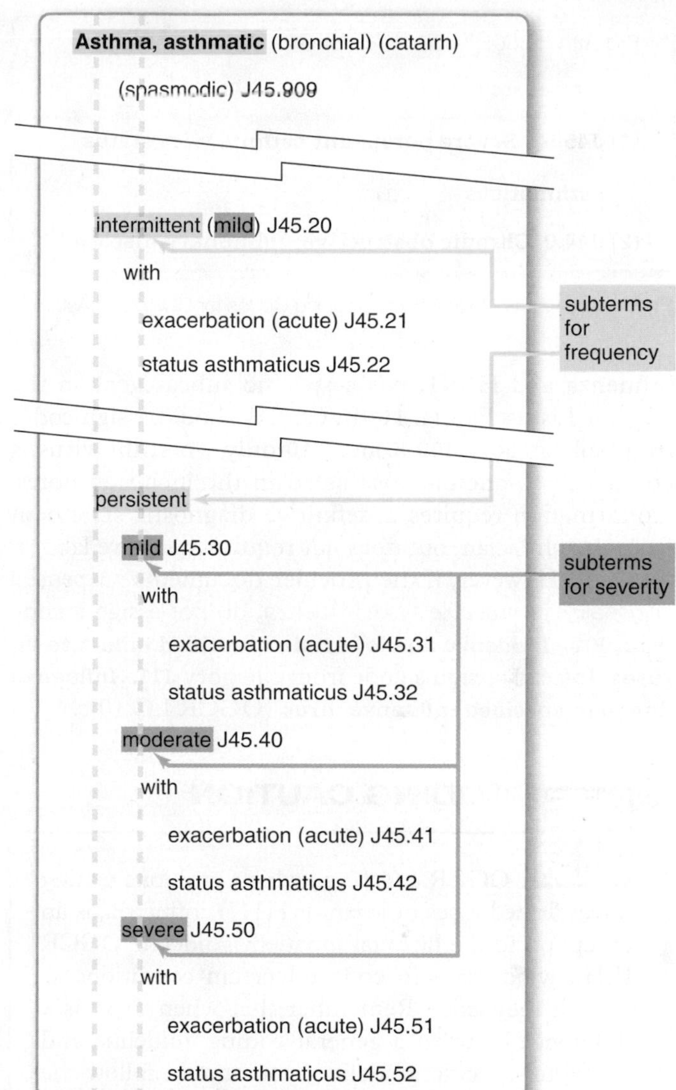

Figure 16-6 ■ Example of the Index Entry for Asthma

subterm **intermittent** contains only one level of severity, **mild,** then provides choices for **with exacerbation** or **with status asthmaticus**. The subterm **persistent** provides additional subterms for **mild, moderate,** or **severe,** then provides choices under each for **with exacerbation** or **with status asthmaticus** (■ FIGURE 16-6).

CODING CAUTION

In ICD-9-CM asthma codes were divided based on whether asthma was extrinsic or intrinsic. In ICD-10-CM, these terms lead you to default codes for unspecified asthma. Instead, you need to locate asthma based on the severity level as mild intermittent, moderate intermittent, moderate persistent, and severe persistent.

Assigning Codes for COPD and Asthma

The codes in categories **J44 Other chronic obstructive pulmonary disease** and **J45 Asthma** distinguish between uncomplicated cases and those in acute exacerbation. An acute exacerbation is a worsening of a chronic condition. An acute exacerbation is not the same as an infection superimposed on a chronic condition, although an exacerbation may be triggered by an infection.

When asthma occurs with COPD, the Index leads to the entry **Asthma, with chronic obstructive pulmonary disease J44.9**, which appears to be a combination code. However, the Tabular List instructs coders to assign an additional code for the type of asthma. The same holds true for chronic obstructive bronchitis with asthma. Sequencing depends on the circumstances of admission. (OGCR I.C.10.a.1)) (■ FIGURE 16-7, page 310).

Assigning Codes for Influenza

When assigning codes for influenza, coders must identify the type of influenza and the manifestations. Influenza codes are divided based on whether the disease is identified as **novel influenza A virus**, other virus, or the virus is unidentified. Novel influenza A, which includes avian

Patient with COPD is admitted for severe persistent asthma with status asthmaticus.

(1) **J45.52 Severe persistent asthma with status asthmaticus**

(2) **J44.0 Chronic obstructive pulmonary disease**

Figure 16-7 ■ Example of Assigning Codes for COPD and Asthma

influenza and H1N1, has a specific subcategory in the Tabular List (■ FIGURE 16-8). Coders should assign codes from subcategory **J09.X** and **J10** only when the virus is confirmed as one of those listed in the inclusion notes. Confirmation requires a definitive diagnostic statement from the physician, but does not require a positive laboratory test. However, if the provider documents *suspected or possible or probable avian influenza*, do not assign a code from **J09.- Influenza due to certain identified influenza viruses**. Instead, assign a code from category **J11.- Influenza due to unspecified influenza virus** (OGCR I.C.10.c.).

CODING CAUTION

OGCR I.C.10.c., which prohibits coding unconfirmed cases of avian or H1N1 influenza, is an exception to the hospital inpatient guideline OGCR II.H., which says to code uncertain conditions as though they exist. Remember that when there is a difference between a general coding guideline and a chapter-specific guideline, you should follow the chapter-specific guideline.

For all types of influenza, assign a combination code that describes the manifestation(s). The choices include the following:

- pneumonia
- other respiratory
- gastrointestinal
- encephalopathy
- myocarditis
- otitis media
- other

Instructional notes in the Tabular List also instruct coders to assign additional codes for lung abscess, **pleural effusion**, perforated **tympanic membrane**, sinusitis, the type of pneumonia, and any additional manifestations.

Guided Example of Assigning Respiratory System Codes

To practice skills for sequencing codes for the respiratory system, continue with the example from earlier in the chapter about patient Jared Hershman, who was admitted to Branton Medical Center due to dehydration.

Follow along in your ICD-10-CM manual as Leanne Riehl, CCS, assigns codes. Check off each step after you complete it.

⇨ First, Leanne reviews all the information she abstracted about the patient. She will tackle each condition, one at a time.

- ❑ The patient was admitted for dehydration.
- ❑ He has COPD.
- ❑ He experienced an acute exacerbation of COPD.

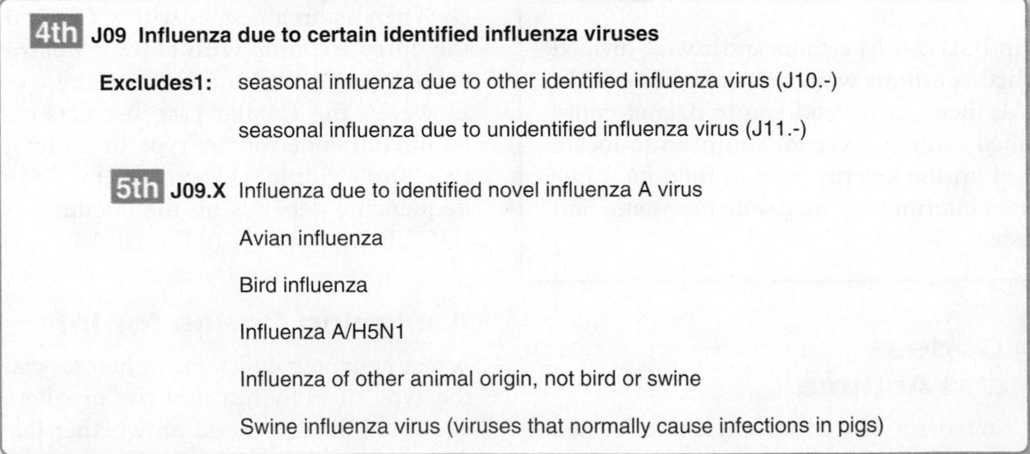

4th **J09 Influenza due to certain identified influenza viruses**

Excludes1: seasonal influenza due to other identified influenza virus (J10.-)

seasonal influenza due to unidentified influenza virus (J11.-)

5th **J09.X** Influenza due to identified novel influenza A virus

Avian influenza

Bird influenza

Influenza A/H5N1

Influenza of other animal origin, not bird or swine

Swine influenza virus (viruses that normally cause infections in pigs)

Figure 16-8 ■ Tabular List Inclusion and Exclusion Notes for Influenza Due to Certain Identified Influenza Viruses

- ❑ He has a history of cigarette smoking.
- ❑ He acquired VAP due to Pseudomonas.

⇨ Leanne searches the Index for the Main Term **Dehydration**.

- ❑ She identifies the default code **E86.0**.
- ❑ She reviews the three subterms and verifies that none of them are documented.

⇨ Leanne verifies code **E86.0** in the Tabular List.

- ❑ She reads the code title for **E86.0, Dehydration** and confirms that this accurately describes the documentation.

⇨ Leanne checks for instructional notes in the Tabular List.

- ❑ She cross-references the beginning of category **E86**, reads the **Excludes1** notes, and verifies that they do not apply to this case.
- ❑ She then cross-references the beginning of the block **E70-E88** and the beginning of the chapter, reads the **Excludes1** notes, and verifies that they do not apply to this case.
- ❑ Leanne finalizes the code **E86.0, Dehydration**.

⇨ Leanne proceeds to assign a code for COPD.

- ❑ She searches the Index for the Main Term **Disease** and subterm **lung**.
- ❑ She locates a second-level subterm **obstructive**.
- ❑ She locates additional subterm levels **with, acute,** and **exacerbation** (■ FIGURE 16-9).

Disease, diseased — *see also* Syndrome

lumbosacral region M53.87

lung J98.4

obstructive (chronic) J44.9

with

acute

bronchitis J44.0

exacerbation NEC J44.1

Figure 16-9 ■ Index Entry for Chronic Obstructive Pulmonary Disease with Acute Exacerbation

- ❑ Now she knows she will have a combination code for COPD and the acute exacerbation. She identifies the code **J44.1**.

⇨ Leanne verifies code **J44.1** in the Tabular List.

- ❑ She reads the code title for **J44.1, Chronic obstructive pulmonary disease with acute exacerbation** and confirms that this accurately describes the documentation.
- ❑ She double-checks to be sure that additional digits are not required.

⇨ Leanne checks for instructional notes in the Tabular List.

- ❑ She reads the **Excludes2** note under code **J44.1** and determines that it does not apply to this case because the patient does not have acute bronchitis.
- ❑ She cross-references the beginning of category **J44** and reads the instructional notes.
  - She determines that the **Excludes1** note does not apply to this case because none of these conditions are documented.
  - She determines that the note **Code also type of asthma, if applicable (J45.-)** does not apply because asthma is not documented.
- ❑ She reads the **Use additional code** notes and determines that **history of tobacco use (Z87.891)** applies to this case, because the patient smoked cigarettes for 50 years. This answers her question as to whether she should code the past nicotine dependence. She verifies this code in the Tabular List. **Z87.891, Personal history of nicotine dependence**.
- ❑ Leanne continues with cross-referencing and turns the page to the beginning of the block **Chronic lower respiratory diseases (J40-J47)**.
  - She reads the **Excludes1** and **Excludes2** notes and determines they do not apply to this case because none of these conditions are documented.
- ❑ She turns to the beginning of **Chapter 10 (J00-J99)** and reads the instructional notes. She locates the same note that appeared under the category heading, **Use additional code for history of tobacco use (Z87.891)**. This confirms that she was correct in assigning the Z code.
- ❑ Leanne reviews her working list of diagnoses and notices that she still needs to assign a code for VAP.

⇨ Leanne searches the Index for the Main Term **Pneumonia**.

- ❑ She locates two possible subterms:
  - **pseudomonas J15.1**
  - **ventilator associated J95.851**

- ❑ In order to determine whether she needs both of the codes or only one, she knows she needs to verify the codes in the Tabular List.
- ❑ She verifies the title for code **J15.1, Pneumonia due to Pseudomonas**, which is classified under the category **J15, Bacterial pneumonia, not elsewhere classified**.
- ❑ She verifies the title for code **J95.851, Ventilator associated pneumonia**, which is classified under the category **J95, Intraoperative and postprocedural complications and disorders of respiratory system, not elsewhere classified**.
- ❑ Leanne refers to OGCR I.C.10.d., which provides guidelines on coding VAP.
    - OGCR I.C.10.d.1) states that code should be used only when the provider has documented VAP. She double-checks the medical record to be certain it is documented.
    - The guideline also states that she should assign an additional code to identify the infectious organism.
    - The guideline also states that a code from **J12** to **J18** should NOT be assigned to identify the type of pneumonia.
- ❑ Leanne now understands that **J15.1** is for pneumonia due to Pseudomonas that patients acquire in the normal course of events and that **J95.851** is specifically for VAP.
- ❑ She returns to the Tabular List for code **J95.851** and reads the instructional note **Use additional code to identify the organism, if known (B95.-, B96.-, B97.-)**. This note is consistent with OGCR I.C.10.d., which she consulted. These codes are located in **Chapter 1, Certain Infectious and Parasitic Diseases (A00-B99)** and are used to identify infectious organisms in diseases classified in other ICD-10-CM chapters.
- ❑ She cross-references the block heading **J95** and sees that it is the same as the category. She sees no further instructional notes.

⇨ Leanne cross-references the codes **B95.-**, **B96.-**, and **B97.-** to locate the code for Pseudomonas, **B96.5**, which has the title **Pseudomonas (aeruginosa) (mallei) (pseudomallei) as the cause of diseases classified elsewhere**.

- ❑ She notices that the terms **(aeruginosa) (mallei) (pseudomallei)** are nonessential modifiers because they are enclosed in parentheses. They describe various forms of Pseudomonas and do not need to be present in the documentation in order to use the code.

⇨ Leanne reviews the codes she has assigned for this case.

- ❑ **J95.851, Ventilator associated pneumonia**
- ❑ **Z87.891, Personal history of nicotine dependence**
- ❑ **J44.1, Chronic obstructive pulmonary disease with acute exacerbation**
- ❑ **E86.0, Dehydration**
- ❑ **B96.5, Pseudomonas (aeruginosa) (mallei) (pseudomallei) as the cause of diseases classified elsewhere**

⇨ Next, Leanne must determine how to sequence the codes.

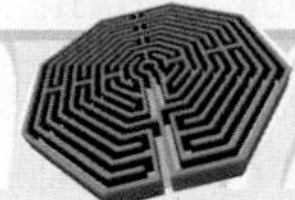

Coding Practice

Now it is your turn to practice assigning codes for diseases of the respiratory system. Refer to the ***Tip*** at the end of the mini-medical-record if you need a little extra help.

Exercise 16.3 Assigning Codes for the Respiratory System

Instructions: Read the mini-medical-record of each patient's encounter, review the information abstracted in Exercise 16.2, and assign ICD-10-CM diagnosis codes (CM) using the Index and Tabular List. Write the code(s) on the line provided.

1. Date: 6/13/yy Location: Branton Family Practice Provider: Kristen Conover, MD

Patient: Allan Westra Gender: M Age: 31

Reason for encounter: patient with previously diagnosed extrinsic asthma presents with increased symptoms of coughing, wheezing, and SOB

Assessment: Symptoms are due to acute exacerbation of mild intermittent asthma.

Plan: oral steroids and quick relief bronchodilator inhaler

Tip: Assign a code for the severity, not extrinsic vs. intrinsic.

1 CM Code ___________

2. Date: 6/13/yy Location: North Side Pulmonology
Provider: Gilbert Stagg, MD
Patient: Noreen Ewers Gender: F Age: 69
Reason for encounter: productive cough and fever, patient is concerned that she may need medication for COPD which she has not needed for several years
Assessment: viral pneumonia unrelated to patient's past history of COPD
Plan: Rx cough medicine with expectorant, take aspirin for fever, drink plenty of fluids to prevent dehydration
1 CM Code __________

3. Date: 6/13/yy Location: Branton Medical Center
Provider: Gilbert Stagg, MD
Patient: Ted Atteberry Gender: M Age: 72
Reason for encounter: management of chronic obstructive pulmonary disease, recent self-administered spirometry results have been declining, increased SOB
Assessment: COPD with chronic bronchitis and emphysema
Plan: nebulizer treatment to administer bronchodilators

Tip: Compare the codes for COPD, COPD with bronchitis, and COPD with emphysema.
1 CM Code __________

ARRANGING CODES FOR THE RESPIRATORY SYSTEM

OGCR provides specific instructions regarding sequencing codes for ventilator associated pneumonia and acute respiratory failure (ARF).

Arranging Codes for Ventilator Associated Pneumonia

VAP is pneumonia that patients acquire as a result of being on a ventilator (■ FIGURE 16-10). The relationship between ventilator use and the pneumonia must be documented by the physician. VAP is a complication of care and is classified separately from other types of pneumonia by ICD-10-CM. OGCR I.C.10.d. provides instructions for how to assign codes for VAP, as follows:

1. Confirm that the provider has documented the relationship between the ventilator use and the pneumonia.
2. Assign code **J95.851 Ventilator associated pneumonia.**
3. Assign an additional code from **B95.-**, **B96.-**, or **B97.-** to identify the infectious organism.
4. Do not assign a code from categories **J12** to **J18** to identify the type of pneumonia.

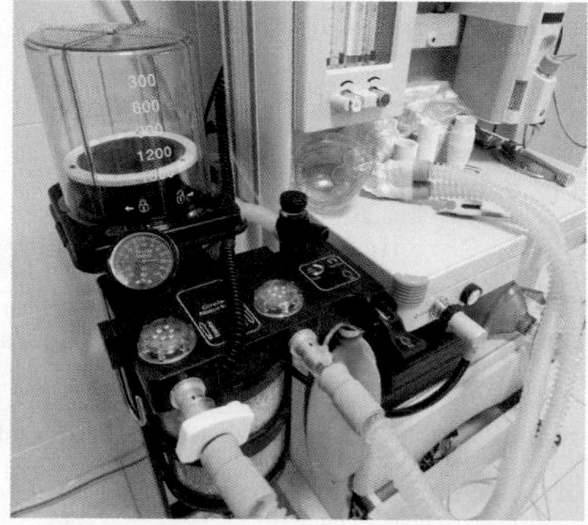

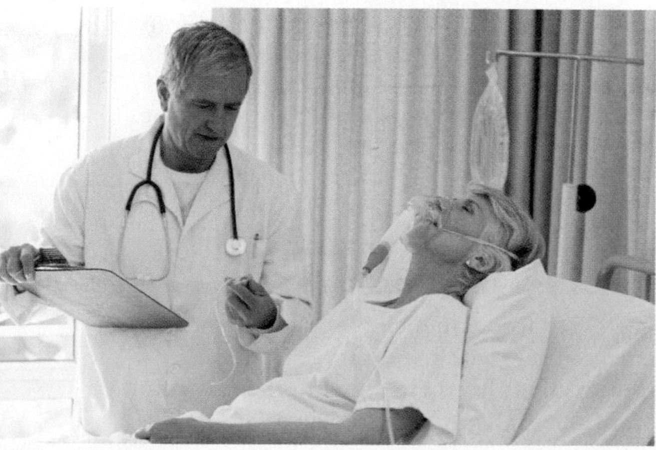

Figure 16-10 ■ Ventilators assist patients with breathing, but can also create an opportunity for pneumonia. *Sources: Paul Vinten/Shutterstock.com (left) and wavebreakmedia ltd/Shutterstock (right).*

Patients may be admitted with one type of pneumonia, then be put on a ventilator and also develop VAP. When this happens, assign and sequence codes as follows:

1. Assign a code from categories **J12** to **J18** to identify the pneumonia the patient had upon admission. Sequence this as the principal diagnosis.
2. Assign code **J95.851 Ventilator associated pneumonia** for VAP.
3. Assign an additional code from **B95.-**, **B96.-**, or **B97.-** to identify the infectious organism.

When patients are on a ventilator and do not have VAP or other ventilator associated complications, assign code **Z99.11 Dependence on respirator [ventilator] status**.

SUCCESS STEP

To locate VAP in the Index, search for the Main Term **Pneumonia** and the subterm **ventilator associated**.

Arranging Codes for Acute Respiratory Failure

Acute respiratory failure (ARF) may be sequenced as either the principal diagnosis or a secondary diagnosis. OGCR I.C.10.b. provides the following guidance:

- When ARF meets the definition of a principal diagnosis, coders should sequence it first, unless another chapter-specific guideline, such as obstetrics, poisoning, HIV, or newborn, provides sequencing direction that takes priority.
- When ARF does not meet the criteria for the principal diagnosis, or arises after admission, coders should sequence it as an additional diagnosis.
- When ARF and another acute condition, such as myocardial infarction, cerebrovascular accident, or aspiration pneumonia, coexist, the circumstances of admission should determine the principal diagnosis.

Guided Example of Arranging Respiratory System Codes

To practice skills for sequencing codes for the respiratory system, continue with the example from earlier in the chapter about patient Jared Hershman, who was admitted to Branton Medical Center due to dehydration.

Follow along in your ICD-10-CM manual as Leanne Riehl, CCS, sequences the codes. Check off each step after you complete it.

⇨ Leanne confirms codes she has assigned.

- ❑ **J95.851, Ventilator associated pneumonia**
- ❑ **Z87.891, Personal history of nicotine dependence**
- ❑ **J44.1, Chronic obstructive pulmonary disease with acute exacerbation**
- ❑ **E86.0, Dehydration**
- ❑ **B96.5, Pseudomonas (aeruginosa) (mallei) (pseudomallei) as the cause of diseases classified elsewhere**

⇨ First, she must determine the principal diagnosis, which the Uniform Hospital Data Discharge Set (UHDDS) defines as "that condition established after study to be chiefly responsible for occasioning the admission of the patient to the hospital for care" (OGCR II).

- ❑ Leanne checks the medical record and confirms that dehydration was the reason for admission. The COPD exacerbation and VAP developed after admission. Although these conditions were responsible for additional services and prolonged the length of stay, they do not meet the criteria for the reason for admission. She sequences **E86.0, Dehydration** as the principal diagnosis.
- ❑ Leanne determines that **J44.1, Chronic obstructive pulmonary disease with acute exacerbation** should be the second code because it was the reason the patient was placed on a ventilator.
- ❑ She sequences **J95.851, Ventilator associated pneumonia** as the third code and **B96.5, Pseudomonas** as the fourth code. The instructional notes and OGCR indicate that the organism is sequenced in addition to or after the code for VAP.
- ❑ The final code is **Z87.891, Personal history of nicotine dependence** because it is required by instructional notes and provides supplementary information.

⇨ Leanne finalizes the code assignment and sequencing for this case:

(1) **E86.0, Dehydration**

(2) **J44.1, Chronic obstructive pulmonary disease with acute exacerbation**

(3) **J95.851, Ventilator associated pneumonia**

(4) **B96.5, Pseudomonas(aeruginosa) (mallei) (pseudomallei) as the cause of diseases classified elsewhere**

(5) **Z87.891, Personal history of nicotine dependence**

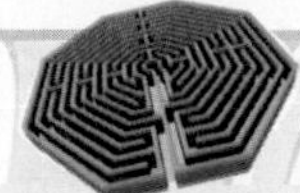

Coding Practice

Now it is your turn to practice sequencing codes for diseases of the respiratory system. Refer to the *Tip* if you need a little extra help.

Exercise 16.4 Arranging Codes for the Respiratory System

Instructions: Read the mini-medical-record of each patient's encounter, review the information abstracted in Exercise 16.2, assign ICD-10-CM diagnosis codes (CM) using the Index and Tabular List, and sequence them correctly.

1. Date: 6/14/yy Location: Branton Medical Center Provider: Gilbert Stagg, MD

Patient: Darren Kaup Gender: M Age: 80

Reason for admission: patient with congestive heart failure admitted from physician's office after presenting with low fever, chills, cough. CHF increases patient risk for complications.

Assessment: lobular pneumonia and acute bronchitis, both due to Mycoplasma pneumoniae

Tip: Be sure to distinguish between lobar pneumonia and lobular pneumonia. Remember to assign a Z code for the supplemental oxygen use.

4 CM Codes __________ __________

__________ __________

2. Date: 6/14/yy Location: Branton Medical Center Provider: Gilbert Stagg, MD

Patient: Penelope Amor Gender: F Age: 76

Reason for admission: COPD with exacerbation

Assessment: COPD with acute bronchitis exacerbation and chronic bronchitis

Plan: antibiotics for the infection, begin oxygen therapy, patient must cease cigarette smoking as it continues to impact her respiratory conditions, counseled her regarding treatment options for tobacco dependence

Tip: Read the instructional notes in the Tabular List for sequencing instructions.

3 CM Codes __________ __________

____

3. Date: 6/14/yy Location: Branton Medical Center Provider: Gilbert Stagg, MD

Patient: Jeanie Emig Gender: F Age: 78

Reason for admission: asbestosis which is thought to be due exposure to asbestos particles brought home by her late husband who worked in the fireproofing industry for many years and died of mesothelioma

Assessment: asbestosis, clubbing of fingers due to the asbestosis, mild persistent asthma

Plan: O_2, thoracentesis, medication, respiratory therapy

3 CM Codes __________ __________

____

CODING NEOPLASMS OF THE RESPIRATORY SYSTEM

Neoplasms of the respiratory system do not appear in ICD-10-CM Chapter 10, Diseases of the Respiratory System (J00-J99). Codes for neoplasms of the respiratory system appear in the block C30 to C39 within the neoplasm chapter.

The most common site for cancer in the respiratory system is the lung. Lung cancer, rare in people under age 45, is the deadliest type of cancer for both men and women, causing more deaths each year than breast, colon, and prostate cancers combined. Most lung cancer is **bronchogenic**, beginning in the cells that line the bronchi. Cigarette smoking is the leading cause of lung cancer; risk increases with how long people have smoked and the number of cigarettes smoked per day (■ FIGURE 16-11).

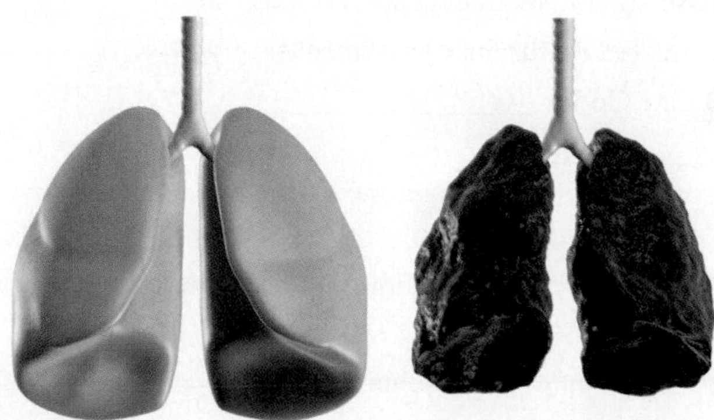

Figure 16-11 ■ Comparison of a Healthy Lung and the Lung of a Smoker. *Source: Sebastian Kaulitzki/Shutterstock.*

However, lung cancer occurs in people who have never smoked. According to the American Cancer Society (ACS), an estimated 3,000 nonsmoking adults die each year from lung cancer related to breathing secondhand smoke. Mesothelioma is lung cancer that is usually caused by exposure to asbestos dust.

Primary lung cancer is divided into non-small cell lung cancer (NSCLC), the most common type; small cell lung cancer (SCLC), which is aggressive and metastasizes quickly; and mixed small cell/large cell, which includes both NSCLC and SCLC. Lung cancer commonly spreads to the liver, adrenal glands, bone, and brain. According to ACS, five-year survival rates depend on the type of lung cancer and stage when discovered, but are lower (16%) compared to other cancers because it is usually not detected until metastasis has occurred. However, NSCLC found in Stage 1 and removed with surgery has a five-year survival rate of 60% to 70%.

The lung is also a common site of metastasis from other types of cancer, the most common being bladder, breast, colon, and kidney cancer. If the lung infiltration is a small area and the original tumor has been cured, then surgery to remove the diseased portion of the lung can be beneficial. However, this is rare and metastasis in the lung usually indicates that the original cancer has spread widely throughout the body and has a poor prognosis.

Although most types of lung cancer are classified in the Table of Neoplasms, coders should always search the Index first for the specific type of malignancy. Mesothelioma is classified in the Index, not the Table of Neoplasms. Codes are divided based on the site within the lung where the tumor is found and also contain laterality.

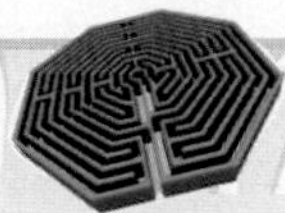

Coding Practice

Now it is your turn to practice coding neoplasms of the respiratory system. Refer to the ***Tip*** at the end of the mini-medical-record if you need a little extra help.

Exercise 16.5 Coding Neoplasms of the Respiratory System

Instructions: Read the mini-medical-record of each patient's encounter, then abstract, assign, and sequence ICD-10-CM diagnosis codes (CM) using the Index and Tabular List. Write the code(s) on the line provided.

1. Date: 6/5/yy Location: Branton Medical Center Provider: Gilbert Stagg, MD

Patient: Lakisha Wirtz Gender: F Age: 51

Reason for encounter: radiotherapy for lung cancer due to cigarette smoking

Assessment: NSCLC, upper left lobe,

Plan: return for daily treatments

3 CM Codes __________ __________ __________

2. Date: 6/5/yy Location: Branton Medical Center

Provider: Gilbert Stagg, MD

Patient: Annabelle Strohm Gender: F Age: 56

Reason for encounter: lung biopsy of mass found on X-ray when patient was treated for pneumonia, CT scan was inconclusive

(continued)

2. (continued)

Assessment: benign neoplasm right inferior lobe

Plan: Patient has been asymptomatic so there is no need to do a resection at this time.

1 CM Code __________

3. Date: 6/5/yy Location: Branton Medical Center

Provider: Gilbert Stagg, MD

Patient: Allan Rahimi Gender: M Age: 55

Reason for encounter: bilateral cervical lymphadenectomy

Assessment: pharyngeal cancer that has spread to lymph nodes, patient is dependent on alcohol and has a past history of nicotine (cigarette) dependence

Plan: radiation therapy

Tip: Lymphadenectomy is the surgical removal of a lymph node.

4 CM Codes __________ __________ __________ __________

4. Date: 6/5/yy Location: Branton Medical Center Provider: Gilbert Stagg, MD

Patient: Christopher Richison Gender: M Age: 68

Reason for encounter: right pulmonectomy

(continued)

4. (continued)

Assessment: bilateral pleural malignant mesothelioma, occupational exposure to asbestosis

Plan: radiotherapy

Tip: Remember to use an external cause code for accidental asbestos poisoning.

2 CM Codes __________ __________

5. Date: 6/5/yy Location: Ear, Nose, and Throat Specialists Provider: Shauna Rotz, MD

Patient: Erik Bucy Gender: M Age: 46

Reason for encounter: sinus pain, facial numbness

Assessment: squamous cell carcinoma (SCCA), maxillary sinus

Plan: surgical removal of tumor, to be followed with radiotherapy and chemotherapy

1 CM Code __________

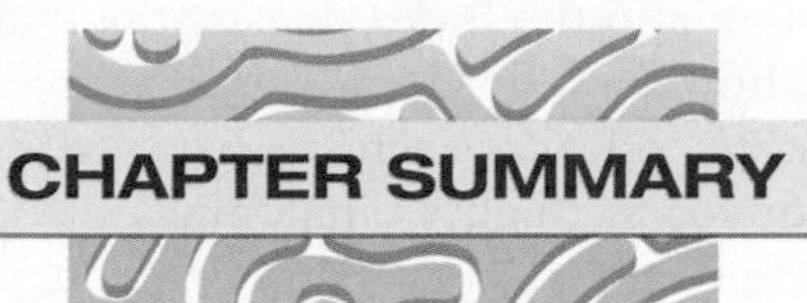

CHAPTER SUMMARY

In this chapter you learned that:

- The function of the respiratory system is to obtain oxygen from the air and deliver it to the lungs and blood for distribution to tissue cells, and to remove the gaseous waste product carbon dioxide from the blood and lungs and expel it.
- ICD-10-CM Chapter 10, Diseases of the Respiratory System (J00-J99), contains 11 blocks or subchapters that are divided by type of disorder and anatomic site.
- Coders should become familiar with chapter-wide coding considerations as well as information specifically for asthma, COPD, and influenza.
- OGCR provides specific instructions regarding sequencing codes for ventilator associated pneumonia and acute respiratory failure.
- Codes for neoplasms of the respiratory system appear in the block C30 to C39 in the neoplasm chapter, with the most common site being the lung.
- ICD-10-CM Official Guidelines for Coding and Reporting (OGCR) for the respiratory system, in OGCR section I.C.10, provide detailed discussion of chronic obstructive pulmonary disease and asthma, acute respiratory failure, influenza, and ventilator associated pneumonia.

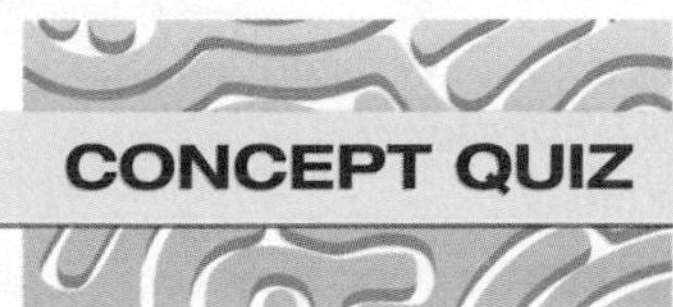

CONCEPT QUIZ

Take a moment to look back at your trip through diseases of the respiratory system and solidify your skills. This is your opportunity to pull together everything you have learned.

Completion

Instructions: Write the term that answers each question based on the information you learned in this chapter. Choose from the list below. Some choices may be used more than once and some choices may not be used at all. Refer to the discussion in this chapter and the Glossary at the end of this book if you need a little extra help.

acute exacerbation	alveoli
acute respiratory failure	asthma
atelectasis	lobular
avian	lower
bronchi	pharyngitis
chronic bronchitis	pleura
emphysema	status asthmaticus
H1N1	tonsillitis
laryngitis	tracheostomy
lobar	upper

1. The ____________________ respiratory tract consists of the nose, pharynx, and larynx.
2. Bronchioles end in small air sacs in the lungs called the ____________________.

3. ____________________ is the collapse of a lung.
4. COPD is the combination of ____________________ and ____________________ as comorbidities.
5. ____________________ is a chronic lung disease that affects the bronchi and is characterized by reversible obstruction and reshaping of the airway.
6. ____________________ pneumonia affects the alveoli and is also called bronchopneumonia.
7. ____________________ is an asthma exacerbation that does not respond to standard treatments.
8. A ____________________ is a surgical opening in the neck leading to the trachea.
9. Codes for ____________________ and ____________________ influenza can be assigned only when the physician documents a confirmed diagnosis.
10. Inflammation of the throat is called ____________________.

Multiple Choice

Instructions: Circle the letter of the best answer to each question based on the information you learned in this chapter. Refer to the discussion in this chapter and the Glossary at the end of this book if you need a little extra help.

1. A collection of air between the chest wall and lungs, which may cause the lung to collapse is
   A. atelectasis.
   B. pneumonia
   C. pneumothorax.
   D. pulmonary edema.
2. Which of the following is NOT one of the four severity levels used to classify asthma?
   A. Mild intermittent
   B. Mild persistent
   C. Moderate intermittent
   D. Moderate persistent
3. A reduction in the amount of inhaled air in each breath, most commonly caused by a reduction in the diameter of the bronchioles due to inflammation, is called
   A. airway obstruction.
   B. asthma.
   C. COPD
   D. status asthmaticus.
4. Ventilator associated pneumonia should be coded
   A. whenever a patient on mechanical ventilation has pneumonia.
   B. when a hospitalized patient acquires pneumonia after admission.
   C. when the physician documents that ventilation was required due to pneumonia.
   D. when the physician documents the relationship between mechanical ventilation and pneumonia.
5. Which of the following is NOT classified in ICD-10-CM Chapter 10, Diseases of the Respiratory System (J00-J99)?
   A. Chronic obstructive diseases
   B. Toxic effects of smoke
   C. Lung diseases due to external agents
   D. Infections of the upper respiratory tract
6. When a condition affects more than one site in the respiratory system and the Index does not provide a separate entry, how should codes be assigned?
   A. Assign separate codes for each site involved.
   B. Assign a code for the highest anatomical site.
   C. Assign a code for the lowest anatomical site.
   D. Assign a code for unspecified site.
7. Which of the following is NOT a key criterion for abstracting conditions of the respiratory system?
   A. Is the cause intrinsic or extrinsic?
   B. Is the condition acute or chronic?
   C. Is the condition in acute exacerbation?
   D. Does a lung abscess exist?
8. What is the correct coding for ventilator assisted pneumonia due to pseudomonas?
   A. J15.1 Pneumonia due to Pseudomonas
   B. J95.851 Ventilator associated pneumonia
   C. J95.851 Ventilator associated pneumonia and J15.1 Pneumonia due to Pseudomonas
   D. J95.851 Ventilator associated pneumonia and J96.5 Pseudomonas
9. Which of the following is NOT generally a manifestation of pneumonia?
   A. Nicotine dependence
   B. Encephalopathy
   C. Myocarditis
   D. Otitis media
10. The instructional note Use additional code, where applicable, to identify exposure to environmental tobacco smoke (Z77.22) applies to
    A. only codes for asthma
    B. only codes for asthma and COPD.
    C. only codes for asthma, COPD, and pneumonia.
    D. all codes in ICD-10-CM Chapter 10.

CODING CHALLENGE

Now it is your turn to demonstrate coding all aspects of diseases of the respiratory system. Refer back to the examples and discussion in this chapter when you need a little extra help. Use your medical dictionary and anatomy references when needed.

Instructions: Read the mini-medical-record of each patient's encounter, then abstract, assign, and sequence ICD-10-CM diagnosis codes (CM) using the Index and Tabular List. Write the code(s) on the line provided.

1. Date: *6/19/yy* Location: North Side Pulmonology Provider: *Gilbert Stagg, MD*

Patient: Emilia Weyandt Gender: F Age: 1

Reason for encounter: *productive cough, SOB, fever*

Assessment: *Chest X-ray and sputum culture positive for acute bronchitis due to Streptococcus pneumonia. Child exposed to cigarette smoke prenatally and currently because her mother smoked during pregnancy and still does.*

Plan: *OTC expectorant, acetaminophen to reduce fever, FU one week or sooner if necessary.*

Tip: Assign one code for the bronchitis and two codes for smoke exposure.

3 ICD-10-CM Codes __________ __________ __________

2. Date: *6/19/yy* Location: North Side Pulmonology Provider: *Gilbert Stagg, MD*

Patient: Eve Maciejewski Gender: F Age: 9

Reason for encounter: *coughing, wheezing, SOB, and chest tightness during and 10 to 15 minutes after exercising during gym at school*

Assessment: *acute exacerbation of mild persistent asthma, intrinsic*

Plan: *Rx bronchodilator, use prior to exercise. FU office visit in one month.*

Tip: Remember to code the severity of the asthma.

1 ICD-10-CM Code __________

3. Date: *6/19/yy* Location: Branton Medical Center Provider: *Gilbert Stagg, MD*

Patient: Brad Matchett Gender: M Age: 82

Reason for admission: *pneumonococcal pneumonia*

Assessment: *COPD with acute exacerbation required ventilation*

Plan: *discharged to skilled nursing facility with oxygen*

2 ICD-10-CM Codes __________ __________

4. Date: *6/19/yy* Location: North Side Pulmonology Provider: *Gilbert Stagg, MD*

Patient: Leslie Viramontes Gender: F Age: 84

Reason for encounter: *cracked tracheostomy tube*

Assessment: *Patient also has sarcoidosis with lung involvement.*

Plan: *replaced tracheostomy tube*

Tip: A cracked tracheostomy tube is a mechanical complication of a tracheostomy.

2 ICD-10-CM Codes __________ __________

5. Date: *6/19/yy* Location: Branton Medical Center Provider: *Gilbert Stagg, MD*

Patient: Roland Yochum Gender: M Age: 33

Reason for encounter: *ethmoidectomy and nasal reconstruction*

Assessment: *ethmoidal polyps and hypertrophy of nasal turbinates due to deviated nasal septum*

Plan: *excised polyps and repaired deviated nasal septum*

3 ICD-10-CM Codes __________ __________ __________

(continued)

(continued from page 319)

6. Date: 6/19/yy Location: North Side Pulmonology Provider: Location: Branton Medical Center Provider: Gilbert, MD

Patient: Mia Morejona Gender: F Age: 23

Reason for encounter: acute sinus pain, toothache, headache

Assessment: acute recurrent sinusitis, right maxillary sinus

Plan: Schedule CT scan of sinuses, analgesic, antihistamine and antibiotic therapy. FU office visit 10 days.

1 CM Code __________

7. Date: 6/19/yy Location: Branton Medical Center Provider: Gilbert Stagg, MD

Patient: Mitchell Krumm Gender: M Age: 89

Reason for admission: admitted from emergency department due to acute respiratory failure

Assessment: ARF is due to aspiration pneumonia due to gastric secretions, lung abscess, diabetes type 2 with gastroparesis

Plan: Discharged to a skilled nursing facility.

4 CM Codes __________ __________ __________ __________

8. Date: 6/19/yy Location: Branton Medical Center Provider: Gilbert Stagg, MD

Patient: Erik Hicklin Gender: M Age: 72

Reason for admission: gram-negative pneumonia

(continued)

8. (continued)

Assessment: Patient's left-sided congestive heart failure and pulmonary edema were managed in addition to the pneumonia. Patient also has chronic back pain with an unknown etiology but it was not a factor during this admission.

Plan: FU with pulmonary clinic and cardiologist in one week

2 CM Codes __________ __________

9. Date: 6/19/yy Location: Branton Medical Center Provider: Gilbert Stagg, MD

Patient: Jared Hershman Gender: M Age: 36

Reason for admission: difficulty breathing

Assessment: spontaneous pneumothorax due to a ruptured bulla

Plan: X-ray confirmed reexpansion of lung, pulmonary clinic FU 1 week

1 CM Code __________

10. Date: 6/19/yy Location: Branton Medical Center Provider: Gilbert Stagg, MD

Patient: Callie Oliveros Gender: F Age: 6

Reason for encounter: **T&A**

Assessment: chronic tonsillitis with adenoiditis

Plan: FU in office 1 week

1 CM Code __________

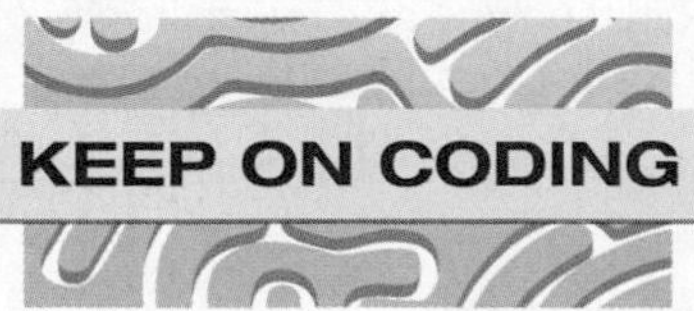

KEEP ON CODING

As a coder, you can never have too much experience. Apply everything you have learned in this chapter to code the following diagnostic statements. Use the OGCR and instructional notes in the Tabular List to help determine how many codes are required.

Instructions: Read the diagnostic statement, then use the Index and Tabular List to assign and sequence ICD-10-CM (CM) diagnosis codes. Write the code(s) on the line provided.

1. Acute pharyngitis: CM Code(s) ____________________
2. Atelectasis: CM Code(s) ____________________

3. Chylous effusion of the pleura: CM Code(s) ____________________
4. Allergic rhinitis due to pollen: CM Code(s) ____________________
5. Malignant neoplasm of the ethmoid sinus, right: CM Code(s) ____________________
6. Stenosis of the larynx: CM Code(s) ____________________
7. Chlamydial pneumonia: CM Code(s) ____________________
8. Acute streptococcal tonsillitis: CM Code(s) ____________________
9. Avian flu: CM Code(s) ____________________
10. Acute bronchiolitis due to respiratory syncytial virus: CM Code(s) ____________________
11. Chronic tonsillitis: CM Code(s) ____________________
12. Exercised induced bronchospasm: CM Code(s) ____________________
13. Postprocedural respiratory failure: CM Code(s) ____________________
14. Hernia of the mediastinum: CM Code(s) ____________________
15. Mixed simple and mucopurulent chronic bronchitis: CM Code(s) ____________________
16. COPD (chronic obstructive pulmonary disease) with acute exacerbation: CM Code(s) ____________________
17. Carcinoma of the trachea: CM Code(s) ____________________
18. Acute respiratory failure with hypoxia: CM Code(s) ____________________
19. Maltworker's lung: CM Code(s) ____________________
20. Personal history of carcinoma of the lung: CM Code(s) ____________________
21. Vocal cord paralysis, bilateral: CM Code(s) ____________________
22. Tracheoesophageal fistula following tracheostomy: CM Code(s) ____________________
23. Ulcer of the left bronchus: CM Code(s) ____________________
24. Exercise induced bronchospasm: CM Code(s) ____________________
25. Pharyngeal abscess: CM Code(s) ____________________

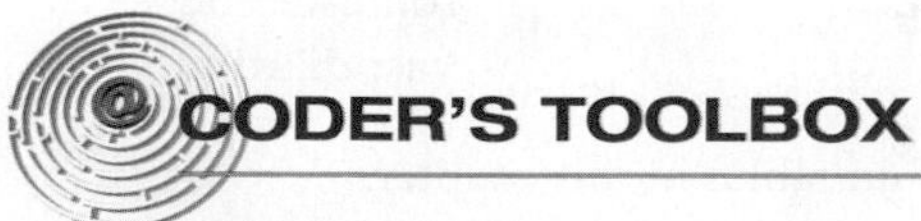

CODER'S TOOLBOX

The following resources are a starting point for learning more about diseases of the respiratory system. The > symbol indicates a menu selection within the website in order to navigate to a specific page.

American Lung Association **http://www.lungusa.org/**

Cancer Care **http://www.lungcancer.org/**

Family Allergy and Asthma > Diseases **http://www.familyallergy.com/diseases/default.asp**

National Heart Blood and Lung Institute (NHBLI) **http://www.nhlbi.nih.gov/**

The American College of Allergy, Asthma, and Immunology (ACAAI) **http://www.acaai.org/allergist/Pages/default.aspx**

Healthline > Videos **http://www.healthline.com/vpvideo/**

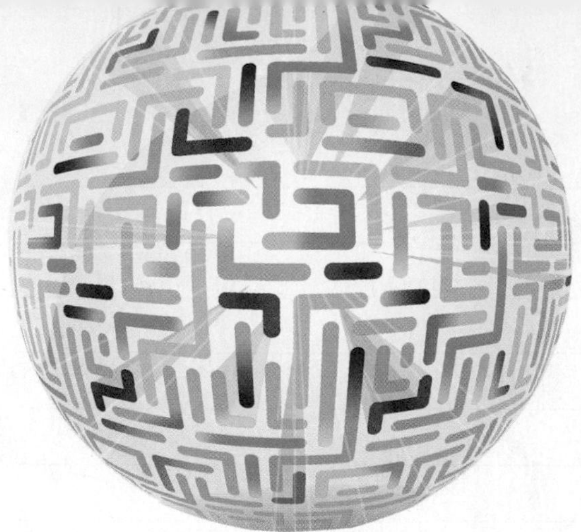

17

Diseases of the Nervous System and Sense Organs (G00-G99)

Learning Objectives

After completing this chapter, you should have the skills to:

- Spell and define the key words, medical terms, and abbreviations related to the nervous system and sense organs.
- Discuss the structure, function, and common conditions of the nervous system and sense organs.
- Identify the main characteristics of coding for the nervous system and sense organs.
- Abstract information from the medical record required for coding the nervous system and sense organs.
- Assign codes for the nervous system and sense organs.
- Arrange codes for the nervous system and sense organs.
- Code neoplasms of the nervous system and sense organs.
- Discuss the Official Guidelines for Coding and Reporting related to the nervous system and sense organs.

Key Terms and Abbreviations

absence seizure
Alzheimer's disease (AD)
atonic
aura
brain
central nervous system (CNS)
clonic
complex partial
dementia
distributed
dominance
early onset
focal
generalized
grand mal
gustatory
hemiplegia
homeostasis
idiopathic
intractable
late onset
localized
monoplegia
myoclonic
nervous system
neurons
olfactory
Parkinson's disease (PD)
Parkinsonian
Parkinsonism
partial
peripheral nervous system (PNS)
petit mal
pharmacoresistant
psychomotor
quadriplegia
reflex sympathetic dystrophy (RSD)
refractory
secondary Parkinsonism
simple partial
spinal cord
status epilepticus
status migrainosus
tonic
tonic-clonic
vasodilation

In addition to the key terms listed here, students should know the terms defined within tables in this chapter.

Chapter Outline

- **Nervous System Refresher**
- **Coding Overview of the Nervous System**
- **Abstracting for the Nervous System**
- **Assigning Codes for the Nervous System**
- **Arranging Codes for the Nervous System**
- **Coding Neoplasms of the Nervous System**

ICD-10-CM codes in this chapter are from the ICD-10-CM 2014 Draft code set from the Department of Health and Human Services, Centers for Disease Control and Prevention.

INTRODUCTION

A properly functioning electrical system in your vehicle is essential for it to run. But anyone who has experienced electrical problems will tell you that they can be among the most difficult car problems to diagnose because they cannot be seen. A defect in the electrical system located in one part of the car can create a problem in a completely different area. The human nervous system is the electrical system in our bodies, sending and receiving messages that enable us to perform all functions.

In your tour of the nervous system and sense organs in this chapter you will learn more about how the nervous system works, why sometimes it does not work as it should, and how physicians treat these conditions. Most importantly, you will practice coding for patient encounters related to nervous diseases and conditions, a skill that requires you to abstract information from the medical record, assign correct codes, and arrange (sequence) the codes in the proper order.

A neurologist specializes in diagnosing and treating conditions of the nervous system. Neurosurgeons specialize in performing surgical procedures on the nervous system. Primary care physicians treat uncomplicated conditions of the nervous system and refer more complex cases to a specialist.

As you read this chapter, open up your medical terminology book to the nervous system and keep a medical dictionary handy to refresh your memory of any unfamiliar terms. Think of these resources as your travel brochures that tell you more about an area. This way, you have the information you need at your fingertips.

NERVOUS SYSTEM REFRESHER

The function of the **nervous system** is to direct the body's response to internal and external stimuli and coordinate the activities of other organ systems. It works with the endocrine system to maintain **homeostasis** (*maintenance of a stable internal physical state*). The nervous system consists of the **central nervous system (CNS)** and **peripheral nervous system (PNS)**. The CNS acts as the control center for the nervous system by processing information and providing short term control over other organ systems. The CNS consists of the **brain** and **spinal cord**. The brain governs perception of the senses, emotions, consciousness, memory, and voluntary movements (■ FIGURE 17-1). The spinal cord relays information to and from the brain. The PNS consists of the 12 nerves that radiate out from the brain and the 31 pairs of nerves that radiate from the spinal cord to all other areas of the body (■ FIGURE 17-2, page 324). The PNS links the CNS with other systems and the sense organs.

In Figures 17-1 and 17-2, each structure in the nervous system is labeled with its name as well as its medical terminology root/combining form where applicable. As you learn about conditions and procedures that affect the nervous system, remember to apply medical terminology skills to use word roots, prefixes, and suffixes you already know to define new terms related to the nervous system. Refer to ■ TABLE 17-1 (page 324) for a refresher on how to build medical terms related to the nervous system.

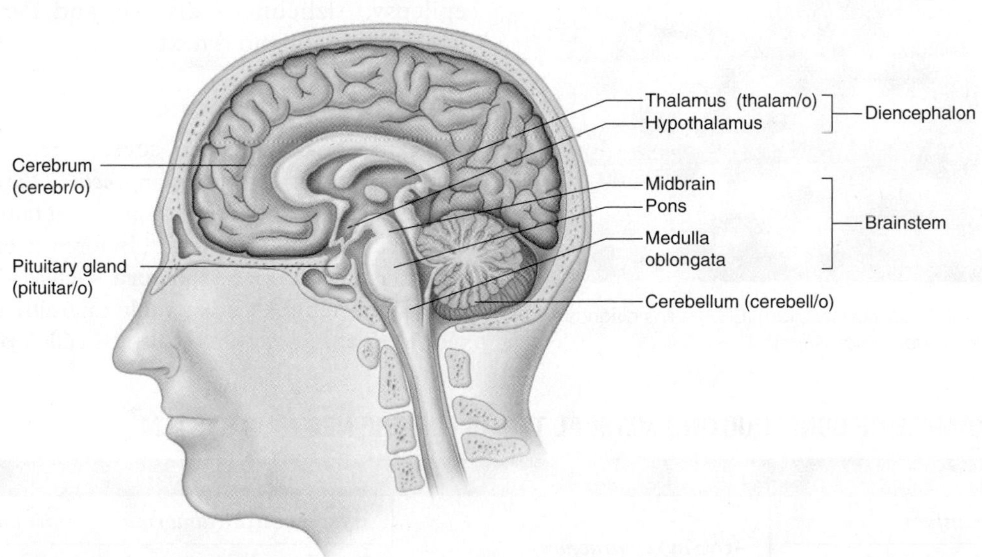

Figure 17-1 ■ The Brain

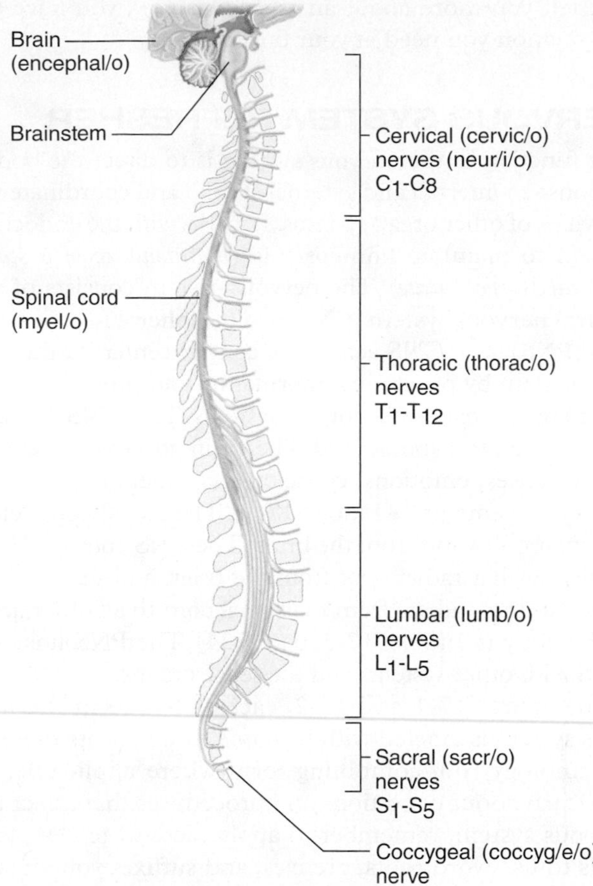

Figure 17-2 ■ The Spinal Cord and Spinal Nerves

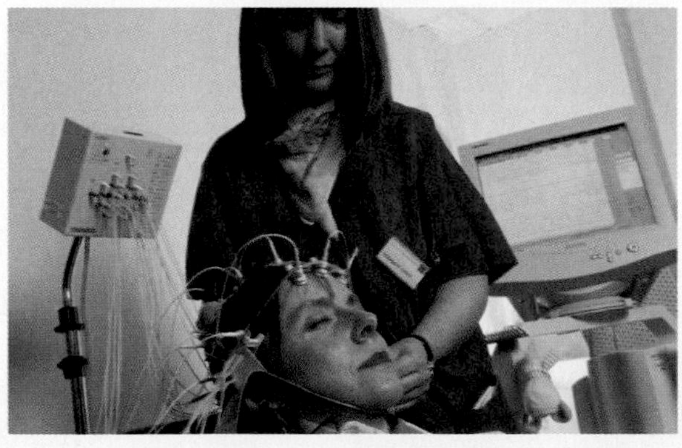

Figure 17-3 ■ An electroencephalogram (EEG) helps diagnose brain disorders. *Source: © doc-stock/Alamy.*

CODING CAUTION

Be alert for medical terms with similar spellings but different meanings:

heme (*word root meaning blood*) and **hemi** (*prefix meaning half*)

cerebrovascular (*pertaining to vessels of the brain*) and **cardiovascular** (*pertaining to vessels of the heart*)

electroencephalogram (EEG) (*recording of the electrical activity of the brain*) (■ FIGURE 17-3) and **electrocardiogram (EKG, ECG)** (*recording of the electrical activity of the heart*)

homeostasis (*maintenance of a stable internal physical state*) and **hemostasis** (*stoppage of bleeding*)

cerebrum (*the largest structure of the brain that controls sensory and motor activity*) and **cerebellum** (*the portion of the brain located below and behind the cerebrum*)

Conditions of the Nervous System

Diseases and disorders of the nervous system include headaches, infectious diseases, CNS disorders, and seizure disorders. Coders use medical resources, such as a reference book on diseases, to understand conditions of the nervous system, diagnostic methods, and common treatments. Refer to ■ TABLE 17-2 for a summary of diseases affecting the nervous system.

In particular, coders must be familiar with specific concepts and terminology related to migraine headaches, epilepsy, Alzheimer's disease, and Parkinson's disease, which are highlighted next.

Migraine Headaches

Migraine headaches are severe, debilitating headaches caused by **vasodilation** (*enlargement of the blood vessels*). They may be accompanied by symptoms of nausea, vomiting, and sensitivity to light and sound. Before the onset of a migraine, patients may experience an **aura**, such as a sensation of voices or colored light. An **intractable** migraine is one that is resistant to treatment and may also be called **pharmacoresistant**

Table 17-1 ■ **EXAMPLE OF CONSTRUCTING MEDICAL TERMS FOR THE NERVOUS SYSTEM**

Prefix/Combining Form	Suffix	Complete Medical Term
dys- (*abnormal, painful*)	**-tonia** (*contraction*) **-plegia** (*paralysis*) **-al** (*pertaining to*)	**dys + tonia** (*abnormal contraction*)
hemi- (*one side*)		**hemi + plegia** (*paralysis on one side of the body*)
neur/i/o (*nerve*)		**neuro + plegia** (*paralysis of a nerve*) **neur + al** (*pertaining to nerves*)

Table 17-2 ■ **COMMON DISEASES OF THE NERVOUS SYSTEM**

Condition	Definition
Alzheimer's disease	A progressive degenerative brain disease
Amyotrophic lateral sclerosis (ALS) or lou gehrig disease	A chronic, terminal neurological disease characterized by a progressive loss of motor neurons and muscle atrophy
Bell's palsy	Inflammation of the seventh (VII) cranial nerve, the facial nerve
Cerebral palsy	A functional disorder of the brain manifested by motor impairment
Chronic pain syndrome (CPS)	A collection of pain conditions lasting more than six months and unresponsive to treatment
Cluster headache	Unilateral pain in the eye or temple
Complex regional pain syndrome	A chronic pain syndrome in which an extremity experiences intense burning pain and changes in skin texture and temperature; also called reflex sympathetic dystrophy (RSD)
Degenerative neural disease	A class of diseases marked by degeneration of nerves and brain tissue, resulting in abnormalities in muscle and sensory functions
Dementia	A loss of brain function that affects memory, thinking, language, judgment, and behavior
Dystonia	Erratic jerky movements due to improperly functioning muscle tension
Encephalitis	A viral inflammation of the brain and meninges
Epilepsy	A brain disorder in which neurons signal abnormally, causing seizures and/or unconsciousness
Huntington's chorea	An inherited progressive, degenerative disease involving loss of muscle control and personality changes
Hydrocephalus	Excess cerebrospinal fluid trapped in the brain
Meningitis	A contagious, acute inflammation of the pia mater and the arachnoid mater in the brain
Migraine headache	A severe, debilitating headache caused by vasodilation
Multiple sclerosis	A chronic, progressive disorder of the CNS characterized by muscle impairment due to patches of hardened tissue in the brain or spinal cord
Narcolepsy	A condition characterized by brief sudden attacks of deep sleep
Parkinson's disease	A degenerative disease that affects muscle control and coordination
Spina bifida	A congenital neural tube defect in which vertebrae do not fuse

(*resistant to medication*) or refractory (*resistant to treatment*). A migraine that lasts more than 72 hours is considered to be status migrainosus.

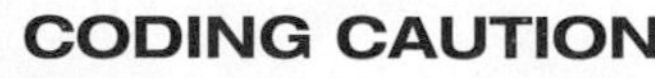

CODING CAUTION

Do not assume that any severe headache is a migraine.

Epilepsy

Epilepsy is a brain disorder in which neurons (*clusters of nerve cells*) signal abnormally, causing seizures and/or unconsciousness. Epilepsy may be due to a medical condition, an injury, or may be idiopathic (*of unknown cause*). Known causes include the following:

- alcoholism
- birth trauma
- depressed skull fracture
- penetrating wound
- infections of the brain
- dementia
- stroke or transient ischemic attack (TIA)
- other traumatic brain injury
- brain tumor

CODING CAUTION

Do not assume that all seizure activity is epilepsy. Seizures may also be caused by high fevers, psychological disorders, or other medical conditions such as narcolepsy, **Tourette syndrome**, or cardiac arrhythmia.

Seizures are classified as localized or generalized based on of the source of the seizure within the brain. Localized, partial, or focal seizures occur in one part of the brain. Localized seizures are further classified based on whether consciousness is affected, as follows:

- A simple partial seizure affects only a small region of the brain and does not cause loss of consciousness.
- A complex partial, or psychomotor, seizure is associated with both sides of the cerebrum and causes a change in or loss of consciousness.

Generalized or distributed seizures are the result of abnormal activity on both sides of the brain and include the following types:

- absence or petit mal—characterized by muscle twitching or jerking for several seconds
- myoclonic—jerking and twitching in upper body, arms, or legs
- tonic—characterized by prolonged muscle contractions or a stiffening
- clonic—characterized by a series of muscle contractions and relaxations on both sides of the body
- tonic-clonic or grand mal—characterized by a sudden loss of consciousness and falling to the floor and affects the entire brain
- atonic—characterized by a brief loss of muscle tone

Epilepsy is classified as to whether or not it is intractable. According to the Centers for Disease Control and Prevention, approximately 70% of epilepsy is responsive to medication and 30% is intractable. Status epilepticus is an epileptic seizure that lasts more than 30 minutes or is a near-constant state of seizures and is a medical emergency.

Alzheimer's Disease

Alzheimer's disease (AD) is a progressive degenerative brain disease that doubles in prevalence with every five years of age. Early onset AD is diagnosed before age 65 and accounts for approximately 10% of all AD cases, according to the Centers for Disease Control and Prevention. Late onset AD is diagnosed after age 65 and affects 30% to 40% of people over age 85. AD is the most common cause of dementia (*a progressive loss of brain function that affects memory, thinking, language, judgment, and behavior*), which is classified in ICD-10-CM Chapter 5, Mental and Behavioral Disorders.

Parkinson's Disease

Parkinson's disease (PD) is a degenerative disease that affects muscle control and coordination, usually occurring in midlife. Symptoms include tremor, rigid muscles, and loss of normal reflexes. Dementia may be caused by PD or it may occur independently of PD. When dementia is diagnosed first, followed at a later time with an additional diagnosis of Parkinson's disease, the combined condition is referred to as Parkinson*ian* dementia or dementia with Parkinson*ism* and assumes the existence of Lewy body disease. When PD is diagnosed first, followed at a later time with an additional diagnosis of dementia, the combined condition is referred to as Parkin*son's* disease with dementia, and the existence of Lewy body disease is not assumed. Secondary Parkinsonism is Parkinson-type abnormal movements that are caused by medication or another condition.

This section provides a general reference to help understand the most common diagnoses of the nervous system, but does not list everything you need to know. Use medical terminology skills discussed earlier in this chapter to learn the meaning of unfamiliar words. Remember to keep standard reference books handy in case you get stuck. Refer to the resources in the Coder's Toolbox at the end of this chapter to learn more about conditions affecting the nervous system.

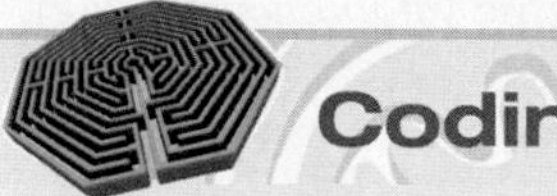

Coding Practice

Refresh your knowledge of terminology related to the nervous system and sense organs. Use a medical terminology text or a website such as GlobalRph.com > Medical Terminology **http://www.globalrph.com/medterm.htm** to identify the meaning of word parts that may not be familiar.

Exercise 17.1 Nervous System Refresher

Instructions: Use your medical terminology skills and resources to define the following conditions related to the nervous system, then assign the default diagnosis code.

Follow these steps:

- Use slash marks "/" to break down each term into its root(s) and suffix.
- Define the meaning of the word, based on the meaning of each word part.
- Assign the default ICD-10-CM diagnosis code (CM) for the condition using the Index and Tabular List.

(continued)

Example: neuropathy neuro/pathy Meaning: abnormal condition of a nerve CM Code: G62.9

1. neuroma Meaning ______________ CM Code ________
2. neuromyelitis Meaning ______________ CM Code ________
3. encephalomyeloradiculitis Meaning ______________ CM Code ________
4. causalgia Meaning ______________ CM Code ________
5. neuromyotonia Meaning ______________ CM Code ________
6. myelinolysis Meaning ______________ CM Code ________
7. hemichorea Meaning ______________ CM Code ________
8. meningoencephalopathy Meaning ______________ CM Code ________
9. myasthenia Meaning ______________ CM Code ________
10. hemiplegia Meaning ______________ CM Code ________

CODING OVERVIEW OF THE NERVOUS SYSTEM

ICD-10-CM Chapter 6, Diseases of the Nervous System and Sense Organs (G00-G99) contains 11 blocks or subchapters that are divided by the type of structure affected. Review the block names and code ranges listed at the beginning of Chapter 6 in the ICD-10-CM manual to become familiar with the content and organization.

ICD-10-CM Chapter 6 is comparable to ICD-9-CM Chapter 6 (320-389). Some codes from other chapters in ICD-9-CM have been moved to the nervous system chapter in ICD-10-CM. For example, ICD-10-CM category G45, Transient cerebral ischemic attacks, includes codes from ICD-9-CM Chapter 7, Diseases of the Circulatory System. Categories for Alzheimer's disease (G30), migraine headaches (G43), secondary Parkinsonism (G21), and dystonia (G24) are examples of categories in which codes have been significantly expanded in ICD-10-CM. Instructional notes have been expanded in ICD-10-CM directing coders to use an external cause code, code first the underlying disease, and code first the underlying neoplasm.

This chapter includes disorders of the central and peripheral nervous systems as well as paralytic syndromes. It also includes the gustatory (*taste*) and olfactory (*smell*) sense organs The eye and the ear, which were both part of Chapter 6 in ICD-9-CM, each has its own chapter in ICD-10-CM. This chapter does not include congenital disorders or injuries, which are classified in other ICD-10-CM chapters. This chapter also does not include cerebrovascular disease, which is classified with the circulatory system in block I60-I69. However, it does include transient ischemic attacks and related syndromes that were classified with the circulatory system in ICD-9-CM.

ICD-10-CM provides Official Guidelines for Coding and Reporting (OGCR) for the nervous system and sense organs in OGCR section I.C.6. OGCR provides detailed discussion of coding for pain, including general coding information, postoperative pain, chronic pain, neoplasm related pain, and chronic pain syndrome. OGCR also discusses the definitions of dominant and nondominant side when coding hemiplegia. OGCR I.C.19.g.2) discusses pain due to devices, implants, and grafts. OGCR I.C.5.a. discusses pain disorders related to psychological factors.

ABSTRACTING FOR THE NERVOUS SYSTEM

When abstracting, coders analyze the medical record to highlight the key facts of the case and to identify details that will be important when assigning and sequencing codes. As coders gain experience in assigning and sequencing codes, they are able to abstract more quickly and more accurately. Review the questions in ■ TABLE 17-3 to learn key questions to ask when analyzing cases related to the nervous system. Remember that the abstracting questions are a guide and that not every question applies to, or can be answered for, every case. Because of the variety of conditions addressed under the nervous system, coders need

Table 17-3 ■ KEY CRITERIA FOR ABSTRACTING CONDITIONS OF THE NERVOUS SYSTEM

- ❑ What is the condition?
- ❑ What is the subtype of the condition?
- ❑ What is the anatomic site?
- ❑ What is the underlying disease, if any?
- ❑ What is external cause, if any?
- ❑ What is the infectious organism, if any?
- ❑ What laterality is documented?
- ❑ Is paralysis documented?

Table 17-4 ■ **KEY CRITERIA FOR ABSTRACTING PAIN**

- ❑ What is the site of the pain?
- ❑ What is the underlying cause of the pain?
- ❑ Is the pain due to a device, implant, graft, or trauma?
- ❑ Is the pain postoperative?
- ❑ Is it related to a specific postoperative complication?
- ❑ Is the pain related to a neoplasm?
- ❑ Is pain management the reason for the encounter?
- ❑ Is treatment of the underlying condition the reason for the encounter?
- ❑ Is the pain documented as chronic?
- ❑ Is chronic pain syndrome documented?
- ❑ Is complex regional pain syndrome documented?
- ❑ What psychological factors are associated with the pain?

Table 17-5 ■ **KEY CRITERIA FOR ABSTRACTING HEADACHES**

- ❑ What specific type of headache is documented?
- ❑ Is it documented as intractable?
- ❑ Is the headache documented as episodic or chronic?
- ❑ Does it affect the entire head or only one side?
- ❑ Is the headache accompanied with aura?
- ❑ Is status migrainosus or duration of 72 hours or more documented?
- ❑ Is the headache associated with another condition, such as trauma, menstruation, cerebral infarction, or drug use?

Table 17-6 ■ **KEY CRITERIA FOR ABSTRACTING EPILEPSY**

- ❑ Is the seizure documented as epilepsy?
- ❑ Is it localized or generalized?
- ❑ Is it documented as intractable?
- ❑ Is status epilepticus or duration of 30 minutes or more documented?
- ❑ Are partial seizures documented as simple or complex?

Table 17-7 ■ **KEY CRITERIA FOR ABSTRACTING PARKINSON'S DISEASE**

- ❑ Is Parkinsonism primary or secondary?
- ❑ Is dementia documented?
- ❑ Is dementia documented as Parkinsonian dementia or Parkinson's disease with dementia?
- ❑ Is secondary Parkinsonism documented?
- ❑ What is the cause?

general criteria for abstracting conditions of the nervous system overall (Table 17-3), as well as specific criteria to abstract pain (■ TABLE 17-4), headaches (■ TABLE 17-5), epilepsy (■ TABLE 17-6), and PD (■ TABLE 17-7).

SUCCESS STEP

Several conditions have been expanded in ICD-10-CM compared to what they were in ICD-9-CM, requiring additional abstracting. The most notable of these are epilepsy, migraines, AD, secondary Parkinsonism, dystonia, and myasthenia gravis. Coders who have mastered ICD-9-CM should review these categories in ICD-10-CM carefully to learn the differences and new elements required.

SUCCESS STEP

Physicians do not need to use the exact word "intractable" in order to abstract a migraine or epilepsy as intractable. Acceptable terms that mean intractable are pharmacoresistant, pharmacologically resistant, treatment resistant, refractory, and poorly controlled.

Guided Example of Abstracting for the Nervous System

Refer to the following example throughout this chapter to practice skills for abstracting, assigning, and sequencing nervous system codes. Angelia Harkey, CPC, is a fictitious coder who guides you through the coding process.

Date: 7/11/yy Location: Branton Medical Center

Provider: Lorene Garman, MD

Patient: Catalina Piatt Gender: F Age: 57

Reason for encounter: patient was admitted from the emergency department where she presented with left sided hemiparesis

Assessment: Imaging studies were negative for CVA, symptoms mitigated within 24 hours leading to a diagnosis of TIA. Patient received Duradrin (*a vasoconstrictor combination medication*) for classical migraine which responded to treatment. She received routine insulin for type 1 diabetes.

Plan: She was discharged to home with no residual weakness. FU in office 1 week.

Follow along as Angelia Harkey, CPC, abstracts the diagnosis. Check off each step after you complete it.

⇨ Angelia reads through the entire record, with special attention to the reason for the encounter and the final assessment.

- ❑ She notes that the presenting symptoms, left sided hemiparesis, were temporary and that imaging studies were negative for CVA, which she knows is a cerebrovascular accident, or a stroke.
- ❑ She reviews Key Criteria for Abstracting Conditions of the Nervous System (Table 17-3).
- ❑ *What is the condition?* She notes there is a definitive diagnosis of TIA, which is a transient ischemic attack. A TIA is a brief episode of ischemia that has temporary symptoms but no permanent damage.
- ❑ *What is the subtype of the condition?* None was listed.
- ❑ *What is the anatomic site?* A TIA by definition is in the brain.
- ❑ *What is the underlying disease if any?* None.
- ❑ *What is the external cause, if any?* None.
- ❑ *What is the infectious organism, if any?* None.
- ❑ *What laterality is documented?* Temporary left-sided hemiparesis.
- ❑ *Is paralysis documented?* Temporary weakness is documented, but no paralysis.
- ❑ Because the left-sided hemiparesis was temporary and the underlying cause was diagnosed as TIA, she knows she should not code for the presenting symptom.
- ❑ She identifies that two additional conditions were treated during the admission: classical migraine and type 1 diabetes.

⇨ At this time, Angelia has a good idea that she will have three diagnoses, but she will not know for certain until she completes the next step of assigning codes.

Coding Practice

Now it is your turn to practice abstracting diagnoses for the nervous system and sense organs. Questions guide your analysis of each scenario.

Exercise 17.2 Abstracting Diagnoses for the Nervous System

Instructions: Read the mini-medical-record of each patient's encounter and answer the abstracting questions. Write the answer on the line provided. Do not assign any codes.

1. Date: 7/13/yy Location: Neurology Associates

Provider: Lorene Garman, MD

Patient: Cherie Holzman Gender: F Age: 31

Reason for encounter: patient comes in today for a migraine which started 2 days ago with aura

Assessment: pharmacoresistant migraine

Plan: Administered injection of sumatriptan and discussed potential side effects and how to manage. Rx oral sumatriptan. Patient to call nurse tomorrow to discuss progress.

a. What condition is documented? ______________

____

b. Is it documented as intractable? ______________

____

(continued)

1. (continued)

c. Is it documented as affecting only one side?

____

d. Is the migraine accompanied with aura?

____

e. Is status migrainosus or duration of 72 hours or more documented? ______________

f. Is the headache associated with another condition: trauma, menstruation, cerebral infarction, or drug use? ______________

2. Date: 7/13/yy Location: Branton Medical Center

Provider: Lorene Garman, MD

Patient: Gordon Blanke Gender: M Age: 9

Reason for encounter: video EEG (*video to monitor brain activity in real time*) as part of ongoing epilepsy evaluation

Assessment: benign childhood epilepsy with EEG spikes, poorly controlled at this time

Plan: we are going to start with Rx gabapentin monotherapy (*single drug therapy*) and reevaluate in 4 weeks, consult with nutritionist re: diet modifications

(continued)

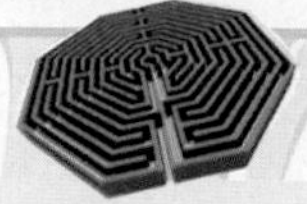

Coding Practice (continued)

2. (continued)

a. What condition is documented? ______________

b. What is the type of epilepsy? ______________

c. Is it documented as intractable? ______________

d. Is status epilepticus or duration of 30 minutes or more documented? ______________

3. Date: 7/13/yy Location: Neurology Associates
Provider: Lorene Garman, MD
Patient: Derek Brannum Gender: M Age: 51
Reason for encounter: management of PD, patient reports increased tremor activity and difficulty walking since last visit
Assessment: PD has progressed
Plan: adjusted medications, referred to physical therapy

a. What symptoms are reported? ______________

b. What condition is documented? ______________

c. Should you code the symptoms? ______________
Why or why not? ______________

d. Is the condition primary or secondary? ______________

e. Is dementia documented? ______________

4. Date: 7/14/yy Location: Branton Medical Center Provider: Lorene Garman, MD
Patient: Patricia Huskins Gender: F Age: 33
Reason for admission: implant neurostimulator (*a device placed under the skin that stimulates the spinal cord by tiny electrical impulses*) for pain control
Assessment: chronic lumbar pain due to displaced disc at L3-L4 which resulted from a back injury two years ago
Plan: FU 2 weeks

(continued)

4. (continued)

a. What is the reason for admission? ______________

b. What is the site of the pain? ______________

c. What is the underlying cause of the pain? ______________

d. Is the pain due to a device, implant, graft, or trauma? ______________

e. Is pain management the reason for the encounter? ______________

f. Is treatment of the underlying condition the reason for the encounter? ______________

g. Is the pain documented as chronic? ______________

h. Is chronic pain syndrome documented? ______________

5. Date: 7/14/yy Location: Branton Medical Center Provider: Lorene Garman, MD
Patient: Darrell Commons Gender: M Age: 86
Reason for encounter: admitted from nursing facility due to generalized weakness
Assessment: weakness is due to hyponatremia, patient presents an elopement risk due to late onset AD, dementia with hallucinations, and wandering
Plan: discharged to nursing facility

a. What symptom is documented? ______________

b. What is the cause of the symptom? ______________

c. What type of AD is documented? ______________

d. What is an elopement risk? ______________

e. Does the dementia have behavioral disturbances? ______________

f. What is the principal diagnosis? ______________

g. What additional diagnosis(es) should be coded? ______________ Why? ______________

(continued)

6. Date: 7/14/yy Location: Branton Medical Center Provider: Lorene Garman, MD

Patient: Leah Caison Gender: F Age: 42

Reason for admission: admitted from emergency department where patient presented with migraine of 4 days duration which has not responded to the usual medication

Assessment: persistent migraine with cerebrovascular infarction, cerebral stenosis of right cerebellar artery, hypertension

a. What specific type of migraine is documented? ______________________

b. Is it documented as intractable? ______________________

(continued)

6. (continued)

c. Is the migraine accompanied with aura? ______________________

d. Is status migrainosus or duration of 72 hours or more documented? ______________________

e. What other conditions are documented? ______________________

f. What is the location of the cerebral stenosis? ______________________

g. What is the principal diagnosis? ______________________

ASSIGNING CODES FOR THE NERVOUS SYSTEM

OGCR contains specific guidelines for assigning codes for hemiplegia and monoplegia, and pain.

Assigning Codes for Hemiplegia and Monoplegia

According to the instructional note at the beginning of categories **G81, G82**, and **G83**, codes for **hemiplegia** (*paralysis of one side of the body*), **quadriplegia** (*paralysis of all limbs*), and **monoplegia** (*paralysis of one limb*) from this ICD-10-CM chapter should be assigned when the paralysis is reported without further specification, or is stated to be old or longstanding but of unspecified cause. Also use these categories in multiple coding to identify these conditions resulting from any cause. When these conditions result from cerebrovascular disease, assign codes from category **I69 Sequelae of cerebrovascular disease.**

Codes for hemiplegia and monoplegia require coders to assign a fifth character to identify a combination of laterality and dominance. **Dominance** refers to the side of the body an individual favors, such as being left-handed or right-handed (■ FIGURE 17-4).

For *right-handed* persons, assign the fifth character as follows:

- **1** identifies that the right side (dominant) of a right-handed person is affected.
- **4** identifies that the left side (nondominant) of a right-handed person is affected.

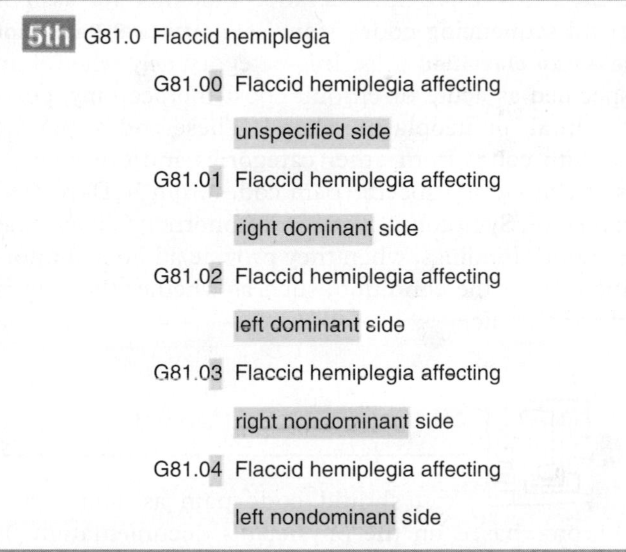

5th G81.0 Flaccid hemiplegia
G81.00 Flaccid hemiplegia affecting unspecified side
G81.01 Flaccid hemiplegia affecting right dominant side
G81.02 Flaccid hemiplegia affecting left dominant side
G81.03 Flaccid hemiplegia affecting right nondominant side
G81.04 Flaccid hemiplegia affecting left nondominant side

Figure 17-4 ■ Tabular List Entry Showing Dominance and Nondominance

For *left-handed* persons, assign the fifth character as follows:

- **2** identifies that the left side (dominant) of a left-handed person is affected (■ FIGURE 17-5, page 332).
- **3** identifies that the right side (nondominant) of a left-handed person is affected.

Assign the fifth character **0** when laterality is not documented.

When laterality is documented, but dominance is not, OGCR I.C.6.a. instructs coders to code the right side as

Patient, who is left-handed, is seen for left side flaccid hemiplegia.

G81.02 Flaccid hemiplegia affecting left dominant side

Figure 17-5 ■ Example of Hemiplegia Affecting Left Dominant Side

Patient is seen for monoplegia of the left arm.

G83.24 Monoplegia of upper limb affecting left nondominant side

Figure 17-6 ■ Example of Monoplegia with Unspecified Dominance

dominant and the left side as nondominant (■ Figure 17-6). For ambidextrous patients, the default is to code the affected side as dominant.

Assigning Codes for Pain

OGCR I.C.6.b. provides detailed guidance for assigning and sequencing codes from category **G89 Pain, not elsewhere classified**. Use this category *only* when pain is specified as acute or chronic, post-thoracotomy, post-procedural, or neoplasm related. These codes may be used with codes from other categories and other chapters, including site-specific pain codes from ICD-10-CM Chapter 18, Symptoms, Signs and Abnormal Clinical and Laboratory Findings, when they provide additional information about the condition, such as whether the pain is acute or chronic.

SUCCESS STEP

You should code pain as acute or chronic based on the physician's documentation. There is no specific timeframe that defines acute or chronic.

Coders must determine if the underlying cause of the pain is known. If it is, assign codes from category **G89** *only* when the purpose of the encounter is to provide pain management (■ Figure 17-7), but not when the purpose of the encounter is to treat the underlying condition (■ Figure 17-8) (OGCR I.C.6.b.1 (a) and (b)).

ICD-10-CM provides a specific code and specific OGCR for neoplasm related pain (OGCR I.C.6.b.5)). Assign code **G89.3 Neoplasm related pain (acute) (chronic)**

Patient with a displaced C4-C5 disk due to trauma and associated severe chronic neck pain presents for a steroid injection in the spinal canal in order to relieve pain.

(1) G89.21 Chronic pain due to trauma

(2) M50.22 Other cervical disc displacement, mid-cervical region

Figure 17-7 ■ Example of an Encounter to Treat Pain

Patient with low back pain due to a wedge compression fracture of lumbar vertebra L4 is seen for balloon kyphoplasty *(a procedure to stabilize the vertebral segments).*

S32.040A Wedge compression fracture of fourth lumbar vertebra

Figure 17-8 ■ Example of an Encounter to Treat the Underlying Condition

when pain is documented as either acute or chronic for any of the following:

- neoplasm related
- cancer associated
- due to malignancy
- tumor associated

Also assign a code(s) for the neoplasm and/or metastases.

Refer to OGCR I.C.6.b.3) for instructions on coding postoperative pain.

CODING CAUTION

Be careful to distinguish codes for chronic pain **(G89.2-)**, chronic pain syndrome **(G89.4)**, and complex regional pain syndrome (CRPS) **(G90.5-)** based on the physician's documentation.

Guided Example of Assigning Nervous System Codes

To practice assigning codes for diseases of the nervous system, continue with the example from earlier in the chapter about patient Catalina Piatt, who was admitted to Branton Medical Center due to left sided hemiparesis.

Follow along in your ICD-10-CM manual as Angelia Harkey, CPC, assigns codes. Check off each step after you complete it.

➪ First, Angelia reviews the conditions she identified during abstracting:

- ❑ TIA
- ❑ *classical migraine*
- ❑ *type 1 diabetes*

➪ Angelia is most concerned about assigning a code for the migraine, so she begins with this diagnosis. She searches the Index for the Main Term **Migraine**.

- ❑ She locates the subterm **classical** and reads the cross-referencing note in the Index, ***see*** **Migraine, with aura**.
- ❑ Staying under the Main Term **Migraine**, she locates the subterm **with aura** (■ FIGURE 17-9).
- ❑ She notices that there are indented third-level subterms for **intractable, not intractable,** and **persistent**.
- ❑ She double-checks the medical record and notes that the physician documented *classical migraine which responded to treatment*. Because intractable means "not responsive to treatment," she determines that she should select a code for not intractable. Although the physician did not use the exact statement "not intractable," she is confident of the meaning of the term and proceeds.
- ❑ Under the entry for **not intractable**, she reads two additional indented subterms for **with** or **without status migrainosus**.
- ❑ She again double-checks the documentation and confirms that status migrainosus is not documented, so she selects the entry for **without status migrainosus, G43.109**.
- ❑ Angelia verifies code **G43.109** in the Tabular List (■ FIGURE 17-10).
- ❑ She reads the code title **G43.109, Migraine with aura, not intractable, without status migrainosus** and is concerned because the documentation did not state that the migraine was accompanied with aura.
- ❑ She reads the inclusion terms under the category heading **G43.1, Migraine with aura** and sees the

Migraine (idiopathic) G43

with aura (acute-onset) (prolonged) (typical)
 (without headache) G43.109

intractable G43.119
 with status migrainosus G43.111
 without status migrainosus G43.119
not intractable G43.109
 with status migrainosus G43.101
 without status migrainosus G43.109

Figure 17-9 ■ Index Entry for Migraine

5th G43.1 Migraine with aura
Basilar migraine
Classical migraine
Migraine equivalents
Migraine preceded or accompanied by transient focal neurological phenomena
Migraine triggered seizures
Migraine with acute-onset aura
Migraine with aura without headache (migraine equivalents)
Migraine with prolonged aura
Migraine with typical aura
Retinal migraine
Code also any associated seizure (G40.-, R56.9)
Excludes1: persistent migraine aura (G43.5-, G43.6-)

6th G43.10 Migraine with aura, not intractable
 G43.101 Migraine with aura, not intractable, with status migrainosus
 G43.109 Migraine with aura, not intractable, without status migrainosus
  Migraine with aura NOS

6th G43.11 Migraine with aura, intractable
 G43.111 Migraine with aura, intractable, with status migrainosus
 G43.119 Migraine with aura, intractable, without status migrainosus

Figure 17-10 ■ Tabular List Entry for G43.1 Migraine with aura

term **Classical migraine**. The inclusion term confirms that this is the correct category to classify a classical migraine.

➪ Angelia checks for instructional notes in the Tabular List.

- ❑ Angelia cross-references the beginning of subcategory **G43.1, Migraine with aura** and reads the instructional notes. The note **Code also any associated seizure** does not apply because no seizure was documented.
- ❑ She cross-references the beginning of category **G43, Migraine** and reads the **NOTE** that defines intractable. She confirms that this case is not intractable.
- ❑ Angelia cross-references the beginning of the block **G40-G47 Episodic and paroxysmal disorders** and verifies that there are no instructional notes that apply to all codes in the block.
- ❑ She cross-references the beginning of **Chapter 6 (G00-G99)** and reviews the **Excludes2** note. She determines that it does not apply to this case because the patient does not have any of the conditions listed.
- ❑ Angelia finalizes the code assignment for the migraine, **G43.109, Migraine with aura, not intractable, without status migrainosus**.

➪ Next, Angelia assigns a code for the TIA. She searches the Index for the Main Term **Transient**.

- ❑ She reads the nonessential modifier **(meaning homeless)** and determines this is not the correct Main Term to use.
- ❑ She searches the Index for the Main Term **Attack**.
- ❑ She locates the subterm **transient ischemic (TIA) G45.9** and determines that this is an appropriate entry.

➪ Angelia verifies code **G45.9** in the Tabular List.

- ❑ She reads the code title **G45.9, Transient cerebral ischemic attack, unspecified**, and confirms that this describes the documentation.
- ❑ She confirms that this is the accurate code by reading the inclusion term **TIA** listed under code **G45.9**.
- ❑ She quickly re-checks the beginning of the category, block, and chapter for instructional notes and finds no notes that apply to this case.
- ❑ Angelia finalizes the code assignment **G45.9, Transient cerebral ischemic attack, unspecified**.

➪ Angelia checks her abstracting notes and identifies that she needs to assign a code for type 1 diabetes because it was treated during this admission.

- ❑ She searches the Index for the Main Term **Diabetes** and the subterm **type 1 E10.9**. No additional complications are documented, so none of the second-level subterms apply.
- ❑ She turns to the Tabular List to verify the code **E10.9, Type 1 diabetes mellitus without complications.**
- ❑ She cross-references the beginning of the category **E10**, the block **E08-E13**, and the chapter to identify that there are no further instructional notes that apply.

➪ Angelia reviews the codes for this case:

- ❑ **E10.9, Type 1 diabetes mellitus without complications**
- ❑ **G45.9, Transient cerebral ischemic attack, unspecified**
- ❑ **G43.109, Migraine with aura, not intractable, without status migrainosus**

➪ Next, Angelia must determine how to sequence the codes.

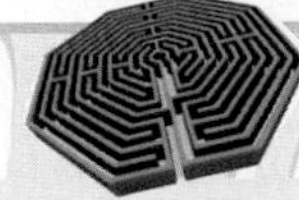

Coding Practice

Now it is your turn to practice assigning codes for diseases of the nervous system and sense organs. Refer to the ***Tip*** at the end of the mini-medical-record if you need a little extra help.

Exercise 17.3 Assigning Codes for the Nervous System

Instructions: Read the mini-medical-record of each patient's encounter, review the information abstracted in Exercise 17.2, and assign ICD-10-CM diagnosis codes (CM) using the Index and Tabular List. Write the code(s) on the line provided.

1. Date: 7/13/yy Location: Neurology Associates
Provider: Lorene Garman, MD
Patient: Cherie Holzman Gender: F Age: 31
Reason for encounter: patient comes in today for a migraine which started 2 days ago with aura
Assessment: pharmacoresistant migraine

(continued)

1. (continued)
Plan: Administered injection of sumatriptan (*a medication used to treat migraines*) and discussed potential side effects and how to manage. Rx oral sumatriptan. Patient to call nurse tomorrow to discuss progress.

Tip: Be sure to review the meaning of intractable.

1 CM Code __________

2. Date: 7/13/yy Location: Branton Medical Center Provider: Lorene Garman, MD

Patient: Gordon Blanke Gender: M Age: 9

Reason for encounter: video EEG as part of ongoing epilepsy evaluation

Assessment: benign childhood epilepsy with EEG spikes, poorly controlled at this time

(continued)

2. (continued)
Plan: we are going to start with Rx gabapentin monotherapy (*single drug therapy*) and reevaluate in 4 weeks, consult with nutritionist re: diet modifications

Tip: Read and follow the cross-referencing instruction in the Index.

1 CM Code __________

3. Date: 7/13/yy Location: Neurology Associates

Provider: Lorene Garman, MD

Patient: Derek Brannum Gender: M Age: 51

Reason for encounter: management of PD, patient reports increased tremor activity and difficulty walking since last visit

Assessment: PD has progressed

Plan: adjusted medications, referred to physical therapy

1 CM Code __________

ARRANGING CODES FOR THE NERVOUS SYSTEM

Sequencing codes that include codes for pain is determined by the circumstances of the encounter. When the purpose of the encounter is to manage the pain, sequence the code for pain first. When the purpose of the encounter is to treat the underlying condition, sequence the code for the condition first. Follow the same procedure when coding neoplasm related pain. Refer to the examples in ■ FIGURE 17-11 and ■ FIGURE 17-12 to learn more about sequencing codes for neoplasm related pain.

Patient is admitted for IV pain control related to metastatic pancreatic cancer.

(1) **G89.3 Neoplasm related pain (acute) (chronic)**

(2) **C25.9 Malignant neoplasm of pancreas, unspecified**

(3) **C79.9 Secondary malignant neoplasm of unspecified site**

Figure 17-11 ■ Example of an Encounter to Treat Neoplasm Related Pain

Patient is admitted for left upper lobectomy for lung cancer and also reports severe neoplasm related pain.

(1) **C34.12 Malignant neoplasm of upper lobe, left bronchus or lung**

(2) **G89.3 Neoplasm related pain (acute) (chronic)**

Figure 17-12 ■ Example of an Encounter to Treat the Neoplasm, with Pain as an Additional Diagnosis

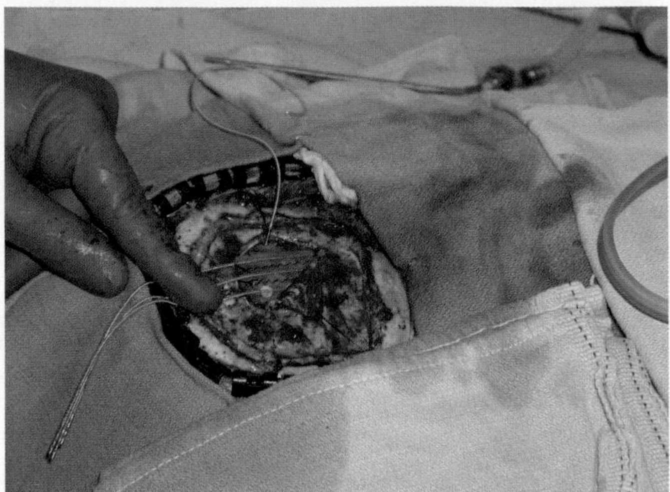

Figure 17-13 ■ A neurostimulator implanted in a patient helps relieve pain. *Source:* © *Travis Hilliard/Shutterstock.*

Guided Example of Arranging Nervous System Codes

To practice skills for sequencing codes for diseases of the nervous system, continue with the example from earlier in the chapter about patient Catalina Piatt, who was admitted to Branton Medical Center due to left sided hemiparesis.

Follow along in your ICD-10-CM manual as Angelia Harkey, CPC, sequences the codes. Check off each step after you complete it.

⇨ Angelia reviews the codes she assigned for this case:

- ❑ **E10.9, Type 1 diabetes mellitus without complications**
- ❑ **G45.9, Transient cerebral ischemic attack, unspecified**
- ❑ **G43.109, Migraine with aura, not intractable, without status migrainosus**

⇨ First, Angelia needs to determine the principal diagnosis.

- ❑ She refers back to the medical record and confirms that the reason established after study for the admission and the services provided is TIA.
- ❑ She sequences **G45.9, Transient cerebral ischemic attack, unspecified**, first, as the principal diagnosis.
- ❑ She refers to the OGCR I.C.4. and 6. to determine if any sequencing guidelines apply for the migraine and diabetes, but finds none.
- ❑ She refers to OGCR Section III, Reporting Additional Diagnoses, and verifies that because the migraine and the diabetes required therapeutic treatment during the admission, she should assign them as additional diagnoses.
- ❑ She determines that the migraine required specific treatment and sequences it as the second code.
- ❑ She determines that the diabetes is a chronic condition and, although routine insulin was administered, there were no diabetic complications requiring attention. She sequences diabetes as the third and final code.

⇨ Angelia finalizes the codes and sequencing for this case:

(1) **G45.9, Transient cerebral ischemic attack, unspecified**

(2) **G43.109, Migraine with aura, not intractable, without status migrainosus**

(3) **E10.9, Type 1 diabetes mellitus without complications**

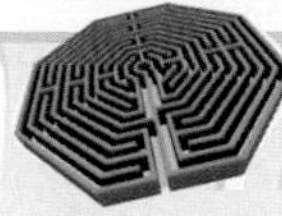

Coding Practice

Now it is your turn to practice sequencing codes for diseases of the nervous system and sense organs. Refer to the ***Tip*** at the end of the mini-medical-record if you need a little extra help.

Exercise 17.4 Arranging Codes for the Nervous System

Instructions: Read the mini-medical-record of each patient's encounter, review the information abstracted in Exercise 17.2, assign ICD-10-CM diagnosis codes (CM) using the Index and Tabular List, and sequence them correctly.

1. Date: 7/14/yy Location: Branton Medical Center Provider: Lorene Garman, MD

Patient: Patricia Huskins Gender: F Age: 29

Reason for admission: implant neurostimulator (*a device placed under the skin that stimulates the spinal cord by tiny electrical impulses*) for pain control (■ FIGURE 17-13)

Assessment: chronic lumbar pain due to displaced disc at L3-L4 which resulted from a back injury two years ago

Plan: FU 2 weeks

Tip: Review OGCR I.C.6.b.1)(a) and (b)(ii) for sequencing instructions.

2 CM Codes __________ __________

(*continued*)

2. Date: 7/14/yy Location: Branton Medical Center Provider: Lorene Garman, MD

Patient: Darrell Commons Gender: M Age: 86

Reason for encounter: admitted from nursing facility due to generalized weakness

Assessment: weakness is due to hyponatremia, patient presents an elopement risk due to late onset AD, dementia with hallucinations, and wandering

Plan: discharged to nursing facility

Tip: Sequencing of the additional diagnoses is indicated in the Index and Tabular List.

3 CM Codes __________ __________ __________

3. Date: 7/14/yy Location: Branton Medical Center Provider: Lorene Garman, MD

Patient: Leah Caison Gender: F Age: 42

Reason for admission: admitted from emergency department where patient presented with migraine of 4 days duration which has not responded to the usual medication

Assessment: persistent migraine with cerebrovascular infarction, cerebral stenosis of right cerebellar artery, hypertension

Tip: Review the subterms in the Index carefully.

3 CM Codes __________ __________ __________

CODING NEOPLASMS OF THE NERVOUS SYSTEM

Neoplasms of the nervous do not appear in ICD-10-CM Chapter 6, Diseases of the Nervous System and Sense Organs (G00-G99). Codes for neoplasms of the nervous system appear in categories C70 to C72 within the neoplasm chapter. Primary malignancies of the nervous system are rare, with the most common being medulloblastoma, an aggressive malignant brain tumor. Benign tumors can cause serious problems, not because they are invasive, but because benign tumors in the brain can apply pressure to the cranial nerves. Benign peripheral tumors can cause nerve damage and loss of muscle control in the extremities.

The brain is a common site of metastases from cancers in other organs, affecting up to 45% of all cancer patients and accounting for 20% of cancer deaths annually, according to the Centers for Disease Control and Prevention. Chemotherapy can have a negative "double effect" on the brain because the treatment itself may not penetrate the brain well, but can weaken the **blood-brain barrier (BBB)**. This weakness allows cancer cells to infiltrate the CNS, enter into the brain, and grow in an environment that is removed from the treatment.

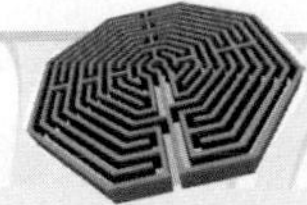

Coding Practice

Now it is your turn to practice coding neoplasms of the nervous system. Refer to the ***Tip*** at the end of the mini-medical-record if you need a little extra help.

Exercise 17.5 Coding Neoplasms of the Nervous System

Instructions: Read the mini-medical-record of each patient's encounter, then abstract, assign, and sequence ICD-10-CM diagnosis codes (CM) using the Index and Tabular List. Write the code(s) on the line provided.

1. Date: 7/15/yy Location: Neurology Associates

Provider: Lorene Garman, MD

Patient: Eva Cantin Gender: F Age: 6

Reason for encounter: review CT scan of head

Assessment: benign hypothalamic astrocytoma (*tumor arising from star shaped cells that form the supportive tissue of the brain*)

Plan: surgery to remove the tumor

1 CM Code __________

(continued)

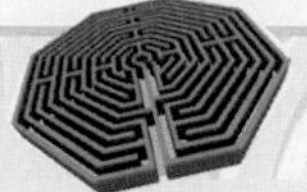

Coding Practice (continued)

2. Date: 7/15/yy Location: Branton Medical Center Provider: Lorene Garman, MD

Patient: Reba Dryden Gender: F Age: 62

Reason for admission: management of pain following pleurectomy of right lung due to non-small cell carcinoma of the right lung (NSCLC)

Assessment: chronic post-thoracotomy (*incision into the chest*) pain

Plan: discharge to home with fentanyl (*a narcotic pain reliever*) transdermal patch and home health follow up

Tip: The principal diagnosis is the condition that is the reason for the admission. Refer to OGCR I.C.6.b.5).

2 CM Codes __________ __________

3. Date: 7/15/yy Location: Branton Medical Center Provider: Lorene Garman, MD

Patient: Trudy Heal Gender: F Age: 71

Reason for admission: pain management

Assessment: nerve root compress d/t stage 4 diffuse large B-cell non-hodgkins lymphoma

Tip: Refer to OGCR I.C.6.b.5).

3 CM Codes __________ __________ __________

4. Date: 7/15/yy Location: Branton Medical Center Provider: Lorene Garman, MD

Patient: Neil Teitelbaum Gender: M Age: 5

Reason for admission: craniotomy with tumor resection

Assessment: primary medulloblastoma of the central cerebellum

Plan: chemotherapy was provided before discharge, follow up in office to establish chemotherapy and radiotherapy plan

Tip: Refer to OGCR I.C.2.e.

2 CM Codes __________ __________

5. Date: 7/15/yy Location: Branton Medical Center Provider: Lorene Garman, MD

Patient: Lenora McDavis Gender: F Age: 67

Reason for admission: anemia due to chemotherapy

Assessment: left ovarian cancer with metastases to the brain, also provided IV pain management

Plan: refer to hospice

Tip: Refer to OGCR I.C.2.c.2) and I.C.2.e.

5 CM Codes __________ __________ __________ __________ __________

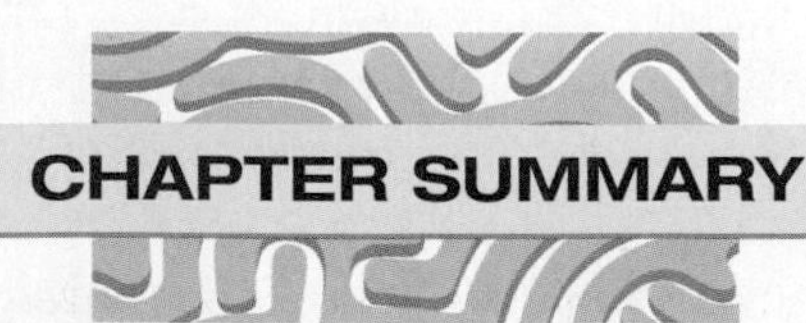

CHAPTER SUMMARY

In this chapter you learned that:

- The function of the nervous system is to direct the body's response to internal and external stimuli and coordinate the activities of other organ systems.
- ICD-10-CM Chapter 6, Diseases of the Nervous System and Sense Organs (G00-G99) contains 11 blocks or subchapters that are divided by the type of structure affected.
- Because of the variety of conditions addressed under the nervous system, coders need general criteria for abstracting conditions of the nervous system overall and specific criteria for abstracting pain, headaches, epilepsy, and Parkinson's disease.
- OGCR contains specific guidelines for assigning codes for hemiplegia, monoplegia, and pain.
- When the purpose of the encounter is to manage the pain, sequence the code for pain first; when the purpose of the encounter is to treat the underlying condition, sequence the code for the condition first.

- Primary malignancies of the nervous system are rare, but the brain is a common site of metastases from other cancers.
- ICD-10-CM provides Official Guidelines for Coding and Reporting (OGCR) for the nervous system and sense organs in OGCR section I.C.6., which provides detailed discussion of coding for pain, including general coding information, postoperative pain, chronic pain, neoplasm related pain, and chronic pain syndrome.

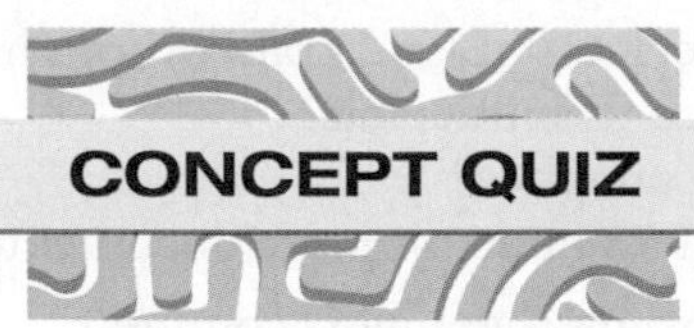

CONCEPT QUIZ

Take a moment to look back at your trip through the nervous system and sense organs and solidify your skills. This is your opportunity to pull together everything you have learned.

Completion

Instructions: Write the term that answers each question based on the information you learned in this chapter. Choose from the list below. Some choices may be used more than once and some choices may not be used at all. Refer to the discussion in this chapter and the Glossary at the end of this book if you need a little extra help.

30	epilepsy
60	hydrocephalus
72	laterality
brain	meningitis
CNS	PNS
dominance	spina bifida
electrocardiogram	spinal cord
electroencephalogram	status epilepticus
encephalitis	status migrainosus

1. The _________________ acts as the control center for the nervous system by processing information and providing short term control over other organ systems
2. _________________ is a viral inflammation of the brain and meninges.
3. _________________ is a brain disorder in which neurons signal abnormally, causing seizures and/or unconsciousness.
4. The _________________ is a common site of metastases from cancers in other organs.
5. The _________________ consists of the 12 nerves that radiate out from the brain and the 31 pairs of nerves that radiate from the spinal cord to all other areas of the body
6. When a condition is _________________, it is resistant to treatment.
7. _________________ refers to the side of the body an individual favors, such as being left-handed or right-handed.
8. _________________ is a recording of the electrical activity of the brain.
9. _________________ is a congenital neural tube defect in which vertebrae do not fuse.
10. Status epilepticus is an epileptic seizure lasting more than _________________ minutes.

Multiple Choice

Instructions: Circle the letter of the best answer to each question based on the information you learned in this chapter. Refer to the discussion in this chapter and the Glossary at the end of this book if you need a little extra help.

1. The maintenance of a stable internal physical state of the body is
   A. hemostasis.
   B. equilibrium.
   C. homeostasis.
   D. intractable.
2. Which of the following terms does NOT mean resistant to treatment?
   A. Poorly controlled
   B. Pharmacoresistant
   C. Refractory
   D. Status migrainosus
3. _________ seizures are the result of abnormal activity on both sides of the brain.
   A. Simple partial
   B. Psychomotor
   C. Status epilepticus
   D. Generalized
4. Parkinson's disease that is followed by a diagnosis of dementia at a later time is
   A. Parkinson's disease with dementia.
   B. Parkinsonian dementia.
   C. Lewy body disease.
   D. secondary Parkinsonism.

5. Which of the following is NOT a key criterion for abstracting headaches?
   A. Is it documented as intractable?
   B. Does it affect the entire head or only one side?
   C. Is a duration of 30 minutes or more documented?
   D. Is it accompanied with aura?
6. Hemiplegia of the right arm in a left-handed person should be coded as
   A. right dominant.
   B. left dominant.
   C. right nondominant.
   D. left nondominant.
7. Codes from category G89 Pain, not elsewhere classified should NOT be assigned when
   A. pain is documented as acute.
   B. the underlying condition is the reason for the encounter.
   C. pain is related to neoplasm.
   D. pain is documented as chronic.
8. Classical migraine is the same as
   A. migraine with aura.
   B. intractable migraine.
   C. cluster headache.
   D. status migrainosus.
9. Which of the following IS a key criterion for abstracting pain?
   A. Is it due to a device, implant, graft, or trauma?
   B. Is it documented as intractable?
   C. Is paralysis documented?
   D. Is a duration of 72 hours or more documented?
10. Which of the following is the most common neoplasm of the nervous system?
   A. Primary malignant neoplasm
   B. Metastasis to the brain
   C. Benign neoplasm of the brain
   D. Benign neoplasm of the PNS

CODING CHALLENGE

Now it is your turn to demonstrate coding all aspects of the nervous system and sense organs. Refer back to the examples and discussion in this chapter when you need a little extra help. Use your medical dictionary and anatomy references when needed.

Instructions: Read the mini-medical-record of each patient's encounter, then abstract, assign, and sequence ICD-10-CM diagnosis codes (CM) using the Index and Tabular List. Write the code(s) on the line provided.

1. Date: 7/19/yy Location: Branton Medical Center Outpatient Infusion Center

Provider: Lorene Garman, MD

Patient: Lewis McAnulty Gender: M Age: 36

Reason for encounter: Patient presents to the infusion center for treatment of meningitis

Assessment: staphylococcal meningitis

Plan: FU in 3 days and 1 week after antibiotic infusions are complete

Tip: Read the instructional notes in the Tabular List.

2 CM Codes __________ __________

2. Date: 7/19/yy Location: Branton Medical Center Provider: Lorene Garman, MD

Patient: Ronald Kraker Gender: M Age: 60

Reason for encounter: acute respiratory distress

Assessment: myasthenia gravis crisis, chronic inflammatory demyelinating polyneuropathy (CIDP) (*an inflammatory disorder of PNS due to abnormal immune activity*)

Plan: Rx cholinesterase inhibitor and immunosuppressant drugs. FU 1 week

2 CM Codes __________ __________

3. Date: 7/19/yy Location: Neurology Associates

Provider: Lorene Garman, MD

Patient: Trisha Adolph Gender: F Age: 13

Reason for encounter: increase in number and intensity of myoclonic seizures.

Assessment: poorly controlled juvenile myoclonic epilepsy (JME)

Plan: valproic acide dosage changes

Tip: Read the cross-reference instruction in the Index.

1 CM Code __________

4. Date: 7/19/yy Location: Neurology Associates
Provider: Lorene Garman, MD
Patient: Dustin Mallon Gender: M Age: 18
Reason for encounter: EEG
Assessment: focal seizures
Plan: Rx Dilantin

Tip: Read the cross-reference instruction in the Index.

1 CM Code __________

5. Date: 7/19/yy Location: Neurology Associates
Provider: Lorene Garman, MD
Patient: Zachary Galyean Gender: M Age: 44
Reason for encounter: Continuing lower back pain with radiating pain in left hip. Patient has had surgical repair of several ruptured discs, and is overweight and sedentary.
Assessment: chronic pain syndrome
Plan: acetaminophen, consult with dietician for weight loss plan, 12 session physical therapy followed by regular exercise, RTO in 4 weeks

2 CM Codes __________ __________

6. Date: 7/19/yy Location: Branton Medical Center Provider: Lorene Garman, MD
Patient: Estella Fox Gender: F Age: 12
Reason for admission: recurring headaches, problems with balance, poor coordination, gait disturbances
Assessment: normal pressure hydrocephalus
Plan: placement of ventriculoperitoneal shunt (*a tube that drains fluid from the brain into the peritoneal cavity*)

1 CM Code __________

7. Date: 7/19/yy Location: Neurology Associates Sleep Study Center Provider: Lorene Garman, MD
Patient: Alvin Morano Gender: M Age: 55
Reason for encounter: sleep study
Assessment: obstructive sleep apnea, nutritional obesity with BMI 33.0,

(continued)

7. (continued)
Plan: Rx **continuous positive airway pressure (CPAP) device**, refer to dietician for weight loss

3 CM Codes __________ __________ __________

8. Date: 7/19/yy Location: Neurology Associates
Provider: Lorene Garman, MD
Patient: Helene Tidd Gender: F Age: 68
Reason for encounter: carpal tunnel release, right hand, endoscopic
Assessment: carpal tunnel syndrome and diabetes type 2 with polyneuropathy
Plan: FU 3 weeks

2 CM Codes __________ __________

9. Date: 7/19/yy Location: Neurology Associates
Provider: Lorene Garman, MD
Patient: Aida Hoerner Gender: F Age: 58
Reason for encounter: pain in the calf muscle, muscle weakness and cramping in thighs and upper arms
Assessment: alcohol dependence with alcoholic myopathy
Plan: referral to alcohol counseling and nutritionist, RTO 1 week

2 CM Codes __________ __________

10. Date: 7/19/yy Location: Neurology Associates
Provider: Lorene Garman, MD
Patient: Candy Ackman Gender: F Age: 43
Reason for encounter: physical therapy
Assessment: long standing left sided hemiplegia due to encephalitis 20 years ago
Plan: return 1 week

Tip: Refer to OGCR I.C.6.a. for coding of hemiplegia. Remember that 20 years ago means that the hemiplegia is a sequela of encephalitis.

2 CM Codes __________ __________

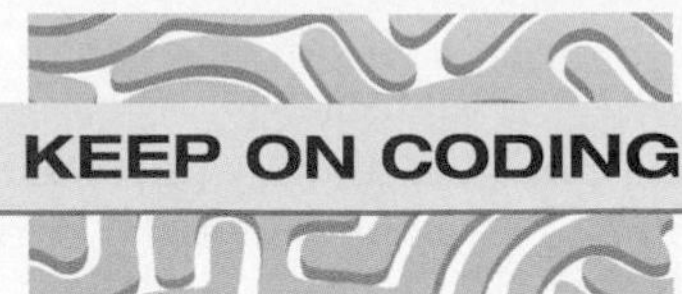

KEEP ON CODING

As a coder, you can never have too much experience. Apply everything you have learned in this chapter to code the following diagnostic statements. Use the OGCR and instructional notes in the Tabular List to help determine how many codes are required.

Instructions: Read the diagnostic statement, then use the Index and Tabular List to assign and sequence ICD-10-CM (CM) diagnosis codes. Write the code(s) on the line provided.

1. Pneumococcal meningitis: CM Code(s) ______
2. Metastatic carcinoma of the thalamus from primary cancer of the right breast: CM Code(s) ______
3. Accidental puncture of the meninges during a nervous system operative procedure: CM Code(s) ______
4. Alper's disease: CM Code(s) ______
5. Migraine with an aura: CM Code(s) ______
6. Restless legs syndrome: CM Code(s) ______
7. Vascular Parkinsonism: CM Code(s) ______
8. Amyotrophic lateral sclerosis: CM Code(s) ______
9. Blepharospasm: CM Code(s) ______
10. Epilepsy due to syphilis: CM Code(s) ______
11. Menstrual migraine, intractable without status migrainosus: CM Code(s) ______
12. Narcolepsy with cataplexy: CM Code(s) ______
13. Huntington's chorea: CM Code(s) ______
14. Headache due to lumbar puncture: CM Code(s) ______
15. Ataxic cerebral palsy: CM Code(s) ______
16. Guillian-Barré syndrome: CM Code(s) ______
17. Myasthenia gravis without exacerbation: CM Code(s) ______
18. Intractable epilepsy with status epilepticus: CM Code(s) ______
19. Primary central sleep apnea: CM Code(s) ______
20. Spasmotic torticollis: CM Code(s) ______
21. Postpolio myelitic syndrome: CM Code(s) ______
22. Tropical spastic paraplegia: CM Code(s) ______
23. Medulloblastoma: CM Code(s) ______
24. Alzheimer's Disease: CM Code(s) ______
25. Episodic tension-type headache: CM Code(s) ______

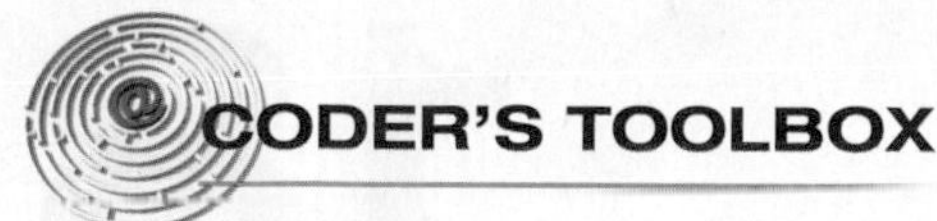

CODER'S TOOLBOX

The following resources are a starting point for learning more about the nervous system and sense organs. The > symbol indicates a menu selection within the website in order to navigate to a specific page.

Alzheimer's Association **http://www.alz.org/index.asp**

Alzheimer's Foundation of America **www.alzfdn.org**

American Academy of Neurology **http://www.aan.com/**

American Association of Neurological Surgeons > Patient Information **http://aans.org/Patient%20Information.aspx**

American Chronic Pain Association **http://www.theacpa.org/default.aspx**

Epilepsy Foundation **www.epilepsyfoundation.org/**

Hydrocephalus Association **www.hydroassoc.org/**

MedicineNet.com > Migraine Center > Cluster Headaches **http://www.medicinenet.com/cluster_headaches/article.htm**

Migraine Awareness Group: A National Understanding for Migraineurs (MAGUM) **http://www.migraines.org/**

National Council of Certified Dementia Practitioners (NCCDP) **http://www.nccdp.org/index.htm**

National Headache Foundation **http://www.headaches.org/**

National Institutes of Health > Alzheimer's Disease Education & Referral (ADEAR) Center **www.nihseniorhealth.gov/alzheimersdisease/toc.html**

National Parkinson Foundation **http://www.parkinson.org**

Neurology Journal **http://www.neurology.org/**

Neurosurgery Journal **http://journals.lww.com/neurosurgery/pages/default.aspx**

Spina Bifida Association **http://www.sbaa.org**

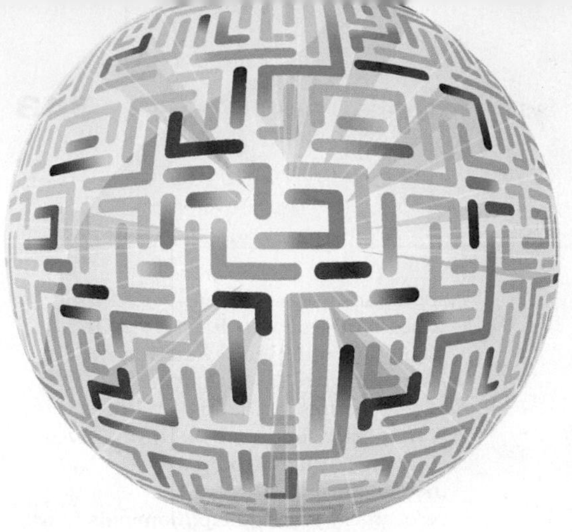

18

Mental, Behavioral, and Neurodevelopmental Disorders (F01-F99)

Learning Objectives

After completing this chapter, you should have the skills to:

- Spell and define the key words, medical terms, and abbreviations related to mental, behavioral, and neurodevelopmental disorders.
- Discuss the common types of mental, behavioral, and neurodevelopmental disorders.
- Identify the main characteristics of coding for mental, behavioral, and neurodevelopmental disorders.
- Abstract diagnostic information from the medical record for coding mental, behavioral, and neurodevelopmental disorders.
- Assign codes for mental, behavioral, and neurodevelopmental disorders.
- Arrange codes for mental, behavioral, and neurodevelopmental disorders.
- Discuss the Official Guidelines for Coding and Reporting related to mental, behavioral, and neurodevelopmental disorders.

Key Terms and Abbreviations

abuse
addiction
behavioral disorder
behavioral disturbances
blood alcohol concentration (BAC)
blood alcohol content
blood alcohol level (BAL)
delirium
delusions
dependence
hallucinations
in remission
intellectual disability
intoxication
Lewy body disease
mental disorders
neurodevelopmental disorder
paranoia
perceptual disturbance
psychoactive substance
psychotherapy
schizophrenia
schizothymia
tolerate
use
vascular dementia

In addition to the key terms listed here, students should know the terms defined within tables in this chapter.

Chapter Outline

- **Psychiatry Refresher**
- **Coding Overview of Psychiatry**
- **Abstracting for Psychiatry**
- **Assigning Codes for Psychiatry**
- **Arranging Codes for Psychiatry**

ICD-10-CM codes in this chapter are from the ICD-10-CM 2014 Draft code set from the Department of Health and Human Services, Centers for Disease Control and Prevention.

INTRODUCTION

While on your road trip, you always want to practice defensive driving—being on the lookout for behavior from other drivers that may endanger you and your vehicle. You are probably all too aware that driving under the influence of alcohol is a major cause of traffic accidents and fatalities. According to the National Highway Traffic Safety Administration (NHTSA), on any given day there are 1,400 injuries and 29 deaths due to drunk driving. Substance abuse is just one of many topics in the ICD-10-CM chapter on mental, behavioral, and neurodevelopmental disorders, but it occupies a significant portion of the codes.

In your tour of the mental, behavioral, and neurodevelopmental disorders in this chapter you will learn more about the types of mental, behavioral, and neurodevelopmental disorders, their causes, and how physicians treat them. Most importantly, you will practice coding for patient encounters related to mental, behavioral, and neurodevelopmental disorders, a skill that requires you to abstract information from the mini-medical-record, assign correct codes, and arrange (sequence) the codes in the correct order. For the sake of brevity, this chapter refers to mental, behavioral, and neurodevelopmental disorders as psychiatry.

A psychiatrist specializes in diagnosing and treating mental, behavioral, and neurodevelopmental disorders and also prescribes medications to treat those disorders. Other providers who may also treat mental, behavioral, and neurodevelopmental disorders are clinical psychologists, social workers, and therapists. However, these non-physician providers cannot prescribe medication. Primary care physicians screen for mental, behavioral, and neurodevelopmental disorders and usually refer patients who need treatment to one of these specialists.

As you read this chapter, open up your medical terminology book and keep a medical dictionary handy to refresh your memory of any unfamiliar terms. Many psychiatric conditions are part of your daily vocabulary, so a reference book will help you understand new terms. Think of these resources as your travel brochures that tell you more about an area.

PSYCHIATRY REFRESHER

Mental, behavioral, and neurodevelopmental disorders are real, not imagined, disorders that have diagnostic criteria and are proven to respond to treatment. Mental disorders are psychological or physical conditions that disrupt an individual's personality, mind, and emotions in such a way that they affect the ability to function and interact with others. Behavioral disorders are manifestations of mental disturbances that result in extreme or disruptive conduct, such as rage, withdrawal, or substance abuse. Neurodevelopmental disorders are conditions that result from impaired development of the nervous system during infancy or childhood. Although mental, behavioral, and neurodevelopmental disorders are not fully understood by scientists, they are believed to be caused by a combination of psychological, environmental, biological, and social factors (■ FIGURE 18-1, page 346).

As you learn about conditions and procedures related to mental, behavioral, and neurodevelopmental disorders, remember to apply medical terminology skills to use word roots, prefixes, and suffixes you already know to define new terms. Refer to ■ TABLE 18-1 (page 346) for a refresher on how to build medical terms related to mental, behavioral, and neurodevelopmental disorders.

Medical terms may seem confusing because the literal meaning of the word parts may not fully describe how the word is used, particularly in the area of mental, behavioral, and neurodevelopmental disorders. For example, **para-** means *beside* or *beyond* and **-noia** means *mind.* The literal meaning of paranoia is beside or beyond the mind, but the word is used to mean a mental condition of delusions of persecution. The suffixes **-thymia** and **-phrenia** both mean *mind*, but schizothymia is a different and less serious condition than schizophrenia. Coders understand that they use medical terminology skills to gain a basic understanding, then they also need to know how a term is actually used within the context of the medical field.

CODING CAUTION

Be alert for medical terms that sound similar but are spelled differently and have different meanings.

thym/o (*thymus gland*) and **-thymia** (*condition of the mind*)

dysthymia (*depression*) and **dysrhythmia** (*abnormal heartbeat*)

Psychiatric Conditions

The National Institutes of Health (NIH) estimates that nearly 25% of adults experience a mental health disorder each year, and 6% of adults and 10% of children live with a serious mental disorder. Mental, behavioral, and neurodevelopmental disorders are classified into broad types (■ TABLE 18-2, page 347). Psychiatrists (*medical doctors, MDs, who diagnose and treat mental disorders*) and psychologists (*non-physicians with advanced training, such as a masters degree or PhD, in psychology*) use written tests, observation, and interviews to diagnose mental, behavioral, and neurodevelopmental disorders. Psychiatrists prescribe medication and provide **electroconvulsive therapy** to treat mental disorders. Both psychiatrists and psychologists use psychotherapy to treat patients. Psychotherapy employs

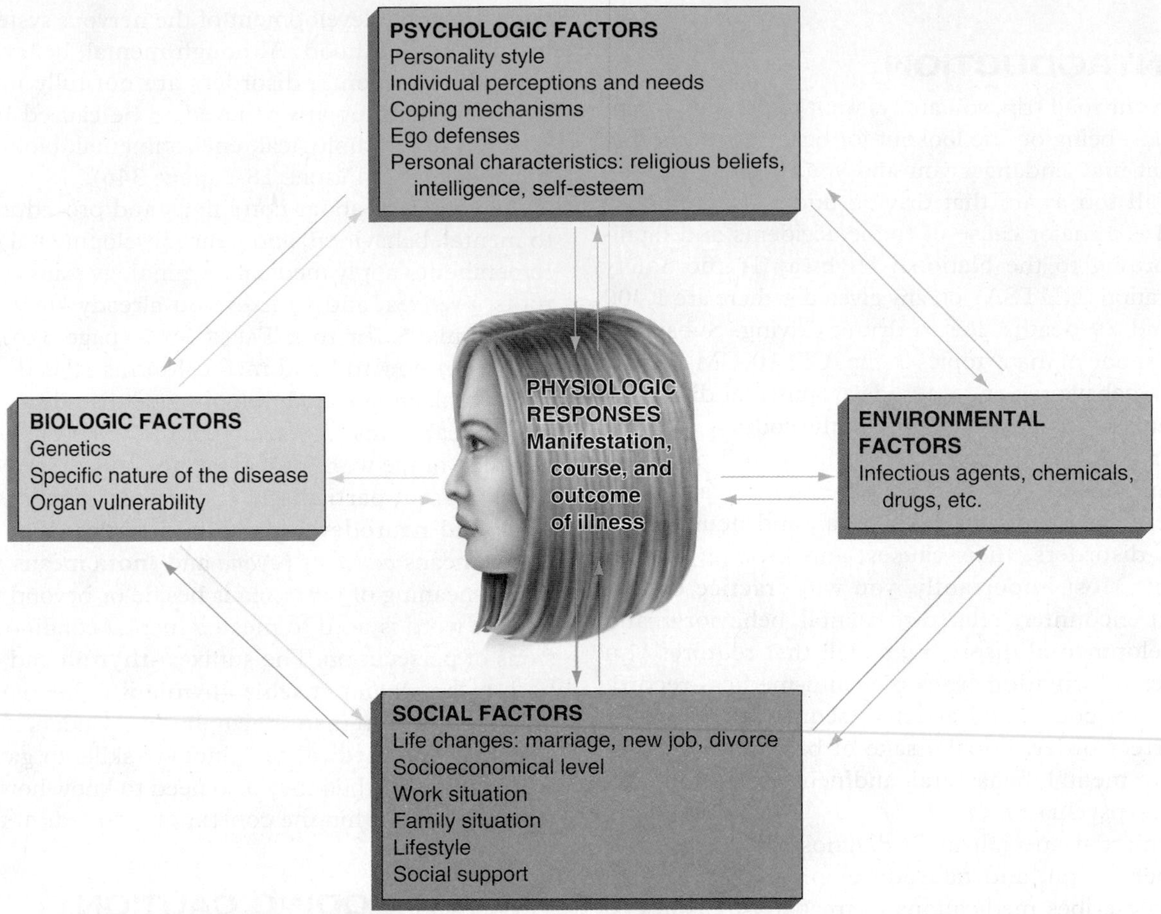

Figure 18-1 ■ Factors Contributing to Mental Health and Mental Illness

Table 18-1 ■ **EXAMPLE OF CONSTRUCTING MEDICAL TERMS FOR PSYCHIATRIC DISORDERS**

Prefix/Combining Form	Suffix	Complete Medical Term
dys- (*abnormal, painful*) **para-** (*beside*)	**-thymia** (*condition of the mind or emotion*) **-phrenia** (*condition of the mind*) **-asthenia** (*lack of strength*)	**dys + thymia** (*abnormal condition of the mind*) **schizo + thymia** (*condition of a split mind*)
schiz/o (*split*)		**schizo + phrenia** (*condition of a split mind*) **para + phrenia** (*condition beside the mind*)
psych/o (*mind*)		**psycho + genic** (*originating in the mind*) **psycho + asthenia** (*lack of strength in the mind*)

non-physical techniques, such as talking, interpreting, listening, rewarding, and role playing, to treat disorders.

In particular, coders must be familiar with the terminology related to psychoactive substance use and dementia in order to code accurately.

Psychoactive Substance Disorders

Psychoactive substances have the ability to alter behavior, impair judgment, or create medical problems. Inappropriate use of such products can create legal, social, employment, family, and medical problems. Psychoactive substance disorders may involve legal substances, such as tobacco and alcohol; illegal substances, such as heroin, cocaine, or cannabis; or prescribed medications, such as pain relievers or tranquilizers, that are used inappropriately. Substances may be taken orally, inhaled through breathing or smoking, injected into veins, or snorted (placed on mucosa of the mouth or nose). They are classified by their effect on the mind and body (■ TABLE 18-3).

Table 18-2 ■ **COMMON MENTAL, BEHAVIORAL, AND NEURODEVELOPMENTAL DISORDERS**

Type of Disorder	Definition	Examples
Adjustment	Abnormal difficulty in responding to life changes	Adjustment disorder with anxiety, adjustment disorder with depressed mood
Anxiety	Abnormal anxiety that interferes with normal activities	Panic disorder, social phobia, obsessive-compulsive, post-traumatic stress disorder (PTSD)
Cognitive	Failure to develop or deterioration of mental comprehension	Autism, dementia, intellectual disability
Dissociative	Disruption in consciousness, memory, identity, or perception	Multiple personality amnesia
Eating	Serious disturbance in eating behavior	Anorexia nervosa, bulimia nervosa
Impulse-control	Extreme difficulty in controlling impulses, despite the negative consequences	Intermittent explosive disorder, **kleptomania**, **pyromania**, pathological gambling
Mood (affective)	Instability of mood	Major depression, mania, bipolar disorder
Personality	Persistent inflexible patterns of behavior that affects interpersonal relationships	Cluster A: Paranoid and schizoid Cluster B: Antisocial, borderline, histrionic, and narcissistic Cluster C: Avoidant, dependent, obsessive-compulsive
Psychotic	**Delusions** (*false beliefs that hinder the ability to function*) and **hallucinations** (*false visual, auditory, olfactory, or* **tactile** *perceptions*)	Schizophrenia (catatonic type, disorganized type, paranoid type, undifferentiated type, residual type), delusional disorder, brief psychotic disorder
Sexual	Repetitive and prolonged sexual activity and sexual dysfunction that interferes with normal relationships or daily activities	Gender identity disorder, pedophilia, voyeurism
Sleeping	Abnormal sleep problems	Insomnia, sleepwalking
Somatoform	Physical symptoms that are not explained by medical conditions	Hypochondriasis, body dysmorphic disorder (BDD), pain disorder
Substance	Drug and alcohol use, abuse, and addiction	Alcoholism, tobacco dependence, illicit drug use

Table 18-3 ■ **COMMONLY ABUSED SUBSTANCES**

Classification	Effect	Examples
Alcohol (ethanol)	Reduces tension, promotes relaxation	Beer, wine, liquor (scotch, gin, vodka, rum)
Barbituate (sedative)	Reduces tension, promotes relaxation	Phenobarbital, tuinal, secobarbital, “downers”
Hallucinogen	Promotes relaxation, changes mood, thoughts, and behavior	Cannabis (marijuana), hashish, LSD, PCP
Narcotic (opiate)	Reduces physical pain and anxiety	Opium, cocaine, heroin, morphine, codeine, meperidine (Demerol), fentanyl, hydrocodone (Vicodin), oxycodone (OxyContin)
Nicotine	Stimulant, increases feelings of confidence and elevates mood	Cigarettes, cigars, pipes, smokeless tobacco, chewing tobacco
Stimulant	Increases feelings of confidence, alertness, and well-being	Amphetamine, “meth” (methamphetamine), Dexedrine, speed, crank
Tranquilizer	Reduces anxiety, induces sleep	Diazepam (Valium), lorazepam (Ativan), alprazolam (Xanax)

Usage patterns of substances are described as use, abuse, dependence, or in remission, as follows:

- use—consuming the substance in moderate amounts that do not create significant legal, social, employment, family, or medical problems.
- abuse—use of the substance in quantity or frequency that creates legal, employment, social, or family problems, or places the individual at physical risk, without causing physical dependence.
- dependence—compulsive reliance on the substance to the extent that it is physically or psychologically difficult to stop, despite the significant problems it creates; also called addiction.
- in remission—a history of past drug or alcohol dependence documented by the physician.

Intoxication occurs when more of the substance is consumed than a person can physically tolerate (*absorb*), resulting in behavioral or physical abnormalities. The level of potential alcohol **impairment** is estimated based on a person's blood alcohol level (BAL), which measures the amount of alcohol present in the blood. BAL is computed as the number of milligrams (mg) of alcohol per 100 milliliters (ml) of blood. BAL may be expressed as a ratio, a percentage, or a number. For example, a BAL of *80 mg per 100 ml* is the same as a BAL of *0.08%*, which may also be written without the percent sign as *.08*. To convert a percentage, such as *0.08%*, to a ratio, simply add a *0* to the end of the percentage and drop the leading decimal point to arrive at *80 mg per 100 ml*.

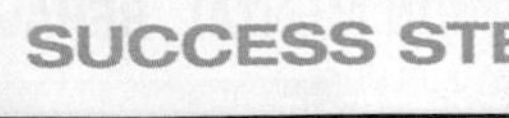

SUCCESS STEP

BAL is also called blood alcohol content or blood alcohol concentration (BAC).

Dementia

Dementia is a progressive loss of brain function that affects memory, thinking, language, judgment, and behavior. A leading cause is Lewy body disease in which patients have abnormal protein structures in certain areas of the brain. Vascular dementia is caused by many small strokes. Dementia may be a manifestation of substance abuse disorders or other nervous systems diseases such as Parkinson's disease, multiple sclerosis, and Alzheimer's disease. Most dementia is accompanied by behavioral disturbances such as aggression, wandering, depression, delusion or hallucinations, sleep disturbances, or poor eating habits.

This section provides a general reference to help understand the most common mental, behavioral, and neurodevelopmental disorders, but does not list everything you need to know. Use medical terminology skills discussed earlier in this chapter to learn the meaning of unfamiliar words. Remember to keep standard reference books handy in case you get stuck. Refer to the resources in the Coder's Toolbox at the end of this chapter to learn more about mental, behavioral, and neurodevelopmental disorders.

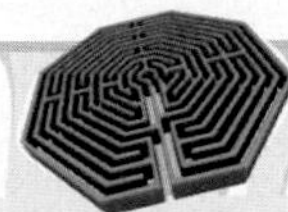

Coding Practice

Refresh your knowledge of terminology related to mental, behavioral, and neurodevelopmental disorders. Use a medical terminology text or a website such as GlobalRph.com > Medical Terminology **http://www.globalrph.com/medterm.htm** to identify the meaning of word parts that may not be familiar.

Exercise 18.1 Psychiatry Refresher

Instructions: Use your medical terminology skills and resources to define the following conditions related to mental, behavioral, and neurodevelopmental disorders, then assign the diagnosis code.

Follow these steps:

- Use slash marks "/" to break down each term into its root(s) and suffix.
- Define the meaning of the word, based on the meaning of each word part.
- Assign the default ICD-10-CM diagnosis code (CM) for the condition using the Index and Tabular List.

Example: arachnophobia arachno/phobia Meaning: fear of spiders CM Code: F40.210

1. agoraphobia Meaning ______ CM Code ______
2. psychasthenia Meaning ______ CM Code ______
3. trichotillomania Meaning ______ CM Code ______

(continued)

4. hypomania Meaning ________________ CM Code ________
5. pedophilia Meaning ________________ CM Code ________
6. hematophobia Meaning ________________ CM Code ________
7. dysmorphophobia Meaning ________________ CM Code ________
8. somnambulism Meaning ________________ CM Code ________
9. paraphrenic Meaning ________________ CM Code ________
10. pseudocyesis Meaning ________________ CM Code ________

CODING OVERVIEW OF PSYCHIATRY

ICD-10-CM Chapter 5, Mental, Behavioral, and Neurodevelopmental Disorders (F01-F99), contains 11 blocks, or subchapters that are divided by the type of disorder. Review the block names and code ranges listed at the beginning of Chapter 5 in the ICD-10-CM manual to become familiar with the content and organization.

ICD-10-CM Chapter 5 is comparable to ICD-9-CM Chapter 4 (290-319). Categories for mental, behavioral, and neurodevelopmental disorders due to psychoactive substance use, F10 through F19, are expanded and more detailed in ICD-10-CM. Codes differentiate between abuse, dependence, and unspecified use and also identify complications, such as delusions, hallucinations, or sleep disturbances. Categories for intellectual disabilities, F70 through F79, provide instructional notes to code first any associated physical or developmental disorder.

This chapter includes mental, behavioral, and neurodevelopmental disorders with physiological causes, personality, mood, and schizophrenic disorders, substance disorders, intellectual disabilities, and developmental disorders. It does not include symptoms and signs, neurological disorders, or congenital conditions.

ICD-10-CM provides Official Guidelines for Coding and Reporting (OGCR) for mental, behavioral, and neurodevelopmental disorders in OGCR section I.C.5. The OGCR provides detailed discussion of pain disorders related to psychological factors and mental, behavioral, and neurodevelopmental disorders due to substance abuse. Additional guidelines related to pain appear in OGCR I.C.6.b.

The American Psychiatric Association (APA) uses the Diagnostic and Statistical Manual of Mental Disorders (DSM) to diagnose and classify mental disorders. In addition to codes, the manual also lists known causes of disorders, statistics regarding gender, age at onset, prognosis, and research concerning optimal approaches. Although the DSM numbering system parallels the one used in ICD-9-CM, the two systems were never completely identical. DSM-5, scheduled for release in 2013, is a major update but does not correspond to the ICD-10-CM numbering system. DSM is not a HIPAA-approved code set and cannot be used for insurance billing.

ABSTRACTING FOR PSYCHIATRY

Many mental, behavioral, and neurodevelopmental disorders have multiple subtypes, so coders must be particularly attentive to the documented wording of the condition. For example, a substance disorder may be stated as use, abuse, or dependence, each of which has a specific meaning and different codes. Some disorders, such as dementia, may have underlying physiological conditions that must be identified and abstracted as well. Diseases and conditions classified in other ICD-10-CM body system chapters, such as digestive, circulatory, and nervous systems, contain frequent instructional notes to assign an additional code for use, abuse, or dependence on alcohol or nicotine.

The table that follows provides general criteria for abstracting mental, behavioral, and neurodevelopmental disorders (■ Table 18-4). Remember that the abstracting

Table 18-4 ■ KEY CRITERIA FOR ABSTRACTING GENERAL PSYCHIATRIC DISORDERS

- ❑ What is the disorder?
- ❑ What is the specific subtype of disorder?
- ❑ Is the disorder due to an underlying physiological condition?
- ❑ Does the patient report symptoms that have no medical cause?
- ❑ What is the severity?
- ❑ Is the condition in remission?

Table 18-5 ■ KEY CRITERIA FOR ABSTRACTING MOOD DISORDERS

- ❑ What is the disorder?
- ❑ Does it have psychotic features?
- ❑ Is the condition current or in remission?
- ❑ Is the current or most recent episode manic, depressed, or mixed?
- ❑ Is the severity mild, moderate, or severe?
- ❑ Is remission partial or full?

Table 18-6 ■ KEY CRITERIA FOR ABSTRACTING PSYCHOACTIVE SUBSTANCE DISORDERS

- ❑ What is the specific substance?
- ❑ What is the class of substance (opioid, sedative, stimulant, hallucinogen, inhalant)?
- ❑ Is the disorder one of use, abuse, or dependence?
- ❑ Does the provider clearly document the relationship between the mental or behavioral disorder and the substance use?
- ❑ What is the blood alcohol level?
- ❑ Is intoxication present?
- ❑ Is withdrawal present?
- ❑ Is **delirium** (*state of confusion, restlessness, and incoherence*) or **perceptual disturbance** (*misinterpretation of surroundings or events*) present?
- ❑ Are any associated hallucinations, delusions, or other psychotic conditions present?
- ❑ Is the condition in remission?

questions are a guide and that not every question applies to, or can be answered for, every case. For example, not every disorder is described based on whether it is in remission. Coders should be alert to the fact that some conditions do have this criterion, so they should always double check the documentation to see if such information is present. Additional tables provide specific criteria for abstracting mood disorders (■ TABLE 18-5) and substance disorders (■ TABLE 18-6).

Guided Example of Abstracting for Psychiatry

Refer to the following example throughout this chapter to learn about abstracting, assigning, and sequencing mental, behavioral, and neurodevelopmental disorder codes. Ladonna Shuck, CPC, is a fictitious coder who will guide you through the coding process.

> Date: 8/11/yy Location: Valley Hospital
>
> Provider: Brett Camden, MD
>
> Patient: Cody Locust Gender: M Age: 58
>
> Reason for admission: admitted from the emergency department with coma
>
> Assessment: Alcoholic liver failure with coma for 4 hours, alcohol dependent abuse for 15 years with intoxication at admission, BAL .23%. Early onset Alzheimer's dementia with behavioral disturbance was managed as well.
>
> Plan: discharge to rehab program

Follow along as Ladonna Shuck, CPC, abstracts the diagnosis. Check off each step after you complete it.

⇨ Ladonna reads through the entire record, with special attention to the reason for the encounter and the final assessment. She notes that the patient was admitted with a coma that lasted for four hours and was later diagnosed with alcoholic liver disease.

⇨ Ladonna refers to the Key Criteria for Abstracting Psychoactive Substance Disorders (Table 18-6).

- ❑ *What is the specific substance?* alcohol
- ❑ *Is the disorder one of use, abuse, or dependence?* dependence
- ❑ *Does the provider clearly document the relationship between the mental or behavioral disorder and the substance use?* Yes, alcoholic liver failure
- ❑ *What is the blood alcohol level?* BAL .23%
- ❑ *Is intoxication present?* Yes, with intoxication at admission
- ❑ *Is withdrawal present?* No.
- ❑ *Is delirium or perceptual disturbance present?* No.
- ❑ *Are any associated hallucinations, delusions, or other psychotic conditions present?* Early onset Alzheimer's dementia with behavioral disturbance
- ❑ *Is the condition in remission?* No.

⇨ At this time, Ladonna does not know which of these conditions may need to be coded, nor how many codes she will end up with. She will learn about this when she moves on to assigning codes.

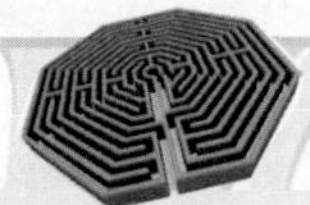

Coding Practice

Now it is your turn to practice abstracting diagnoses for mental, behavioral, and neurodevelopmental disorders. Questions guide your analysis of each scenario.

Exercise 18.2 Abstracting Diagnoses for Psychiatry

Instructions: Read the mini-medical-record of each patient's encounter and answer the abstracting questions. Write the answer on the line provided. Do not assign any codes.

1. Date: 8/13/yy Location: Behavioral Health Associates Provider: Brett Camden, MD

Patient: Lisa Klingler Gender: F Age: 9

Reason for encounter: referred by pediatrician for hyperactivity, short attention span, and irritability

Assessment: after testing, symptoms are due to attention deficit hyperactive disorder, predominately hyperactive type

Plan: Start medication and behavior therapy

a. What symptoms are reported? ______________

b. What is the disorder? ______________

c. What is the specific subtype of the disorder? ______________

d. What symptoms should you report? ______________ Why? ______________

2. Date: 8/13/yy Location: Valley Hospital Provider: Brett Camden, MD

Patient: Lance Charboneau Gender: M Age: 31

Reason for encounter: extreme delusions of paranoia

Assessment: dependent continual user of coke, psychosis with delusions due to dependence and long term use of cocaine

Plan: Rx to help manage delusions, transfer to rehab

a. What is the specific substance? ______________

b. Is the disorder one of use, abuse, or dependence? ______________

c. Does the provider clearly document the relationship between the mental or behavioral disorder and the substance use? ______________

d. Is withdrawal present? ______________

(continued)

2. (continued)

e. Is delirium or perceptual disturbance present? ______________

f. Are any associated hallucinations, delusions, or other psychotic conditions present? ______________

3. Date: 8/13/yy Location: Behavioral Health Associates Provider: Brett Camden, MD

Patient: Kelly Tanouye Gender: F Age: 21

Reason for encounter: ongoing medical management (*evaluation and renewal of prescription*) of schizophrenia

Assessment: paranoid schizophrenia

Plan: medication is managing the condition well and patient is interested in getting a job. Referred to a supported employment service (*a program that assists in locating community-based employment*)

a. What is the reason for the encounter? ______________

b. What condition does the medication treat? ______________

c. What is the specific subtype of disorder? ______________

d. Is the disorder due to an underlying physiological condition? ______________

4. Date: 8/14/yy Location: Behavioral Health Associates Provider: Brett Camden, MD

Patient: Dwayne Angelle Gender: M Age: 10

Reason for encounter: I have been seeing this child for autism, but today his mother is concerned about continuing "fussing and worry about his private parts" that has been going on for quite awhile and his "desire to be like his sister."

Assessment: gender identity disorder

Plan: adjusted medications for current autism.

a. What concerns did the mother express? ______________

b. What is the disorder? ______________

c. What other conditions were managed? ______________

d. What condition is the main reason for the encounter? ______________

(continued)

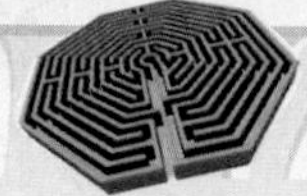

Coding Practice (continued)

5. Date: 8/14/yy Location: Valley Hospital
Provider: Brett Camden, MD
Patient: Marcus Evitt Gender: M Age: 48
Reason for encounter: admitted from emergency department for alcohol-induced gastritis with hemorrhaging and intoxication with BAL of .09%
Assessment: patient has long-term alcohol use with dependence, prior cocaine abuser but states he no longer uses
Plan: patient agreed to counseling after discharge

a. What is the medical condition? ______________

b. What substance is the cause? ______________

c. Does the provider clearly document the relationship between the mental or behavioral disorder and the substance use? ______________

d. Is the disorder one of use, abuse, or dependence? ______________

e. Is intoxication present? ______________

f. What is the blood alcohol level? ______________
How do you write this number as a ratio? ______________ mg per 100 ml

g. Is delirium or perceptual disturbance present? ______________

h. What substance abuse is in remission? ______________

6. Date: 8/14/yy Location: Valley Hospital
Provider: Brett Camden, MD
Patient: Wallace Bosque Gender: M Age: 56
Reason for encounter: severe depression due to bipolar disorder
Assessment: patient is also being treated for liver cirrhosis with ascites due to chronic continuous alcoholism
Plan: patient has stable living situation so we are going to discharge him to a partial hospitalization program (*a treatment program that participants attend during the day and return home at night*)

a. What is the mood disorder? ______________

b. Is the current or most recent episode manic, depressed, or mixed? ______________

c. Does it have psychotic features? ______________

d. Is the severity mild, moderate, or severe? ______________

e. What physical condition exists? ______________

f. What substance disorder is documented? ______________

g. Is the disorder one of use, abuse, or dependence? ______________

h. Are any associated hallucinations, delusions, or other psychotic conditions present? ______________

i. What condition was chiefly responsible for the admission and services? ______________

ASSIGNING CODES FOR PSYCHIATRY

Three types of conditions in this ICD-10-CM chapter present challenges in assigning codes due to the level of detail that must be reported: bipolar disorder, schizophrenic disorders, and substance disorders.

Assigning Codes for Bipolar Disorder

Bipolar disorder has numerous variations based on the episode, severity, and psychotic disturbances that may accompany it. Follow these steps to assign codes for bipolar disorder (■ FIGURES 18-2 and 18-3):

1. Locate the Main Term **Disorder** in the Index.
2. Locate the subterm **bipolar (I)**.
   - For bipolar II disorder, locate the subterm **bipolar II**, which follows the subterm entry for **bipolar (I)**.
3. Determine if the disorder is documented as **current** or **in remission** and locate the corresponding second-level subterm.
4. For current bipolar disorder, identify if the current episode is **depressed**, **hypomanic**, **manic**, or **mixed** and locate the corresponding third-level subterm.

Dr. Camden saw a patient for medication management of bipolar I disorder. After questioning, Dr. Camden documented that the patient reported experiencing severe manic episodes during the past several days.

F31.13 Bipolar disorder, current episode manic without psychotic features, severe

Figure 18-2 ■ Example of Assigning Codes for Bipolar Disorder

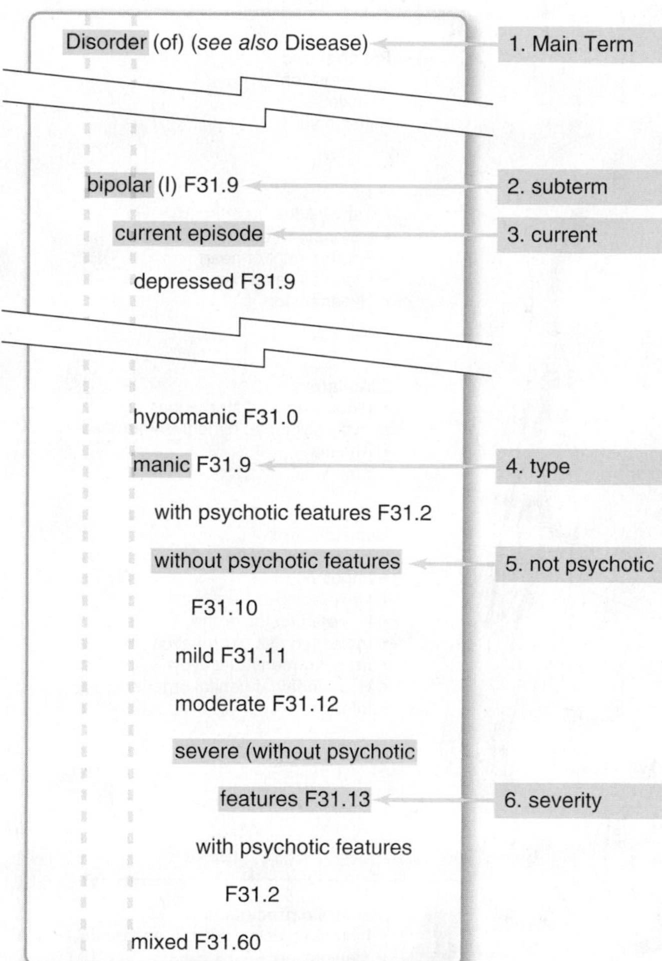

Figure 18-3 ■ Index Entry for the Bipolar Disorder

5. Identify whether the disorder is **with psychotic features** or **without psychotic features** and locate the corresponding fourth-level subterm.
6. For cases **without psychotic features**, select the fifth-level subterm that describes the severity as **mild, moderate**, or **severe**. Verify the code in the Tabular List.
7. For bipolar **in remission**, locate the corresponding second-level subterm, then identify if the remission is **full** or **partial**. Under the corresponding third-level subterm, select the additional subterm that describes the severity. Verify the code in the Tabular List.

SUCCESS STEP

If a patient has a **single manic episode,** locate the corresponding subterm under **Disorder, bipolar.**

Assigning Codes for Schizophrenic Spectrum Disorders

Schizophrenic spectrum disorders (SSD) include several different disorders, each with different characteristics and diagnostic criteria. Coders must be careful to identify the specific terminology documented in order to assign the correct code. Refer to ■ TABLE 18-7 for a summary of SSD and associated codes.

Table 18-7 ■ **ASSIGNING CODES FOR SCHIZOPHRENIC SPECTRUM DISORDERS**

Condition	Description	Code(s)
Schizoaffective disorder	Characterized by an extended period in which schizophrenia is accompanied by major depressive, manic, or mixed episodes	F25.-
Schizoid of childhood (Asperger's syndrome)	Severe and sustained impairment in social interactions and restricted, repetitive patterns of behaviors, interests, and activities.	F84.5
Schizoid personality disorder, schizothymia	Persistent withdrawal from social relationships and lack of emotional responsiveness in most situations	F60.1
Schizophrenia	Inability to distinguish between thoughts and reality, think logically, and have normal emotional and social relationships	F20.0 through F20.5
Schizophreniform disorder	Identical to schizophrenia except that the total duration is greater than one month but less than six months; impaired social or occupational functioning may not be apparent	F20.81
Schizotypal personality disorder	Trouble with relationships and disturbances in thought patterns, appearance, and behavior	F21

Assigning Codes for Psychoactive Substance Disorders

When mental, behavioral, and neurodevelopmental disorders are documented as being due to or associated with psychoactive substance use, coders need to review their abstracting results carefully in order to assign accurate codes (Table 18-6). Assign codes for substance disorders *only* when the *relationship* between the mental or behavioral disorder and the substance use is clearly documented (OGCR I.C.5.b.1)). To better understand the effect of substance abuse on the rest of the body, refer to ■ FIGURE 18-4.

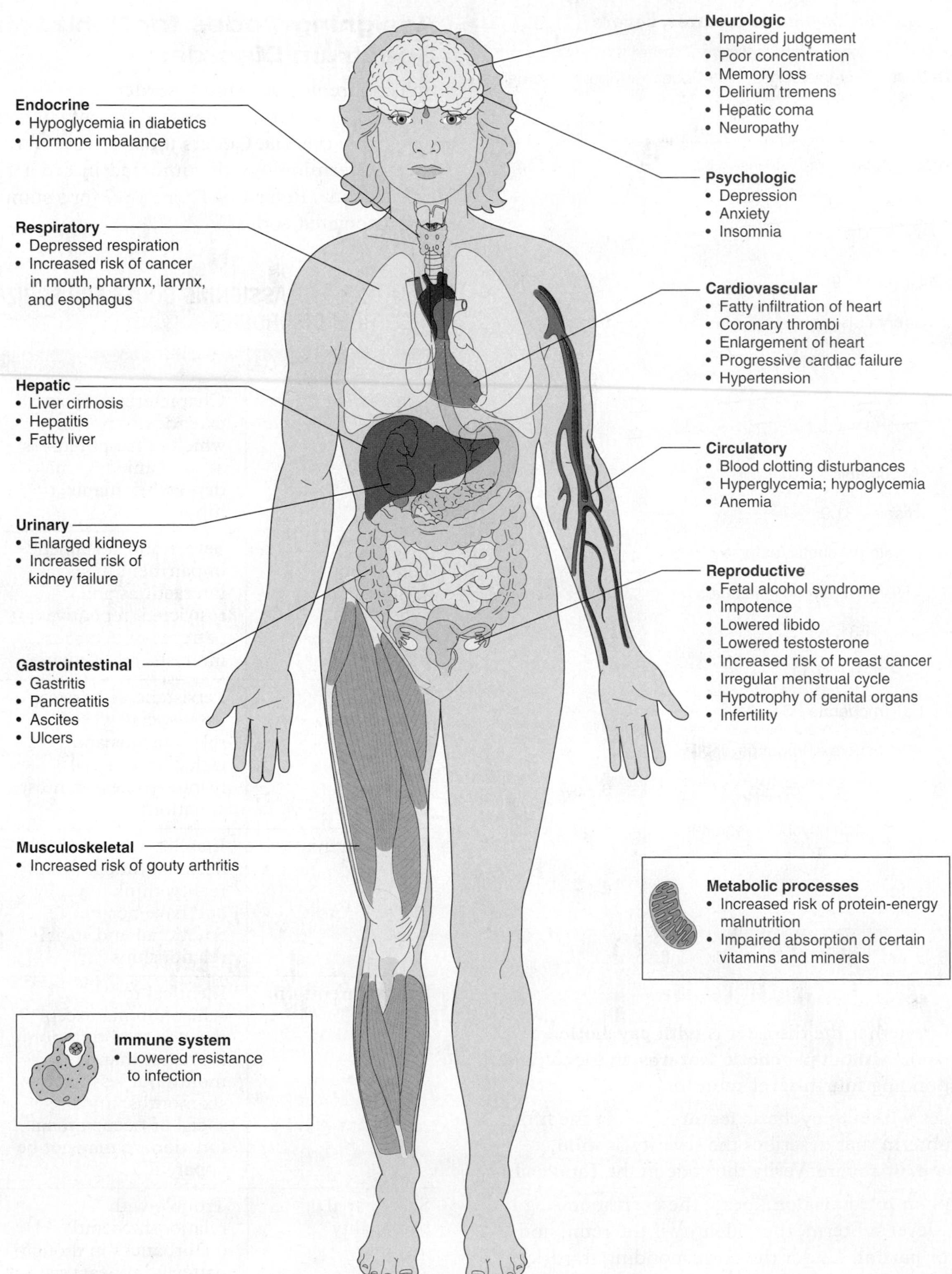

Figure 18-4 ■ The Multisystem Effects of Alcohol Use, Abuse, and Dependence

SUCCESS STEP

Alcoholism is indexed under the Main Term **Dependence** and the subterm **alcohol**.

Most codes related to substance disorders contain six characters that identify several pieces of specific information. To assign codes accurately, follow these steps:

1. Determine if the condition is **use, abuse**, or **dependence**. Use this word as the Main Term in the Index.
   - When the documentation mentions both use and abuse, assign a code for abuse. When it mentions both abuse and dependence, assign a code for dependence (OGCR I.C.5.b.2)).
2. Locate the subterm **drug**, if the substance is other than alcohol.
   - When the substance is alcohol, go directly to the subterm **alcohol**.
3. Locate a second-level subterm for the specific substance or class of substance.
   - **Cannabis, cocaine,** and **nicotine** are seperate subterms.
   - **Nicotine** has additional subterms for **chewing tobacco** and **cigarettes**.
   - Other substances are classified under subterms for the class of substance: **hallucinogen, inhalant, opioid, sedative, stimulant,** or **psychoactive substance NEC** (Table 18-3).
4. Review the entries under the third-level subterm **with** in order to locate a combination code for the substance and any manifestations.
5. When the condition is stated as in remission, select the subterm **in remission**.
6. Verify the code in the Tabular List, being certain that all aspects of code title correctly describe the documented diagnosis.

SUCCESS STEP

ICD-10-CM codes do not identify continuous or episodic substance use as ICD-9-CM did.

Guided Example of Assigning Psychiatry Codes

To learn more about assigning codes for mental, behavioral, and neurodevelopmental disorders, continue with the example from earlier in the chapter about patient Cody Locust, who was admitted to Valley Hospital with a coma.

Follow along in your ICD-10-CM manual as Ladonna Shuck, CPC, assigns codes. Check off each step after you complete it.

⇨ First, Ladonna confirms the conditions she abstracted:

- ❑ coma that lasted for four hours
- ❑ alcoholic liver disease
- ❑ alcohol dependence of 15 years
- ❑ alcohol intoxication with BAL of .23%
- ❑ dementia with behavioral disturbance due to Alzheimer's

⇨ Ladonna reads the medical record again to determine the main reason for the admission and the services provided, as determined after tests and studies were done.

- ❑ Although the patient was admitted with a coma, the physician linked the coma to alcoholic liver disease.
- ❑ Ladonna decides to begin assigning codes with alcoholic liver disease. Depending on what she finds for that condition, she will determine if she needs to go back and also assign a code for the coma.

⇨ Ladonna searches the Index for the Main Term **Disease**.

- ❑ She searches for a subterm for alcoholic, but does not find one. So she then searches for the subterm that describes the anatomic site, **liver**.
- ❑ Under **liver**, she locates a second-level subterm **alcoholic**.
- ❑ Under **alcoholic**, she locates a third-level subterm **failure**.
- ❑ Under **failure**, she locates a fourth-level subterm **with coma K70.41**.
- ❑ This code appears to be a combination code that includes both alcoholic liver failure and the coma.

⇨ Ladonna verifies code **K70.41** in the Tabular List.

- ❑ She reads the code title for **K70.41, Alcoholic hepatic failure with coma**. She knows that hepatic means liver and confirms that this accurately describes the diagnosis.

⇨ Ladonna checks for instructional notes in the Tabular List.

- ❑ She cross-references the beginning of category **K70** and reads the instructional note, **Use additional code to identify: alcohol abuse and dependence (F10.-)**.
- ❑ She cross-references the beginning of the block **Diseases of liver (K70-K77)** and reads the **Excludes1** and **Excludes2** notes. She determines that they do not apply to her because they do not include any of the conditions she abstracted.
- ❑ She cross-references the beginning of **Chapter 11 (K00-K94)** and reads the **Excludes1** and **Excludes2** notes. She determines that they do not apply to her because they do not include any of the conditions she abstracted.

- ❑ She has finished verifying the code **K70.41, Alcoholic hepatic failure with coma**.

➪ Next, Ladonna assigns a code for alcohol dependence.

- ❑ She searches the Index for the Main Term **Dependence** (■ FIGURE 18-5).

Dependence (on) (syndrome) F19.20
  with remission F19.21
  alcohol (ethyl) (methyl) (without remission) F10.20
    with
      amnestic disorder, persisting F10.26
      anxiety disorder F10.280
      dementia, persisting F10.27
      intoxication F10.229
        with delirium F10.221
        uncomplicated F10.220
      mood disorder F10.24
      psychotic disorder F10.259

Figure 18-5 ■ Index Entry for Alcohol Dependence

- ❑ She locates a subterm for **alcohol**.
- ❑ Under the subterm alcohol, she locates a second-level subterm, **with, dementia, persisting F10.27**.
- ❑ She also locates another second-level subterm, **with, intoxication F10.229**.
- ❑ Under intoxication, she locates another set of choices: **with delirium** or **uncomplicated**. Because neither **with delirium** or **uncomplicated** are documented, she must use the default code next to **intoxication**.
- ❑ She selects the entry **intoxication, F10.229**.
- ❑ She also decides to check out the code **with, dementia, persisting F10.27** to see if that will work for the patient's dementia. So, she will verify both codes at the same time in the Tabular List.

➪ Ladonna verifies code **F10.229** in the Tabular List (■ FIGURE 18-6).

- ❑ She reads the code title **F10.229, Alcohol dependence with intoxication, unspecified** and determines it accurately describes the diagnosis.

4th F10 Alcohol related disorders
  Use additional code for blood alcohol level, if applicable (Y90.-)
  5th F10.1 Alcohol abuse

  5th F10.2 Alcohol dependence
    Excludes1: alcohol abuse (F10.1-)
      alcohol use, unspecified (F10.9-)
    Excludes2: toxic effect of alcohol (T51.0-)
    F10.20 Alcohol dependence, uncomplicated
    F10.21 Alcohol dependence, in remission
    6th F10.22 Alcohol dependence with intoxication
      Acute drunkenness (in alcoholism)
      Excludes1: alcohol dependence with withdrawal (F10.23-)
      F10.220 Alcohol dependence with intoxication, uncomplicated
      F10.221 Alcohol dependence with intoxication delirium
      F10.229 Alcohol dependence with intoxication, unspecified

Figure 18-6 ■ Tabular List Entry for F10 Alcohol Related Disorders

- ❑ Next, she verifies the code **F10.27** and reads the code title **Alcohol dependence with alcohol-induced persisting dementia.**
    - She determines that this code does NOT accurately describe the dementia diagnosis.
    - This code describes alcohol-induced dementia, but the medical record does not state the dementia is due to alcohol. The medical record documents *Alzheimer's dementia*.
    - She eliminates code **F10.27** from consideration.
- ❑ Ladonna still needs to check the instructional notes that apply to code **F10.229, Alcohol dependence with intoxication, unspecified**.
- ❑ She cross-references the beginning of the category **F10 Alcohol related disorders** and reads the instructional note that states, **Use additional code for blood alcohol level, if applicable (Y90.-)**.
    - This instructional note applies to this case because the patient was intoxicated and the BAL is documented.
- ❑ She cross-references the beginning of the block **Mental and behavioral disorders due to psychoactive substance use (F10-F19)** and does not see any instructional notes.
- ❑ She cross-references the beginning of **Chapter 5 (F01-F99)**. The only notes are an **Includes** note and an **Excludes2** note, neither of which applies to this case.
- ❑ She has finished verifying the code **F10.229, Alcohol dependence with intoxication, unspecified.**

⇨ Next, Ladonna assigns the code for BAL, which the instructional note lists as **Y90.-**.

- ❑ She locates the entry for **Y90** and reads the category title **Y90, Evidence of alcohol involvement determined by blood alcohol level** (■ FIGURE 18-7).
- ❑ She notices the symbol **4th** next to the entry, so she knows she must assign an additional character.
- ❑ She double checks the medical record and identifies the BAL as *0.23%*.
- ❑ She notices that the codes in the Tabular List do not list percentages. They list the ratio per 100 ml. To convert the percentage to mg, she knows she simply adds a 0 to the percentage and drops the leading decimal point to arrive at 230 mg.
- ❑ She locates the code with the range that includes 230 mg, **Y90.7, Blood alcohol level of 200-239 mg/100 ml.**
- ❑ She also makes a note of the instructional note at the beginning of the category, **Code first any associated alcohol related disorders (F10)**. This note will guide her when she has to sequence the codes.
- ❑ She reads the instructional note at the beginning of the block **Supplementary factors related to causes of morbidity classified elsewhere (Y90-Y99)** that states: **These categories may be used to provide**

Supplementary factors related to causes of morbidity classified elsewhere (Y90-Y99)

NOTE: These categories may be used to provide supplementary information concerning causes of morbidity. They are not to be used for single-condition coding.

4th Y90 Evidence of alcohol involvement determined by blood alcohol level

Code first any associated alcohol related disorders (F10)

Y90.0 Blood alcohol level of less than 20 mg/100 ml

Y90.1 Blood alcohol level of 20–39 mg/100 ml

Y90.2 Blood alcohol level of 40–59 mg/100 ml

Y90.3 Blood alcohol level of 60–79 mg/100 ml

Y90.4 Blood alcohol level of 80–99 mg/100 ml

Y90.5 Blood alcohol level of 100–119 mg/100 ml

Y90.6 Blood alcohol level of 120–199 mg/100 ml

Y90.7 Blood alcohol level of 200–239 mg/100 ml

Y90.8 Blood alcohol level of 240 mg/100 ml or more

Y90.9 Presence of alcohol in blood, level not specified

Figure 18-7 ■ Tabular List Entry for Y90 Blood Alcohol Level

supplementary information concerning causes of morbidity. They are not to be used for single-condition coding. This note confirms that BAL is NOT a diagnosis that can stand alone; it must always be assigned in conjunction with other codes that describe the condition.

- ❑ She has finished verifying the code **Y90.7, Blood alcohol level of 200-239 mg/100 ml.**

SUCCESS STEP

BAL is indexed in the Index to External Causes under the Main Term **Blood alcohol level.**

⇨ Next, Ladonna must determine the code for Alzheimer's with dementia.

⇨ Ladonna searches the Index for the Main Term **Disease.**

- ❑ She locates the subterm **Alzheimer's.**
- ❑ She checks the medical record for details, then locates the second-level subterm **late onset.**
- ❑ Under **late onset,** she locates the third-level subterm **with behavioral disturbance G30.1 [F02.80].**
- ❑ She notices that two codes are provided. She knows that the *[slanted brackets]* are a coding manual convention that identifies the second code as a manifestation that must be sequenced second.

⇨ Ladonna verifies code **G30.1** in the Tabular List.

- ❑ She reads the code title **G30.1, Alzheimer's disease with late onset** and confirms that it accurately describes the documented diagnosis.
- ❑ She cross-references the instructional notes under the heading for category **G30, Alzheimer's disease.**
- ❑ She reads the **Includes** and **Excludes1** notes. The conditions listed under **Excludes1** do not describe this case, so this note does not apply.
- ❑ She checks the beginning of the block and chapter for instructional notes, but does not find any that apply to this case.
- ❑ She has finished verifying the code **G30.1, Alzheimer's disease with late onset.**

⇨ Ladonna verifies the second code that was listed in the Index for late onset Alzheimer's disease with behavioral disturbance, code **F02.80,** in the Tabular List.

- ❑ She reads the code title **F02.80, Dementia in other diseases classified elsewhere, with behavioral disturbance** and confirms that it accurately describes the documented diagnosis.
- ❑ She notes that the blue highlighting of the code title indicates that this is a manifestation code that should be sequenced after the etiology code.
- ❑ She cross-references the instructional notes under the heading for category **F02, Dementia in other diseases classified elsewhere.**
- ❑ She reads the **Excludes1** note and determines that the conditions do not describe this case, so this note does not apply.
- ❑ She reads the note **Code first the underlying physiological condition, such as:** and locates the entry for **Alzheimer's (G30.-).** This instruction confirms the sequencing order. The code for Alzheimer's should be sequenced before the code for dementia because it is the etiology.
- ❑ She reads the instructional note at the beginning of the block **Mental disorders due to known physiological conditions (F01-F09)** that describes the purpose of this category, but the note does not change the code assigned.
- ❑ She cross-references the beginning of **Chapter 5 (F01-F99)** for instructional notes, but does not find any that relate to this case.
- ❑ She has finished verifying the code **F02, Dementia in other diseases classified elsewhere.**

⇨ Ladonna reviews the codes she has assigned for this case.

- ❑ **K70.41, Alcoholic hepatic failure with coma**
- ❑ **F10.229, Alcohol dependence with intoxication, unspecified**
- ❑ **Y90.7, Blood alcohol level, 220-239 mg/100ml**
- ❑ **G30.0, Late onset Alzheimer's**
- ❑ **F02.81, Dementia in diseases classified elsewhere, with behavioral disturbance**

⇨ Next, Ladonna must determine how to sequence the codes.

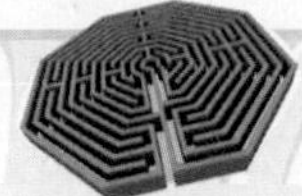

Coding Practice

Now it is your turn to practice assigning codes for mental, behavioral, and neurodevelopmental disorders. Refer to the *Tip* at the end of the mini-medical-record if you need a little extra help.

Exercise 18.3 Assigning Codes for Psychiatry

Instructions: Read the mini-medical-record of each patient's encounter, review the information abstracted in Exercise 18.2, and assign ICD-10-CM diagnosis codes (CM) using the Index and Tabular List. Write the code(s) on the line provided.

1. Date: 8/13/yy Location: Behavioral Health Associates Provider: Brett Camden, MD

Patient: Lisa Klingler Gender: F Age: 9

Reason for encounter: referred by pediatrician for hyperactivity, short attention span, and irritability

Assessment: after testing, symptoms are due to attention deficit hyperactive disorder, predominately hyperactive type

Plan: start medication and behavior therapy

1 CM Code ___________

2. Date: 8/13/yy Location: Valley Hospital

Provider: Brett Camden, MD

Patient: Lance Charboneau Gender: M Age: 31

Reason for encounter: extreme delusions of paranoia

Assessment: dependent continual user of coke, psychosis with delusions due to dependence and long-term use of cocaine

Plan: Rx to help manage delusions, transfer to rehab

1 CM Code ___________

3. Date: 8/13/yy Location: Behavioral Health Associates Provider: Brett Camden, MD

Patient: Kelly Tanouye Gender: F Age: 21

Reason for encounter: ongoing medical management of schizophrenia

Assessment: paranoid schizophrenia

Plan: Medication is managing the condition well. Renewed Rx. Patient is interested in getting a job. Referred to a supported employment service

Tip: The first code is a Z code to issue a repeat prescription.

2 CM Codes ___________ ___________

ARRANGING CODES FOR PSYCHIATRY

Sequencing of codes for mental, behavioral, and neurodevelopmental disorders is determined by instructional notes in the Tabular List. When mental disorders are associated with underlying physical conditions, the Tabular List provides an instructional note, **Code first the underlying physiological condition**. Coders must read the documentation carefully to identify when the physician documents a relationship between a mental disorder and a physiological condition.

Arranging Codes for Pain

ICD-10-CM provides codes to use when pain is documented as exclusively or partially psychological. The guidelines for coding pain are summarized next.

When pain is exclusively psychological with no identifiable medical condition and no documentation of acute or chronic pain, assign **F45.41 Pain disorder exclusively related to psychological factors**.

When pain is exclusively psychological and there is also documentation of acute or chronic pain, assign only code F45.41. (OGCR I.C.5.a.):

When the documentation reports pain with related psychological factors, assign and sequence codes as follows:

1. Assign the appropriate code from category **G89.- Pain, not elsewhere classified.**
2. Assign code **F45.42 Pain disorder with related psychological factors.**

Patient with moderate intellectual disabilities is seen for neurological endemic cretinism. Patient also has associated overactive disorder and difficulty with verbal expression. Patient is dependent on assistance with personal care.

(1) **E00.0 Congenital iodine-deficiency syndrome, neurological type**

(2) **F80.1 Expressive language disorder**

(3) **F84.8 Other pervasive developmental disorders**

(4) **Z74.1 Need for assistance with personal care**

(5) **F70 Mild intellectual disabilities**

Figure 18-8 ■ Example of Sequencing Codes for Intellectual Disabilities

Arranging Codes for Intellectual Disabilities

A new instructional note in ICD-10-CM for intellectual disabilities (F70 through F79) directs coders to **Code first any associated physical or developmental disorders.** According to the Diagnostic and Statistical Manual of Mental Disorders (DSM-IV), the following criteria must be met for a diagnosis of intellectual disabilities:

- an IQ below 70
- significant limitations in two or more areas of adaptive behavior
- evidence that the limitations became apparent before the age of 18

Refer to ■ FIGURE 18-8 to learn more about sequencing codes for intellectual disabilities.

SUCCESS STEP

The American Association on Intellectual and Developmental Disabilities (AAIDD), formerly the Association on Mental Retardation, advocates the use of the term intellectual disability instead of mental retardation.

Guided Example of Arranging Psychiatry Codes

To learn more about sequencing codes for mental, behavioral, and neurodevelopmental disorders, continue with the example from earlier in the chapter about patient Cody Locust, who was admitted to Valley Hospital with a coma.

Follow along in your ICD-10-CM manual as Ladonna Shuck, CPC, sequences the codes. Check off each step after you complete it.

⇨ First, Ladonna confirms the codes she assigned for this case.

- ❑ **K70.41, Alcoholic hepatic failure with coma**
- ❑ **F10.229, Alcohol dependence with intoxication, unspecified**
- ❑ **Y90.7, Blood alcohol level, 220-239 mg/100 ml**
- ❑ **G30.0, Late onset Alzheimer's**
- ❑ **F02.81, Dementia in diseases classified elsewhere, with behavioral disturbance**

⇨ Ladonna takes a moment to read the medical record to review the details of the case.

- ❑ She confirms that the principal diagnosis is **K70.41, Alcoholic hepatic failure with coma** because it meets the definition of principal diagnosis defined by the Uniform Hospital Data Discharge Set (UHDDS) (OGCR II).
- ❑ She determines that the second code should be **F10.2209, Alcohol dependence with intoxication, unspecified** because it further describes the principal diagnosis.
- ❑ Although the code for BAL relates to code **F10.229,** she decides to sequence it as the last code because it is a supplemental code.
- ❑ She determines that the third code should be **G30.0, Late onset Alzheimer's** because the documentation states that the condition was managed during the admission, but does not qualify as the principal diagnosis.
- ❑ She sequences **F02.81, Dementia in diseases classified elsewhere, with behavioral disturbance** as the fourth code because it is a manifestation code for Alzheimer's and must be sequenced after **G30.0.** During the process of assigning codes, she found four instructional codes directing her to sequence the dementia code after the Alzheimer's code:
  - the *[slanted brackets]* convention in the Index
  - the instructional note in the Tabular List under category G30 to **Use additional code** to identify the dementia
  - the blue highlighting of code **F02.81** in the Tabular List that identified it as a manifestation
  - the instructional note in the Tabular List under category F02 to **Code first the underlying condition,** Alzheimer's
- ❑ She sequences the final code as **Y90.7, Blood alcohol level, 220-239 mg/100 ml** because it is a supplemental code that provides added information, but is not a diagnosis code on its own.

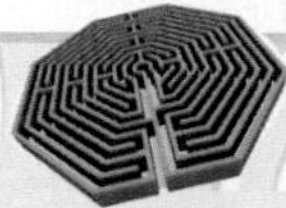

CODING CAUTION

When the Tabular List provides the instructional note to **Code first the underlying condition**, it does not mean that Alzheimer's should always be the principal diagnosis. The note describes the relationship between Alzheimer's (the etiology) and dementia (the manifestation) (OGCR I.A.13). The principal diagnosis is determined based on the criteria in OGCR II.

➩ Ladonna finalizes the codes and sequencing for this case:

(1) **K70.41, Alcoholic hepatic failure with coma**

(2) **F10.229, Alcohol dependence with intoxication, unspecified**

(3) **G30.0, Late onset Alzheimer's**

(4) **F02.81, Dementia in diseases classified elsewhere, with behavioral disturbance**

(5) **Y90.7, Blood alcohol level, 220–239 mg/100 ml**

Coding Practice

Now it is your turn to practice sequencing codes for mental, behavioral, and neurodevelopmental disorders. Refer to the ***Tip*** at the end of the mini-medical-record if you need a little extra help.

Exercise 18.4 Arranging Codes for Psychiatry

Instructions: Read the mini-medical-record of each patient's encounter, review the information abstracted in Exercise 18.2, assign ICD-10-CM diagnosis codes (CM) using the Index and Tabular List, and sequence them correctly.

1. Date: 8/14/yy Location: Behavioral Health Associates Provider: Brett Camden, MD

Patient: Dwayne Angelle Gender: M Age: 10

Reason for encounter: I have been seeing this child for autism, but today his mother is concerned about continuing "fussing and worry about his private parts" that has been going on for quite awhile and his "desire to be like his sister."

Assessment: gender identity disorder

Plan: adjusted medications for current autism.

2 CM Codes __________ __________

2. Date: 8/14/yy Location: Valley Hospital

Provider: Brett Camden, MD

Patient: Marcus Evitt Gender: M Age: 48

Reason for encounter: admitted from emergency department for alcohol-induced gastritis with hemorrhaging and intoxication with BAL of .09

(continued)

2. (continued)

Assessment: patient has long-term alcohol use with dependence, prior cocaine abuser but states he no longer uses

Plan: patient agreed to counseling after discharge

***Tip*:** Follow instructional notes in the Tabular List to help determine sequencing.

4 CM Codes __________ __________ __________ __________

3. Date: 8/14/yy Location: Valley Hospital

Provider: Brett Camden, MD

Patient: Wallace Bosque Gender: M Age: 56

Reason for encounter: severe depression due to bipolar disorder

Assessment: patient is also being treated for liver cirrhosis with ascites due to chronic continuous alcoholism

Plan: patient has stable living situation so we are going to discharge him to a partial hospitalization program

3 CM Codes __________ __________ __________

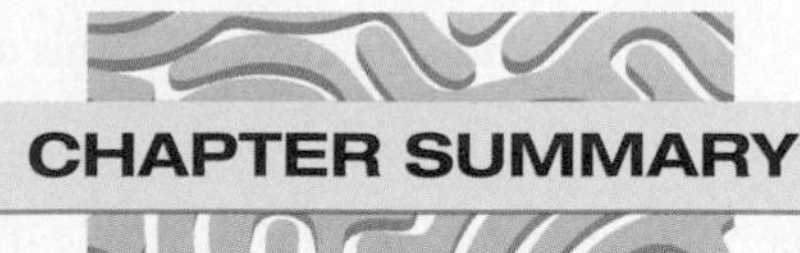

CHAPTER SUMMARY

In this chapter you learned that:

- Mental, behavioral, and neurodevelopmental disorders are real, not imagined, disorders that have diagnostic criteria and are proven to respond to treatment.
- ICD-10-CM Chapter 5, Mental, Behavioral, and Neurodevelopmental Disorders (F01-F99), contains 11 blocks or subchapters that are divided by the type of disorder.
- Many mental, behavioral, and neurodevelopmental disorders have multiple subtypes, so coders must be particularly attentive to the documented wording of the condition.
- Three types of conditions in this ICD-10-CM chapter present challenges in assigning codes due to the level of detail that must be reported: bipolar disorder, schizophrenic disorders, and substance disorders.
- When mental disorders are associated with underlying physical conditions, the Tabular List provides an instructional note to code the underlying physiological condition first.
- ICD-10-CM Official Guidelines for Coding and Reporting (OGCR) section I.C.5. provides detailed discussion of pain disorders related to psychological factors and mental, behavioral, and neurodevelopmental disorders due to substance abuse.

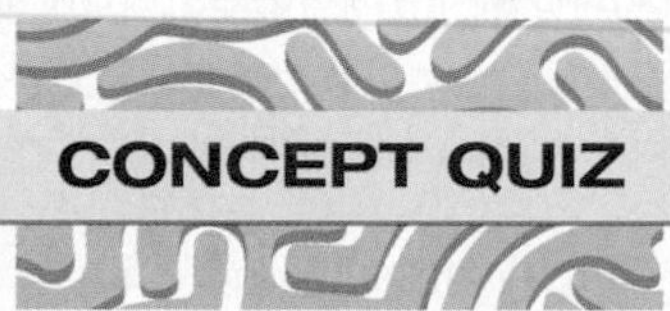

CONCEPT QUIZ

Take a moment to look back at your trip through mental, behavioral, and neurodevelopmental disorders and solidify your skills. This is your opportunity to pull together everything you have learned.

Completion

Instructions: Write the term that answers each question based on the information you learned in this chapter. Choose from the list below. Some choices may be used more than once and some choices may not be used at all. Refer to the discussion in this chapter and the Glossary at the end of this book if you need a little extra help.

abuse	intoxication
barbiturate	mood
cognitive	narcotic
dependence	personality
dissociative	psychotic
hallucinogen	sexual
impulse-control	use
in remission	

1. Dementia is an example of a/an _______________ disorder.
2. Voyeurism is an example of a/an _______________ disorder.
3. Kleptomania is an example of a/an _______________ disorder.
4. Bipolar is an example of a/an _______________ disorder.
5. Phenobarbital is an example of the _______________ class of drugs.
6. Fentanyl is an example of the _______________ class of drugs.
7. LSD is an example of the _______________ class of drugs.
8. _______________ occurs when more of a substance is consumed than a person can physically tolerate, resulting in behavioral or physical abnormalities.
9. Past history of a substance disorder is _______________.
10. _______________ of a substance is consuming it in moderate amounts that do not create significant legal, social, employment, family, or medical problems.

Multiple Choice

Instructions: Circle the letter of the best answer to each question based on the information you learned in this chapter.

Refer to the discussion in this chapter and the Glossary at the end of this book if you need a little extra help.

1. Psychotic disorders consist of
   A. depression and mania.
   B. delusions and hallucinations.
   C. impulse and control behaviors.
   D. obsessive and compulsive behaviors.
2. Physical symptoms that are not explained by medical conditions are
   A. affective disorders.
   B. dissociative disorders.
   C. adjustment disorders.
   D. somatoform disorders.
3. Which of the following substances is a narcotic?
   A. Secobarbital
   B. PCP
   C. Heroin
   D. Amphetamine
4. Which of the following is NOT a behavioral disturbance of dementia?
   A. Memory loss
   B. Aggression
   C. Wandering
   D. Depression
5. Which of the following is NOT a key criterion for abstracting psychoactive substance disorders?
   A. What is the class of substance?
   B. Is use episodic or continuous?
   C. Is withdrawal present?
   D. Is delirium or perceptual disturbance present?
6. A BAL of 0.08% may also be expressed as
   A. 08 mg per 100 ml.
   B. 8 mg per 100 ml.
   C. 80 mg per 100 ml.
   D. 800 mg per 100 ml.
7. When substance abuse and dependence are both documented, how should the condition be coded?
   A. Assign a code for abuse only.
   B. Assign a code for dependence only.
   C. Assign two codes, one for abuse and one for dependence.
   D. Assign a combination code for abuse with dependence.
8. Which of the following is coded under category F20 Schizophrenia?
   A. Paranoid schizophrenia
   B. Schizoaffective disorder
   C. Schizothymia
   D. Schizophreniform disorder
9. How should alcoholic liver disease with coma be coded?
   A. Assign the code for coma followed by the code for alcoholic liver disease.
   B. Assign the code for alcoholic liver disease followed by the code for coma.
   C. Assign a combination code for coma due to alcoholic liver disease.
   D. Assign a combination code for alcoholic liver disease with coma.
10. A new instructional note in ICD-10-CM for intellectual disabilities (F70 through F79) directs coders to
   A. code first any associated physical or developmental disorders.
   B. use additional code for any associated physical or developmental disorders.
   C. assign combination codes for the intellectual disability and any associated physical or developmental disorders.
   D. not code any associated physical or developmental disorders.

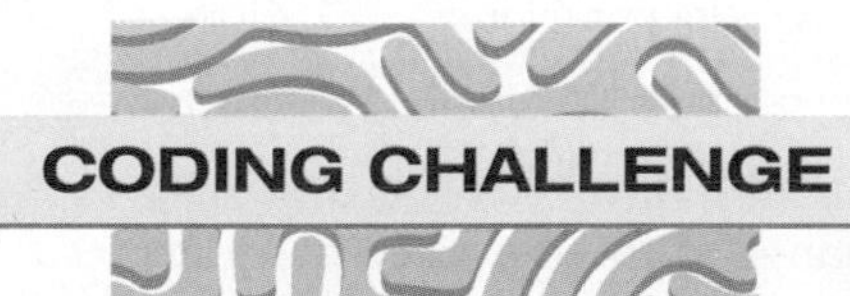

CODING CHALLENGE

Now it is your turn to demonstrate coding all aspects of mental, behavioral, and neurodevelopmental disorders. Refer back to the examples and discussion in this chapter when you need a little extra help. Use your medical dictionary and anatomy references when needed.

Instructions: Read the mini-medical-record of each patient's encounter, then abstract, assign, and sequence ICD-10-CM diagnosis codes (CM) using the Index and Tabular List. Write the code(s) on the line provided.

1. Date: 8/19/yy Location: North Side Pulmonology Provider: Gilbert Stagg, MD

Patient: Max Holdaway Gender: M Age: 19

Reason for encounter: pattern of exacerbation of asthma attacks on the weekends

Assessment: psychogenic moderate persistent asthma

(continued)

(continued from page 363)

1. (continued)

Plan: *allergy studies are scheduled in addition to follow-up with a family systems therapist to address the psychogenic component*

***Tip*:** Read the instructional notes in the Tabular List to determine the codes and sequencing.

2 CM Codes __________ __________

2. Date: *8/19/yy* Location: *Behavioral Health Associates* Provider: *Brett Camden, MD*

Patient: *Jaime Waldow* Gender: *F* Age: *20*

Reason for encounter: *veteran experiencing flashbacks accompanied by nightmares, angry outbursts, hypervigilance, and anxiousness*

Assessment: *chronic posttraumatic stress disorder*

Plan: *trauma-focused cognitive-behavioral (TFCBT) treatments 12 weeks*

1 CM Code __________

3. Date: *8/19/yy* Location: *Branton Family Practice* Provider: *Kristen Conover, MD*

Patient: *Ken Pagani* Gender: *M* Age: *52*

Reason for encounter: *review results of brain MRI, ordered after he complained at a previous visit of episodes of sleepwalking*

Assessment: *MRI shows brain metastasis from pancreatic cancer; patient has secondary diabetes d/t pancreatic cancer and is on long-term insulin*

Plan: *refer to neurologist for further workup on sleep walking*

***Tip*:** Review OGCR I.C.2.a. and b. for sequencing of neoplasm codes. Review OGCR I.C.4.a.6) regarding secondary diabetes.

5 CM Codes __________ __________

__________ __________ __________

4. Date: *8/19/yy* Location: *Behavioral Health Associates* Provider: *Brett Camden, MD*

Patient: *Armando Riehle* Gender: *M* Age: *26*

Reason for encounter: *Patient reports feeling extremely irritable, having cold sweats, and headaches. He went cold turkey for 4 days to try and get off heroin.*

(continued)

4. (continued)

Assessment: *symptoms are due to drug withdrawal with heroin dependence*

Plan: *the patient met with a drug counselor to discuss a more appropriate way to address his addiction, started patient on methadone (opiate substitute) treatment*

***Tip*:** Review OGCR I.C.21.c.10) regarding the use of a Z code for the drug counseling.

1 CM Code __________

5. Date: *8/19/yy* Location: *Valley Hospital* Provider: *Brett Camden, MD*

Patient: *Chrystal Touchton* Gender: *F* Age: *36*

Reason for encounter: *severe depression, has considered suicide*

Assessment: *depression and suicide ideation due to persistent anxiety regarding being unemployed for the past year*

Plan: *psychotherapy with no-suicide contract, antidepressant medication, refer to unemployment support group*

3 CM Codes __________ __________

____

6. Date: *8/19/yy* Location: *Behavioral Health Associates* Provider: *Brett Camden, MD*

Patient: *Casey Dease* Gender: *M* Age: *43*

Reason for encounter: *depressed mood (3 week duration), excessive sleep, fatigue*

Assessment: *depressive episode due to bipolar disorder which is in partial remission*

Plan: *dosage change of present mood stabilizer, psychotherapy*

1 CM Code __________

7. Date: *8/19/yy* Location: *Behavioral Health Associates* Provider: *Brett Camden, MD*

Patient: *Jamie Geren* Gender: *F* Age: *22*

Reason for encounter: *excessive sadness, crying and, sleeping, lethargy, feeling emotionally numb. Gave birth 3 weeks ago*

Assessment: *postpartum depression*

(continued)

7. (continued)

Plan: interpersonal relationship counseling, Rx SSRI (selective serotonin reuptake inhibitor) antidepressant meds, obtain part time mother's helper

1 CM Code ___________

8. Date: 8/19/yy Location: Behavioral Health Associates Provider: Brett Camden, MD

Patient: Roxie Piccoli Gender: F Age: 10

Reason for encounter: struggling in school with reading and spelling

Assessment: developmental dyslexia, spelling disorder

Plan: special ed schooling, teach compensating and coping skills

2 CM Codes ___________ ___________

9. Date: 8/19/yy Location: Valley Hospital

Provider: Brett Camden, MD

Patient: Ophelia Hachey Gender: F Age: 16

Reason for encounter: admitted from psychiatrist's office for multiple personality disorder

Assessment: Multiple personality disorder and mild intellectual disability. Patient presents with learning deficiencies (IQ 65) and with physical disability of anemia due to poor nutrition.

(continued)

9. (continued)

Plan: psychotherapy weekly, transfer patient into special education program at school, home visit by social services to address nutritional issues

***Tip*:** Assign codes for the personality disorder, the cognitive disorder, and the physical disability.

3 CM Codes ___________ ___________ ___________

10. Date: 8/19/yy Location: Behavioral Health Associates Provider: Brett Camden, MD

Patient: Amie Cubbage Gender: F Age: 25

Reason for encounter: chewing tobacco since age 13 and wants to quit

Assessment: counseling to address dependence on tobacco

Plan: RTO 1 week

***Tip*:** Read the instructional note in the Tabular List that indicates sequencing.

2 CM Codes ___________ ___________

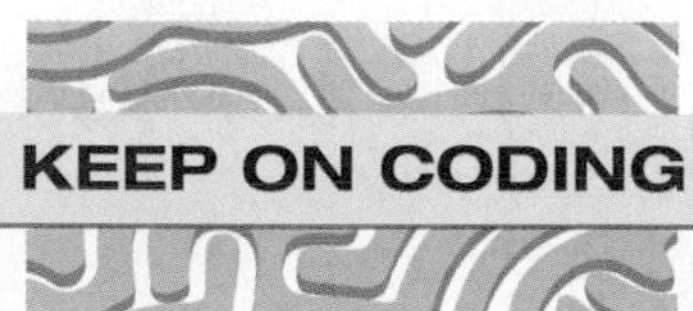

KEEP ON CODING

As a coder, you can never have too much experience. Apply everything you have learned in this chapter to code the following diagnostic statements. Use the OGCR and instructional notes in the Tabular List to help determine how many codes are required.

Instructions: Read the diagnostic statement, then use the Index and Tabular List to assign and sequence ICD-10-CM (CM) diagnosis codes. Write the code(s) on the line provided.

1. Acute brain syndrome: CM Code(s) ___________
2. Catatonic schizophrenia: CM Code(s) ___________
3. Thumb sucking: CM Code(s) ___________
4. Bulimia nervosa: CM Code(s) ___________

5. Fear of flying: CM Code(s) ______
6. Nicotine dependence with withdrawal: CM Code(s) ______
7. Alcohol abuse with alcohol-induced sleep disorder: CM Code(s) ______
8. Bipolar II disorder: CM Code(s) ______
9. Adjustment disorder with anxiety: CM Code(s) ______
10. Primary hypersomnia: CM Code(s) ______
11. Voyeurism: CM Code(s) ______
12. Autistic disorder: CM Code(s) ______
13. Intellectual disability with IQ level 19: CM Code(s) ______
14. Psychogenic encopresis: CM Code(s) ______
15. Trichotillomania: CM Code(s) ______
16. Abuse of antacids: CM Code(s) ______
17. Dissociative stupor: CM Code(s) ______
18. Sleepwalking: CM Code(s) ______
19. Selective mutism: CM Code(s) ______
20. Psychogenic torticollis: CM Code(s) ______
21. Dysthymic disorder: CM Code(s) ______
22. Hypochondria: CM Code(s) ______
23. Clumsy child syndrome: CM Code(s) ______
24. Premature ejaculation: CM Code(s) ______
25. Cocaine dependence with withdrawal: CM Code(s) ______

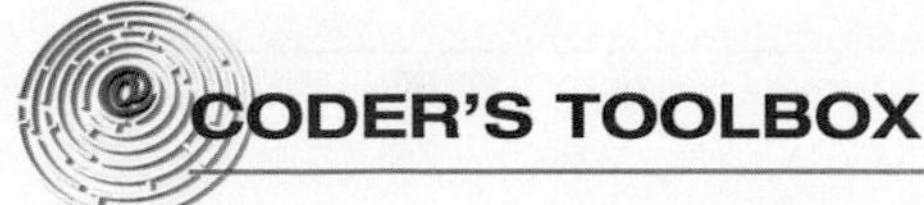

CODER'S TOOLBOX

The following resources are a starting point for learning more about mental, behavioral, and neurodevelopmental disorders.

Addictions and Recovery **http://www.addictionsandrecovery.org/index.html**
AllPsych Online, the Virtual Psychology Classroom **http://allpsych.com/**
American Association on Intellectual and Developmental Disabilities (AAIDD) **http://www.aamr.org/**
American Psychiatric Association > DSM-5 Development > Proposed Revisions **http://www.dsm5.org/proposedrevision/Pages/Default.aspx**
American Society of Addiction Medicine **http://www.asam.org/**
Council for Exceptional Children (CEC) **http://www.cec.sped.org/AM/Template.cfm?Section=Home&Template=/templates/CECHomePage.cfm**
Drug And Alcohol Rehab Services **http://www.drugandalcoholrehab.net/**
Mental Health America **http://www.nmha.org**
Mothers Against Drunk Driving **http://www.madd.org/**
National Alliance on Mental Illness **http://www.nami.org/**
Schizophrenia **http://www.schizophrenia.com/family/sz.overview.htm**

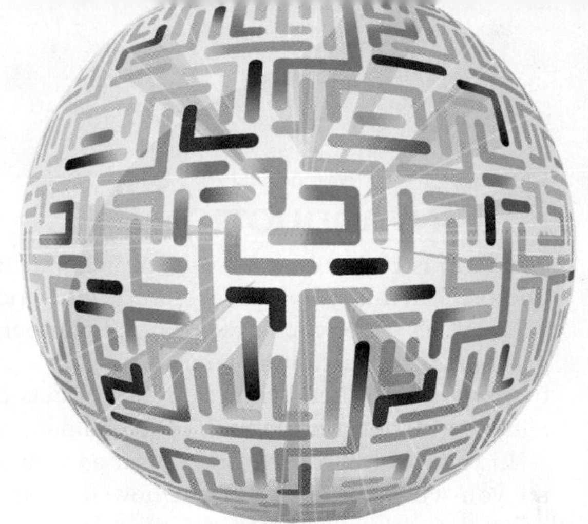

19 Diseases of the Eye and Adnexa (H00-H59)

Learning Objectives

After completing this chapter, you should have the skills to:

- Spell and define the key words, medical terms, and abbreviations related to diseases of the eye and ocular adnexa.
- Discuss the structure, function, and common conditions of the eye and ocular adnexa.
- Identify the main characteristics of coding for diseases of the eye and ocular adnexa.
- Abstract diagnostic information from the medical record for conditions of the eye and ocular adnexa.
- Assign codes for diseases of the eye and ocular adnexa.
- Arrange codes for diseases of the eye and ocular adnexa.
- Code neoplasms of the eye and ocular adnexa.
- Discuss the Official Guidelines for Coding and Reporting related to diseases of the eye and ocular adnexa.

Key Terms and Abbreviations

adnexa
choroid
colloid
cone
conjunctiva
cornea
lens
ocular globe
optic nerve
orbital cavity
pupil
retina
rod
sclera
vitreous body

In addition to the key terms listed here, students should know the terms defined within tables in this chapter.

Chapter Outline

- **Eye Refresher**
- **Coding Overview of the Eye**
- **Abstracting for the Eye**
- **Assigning Codes for the Eye**
- **Arranging Codes for the Eye**
- **Coding Neoplasms of the Eye**

ICD-10-CM codes in this chapter are from the ICD-10-CM 2014 Draft code set from the Department of Health and Human Services, Centers for Disease Control and Prevention.

INTRODUCTION

Your trip is probably not complete without taking a few photos. Whether your camera use begins and ends with your cell phone or you have advanced photographic skills, photographs help capture your memories. A camera, particularly a traditional film camera, collects and focuses light in a manner very similar to the human eye.

In your tour of the eye and ocular adnexa in this chapter you will learn more about how the eye and ocular adnexa works, why sometimes they do not work as they should, and how physicians treat these conditions. Most importantly, you will practice coding for patient encounters related to eye and ocular adnexa diseases and conditions, a skill that requires you to abstract information from the mini-medical-record, assign correct codes, and arrange (sequence) the codes in the correct order.

An ophthalmologist is a physician (MD) who specializes in diagnosing and treating diseases of the eye. Ophthalmologists may specialize in a specific part of the eye, such as the cornea or the retina. An optometrist is a doctor of optometry (OD) who specializes in examining the eyes and prescribing corrective lenses. Optometrists screen patients for certain eye diseases, such as glaucoma, and refer patients to an ophthalmologist if there are any concerns.

As you read this chapter, open up your medical terminology book to the chapter on the eye and keep a medical dictionary handy to refresh your memory of any unfamiliar terms. Coders do not know every detail of every body system, but they should know how to find the answers to ensure accurate coding. These resources ensure that you have the information you need at your fingertips.

EYE REFRESHER

The eye and ocular **adnexa** (*associated anatomic structures*) make vision possible by receiving light from the external world and converting it into impulses that are transmitted to the brain through the **optic nerve**, which is cranial nerve II. The **ocular globe** refers to the eyeball itself. The eyeball consists of three layers: the **sclera** (*tough, white outer layer*), the **choroid** (*opaque middle layer that supplies blood to the eye*), and the **retina** (*the innermost layer that contains sensory receptor cells*). The **orbital cavity** is the bony structure around the eye, commonly known as the eye socket. The adnexa are the surrounding ocular muscles, eyelids, and **conjunctiva** (*membrane that lines the eyelids*) (■ Figure 19-1).

Light rays pass through the **cornea** (*the clear hard portion of the sclera that protects the lens*), **pupil** (*the black central part of eye that opens and closes in response to light*), **lens** (*the clear part of the front of the eye that focuses light rays on the retina*), and **vitreous body** (*the transparent jelly that fills the eyeball*

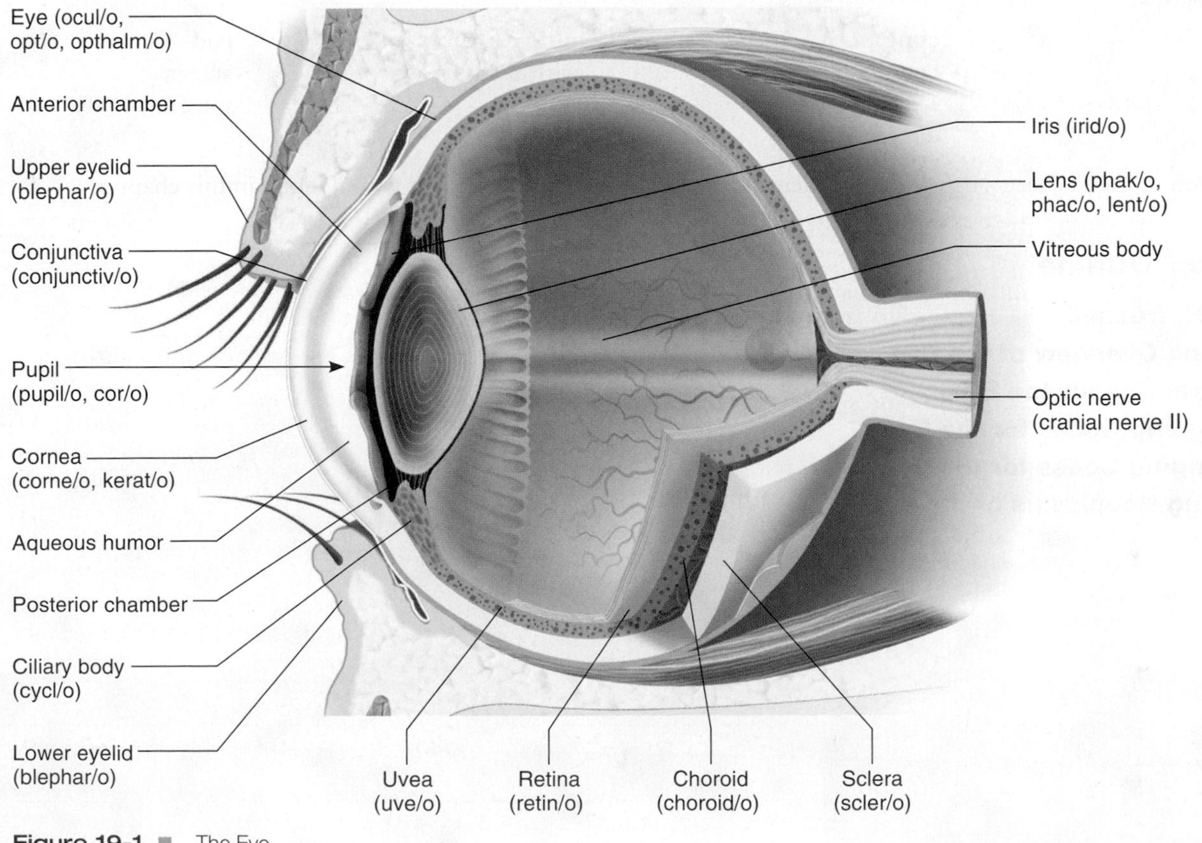

Figure 19-1 ■ The Eye

and is surrounded by a membrane) to focus on the retina. Rods and cones (*light sensitive receptor cells*) in the retina are stimulated and transmit sensory impulses to the brain, which interprets the impulses as a visual image.

In Figure 19-1, each structure in the eye is labeled with its name as well as its medical terminology root/combining form where applicable. As you learn about conditions and procedures that affect the eye, remember to apply medical terminology skills to use word roots, prefixes, and suffixes you already know to define new terms. Refer to ■ TABLE 19-1 for a refresher on how to build medical terms related to the eye and ocular adnexa.

Conditions of the Eye

Refer to ■ TABLE 19-2 for a summary of diseases affecting the eye and ocular adnexa.

CODING CAUTION

Be alert for medical words that sound and are spelled similarly but have different meanings.

uvea (*the middle layer of eye consisting of the iris, ciliary body, and choroid*) and **uvula** (*a pendant fleshy lobe, most commonly referred to as the one in the back of the mount*)

keratitis (*inflammation of the cornea*) and **keratin** (*horny tissues found in the epidermis, hair, and nails*)

choroid (*the middle layer of the eye*) and **colloid** (*gelatin-like or mucous substance found in tissues*)

Table 19-1 ■ **EXAMPLE OF CONSTRUCTING MEDICAL TERMS FOR THE EYE AND OCULAR ADNEXA**

Combining Form	Suffix	Complete Medical Term
retin/o (*retina*)	**-itis** (*inflammation*) **-ptosis** (*drooping*) **-pathy** (*abnormal condition*)	**retin + itis** (*inflammation of the retina*) **retino + pathy** (*abnormal condition of the retina*)
blephar/o (*eyelid*)		**blephar + itis** (*inflammation of the eyelid*) **blephar + optosis** (*drooping eyelid*)
choroid/o (*vascular coat of the eye*)		**choroid + itis** (*inflammation of the vascular coat of the eye*)

Table 19-2 ■ **COMMON DISEASES OF THE EYE AND OCULAR ADNEXA**

Condition	Definition
Blepharitis	An inflammation and infection of hair follicles and glands at the margins of the eyelids, due to virus, bacteria, allergic response, or exposure to irritants
Cataract	A cloudiness of the lens that usually develops slowly over time due to aging
Chalazion	A small hard cyst on the eyelid caused by blockage of a gland on the eyelid
Conjunctivitis	A viral or bacterial inflammation and infection of the conjunctiva
Diabetic retinopathy	The abnormal expansion of blood vessels and hemorrhaging in the vessels of the retina, caused by diabetes
Glaucoma	An increased fluid pressure within the eye that damages the optic nerve and can cause blindness
Hordeolum	A bacterial inflammation of an sebaceous gland on the edge or lining of the eyelid; also called a stye
Keratitis	An inflammation and ulceration of the surface of the cornea
Macular degeneration	The gradual loss of central vision due to aging, with no cure (■ FIGURE 19-2 and ■ FIGURE 19-3, page 370)
Retinal detachment	The separation of the retina from the choroid layer of the eye

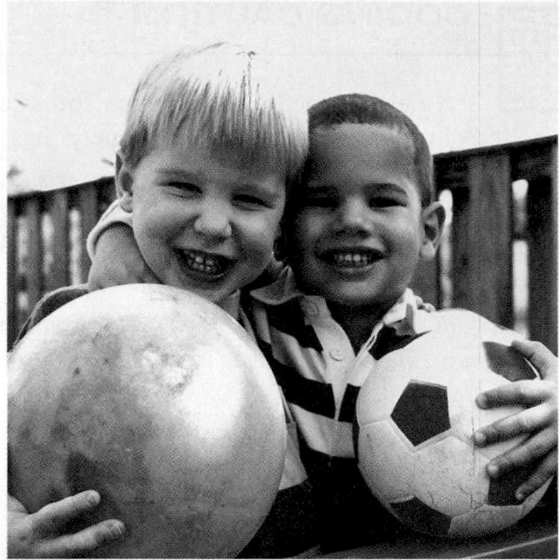

Figure 19-2 ■ Image Seen by a Person with Normal Vision. *Source: National Eye Institute, National Institutes of Health.*

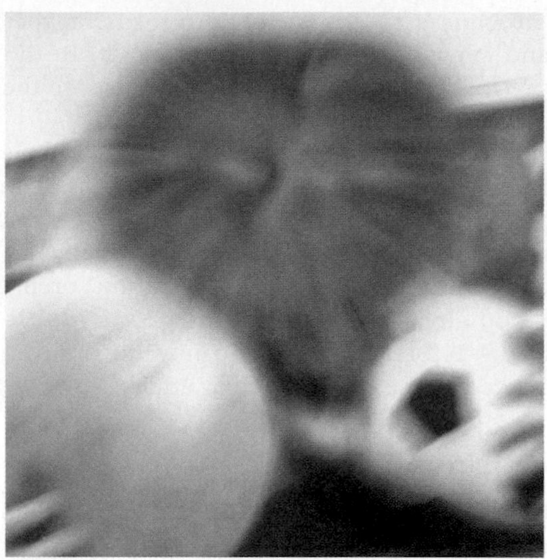

Figure 19-3 ■ Image with Loss of Central Vision Seen by a Person with Macular Degeneration. *Source: National Eye Institute, National Institutes of Health.*

This section provides a general reference to help understand the most common diagnoses of the eye and ocular adnexa, but does not list everything you need to know. Use medical terminology skills discussed earlier in this chapter to learn the meaning of unfamiliar words. Remember to keep standard reference books handy in case you get stuck. Refer to the resources in the Coder's Toolbox at the end of this chapter to learn more about conditions affecting the eye and ocular adnexa.

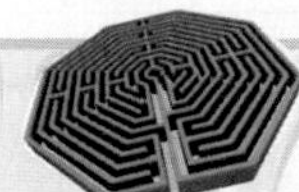

Coding Practice

Refresh your knowledge of terminology related to the eye and ocular adnexa. Use a medical terminology text or a website such as GlobalRph.com > Medical Terminology **http://www.globalrph.com/medterm.htm** to identify the meaning of word parts that may not be familiar.

Exercise 19.1 Eye Refresher

Instructions: Use your medical terminology skills and resources to define the following conditions related to the eye and ocular adnexa, then assign the default diagnosis code.

Follow these steps:

- Use slash marks "/" to break down each term into its root(s) and suffix.
- Define the meaning of the word, based on the meaning of each word part.
- Assign the default ICD-10-CM diagnosis code for the condition, including laterality, using the Index and Tabular List.

Example: conjunctivitis (right eye) conjunctiv/itis — Meaning: *inflammation of the lining of the eye* — CM Code: *H10.31*

1. photokeratitis (right eye) Meaning ____________ CM Code ________
2. retinoblastoma (left eye) Meaning ____________ CM Code ________
3. lagophthalmos Meaning ____________ CM Code ________
4. blepharoptosis (bilateral) Meaning ____________ CM Code ________
5. dacryoadenitis (right eye) Meaning ____________ CM Code ________
6. keratomalacia (bilateral) Meaning ____________ CM Code ________
7. retinoschisis (left eye) Meaning ____________ CM Code ________
8. amblyopia (bilateral) Meaning ____________ CM Code ________
9. iridocyclitis Meaning ____________ CM Code ________
10. aphakia (right eye) Meaning ____________ CM Code ________

CODING OVERVIEW OF THE EYE

ICD-10-CM Chapter 7, Diseases of the Eye and Adnexa (H00-H59), is a new chapter that did not exist in ICD-9-CM. In ICD-9-CM, the eye and ocular adnexa were included in Chapter 6 (360-379) for the nervous system and special senses. This is one of two chapters in which codes begin with the letter H; codes for the ear and mastoid process occupy codes H60 through H95.This chapter contains 12 blocks or subchapters that are divided by anatomical site within the eye. Review the block names and code ranges listed at the beginning of Chapter 7 in the ICD-10-CM manual to become familiar with the content and organization.

ICD-10-CM uses the term *age-related cataract* in place of *senile cataract*, which was used in ICD-9-CM. Most codes have been expanded to include greater specificity of anatomic site and laterality.

This chapter includes disorders affecting each structure within the eye, glaucoma, and visual disturbances and blindness. It does not include injuries to the eye, congenital conditions, infectious, parasitic, or syphilis-related eye disorders, which are classified in other ICD-10-CM chapters. It also does not include diabetic or many other endocrine eye disorders, which are reported with combination codes in ICD-10-CM Chapter 4, Endocrine, Nutritional, and Metabolic Diseases (E00-E89).

ICD-10-CM provides Official Guidelines for Coding and Reporting (OGCR) in OGCR section I.C.7 regarding assigning codes for the stages of glaucoma. General OGCR in sections I.A., I.B., II, III, and IV direct the coder. Instructional notes in the Tabular List guide the coder when additional codes are required. An instructional note at the beginning of the chapter directs coders to use an external cause code following the code for the eye condition when an external cause is involved in creating the eye condition. This note applies to all codes in ICD-10-CM Chapter 7.

Table 19-3 ■ KEY CRITERIA FOR ABSTRACTING CONDITIONS OF THE EYE AND OCULAR ADNEXA

- ❑ What is the condition?
- ❑ What is the subtype of the condition?
- ❑ Is a more specific subtype documented?
- ❑ What is the stage (certain types of glaucoma)?
- ❑ Is laterality right, left, bilateral, or unspecified?
- ❑ For conditions affecting the eyelid, is the upper or lower lid involved?
- ❑ Is the condition acute or chronic?
- ❑ Is the eye condition secondary to diabetes or a condition from another body system?
- ❑ Do any additional eye conditions exist?
- ❑ Is the condition due to an external cause?

Table 19-4 ■ KEY CRITERIA FOR ABSTRACTING OPHTHALMIC MANIFESTATIONS OF DIABETES

- ❑ Is the diabetes type 1 or type 2?
- ❑ Is the eye condition documented as related to diabetes?
- ❑ Is the condition retinopathy, cataracts, or other?
- ❑ What is the laterality?

For retinopathy:

- ❑ Is retinopathy proliferative or nonproliferative?
- ❑ Is nonproliferative retinopathy mild, moderate, or severe?
- ❑ Is retinopathy accompanied by macular edema?

ABSTRACTING FOR THE EYE

The main concerns when abstracting eye conditions are identifying laterality and the presence of underlying conditions, particularly diabetes. The majority of eye conditions require that the laterality be identified. Laterality is expressed at the following levels:

- right, left, or unspecified eye
- bilateral, for applicable conditions
- upper, lower, or unspecified lid of each eye, for applicable conditions

Refer to ■ TABLE 19-3 for guidance on how to abstract conditions of the eye and ocular adnexa. Remember that the abstracting questions are a guide and that not every question applies to, or can be answered for, every case. For example, some conditions, such as glaucoma and conjunctivitis, are designated as acute or chronic, while other conditions, such as cataracts, are not.

Abstracting Diabetic Eye Conditions

Retinopathy and cataracts are common diabetic manifestations. Even though diabetic eye conditions are not classified to ICD-10-CM Chapter 7, coders must know how to abstract them. Laterality is not a requirement for diabetic manifestations. Refer to ■ TABLE 19-4 to learn key criteria for abstracting ophthalmic manifestation of diabetes.

Guided Example of Abstracting for the Eye

Refer to the following example throughout this chapter to learn about abstracting, assigning, and sequencing eye and ocular adnexa codes. Megan Scheidler, CCS-P, is a fictitious coder who guides you through the coding process.

Date: 9/1/yy Location: Branton Eye Care

Provider: Margo Bittinger, MD

Patient: Jaclyn Vandeventer Gender: F Age: 71

Reason for encounter: referred by optometrist after abnormal findings on a routine vision exam

Assessment: right normal tension glaucoma, mild stage (*damage to the optic nerve despite normal pressure in the eye*), age related nuclear (*centrally located*) cataracts bilaterally that are interfering with vision

Plan: drops and medication for glaucoma, we will see how that does, then see if surgery is needed, we will wait on cataract removal until the glaucoma is controlled

Follow along as Megan Scheidler, CCS-P, abstracts the diagnosis. Check off each step after you complete it.

⇨ Megan reads through the entire record, with special attention to the reason for the encounter and the final assessment.

- ❑ She notes that the patient was seen at a clinic by an optometrist who identified some concerns that required the attention of an ophthalmologist.

⇨ Megan refers to Key Criteria for Abstracting Conditions of the Eye and Ocular Adnexa (Table 19-3) and begins with glaucoma.

- ❑ *What is the condition?* glaucoma (■ FIGURE 19-4).
- ❑ *What is the subtype of the condition?* normal tension glaucoma
- ❑ *Is laterality right, left, bilateral, or unspecified?* right eye
- ❑ *What is the stage?* mild
- ❑ *Is the condition acute or chronic?* She notes that acute or chronic does not apply to glaucoma.
- ❑ *Is the eye condition secondary to diabetes or a condition from another body system?* No.
- ❑ *Do any additional eye conditions exist?* Yes, cataracts are documented.
- ❑ *Is the condition due to an external cause?* No.

⇨ Next, Megan abstracts for cataracts (■ FIGURE 19-5).

- ❑ *What is the condition?* cataracts
- ❑ *What is the subtype of the condition?* age related
- ❑ *Is a more specific subtype documented?* nuclear
- ❑ *Is laterality right, left, bilateral, or unspecified?* The laterality is both eyes. She notes that although the glaucoma affects only the right eye, the cataracts are bilateral.
- ❑ *Is the condition acute or chronic?* Acute or chronic is not applicable to cataracts.
- ❑ *Is the eye condition secondary to diabetes or a condition from another body system?* No.
- ❑ *Do any additional eye conditions exist?* No.
- ❑ *Is the condition due to an external cause?* No.

⇨ At this time, Megan thinks she will need a code for glaucoma and a code for cataracts, but she will not know for certain until she moves on to assigning codes.

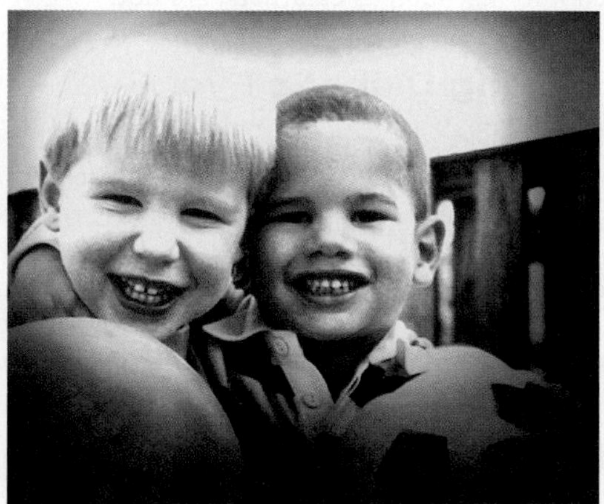

Figure 19-4 ■ Image with Tunnel Vision Seen by a Person with Glaucoma. *Source: National Eye Institute, National Institutes of Health.*

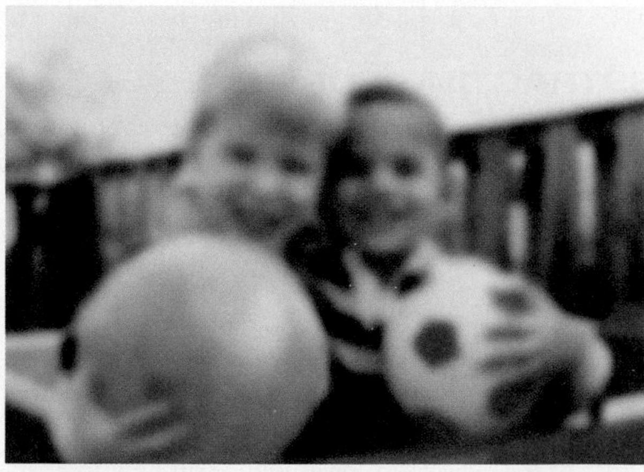

Figure 19-5 ■ Blurry Image Seen by a Person with Cataracts. *Source: National Eye Institute, National Institutes of Health.*

Coding Practice

Now it is your turn to practice abstracting diagnoses for the eye and ocular adnexa. Questions guide your analysis of each scenario.

Exercise 19.2 Abstracting for the Eye

Instructions: Read the mini-medical-record of each patient's encounter and answer the abstracting questions. Write the answer on the line provided. Do not assign any codes.

1. Date: 9/13/yy Location: Branton Eye Care
Provider: Margo Bittinger, MD
Patient: Morris Marcilus Gender: M Age: 76
Reason for encounter: phacoemulsification of cataract and intraocular lens (IOL) implant
Assessment: age related nuclear cataract, left eye
Plan: FU in office, 2 days

a. Define the procedures that are the reason for the encounter. ____________

b. What is the condition? ____________

c. What is the subtype of the condition? ____________

d. What is the laterality? ____________

2. Date: 9/13/yy Location: Branton Eye Care
Provider: Margo Bittinger, MD
Patient: Juliette Pardon Gender: F Age: 84
Reason for encounter: monthly retinal injections
Assessment: wet macular degeneration, in both eyes
Plan: return, 1 month

a. Define the procedure that is the reason for the encounter. ____________

b. What is the condition? ____________

c. What is the subtype of the condition? ____________

d. What is the laterality? ____________

3. Date: 9/14/yy Location: Branton Eye Care
Provider: Margo Bittinger, MD
Patient: Sheree Shambo Gender: F Age: 69
Reason for encounter: crusty eyelids
Assessment: nonulcerative blepharitis on both upper lids
Plan: keep clean, Rx topical antibiotic

a. What is the condition? ____________

b. What is the subtype of the condition? ____________

c. What is the laterality? ____________

d. Is the upper or lower lid involved on the right side? ____________

On the left side? ____________

4. Date: 9/13/yy Location: Branton Eye Care
Provider: Margo Bittinger, MD
Patient: Ken Rocker Gender: M Age: 61
Reason for encounter: routine eye exam as part of diabetic monitoring
Assessment: moderate diabetic nonproliferative retinopathy with no macular edema
Plan: be diligent about keeping sugar and BP well controlled, to slow progression of condition

a. What is the reason for the encounter? ____________

b. Are there abnormal findings? ____________

c. What eye condition is diagnosed? ____________

e. Is it proliferative or nonproliferative? ____________

e. Is it mild, moderate, or severe? ____________

f. Is it accompanied by macular edema? ____________

g. What is the underlying condition? ____________

h. What is the type? ____________

(continued)

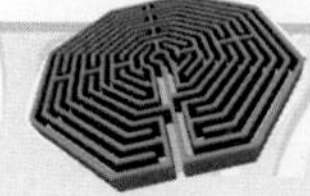

Coding Practice (continued)

5. Date: 9/14/yy Location: Branton Eye Care
Provider: Margo Bittinger, MD
Patient: Corine Propes Gender: F Age 53
Reason for encounter: blurred vision, eye pain, floaters in both eyes
Assessment: bilateral anterior uveitis due to juvenile rheumatoid arthritis, associated cataracts with neovascularization in left eye also noted
Plan: eye drops, dark glasses

a. What is the condition? ____________
b. What is the laterality? ____________
c. What additional eye condition exists? ____________
d. What is the subtype of the condition? ____________
e. What is the laterality? ____________
f. Is the eye condition secondary to a condition from another body system? ____________
g. What is the underlying condition? ____________
h. What is the subtype? ____________

6. Date: 9/14/yy Location: Branton Eye Care
Provider: Margo Bittinger, MD
Patient: Briana Effinger Gender: F Age: 54
Reason for encounter: difficulty seeing, gritty feeling in eyes, ocular hyperemia (*blood-shot eye*)
Assessment: bilateral grade 2 corneal and conjunctival deposits, likely due to stage 5 renal failure, patient has been on dialysis for about 18 months
Plan: schedule cornea scraping to remove deposits

a. What are the symptoms and signs? ____________
b. What two eye conditions are diagnosed? ____________
c. What is the laterality? ____________
d. Are the symptoms integral to the condition(s)? ____________
e. What is the underlying condition? ____________
What stage? ____________
f. How is the underlying condition being treated? ____________

ASSIGNING CODES FOR THE EYE

Coders need to be attentive when assigning codes that involve laterality. The fifth or sixth character of the code identifies laterality. Always verify the character for laterality in the Tabular List. Although *often* the right side is **1**, the left side is **2**, and bilateral is **3**, this is not *always* the case. In some categories, laterality designations use characters other than **1**, **2**, or **3**. Some codes that have laterality do not provide an option for bilateral because the condition is commonly unilateral.

When a condition affects both eyes, but no code is provided for bilateral, assign two codes: one for the right eye and a second one for the left eye (OGCR I.B.13). For example, disorders of the eyelid have codes for right and left laterality as well as upper and lower, but do not usually have codes for bilateral. (■ FIGURE 19-6).

When coding glaucoma, assign a seventh-character extension to identify the stage of glaucoma as **unspecified, mild, moderate, severe, or indeterminate**. Assign as many codes as necessary from category **H40 Glaucoma** as needed to fully describe the type of glaucoma, the affected eye, and the stage (OGCR I.C.7.a).

Patient is seen for senile entropion (*turning inward*) of both upper eyelids.

H02.031 Senile entropion of right upper eyelid

H02.034 Senile entropion of left upper eyelid

Figure 19-6 ■ Example of Assigning Codes for a Bilateral Condition When No Code Option for Bilaterality Exists

Assigning Codes for Diabetic Eye Conditions

Codes for diabetic ophthalmic manifestations are not indexed under the Main Term for the eye condition, such as retinopathy. They are indexed under the Main Term **Diabetes**, then a subterm for the type of diabetes, then a

E08.3- Diabetes mellitus due to underlying condition with ophthalmic complications

E09.3- Drug or chemical induced diabetes mellitus with ophthalmic complications

E10.3- Type 1 diabetes mellitus with ophthalmic complications

E11.3- Type 2 diabetes mellitus with ophthalmic complications

E13.3- Other specified diabetes mellitus with ophthalmic complications

Figure 19-7 ■ Tabular List Subcategories for Diabetes with Ophthalmic Manifestations

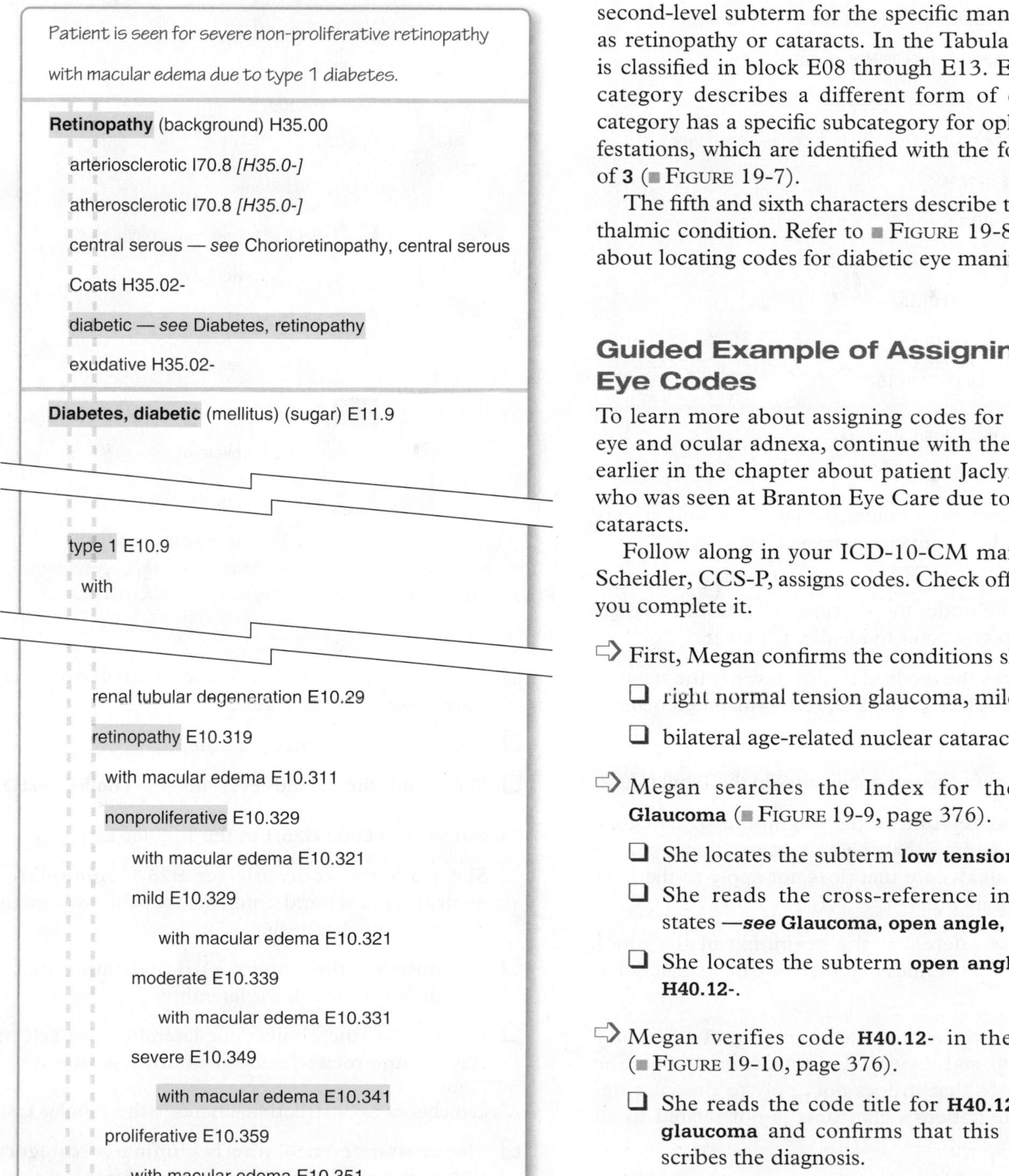

Patient is seen for severe non-proliferative retinopathy with macular edema due to type 1 diabetes.

Retinopathy (background) H35.00
 arteriosclerotic I70.8 *[H35.0-]*
 atherosclerotic I70.8 *[H35.0-]*
 central serous — *see* Chorioretinopathy, central serous
 Coats H35.02-
 diabetic — *see* Diabetes, retinopathy
 exudative H35.02-

Diabetes, diabetic (mellitus) (sugar) E11.9

 type 1 E10.9
  with

  renal tubular degeneration E10.29
  retinopathy E10.319
   with macular edema E10.311
   nonproliferative E10.329
    with macular edema E10.321
    mild E10.329
     with macular edema E10.321
    moderate E10.339
     with macular edema E10.331
    severe E10.349
     with macular edema E10.341
   proliferative E10.359
    with macular edema E10.351

Figure 19-8 ■ Example of Index Entry for Diabetic Retinopathy

second-level subterm for the specific manifestation, such as retinopathy or cataracts. In the Tabular List, diabetes is classified in block E08 through E13. Each three-digit category describes a different form of diabetes. Each category has a specific subcategory for ophthalmic manifestations, which are identified with the fourth character of **3** (■ FIGURE 19-7).

The fifth and sixth characters describe the type of ophthalmic condition. Refer to ■ FIGURE 19-8 to learn more about locating codes for diabetic eye manifestations.

Guided Example of Assigning Eye Codes

To learn more about assigning codes for diseases of the eye and ocular adnexa, continue with the example from earlier in the chapter about patient Jaclyn Vandeventer, who was seen at Branton Eye Care due to glaucoma and cataracts.

Follow along in your ICD-10-CM manual as Megan Scheidler, CCS-P, assigns codes. Check off each step after you complete it.

⇨ First, Megan confirms the conditions she abstracted.

- ❑ right normal tension glaucoma, mild stage
- ❑ bilateral age-related nuclear cataracts

⇨ Megan searches the Index for the Main Term **Glaucoma** (■ FIGURE 19-9, page 376).

- ❑ She locates the subterm **low tension.**
- ❑ She reads the cross-reference instruction that states ***—see* Glaucoma, open angle, low-tension.**
- ❑ She locates the subterm **open angle, low-tension H40.12-.**

⇨ Megan verifies code **H40.12-** in the Tabular List (■ FIGURE 19-10, page 376).

- ❑ She reads the code title for **H40.12, Low-tension glaucoma** and confirms that this accurately describes the diagnosis.
- ❑ She observes the symbol **6th**, indicating that a sixth digit is required for laterality.

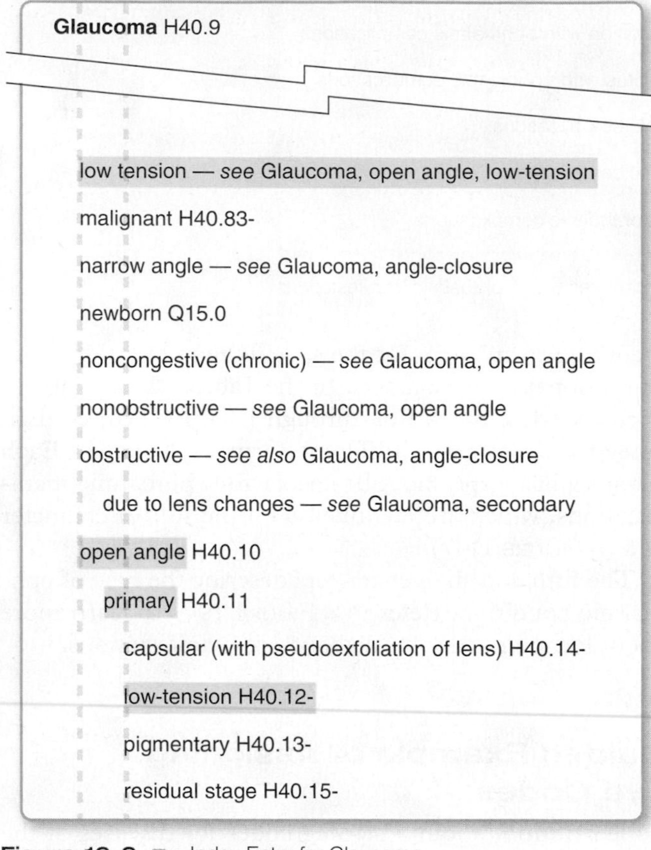

Figure 19-9 ■ Index Entry for Glaucoma

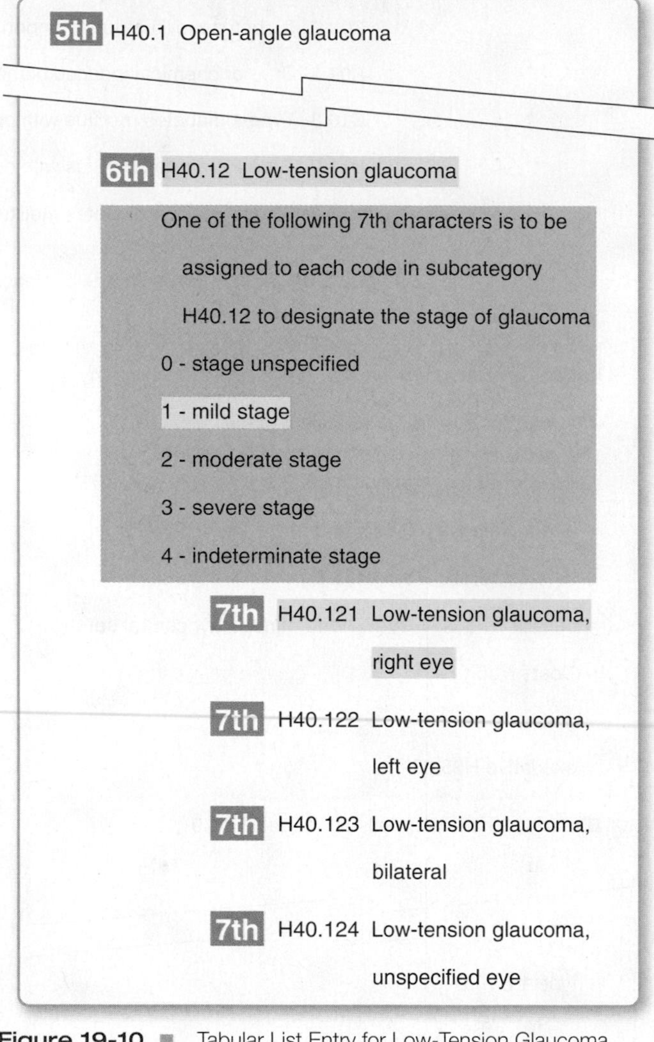

Figure 19-10 ■ Tabular List Entry for Low-Tension Glaucoma

- ❑ She reviews the choices for laterality and selects **H40.121, Low-tension glaucoma, right eye.**
- ❑ She notices the 7th symbol and reads the instructional note under the subcategory **H40.12** to assign a seventh character to identify the stage.
- ❑ She checks the medical record to verify the stage as mild and selects **H40.1211, Low-tension glaucoma, right eye, mild stage.**

⇨ Megan checks for instructional notes in the Tabular List.

- ❑ She cross-references the beginning of category **H40** and verifies that the only instructional note is an **Excludes1** note that does not apply to the low-tension glaucoma.
- ❑ She cross-references the beginning of the block **H40-H42** and verifies that there are no instructional notes.
- ❑ She cross-references the beginning of **Chapter 7 (H00-H89)** and reviews the instructional note. She determines that it does not apply to this case because the patient's glaucoma is not related to an external cause.

⇨ Megan searches the Index for the Main Term **Cataract.**

- ❑ She locates the subterm **age-related.**
- ❑ She reads the cross-reference instruction that states —***see* Cataract, senile.**
- ❑ She locates the subterm **senile.**
- ❑ She locates the second-level subterm **nuclear H25.1.**

⇨ Megan verifies code **H25.1** in the Tabular List.

- ❑ She reads the code title for **H25.1, Age-related nuclear cataract** and confirms that this accurately describes the diagnosis.
- ❑ She observes the symbol 5th, indicating that a fifth digit is required for laterality.
- ❑ She reviews the choices for laterality and selects **H25.13, Age-related nuclear cataract, bilateral.**

⇨ Megan checks for instructional notes in the Tabular List.

- ❑ She cross-references the beginning of category **H25** and verifies that the only instructional note is an **Excludes1** note that does not apply to the low-tension glaucoma.

- ❑ She cross-references the beginning of the block **H25-H28** and verifies that there are no instructional notes.
- ❑ She previously checked the beginning of **Chapter 7 (H00-H89)** and knows that the note does not apply because the cataract is not related to an external cause.

⇨ Megan reviews the codes she has assigned for this case.

- ❑ **H40.1211, Low-tension glaucoma, right eye, mild stage**
- ❑ **H25.13, Age-related nuclear cataract, bilateral**

⇨ Next, Megan must determine how to sequence the codes.

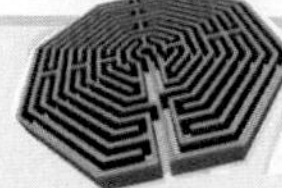

Coding Practice

Now it is your turn to practice assigning codes for diseases of the eye and ocular adnexa. Refer to the ***Tip*** at the end of the mini-medical-record if you need a little extra help.

Exercise 19.3 Assigning Codes for the Eye

Instructions: Read the mini-medical-record of each patient's encounter, review the information abstracted in Exercise 19.2, and assign ICD-10-CM diagnosis codes (CM) using the Index and Tabular List. Write the code(s) on the line provided.

1. Date: 9/13/yy Location: Branton Eye Care
Provider: Margo Bittinger, MD
Patient: Morris Marcilus Gender: M Age: 76
Reason for encounter: phacoemulsification of cataract and intraocular lens (IOL) implant
Assessment: age related nuclear cataract, left eye
Plan: FU in office, 2 days

Tip: Follow cross-referencing instructions in the Index.
1 CM Code ___________

2. Date: 9/13/yy Location: Branton Eye Care
Provider: Margo Bittinger, MD
Patient: Juliette Pardon Gender: F Age: 84
Reason for encounter: monthly retinal injections
Assessment: wet macular degeneration, in both eyes
Plan: return, 1 month
1 CM Code ___________

3. Date: 9/14/yy Location: Branton Eye Care
Provider: Margo Bittinger, MD
Patient: Sheree Shambo Gender: F Age: 69
Reason for encounter: crusty eyelids
Assessment: nonulcerative blepharitis on both upper lids
Plan: keep clean, Rx topical antibiotic

Tip: Either code can be sequenced first.
2 CM Codes ___________ ___________

ARRANGING CODES FOR THE EYE

ICD-10-CM does not provide any unique instructions for sequencing codes related to diseases of the eye. Coders follow the general OGCR for selecting the principal or first-listed diagnosis. They also follow instructional notes within the Tabular List. The most common situations when coders will see instructional notes in this ICD-10-CM chapter are the following:

- When the eye condition is secondary to another condition, sequence the underlying condition first.
- When the condition is due to a drug, sequence a code for the drug first. Use the Table of Drugs and Chemicals to identify the drug.
- When another associated condition is documented, such as hypertension or glaucoma, assign codes for both conditions and sequence them according to the circumstances of the encounter.
- When the eye condition is due to an external cause, sequence the eye condition first, followed by the external cause code.

Guided Example of Arranging Eye Codes

To learn more about sequencing codes for diseases of the eye and ocular adnexa, continue with the example from earlier in the chapter about patient Jaclyn Vandeventer, who was seen at Branton Eye Care due to glaucoma and cataracts.

Follow along in your ICD-10-CM manual as Megan Scheidler, CCS-P, sequences the codes. Check off each step after you complete it.

⇨ First, Megan confirms the codes she assigned.

- ❑ **H40.1211, Low-tension glaucoma, right eye, mild stage**
- ❑ **H25.13, Age-related nuclear cataract, bilateral**

⇨ Megan reviews the medical record to determine which condition was the main reason for the visit.

- ❑ The encounter was due to a referral from the optometrist.
- ❑ Both conditions were evaluated during the visit.
- ❑ The Tabular List provides no instructional notes regarding sequencing.

⇨ Megan evaluates the relative severity of the glaucoma compared to cataracts.

- ❑ Glaucoma has already damaged the optic nerve and has potential of permanent damage to vision.
- ❑ Cataracts, while annoying, do not present a risk of permanent damage.
- ❑ The physician documents that glaucoma will be treated first, followed by cataract surgery at a later time.
- ❑ Based on these considerations, Megan sequences the glaucoma first.

⇨ Megan finalizes the codes and sequencing for this case:

(1) **H40.1211, Low-tension glaucoma, right eye, mild stage**

(2) **H25.13, Age-related nuclear cataract, bilateral**

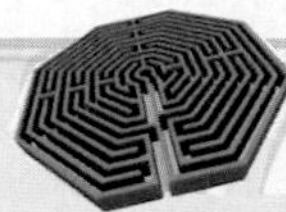

Coding Practice

Now it is your turn to practice sequencing codes for diseases of the eye and ocular adnexa. Refer to the ***Tip*** at the end of the mini-medical-record if you need a little extra help.

Exercise 19.4 Arranging Codes for the Eye

Instructions: Read the mini-medical-record of each patient's encounter, review the information abstracted in Exercise 19.2, assign ICD-10-CM diagnosis codes (CM) using the Index and Tabular List, and sequence them correctly.

1. Date: 9/13/yy Location: Branton Eye Care

Provider: Margo Bittinger, MD

Patient: Ken Rocker Gender: M Age: 61

Reason for encounter: routine eye exam as part of diabetic monitoring

Assessment: moderate diabetic nonproliferative retinopathy with no macular edema

Plan: be diligent about keeping sugar and BP well controlled, to slow progression of condition

Tip: Assign a Z code for the reason for the encounter. Follow sequencing instructions in the Tabular List.

2 CM Codes __________ __________

2. Date: 9/14/yy Location: Branton Eye Care

Provider: Margo Bittinger, MD

(continued)

2. (continued)

Patient: Corine Propes Gender: F Age 53

Reason for encounter: blurred vision, eye pain, floaters in both eyes

Assessment: bilateral anterior uveitis due to juvenile rheumatoid arthritis, associated cataract with neovascularization in left eye also noted

Plan: eye drops, dark glasses

Tip: Follow cross-referencing instructions in the Index.

3 CM Codes __________ __________ __________

3. Date: 9/14/yy Location: Branton Eye Care Provider: Margo Bittinger, MD

Patient: Briana Effinger Gender: F Age: 54

Reason for encounter: difficulty seeing, gritty feeling in eyes, ocular hyperemia (blood-shot eyes)

Assessment: bilateral grade 2 corneal and conjunctival deposits, likely due to stage 5 renal failure, patient has been on dialysis for about 18 months

Plan: schedule cornea scraping to remove deposits

Tip: Instructional notes in the Tabular List guide you to the additional codes and sequencing.

4 CM Codes __________ __________ __________ __________

CODING NEOPLASMS OF THE EYE

Neoplasms of the eye and ocular adnexa do not appear in ICD-10-CM Chapter 7, Diseases of the Eye and Adnexa (H00-H59). Codes for neoplasms of the eye and ocular adnexa appear in category **C69 Malignant Neoplasm of eye and adnexa** within the neoplasm chapter.

The most common primary malignant neoplasm for adults in the eye is intraocular melanoma, followed by intraocular lymphoma, although both are relatively rare. In children, the most common eye cancers are retinoblastoma (cancer arising from cells in the retina).

Metastatic neoplasms are more common than primary neoplasms of the eye. The most common cancers that spread to the eye are breast and lung cancers. Most often, these cancers spread to the uvea. Metastatic breast cancer usually appears in the eye several years after breast cancer treatment has been completed. Metastatic lung cancer to the eye is often the first sign that lung cancer exists. Patients may be surprised to learn that a vision problem is a manifestation of breast or lung cancer.

Cancers of the orbit and ocular adnexa develop from tissues such as muscle, nerve, and skin around the eyeball and are classified as neoplasms of the type of tissue they arise in. For example, cancers of the eyelid are usually skin cancers and cancers of the eye muscles are usually rhabdomyosarcoma.

When eye cancer needs specific treatment, physicians use targeted radiation therapy to the eye or eye injections of chemotherapeutic drugs. Unfortunately, by the time cancer has metastasized to the eye, patients often have more serious problems to address, and the eye metastasis may not be a high treatment priority.

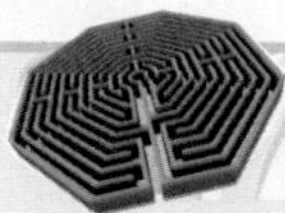

Coding Practice

Now it is your turn to practice coding neoplasms of the eye and ocular adnexa.

Exercise 19.5 Coding Neoplasms of the Eye

Instructions: Read the mini-medical-record of each patient's encounter, then abstract, assign, and sequence ICD-10-CM diagnosis codes (CM) using the Index and Tabular List. Write the code(s) on the line provided.

1. Date: 9/15/yy Location: Branton Eye Care Provider: Margo Bittinger, MD

Patient: Craig Henning Gender: M Age: 8

Reason for encounter: mother is concerned about a white spot in her son's right eye and says he seems to be cross-eyed

Assessment: retinoblastoma

Plan: schedule a consultation with ophthalmologic oncologist, pediatric oncologist, and radiation oncologist to determine treatment options

1 CM Code __________

2. Date: 9/15/yy Location: Branton Eye Care

Provider: Margo Bittinger, MD

Patient: Alberta Littlejohn Gender: F Age: 58

Reason for encounter: patient is concerned because she can see a dark spot on the left iris and has been having headaches

Assessment: melanocytoma with secondary glaucoma

Plan: this is benign and does not require treatment at this time, but we need to monitor the glaucoma

2 CM Codes __________ __________

3. Date: 9/15/yy Location: Branton Eye Care

Provider: Margo Bittinger, MD

Patient: Stephany Comeau Gender: F Age: 49

Reason for encounter: blurry vision

Assessment: metastatic cancer to choroid in both eyes, history of right breast cancer 5 years ago which is no longer under treatment, status post right mastectomy

Plan: targeted radiotherapy, referred back to her oncologist for detection of other possible metastases

3 CM Codes __________ __________ __________

4. Date: 9/15/yy Location: Branton Eye Care

Provider: Margo Bittinger, MD

Patient: Sandra Lowe Gender: F Age: 56

Reason for encounter: removal of lesion from right upper eyelid

Assessment: basal cell carcinoma

1 CM Code __________

(continued)

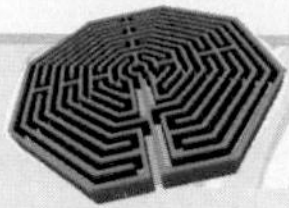

Coding Practice (continued)

5. Date: 9/15/yy Location: Branton Eye Care
Provider: Margo Bittinger, MD
Patient: Alma Fuentes Gender: F Age: 54
Reason for encounter: review biopsy and consultation results for salmon colored patch on right conjunctiva

(continued)

5. (continued)
Assessment: malignant conjunctival lymphoma mucosa associated lymphoid tissue (MALT)
Plan: refer to oncologist for evaluation for possible systemic lymphoma, then determine course of treatment
1 CM Code ___________

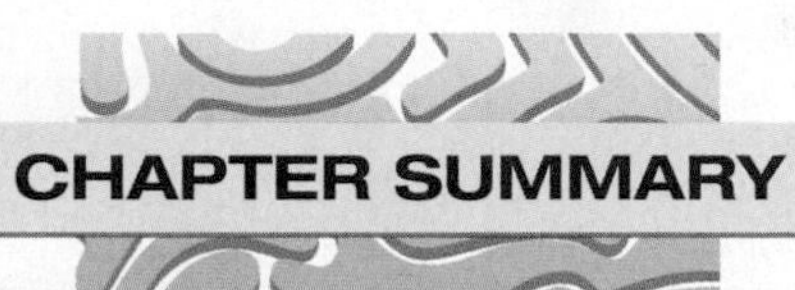

CHAPTER SUMMARY

In this chapter you learned that:

- The eye and ocular adnexa make vision possible by receiving light from the external world and converting it into impulses that are transmitted to the brain through the optic nerve.
- The majority of conditions in this chapter require that the laterality be identified.
- When a condition affects both eyes but there is no option for bilateral, assign two codes, one for the right eye and a second one for the left eye.
- ICD-10-CM does not provide any unique instructions for arranging codes related to diseases of the eye, so coders follow the general OGCR for selecting the principal or first-listed diagnosis.
- Metastatic neoplasms are more common than primary neoplasms of the eye with the most common being metastatic breast and lung cancers.
- ICD-10-CM provides no Official Guidelines for Coding and Reporting (OGCR) for Chapter 7.

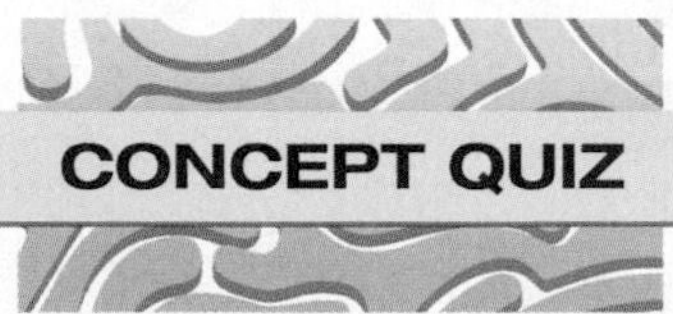

CONCEPT QUIZ

Take a moment to look back at your trip through the eye and ocular adnexa and solidify your skills. This is your opportunity to pull together everything you have learned.

Completion

Instructions: Write the term that answers each question based on the information you learned in this chapter. Choose from the list below. Some choices may be used more than once and some choices may not be used at all. Refer to the discussion in this chapter and the Glossary at the end of this book if you need a little extra help.

adnexa	chalazion
cataract	conjunctivitis
diabetic retinopathy	ocular globe
glaucoma	optic nerve
hordeolum	orbital cavity
keratin	uvea
keratitis	uvula
macular degeneration	vitreous body

1. The ocular muscles, eyelids, and conjunctiva make up the ________________________________.
2. A(an) ________________________________ is a small hard cyst on the eyelid caused by blockage of a gland on the eyelid.

3. The transparent jelly that fills the eyeball and is surrounded by a membrane is the ______________ ______________.
4. The condition of ______________ may be proliferative or non-proliferative.
5. The middle layer of eye consisting of the iris, ciliary body, and choroid is the ______________ ______________.
6. The gradual loss of central vision due to aging with no cure is ______________.
7. A(an) ______________ is a bacterial inflammation of a sebaceous gland on the edge or lining of the eyelid.
8. The eye socket is also called the ______________ ______________.
9. ______________ is a viral or bacterial inflammation and infection of the lining of the eyelid.
10. ______________ is an inflammation and ulceration of the surface of the cornea.

Multiple Choice

Instructions: Circle the letter of the best answer to each question based on the information you learned in this chapter. Refer to the discussion in this chapter and the Glossary at the end of this book if you need a little extra help.

1. The separation of the retina from the choroid layer of the eye is
   A. choroiditis.
   B. macular degeneration.
   C. diabetic retinopathy.
   D. retinal detachment.
2. ICD-10-CM Chapter 7 includes codes for
   A. syphilis-related eye disorders.
   B. injuries to the eye.
   C. visual disturbances and blindness.
   D. diabetic eye disorders.
3. Which of the following is NOT a key criterion for abstracting conditions of the eye and ocular adnexa?
   A. Is the condition malignant or benign?
   B. Is laterality right, left, bilateral, or unspecified?
   C. Is the condition acute or chronic?
   D. Is the condition due to an external cause?
4. Which character(s) of a code indicates laterality?
   A. First
   B. Second or third
   C. Fifth or sixth
   D. Seventh-character extension
5. When a condition affects both eyes but there is no option for bilateral, the coder should assign
   A. a code for unspecified eye.
   B. one code for the right eye and a second code for the left eye.
   C. a code for the dominant eye.
   D. does not apply because all eye codes have an option for bilateral.
6. The codes for diabetic retinopathy are indexed under the Main Term
   A. Diabetes.
   B. Retinopathy.
   C. either Diabetes or Retinopathy.
   D. Manifestation, diabetic.
7. The codes for age-related cataracts are located under Cataract and which subterm?
   A. Age
   B. Old
   C. Nuclear
   D. Senile
8. When the eye condition is due to an external cause, which should be sequenced first?
   A. The place of occurrence
   B. The laterality
   C. The eye condition
   D. The external cause
9. A nuclear cataract is
   A. located in the center of the eye.
   B. the result of exposure to radiation.
   C. beginning to become apparent.
   D. caused by diabetes.
10. The most common neoplasm that affects the eye is
    A. intraocular melanoma.
    B. retinoblastoma.
    C. metastasis.
    D. rhabdomyosarcoma.

CODING CHALLENGE

Now it is your turn to demonstrate coding all aspects of diseases of the eye and ocular adnexa. Refer back to the examples and discussion in this chapter when you need a little extra help. Use your medical dictionary and anatomy references when needed.

Instructions: Read the mini-medical-record of each patient's encounter, then abstract, assign, and sequence ICD-10-CM diagnosis codes (CM) using the Index and Tabular List. Write the code(s) on the line provided.

1. Date: 9/19/yy Location: Branton Eye Care
Provider: Margo Bittinger, MD
Patient: Miriam Latham Gender: F Age: 28
Reason for encounter: routine vision examination
Assessment: latent nystagmus, right eye
Plan: prescription contact lenses

Tip: Assign one code for the eye exam and a second code for the finding.

2 CM Codes __________ __________

2. Date: 9/19/yy Location: Branton Eye Care
Provider: Margo Bittinger, MD
Patient: Carlos Dias Gender: M Age: 48
Reason for encounter: light flashes for 2 months, dense shadow/curtain progressing towards central vision this morning
Assessment: detachment of retina with one break, right eye
Plan: scleral buckle surgery

1 CM Code __________

3. Date: 9/19/yy Location: Branton Eye Care
Provider: Margo Bittinger, MD
Patient: Nicole Driver Gender: F Age: 42
Reason for encounter: pain and redness in R eye
Assessment: R eye marginal corneal ulcer due to dry eye syndrome which is bilateral, so we will keep watch on the other eye as well
Plan: pain medication, tear substitute drops, discontinue contact use, RTO tomorrow

2 CM Codes __________ __________

4. Date: 9/19/yy Location: Branton Eye Care
Provider: Margo Bittinger, MD
Patient: Jason Walther Gender: M Age: 57
Reason for encounter: noticing mild impairment of vision, redness of eyes, foreign body sensation in eyes
Assessment: recurrent pterygium, bilateral
Plan: artificial tears, anti-inflammatory drops, RTO one month

1 CM Code __________

5. Date: 9/19/yy Location: Branton Eye Care
Provider: Margo Bittinger, MD
Patient: Inez Arcena Gender: F Age: 2
Reason for encounter: scheduled cataract removal
Assessment: subcapsular posterior juvenile cataract, cerebrotendinous xanthomatosis (*a metabolic disorder related to fat storage*)
Plan: RTO tomorrow, genetic counseling for family, referral to pediatric endocrinologist for FU

2 CM Codes __________ __________

6. Date: 9/19/yy Location: Branton Eye Care
Provider: Margo Bittinger, MD
Patient: Patrick Henninger Gender: M Age: 66
Reason for encounter: sudden painless loss of vision
Assessment: occlusion of left central retinal artery. Pt has hypertension and CAD which place her at risk for embolism
Plan: aspirin and Plavix, ocular-digital massage, admit for angiogram to evaluate carotid circulation

3 CM Codes __________ __________ __________

7. Date: 9/19/yy Location: Branton Eye Care
Provider: Charles Bragdon, OD
Patient: Douglas Wolf Gender: M Age: 9
Reason for encounter: Child referred to clinic by school teacher. Child unable to distinguish the color red from green.

(*continued*)

7. (continued)
Assessment: *acquired color blindness*
Plan: *teach coping skills to distinguish colors*
1 CM Code __________

8. Date: *9/19/yy* Location: *Branton Eye Care*
Provider: *Margo Bittinger, MD*
Patient: *Priscilla Teter* Gender: *F* Age: *31*
Reason for encounter: *cloudy blurred vision*
Assessment: *idiopathic corneal edema*
Plan: *hypertonic eye drops and ointment*
1 CM Code __________

9. Date: *9/19/yy* Location: *Branton Eye Care*
Provider: *Margo Bittinger, MD*
Patient: *Beulah Burnell* Gender: *F* Age: *68*
Reason for encounter: *swelling of lower right eyelid, tenderness, increased tearing*

(continued)

9. (continued)
Assessment: *chalazion on right lower eyelid*
Plan: *topical antibiotic eye drops for initial infection. RTO 2 months to inject with a corticosteroid if chalazion has not disappeared*
1 CM Code __________

10. Date: *9/19/yy* Location: *Branton Eye Care*
Provider: *Margo Bittinger, MD*
Patient: *Krista Steelman* Gender: *F* Age: *16*
Reason for encounter: *pink eye, ocular itching, tearing, photophobia, watery discharge, painful socialized swelling on lid*
Assessment: *bilateral chronic conjunctivitis due to allergies and a stye on the edge of the right upper lid*
Plan: *cold compresses, NSAIDs, mast cell stabilizers, antihistamine, RTO 1 week*
2 CM Codes __________ __________

KEEP ON CODING

As a coder, you can never have too much experience. Apply everything you have learned in this chapter to code the following diagnostic statements. Use the OGCR and instructional notes in the Tabular List to help determine how many codes are required.

Instructions: Read the diagnostic statement, then use the Index and Tabular List to assign and sequence ICD-10-CM (CM) diagnosis codes. Write the code(s) on the line provided.

1. Abscess of both upper eyelids: CM Code(s) __________
2. Acute atopic conjunctivitis, both eyes: CM Code(s) __________
3. Kayser-Fleischer ring, left eye: CM Code(s) __________
4. Stable keratoconus, right eye: CM Code(s) __________
5. Anterior subcapsular polar age-related cataract, both eyes: CM Code(s) __________
6. Retinopathy of prematurity, stage 1, right eye: CM Code(s) __________
7. Low-tension glaucoma: CM Code(s) __________
8. Malignant melanoma of choroid, right eye: CM Code(s) __________

9. Optic nerve hypoplasia, left eye: CM Code(s) ________________
10. Vertical strabismus, right eye: CM Code(s) ________________
11. Sebaceous cyst of right lower eyelid: CM Code(s) ________________
12. Low vision, both eyes: CM Code(s) ________________
13. Cystoid macular edema post cataract surgery, left eye: CM Code(s) ________________
14. Convergence insufficiency: CM Code(s) ________________
15. Epiphora due to excessive discharge of tears, bilateral: CM Code(s) ________________
16. Progressive external ophthalmoplegia, right eye: CM Code(s) ________________
17. Horseshoe tear of retina without detachment, left eye: CM Code(s) ________________
18. Harada's disease, both eyes: CM Code(s) ________________
19. Cortical age-related cataract, right eye: CM Code(s) ________________
20. Staphyloma posticum: CM Code(s) ________________
21. Pseudotumor of the left orbit: CM Code(s) ________________
22. Ptosis of both eyelids: CM Code(s) ________________
23. Diplopia: CM Code(s) ________________
24. Ghost vessels in the cornea of the left eye: CM Code(s) ________________
25. Postprocedural blebitis, stage 2: CM Code(s) ________________

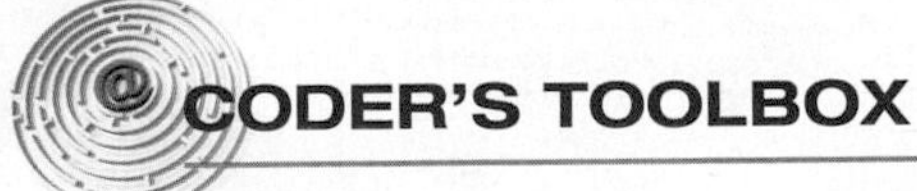

CODER'S TOOLBOX

The following resources are a starting point for learning more about diseases of the eye and ocular adnexa.

American Association of the Deaf-Blind (AADB) **http://www.aadb.org/**

American Foundation for the Blind
http://www.afb.org/

American Optometric Association
http://www.aoa.org

Eye Cancer Network
http://www.eyecancer.com/

Foundation Fighting Blindness
http://www.blindness.org/

Glaucoma Foundation
http://www.glaucoma.org/

Ophthalmology Textbook
http://www.ophthobook.com/

20

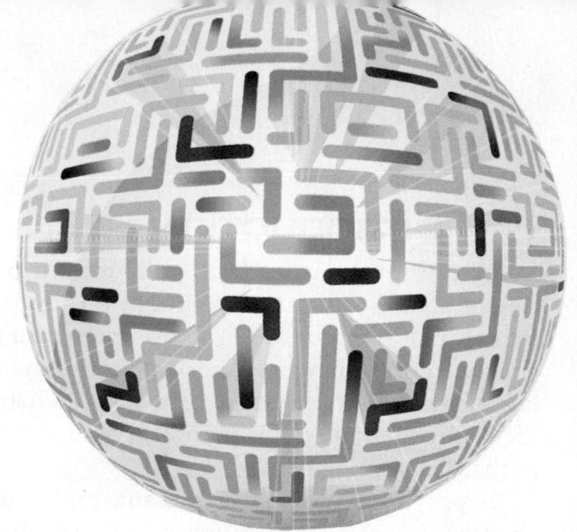

Diseases of the Ear and Mastoid Process (H60-H95)

Learning Objectives

After completing this chapter, you should have the skills to:

- Spell and define the key words, medical terms, and abbreviations related to the ear and mastoid process.
- Discuss the structure, function, and common conditions of the ear and mastoid process.
- Identify the main characteristics of coding for the ear and mastoid process.
- Abstract diagnostic information from the medical record for conditions of the ear and mastoid process.
- Assign codes for diseases of the ear and mastoid process.
- Arrange codes for diseases of the ear and mastoid process.
- Code neoplasms of the ear and mastoid process.
- Discuss the Official Guidelines for Coding and Reporting related to diseases of the ear and mastoid process.

Key Terms and Abbreviations

auditory canal
auricle
cerumen
cochlea
eardrum
equilibrium
external ear
incus
inner ear
labyrinth
malleus
mastoid process
middle ear
ossicles
otitis media (OM)
oval window
pinna
purulent otitis media
saccule
semicircular canals
stapes
tympanic membrane
tympanic membrane perforation (TMP)
tympanum
utricle
vestibulocochlear nerve

In addition to the key terms listed here, students should know the terms defined within tables in this chapter.

Chapter Outline

- **Ear Refresher**
- **Coding Overview of the Ear**
- **Abstracting for the Ear**
- **Assigning Codes for the Ear**
- **Arranging Codes for the Ear**

ICD-10-CM codes in this chapter are from the ICD-10-CM 2014 Draft code set from the Department of Health and Human Services, Centers for Disease Control and Prevention.

INTRODUCTION

Many of the memories from your road trip are memories of sounds—a trickling brook, a thundering waterfall, or a chirping bird. If you are more of a city person, your memories may be the clacking of a train, the honking of traffic, or the music of a show. Whatever sounds are imbedded in your memory, you have your ears to thank.

In your tour of the ear and mastoid process in this chapter you will learn more about how the ear works, why sometimes it does not work as it should, and how physicians treat these conditions. Most importantly, you will practice coding for patient encounters related to diseases and conditions of the ear and mastoid process, a skill that requires you to abstract information from the mini-medical-record, assign correct codes, and arrange (sequence) the codes in the correct order.

An otolaryngologist is a physician who specializes in diagnosing and treating conditions of the ear, nose, and throat (ENT). Primary care physicians treat uncomplicated conditions of the ear, nose, and throat. They refer patients with more complex conditions to otolaryngologists.

As you read this chapter, open up your medical terminology book to the chapter on the ear and keep a medical dictionary handy to refresh your memory of any unfamiliar terms. The ear contains some of the smallest structures in the human body and it is important to understand the function of each. Experienced coders keep the information they need at their fingertips.

EAR REFRESHER

The ear makes hearing possible by collecting sound waves from the external world and converting them into impulses that are transmitted to the brain through the **vestibulocochlear nerve**, cranial nerve VIII. The ear also maintains **equilibrium**, the sense of balance. The **mastoid process** is the portion of the temporal bone of the skull that juts forward behind the ear.

The ear is divided into three sections: the **external ear**, **middle ear**, and **inner ear** (■ Figure 20-1). The external ear consists of the **auricle** or **pinna**, the visible part of the ear, which collects sound waves; the **auditory canal**, which funnels the sound waves; and the **tympanic membrane**, also called the **tympanum** or **eardrum**, which separates the external ear from the middle ear. Glands in the auditory canal produce **cerumen** (*ear wax*) that protects and lubricates the ear.

The middle ear is a small air-filled cavity in the temporal bone that contains the **ossicles**, three small bones that are critical to the hearing process. The ossicles amplify vibrations in the middle ear and transmit them to the inner ear, from the **malleus** (*hammer*) to the **incus** (*anvil*) to the **stapes** (*stirrup*). The stapes is attached to the **oval window**, a thin membrane that covers the opening to the inner ear and passes vibrations to the cochlea.

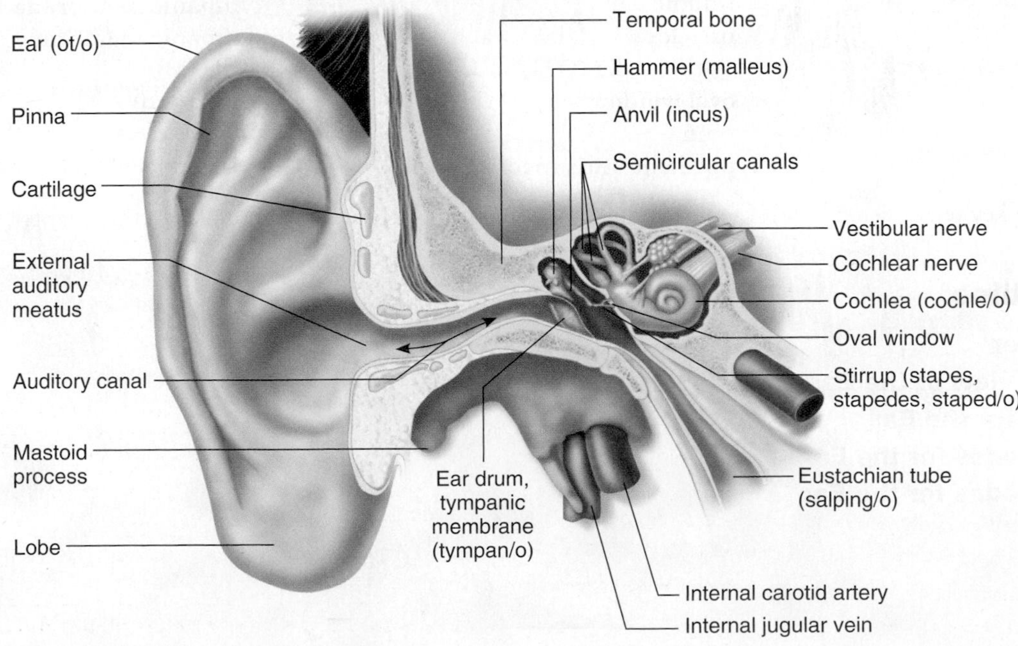

Figure 20-1 ■ The Ear and Mastoid Process

SUCCESS STEP

The stapes is the smallest named bone in the human body. Without it, you would be unable to hear.

The inner ear, or **labyrinth**, is a fluid-filled cavity in the temporal bone that contains the **cochlea**, a snail-shaped organ that makes hearing possible, and the sensors for equilibrium, which are the **semicircular canals**, **utricle**, and **saccule**.

In Figure 20-1, each structure in the ear and mastoid process is labeled with its name as well as its medical terminology root/combining form where applicable. As you learn about conditions and procedures that affect the ear, remember to apply medical terminology skills to use word roots, prefixes, and suffixes you already know to define new terms related to the ear and mastoid process. Refer to ■ TABLE 20-1 for a refresher on how to build medical terms related to the ear and mastoid process.

CODING CAUTION

Be alert for medical word roots that sound and are spelled similarly but have different meanings.

ot/o (*ear*) and **opt/o** (*vision, eye*)

mastoid/o (*the combining form for the mastoid process, which is "breast shaped"*) and **mast/o** (*the combining form for the breast*)

tinnitus (*ringing in the ears*) and **tinea** (*a skin fungus*)

serous (*a clear fluid*) and **serious** (*important or somber*)

Conditions of the Ear

Coders must be familiar with the most common conditions of the ear: hearing loss, or deafness, and **otitis media (OM)** (*infection of the middle ear*). Approximately 17% of American adults report some degree of hearing loss and 47% of adults age 75 or older have a hearing impairment, according to the National Institute on Deafness and Other Communication Disorders (NIDCD).

Three out of four children experience OM by the time they are three years old, according to NIDCD. Ear infections are the second most common reason for trips to the pediatrician, after wellness visits; almost half of all antibiotic prescriptions written for children are for ear infections. Untreated OM can lead to complications, such as mastoiditis, hearing loss, perforation of the tympanum, meningitis, facial nerve paralysis, and Meniere's disease. Refer to ■ TABLE 20-2 (page 388) for a summary of diseases affecting the ear and mastoid process.

Neoplasms of the Ear

Neoplasms of the ear are rare. Basal cell carcinoma and malignant melanoma may occur on the skin of the external ear; these are classified under malignant neoplasms of the skin. Squamous cell carcinoma may occur in the ear canal; adenoid cystic carcinoma may occur in the ear glands. Acoustic neuroma, also called vestibular schwannoma, is a benign tumor of the vestibular cochlear nerve, which connects the ear to the brain. It grows slowly, not showing symptoms until after age 30.

This section provides a general reference to help understand the most common diagnoses of the ear and mastoid process, but does not list everything you need to know. Use medical terminology skills discussed earlier in this chapter to learn the meaning of unfamiliar words. Remember to keep standard reference books handy in case you get stuck. Refer to the resources in the Coder's Toolbox at the end of this chapter to learn more about conditions affecting the ear and mastoid process.

Table 20-1 ■ EXAMPLE OF CONSTRUCTING MEDICAL TERMS FOR THE EAR AND MASTOID PROCESS

Combining Form	Suffix	Complete Medical Term
ot/o (*ear*)	**-itis** (*inflammation*) **-plasty** (*surgical repair*) **-tomy** (*make an incision into*)	**ot + itis** (*inflammation of the ear*) **oto + plasty** (*surgical repair of the ear*)
myring/o (*eardrum*) **tympan/o** (*eardrum, tympanic membrane*)		**myring + itis** (*inflammation of the eardrum*) **myringo + tomy** (*making an incision in the eardrum*) **tympano + plasty** (*surgical repair of the tympanic membrane*)
staped/o (*stapes bone*)		**stapedo + tomy** (*make an incision in the stapes bone*)
mastoid/o (*mastoid process bone, breast shaped*)		**mastoid + itis** (*inflammation of the mastoid process bone*)

Table 20-2 ■ **COMMON DISEASES OF THE EAR AND MASTOID PROCESS**

Condition	Definition
Ceruminoma	Excessive accumulation of ear wax, also called impacted cerumen
Cholesteatoma	A cyst or benign tumor consisting of epithelial cells and fat
Hearing loss—conductive	Hearing loss due to abnormal formation of the external or middle ear
Hearing loss—sensorineural	Hearing loss due to abnormal formation of the cochlea or cochlear nerve
Labrynthitis	A viral or bacterial inflammation or infection of the semicircular canals of the inner ear
Mastoiditis	A serious infection of the mastoid process that carries the risk of infecting the brain
Meniere's disease	An abnormality of the fluid of the inner ear that can lead to a progressive hearing loss
Otitis externa	An inflammation of the external ear (pinna)
Otitis media (OM)—nonsuppurative	An inflammation of the middle ear that does not produce pus
Otitis media (OM)—serous	A subtype of nonsuppurative otitis media involving clear fluid in the middle ear
Otitis media (OM)—suppurative	An infection of the middle ear, usually bacterial, involving the discharge of pus, also called **purulent otitis media**
Otosclerosis	A loss of mobility of the stapes bone
Ruptured tympanic membrane	A hole or break in the eardrum, also called **tympanic membrane perforation (TMP)**
Tinnitus	Ringing of the ear that may be subjective (*heard only by the patient*) or objective (*audible to the physician*)
Vertigo	A sensation of motion or dizziness

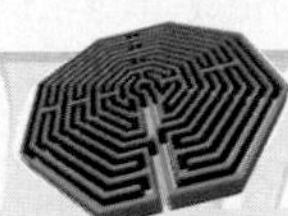

Coding Practice

Refresh your knowledge of terminology related to the ear and mastoid process. Use a medical terminology text or a website such as GlobalRph.com > Medical Terminology http://www.globalrph.com/medterm.htm to identify the meaning of word parts that may not be familiar.

Exercise 20.1 Ear Refresher

Instructions: Use your medical terminology skills and resources to define the following conditions related to the ear and mastoid process, then assign the default diagnosis code.

Follow these steps:

- Use slash marks "/" to break down each term into its root(s) and suffix.
- Define the meaning of the word, based on the meaning of each word part.
- Assign the default ICD-10-CM diagnosis code (CM) and laterality for the condition using the Index and Tabular List.

Example: otitis (right) ot/itis Meaning: *inflammation of the right ear* CM Code: *H66.901*

1. labyrnthitis (bilateral) Meaning ______________ CM Code ________
2. otosclerosis (right) Meaning ______________ CM Code ________
3. cholesteatoma (left) Meaning ______________ CM Code ________
4. mastoiditis Meaning ______________ CM Code ________
5. presbycusis (bilateral) Meaning ______________ CM Code ________
6. otolith (left) Meaning ______________ CM Code ________
7. otorrhagia (left) Meaning ______________ CM Code ________

8. otorrhea	Meaning ______	CM Code ______
9. mastoidalgia (right)	Meaning ______	CM Code ______
10. tympanosclerosis (bilateral)	Meaning ______	CM Code ______

CODING OVERVIEW OF THE EAR

ICD-10-CM Chapter 8, Diseases of the Ear and Mastoid Process (H60-H95), is a new chapter that did not exist in ICD-9-CM. In ICD-9-CM, the ear and mastoid process were included in Chapter 6 (380-389) for the nervous system and special senses. This is the second of two ICD-10-CM chapters in which codes begin with the letter H; codes for the eye and adnexa occupy codes H00 through H59. This chapter contains five blocks or subchapters that are divided by external, middle, and internal ear. Review the block names and code ranges listed at the beginning of Chapter 8 in the ICD-10-CM manual to become familiar with the content and organization.

ICD-10-CM has expanded numerous codes in this chapter, compared to ICD-9-CM. Additional codes identify laterality and greater anatomic specificity. Some categories have been reorganized. Instructional notes to code first the underlying condition have been added throughout the chapter.

This chapter includes disorders affecting the external, middle, and inner ear, as well as the mastoid process. It does not include injuries to the ear, which are classified in ICD-10-CM Chapter 19.

ICD-10-CM does not provide any Official Guidelines for Coding and Reporting (OGCR) specific to this chapter. General OGCR in sections I.A., I.B., II, III, and IV direct the coder. Instructional notes in the Tabular List guide coders when additional codes are required. An instructional note at the beginning of the chapter directs coders to use an external cause code following the code for the ear condition when an external cause is involved in created the ear condition. This note applies to all codes in ICD-10-CM Chapter 8.

ABSTRACTING FOR THE EAR

The primary concerns in abstracting for diagnoses of the ear and mastoid process are laterality, external causes, and tobacco use or exposure. In addition, coders should be aware of the many variations of OM in order to abstract all the needed details.

Abstracting Laterality

The majority of ear conditions require that the laterality be identified. Laterality is expressed at the following levels:

- right, left, or unspecified ear
- bilateral, for applicable conditions

When a patient has more than one ear condition, the laterality for *each* condition must be identified separately. For example, a patient may have *bilateral* OM, but *unilateral* TMP in the right or left ear only.

Refer to ■ Table 20-3 for guidance on how to abstract conditions of the ear and mastoid process. Remember that abstracting questions are a guide and that not every question applies to, or can be answered for, every case. For example, tinnitus does not have subtype conditions.

Abstracting for Otitis Media

Otitis media requires that coders abstract the basic information required for all ear conditions, plus additional details unique to OM. Coders need to abstract the specific subtype of OM. The two most common are suppurative and serous. Serous is one form of nonsuppurative OM, but coders may occasionally encounter other nonsuppurative types, such as **mucoid**, **allergic**, **secretory**, and **seromucinous**.

CODING CAUTION

Do not assume that all conditions named *otitis* are otitis media. You need to distinguish between otitis *media*, inflammation of the middle ear, and otitis *externa*, inflammation of the external ear. These are separate conditions with different codes.

Table 20-3 ■ KEY CRITERIA FOR ABSTRACTING CONDITIONS OF THE EAR AND MASTOID PROCESS

- ❑ What is the condition?
- ❑ What is the subtype of the condition?
- ❑ Is a more specific subtype documented?
- ❑ What part of the ear is affected?
- ❑ What is the laterality?
- ❑ What other conditions coexist?
- ❑ Is there an underlying disease?
- ❑ Is the condition due to a drug or external cause?
- ❑ Is there documentation of current or past use of tobacco or exposure to tobacco smoke?

Table 20-4 ■ KEY CRITERIA FOR ABSTRACTING OTITIS MEDIA

- ❑ What is the subtype of otitis media?
- ❑ Is it suppurative/purulent, nonsuppurative/serous, or another subtype?
- ❑ Is it acute, acute recurrent, or chronic?
- ❑ What is the laterality?
- ❑ Is there associated rupture of the tympanic membrane?
- ❑ What is the type or extent of rupture?
- ❑ What is the laterality of the rupture?
- ❑ Is it a manifestation of another disease?
- ❑ Is there documentation of current or past use of tobacco or exposure to tobacco smoke?

OM is classified as acute, acute recurrent, and chronic. Although there are no universal definitions of these stages, a common practice is to classify recurrent acute otitis media as chronic when it persists for longer than three months and is accompanied by changes in the lining of the middle ear. Coders abstract this information based on how physicians describe the condition in the documentation. When in doubt, query the physician for clarification. Refer to ■ TABLE 20-4 for guidance on how to abstract for otitis media, then work through the detailed example that follows.

Guided Example of Abstracting for the Ear

Refer to the following example throughout this chapter to learn about abstracting, assigning, and sequencing codes for the ear and mastoid process. Gabrielle Javiera, CPC, is a fictitious coder who guides you through the coding process.

> Date: 10/21/yy Location: Ear, Nose, and Throat Specialists
>
> Provider: Shauna Rotz, MD
>
> Patient: Estela Nuno Gender: F Age: 4
>
> Reason for encounter: ear pain, fever
>
> Assessment: bilateral acute serous otitis media with total rupture of tympanic membrane of the right ear, no one in the household smokes
>
> Plan: antibiotics, **fat-plug tympanoplasty**

Follow along as Gabrielle Javiera, CPC, abstracts the diagnosis. Check off each step after you complete it.

⇨ Gabrielle reads through the entire record, with special attention to the reason for the encounter and the final assessment. She refers to the Key Criteria for Abstracting Otitis Media (Table 20-4).

- ❑ She notes the presenting symptoms: ear pain, fever
- ❑ *What is the condition?* otitis media
- ❑ *What is the subtype of the condition?* acute serous
- ❑ *Is it suppurative/purulent, nonsuppurative/serous, or another subtype?* serous, which is a type of nonsuppurative
- ❑ *What is the laterality?* bilateral
- ❑ *Is it acute, acute recurrent, or chronic?* acute
- ❑ *Is there associated rupture of the tympanic membrane?* Yes.
- ❑ *What is the type or extent of rupture?* total
- ❑ *What is the laterality of the rupture?* She notes that laterality of the rupture is right, although the otitis media is bilateral.
- ❑ *Is it a manifestation of another disease?* No.
- ❑ *Is there documentation of current or past use of tobacco or exposure to tobacco smoke?* no one in the household smokes
- ❑ Now that she has identified the conditions, she reviews the symptoms again. She determines that ear pain and fever are integral to otitis media and should not be coded (■ FIGURE 20-2).
- ❑ She reviews the planned treatments and concludes that they are consistent with the condition she abstracted.

⇨ At this time, Gabrielle does not know how many codes she will need. She will learn about this when she moves on to assigning codes.

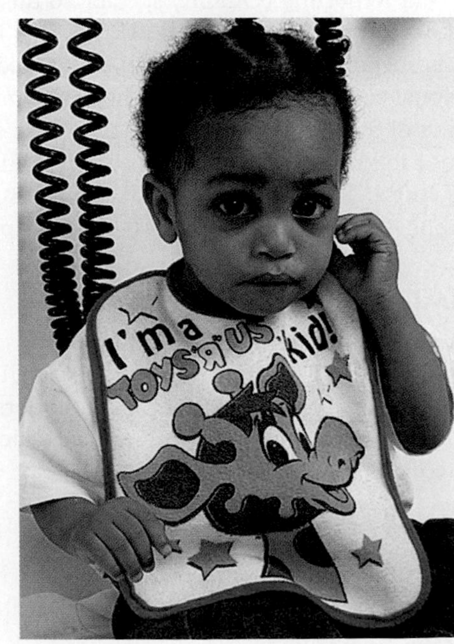

Figure 20-2 ■ Common signs of otitis media are fussiness and pulling at the ear. *Source: Pearson Education.*

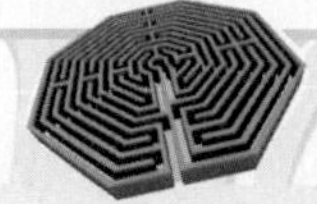

Coding Practice

Now it is your turn to practice abstracting diagnoses for the ear and mastoid process. Questions guide your analysis of each scenario.

Exercise 20.2 Abstracting for the Ear

Instructions: Read the mini-medical-record of each patient's encounter and answer the abstracting questions. Write the answer on the line provided. Do not assign any codes.

1. Date: 10/23/yy Location: Branton Medical Center Outpatient Procedure Center

Provider: Shauna Rotz, MD

Patient: Chester Suttle Gender: M Age: 7

Reason for encounter: bilateral tympanoplasty

Assessment: bilateral chronic serous otitis media

Plan: FU in office, 2 weeks

a. What is tympanoplasty? ______

b. What is the condition? ______

c. Is it suppurative or nonsuppurative? ______

d. What is the laterality? ______

e. Is the condition acute or chronic? ______

2. Date: 10/23/yy Location: Ear, Nose, and Throat Specialists Provider: Shauna Rotz, MD

Patient: Hilary Reasor Gender: F Age: 23

Chief complaint: severe nausea, vomiting, sweating, vertigo

Assessment: symptoms are due to Meniere's disease, left ear

Plan: diazepam (*a sedative*) for vertigo, it may get better on its own or it may not, will consider surgery if necessary, but we want to follow it for awhile

a. What are the symptoms? ______

b. Will you code the symptoms? ______

Why or why not? ______

c. What condition is diagnosed? ______

d. What is the laterality? ______

3. Date: 10/23/yy Location: Ear, Nose, and Throat Specialists Provider: Shauna Rotz, MD

Patient: Bettye Neer Gender: F Age: 32

Chief complaint: ringing and buzzing in right ear, difficulty hearing in right ear

Assessment: objective tinnitus

Plan: We will try electrical stimulation treatments and see how the condition responds before considering surgery.

a. What are the symptoms? ______

b. Will you code the symptoms? ______

Why or why not? ______

c. What condition is diagnosed? ______

What does objective mean? ______

d. What is the laterality? ______

4. Date: 10/24/yy Location: Branton Medical Center Outpatient Procedure Center

Provider: Shauna Rotz, MD

Patient: Milton Hern Gender: M Age: 58

Reason for encounter: bilateral stapedotomy (*making an incision in the stapes bone*) and placement of prosthesis

Assessment: bilateral conductive hearing loss due to bilateral nonobliterative otosclerosis of the stapes at the oval window

Plan: FU in office, 2 weeks

a. What is stapedotomy? ______

b. What type of hearing loss is documented? ______

c. What is the laterality of the hearing loss? ______

d. What is otosclerosis? ______

e. What is the type of otosclerosis? ______

f. What bone is affected by the otosclerosis? ______

g. What is the laterality of the otosclerosis ______

(*continued*)

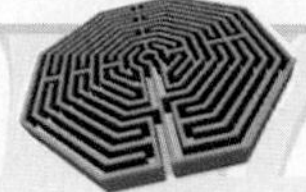

Coding Practice (continued)

5. Date: 10/24/yy Location: Ear, Nose, and Throat Specialists Provider: Shauna Rotz, MD

Patient: Deana Kurland Gender: F Age: 12

Reason for encounter: left earache, fever, head congestion

Assessment: acute recurrent suppurative otitis media and acute recurrent sinusitis, mother is a heavy cigarette smoker

Plan: antibiotics for OM, decongestant, and fluids

a. What are the symptoms? __________

b. What condition is the first condition diagnosed? __________

c. Is it suppurative or nonsuppurative? __________

d. Is it acute or chronic? __________

e. Is it recurrent? __________

f. Which symptoms relate to the first condition? __________

g. What is the laterality of the first condition? __________

h. What condition is the second condition diagnosed? __________

i. Is it acute or chronic? __________

j. Is it recurrent? __________

(continued)

5. (continued)

k. Which symptoms relate to the second condition? __________

l. Which condition should you sequence first? __________

Why? __________

m. Is tobacco use or exposure documented? __________

6. Date: 10/24/yy Location: Ear, Nose, and Throat Specialists Provider: Shauna Rotz, MD

Patient: Ben Stogner Gender: M Age: 19

Reason for encounter: dizziness, nausea, low back pain, headache on right side

Assessment: dizziness, nausea, and headache due to labyrinthitis, right

Plan: refer to physical therapy for balance and for LBP

a. What are the symptoms? __________

b. What is labyrinthitis? __________

c. What is the laterality? __________

d. Which symptoms relate to the labyrinthitis? __________

e. What symptom does not relate to labyrinthitis? __________

Should it be coded? __________

Why or why not? __________

ASSIGNING CODES FOR THE EAR

The Index provides cross-referencing instructions that redirect coders to alternative Main Terms for many ear conditions. When a condition cannot be located under a Main Term, remember to refer to any alternative Main Terms provided in the cross-reference notes. This is especially helpful when assigning codes for hearing loss and OM.

Assigning Codes for Hearing Loss

Coders may use the Main Term **Deafness** for any condition described as hearing loss or deafness. Hearing loss is indexed under the Main Term **Loss** and the subterm **hearing**. Five second-level subterms direct coders to the same code, **H90.5 Unspecified sensorineural hearing loss**. A cross-reference note states ***see also*** **Deafness**. The Main Term **Deafness** provides over 40 subterms, which direct coders to specific codes, including the ones listed under the Main Term **Loss, hearing**. Therefore, it is most efficient for coders to go directly to **Deafness** when assigning codes for hearing loss or deafness (■ FIGURE 20-3).

Assigning Codes for Otitis Media

The Index entry **Otitis, media** contains numerous cross-references between second-level subterms, which may seem confusing. Nearly all types of OM can be located

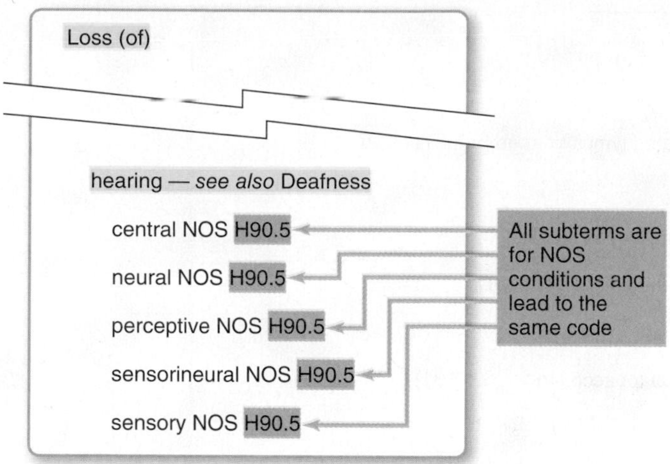

Figure 20-3 ■ Index Entry for Hearing Loss with a Cross-Reference to Deafness

under the two second-level subterms **nonsuppurative** and **suppurative**. Third- and fourth-level subterms further identify the specific subtype of OM.

SUCCESS STEP

To make navigating the Index for OM easier, highlight the subterm entries for **nonsuppurative** and **suppurative**.

Guided Example of Assigning Codes for the Ear

To learn more about assigning codes for the ear and mastoid process, continue with the example from earlier in the chapter about patient Estela Nuno, who was seen at Ear, Nose, and Throat Specialists due to ear pain and fever.

Follow along in your ICD-10-CM manual as Gabrielle Javiera, CPC, assigns codes. Check off each step after you complete it.

➪ First, Gabrielle confirms the diagnoses.

- ❑ *bilateral acute serous otitis media*
- ❑ *total rupture of tympanic membrane of the right ear*

➪ Gabrielle searches the Index for the Main Term **Otitis** (■ FIGURE 20-4).

- ❑ She locates the subterm **media**.
- ❑ She knows that serous otitis media is a type of nonsuppurative otitis media, so she locates the second-level subterm, **nonsuppurative**.
- ❑ She locates the third-level subterm **acute**.
- ❑ She locates the fourth-level subterm **serous H65.0-**.

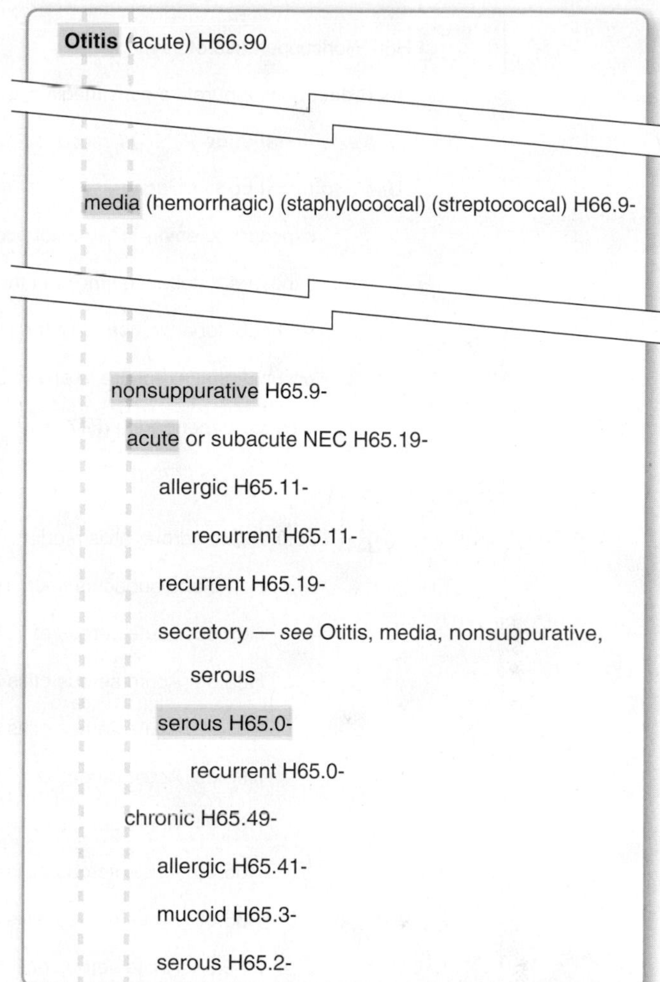

Figure 20-4 ■ Index Entry for Nonsuppurative Otitis Media

➪ Gabrielle verifies **H65.0-** in the Tabular List (■ FIGURE 20-5, page 394).

- ❑ She reads the subcategory title for **H65.0, Acute serous otitis media** and confirms that this accurately describes the condition.
- ❑ She identifies the symbol **5th** in front of the subcategory number, telling her that a fifth digit is required to identify the laterality.
- ❑ She notices that there eight codes in this category, four for acute serous otitis media and four for acute serous otitis media, *recurrent*.
- ❑ She verifies that the documentation does not state recurrent, so she selects the code **H65.03, Acute serous otitis media, bilateral**.

➪ Gabrielle checks for instructional notes in the Tabular List.

- ❑ She cross-references the beginning of subcategory **H65.0** and verifies that there are no instructional notes.

4th H65 Nonsuppurative otitis media

Includes: nonsuppurative otitis media with myringitis

Use additional code for any associated perforated tympanic membrane (H72.-)

Use additional code to identify:

exposure to environmental tobacco smoke (Z77.22)

exposure to tobacco smoke in the perinatal period (P96.81)

history of tobacco use (Z87.891)

occupational exposure to environmental tobacco smoke (Z57.31)

tobacco dependence (F17.-)

tobacco use (Z72.0)

5th H65.0 Acute serous otitis media

Acute and subacute secretory otitis

H65.00 Acute serous otitis media, unspecified ear

H65.01 Acute serous otitis media, right ear

H65.02 Acute serous otitis media, left ear

H65.03 Acute serous otitis media, bilateral

H65.04 Acute serous otitis media, recurrent, right ear

H65.05 Acute serous otitis media, recurrent, left ear

H65.06 Acute serous otitis media, recurrent, bilateral

H65.07 Acute serous otitis media, recurrent, unspecified ear

Figure 20-5 ■ Tabular List Entry for Acute Serous Otitis Media

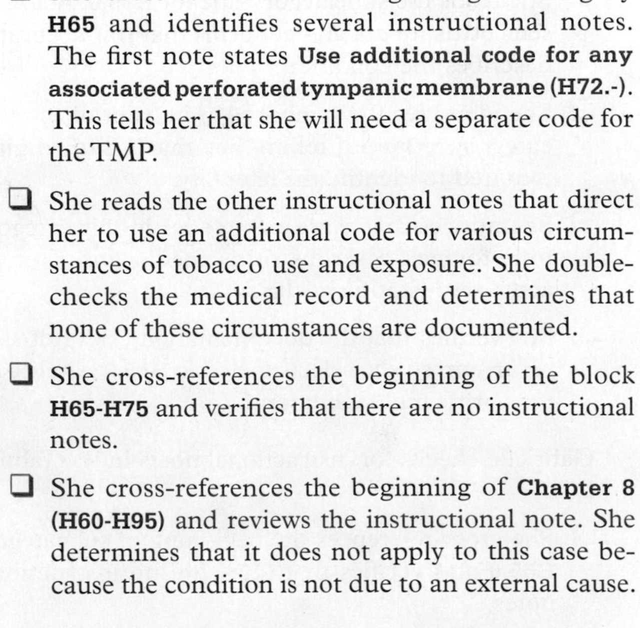

- ❑ She cross-references the beginning of category **H65** and identifies several instructional notes. The first note states **Use additional code for any associated perforated tympanic membrane (H72.-)**. This tells her that she will need a separate code for the TMP.
- ❑ She reads the other instructional notes that direct her to use an additional code for various circumstances of tobacco use and exposure. She double-checks the medical record and determines that none of these circumstances are documented.
- ❑ She cross-references the beginning of the block **H65-H75** and verifies that there are no instructional notes.
- ❑ She cross-references the beginning of **Chapter 8 (H60-H95)** and reviews the instructional note. She determines that it does not apply to this case because the condition is not due to an external cause.

➩ Gabrielle proceeds to code the *ruptured tympanic membrane*.

- ❑ She cross-references the Tabular List entry for **H72.-** that is listed in the instructional note.
- ❑ She notices there are a lot of codes under category **H72**.
- ❑ She reviews the subcategory headings until she locates subcategory **H72.82, Total perforation of tympanic membrane**.
- ❑ She identifies the symbol **6th** in front of the subcategory number, telling her that a sixth digit is required to identify the laterality.
- ❑ She double-checks the medical record to confirm that laterality for the TMP is right.
- ❑ She reviews the available code options and selects the code **H72.821, Total perforation of tympanic membrane, right ear**.

➪ Gabrielle checks for instructional notes in the Tabular List.

- ❑ She cross-references the beginning of category **H72** and identifies the instructional note that states **Code first any associated otitis media**.
- ❑ She already checked the instructional notes for the block and chapter, so she does not check them again because she knows they do not apply to this case.

➪ Gabrielle reviews the codes she has assigned for this case.

- ❑ **H72.821, Total perforation of tympanic membrane, right ear**
- ❑ **H65.03, Acute serous otitis media, bilateral**

➪ Next, Gabrielle must decide how to sequence the codes.

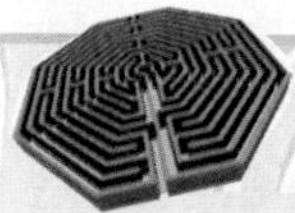

Coding Practice

Now it is your turn to practice assigning codes for the ear and mastoid process.

Exercise 20.3 Assigning Codes for the Ear

Instructions: Read the mini-medical-record of each patient's encounter, review the information abstracted in Exercise 20.2, and assign ICD-10-CM diagnosis codes (CM) using the Index and Tabular List. Write the code(s) on the line provided.

1. Date: 10/23/yy Location: Branton Medical Center Outpatient Procedure Center
Provider: Shauna Rotz, MD
Patient: Chester Suttle Gender: M Age: 7
Reason for encounter: bilateral tympanoplasty
Assessment: bilateral chronic serous otitis media
Plan: FU in office, 2 weeks
1 CM Code __________

2. Date: 10/23/yy Location: Ear, Nose, and Throat Specialists Provider: Shauna Rotz, MD
Patient: Hilary Reasor Gender: F Age: 23
Chief complaint: severe nausea, vomiting, sweating, vertigo
Assessment: symptoms are due to Meniere's disease, left ear
Plan: diazepam for vertigo, it may get better on its own or it may not, will consider surgery if necessary, but we want to follow it for awhile
1 CM Code __________

3. Date: 10/23/yy Location: Ear, Nose, and Throat Specialists Provider: Shauna Rotz, MD
Patient: Bettye Neer Gender: F Age: 32
Chief complaint: ringing and buzzing in right ear, difficulty hearing in right ear
Assessment: objective tinnitus
Plan: We will try electrical stimulation treatments and see how the condition responds before considering surgery.
1 CM Code __________

ARRANGING CODES FOR THE EAR

ICD-10-CM does not provide any unique instructions for sequencing codes related to diseases of the ear. Coders follow the general OGCR for selecting the principal or first-listed diagnosis. They also follow instructional notes within the Tabular List. The most common situations in which coders will see instructional notes in this ICD-10-CM chapter are the following.

- When the ear condition is secondary to another condition, sequence the underlying condition first.
- When the ear condition is due to a poisoning from a drug or toxin, sequence the code from the Table of Drugs and Chemicals first.
- When OM is accompanied by a perforated tympanic membrane, sequence the OM first and the perforated membrane second.

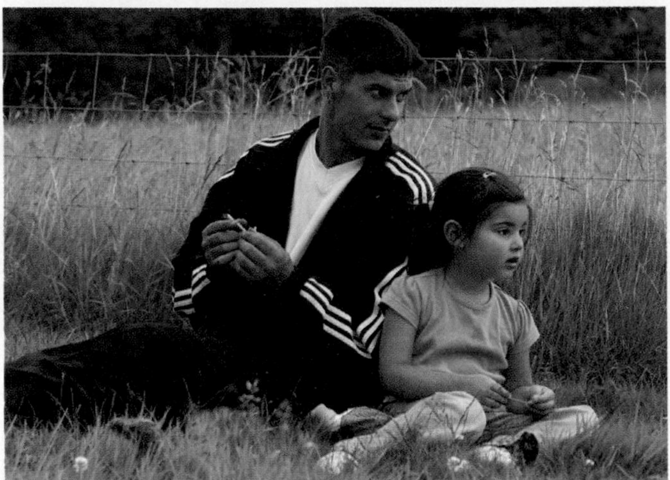

Figure 20-6 ■ Exposure to tobacco smoke is a risk factor for ear infections that should be coded. *Source: marliyn barbone/Shutterstock.*

- When the ear condition is due to an external cause, sequence the ear condition first, followed by the external cause code.
- Sequence codes describing tobacco use or exposure as secondary codes (■ FIGURE 20-6).

Guided Example of Arranging Codes for the Ear

To learn more about sequencing codes for the ear and mastoid process, continue with the example from earlier in the chapter about patient Estela Nuno, who was seen at Ear, Nose, and Throat Specialists due to ear pain and fever.

Follow along in your ICD-10-CM manual as Gabrielle Javiera, CPC, sequences the codes. Check off each step after you complete it.

⇨ First, Gabrielle confirms the codes she assigned.

❑ **H72.821, Total perforation of tympanic membrane, right ear**

❑ **H65.03, Acute serous otitis media, bilateral**

⇨ Gabrielle reviews the instructional notes in the Tabular List to determine how to sequence the codes.

❑ The instructional note for code **H72.821** directs her to **Code first any associated otitis media**. This tells her that the code for otitis media, **H65.03**, should be sequenced first.

❑ The instructional note for code **H65.03** directs her to **Use additional code for any associated perforated tympanic membrane**. This confirms that the code for TMP, **H72.821**, should be sequenced second.

⇨ Gabrielle finalizes the codes and sequencing for this case:

(1) **H65.03, Acute serous otitis media, bilateral**

(2) **H72.821, Total perforation of tympanic membrane, right ear**

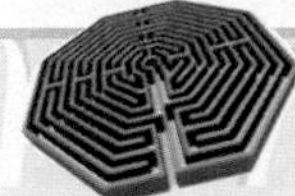

Coding Practice

Now it is your turn to practice sequencing codes for the ear and mastoid process. Refer to the ***Tip*** at the end of the mini-medical-record if you need a little extra help.

Exercise 20.4 Arranging Codes for the Ear

Instructions: Read the mini-medical-record of each patient's encounter, review the information abstracted in Exercise 20.2, assign ICD-10-CM diagnosis codes (CM) using the Index and Tabular List, and sequence them correctly.

1. Date: 10/24/yy Location: Branton Medical Center Outpatient Procedure Center

Provider: Shauna Rotz, MD

Patient: Milton Hern Gender: M Age: 58

Reason for encounter: bilateral stapedotomy and placement of prosthesis

Assessment: bilateral conductive hearing loss due to bilateral nonobliterative otosclerosis of the stapes at the oval window

Plan: FU in office, 2 weeks

***Tip*:** Nonobliterative means nonblocking. Sequence the underlying condition first because it is the reason for the procedure.

2 CM Codes __________ __________

2. Date: 10/24/yy Location: Ear, Nose, and Throat Specialists Provider: Shauna Rotz, MD

Patient: Deana Kurland Gender: F Age: 12

Reason for encounter: left earache, fever, head congestion

Assessment: acute recurrent suppurative otitis media and acute recurrent sinusitis, mother is a heavy cigarette smoker in the home

Plan: antibiotics for OM, decongestant, and fluids

3 CM Codes ___________ ___________ ___________

3. Date: 10/24/yy Location: Ear, Nose, and Throat Specialists Provider: Shauna Rotz, MD

Patient: Ben Stogner Gender: M Age: 19

Reason for encounter: dizziness, nausea, low back pain, headache on right side

Assessment: dizziness, nausea, and headache due to labyrinthitis, right

Plan: refer to physical therapy for balance and for LBP

2 CM Codes ___________ ___________

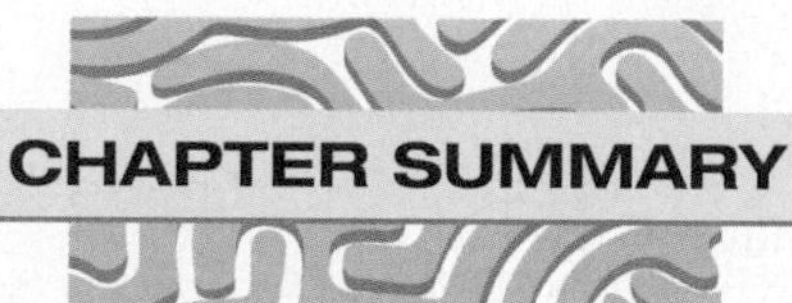

CHAPTER SUMMARY

In this chapter you learned that:

- The ear makes hearing possible by collecting sound waves from the external world and converting them into impulses that are transmitted to the brain through the vestibulocochlear nerve, cranial nerve VIII.
- ICD-10-CM Chapter 8, Diseases of the Ear and Mastoid Process (H60-H95), is a new chapter that did not exist in ICD-9-CM.
- The primary concerns in abstracting for diagnoses of the ear and mastoid process are laterality, external causes, tobacco use or exposure, and the many variations of otitis media.
- The Index provides cross-references that redirect coders to alternative Main Terms for many ear conditions.
- ICD-10-CM does not provide any unique instructions for sequencing codes related to diseases of the ear.
- ICD-10-CM provides no Official Guidelines for Coding and Reporting (OGCR) for Chapter 8.

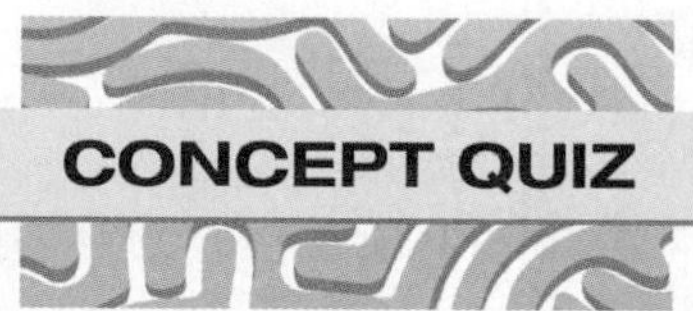

CONCEPT QUIZ

Take a moment to look back at your trip through the ear and mastoid process and solidify your skills. This is your opportunity to pull together everything you have learned.

Completion

Instructions: Write the term that answers each question based on the information you learned in this chapter. Choose from the list below. Some choices may be used more than once and some choices may not be used at all. Refer to the discussion in this chapter and the Glossary at the end of this book if you need a little extra help.

ceruminoma	labrynthitis	recurrent
cholesteatoma	mastoid	sensorineural
chronic	Meniere's disease	serous
conductive	middle	suppurative
external	nonsuppurative	tinnitus
inner		vertigo

1. The tympanic membrane is part of the _________________ ear.
2. _________________ is excessive accumulation of ear wax.

3. ________________ hearing loss is due to abnormal formation of the cochlea or cochlear nerve.
4. Otitis media is an infection of the ________________ ear.
5. The ossicles are part of the ________________ ear.
6. ________________ OM involves the discharge of pus.
7. The cochlea is part of the ________________ ear.
8. ________________ is a viral or bacterial inflammation or infection of the semicircular canals of the inner ear.
9. ________________ is a sensation of motion or dizziness.
10. A common practice is to classify recurrent acute otitis media as ________________ when it persists for longer than three months and is accompanied by changes in the lining of the middle ear.

Multiple Choice

Instructions: Circle the letter of the best answer to each question based on the information you learned in this chapter. Refer to the discussion in this chapter and the Glossary at the end of this book if you need a little extra help.

1. When a patient has more than one ear condition
   A. the laterality for each condition must be the same.
   B. the laterality for each condition must be different.
   C. the laterality for each condition must be bilateral.
   D. the laterality for each condition must be identified separately.
2. Laterality for the ear designates all of the following EXCEPT
   A. right.
   B. left.
   C. bilateral.
   D. inner.
3. An instructional note at the beginning of Chapter 8 directs coders to assign an additional code for
   A. external cause.
   B. alcohol use.
   C. tobacco use.
   D. exposure to loud music.
4. Which is NOT a subtype of otitis media?
   A. Suppurative
   B. Serous
   C. Sensorineural
   D. Allergic
5. Untreated OM can lead to all of the following EXCEPT
   A. strep throat.
   B. meningitis.
   C. mastoiditis.
   D. facial nerve paralysis.
6. What is the focus of OGCR for Chapter 8?
   A. Otitis media
   B. Laterality
   C. Hearing loss
   D. There are no OGCR for Chapter 8.
7. Serous OM is the most common type of ________ OM.
   A. suppurative
   B. nonsuppurative
   C. chronic
   D. allergic
8. The Index entry for Loss, hearing cross-references coders to the Main Term
   A. sensorineural.
   B. conductive.
   C. deafness.
   D. hearing.
9. Nearly all types of OM can be located under the second-level subterms
   A. nonsuppurative and suppurative.
   B. acute and chronic.
   C. otitis and media.
   D. serous and recurrent.
10. How should acute serous OM with TMP be coded?
    A. Assign a combination code for both OM and TMP.
    B. Assign a code for OM first, with TMP as an additional code.
    C. Assign a code for TMP first, with OM as an additional code.
    D. Assign a code for OM and do not code TMP.

CODING CHALLENGE

Now it is your turn to demonstrate coding all aspects of the ear and mastoid process. Refer back to the examples and discussion in this chapter when you need a little extra help. Use your medical dictionary and anatomy references when needed.

Instructions: Read the mini-medical-record of each patient's encounter, then abstract, assign, and sequence ICD-10-CM diagnosis codes (CM) using the Index and Tabular List. Write the code(s) on the line provided.

1. Date: 10/29/yy Location: Ear, Nose, and Throat Specialists Provider: Shauna Rotz, MD

Patient: Arnold Cornelison Gender: M Age: 6

Reason for encounter: Earache in left ear and fever

Assessment: acute bullous myringitis, left ear

Plan: antipyrine and benzocaine ear drops for pain, amoxillin, RTO 1 week

1 CM Code __________

2. Date: 10/29/yy Location: Ear, Nose, and Throat Specialists Provider: Shauna Rotz, MD

Patient: Letha Trabert Gender: F Age: 41

Reason for encounter: sudden loss of hearing after taking Tobramycin as prescribed for an infection

Assessment: ototoxic bilateral sensorineural hearing loss

Plan: hearing workup for hearing aids

Tip: Follow any cross-reference notes you find in the Index. Remember to code for the drug using the Table of Drugs and Chemicals.

2 CM Codes __________ __________

3. Date: 10/29/yy Location: Ear, Nose, and Throat Specialists Provider: Shauna Rotz, MD

Patient: Mavis Rozman Beaufort Gender: M Age: 21

Reason for encounter: right ear pain and otorrhagia

Assessment: polyp of right middle ear and associated cholesteatoma in middle ear

Plan: removed cholesteatoma, Rx antibiotics, RTO 3 weeks

2 CM Codes __________ __________

4. Date: 10/29/yy Location: Ear, Nose, and Throat Specialists Provider: Shauna Rotz, MD

Patient: Raul Suitt Gender: M Age: 11

Reason for encounter: frequent ear aches

Assessment: chronic serous otitis media (CSOM), bilateral, with attic rupture of left eardrum

Plan: Rx antibiotics

1 CM Code __________

5. Date: 10/29/yy Location: Ear, Nose, and Throat Specialists Provider: Shauna Rotz, MD

Patient: Philip Tetreault Gender: M Age: 58

Reason for encounter: patient had URI followed by feeling of fullness, popping ears, intermittent sharp ear pain and mild disequilibrium

Assessment: acute Eustachian salpingitis, left ear, URI

Plan: 10 day course of amoxillin, nasal decongestant limited to short term and only 3-4 times daily

2 CM Codes __________ __________

6. Date: 10/29/yy Location: Ear, Nose, and Throat Specialists Provider: Shauna Rotz, MD

Patient: Leann Aschenbrenner Gender: F Age: 16

Reason for encounter: ear pain, recurrent upper respiratory infections (URI)

Assessment: acute and subacute allergic serous otitis media, bilateral, recurrent; the patient smokes cigarettes and both parents smoke at home

Plan: ear drops to control pain, refer patient and parents to stop smoking clinic

2 CM Codes __________ __________

(continued)

(continued from page 399)

7. Date: 10/29/yy Location: Ear, Nose, and Throat Specialists Provider: Shauna Rotz, MD

Patient: Duane Lathem Gender: M Age: 17

Reason for encounter: mild hearing impairment, R ear; has been using q-tips to clean ears

Assessment: impacted cerumen, right ear

Plan: removed cerumen with curette, call if any further problems

1 CM Code __________

8. Date: 10/29/yy Location: Ear, Nose, and Throat Specialists Provider: Shauna Rotz, MD

Patient: Eliza Aube Gender: F Age: 22

Reason for encounter: pain, swelling, discharge and itchiness of outer ear

Assessment: malignant bilateral otitis externa due to pseudomonas aeruginosa, diabetes type 1

Plan: schedule for surgical debridement of necrotic tissue, antipseudomonal antibiotic course of 4–6 weeks, RTO in one week

3 CM Codes __________ __________ __________

9. Date: 10/29/yy Location: Ear, Nose, and Throat Specialists Provider: Shauna Rotz, MD

Patient: Callie Rega Gender: F Age: 9

Reason for encounter: yellow discharge, redness, and some swelling on left ear lobe after getting her ears pierced

Assessment: abscess of external ear

Plan: instruct patient on cleaning area with saline, warm salt water compresses to be performed 4x daily, RTO in 2 days if infection has not mitigated

Tip: Code for the condition only. Do not assign external cause codes.

1 CM Codes __________

10. Date: 10/29/yy Location: Ear, Nose, and Throat Specialists Provider: Shauna Rotz, MD

Patient: Mitchell Janco Gender: M Age: 4

Reason for encounter: admitted for intravenous antibiotics and mastoidectomy d/t. fever, mastoid swelling, deep ear pain at physician's office

Assessment: left subperiosteal mastoiditis

Plan: oral antibiotic, RTO in 1 week

1 CM Code __________

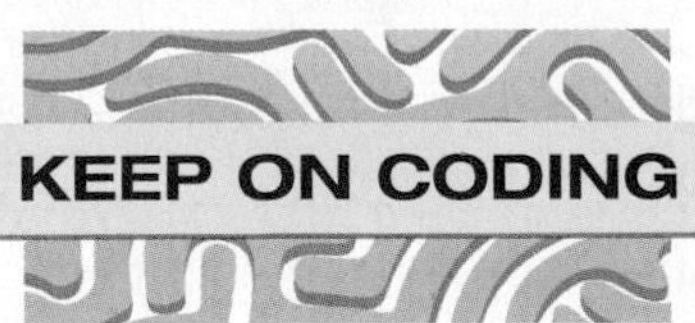

KEEP ON CODING

As a coder, you can never have too much experience. Apply everything you have learned in this chapter to code the following diagnostic statements. Use the OGCR and instructional notes in the Tabular List to help determine how many codes are required.

Instructions: Read the diagnostic statement, then use the Index and Tabular List to assign and sequence ICD-10-CM (CM) diagnosis codes. Write the code(s) on the line provided.

1. Diffuse cholesteatosis, right ear: CM Code(s) __________
2. Noise-induced hearing loss of bilateral inner ears: CM Code(s) __________
3. Mucosal cyst of postmastoidectomy cavity, both ears: CM Code(s) __________
4. Swimmer's ear, left: CM Code(s) __________
5. Exostosis, right external ear canal: CM Code(s) __________
6. Postauricular fistula, both ears: CM Code(s) __________

7. Aural vertigo: CM Code(s) ____________________

8. Conductive deafness: CM Code(s) ____________________

9. Cochlear otosclerosis, right ear: CM Code(s) ____________________

10. Partial loss of ear ossicles, left ear: CM Code(s) ____________________

11. Acute petrositis, both ears: CM Code(s) ____________________

12. Post-operative stenosis of right external ear canal: CM Code(s) ____________________

13. Otorrhea, left ear: CM Code(s) ____________________

14. Basal cell carcinoma of pinna of right ear: CM Code(s) ____________________

15. Chronic allergic otitis media: CM Code(s) ____________________

16. Hyperacusis, right ear: CM Code(s) ____________________

17. Adhesive otitis, left middle ear: CM Code(s) ____________________

18. Patulous Eustachian tube, both ears: CM Code(s) ____________________

19. Acute reactive otitis externa, left ear: CM Code(s) ____________________

20. Acute myringitis, bilateral: CM Code(s) ____________________

21. Labyrinthine hydrops: CM Code(s) ____________________

22. Perforation of tympanic membrane, left: CM Code(s) ____________________

23. Transient ischemic deafness, left: CM Code(s) ____________________

24. Otitic barotrauma, both ears: CM Code(s) ____________________

25. Hematoma of pinna, right ear: CM Code(s) ____________________

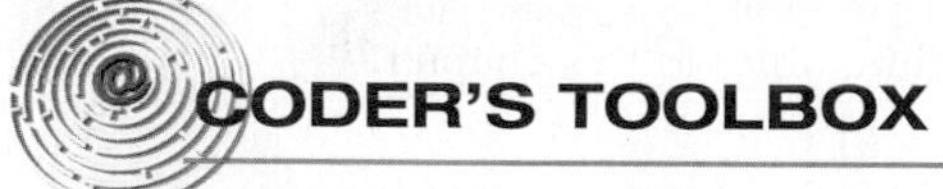

CODER'S TOOLBOX

The following resources are a starting point for learning more about the ear and mastoid process.

American Academy of Audiology **http://www.audiology.org**

American Academy of Otolaryngology-Head and Neck Surgery **http://www.entnet.org/**

American Academy of Pediatrics **http://www.aap.org/**

American Board of Pediatrics **https://www.abp.org/**

American Speech-Language-Hearing Association **http://www.asha.org**

Meniere's Disease Foundation **http://www.menieresfoundation.org/**

National Association of the Deaf (NAD) **http://www.nad.org/**

National Institute on Deafness and Other Communication Disorders (NIDCD) **http://www.nidcd.nih.gov/**

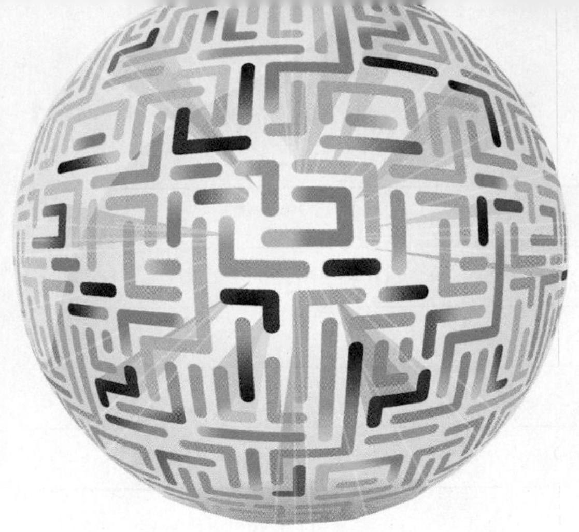

21

Certain Infectious and Parasitic Diseases (A00-B99)

Learning Objectives

After completing this chapter, you should have the skills to:

- Spell and define the key words, medical terms, and abbreviations related to infectious and parasitic diseases.
- Discuss the nature of infectious and parasitic diseases.
- Identify the main characteristics of coding for infectious and parasitic diseases.
- Abstract diagnostic information from the medical record for coding infectious and parasitic diseases.
- Assign codes for infectious and parasitic diseases.
- Arrange codes for infectious and parasitic diseases.
- Discuss the Official Guidelines for Coding and Reporting related to infectious and parasitic diseases.

Key Terms and Abbreviations

acquired immunodeficiency syndrome (AIDS)
asymptomatic
bacteria
Candida
Escherichia coli
fungi
Giardia
helminths
herpes
human immunodeficiency virus (HIV)
inconclusive HIV
indeterminate HIV
localized
multiple organ dysfunction
opportunistic infection
pandemic
parasites
protozoa
Pseudomonas aeruginosa
serology
smallpox
systemic
varicella
viruses

In addition to the key terms listed here, students should know the terms defined within tables in this chapter.

Chapter Outline

- **Infectious Disease Refresher**
- **Coding Overview of Infectious Diseases**
- **Abstracting for Infectious Diseases**
- **Assigning Codes for Infectious Diseases**
- **Arranging Codes for Infectious Diseases**

ICD-10-CM codes in this chapter are from the ICD-10-CM 2014 Draft code set from the Department of Health and Human Services, Centers for Disease Control and Prevention.

INTRODUCTION

When you travel out of the United States or Canada, you will most likely be required to get some vaccinations. These "travel shots" help protect you from contracting an infectious disease and, as importantly, prevent you from spreading it to others. Most such infectious diseases are classified in ICD-10-CM Chapter 1.

In your tour of infectious and parasitic diseases in this chapter you will learn more about what these conditions are, what causes them, and how physicians treat these conditions. Most importantly, you will practice coding for patient encounters related to infectious and parasitic diseases, a skill that requires you to abstract information from the medical record, assign correct codes, and arrange (sequence) the codes in the correct order.

An infectious disease physician specializes in diagnosing and treating infectious diseases. Primary care physicians treat common infectious diseases, but refer patients with more complex conditions to an infectious disease specialist.

As you read this chapter, open up your medical terminology book to the chapter on infectious disease and keep a medical dictionary handy to refresh your memory of any unfamiliar terms. Think of these resources as your travel brochures that tell you more about an area. Coding infectious diseases requires working with the scientific names of microorganisms. Rather than feeling confused by these terms, rely on your resources so you have the information you need at your fingertips.

INFECTIOUS DISEASE REFRESHER

Infectious and parasitic diseases are not a body system; they are a class of diseases that affect the entire body, called systemic diseases. This is in contrast to localized infections, which primarily affect a single organ or body system, such as pneumonia or pharyngitis. Infectious organisms (germs) live in the environment, in the air, on the skin, and inside the body. When the body's immune defenses are weaker than the organism, the organism multiplies to the extent that it causes illness. Infectious organisms are classified by scientists based on the type of cell, shape, and behavior (■ FIGURE 21-1). There are four main types of infectious organisms, as follows:

- bacteria—one-celled germs that multiply quickly and may release toxins that create illness. Examples are *Escherichia coli* (*E.coli*) and *Pseudomonas aeruginosa* (*P. aeruginosa*).

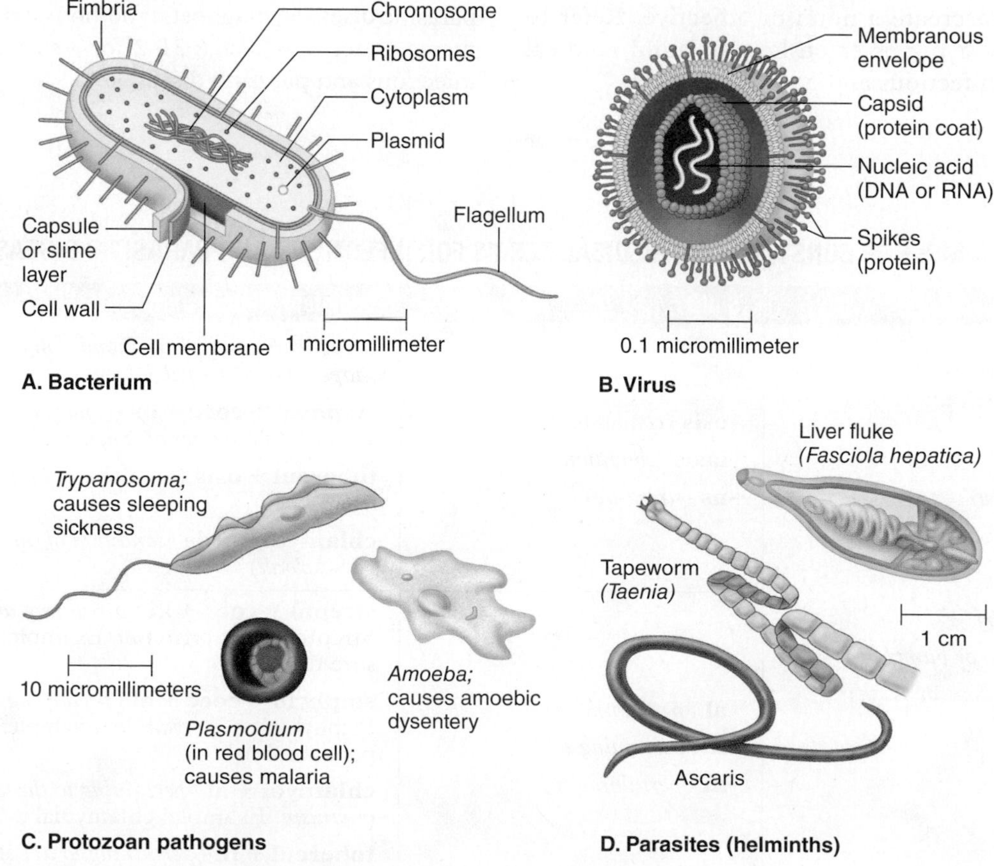

Figure 21-1 ■ Pathogens Causing Infectious and Parasitic Diseases

- viruses—capsules that contain genetic material and use the body's own cells to multiply. Examples are varicella (*chicken pox*) and herpes (*shingles*).
- protozoa—one-celled beings, more complex than bacteria, that use other living things as a source of food and a place to live. Examples are *Trichomonas vaginalis* (the cause of trichomoniases, a sexually transmitted disease) and *Giardia* (*the cause of giardiasis, an intestinal tract infection*).
- fungi—primitive vegetables that reproduce through spores. Examples include *Candida* (*yeast*) and *Trichophyton rubrum* (the cause of athlete's foot).

The type of infectious organism also determines how physicians treat it. For example, antibiotics treat many bacterial infections but are useless against viruses.

Parasites, also called helminths, are plants or animals that live in or on another living organism, or host, and often cause damage to the host. Examples are tapeworm and head lice.

Medical terms related to infectious diseases are built on the word root for the causal organism, which is often named after its shape. As you learn about infectious and parasitic diseases, remember to use medical terminology skills to distinguish between word roots for organisms, nouns that describe conditions, and adjectives that mean *pertaining to*. When the organism causes a condition, a suffix is added to create a noun or adjective. Refer to ■ TABLE 21-1 for a refresher on how to build medical terms related to infectious and parasitic diseases.

CODING CAUTION

Be alert for medical word roots that are spelled similarly but have different meanings.

HIV (*human immunodeficiency virus*) and **HPV** (*human papilloma virus*, which causes cervical cancer)

candidiasis (*a yeast infection*) and **chlamydia** (*a sexually transmitted disease*)

trichomoniasis (*a sexually transmitted disease*) and **trichinosis** (*a roundworm infection caused by eating raw pork or certain other meats*)

Common Infectious Diseases

Smallpox is the only infectious disease of humans that the World Health Organization (WHO) has declared to have been eradicated, with the last known case in 1977. Some infectious diseases that once were common, such as poliomyelitis, are now quite rare in the United States. However, new diseases, such as HIV and Lyme disease, have taken their places. Coders use medical resources, such as reference books on diseases, to understand infectious and parasitic diseases, diagnostic methods, and common treatments. Refer to ■ TABLE 21-2 for a summary of common infectious and parasitic diseases.

Table 21-1 ■ **EXAMPLE OF CONSTRUCTING MEDICAL TERMS FOR INFECTIOUS AND PARASITIC DISEASES**

Combining Form	Suffix	Complete Medical Term
cocc/o (*sphere*) **strept/o** (*twisted*) **staphyl/o** (*cluster*) **tubercul/o** (*knob or bump*) **chlamyd/o** (*envelope or cloak*)	**-osis** (*condition of*) **-iasis** (*condition of*) **-us** (*structure*)	**strepto + cocc + us** (*condition of an organism shaped like a twisted sphere*) **staphylo + cocc + us** (*condition of an organism shaped like a cluster of spheres*) **tubercul + osis** (*condition of an organism shaped like a knob*) **chlamydi + osis** (*condition of an organism shaped like a cloak*)
	-al (*pertaining to*) **-ic** (*pertaining to*) **-in** (*pertaining to*)	**strepto + cocc + al** (*pertaining to the* Streptococcus *organism*. Example: streptococcal sore throat) **staphylo + cocc + al** (*pertaining to the* Staphylococcus *organism*. Example: staphylococcal pneumonia) **chlamydi + al** (*pertaining to the* Chlamydia *organism*. Example: chlamydial cystitis) **tubercul + in** (*pertaining to a* Tuberculosis *organism*. Example: tuberculin test)

Table 21-2 ■ **COMMON INFECTIOUS AND PARASITIC DISEASES**

Condition	Definition
Acquired immunodeficiency syndrome (AIDS)	A disease caused by the HIV virus that weakens and paralyzes the immune system
Hepatitis	A viral inflammation of the liver
Herpes zoster	A painful, blistering skin rash due to the varicella-zoster virus that causes chickenpox; also called shingles
Human immunodeficiency virus (HIV)	A virus that infects and destroys helper T cells of the immune system and causes AIDS
Human papilloma virus (HPV)	A virus that causes cervical cancer
leprosy	A chronic bacterial disease characterized by the formation of nodules on the surface of the body
Malaria	An acute or chronic disease caused by parasites and characterized by high fevers, shaking chills, flu-like symptoms, and anemia
Methicillin-susceptible *Staphylococcus aureus* infection (MSSA)	A type of staph infection that responds to commonly used antibiotics
Methicillin-resistant *Staphylococcus aureus* infection (MRSA)	A type of staph infection that does not respond to commonly used antibiotics
Mononucleosis	A viral infection causing fever, sore throat, and swollen lymph glands
Multiple drug resistant organism (MDRO)	A bacteria that survives exposure to many different antibiotics
Nosocomial	Any hospital-acquired infection
Sepsis	A severe, life-threatening, system-wide reaction to infection caused by disease-causing organisms, especially bacteria, in the blood or tissues
Septic shock	Life-threatening low blood pressure due to sepsis
Septicemia	A systemic disease associated with the presence and persistence of bacteria, viruses, fungi, or other organisms or toxins in the blood
Severe sepsis	Acute or multiple organ dysfunction (MOD) due to sepsis
Syphilis	A sexually transmitted disease (STD) caused by bacteria that produces chancres, rashes, and systemic lesions
Systemic inflammatory response syndrome (SIRS)	An acute, system-wide inflammatory reaction with at least two manifestations: fever, tachycardia, tachypnea, leukocytosis, or leukopenia
Tuberculosis (TB)	A contagious bacterial infection that involves the lungs, but may spread to other organs

In particular, coders must be familiar with the terminology related to HIV/AIDS and sepsis/septic shock, which are highlighted next.

HIV and AIDS

Human immunodeficiency virus (HIV) was first identified in 1983 and has spread so rapidly that it is now considered a **pandemic** by the WHO. HIV is the virus that causes **acquired immunodeficiency syndrome (AIDS)**. It is transmitted through unsafe sex, contaminated needles, blood products, breast milk, and perinatal means (the birth process). Screening of blood products for HIV has nearly eliminated the transmission of HIV through blood transfusions in developed countries.

HIV invades T4 lymphocytes and eventually paralyzes the body's immune system. People can be infected with the HIV virus and be **asymptomatic** (*have no symptoms*) for many years. During this time **serology** (*blood tests*) will be positive for the virus.

An **indeterminate** or **inconclusive HIV** test result means that the antibody test was neither positive nor negative. This may be due to a variety of causes and the test should be repeated.

AIDS is the final stage of the HIV infection and is diagnosed based on blood cell counts. The symptoms of AIDS are **opportunistic infections**, diseases that attack those with weakened immune systems but do not develop in those with healthy immune systems

Table 21-3 ■ **CONDITIONS COMMON TO AIDS**

Type of Complication	Conditions
Malignancies	Kaposi's sarcoma (malignant neoplasm of the connective tissue) lymphoma
Infections	Candidiasis Herpes simplex Herpes zoster (shingles) Pneumonia (*Pneumocystis carinii* pneumonia [PCP]) Toxoplasmosis Tuberculosis
Gastrointestinal symptoms	Diarrhea Lack of appetite Nausea and vomiting
Neurological symptoms	Confusion and memory loss Headaches and visual changes

(■ TABLE 21-3). Patients with AIDS usually die from an opportunistic infection, such as Kaposi's sarcoma or pneumonia. There is no cure for HIV or AIDS, although researchers have made immense progress in developing drugs that slow the rate at which the disease progresses.

Sepsis, Severe Sepsis, and Septic Shock

Sepsis is the presence of bacteria or their toxins in the blood. Usually, the body's response to infection is limited to the specific area infected. In sepsis, the body has a systemic response, in which all body systems try to fight the infection. The invasive bacteria cause cells in the body to release cytokines, substances that trigger inflammation. An abnormally high release of cytokines causes blood vessels to dilate, which decreases blood pressure and causes blood to clot within vital organs. Signs of sepsis include either an abnormally high fever or hypothermia, as well as rapid heart rate, rapid breathing rate, or an abnormally high or low number of white blood cells.

As sepsis worsens, organs begin to malfunction and blood pressure may decrease. Septic shock is diagnosed when blood pressure remains low despite intensive treatment. Severe sepsis is organ malfunction, which results from a blockage of blood flow to vital organs due to blood clots.

Infants, the elderly, and those with weakened immune systems are most likely to get sepsis. Physicians treat sepsis with antibiotics to kill the bacteria, fluids to maintain adequate blood pressure, and mechanical ventilation to aid in breathing. Sepsis progresses rapidly, causing death in one-third of those who get sepsis, according to the Centers for Disease Control and Prevention (CDC).

This section provides a general reference to help understand the most common infectious and parasitic diseases, but does not list everything you need to know. Use medical terminology skills discussed earlier in this chapter to learn the meaning of unfamiliar words. Remember to keep standard reference books handy in case you get stuck. Refer to the resources in the Coder's Toolbox at the end of this chapter to learn more about infectious and parasitic diseases.

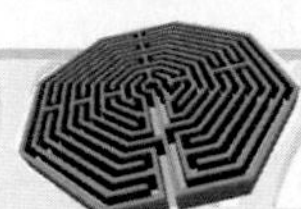

Coding Practice

Refresh your knowledge of terminology related to infectious and parasitic diseases. Use a medical terminology text or a website such as GlobalRph.com > Medical Terminology http://www.globalrph.com/medterm.htm to identify the meaning of word parts that may not be familiar.

Follow these steps:

- Identify the infectious organism.
- Define the meaning of the condition.
- Assign the diagnosis code for the condition using the Index and Tabular List.

Exercise 21.1 Infectious Disease Refresher

Instructions: Use your medical terminology skills and resources to define the following conditions related to infectious and parasitic diseases, then assign the default diagnosis code.

Example: chlamydial cervicitis Organism: *Chlamydia* Meaning: *inflammation of the cervix due to Chlamydia* CM Code: *A56.09*

1. candidiasis bronchitis Organism ______ Meaning ______ CM Code ______
2. syphilitic endocarditis Organism ______ Meaning ______ CM Code ______
3. herpetic eyelid Organism ______ Meaning ______ CM Code ______
4. typhoid meningitis Organism ______ Meaning ______ CM Code ______

5. amebiasis cutaneous Organism ____________ Meaning ____________ CM Code ________
6. parasitic stomatitis Organism ____________ Meaning ____________ CM Code ________
7. Rickettsialpox (pox is a disease manifested through eruptions or pustules) Organism ____________ Meaning ____________ CM Code ________
8. trichomoniasis prostate Organism ____________ Meaning ____________ CM Code ________
9. tubercular anus Organism ____________ Meaning ____________ CM Code ________
10. gonococcal pharyngitis Organism ____________ Meaning ____________ CM Code ________

CODING OVERVIEW OF INFECTIOUS DISEASES

ICD-10-CM Chapter 1, Certain Infectious and Parasitic Diseases (A00-B99), contains 22 blocks or subchapters that are divided by the type of infection. Review the block names and code ranges listed at the beginning of Chapter 1 in the ICD-10-CM manual to become familiar with the content and organization. Two letters of the alphabet, A or B, are used as the first letter of codes.

Chapter 1 is comparable to ICD-9-CM Chapter 1 (001-139) and has been reorganized in some areas compared to ICD-9-CM. Certain diseases, such as malaria, leprosy, hepatitis, and mononucleosis, contain expanded or redefined codes. Codes for bacterial and viral infectious agents have been expanded for increased specificity.

This chapter includes parasitic infestations and systemic infections due to viruses, bacteria, protozoa, and fungi. It also includes the named organisms that cause localized infections. This chapter does not include localized infections, which are classified in the body system chapter. Localized infections may be assigned a combination code that identifies the condition and the causal organism, or they may require one code for the condition and a second code from Chapter 1 to identify the causal organism. Instructional notes in the Tabular List, under the code for the localized infection, identify when to assign an additional code for the infectious organism. This chapter also does not include obstetric- or newborn-related conditions, which are classified in ICD-10-CM Chapters 15 and 16, respectively.

ICD-10-CM provides Official Guidelines for Coding and Reporting (OGCR) infectious and parasitic diseases in OGCR section I.C.1. OGCR provides a detailed discussion of assigning and sequencing codes for HIV, sepsis, and septic shock. An instructional note at the beginning of Chapter 1 in the Tabular List instructs coders to assign an additional code when an infection is drug resistant. This instruction applies to all codes in Chapter 1.

SUCCESS STEP

Experienced coders will notice that this chapter has been reorganized and expanded compared to Chapter 1 in ICD-9-CM. However, as long you follow standard coding practices for using the Index, you should have little problem locating new or changed codes.

ABSTRACTING FOR INFECTIOUS DISEASES

Coders always need to identify the scientific name of the infectious organism and subtype, as well as associated complications or manifestations. Additional details are needed when abstracting HIV/AIDS and sepsis. Refer to ■ Table 21-4 for guidance on how to abstract infectious and parasitic diseases. Remember that the

Table 21-4 ■ KEY CRITERIA FOR ABSTRACTING INFECTIOUS AND PARASITIC DISEASES

- ❑ What is the named organism responsible for the patient's condition?
- ❑ What type of organism is it (bacteria, virus, etc.)?
- ❑ What is the subtype of the condition?
- ❑ Is a more specific subtype documented?
- ❑ Does the patient have a condition that is due to *Streptococcus*, *Staphylococcus*, or *Enterococcus*?
- ❑ Is the infection systemic or localized (organ specific)?
- ❑ Is the organism the cause of a condition that exists in a specific body system?
- ❑ Does the documentation state that the infection is resistant to antibiotics?

abstracting questions are a guide and that not every question applies to, or can be answered for, every case. For example, the hepatitis virus has subtypes A, B, or C, but not every organism does. Also remember to abstract for symptoms and determine if they are integral to the confirmed diagnoses.

Abstracting HIV and AIDS

When abstracting cases involving HIV and AIDS, coders must determine whether or not physician documentation confirms HIV infection. In addition, coders must determine whether HIV is asymptomatic or if it manifests itself in AIDS-related conditions. For any encounter with an HIV or AIDS patient, coders must also determine if the reason for the encounter is related to HIV or AIDS, or if it is unrelated, such as an accident that causes a fracture. Refer to ■ TABLE 21-5 for guidance in abstracting HIV and AIDS cases, then refer to the example that follows (■ FIGURE 21-2).

Table 21-5 ■ KEY CRITERIA FOR ABSTRACTING HIV AND AIDS

- ❑ Does the physician clearly document a confirmed diagnosis of HIV positive?
- ❑ Does the patient have symptoms or complications?
- ❑ Is the patient being seen (or admitted) for an HIV-related condition?
- ❑ Is the patient being seen (or admitted) for a condition *un*related to HIV?
- ❑ Has the patient been previously diagnosed with an HIV-related illness?
- ❑ Is the purpose of the encounter HIV testing?
- ❑ Did the patient receive HIV counseling?
- ❑ Is HIV serology inconclusive?

Abstracting Sepsis, Severe Sepsis, and Septic Shock

When abstracting sepsis, severe sepsis, and septic shock, coders must have a clear understanding of the definitions of these conditions. For example, patients with sepsis and associated acute organ dysfunction are classified as severe sepsis even if the documentation does not contain the precise word *severe* (OGCR I.C.1.d.1)(a)). When the documentation is unclear regarding the status of the patient, query the physician for clarification. Coders also abstract the underlying systemic infection, such as *Pseudomonas aeruginosa* or *Escherichia coli*. Refer to ■ TABLE 21-6 for guidance in abstracting these cases, then work through the detailed example that follows.

Table 21-6 ■ KEY CRITERIA FOR ABSTRACTING SEPSIS AND SEPTIC SHOCK

- ❑ What is the systemic infection underlying the sepsis?
- ❑ Is a more specific subtype documented?
- ❑ Is sepsis documented as severe?
- ❑ Is an associated acute organ dysfunction documented?
- ❑ Is septic shock documented?
- ❑ Was the severe sepsis present on admission or did it develop after admission?
- ❑ Does a localized (organ-specific) infection exist in addition to sepsis?
- ❑ Is the sepsis the complication of a procedure that was performed?
- ❑ Is the sepsis associated with a wound?
- ❑ Is the sepsis associated with a noninfectious condition (such as trauma)?

Patient with known AIDS is admitted for AIDS-related pneumocystis carinii pneumonia (PCP).

Does the physician clearly document a confirmed diagnosis of HIV positive? **Yes, a diagnosis of AIDS presumes HIV positive.**

Does the patient have symptoms or complications? **Yes, pneumonia.**

Is the patient being seen (or admitted) for an HIV-related condition? **Yes, PCP.**

Is the patient being seen (or admitted) for a condition unrelated to HIV? **No.**

Has the patient been previously diagnosed with an HIV-related illness? **Yes, patient is known to have AIDS at the time of admission.**

Is the purpose of the encounter HIV testing? **No.**

Did the patient receive HIV counseling? **No.**

Is HIV serology inconclusive? **No.**

Figure 21-2 ■ Example of Abstracting HIV/AIDS

Guided Example of Abstracting for Infectious Diseases

Refer to the following example throughout this chapter to practice skills for abstracting, assigning, and sequencing infectious and parasitic disease codes. Susanna Vannote, CPC, is a fictitious coder who guides you through the coding process.

Date: 02/11/yy Location: Branton Medical Center
Provider: James Cruickshank, MD
Patient: Faye Gillis Gender: F Age: 81
Reason for admission: admitted to ICU from the emergency department due to acute respiratory failure
Assessment: E. coli sepsis with organ failure
Plan: discharged to skilled nursing facility

Follow along as Susanna Vannote, CPC, abstracts the diagnosis. Check off each step after you complete it.

⇨ Susanna reads through the entire record, with special attention to the reason for the encounter and the final assessment. She refers to the Key Criteria for Abstracting Sepsis and Septic Shock (Table 21-6).

- ❑ *What is the systemic infection underlying the sepsis?* E. coli
- ❑ *Is sepsis documented as severe?* No.
- ❑ *Is an associated acute organ dysfunction documented?* Yes, respiratory
- ❑ *Is septic shock documented?* No.
- ❑ *Was the severe sepsis present on admission or did it develop after admission?* present on admission
- ❑ *Does a localized (organ-specific) infection exist in addition to sepsis?* No.
- ❑ *Is the sepsis the complication of a procedure that was performed?* No.
- ❑ *Is the sepsis associated with a wound?* No.
- ❑ *Is the sepsis associated with a noninfectious condition (such as trauma)?* No.

⇨ At this time, Susanna does not know which of these conditions may need to be coded, nor how many codes she will end up with. She will learn about this when she moves on to assigning codes.

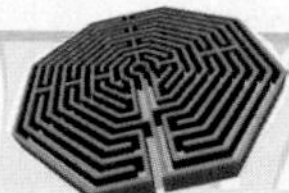

Coding Practice

Now it is your turn to practice abstracting diagnoses for infectious and parasitic diseases. Questions guide your analysis of each scenario.

Exercise 21.2 Abstracting for Infectious Diseases

Instructions: Read the mini-medical-record of each patient's encounter and answer the abstracting questions. Write the answer on the line provided. Do not assign any codes.

1. Date: 2/13/yy Location: Branton Medical Group
Provider: James Cruickshank, MD
Patient: Otis Kinsel Gender: M Age: 18
Chief complains: general lack of energy, fatigue, loss of appetite, fever, and chills
Assessment: suspected Epstein-Barr mononucleosis, which was confirmed by a blood test
Plan: drink fluids, get rest, acetaminophen or ibuprofen for pain and fever, recovery can take several weeks, call if abdominal pain, difficulty breathing, severe weakness, or persistent high fever

(continued)

1. (continued)

a. What are the symptoms? ______________________

____

b. Is the condition uncertain or confirmed? ______

____

c. What is the named organism? ______________

____

d. Should the symptoms be coded? ______________
Why or why not? ______________________

2. Date: 2/13/yy Location: Branton Medical Group
Provider: James Cruickshank, MD
Patient: Lolita Hemstreet Gender: F Age: 46
Reason for encounter: annual work related PPD tuberculin test (*Purified Protein Derivative*)
Assessment: PPD positive for TB, X-ray of lung positive for nodules in lung
Plan: order sputum culture, begin pharmacotherapy

(continued)

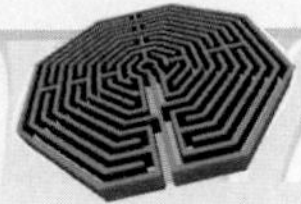

Coding Practice (continued)

2. (continued)

a. What is the named organism responsible for the patient's condition? ____________

b. Does the documentation state that the infection is resistant to antibiotics? ____________

c. What anatomic site is involved? ____________

3. Date: 2/14/yy Location: Branton Medical Center Provider: James Cruickshank, MD

Patient: Liz Spagnola Gender: F Age: 70

Reason for encounter: called in for a consult on Staphylococcus aureus pneumonia

Assessment: culture result shows MSSA

Plan: IV teicoplanin (*an antibiotic*) was successful and patient was discharged with instructions to help prevent recurrence

a. What is the named organism responsible for the patient's condition? ____________

b. Does the patient have a condition that is due to *Streptococcus, Staphylococcus*, or *Enterococcus*? ____________

c. Does the documentation state that the infection is resistant to antibiotics? ____________

4. Date: 2/13/yy Location: Branton Medical Group Provider: James Cruickshank, MD

Patient: Arturo Wedge Gender: M Age: 27

Reason for encounter: genital chancre (*a firm, non-itchy skin ulcer*)

Assessment: primary syphilis

Plan: antibiotics

a. What is the named organism responsible for the patient's condition? ____________

(continued)

4. (continued)

b. What is the subtype of the condition? ____________

c. Does the patient have a condition that is due to Streptococcus, Staphylococcus, or Enterococcus? ____________

d. Does the documentation state that the infection is resistant to antibiotics? ____________

5. Date: 2/13/yy Location: Branton Medical Center Provider: James Cruickshank, MD

Patient: Brandie Golson Gender: F Age: 35

Reason for encounter: admitted from emergency department due to septicemia

Assessment: Staphylococcus aureus septicemia, cause unknown, responsive to antibiotics

Plan: after O2 and IV fluids and antibiotics, patient was discharged home in good condition

a. What is the systemic infection underlying the sepsis? ____________

b. Does the documentation state that the infection is resistant to antibiotics? ____________

c. Is sepsis documented as severe? ____________

d. Is an associated acute organ dysfunction documented? ____________

e. Is the sepsis the complication of a procedure or a wound? ____________

6. Date: 2/14/yy Location: Branton Medical Group Provider: James Cruickshank, MD

Patient: Terrence Kestler Gender: M Age: 26

Reason for encounter: lesions on the skin of this HIV positive patient

Assessment: Kaposi's sarcoma of the skin

(continued)

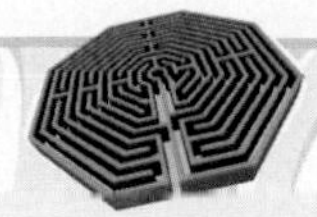

Coding Practice (continued)

6. (continued)

Plan: *refer to oncologist to evaluate extent of the cancer and determine treatment plan*

a. Does the physician clearly document a confirmed diagnosis of HIV positive?______________

b. Does the patient have symptoms or complications?
____

c. Is the patient being seen (or admitted) for an HIV-related condition? ______________
____

7. Date: *2/14/yy* Location: *Branton Medical Center Emergency Department*

Provider: *James Cruickshank, MD*

Patient: *Terrence Kestler* Gender: *M* Age: *26*

Reason for encounter: *toe pain after a horse stepped on his foot*

Assessment: *fractured distal phalanx of great toe on the right foot, AIDS patient with Kaposi's sarcoma of the lymph nodes which was not treated at this encounter*

Plan: *reduced fracture and applied cast, crutches, FU office 2 weeks*

a. What is the reason for the encounter? ______________
____

b. What bone was fractured? ______________
____

c. What is the laterality? ______________
____

d. What is the episode of care? ______________
____

e. Does the physician clearly document a confirmed diagnosis of HIV positive? ______________
____

f. Does the patient have symptoms or complications? ______________

g. Is the patient being seen (or admitted) for an HIV-related condition? ______________
____

8. Date: *2/13/yy* Location: *Branton Medical Group*

Provider: *James Cruickshank, MD*

Patient: *Deanna Hentz* Gender: *F* Age: *31*

Reason for encounter: *follow up on HIV test results*

Assessment: *positive for HIV, asymptomatic, counseled patient on managing the infection*

Plan: *refer to HIV support group*

a. Did the physician clearly document a confirmed diagnosis of HIV positive? ______________
____

b. Does the patient have symptoms or complications?
____

c. Is the purpose of the encounter HIV testing?
____

d. Did the patient receive HIV counseling? ______________
____

9. Date: *2/14/yy* Location: *Branton Medical Group*

Provider: *James Cruickshank, MD*

Patient: *Donald Plewa* Gender: *M* Age: *45*

Reason for encounter: *HIV positive patient with no related conditions presents with dysuria, weakness, and fever*

Assessment: *urosepsis (UTI) d/t E.coli (non-Shiga toxin-producing)*

Plan: *antibiotics*

a. What are the symptoms? ______________
____

b. What condition is diagnosed? ______________
____

c. What is the infectious organism? ______________
____

What is the subtype? ______________
____

d. Does the documentation state that the infection is resistant to antibiotics? ______________
____

(continued)

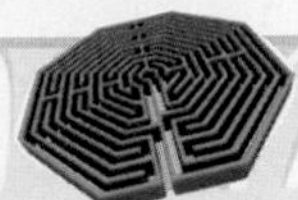

Coding Practice (continued)

9. (continued)

e. Does the physician clearly document a confirmed diagnosis of HIV positive? ______________________

f. Is the urosepsis documented as HIV related? ______________________

g. What condition is the reason for the encounter? ______________________

10. Date: 2/14/yy Location: Branton Medical Center Provider: James Cruickshank, MD

Patient: Rhea Niederhauser Gender: F Age: 77

Reason for admission: *admitted from SNF 1 day post-hospital-discharge with 102 F fever, dyspnea, heart rate 100 per minute, low BP*

Assessment: *severe sepsis d/t nosocomial MRSA and associated heart failure*

(continued)

10. (continued)

Plan: *deceased*

a. What is the systemic infection underlying the sepsis? ______________________

b. Does the documentation state that the infection is resistant to antibiotics? ______________________

c. Is sepsis documented as severe? ______________________

d. Is septic shock present? ______________________
Why or why not? ______________________

e. Is an associated acute organ dysfunction documented? ______________________

ASSIGNING CODES FOR INFECTIOUS DISEASES

OGCR provides many detailed guidelines for coding infectious organisms; HIV and AIDS; and sepsis, severe sepsis, and septic shock. Although coders do not need to memorize every guideline, they should memorize the *fact* that OGCR exist for these conditions and refer to OGCR every time they code these conditions.

Assigning Codes for Infectious Organisms

Guidelines describe how to code infectious organisms that are the cause of localized infections and organisms that are resistant to drugs.

Infectious Organisms in Diseases Classified Elsewhere

As discussed earlier in this chapter, localized infections are classified in body system chapters. In some cases, a combination code describes the condition and the infectious organism. In other cases, the body system chapter provides a code for the condition with an instructional note to assign an additional code for the causal agent. Assign a code from one of the following categories:

- **B95 Streptococcus, Staphylococcus, and Enterococcus as the cause of diseases classified to other chapters**
- **B96 Other bacterial agents as the cause of diseases classified to other chapters**
- **B97 Viral agents as the cause of diseases classified to other chapters**

These are causal agent codes and should be assigned only as a secondary code, in conjunction with a principal or first-listed diagnosis code for the localized infection (OGCR I.C.1.b.). When an infectious organism causes a systemic infection, assign a code from elsewhere in ICD-10-CM Chapter 1 based on guidance from the Index and OGCR.

SUCCESS STEP

E. coli is classified by its strain. O157 is a strain that produces potentially harmful Shiga toxins. Shiga toxins can also be present in other strains of *E. coli*. Review the code selections under category **B96.2** to identify codes for the various strains of *E. coli*.

Drug-Resistant Organisms

When an organism is stated as resistant to antibiotics or other drugs, report the resistance with a combination code that identifies the organism and its resistance, if one is available. *Staphylococcus aureus* is classified as either susceptible (responsive) to methicillin, described as methicillin-susceptible *Staphylococcus aureus* (MSSA), or resistant to methicillin, described as methicillin-resistant *Staphylococcus aureus* (MRSA). Combination codes for both MSSA and MRSA are located in the Index under the Main Term **MSSA** and **MRSA**, respectively, and also under the Main Term **Staphylococcus**. Read the documentation carefully to identify the correct type of *Staphylococcus aureus*.

When a combination code is not available, report the resistance with two codes: (1) the infection code and (2) a code from category **Z16 Resistance to antimicrobial drugs** (OGCR I.C.1.c.). Locate the code for resistance in the Index under the Main Term **Resistance** and subterms **organism, to, drug** with a final subterm for the class of drug. When an organism is resistance to multiple drugs, select the subterm **multiple drugs (MDRO)** (■ FIGURE 21-3).

Assigning Codes for HIV and AIDS

ICD-10-CM provides detailed guidelines for assigning codes related to HIV and AIDS. Coders must be careful to use the terminology for HIV and AIDS correctly and precisely, as discussed earlier in this chapter. The codes for a patient with HIV or AIDS change as the disease progresses (■ FIGURE 21-4, page 414).

Asymptomatic HIV

Assign code **Z21 Asymptomatic human immunodeficiency virus [HIV] infection status** when the documentation describes the following circumstances (OGCR I.C.1.a.2)(d)):

- HIV positive
- known HIV
- HIV test positive
- asymptomatic HIV

To locate the code, search the Index for the Main Term **HIV** and the subterm **positive, seropositive** (■ FIGURE 21-5, page 415). Do not assign code **Z21** when the test results are documented as inconclusive or when terms AIDS or HIV disease are documented. These situations are discussed next.

Patient is treated for Klebsiella pneumoniae pneumonia which is not responding to multiple antibiotics.
(1) **J15.0 Pneumonia due to Klebsiella pneumoniae**
(2) **Z16.24 Resistance to multiple antibiotics**

Figure 21-3 ■ Example of Coding Multiple Drug-Resistant Organisms

AIDS

Assign code **B20 Human immunodeficiency virus [HIV] disease** in the following documented circumstances:

- documentation uses the terms AIDS or HIV *disease*
- the patient is treated for any HIV-related illness
- the patient is described as having any condition resulting from HIV positive status
- the patient has been previously diagnosed with AIDS (OGCR I.C.1.a.2)(f))

To locate the code, search the Index for the Main Term **HIV** and use the default code (Figure 21-5), or search for the Main Term **AIDS** and use the default code (■ FIGURE 21-6, page 415).

SUCCESS STEP

The ICD-10-CM code description for AIDS is **HIV disease**. Remember to distinguish between the term *HIV disease* and the terms *HIV virus*, *HIV positive*, or *asymptomatic HIV*, which describe a different aspect of the HIV/AIDS cycle.

Inconclusive HIV Test Results

Assign code **R75 Inconclusive laboratory evidence of human immunodeficiency virus [HIV]** for patients with inconclusive HIV serology, but no definitive diagnosis or manifestations of the illness (OGCR I.C.1.a.2)(e)). Locate this code under the Main Term **HIV** and the subterm **nonconclusive** (Figure 21-5).

CODING CAUTION

Once a patient has developed an HIV-related illness, you should assign code **B20** on *every* encounter. Patients previously diagnosed with any HIV illness (**B20**) should *never* be assigned to **R75** or **Z21**.

Other HIV-Related Encounters

OGCR I.C.1.a.2)(h) provides additional guidelines for coding encounters for testing for HIV, exposure to HIV, HIV counseling, and high risk behavior. These and other HIV-related codes can be located in the Index under the Main Term **Human** and subterm **immunodeficiency**. The codes for asymptomatic HIV, inconclusive HIV results, and HIV infection are also located under this entry (■ FIGURE 21-7, page 415).

Refer to ■ FIGURE 21-8 (page 415) to learn more about assigning codes for HIV and AIDS. Sequencing of codes for AIDS patients is discussed later in this chapter.

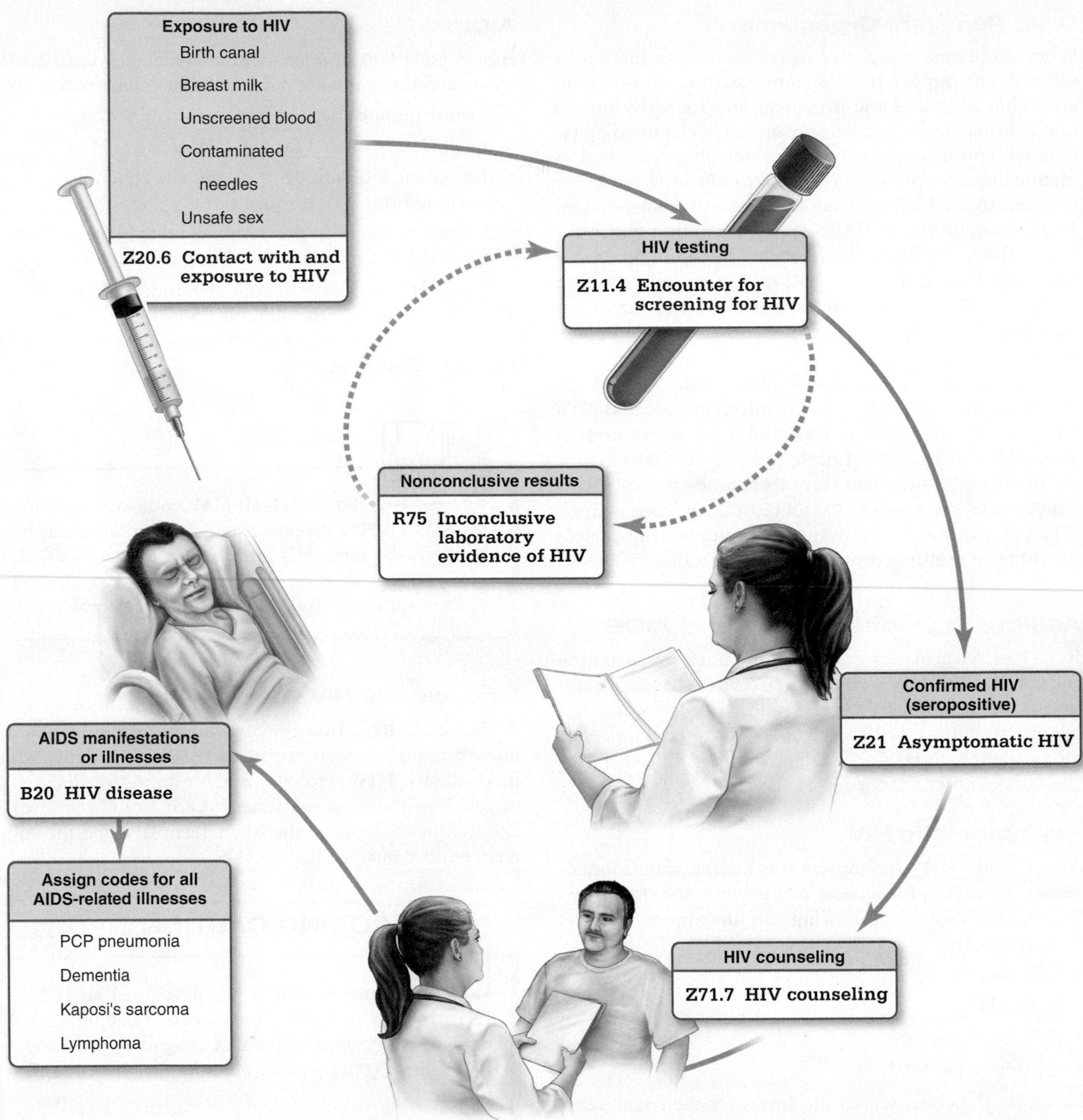

Figure 21-4 ■ Each stage of HIV and AIDS requires unique codes.

Assigning Codes for Sepsis and Severe Sepsis

ICD-10-CM provides different OGCR for sepsis and severe sepsis, which are discussed next.

Sepsis

For a diagnosis of sepsis, assign the appropriate code for the underlying systemic infection, which corresponds to the scientific name of the causal organism. If the type of infection or causal organism is not specified, assign code **A41.9 Sepsis, unspecified** (OGCR I.C.1.d.1)(a)). Do not assign a code from subcategory **R65.2 Severe sepsis** unless severe sepsis or an associated acute organ dysfunction is documented.

CODING CAUTION

ICD-9-CM provided over 50 Index entries for septicemia. ICD-10-CM provides only one Index entry, which directs coders to category **A41 Other sepsis**.

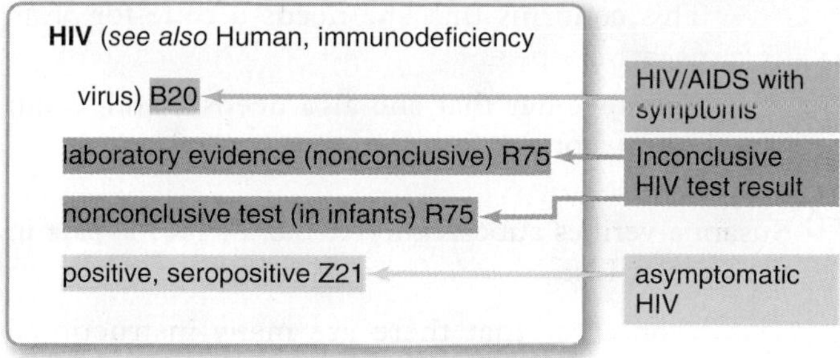

Figure 21-5 ■ Index Entry for HIV

AIDS (related complex) B20

Figure 21-6 ■ Index Entry for AIDS

Human
- bite (open wound) — *see also* Bite
  - intact skin surface — *see* Bite, superficial
- herpesvirus — *see* Herpes
- immunodeficiency virus (HIV) disease (infection) B20
  - asymptomatic status Z21
  - contact Z20.6
  - counseling Z71.7
  - dementia B20 *[F02.80]*
    - with behavioral disturbance B20 *[F02.81]*
  - exposure to Z20.6
  - laboratory evidence R75
  - type-2 (HIV 2) as cause of disease classified elsewhere B97.35

Figure 21-7 ■ Index Entry for Main Term Human with Subterm Immunodeficiency Virus

Patient with known AIDS is admitted for AIDS-related pneumocystis carinii pneumonia (PCP).

(1) **B20 Human immunodeficiency virus [HIV] disease**

(2) **B59 Pneumocystosis**

Figure 21-8 ■ Example of Assigning Codes for HIV/AIDS

Severe Sepsis

When severe sepsis or sepsis *with* organ dysfunction are specifically documented, assign a code from category **R65.2 Severe sepsis** in addition to codes for the infection and organ dysfunction. Assign the fifth character **0** for **without septic shock** or the fifth character **1** for **with septic shock**. When patients have sepsis and *associated* acute organ dysfunction or **multiple organ dysfunction**, follow these instructions for coding severe sepsis (OGCR I.C.1.d.1)(a)(iii)). Documentation must state the association between sepsis and the organ dysfunction through the use of the word *with*, *associated*, or similar terminology. The word *and* does *not* indicate a relationship (OGCR I.C.1.d.1)(a)(iv)). Sequencing of the codes is discussed later in this chapter.

SUCCESS STEP

Review the OGCR for additional guidelines regarding the following:

- Sepsis and severe sepsis with a localized infection (OGCR I.C.1.d.4)).
- Sepsis due to a postprocedural infection (OGCR I.C.1.d.5)).
- Sepsis and severe sepsis associated with a noninfectious process (OGCR I.C.1.d.6)).

Septic Shock

Septic shock, by definition, includes severe sepsis. Therefore, whenever septic shock is documented, assign a code for the systemic infection and also code **R65.21 Severe sepsis with septic shock.**

Guided Example of Assigning Infectious Disease Codes

To practice skills for assigning codes for infectious and parasitic diseases, continue with the example from earlier in the chapter about patient Faye Gillis, who was admitted to Branton Medical Center due to acute respiratory failure.

Follow along in your ICD-10-CM manual as Susanna Vannote, CPC, assigns codes. Check off each step after you complete it.

⇨ First, Susanna confirms the diagnoses.

- ❑ *gram negative sepsis*
- ❑ *acute respiratory failure*

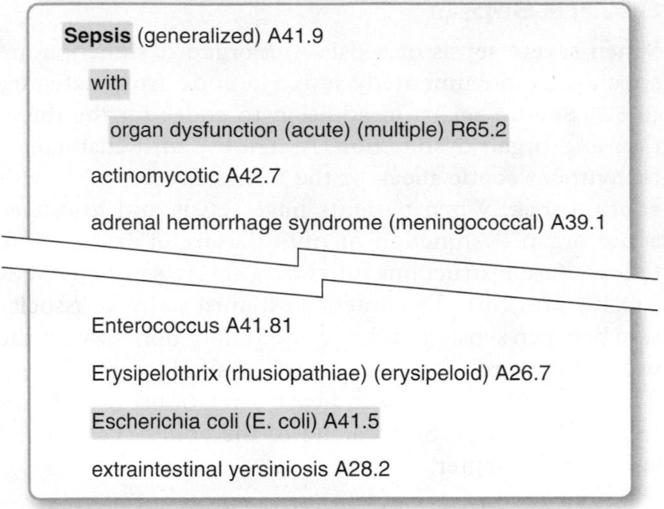
Sepsis (generalized) A41.9
with
organ dysfunction (acute) (multiple) R65.2
actinomycotic A42.7
adrenal hemorrhage syndrome (meningococcal) A39.1
Enterococcus A41.81
Erysipelothrix (rhusiopathiae) (erysipeloid) A26.7
Escherichia coli (E. coli) A41.5
extraintestinal yersiniosis A28.2

Figure 21-9 ■ Index Entry for Sepsis

➩ Susanna searches the Index for the Main Term **Sepsis** (■ FIGURE 21-9).

- ❑ She locates the subterm for the type of sepsis, **Escherichia coli A41.51**.
- ❑ As Susanna continues to review all the subterms under **Sepsis**, she notes an additional subterm that may apply.
  - Immediately under **Sepsis**, she sees the subterm, **with, acute organ dysfunction R65.2**.

➩ Susanna feels confused with so many choices. She remembers that the OGCR contains several guidelines regarding sepsis, so turns to OGCR I.C.1. near the front of her ICD-10-CM manual for more information.

- ❑ OGCR I.C.1.d.1)(a) states **For a diagnosis of sepsis, assign the appropriate code for the underlying systemic infection**.
  - This tells her she needs a code for gram negative sepsis because it is the underlying systemic infection.
- ❑ OGCR I.C.1.d.1)(a)(iii) states **If a patient has sepsis and associated acute organ dysfunction or multiple organ dysfunction (MOD), follow the instructions for coding severe sepsis.**
  - This tells her that **acute organ dysfunction** follows the same guidelines as **severe sepsis**, even though the word *severe* was not specifically documented.
- ❑ OGCR I.C.1.d.1)(b) states **The coding of severe sepsis requires a minimum of 2 codes: first a code for the underlying systemic infection, followed by a code from subcategory R65.2.**
  - This confirms that she needs a code for gram negative sepsis.
  - This tells her that she also needs a code from subcategory **R65.2.**

➩ Susanna verifies subcategory **R65.2, Severe sepsis** in the Tabular List.

- ❑ She observes that there are many instructional notes under the subcategory title.
- ❑ She identifies the symbol **5th** in front of the subcategory title, which tells her that a fifth character is required to complete the code.
- ❑ She locates the fifth-character codes below the instructional notes and determines that code **R65.20, Severe sepsis without septic shock** describes this case because septic shock was not documented.

➩ Susanna reviews the instructional notes in the Tabular List for **R65.20** (■ FIGURE 21-10).

- ❑ She cross-references the notes at the beginning of subcategory **R65.2.**
- ❑ The inclusion notes state **Sepsis with acute organ dysfunction**. This accurately describes the case.
- ❑ She reviews the note **Code first underlying infection, such as:**.
- ❑ None of the conditions listed include the code she assigned for gram negative sepsis. However, she recalls that OGCR I.C.1.d.1)(b) already gave her sequencing instructions, which she will review later.
- ❑ She reviews the note **Use additional code to identify specific acute organ dysfunction, such as:**.
- ❑ She determines that this note applies because the patient had acute respiratory failure, which is listed in the instruction as **acute respiratory failure (J96.0-)**. She will finish verifying the instructional notes for **R65.20**, then will assign and verify code for acute respiratory failure.
- ❑ She cross-references the beginning of the category **R65** and verifies that there are no instructional notes that apply to all codes in the category.
- ❑ She cross-references the beginning of the block **R50-R69** and verifies that there are no instructional notes that apply to all codes in the block.
- ❑ She cross-references the beginning of **Chapter 18 (R00-R99)** and reviews the instructional notes. These notes apply to assigning codes for symptoms and signs when a more specific diagnosis cannot be established. She determines that she

should assign **R65.20** from this chapter, although a more specific diagnosis code is available, because the OGCR specifically directs her to assign a code from category **R65.2**.

5th **R65.2 Severe sepsis**

Infection with associated acute organ dysfunction

Sepsis with acute organ dysfunction

Sepsis with multiple organ dysfunction

Systemic inflammatory response syndrome due to infectious process with acute organ dysfunction

Code first underlying infection, such as:

Infection following a procedure (T81.4)

Infections following infusion, transfusion and therapeutic injection (T80.2)

Puerperal sepsis (O85)

Sepsis following complete or unspecified spontaneous abortion (O03.87)

Sepsis following ectopic and molar pregnancy (O08.82)

Sepsis following incomplete spontaneous abortion (O03.37)

Sepsis following (induced) termination of pregnancy (O04.87)

Sepsis NOS A41.9

Use additional code to identify specific acute organ dysfunction, such as:

acute kidney failure (N17.-)

acute respiratory failure (J96.0-)

critical illness myopathy (G72.81)

critical illness polyneuropathy (G62.81)

disseminated intravascular coagulopathy [DIC] (D65)

encephalopathy (metabolic) (septic) (G93.41)

hepatic failure (K72.0-)

R65.20 Severe sepsis without septic shock

Severe sepsis NOS

R65.21 Severe sepsis with septic shock

Figure 21-10 ■ Tabular List Entry for Severe Sepsis

➪ Next, Susanna wants to assign a code for acute respiratory failure. She locates the cross-referenced subcategory **J96.0, Acute respiratory failure** in the Tabular List.

- ❑ She identifies the symbol 5th in front of the subcategory title, which tells her that a fifth character is required to complete the code.
- ❑ She reviews the fifth-digit options and determines that the code that best describes the case is **J96.00, Acute respiratory failure, unspecified whether with hypoxia or hypercapnia** because neither hypoxia for hypercapnia were documented.
- ❑ Susanna cross-references the beginning of the category **J96**, the beginning of the block **J96-J99** and the beginning of **Chapter 10 (J00-J99)** for additional instructional notes, and finds none that apply to this case.

➪ Susanna checks her notes and realizes she still needs to verify the code she located in the Index for the underlying infection, **Sepsis, Escherichia coli A41.51.**

- ❑ She locates the code in the Tabular List and reads the code title **A41.51, Sepsis due to Escherichia coli [E. coli].**
- ❑ She confirms that this accurately describes the documented organism.
- ❑ She confirms that no additional characters apply.
- ❑ She cross-references the instructional notes at the beginning of category **A41, Other sepsis.** She determines that the conditions listed do not apply to this case.
- ❑ She cross-references the beginning of the block **A30-A49** and verifies that there are no instructional notes for this block.
- ❑ She cross-references the beginning of **Chapter 1 (A00-B99)** and reviews the instructional note that applies to all codes in this chapter. She determines that it does not apply to this case because the infection is not due to an external cause.

➪ Susanna reviews the codes she has assigned for this case.

- ❑ **R65.20, Severe sepsis without septic shock**
- ❑ **J96.00, Acute respiratory failure, unspecified whether with hypoxia or hypercapnia**
- ❑ **A41.51, Sepsis due to Escherichia coli [E. coli]**

➪ Next, Susanna must determine how to sequence the codes.

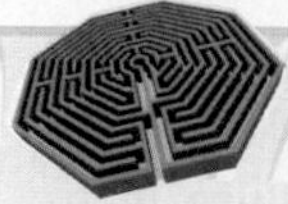

Coding Practice

Now it is your turn to practice assigning codes for infectious and parasitic diseases. Refer to the ***Tip*** at the end of the mini-medical-record if you need a little extra help.

Exercise 21.3 Assigning Codes for Infectious Diseases

Instructions: Read the mini-medical-record of each patient's encounter, review the information abstracted in Exercise 21.2, and assign ICD-10-CM diagnosis codes (CM) using the Index and Tabular List. Write the code(s) on the line provided.

1. Date: 2/13/yy Location: Branton Medical Group
Provider: James Cruickshank, MD
Patient: Otis Kinsel Gender: M Age: 18
Chief complains: general lack of energy, fatigue, loss of appetite, fever, and chills
Assessment: suspected Epstein-Barr mononucleosis, which was confirmed by a blood test
Plan: drink fluids, get rest, acetaminophen or ibuprofen for pain and fever, recovery can take several weeks, call if abdominal pain, difficulty breathing, severe weakness, or persistent high fever
1 CM Code __________

2. Date: 2/13/yy Location: Branton Medical Group
Provider: James Cruickshank, MD
Patient: Lolita Hemstreet Gender: F Age: 46
Reason for encounter: annual work related PPD tuberculin test
Assessment: PPD positive for TB, X-ray of lung positive for nodules in lung
Plan: order sputum culture, begin pharmacotherapy
1 CM Code __________

3. Date: 2/13/yy Location: Branton Medical Group
Provider: James Cruickshank, MD
Patient: Deanna Hentz Gender: F Age: 31
Reason for encounter: follow up on HIV test results
Assessment: positive for HIV, asymptomatic, counseled patient on managing the infection
Plan: refer to HIV support group

***Tip*:** Refer to OGCR I.C.1.a.2)(d). The second code is for HIV counseling.
2 CM Codes __________ __________

4. Date: 2/13/yy Location: Branton Medical Group
Provider: James Cruickshank, MD
Patient: Arturo Wedge Gender: M Age: 27
Reason for encounter: genital chancre
Assessment: primary syphilis
Plan: antibiotics
1 CM Code __________

5. Date: 2/13/yy Location: Branton Medical Center Provider: James Cruickshank, MD
Patient: Brandie Golson Gender: F Age: 35
Reason for encounter: admitted from emergency department due to septicemia
Assessment: Staphylococcus aureus septicemia, cause unknown, responsive to antibiotics
Plan: after O2 and IV fluids and antibiotics, patient was discharged home in good condition

***Tip*:** Refer to OGCR I.C.1.d.1)(a).
1 CM Code __________

ARRANGING CODES FOR INFECTIOUS DISEASES

Codes from this ICD-10-CM chapter are sequenced first when the systemic infection qualifies as the principal or first-listed diagnosis. Manifestations or conditions associated with the infection are sequenced after the systemic infection code. This order is indicated in the Tabular List through the use of the instructional notes **Code first** for the systemic infection and **Use additional code** for the associated condition (■ FIGURE 21-11).

Patient is seen for Q fever and associated endocarditis.

(1) **A78 Q fever**

(2) **I39 Endocarditis and heart valve disorders in diseases classified elsewhere**

Figure 21-11 ■ Example of Body System Disease Associated with an Infection

CODING CAUTION

Do not confuse the guidelines for sequencing of codes for causal organisms with the sequencing guidelines for etiology and manifestation. When an etiology/manifestation relationship exists, sequencing is specifically designated in ICD-10-CM through the use of conventions, such as brackets in the Index and highlighting in the Tabular List. These conventions direct coders to sequence the etiology first and the manifestation second.

The exception to this guideline is when a localized infection is described with a code from a body system chapter but the causal organism is *not* identified with a combination code. Assign the localized infection from the body system chapter as the first code. Assign a secondary code from the block **Bacterial and viral infectious agents (B95-B97)**, which contains codes to identify the infectious agent in diseases classified elsewhere. This order is indicated in the Tabular List through the use of the instructional notes **Code first** for the primary disease and **Use additional code** for the infectious organism (■ Figure 21-12).

OGCR provides specific guidelines for sequencing codes related to HIV/AIDS and sepsis/severe sepsis/septic shock. These are discussed next.

Arranging Codes for HIV and AIDS

Sequencing of codes for HIV and AIDS depends on the circumstances of admission. Review the documentation and abstracting notes carefully to determine whether the patient was seen or admitted for treatment related directly to HIV or if the reason for the encounter was an unrelated condition, such as a traumatic injury.

Patient is seen for infective myocarditis due to methicillin-resistant staphylococcal aureus.

(1) **I40.0 Infective myocarditis**

(2) **B95.62 Methicillin resistant Staphylococcal aureus as the cause of diseases classified elsewhere**

Figure 21-12 ■ Example of Sequencing for a Body System Disease Due to an Infectious Organism

Admission for HIV

When a patient is admitted for an HIV-related condition, assign and sequence codes as follows (OGCR I.C.1.a.2)(a)) (see Figure 21-8):

1. Assign code **B20 Human immunodeficiency virus [HIV] disease.**
2. Assign code(s) for all reported HIV-related condition(s).

Admission for a Condition Not Related to HIV

When a patient with HIV disease is admitted for an unrelated condition, assign and sequence codes as follows (OGCR I.C.1.a.2)(b)) (■ Figure 21-13):

1. Assign code(s) for the unrelated condition(s).
2. Assign code **B20 Human immunodeficiency virus [HIV] disease.**
3. Assign code(s) for all reported HIV-related condition(s).

Arranging Codes for Severe Sepsis and Septic Shock

Sequencing of codes for severe sepsis and septic shock is dependent on the circumstances of admission and when the condition develops.

Severe Sepsis

OGCR provide specific sequencing guidelines based on whether severe sepsis is the reason for admission or develops after admission.

Patient is admitted for repair of a partial right rotator cuff tear.

Patient also has AIDS with Kaposi's sarcoma of the skin.

(1) **M75.111 Incomplete rotator cuff tear or rupture of right shoulder, not specified as traumatic**

(2) **B20 Human immunodeficiency virus [HIV] disease**

(3) **C46.0 Kaposi's sarcoma of skin**

Figure 21-13 ■ Example of Sequencing for an AIDS Patient Admitted with a Non-related Condition

Severe Sepsis Present at Admission. When severe sepsis meets the requirements of principal diagnosis, assign and sequence codes as follows (OGCR I.C.1.d.1)(b) and OGCR I.C.1.d.3)):

1. Assign a code for the underlying systemic infection or assign **A41.9 Sepsis, unspecified** if the infection is not specified.
2. Assign either **R65.20 Severe sepsis without septic shock** or **R65.21 Severe sepsis with septic shock**, as appropriate.
3. Assign code(s) for acute organ dysfunction.

Severe Sepsis That Develops after Admission. When severe sepsis develops after admission, assign and sequence codes as follows:

1. Assign code(s) for the condition(s) that meet the requirements of principal diagnosis.
2. Assign a code for the underlying systemic infection or assign **A41.9 Sepsis, unspecified** if the infection is not specified.
3. Assign either **R65.20 Severe sepsis without septic shock** or **R65.21 Severe sepsis with septic shock**, as appropriate.
4. Assign code(s) for acute organ dysfunction.

Septic Shock

OGCR provide specific sequencing guidelines based on whether septic shock is the reason for admission or develops after admission.

Septic Shock Present at Admission. When septic shock meets the requirements of principal diagnosis, assign and sequence codes as follows (OGCR I.C.1.d.2)):

1. Assign a code for the underlying systemic infection or assign **A41.9 Sepsis, unspecified** if the infection is not specified.
2. Assign code **R65.21 Severe sepsis with septic shock.**
3. Assign code(s) for acute organ dysfunction, when applicable.

Septic Shock That Develops after Admission. When septic shock develops after admission, assign and sequence codes as follows (OGCR I.C.1.d.3)) (■ FIGURE 21-14):

1. Assign code(s) for the condition(s) that meet the requirements of principal diagnosis.
2. Assign a code for the underlying systemic infection or assign **A41.9 Sepsis, unspecified** if the infection is not specified.
3. Assign code **R65.21 Severe sepsis with septic shock.**
4. Assign code(s) for acute organ dysfunction, when applicable.

Patient is admitted for repair of mitral valve stenosis. Two days after the procedure, the patient experiences septic shock due to methicillin-resistant staphylococcus aureus.

(1) **I05.0 Rheumatic mitral stenosis**

(2) **T81.4 Infection following a procedure**

(3) **A41.02 Sepsis due to methicillin resistant Staphylococcus aureus**

(4) **R65.21 Severe sepsis with septic shock**

Figure 21-14 ■ Example of Sequencing for a Patient Who Develops Septic Shock Following a Procedure

Guided Example of Arranging Infectious Disease Codes

To practice skills for sequencing codes for infectious and parasitic diseases, continue with the example from earlier in the chapter about patient Faye Gillis, who was admitted to Branton Medical Center due to acute respiratory failure.

Follow along in your ICD-10-CM manual as Susanna Vannote, CPC, sequences the codes. Check off each step after you complete it.

⇨ First, Susanna confirms codes she has assigned.

- ❑ **R65.20, Severe sepsis without septic shock**
- ❑ **J96.00, Acute respiratory failure, unspecified whether with hypoxia or hypercapnia**
- ❑ **A41.51, Sepsis due to Escherichia coli [E. coli]**

⇨ Susanna refers back to the OGCR and instructional notes she read earlier.

- ❑ OGCR I.C.1.d.1)(b) states **The coding of severe sepsis requires a minimum of 2 codes: first a code for the underlying systemic infection, followed by a code from subcategory R65.2.**
- ❑ This tells her that the code **A41.51** for the systemic infection should be sequenced before **R65.20**.
- ❑ She is still unsure if **R65.20** should be sequenced before or after **J96.00**.
- ❑ She refers back to the instructional note under subcategory **R65.2** that states **Use additional code to identify specific acute organ dysfunction, such as: acute respiratory failure (J96.0-).**
- ❑ This tells her that **J96.00** should be sequenced after **R65.20**, because it says that **J96.00-** is an additional code.

Susanna finalizes the codes and sequencing for this case:

(1) **A41.51, Sepsis due to Escherichia coli [E. coli]**

(2) **R65.20, Severe sepsis without septic shock**

(3) **J96.00, Acute respiratory failure, unspecified whether with hypoxia or hypercapnia**

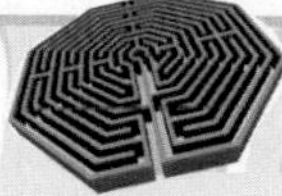

Coding Practice

Now it is your turn to practice sequencing codes for infectious and parasitic diseases. Refer to the ***Tip*** at the end of the mini-medical-record if you need a little extra help.

Exercise 21.4 Arranging Codes for Infectious Diseases

Instructions: Read the mini-medical-record of each patient's encounter, review the information abstracted in Exercise 21.2, assign ICD-10-CM diagnosis codes (CM) using the Index and Tabular List, and sequence them correctly.

1. Date: 2/14/yy Location: Branton Medical Group
Provider: James Cruickshank, MD
Patient: Terrence Kestler Gender: M Age: 26
Reason for encounter: lesions on the skin of this HIV positive patient
Assessment: Kaposi's sarcoma of the skin
Plan: refer to oncologist to evaluate extent of the cancer and determine treatment plan

Tip: Refer to OGCR I.C.1.a.2)(a) for sequencing instructions.

2 CM Codes __________ __________

2. Date: 2/14/yy Location: Branton Medical Center Emergency Department
Provider: Cynthia Hiatt, MD
Patient: Terrence Kestler Gender: M Age: 26
Reason for encounter: toe pain after a horse stepped on his foot
Assessment: fractured distal phalanx of great toe on the right foot, AIDS patient with Kaposi's sarcoma of the lymph nodes which was not treated at this encounter
Plan: reduced fracture and applied cast, crutches, FU office 2 weeks

(continued)

2. (continued)

Tip: Refer to OGCR I.C.1.a.2)(b) and (f) for coding and sequencing instructions. Also, remember to assign an external cause code.

4 CM Codes __________ __________ __________ __________

3. Date: 2/14/yy Location: Branton Medical Center Provider: James Cruickshank, MD
Patient: Liz Spagnola Gender: F Age: 70
Reason for encounter: called in for a consult on Staphylococcus aureus pneumonia
Assessment: culture result shows MSSA
Plan: IV teicoplanin was successful and patient was discharged with instructions to help prevent recurrence

Tip: Refer to OGCR I.C.1.c.

1 CM Code __________

4. Date: 2/14/yy Location: Branton Medical Group
Provider: James Cruickshank, MD
Patient: Donald Plewa Gender: M Age: 45
Reason for encounter: HIV positive patient with no related conditions presents with dysuria, weakness, and fever
Assessment: urosepsis (UTI) d/t E.coli (non-Shiga toxin-producing)
Plan: antibiotics

Tip: Urosepsis is not sepsis or septicemia. Refer to OGCR I.C.1.a.2)(d) and I.C.1.b.

3 CM Codes __________ __________ __________

(continued)

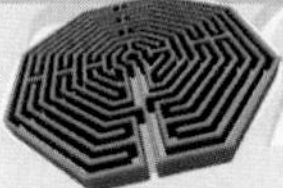

Coding Practice (continued)

5. Date: 2/14/yy Location: Branton Medical Center Provider: James Cruickshank, MD

Patient: Rhea Niederhauser Gender: F Age: 77

Reason for encounter: admitted from SNF 1 day post-hospital-discharge with 102 F fever, dyspnea, heart rate 100 per minute, low BP

(continued)

5. (continued)

Assessment: *severe sepsis d/t nosocomial MRSA aureus and has associated heart failure*

Plan: *deceased*

Tip: Refer to OGCR I.C.1.d.1) and 2).

3 CM Codes __________ __________ __________

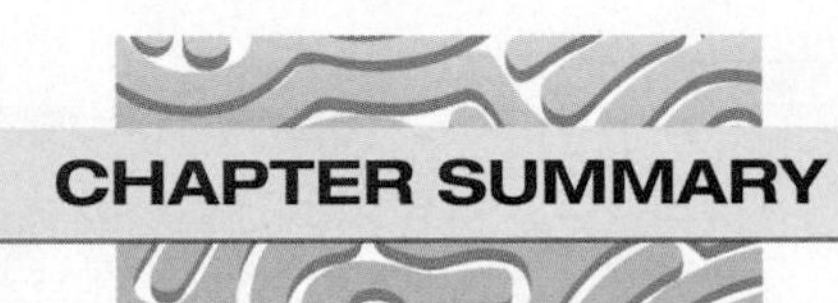

CHAPTER SUMMARY

In this chapter you learned that:

- Infectious and parasitic diseases are not a body system; they are systemic diseases that affect the entire body.
- ICD-10-CM Chapter 1, Certain Infectious and Parasitic Diseases (A00-B99), contains 22 blocks or subchapters that are divided by the type of infection.
- Coders always need to identify the scientific name of the infectious organism and subtype, as well as associated complications or manifestations.
- Although coders do not need to memorize every guideline, they should memorize the *fact* that OGCR exist for HIV and AIDS and sepsis, severe sepsis, and septic shock; they should refer to OGCR every time they code these conditions.
- Codes from this ICD-10-CM chapter are sequenced first when the systemic infection qualifies as the principal or first-listed diagnosis, followed by codes for associated conditions.
- OGCR I.C.1. provides detailed discussion of assigning and sequencing codes for HIV, sepsis, and septic shock.

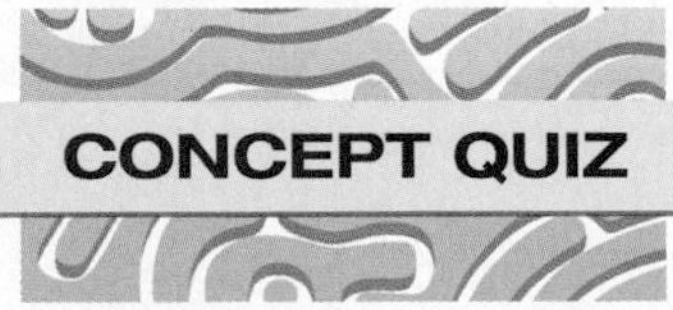

CONCEPT QUIZ

Take a moment to look back at your trip through infectious and parasitic diseases and solidify your skills. This is your opportunity to pull together everything you have learned.

Completion

Instructions: Write the term that answers each question based on the information you learned in this chapter. Choose from the list below. Some choices may be used more than once and some choices may not be used at all. Refer to the discussion in this chapter and the Glossary at the end of this book if you need a little extra help.

asymptomatic
bacteria
herpes zoster
HIV
HPV
inconclusive
leprosy
opportunistic
parasites
septic shock
severe sepsis
smallpox
trichinosis
tuberculosis
viruses

1. ______________ is a virus that causes cervical cancer.
2. ______________ is a roundworm infestation caused by eating raw pork.
3. ______________ is a chronic bacterial disease characterized by the formation of nodules on the surface of the body.

4. _______________ is organ malfunction due to sepsis.

5. _______________ is a virus that causes AIDS.

6. A disease that attacks people with weakened immune systems but does not develop in those with healthy immune systems is a(an) _______________ infection.

7. _______________ is a painful, blistering skin rash due to the varicella-zoster virus that causes chickenpox.

8. HIV serology that is neither positive or negative is _______________.

9. *Escherichia coli* is an example of _______________.

10. _______________ is diagnosed when blood pressure remains low despite intensive treatment.

Multiple Choice

Instructions: Circle the letter of the best answer to each question based on the information you learned in this chapter. Refer to the discussion in this chapter and the Glossary at the end of this book if you need a little extra help.

1. Examples of protozoa include
   A. *Trichomonas vaginalis* and *Giardia*.
   B. varicella and herpes.
   C. HIV and AIDS.
   D. *Escherichia coli* and *Pseudomonas aeruginosa*.
2. Pneumonia and pharyngitis are examples of
   A. systemic diseases.
   B. infectious agents.
   C. localized infections.
   D. bacteria.
3. The word roots for causal organisms often describe their
   A. frequency.
   B. shape.
   C. toxicity.
   D. immunity.
4. AIDS is
   A. the cause of HIV.
   B. asymptomatic HIV.
   C. an opportunistic infection.
   D. the final stage of HIV.
5. Which of the following is a key criterion for abstracting HIV/AIDS?
   A. Is HIV acute or chronic?
   B. Is HIV serology inconclusive?
   C. Is HIV shock documented?
   D. Is it considered curable?
6. What code should be assigned for a patient who is HIV positive with no symptoms?
   A. B20, HIV disease
   B. R75, Inconclusive laboratory evidence of HIV
   C. Z0.6, Exposure to HIV
   D. Z21, Asymptomatic HIV
7. *E. coli* sepsis with organ failure should be coded as
   A. sepsis.
   B. severe sepsis.
   C. septic shock.
   D. two unrelated infections.
8. When a patient is treated for any HIV-related illness, assign code
   A. B20, HIV disease.
   B. B97.35 HIV 2 as the cause of diseases classified elsewhere.
   C. Z0.6, Exposure to HIV.
   D. Z71.7, HIV counseling.
9. When septic shock develops after admission, what should the principal diagnosis code be?
   A. The condition that is responsible for the admission and the services provided
   B. A code for the systemic infection
   C. R65.21 Severe sepsis with septic shock
   D. A41.9 Sepsis, unspecified
10. A patient with AIDS and associated Kaposi's sarcoma is admitted for repair of a torn rotator cuff. What condition is the principal diagnosis?
    A. HIV disease
    B. Kaposi's sarcoma
    C. HIV as the cause of diseases classified elsewhere
    D. rotator cuff tear

CODING CHALLENGE

Now it is your turn to demonstrate coding all aspects of infectious and parasitic diseases. Refer back to the examples and discussion in this chapter when you need a little extra help. Use your medical dictionary and anatomy references when needed.

Instructions: Read the mini-medical-record of each patient's encounter, then abstract, assign, and sequence ICD-10-CM diagnosis codes (CM) using the Index and Tabular List. Write the code(s) on the line provided.

1. Date: 2/19/yy Location: Branton Medical Group Provider: James Cruickshank, MD

Patient: Dana Slaybaugh Gender: F Age: 52

Reason for encounter: bloody diarrhea, patient states she is worried she might have cancer

Assessment: Symptoms started a few days after eating hamburgers at a cookout. Hemorrhagic colitis (*inflammation and bleeding of the colon*) due to E. coli.

Plan: call back if it does not improve within 1 week

Tip: Follow the cross-references in the Index.

1 CM Code __________

2. Date: 2/19/yy Location: Branton Medical Group Provider: James Cruickshank, MD

Patient: Alejandro Jarvia Gender: M Age: 44

Reason for encounter: blisters and scabs on face and left side of body, unexplained pain

Assessment: disseminated herpes zoster

Plan: Rx pain management medication, Calamine lotion applied topically to blisters and rash, RTO 1 week.

1 CM Code __________

3. Date: 2/19/yy Location: Branton Medical Group Provider: James Cruickshank, MD

Patient: Wendell Kochan Gender: M Age: 23

Reason for encounter: HIV testing (screening) after unprotected sex with an infected partner

(continued)

3. (continued)

Assessment: exposure to HIV

Plan: FU in 1 week for results

Tip: You need two Z codes, one for the reason for the encounter and a second for the exposure.

2 CM Codes __________ __________

4. Date: 2/19/yy Location: Branton Medical Center Provider: James Cruickshank, MD

Patient: Corine Guan Gender: F Age: 43

Reason for encounter: antiviral therapy

Assessment: chronic hepatitis due to hepatitis B

Plan: RTO as protocol for antiviral therapy stipulates, FU liver function tests at next office visit

1 CM Code __________

5. Date: 2/19/yy Location: Branton Medical Center Provider: James Cruickshank, MD

Patient: Sasha Fleckenstein Gender: F Age: 22

Reason for encounter: diarrhea and vomiting, fever

Assessment: gastroenteritis d/t salmonella food poisoning

Plan: Rx antibiotics. RTO 1 week following discharge

1 CM Code __________

6. Date: 2/19/yy Location: Branton Medical Center Provider: James Cruickshank, MD

Patient: Byron Forness Gender: M Age: 84

Reason for encounter: redness on neck is spreading

Assessment: cellulitis due to group F streptococcus infection of tracheostomy tube

Plan: Discharge to skilled nursing facility. Rx oral antibiotics and antibiotic cream.

3 CM Codes __________ __________ __________

7. Date: 2/19/yy Location: Branton Medical Center Provider: James Cruickshank, MD

Patient: Tessa Slaybaugh Gender: F Age: 58

Reason for encounter: recent trip to Sumatra without malaria prophylaxis, 4 day history of fever, sudden onset (SO) left upper quadrant (LUQ) pain and tenderness

Assessment: plasmodium vivax malaria with splenic rupture

Plan: post ICU discharge: 14 day course of Chloroquine to be taken with food, RTO in 1 week

Tip: *Plasmodium vivax* is the type of malaria.

1 CM Code __________

8. Date: 2/19/yy Location: Branton Medical Group

Provider: James Cruickshank, MD

Patient: Clifton Parlin Gender: M Age: 7

Reason for encounter: itchy scalp and rash on the child's neck. Parent suspects that they have identified nits in the patient's hair.

Assessment: head lice infestation

Plan: Advise head lice shampoo, (Rid, Nix).

Tip: Read and follow the cross-reference in the Index.

1 CM Code __________

9. Date: 2/19/yy Location: Branton Medical Group

Provider: James Cruickshank, MD

Patient: Rudy Koepsell Gender: M Age: 29

Reason for encounter: numbness (temperature sensations), multiple, pale, diffuse cutaneous lesions

Assessment: BL leprosy (borderline lepromatous leprosy)

Plan: multidrug therapy (Dapsone, Rifampin, and Clofazimine) regime initiated, RTO in 3 months

1 CM Code __________

10. Date: 2/19/yy Location: Branton Medical Center Provider: James Cruickshank, MD

Patient: Kenneth Dudney Gender: M Age: 30

Reason for encounter: admitted from emergency department due to septic shock

Assessment: sepsis is due to an infected tooth that patient has had for six months

Plan: Rx antibiotic, FU with dentist for extraction when patient is organism free.

Tip: Because the infectious organism is not identified, you need to assign a default NOS code for sepsis. Refer also to OGCR I.C.1.d.1) and 2).

3 CM Codes __________ __________ __________

KEEP ON CODING

As a coder, you can never have too much experience. Apply everything you have learned in this chapter to code the following diagnostic statements. Use the OGCR and instructional notes in the Tabular List to help determine how many codes are required.

Instructions: Read the diagnostic statement, then use the Index and Tabular List to assign and sequence ICD-10-CM (CM) diagnosis codes. Write the code(s) on the line provided.

1. Salmonella pyelonephritis: CM Code(s) __________
2. Glanders: CM Code(s) __________
3. Infant botulism: CM Code(s) __________
4. Gonococcal orchitis: CM Code(s) __________
5. Fatal familial insomnia: CM Code(s) __________

6. Postmeasles otitis media: CM Code(s) ____________________
7. Thrush: CM Code(s) ____________________
8. Meningococcal meningitis: CM Code(s) ____________________
9. Acute military tuberculosis: CM Code(s) ____________________
10. Monkeypox: CM Code(s) ____________________
11. Cat scratch fever: CM Code(s) ____________________
12. Postherpetic trigeminal neuralgia: CM Code(s) ____________________
13. Eczema herpeticum: CM Code(s) ____________________
14. Viral pericarditis, coxsackie: CM Code(s) ____________________
15. Toxoplasma myositis: CM Code(s) ____________________
16. Rhodesiense trypanosomiasis: CM Code(s) ____________________
17. Whooping cough due to *Bordetella pertussis* with pneumonia: CM Code(s) ____________________
18. Acute hepatitis E: CM Code(s) ____________________
19. Sepsis due to *Escherichia coli*: CM Code(s) ____________________
20. Jungle yellow fever: CM Code(s) ____________________
21. African histoplasmosis: CM Code(s) ____________________
22. Sequelae of leprosy: CM Code(s) ____________________
23. Rabies: CM Code(s) ____________________
24. Chlamydial conjunctivitis: CM Code(s) ____________________
25. West Nile fever: CM Code(s) ____________________

CODER'S TOOLBOX

The following resources are a starting point for learning more about infectious and parasitic diseases. The > symbol indicates a menu selection within the website in order to navigate to a specific page.

AIDS.gov **http://aids.gov/**

American Academy of Pediatrics (AAP) > Health Topics > Immunization **http://www.aap.org/immunization/izschedule.html**

Centers for Disease Control and Prevention > HIV **http://www.cdc.gov/hiv/default.htm**

Healthy Kids > Health Issues > Infections **http://www.healthychildren.org/English/health-issues/conditions/infections/Pages/default.aspx**

Infectious Disease Research Institute (IDRI) **http://www.idri.org/**

Infectious Diseases Society of America (IDSA) **http://www.idsociety.org/Index.aspx**

KidsHealth > Parents > Infections **http://kidshealth.org/parent/infections/index.html**

New York State > Department of Health > Communicable Disease Fact Sheets **http://www.health.ny.gov/diseases/communicable/**

Parasites In Humans **http://www.parasitesinhumans.org/**

Surviving Septicemia Campaign (SCC) **http://ssc.sccm.org/**

University of California, San Francisco > HIV **http://hivinsite.ucsf.edu/**

22

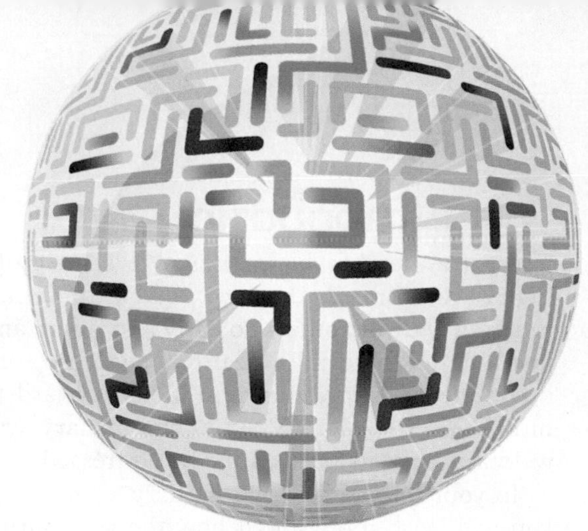

Diseases of the Genitourinary System (N00-N99)

Learning Objectives

After completing this chapter, you should have the skills to:

- Spell and define the key words, medical terms, and abbreviations related to the urinary system and male and female reproductive systems.
- Discuss the structure, function, and common conditions of the urinary system and male and female reproductive systems.
- Identify the main characteristics of coding for diseases of the urinary system and male and female reproductive systems.
- Abstract diagnostic information from the medical record for conditions of the urinary system and male and female reproductive systems.
- Assign codes for diseases of the urinary system and male and female reproductive systems.
- Arrange codes for diseases of the urinary system and male and female reproductive systems.
- Code neoplasms of the urinary system and male and female reproductive systems.
- Discuss the Official Guidelines for Coding and Reporting related to diseases of the genitourinary system.

Key Terms and Abbreviations

Bartholin's gland
blood creatinine
benign prostatic hyperplasia (BPH)
benign prostatic hypertrophy (BPH)
bulbo-urethral gland
clitoris
dialysis
dialysis-related amyloidosis (DRA)
ductal
electrolytes
fallopian tubes
genitourinary (GU) system
glomerular filtration rate (GFR)
glomerulus
hematuria
hemodialysis (HD)
impotence
kidneys
labia major
labia minor
lobular
lower urinary tract symptoms (LUTS)
nephrons
ovaries
penis
peritoneal dialysis (PD)
peritoneal membrane
polycystic kidney disease
polynephritis
prostate
prostate specific antigen (PSA)
reflux nephropathy
renal pelvis
reproductive ducts
salpingitis
testes
ureter
urethra
urinary bladder
urinary tract infection (UTI)
uterus
vagina

In addition to the key terms listed here, students should know the terms defined within tables in this chapter.

Chapter Outline

- **Genitourinary System Refresher**
- **Coding Overview of the Genitourinary System**
- **Abstracting for the Genitourinary System**
- **Assigning Codes for the Genitourinary System**
- **Arranging Codes for the Genitourinary System**
- **Coding Neoplasms of the Genitourinary System**

ICD-10-CM codes in this chapter are from the ICD-10-CM 2014 Draft code set from the Department of Health and Human Services, Centers for Disease Control and Prevention.

INTRODUCTION

Every traveler has his or her own strategy for managing restroom needs during a road trip. Some limit how much they drink, others go early and often, and some are just able to "hold it." Regardless, when travelling on an interstate highway, everyone looks forward to the next blue Rest Area sign. Whether the urinary system works well or poorly, its needs must be addressed.

In your tour of the genitourinary system in this chapter you will learn more about how the genitourinary system works, why sometimes it does not work as it should, and how physicians treat these conditions. Most importantly, you will practice coding for patient encounters related to genitourinary diseases and conditions, a skill that requires you to abstract information from the medical record, assign correct codes, and arrange the codes in the proper order.

A urologist specializes in diagnosing and treating conditions of the urinary tract and male reproductive organs, and a nephrologist specializes in diagnosing and treating conditions of the kidney. A gynecologist specializes in diagnosing and treating conditions of the female reproductive organs. Primary care physicians treat common conditions affecting the genitourinary system and refer more complex cases to a specialist.

Although you may already be familiar with many of the structures in this system, do not be surprised if you encounter new terms. As you read this chapter, open up your medical terminology book to the chapters on the urinary system and the male and female reproductive systems. Keep a medical dictionary handy to refresh your memory of any unfamiliar terms. Think of these resources as your travel brochures that tell you more about an area. This way, you have the information you need at your fingertips.

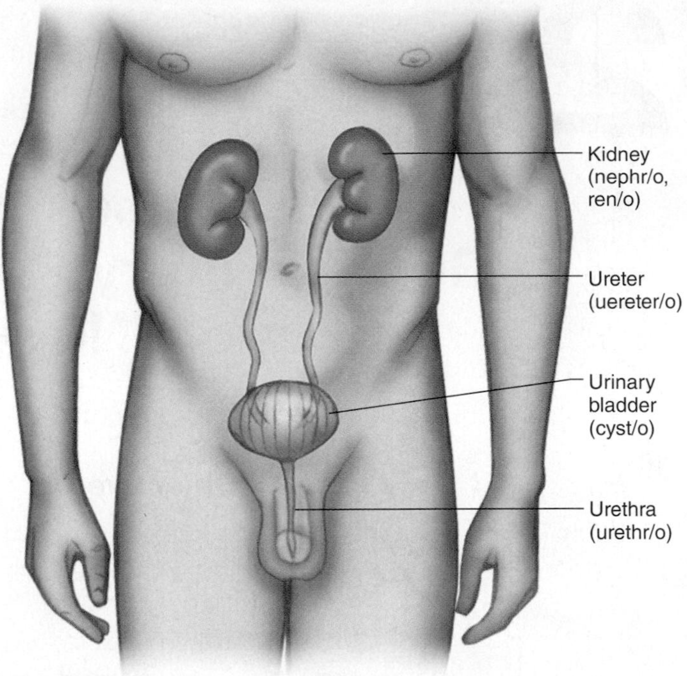

Figure 22-1 ■ The Urinary System

GENITOURINARY SYSTEM REFRESHER

The **genitourinary (GU) system** includes the urinary system and the male and female genital, or reproductive, systems. The function of the urinary system is to filter, store, and remove waste products from the blood and maintain homeostasis. The function of the genital system is sexual reproduction. The urinary and reproductive systems are grouped together in the coding manual because they arise from the same embryonic tissue, use common structures, and are in close physical proximity. Each major section of this chapter is divided into subsections on the urinary, male reproductive, and female reproductive systems.

Urinary System Refresher

The urinary system consists of two kidneys, two ureters, the urinary bladder, and the urethra (■ FIGURE 22-1). The **kidneys** produce urine and regulate the level of **electrolytes** and body fluid (■ FIGURE 22-2). The **nephrons** are the functioning part of each kidney and filter waste from the blood, beginning with the **glomerulus**, a cluster of capillaries that separates the urinary space from the blood. The **renal pelvis** of each kidney collects urine, which then passes through the **ureter** (*a tube that drains each kidney*) to the **urinary bladder**, a muscular sac that holds urine until it is expelled through the **urethra** (*the tube that carries urine out of the body*).

Male Reproductive System Refresher

The male reproductive system consists of the external genital organ, internal genital organs, and associated glands (■ FIGURE 22-3). The **penis**, the external male sex organ, is a conduit for the urethra, which carries urine and semen out of the body. The male urethra is approximately eight inches long. Internal genital organs are the **testes** and the **reproductive ducts**. Associated glands are the **prostate** and **bulbo-urethral glands**. The testes also function as part of the endocrine system.

Female Reproductive System Refresher

The female reproductive system also consists of external and internal genital organs (■ FIGURE 22-4, page 430). The external genital organs are the **labia major** and **labia minor** (*folds of flesh that surround and protect the opening to the vagina and urethra*), **Bartholin's gland** (*a gland that secretes mucus*), and the **clitoris** (*a small sensitive protrusion*). The internal genital organs consist of two **ovaries**, which produce

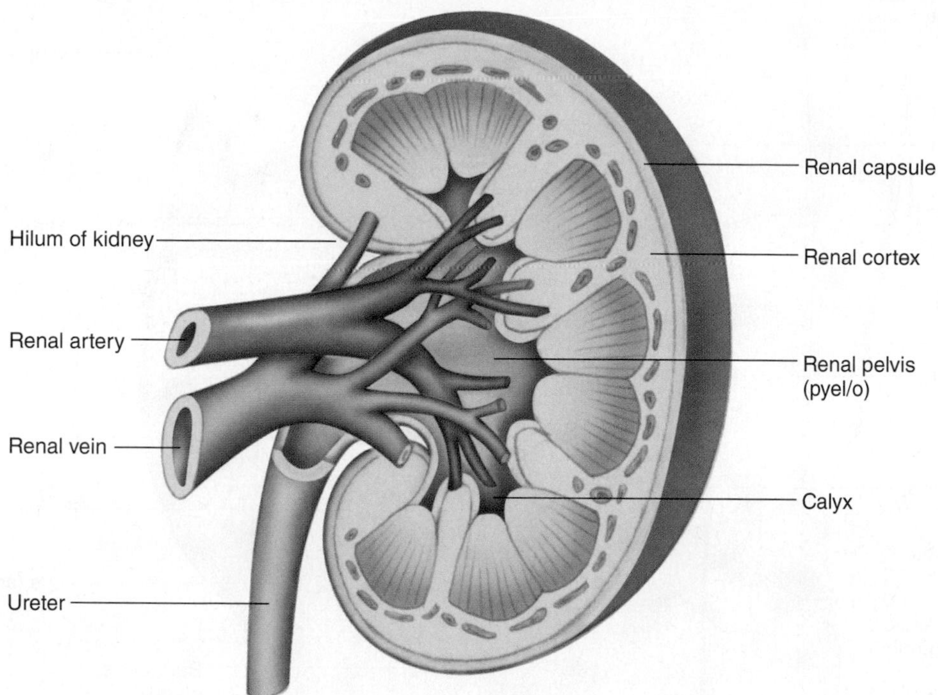

Figure 22-2 ■ The Kidney

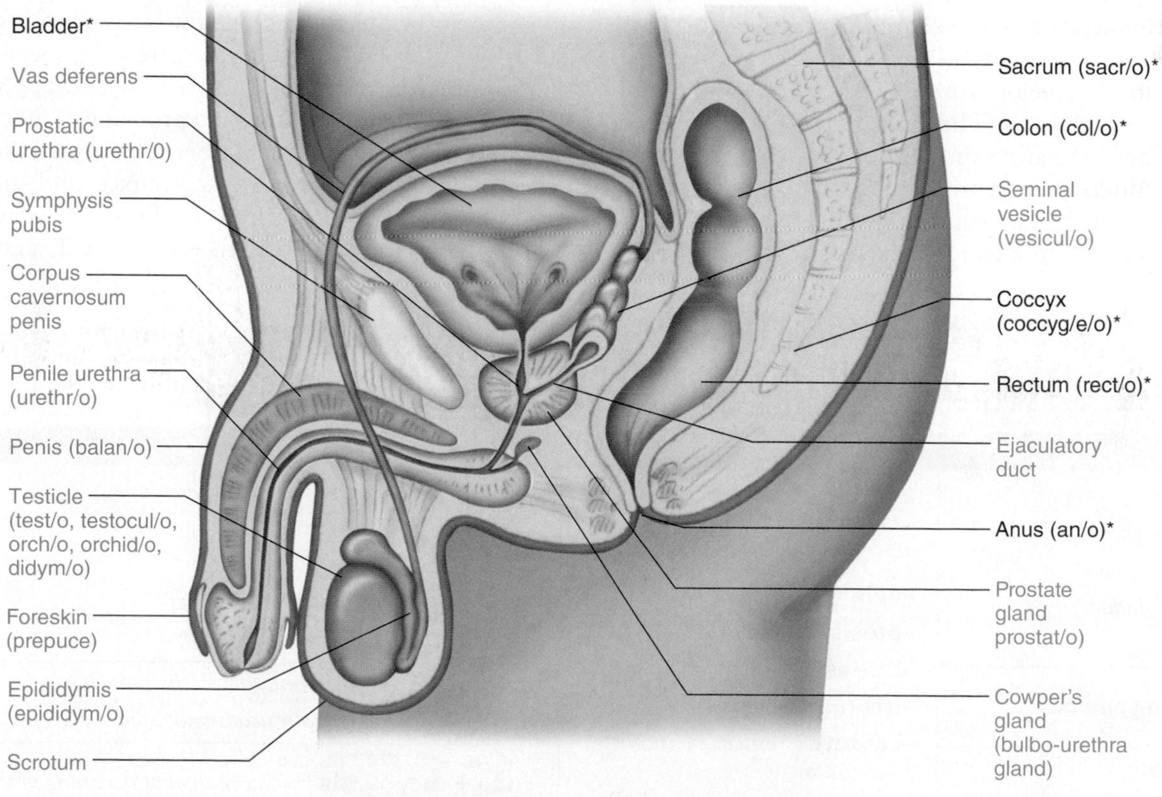

Figure 22-3 ■ The Male Reproductive System

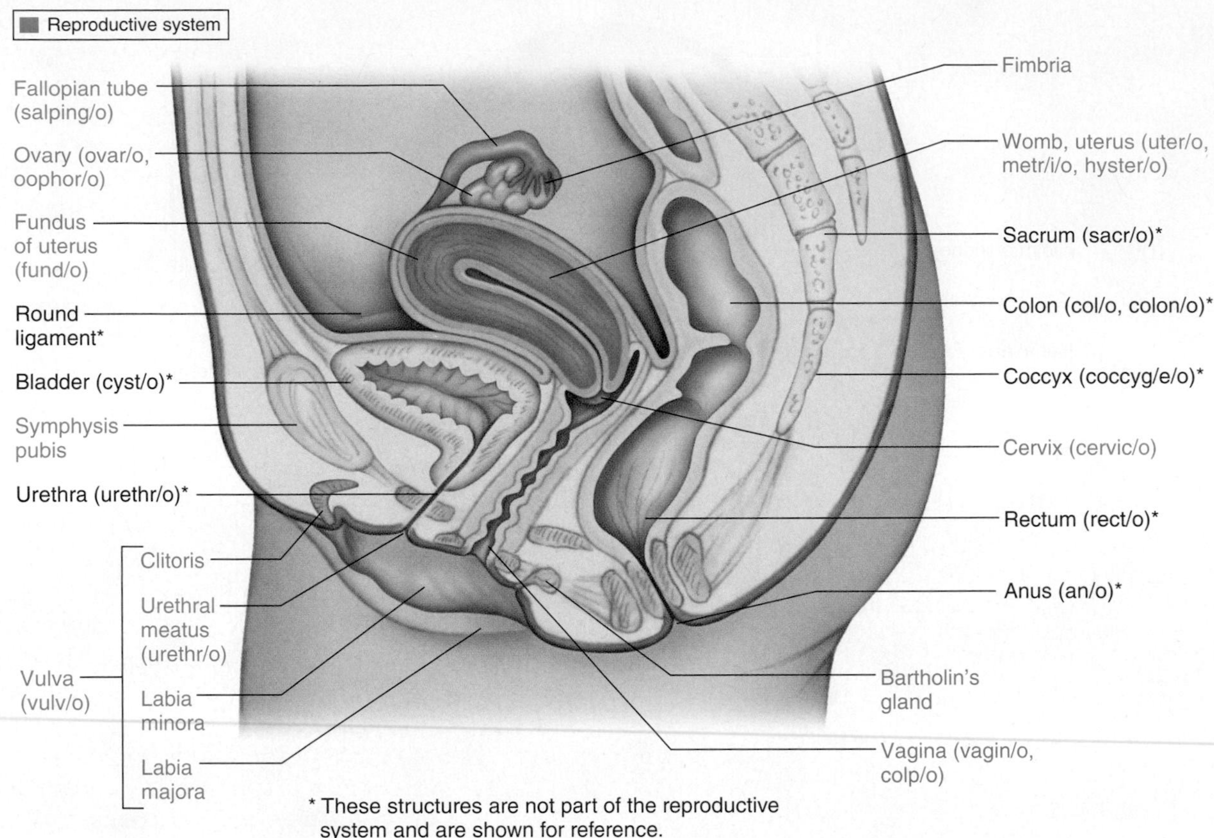

Figure 22-4 ■ The Female Reproductive System

eggs; two **fallopian tubes**, which transport eggs for fertilization and implantation in the uterus; the **uterus**, which is the womb for development of the fetus; and the **vagina**, which is the birth canal. The female urethra, which is one to two inches long and exits the body in front the vagina, does not function in reproduction. The female breasts are also part of the reproductive system. The ovaries also function as part of the endocrine system.

In the previous figures, each structure in the genitourinary system is labeled with its name as well as its medical terminology root/combining form, where applicable. As you learn about conditions and procedures that affect the genitourinary system, remember to apply medical terminology skills to use word roots, prefixes, and suffixes that you already know in order to define new terms related to the genitourinary system. Refer to ■ Table 22-1 for

Table 22-1 ■ **EXAMPLE OF CONSTRUCTING MEDICAL TERMS FOR GENITOURINARY SYSTEM**

Combining Form	Suffix	Complete Medical Term
nephr/o- (*kidney*) **hemat/o** (*blood*) **cyst/o-** (*bladder*)	**-uria** (*condition of urine*) **-ptosis** (*to droop*) **-lithiasis** (*condition of stones*) **-itis** (*inflammation*) **-ectomy** (*surgical excision*)	**nephro + ptosis** (*drooping of the kidney*) **cyst + ptosis** (*drooping of the bladder*) **hemat + uria** (*blood in urine*) **nephro + lithiasis** (*kidney stones*) **cysto + lithiasis** (*bladder stones*)
prostat/o (*prostate*)		**prostat + itis** (*inflammation of the prostate*) **prostat + ectomy** (*surgical removal of the prostate*)
end/o (*within*) **metr/i** (*uterus*) **hyster/o** (*uterus*)		**endo + metr + itis** (*inflammation of the lining of the uterus*) **hyster + ectomy** (*surgical removal of the uterus*)

a refresher on how to build medical terms related to the genitourinary system.

CODING CAUTION

Be alert for medical word terms that are spelled similarly but have different meanings.

prostat/o (*prostate*) and **proct/o** (*anus and rectum*)

salpingitis of the **fallopian tube** (*part of the female reproductive system*) and salpingitis of **Eustachian tube** (*located between the ear and the nasopharynx*)

ureter (*the two tubes that drain the kidneys into the bladder*) and **urethra** (*a single tube that carries urine from the bladder to the outside of the body*)

colp/o (*vagina*) and **col/o** or **colon/o** (*colon or large intestine*)

Conditions of the Urinary System

Urologic and kidney conditions are among the most common reasons for doctor visits and hospital admissions. Over 13% of women have a urinary tract infection each year; more than 10% of the population over age 20 has chronic kidney disease, according to the National Institutes of Health (NIH).

Diseases and disorders of the urinary system include infections and inflammations of nearly any anatomic site, glomerular diseases that attack the kidneys' filtering ability, kidney failure, and obstructions. Coders use medical resources, such as reference books on diseases, to understand conditions of the genitourinary system, diagnostic methods, and common treatments. Refer to ■ TABLE 22-2 for a summary of diseases affecting the urinary system.

In particular, coders must be familiar with the terminology related to chronic kidney disease.

Chronic Kidney Disease

Chronic kidney disease (CKD), also called chronic renal failure, is the slow loss of kidney function over a period of months or years. People are able to live long periods of time with decreased kidney function; symptoms of the disease may not appear until as little as 10% of kidney function remains. However, the loss of kidney function results in the build up of toxins in the body, which can have serious effects on most body functions, especially red

Table 22-2 ■ **COMMON DISEASES OF THE URINARY SYSTEM**

Condition	Definition
Acute kidney failure	The rapid loss of kidney function over a period of days or weeks
Acute tubular necrosis	Damage to the renal tubules due to reduced blood flow or toxins in the urine
Calculi	Stones that may accumulate in the kidneys, bladder, or ureters
Chronic kidney disease (CKD)	The slow loss of kidney function over a period of months or years
Cystitis	Bacterial infection of the urinary bladder; also called urinary tract infection (UTI)
Diabetic nephropathy	Accumulated damage to the glomerulus capillaries due to chronic high blood sugar
Glomerulonephritis	Inflammation of the glomerulus of the kidney, allowing protein and blood into the urine
Hydronephrosis	Distention of the renal pelvis due to excessive urine collection in the kidney, often due to ureteral obstruction (■ FIGURE 22-5, page 432)
Incontinence	The inability to control bladder muscles
Nephritic syndrome	A collection of disorders affecting the kidneys, characterized by nonpurulent inflammatory glomerular disorders that allow proteins and red blood cells to pass into the urine, resulting in proteinuria and hematuria (*blood in the urine*)
Nephroptosis	Downward placement of the kidney from its normal location
Nephrotic syndrome	A collection of disorders affecting the kidneys, characterized by proteinuria, but not hematuria
Pyelonephritis	Acute or chronic infection of the renal medulla and upper urinary tract as a result of untreated cystitis, also called polynephritis
Uremia	Toxic blood condition due to the inability of the kidneys to remove nitrogenous substances from the blood

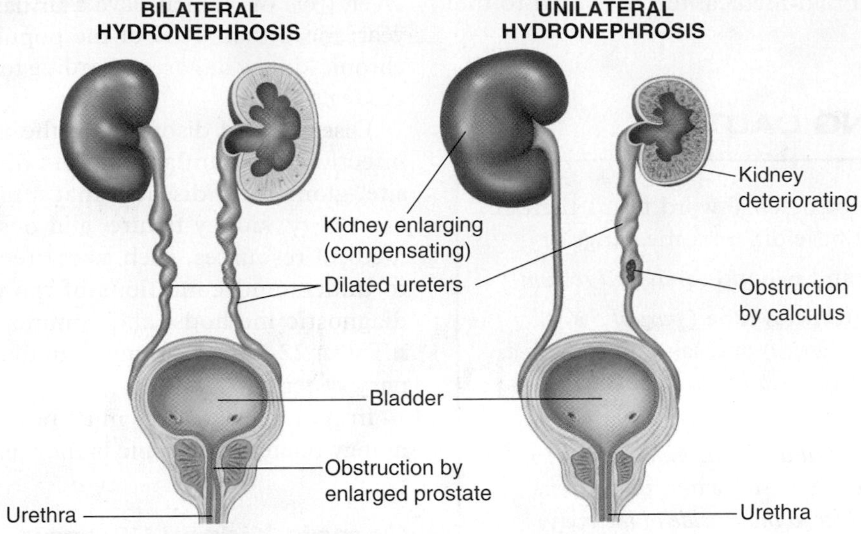

Figure 22-5 ■ Hydronephrosis: Bilateral and Unilateral

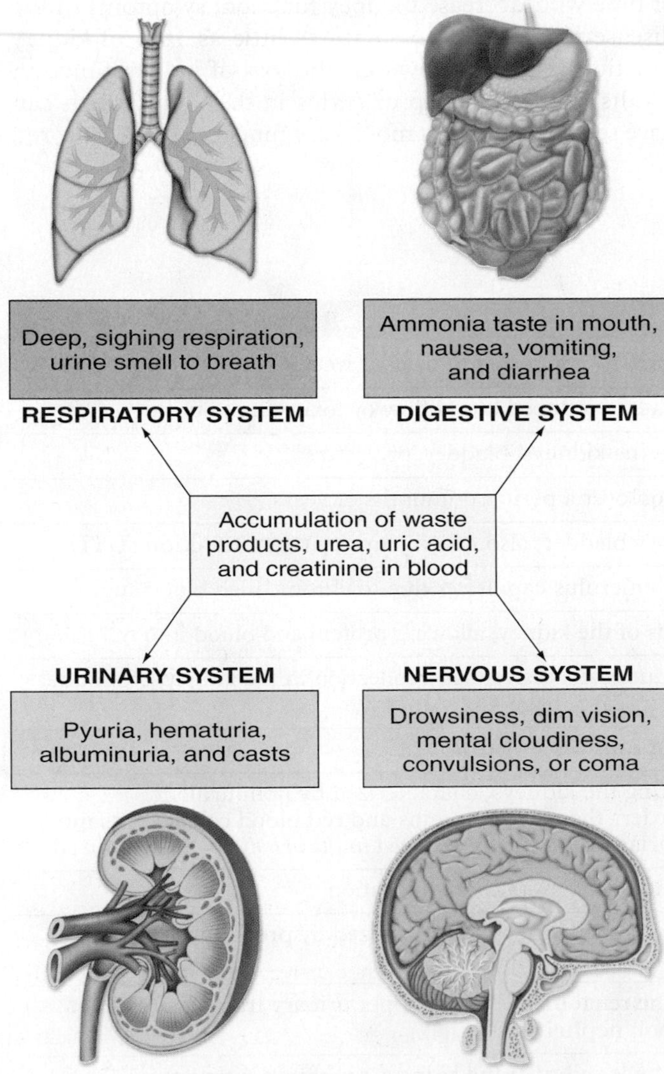

Figure 22-6 ■ Manifestations of Chronic Kidney Disease

blood cell production, blood pressure control, vitamin D, and bone health (■ FIGURE 22-6).

Diabetes and high blood pressure account for two-thirds of the cases of CKD, according to the National Kidney Foundation. Other conditions that cause CKD include **polycystic kidney disease**, glomerulonephritis, medications, autoimmune disorders such as lupus erythematosus and scleroderma, kidney stones, recurrent UTIs, and **reflux nephropathy**.

Kidney health is monitored through a wide range of blood tests that are included as part of most routine physical examinations. Persistent protein in the urine is an early sign of possible CKD. **Glomerular filtration rate (GFR)** is the preferred way to measure kidney function and determine the stage of kidney disease (■ TABLE 22-3). Physicians calculate GFR from the results of a **blood creatinine** test, the patient's age, race, gender, and other factors. They also use CT scans, ultrasounds, and kidney biopsies to help evaluate kidney disease.

CKD is not curable, but its progress can be slowed through diet, lifestyle, and medication. When CKD reaches

Table 22-3 ■ THE STAGES OF CHRONIC KIDNEY DISEASE

Stage	GFR	Description
1	130-90	Kidney damage with normal or slightly diminished kidney function
2	90-60	Kidney damage with mild reduction in kidney function
3	60-30	Moderate reduction kidney function
4	30-15	Severe reduction kidney function
5	15-0	Kidney failure; End Stage Renal Disease (ESRD)

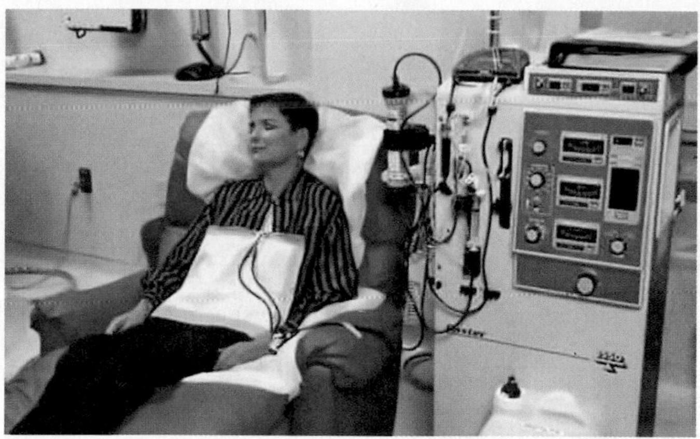

Figure 22-7 ■ A Patient Undergoing Hemodialysis. *Source: Michal Heron/Pearson Education.*

stage 5, the kidneys cease to function, and patients must receive dialysis or a kidney transplant in order to survive.

Dialysis is a treatment that filters the blood to remove waste, excess salt, and water. Over a half-million Americans are on dialysis, according to NIH. In hemodialysis (HD) the blood is processed through a machine (■ FIGURE 22-7). In peritoneal dialysis (PD), the peritoneal membrane (*the lining of the abdomen*) is used to filter the blood. Although 99% of dialysis is performed at centralized dialysis centers, according to Home Dialysis Central, it can be done at home with proper training and support. Medicare, which covers dialysis services for ESRD, requires that all patients be offered all dialysis options. Dialysis brings on its own complications as well, including infections and hemorrhaging through the dialysis port access site, electrolyte abnormalities, anemia, cardiac dysfunction, and dialysis-related amyloidosis (DRA) (*deposits of the starchy substance amyloid in the joints*) in long term dialysis patients. Kidney transplants are an option to treat ESRD, making the kidney one of the most frequently transplanted organs.

SUCCESS STEP

ESRD is the only specific disease that Medicare covers for the entire population, regardless of age. Individuals, their guardians, or spouses must meet Medicare eligibility requirement of 40 quarters of employment and are responsible for the usual Medicare deductibles and coinsurance. Medicare covers dialysis services and transplants.

Conditions of the Male Reproductive System

Conditions of the male reproductive system relate to both the structure and function of the organs. Components may be misshaped or out of place. When portions of the system malfunction, fertility and reproduction are affected. ■ TABLE 22-4 summarizes conditions of the male reproductive system covered in ICD-10-CM Chapter 14. Sexually transmitted diseases are classified in ICD-10-CM Chapter 1, Certain Infections and Parasitic Diseases (A00-B99).

Table 22-4 ■ **COMMON DISEASES OF THE MALE REPRODUCTIVE SYSTEM**

Condition	Definition
Enlarged prostate (EP)	The abnormal growth of epithelial cells of the prostate, causing compression or obstruction of the urethra; also called benign prostatic hypertrophy or hyperplasia (BPH)
Erectile dysfunction (ED)	The chronic inability to achieve or maintain a penile erection until ejaculation; also called impotence
Hydrocele	A fluid-filled sack in the scrotum caused by abnormal fetal development, injury, hernia, or blockages
Male factor infertility	A problem in the male genital system that diminishes reproduction, such as inability to ejaculate, lack of sperm production, or lack of live sperm
Prostatic intraepithelial neoplasia (PIN)	Neoplastic changes in the epithelial cells of the prostate ducts showing some features of cancer, but not invasive; a potential precursor of carcinoma or adenocarcinoma
Spermatocele	Benign cystic swelling of sperm in the ducts of of the epididymis

Conditions of the Female Reproductive System

Conditions of the female reproductive system are related to organ position, fertility, and reproduction; they include disorders of the breast in addition to the reproductive organs located in the pelvic region (■ TABLE 22-5, page 434). Sexually transmitted diseases are classified in ICD-10-CM Chapter 1, Certain Infections and Parasitic Diseases (A00-B99).

This section provides a general reference to help understand the most common diagnoses of the genitourinary system, but does not list everything you need to know. Use medical terminology skills discussed earlier in this chapter to learn the meaning of unfamiliar words. Remember to keep standard reference books handy in case you get stuck. Refer to the resources in the Coder's Toolbox at the end of this chapter to learn more about conditions affecting the genitourinary system.

Table 22-5 ■ **COMMON DISEASES OF THE FEMALE REPRODUCTIVE SYSTEM**

Condition	Definition
Cervical dysplasia	Abnormal changes in the cells on the surface of the cervix that may lead to cancer if not treated
Cervical intraepithelial neoplasia (CIN)	Cervical dysplasia seen on a cervical biopsy, classified as mild dysplasia (CIN I), moderate to marked dysplasia (CIN II), and sever dysplasia to cancer in situ (CIN III)
Endometriosis	The growth of endometrial tissue in any area other than the uterus
Female factor infertility	A problem in the female genital system that diminishes reproduction, such as scarring or obstruction of the fallopian tubes or abnormal interaction between the sperm and the mucous membrane in the cervix
Fibrocystic breast disease	Lumps of benign fibrous tissue in the breast
Genital prolapse	Downward displacement of the uterus or vagina to an abnormal position
Pelvic inflammatory disease (PID)	Inflammation of the female reproductive tract above the cervix
Squamous intraepithelial lesion (SIL)	Cervical dysplasia seen on a **PAP** smear, graded as low-grade (LSIL), high-grade (HSIL), and possibly cancerous or malignant
Vulvovaginitis	Inflammation of the vulva and vagina due to yeast, bacteria, viruses, parasites, or skin care products

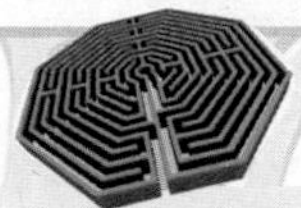

Coding Practice

Refresh your knowledge of terminology related to the genitourinary system. Use a medical terminology text or a website such as GlobalRph.com > Medical Terminology **http://www.globalrph.com/medterm.htm** to identify the meaning of word parts that may not be familiar.

Exercise 22.1 Genitourinary System Refresher

Instructions: Use your medical terminology skills and resources to define the following conditions related to the genitourinary system, then assign the default diagnosis code. Follow these steps:

- Use slash marks "/" to break down each term into its root(s) and suffix.
- Define the meaning of the word, based on the meaning of each word part.
- Assign the default ICD-10-CM diagnosis code for the condition using the Index and Tabular List.

Example: cystitis cyst/itis — Meaning: *inflammation of the bladder* — CM Code: *N30.90*

1. amenorrhea — Meaning ____________ CM Code ________
2. cystolithiasis — Meaning ____________ CM Code ________
3. dyspareunia — Meaning ____________ CM Code ________
4. hydrocele — Meaning ____________ CM Code ________
5. cystoptosis — Meaning ____________ CM Code ________
6. nephralgia — Meaning ____________ CM Code ________
7. urethrorrhagia — Meaning ____________ CM Code ________
8. nephrosis — Meaning ____________ CM Code ________
9. ureterocele — Meaning ____________ CM Code ________
10. pyelonephrosis — Meaning ____________ CM Code ________

CODING OVERVIEW OF THE GENITOURINARY SYSTEM

ICD-10-CM Chapter 14, Diseases of the Genitourinary System (N00-N99) contains 11 blocks or subchapters that are divided by anatomical site. Review the block names and code ranges listed at the beginning of Chapter 14 in the ICD-10-CM manual to become familiar with the content and organization.

ICD-10-CM Chapter 14 corresponds to ICD-9-CM Chapter 10 (580-629). Many codes have been added, deleted, expanded, combined, or moved. Codes for stress incontinence, nonspecific urethritis, and other ovarian hyperfunction have been moved to this chapter from other chapters in ICD-9-CM. Codes for vesicoureteral reflux, hematuria, salpingitis, and oophoritis are expanded and restructured in ICD-10-CM.

This chapter includes conditions of the male and female urinary system, the male reproductive system, the female breast, and disorders of the female genital tract. It does not include disorders related to pregnancy, which are classified in Chapter 15, Pregnancy, Childbirth and the Puerperium (O00-O9A). It also does not include injuries or congenital conditions of the genitourinary system.

ICD-10-CM provides Official Guidelines for Coding and Reporting (OGCR) diseases of the genitourinary system in OGCR section I.C.14. OGCR provides detailed discussion of chronic kidney disease. Additional OGCR related to hypertensive chronic kidney disease appear in OGCR I.C.9.a.2) and 3).

ABSTRACTING FOR THE GENITOURINARY SYSTEM

Disorders in this chapter have a wide range of abstracting criteria because there is a wide range of organs and types of disorders. Most conditions can be adequately abstracted by being attentive to the specific type and subtype of condition. Certain conditions require additional specific criteria, such as CKD and BPH. Refer to the following tables for guidance on how to abstract conditions of the urinary system (■ TABLE 22-6), male reproductive system (■ TABLE 22-7), and female reproductive system (■ TABLE 22-8), then work through the detailed example that follows. Remember that the abstracting questions are a guide and that not every question applies to, or can be answered for, every case. For example, laterality applies to many, but not all, disorders of the breast, but not to most disorders of the kidneys, ureters, ovaries, or fallopian tubes, all of which are paired organs. Also remember to abstract for symptoms and determine if they are integral to the confirmed diagnoses.

Table 22-6 ■ KEY CRITERIA FOR ABSTRACTING CONDITIONS OF THE URINARY SYSTEM

- ❑ What is the condition?
- ❑ What is the subtype or anatomic site?
- ❑ Does laterality apply?
- ❑ Is the condition acute or chronic?
- ❑ Is an obstruction documented?
- ❑ What is the infectious organism?
- ❑ Is there a history of recurrent UTIs?
- ❑ What stage is the chronic kidney disease?
- ❑ Does the patient receive dialysis?
- ❑ Is the patient on a transplant waiting list or the recipient of a transplant?
- ❑ Do any additional conditions coexist?

CODING CAUTION

Checking patients' gender helps prevent coding errors, such as picking up a code for the wrong gender, and also helps identify potential keying errors. Never assume a patient's gender based on the name because many common names are androgynous, such as Terry, Taylor, Lynn, or Pat. In addition, if ethnic names are unfamiliar, it is impossible to "guess." Examples are Shing, which is Chinese (male); Iffat, which is Muslim (female); or Gwandoya, which is African (male).

Table 22-7 ■ KEY CRITERIA FOR ABSTRACTING CONDITIONS OF THE MALE REPRODUCTIVE SYSTEM

- ❑ Verify the patient's gender.
- ❑ What is the condition?
- ❑ What is the subtype or anatomic site?
- ❑ Does laterality apply?
- ❑ Is the condition acute or chronic?
- ❑ Is an obstruction documented?
- ❑ What is the infectious organism?
- ❑ What symptoms are associated with prostatic hypertrophy?
- ❑ Do any additional conditions coexist?

Table 22-8 ■ KEY CRITERIA FOR ABSTRACTING CONDITIONS OF THE FEMALE REPRODUCTIVE SYSTEM

- ❑ Verify the patient's gender.
- ❑ What is the condition?
- ❑ What is the subtype or anatomic site?
- ❑ Does laterality apply?
- ❑ Is the condition acute or chronic?
- ❑ What is the infectious organism?
- ❑ Do any additional conditions coexist?

Guided Example of Abstracting for the Urinary System

Refer to the following example throughout this chapter to learn skills for abstracting, assigning, and sequencing urinary system codes. Chrystal Crago, CCA, is a fictitious coder who guides you through the coding process.

> Date: 02/21/yy Location: Branton Professional Group Provider: Ann Colyer, MD
>
> Patient: Ronald Coffield Gender: M Age: 53
>
> Reason for encounter: ESRD patient presents with ongoing complaints of extreme joint pain
>
> Assessment: joint pain is due to dialysis-related amyloidosis (DRA), ESRD, HD, on kidney transplant waiting list
>
> Plan: begin medication regimen despite side effects, and consider surgical intervention

Follow along as Chrystal Crago, CCA, abstracts the diagnosis. Check off each step after you complete it.

⇨ Chrystal reads through the entire record, with special attention to the reason for the encounter and the final assessment. She refers to the Key Criteria for Abstracting Conditions of the Urinary System (Table 22-6).

- ❑ She notes that the reason for the encounter is ongoing complaints extreme joint pain for an ESRD patient.
- ❑ *Which system does this case relate to: urinary, male reproductive, or female reproductive?* Urinary.
- ❑ *What are the presenting symptom(s)?* ongoing extreme joint pain
- ❑ *What is the condition?* amyloidosis
- ❑ *What is the subtype?* ESRD dialysis-related (DRA)
- ❑ *What stage is the chronic kidney disease?* By definition, ESRD is stage 5.
- ❑ *Does the patient receive dialysis?* Yes, HD is documented.
- ❑ *Is the patient on a transplant waiting list or the recipient of a transplant?* Yes.

⇨ At this time, Chrystal does not how many codes she will end up with. She will learn about this when she moves on to assigning codes.

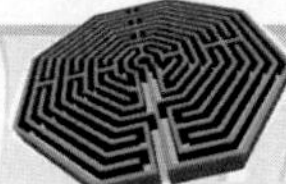

Coding Practice

Now it is your turn to practice abstracting diagnoses for the genitourinary system. Questions guide your analysis of each scenario.

Exercise 22.2 Abstracting for the Genitourinary System

Instructions: Read the mini-medical-record of each patient's encounter and answer the abstracting questions. Write the answer on the line provided. Do not assign any codes.

> **1.** Date: 2/23/yy Location: Branton Professional Group Provider: Ann Colyer, MD
>
> Patient: Wing Kwan Gender: F Age: 42
>
> Reason for encounter: surgery for endometriosis
>
> Assessment: endometriosis of the uterus
>
> Plan: FU in office 2 weeks
>
> a. Which system does this case relate to: urinary, male reproductive, or female reproductive?
>
> ______________________________
>
> *(continued)*

> **1.** (continued)
>
> b. What is the condition? ______________________________
>
> c. What is the subtype or anatomic site?
>
> ______________________________
>
> d. Is an infectious organism named? ______________________________

> **2.** Date: 2/23/yy Location: Branton Family Practice Provider: Kristen Conover, MD
>
> Patient: Robyn Lemmon Gender: F Age: 46
>
> Reason for encounter: painful lumps in both breasts
>
> Assessment: fibrocystic breast changes
>
> Plan: OTC acetaminophen, heat and ice as needed to relieve local pain
>
> *(continued)*

2. (continued)

Tip: Physicians use the term "changes" rather than the more traditional "disease" to avoid alarming patients.

a. Which system does this case relate to: urinary, male reproductive, or female reproductive?

____

b. What is the condition? _______________

c. What is the anatomic site? _______________

d. Does laterality apply? _______________

e. Is an obstruction documented? _______________

f. Do any additional conditions coexist? _______________

3. Date: 2/23/yy Location: Branton Professional Group Provider: Brent Eberhart, MD

Patient: Shawn Spates Gender: M Age: 61

Reason for encounter: occasional excruciating low back pain

Assessment: renal and ureteral calculi

Plan: medical expulsive therapy (MET) (*treatment with drugs to expel the calculi*) with tamsulosin (*an alpha blocker*)

a. Which system does this case relate to: urinary, male reproductive, or female reproductive?

____

b. What are the symptoms? _______________

c. What is the condition? _______________

d. Does the condition account for the symptom?

____

e. What is the anatomic site? _______________

f. Does laterality apply? _______________

g. Is an obstruction documented? _______________

4. Date: 2/24/yy Location: Branton Professional Group Provider: Brent Eberhart, MD

Patient: Dale Viera Gender: M Age: 81

Reason for encounter: FU on EP with obstruction and urinary retention

Assessment: little improvement seen despite multiple medication adjustments

Plan: schedule transurethral resection of the prostate (TURP)

a. Which system does this case relate to: urinary, male reproductive, or female reproductive?

____

b. What is the condition? _______________

c. Is an obstruction documented? _______________

d. What symptoms are associated with prostatic hypertrophy? _______________

5. Date: 2/24/yy Location: Branton Family Practice Provider: Kristen Conover, MD

Patient: Lyn Bowes Gender: F Age: 37

Reason for encounter: vaginal discharge, burning, redness in perineal area

Assessment: lab results show bacterial vaginitis due to staphylococcus, which is treatable

Plan: antibiotics

a. Which system does this case relate to: urinary, male reproductive, or female reproductive?

____

b. What are the symptoms? _______________

c. What is the condition? _______________

d. What is the subtype of the condition? _______________

e. What is the infectious organism? _______________

f. Is the organism resistant to antibiotic treatment?

____

(continued)

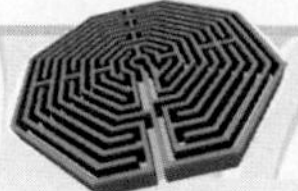

Coding Practice (continued)

6. Date: 2/24/yy Location: Branton Medical Center Provider: Ann Colyer, MD

Patient: Clare Browder Gender: F Age: 83

Reason for admission: skilled nursing facility (SNF) patient brought to emergency department with suspected UTI due to confusion and lack of cooperation; history of UTI over the past 2 years

Assessment: UTI due to E. coli, (non-Shiga toxin-producing)

Plan: administered IV antibiotics, discharged after 2 days to SNF with Rx

(continued)

6. (continued)

a. Which system does this case relate to: urinary, male reproductive, or female reproductive? ______

b. What is the condition? ______

c. Is an obstruction documented? ______

d. What is the infectious organism? ______
What is the subtype? ______

e. Is there a history of recurrent UTIs? ______

ASSIGNING CODES FOR THE GENITOURINARY SYSTEM

Two similar urinary system conditions, nephritic syndrome and nephrotic syndrome, demonstrate the importance of checking cross-referencing instructions in the Index in order to assign the most specific code available.

Assigning Codes for Nephritic Syndrome and Nephrotic Syndrome

An analysis of word roots and suffixes leads to similar descriptions of nephritis (inflammation of the kidney) and nephrosis (abnormal condition of the kidney), but, clinically, they are distinct conditions with distinct diagnostic criteria (Table 22-2).

Nephritic syndrome is a collection of disorders affecting the kidneys, characterized by nonpurulent inflammatory glomerular disorders that allow proteins and red blood cells to pass into the urine, resulting in proteinuria and hematuria. The Index entry for the Main Term **Syndrome** and the subterm **nephritic** provides a cross-referencing instruction, ***see also*** **Nephritis**. It provides additional subterms for **acute**, **chronic**, and **rapidly progressive** (■ Figure 22-8). The subterm **with edema** provides a cross-reference **see Nephrosis** because edema is characteristic of nephrosis.

Coders may feel confused whether they should assign one of the codes listed under **Syndrome, nephritic**, or whether they must follow the cross-reference. Remember the following tips:

- When the condition is *not specified any further* in the documentation, assign the code that follows the appropriate subterm.
- When documentation *provides more details than appear in the Index entry*, follow the cross-referenced Main Term to search for a more specific code.

SUCCESS STEP

Whenever you are in doubt if you have the correct code, follow the cross-reference. It only takes a moment and either confirms your initial choice or leads you to a more specific code. Either way, cross-referencing gives you confidence in your coding skills.

Nephrotic syndrome is a collection of disorders affecting the kidneys, characterized by proteinuria and edema, but *not* hematuria. The Index entry for the Main Term **Syndrome** and the subterm **nephrotic** provides a cross-referencing instruction, ***see also*** **Nephrosis**. It provides additional subterms for certain subtypes of the condition.

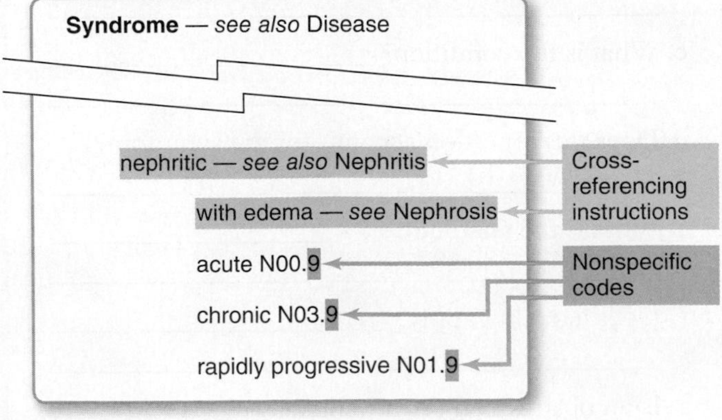

Figure 22-8 ■ Index Entry for Nephritic Syndrome

Refer to ■ FIGURE 22-9 to learn more about when to follow the cross-referencing instructions in the Index.

When coders search only under **Syndrome, nephritic, acute**, they identify the code **N00.9 Acute nephritic syndrome with unspecified morphologic changes** (■ FIGURE 22-10). When they follow the cross-reference to **Nephritis,** then follow the subterms that describe the specific subtype, they identify code **N00.3 Acute nephritic syndrome with diffuse mesangial proliferative glomerulonephritis** (Figure 22-10). Because **N00.3** is a specific code, it is the correct code for this example.

A mother presents with her 6 year old daughter who has blood in her urine. Urinalysis testing shows albuminuria, hematuria, and proteinuria. A kidney biopsy is also done and after results come back, the physician diagnoses her with acute nephritic syndrome with mesangial proliferative glomerulonephritis.

Index: **Nephritis, acute, diffuse, mesangial proliferative glomerulonephritis**

Tabular List: **N00.3 Acute nephritic syndrome with diffuse mesangial proliferative glomerulonephritis**

Figure 22-9 ■ Example of Assigning Codes for Nephritic Syndrome

Nephritis, nephritic (albuminuric) (azotemic) (congenital) (disseminated) (epithelial) (familial) (focal) (granulomatous) (hemorrhagic) (infantile) (nonsuppurative, excretory) (uremic) N05.9

acute N00.9
with
dense deposit disease N00.6
diffuse
crescentic glomerulonephritis N00.7
endocapillary proliferative glomerulonephritis N00.4
membranous glomerulonephritis N00.2
mesangial proliferative glomerulonephritis N00.3
mesangiocapillary glomerulonephritis N00.5
focal and segmental glomerular lesions N00.1
minor glomerular abnormality N00.0
specified morphological changes NEC N00.8

Figure 22-10 ■ Index Entry for the Main Term Nephritis

Guided Example of Assigning Urinary System Codes

To practice skills for assigning codes for diseases of the urinary system, continue with the example from earlier in the chapter about patient Ronald Coffield, who was seen at Branton Professional Group for ESRD and joint pain.

Follow along in your ICD-10-CM manual as Chrystal Crago, CCA, assigns codes. Check off each step after you complete it.

⇨ First, Chrystal confirms the information she abstracted:

- ❑ ESRD
- ❑ HD
- ❑ DRA
- ❑ on transplant waiting list

⇨ Chrystal begins with ESRD and searches the Index for the Main Term **Disease.**

- ❑ She locates the subterm **renal.**
- ❑ She locates the second-level subterm **end stage (failure) N18.6.**
- ❑ She notes an additional level subterm **due to hypertension,** but concludes it does not describe this case because the patient's ESRD is not documented as due to hypertension.

⇨ Chrystal verifies code **N18.6** in the Tabular List (■ FIGURE 22-11, page 440).

- ❑ She reads the code title for **N18.6, End stage renal disease** and confirms that this accurately describes the diagnosis.
- ❑ She reads the inclusion note under the code title that states **Chronic kidney disease requiring chronic dialysis.**
- ❑ She reads the instructional note under the code title that states **Use additional code to identify dialysis status (Z99.2).**
- ❑ This tells her to assign a code for dialysis and that it should be a secondary code.

⇨ Chrystal checks for other instructional notes in the Tabular List.

- ❑ She cross-references the beginning of category **N18** and reads the instructional notes.
- ❑ This patient does not have diabetes or hypertension, so the first two notes do not apply.

4th N18 Chronic kidney disease (CKD)

Code first any associated:

diabetic chronic kidney disease (E08.22, E09.22, E10.22, E11.22, E13.22)

hypertensive chronic kidney disease (I12.-, I13.-)

Use additional code to identify kidney transplant status, if applicable, (Z94.0)

N18.1 Chronic kidney disease, stage 1

N18.2 Chronic kidney disease, stage 2 (mild)

N18.3 Chronic kidney disease, stage 3 (moderate)

N18.4 Chronic kidney disease, stage 4 (severe)

N18.5 Chronic kidney disease, stage 5

Excludes1: chronic kidney disease, stage 5 requiring chronic dialysis (N18.6)

N18.6 End stage renal disease

Chronic kidney disease requiring chronic dialysis

Use additional code to identify dialysis status (Z99.2)

N18.9 Chronic kidney disease, unspecified

Figure 22-11 ■ Tabular List Entry for Chronic Kidney Disease

- ❑ The third note that states **Use additional code to identify kidney transplant status, if applicable, (Z94.0)** also does not apply because the patient has not yet received a transplant.
- ❑ She cross-references the beginning of the block **(N17-N19)** and reviews the **Excludes2** notes. None of them apply because they do not describe ESRD.
- ❑ She cross-references the beginning of **Chapter 14 (N00-N99)** and reviews the **Excludes2** notes. None of them apply.

⇨ Chrystal moves on to HD and searches the Index for the Main Term **Dialysis.**

- ❑ She locates the subterm **renal Z99.2.**
- ❑ This code is the same as the one cross-referenced by the Tabular List under code **N18.6.**
- ❑ She reviews the rest of the subterms and does not see any others that apply.

⇨ Chrystal verifies code **Z99.2** in the Tabular List.

- ❑ She reads the code title for **Z99.2, Dependence on renal dialysis** and confirms that this accurately describes the diagnosis.
- ❑ She reads the inclusion items under the code title and learns that this code describes both hemodialysis and peritoneal dialysis.
- ❑ She reads the **Excludes1** notes, which do not apply.

⇨ Chrystal checks for instructional notes in the Tabular List.

- ❑ She cross-references the beginning of category **Z99.2** and verifies that there are no instructional notes.
- ❑ She cross-references the beginning of the block **Z77-Z99** and reads the instructional note. It does not apply because there was no follow-up examination.
- ❑ She cross-references the beginning of **Chapter 21 (Z00-Z99)** and reviews the instructional notes, which describe the general use and purpose of Z codes. Nothing she reads changes the code assigned.

⇨ Next, Chrystal works on DRA *dialysis-related amyloidosis* and searches the Index for the Main Term **Amyloidosis.**

- ❑ She locates the subterm **hemodialysis-associated E85.3.**
- ❑ She reviews the rest of the subterms and does not see any others that apply.

⇨ Chrystal verifies code **E85.3** in the Tabular List.

- ❑ She reads the code title for **E85.3, Secondary systemic amyloidosis** and confirms that this accurately describes the diagnosis.
- ❑ She reads the inclusion item under the code title and confirms that this code describes **Hemodialysis-associated amyloidosis.**

⇨ Chrystal checks for instructional notes in the Tabular List.

- ❑ She cross-references the beginning of category **E85** and verifies that the **Excludes1** note regarding Alzheimer's disease does not apply.
- ❑ She cross-references the beginning of the block **E70-E88** and verifies that the **Excludes1** notes do not apply.
- ❑ She cross-references the beginning of **Chapter 14 (E00-E89)** and determines that the notes do not apply to this case because the patient does not have any of the conditions listed.

⇨ Chrystal finishes with *on kidney transplant waiting list* and searches the Index for the Main Term **Waiting.**

- ❑ She locates the subterm **for organ transplant Z76.82.**

⇨ Chrystal verifies code **Z76.82** in the Tabular List.

- ❑ She reads the code title for **Z76.82, Awaiting organ transplant status** and confirms that this accurately describes the diagnosis. She searches for, but does not find, a code specifically for kidney transplant waiting list.

⇨ Chrystal checks for instructional notes in the Tabular List.

- ❑ She cross-references the beginning of category **Z76** and verifies that there are no instructional notes.
- ❑ She cross-references the beginning of the block **Z69-Z76** and verifies that there are no instructional notes.
- ❑ She previously cross-referenced the beginning of **Chapter 21 (Z00-Z99)** and remembers that there are not chapter-wide instructional notes that apply to this case.

⇨ Chrystal reviews the codes she has assigned for this case.

- ❑ **N18.6, End stage renal disease**
- ❑ **Z99.2, Dependence on renal dialysis**
- ❑ **E85.3, Secondary systemic amyloidosis**
- ❑ **Z76.82, Awaiting organ transplant status**

⇨ Next, Chrystal must determine how to sequence the codes.

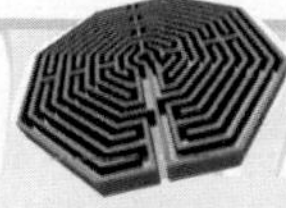

Coding Practice

Now it is your turn to practice assigning codes for diseases of the genitourinary system. Refer to the ***Tip*** at the end of the mini-medical-record if you need a little extra help.

Exercise 22.3 Assigning Codes for the Genitourinary System

Instructions: Read the mini-medical-record of each patient's encounter, review the information abstracted in Exercise 22.2, and assign ICD-10-CM diagnosis codes (CM) using the Index and Tabular List. Write the code(s) on the line provided.

1. Date: 2/23/yy Location: Branton Professional Group Provider: Ann Colyer, MD

Patient: Wing Kwan Gender: F Age: 42

Reason for encounter: surgery for endometriosis

Assessment: endometriosis of the uterus

Plan: FU in office 2 weeks

1 CM Code ___________

2. Date: 2/23/yy Location: Branton Family Practice Provider: Kristen Conover, MD

Patient: Robyn Lemmon Gender: F Age: 46

Reason for encounter: painful lumps in both breasts

Assessment: fibrocystic breast changes

Plan: OTC acetaminophen, heat and ice as needed to relieve local pain

***Tip*:** Physicians use the term "changes" rather than the more traditional "disease" to avoid alarming patients.

2 CM Codes ___________ ___________

3. Date: 2/23/yy Location: Branton Professional Group Provider: Brent Eberhart, MD

Patient: Shawn Spates Gender: M Age: 61

Reason for encounter: occasional excruciating low back pain

Assessment: ureteral calculi

Plan: medical expulsive therapy (MET) with tamsulosin

***Tip*:** The presence of calculi accounts for the low back pain.

1 CM Code ___________

ARRANGING CODES FOR THE GENITOURINARY SYSTEM

Coders should be attentive to instructional notes in the Tabular List regarding how to sequence codes for genitourinary conditions due to infections and codes for enlarged prostate (EP) and associated symptoms.

Arranging Codes for Genitourinary Conditions Due to Infections

Because many disorders of the genitourinary system are infections, the Tabular List provides frequent instructional notes directing coders to assign an additional code to identify the infectious organism or underlying condition. Sequence the genitourinary condition first and the infectious organism second (■ FIGURE 22-12).

Arranging Codes for Enlarged Prostate

An enlarged prostate (EP), or benign prostatic hypertrophy (BPH), is the abnormal growth of epithelial cells of the prostate, causing compression or obstruction of the urethra. The condition is a common condition in men over 50 years old and may be accompanied by a variety of **lower urinary tract symptoms (LUTS)** (*symptoms relating to urine storage and voiding disturbances*). ICD-10-CM provides separate codes for EP based on whether LUTS exist. When EP is accompanied with LUTS, coders must assign codes for LUTS and sequence them after the code for the EP (■ FIGURE 22-13).

CODING CAUTION

Do not confuse the abbreviation EP, which is an enlarged prostate, with the abbreviation ED, which is erectile dysfunction.

Refer to ■ FIGURE 22-14 to learn more about assigning and sequencing codes for EP with LUTS. The code for EP must be sequenced first, followed by the two symptoms. The order of the symptoms does not matter, unless the physician indicates that one is of greater importance.

Patient is seen for acute vaginitis due to Candida.

(1) **N76.0 Acute vaginitis**

(2) **B37.3 Candidiasis of vulva and vagina**

Figure 22-12 ■ Example of Arranging Codes for a Genitourinary Condition Due to an Infectious Organism

4th N40 Enlarged prostate (EP)

Includes: adenofibromatous hypertrophy of prostate
benign hypertrophy of the prostate
benign prostatic hyperplasia
benign prostatic hypertrophy (BPH)
nodular prostate
polyp of prostate

Excludes1: benign neoplasms of prostate (adenoma, benign) (fibroadenoma) (fibroma) (myoma) (D29.1)

Excludes2: malignant neoplasm of prostate (C61)

N40.0 Enlarged prostate without lower urinary tract symptoms (LUTS)
Enlarged prostate NOS

N40.1 Enlarged prostate with lower urinary tract symptoms (LUTS)
Use additional code for associated symptoms, when specified:
incomplete bladder emptying (R39.14)
nocturia (R35.1)
straining on urination (R39.16)
urinary frequency (R35.0)
urinary hesitancy (R39.11)
urinary incontinence (N39.4-)
urinary obstruction (N13.8)
urinary retention (R33.8)
urinary urgency (R39.15)
weak urinary stream (R39.12)

Figure 22-13 ■ Tabular List Entry for Enlarged Prostate

Patient is seen due to complaints of a weak urine stream and straining to urinate. The physician determines these symptoms are due to an enlarged prostate.

(1) **N40.1 Enlarged prostate with lower urinary tract symptoms (LUTS)**

(2) **R39.16 Straining to void**

(3) **R39.12 Poor urinary stream**

Figure 22-14 ■ Example of Arranging Codes for Enlarged Prostate with Lower Urinary Tract Symptoms

Guided Example of Arranging Urinary System Codes

To practice skills for sequencing codes for diseases of the urinary system, continue with the example from earlier in the chapter about patient Ronald Coffield, who was seen at Branton Professional Group for ESRD and joint pain.

Follow along in your ICD-10-CM manual as Chrystal Crago, CCA, sequences the codes. Check off each step after you complete it.

⇨ First, Chrystal confirms the codes she assigned.

- ☐ **N18.6, End stage renal disease**
- ☐ **Z99.2, Dependence on renal dialysis**
- ☐ **E85.3, Secondary systemic amyloidosis**
- ☐ **Z76.82, Awaiting organ transplant status**

⇨ Chrystal must determine the first-listed diagnosis because this was an outpatient office visit.

- ☐ She reviews OGCR IV.G., which states the following:
  - **List first the ICD-10-CM code for the diagnosis, condition, problem, or other reason for encounter/visit shown in the medical record to be chiefly responsible for the services provided. List additional codes that describe any coexisting conditions.**
- ☐ She reviews the medical record and determines that the diagnosis that best meets this definition is DRA. The patient's ongoing complaints of severe joint pain were the main reason for the visit and the services.
- ☐ She assigns DRA as the first-listed diagnosis.
  - Although the DRA is secondary to the ESRD, she did not see any instructional notes that directed her to sequence ESRD first.

⇨ Chrystal determines that ESRD should be the second sequenced diagnosis because it is responsible for the DRA. It takes priority over the Z codes, which describe the status of the patient but not specific conditions.

⇨ Chrystal sequences HD status as the third code because it is required by the instructional note under code **N18.6**. The instructional note also indicates that HD should be sequenced secondary to ESRD.

⇨ Chrystal sequences the code for awaiting organ transplant as the final code.

⇨ Chrystal reviews the medical record one final time to assure that she has captured all the details and that the final codes are consistent with the medical record.

⇨ Chrystal finalizes the codes and sequencing for this case:

(1) **E85.3, Secondary systemic amyloidosis**

(2) **N18.6, End stage renal disease**

(3) **Z99.2, Dependence on renal dialysis**

(4) **Z76.82, Awaiting organ transplant status**

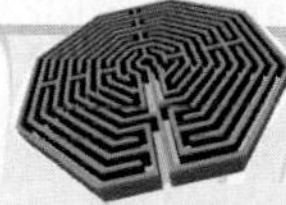

Coding Practice

Now it is your turn to practice sequencing codes for disease of the genitourinary system. Refer to the ***Tip*** at the end of the mini-medical-record if you need a little extra help.

Exercise 22.4 Arranging Codes for the Genitourinary System

Instructions: Read the mini-medical-record of each patient's encounter, review the information abstracted in Exercise 22.2, assign ICD-10-CM diagnosis codes (CM) using the Index and Tabular List, and sequence them correctly.

1. Date: 2/24/yy Location: Branton Professional Group Provider: Brent Eberhart, MD

Patient: Dale Viera Gender: M Age: 81

Reason for encounter: FU on EP with obstruction and urinary retention

Assessment: little improvement seen despite multiple medication adjustments

Plan: schedule transurethral resection of the prostate (TURP)

***Tip*:** Follow instructional notes in the Tabular List for additional codes and sequencing.

3 CM Codes ______ ______ ______

(*continued*)

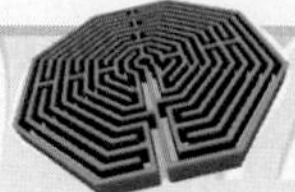

Coding Practice (continued)

2. Date: 2/24/yy Location: Branton Family Practice Provider: Kristen Conover, MD

Patient: Lyn Bowes Gender: F Age: 37

Reason for encounter: *vaginal discharge, burning, redness in perineal area*

Assessment: lab results show bacterial vaginitis due to staphylococcus, which is treatable

Plan: antibiotics

Tip: The type of *Staphylococcus* is not specified.

2 CM Codes __________ __________

3. Date: 2/24/yy Location: Branton Medical Center Provider: Ann Colyer, MD

Patient: Clare Browder Gender: F Age: 83

Reason for admission: skilled nursing facility (SNF) patient brought to emergency department with suspected UTI due to confusion and lack of cooperation; history of UTI over the past 2 years

Assessment: UTI due to E.coli (non-Shiga toxin-producing)

Plan: administered IV antibiotics, discharged after 2 days to SNF with Rx

Tip: In the elderly, confusion and cooperation may be the only symptoms of UTI.

3 CM Codes __________ __________ __________

CODING NEOPLASMS OF THE GENITOURINARY SYSTEM

Neoplasms of the genitourinary system do not appear in ICD-10-CM Chapter 14 Diseases of the Genitourinary System (N00-N99). Codes for neoplasms of the genitourinary system appear in the following blocks within the neoplasm chapter:

- **C50 Malignant neoplasm of breast**
- **C51-C58 Malignant neoplasm of female genital organs**
- **C60-C63 Malignant neoplasms of male genital organs**
- **C64-C68 Malignant neoplasm of urinary tract**

The most common cancer of the urinary system is bladder cancer, which is the sixth most common cancer in the United States, according to NIH. Most bladder cancer is transitional cell carcinoma, which starts from the cells lining the bladder. The tumors are classified based on the way they grow. Papillary tumors have a wart-like appearance and are attached to a stalk. Nonpapillary tumors are less common but more invasive, with a poorer outcome. Smoking is a major risk factor for bladder cancer. Other risk factors are a family history of bladder cancer, advanced age, Caucasian race, and male gender.

The most common sites for cancer in the reproductive system are the prostate in males and the breast and ovaries in females, according to NIH.

Prostate cancer is the most common cancer in men and third most common cause of death from cancer in men of all ages. It is the most common cause of death from cancer in men over age 75. Prostate cancer is rarely found in men younger than 40. The **prostate specific antigen (PSA)** blood test is performed to screen for prostate cancer, enabling physicians to detect prostate cancer before it causes symptoms. At an early stage, prostate cancer is very treatable through surgery and radiation.

Breast cancer is the most common cancer in women, affecting one in eight women at some point during their lifetime. Most occurrences of breast cancer are **ductal**, starting in the milk ducts. **Lobular** breast cancer starts in the lobules that produce milk. Screening mammograms are proven to be effective at identifying breast cancer in early stages (■ FIGURE 22-15). Treatment of breast cancer in the early stages, through surgery and radiation, has a high success rate.

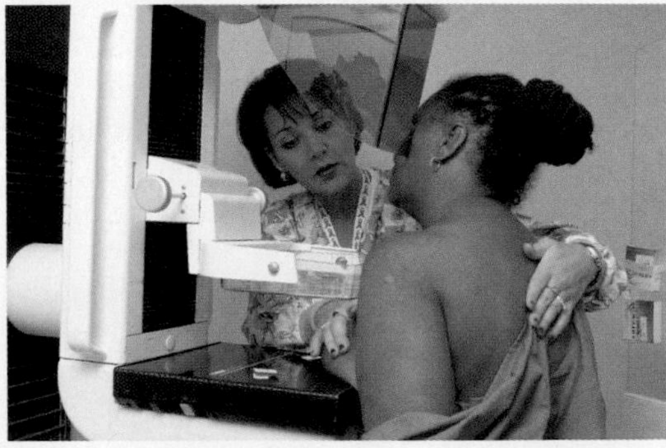

Figure 22-15 ■ Screening mammograms aid in the early detection of breast cancer. *Source: Robin Nelson/PhotoEdit.*

Ovarian cancer is the fifth most common cancer among women, according to NIH. It causes more deaths than any other type of female genital cancer, largely because its symptoms of bloating, pain, and the feeling of fullness are often attributed to other causes. Ovarian cancer usually is not diagnosed until after it has metastasized, making it difficult to treat.

Genetic testing for mutations in the genes BRCA1 and BRCA2 can be helpful in identifying women who are at greater risk of breast or ovarian cancer and men who are at greater risk of breast cancer, prostate cancer, and several other cancers.

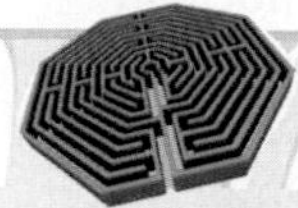

Coding Practice

Now it is your turn to practice coding neoplasms of the genitourinary system. Refer to the ***Tip*** at the end of the mini-medical-record if you need a little extra help.

Exercise 22.5 Coding Neoplasms of the Genitourinary System

Instructions: Read the mini-medical-record of each patient's encounter, then abstract, assign, and sequence ICD-10-CM diagnosis codes (CM) using the Index and Tabular List. Write the code(s) on the line provided.

1. Date: 2/25/yy Location: Branton Professional Group Provider: Brent Eberhart, MD

Patient: Manuel Vinson Gender: M Age: 62

Reason for encounter: review results of needle biopsy which was performed due to elevated PSA

Assessment: stage 1 adenocarcinoma of the prostate which affects less than 5% of the prostate

Plan: brachytherapy (*placing radioactive seeds inside the prostate gland*)

1 CM Code __________

2. Date: 2/25/yy Location: Branton Medical Center Outpatient Radiology

Provider: Brent Eberhart, MD

Patient: Peter Breunig Gender: M Age: 64

Reason for encounter: radiation therapy

Assessment: transitional cell carcinoma bladder cancer with overlapping lesions of the orifice and metastasis to the prostate

Plan: daily treatments for 3 more weeks

3 CM Codes __________ __________ __________

3. Date: 2/25/yy Location: Branton Professional Group Provider: Ann Colyer, MD

Patient: Kendra Converse Gender: F Age: 60

Reason for encounter: painful and frequent urination, blood in urine

Assessment: radiation cystitis as a result of external beam radiotherapy for metastatic ovarian cancer

Tip: The fourth code is an external cause code for a complication of radiotherapy.

4 CM Codes __________ __________ __________ __________

4. Date: 2/25/yy Location: Branton Professional Group Provider: Ann Colyer, MD

Patient: Alma Hilburn Gender: F Age: 44

Reason for encounter: FU on imaging for pain and hematuria

Assessment: angiomyolipoma, right kidney

Plan: embolization to reduce risk of hemorrhage and shrink the tumor

1 CM Code __________

5. Date: 2/25/yy Location: Branton Medical Center Outpatient Procedure Center

Provider: Brent Eberhart, MD

Patient: Tami Welborn Gender: F Age: 58

Reason for encounter: lumpectomy

Assessment: ductal cancer in situ (DCIS) of the left breast, upper inner quadrant

1 CM Code __________

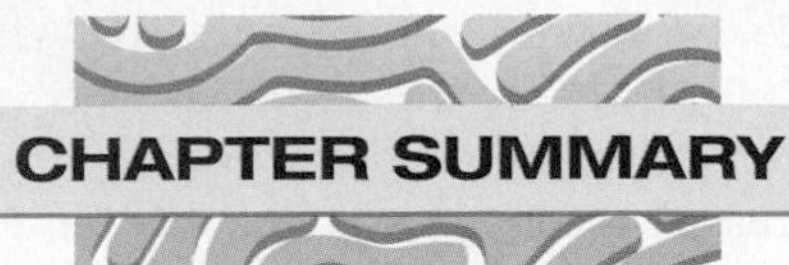

CHAPTER SUMMARY

In this chapter you learned that:

- The genitourinary (GU) system includes the urinary system and male and female genital, or reproductive, systems. The function of the urinary system is to filter, store, and remove waste products from the blood and maintain homeostasis. The function of the genital system is sexual reproduction.
- ICD-10-CM Chapter 14 Diseases of the Genitourinary System (N00-N99) contains 11 blocks or subchapters that are divided by anatomical site.
- Disorders in this chapter have a wide range of abstracting criteria because there is a wide range of organs and types of disorders.
- Two similar genitourinary conditions, nephritic syndrome and nephrotic syndrome, demonstrate the importance of checking cross-referencing instructions in the Index in order to assign the most specific code available.
- Coders should be attentive to instructional notes in the Tabular List regarding how to sequence codes for genitourinary conditions due to infections and codes for enlarged prostate (EP) and associated symptoms.
- The most common sites for cancer in the genital system are the prostate in males and the breast and ovaries in females, according to NIH.
- ICD-10-CM Official Guidelines for Coding and Reporting (OGCR) OGCR I.C.14. provides detailed discussion of chronic kidney disease.

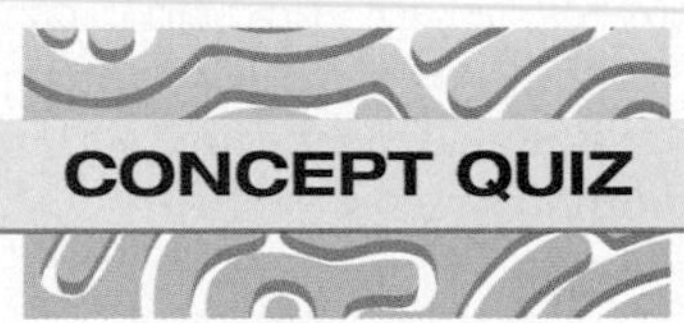

CONCEPT QUIZ

Take a moment to look back at your trip through diseases of the genitourinary system and solidify your skills. This is your opportunity to pull together everything you have learned.

Completion

Instructions: Write the term that answers each question based on the information you learned in this chapter. Choose from the list below. Some choices may be used more than once and some choices may not be used at all. Refer to the discussion in this chapter and the Glossary at the end of this book if you need a little extra help.

calculi	glomerulonephritis
cervical dysplasia	glomerulus
cervical intraepithelial neoplasia	nephritic
CKD	nephron
diabetic nephropathy	nephroptosis
dialysis	nephrotic
ED	renal pelvis
endometriosis	transplant
EP	ureter
ESRD	urethra

1. Urine passes from the renal pelvis through the ____________________ to the urinary bladder.
2. ____________________ syndrome is a collection of disorders affecting the kidneys, characterized by nonpurulent inflammatory glomerular disorders that allow proteins and red blood cells to pass into the urine, resulting in proteinuria and hematuria
3. The ____________________ is a cluster of capillaries in the kidney that separates the urinary space from the blood.
4. ____________________ is accumulated damage to the glomerulus capillaries due to chronic high blood sugar.
5. BPH is also called ____________________.
6. Diseases of the ____________________ attack the kidneys' filtering ability.
7. ____________________ is abnormal changes in the cells on the surface of the cervix that may lead to cancer if not treated.
8. ____________________ is stage 5 chronic kidney disease.
9. Stones that may accumulate in the kidneys, bladder, or ureters are called ____________________.
10. ____________________ is a treatment that filters the blood to remove waste, excess salt, and water.

Multiple Choice

Instructions: Circle the letter of the best answer to each question based on the information you learned in this chapter. Refer to the discussion in this chapter and the Glossary at the end of this book if you need a little extra help.

1. The kidneys cease to function and patients must receive dialysis or a kidney transplant in order to survive when CKD reaches stage
   A. 1.
   B. 3.
   C. 4.
   D. 5.
2. Long term dialysis patients may accumulate deposits of the starchy substance amyloid in the joints called
   A. dialysis-related amyloidosis.
   B. end stage renal disease.
   C. nephritic syndrome.
   D. nephrolithiasis.
3. The only specific disease that Medicare covers for the entire population, regardless of age, is
   A. BPH.
   B. ED.
   C. CKD.
   D. ESRD.
4. Which of the following is NOT included in ICD-10-CM Chapter 14?
   A. Conditions of the urinary system
   B. Conditions of the female breast
   C. Conditions of the kidney related to pregnancy
   D. Conditions of the male reproductive system
5. OGCR I.C.14. provides detailed discussion of
   A. hypertensive kidney disease.
   B. chronic kidney disease.
   C. nephritic and nephrotic syndrome.
   D. enlarged prostate.
6. When documentation provides more details than appear in the Index entry, search for a more specific code by
   A. browsing through the Tabular List.
   B. assigning the default code next to the Main Term.
   C. following the cross-referenced Main Term.
   D. reading the OGCR.
7. What code should be assigned when an ESRD patient is receiving dialysis?
   A. N18.5, Chronic kidney disease, stage 5
   B. Z99.2, Dependence on renal dialysis
   C. I12.0, Hypertensive chronic kidney disease with end stage renal disease
   D. Z76.82, Awaiting organ transplant status
8. What codes should be sequenced after code N40.1 Enlarged prostate with lower urinary tract symptoms (LUTS)?
   A. Associated symptoms
   B. With or without obstruction
   C. Infectious organism
   D. Acute or chronic
9. Which type of cancer is often not diagnosed until after it has metastasized, making it more difficult to treat?
   A. Prostate
   B. Ovarian
   C. Breast
   D. Bladder
10. PSA is a blood test performed to screen for
    A. cervical cancer.
    B. enlarged prostate.
    C. prostate cancer.
    D. pyelonephritis.

CODING CHALLENGE

Now it is your turn to demonstrate coding all aspects diseases of the genitourinary system. The coders who have helped you during this trip are confident in the skills you have developed and give you only a few tips. Refer back to the examples and discussion in this chapter when you need a little extra help. Use your medical dictionary and anatomy references when needed.

Instructions: Read the mini-medical-record of each patient's encounter, then abstract, assign, and arrange ICD-10-CM diagnosis codes (CM) using the Index and Tabular List. Write the code(s) on the line provided.

(*continued*)

(continued from page 447)

Urinary System

1. Date: 2/19/yy Location: Branton Medical Center
Provider: Ann Colyer, MD
Patient: Edwin Armes Gender: M Age: 46
Reason for encounter: oliguria, drowsy and lethargic, edema
Assessment: acute renal failure with tubular necrosis and hypertension
Plan: fluid restriction, diuretics, restrict mineral intake, dialysis if serum potassium remains high

Tip: Only chronic renal failure is assumed to be related to hypertension.

2 CM Codes __________ __________

2. Date: 2/19/yy Location: Branton Medical Center
Provider: Ann Colyer, MD
Patient: Bruce Jaynes Gender: M Age: 37
Reason for encounter: bloody urine, edema of feet, ankles, and legs, uncontrolled high BP, upper abdominal pain, general malaise
Assessment: glomerulonephrosis due to secondary DM which is a result of alcohol dependent chronic pancreatitis, 2 years on insulin
Plan: adjust BP meds, diuretics, angiotension-converting enzyme inhibitors

4 CM Codes __________ __________ __________ __________

3. Date: 2/19/yy Location: Branton Professional Group Provider: Ann Colyer, MD
Patient: Katherine Manzano Gender: F Age: 56
Reason for encounter: renal dialysis
Assessment: stage V CKD due to autosomal recessive polycystic kidney disease
Plan: return in 2 days

Tip: Patients typically receive dialysis three times per week.

3 CM Codes __________ __________ __________

Male Reproductive System

4. Date: 2/19/yy Location: Branton Medical Center
Provider: Brent Eberhart, MD
Patient: Randall Corum Gender: M Age: 63
Reason for encounter: painful urination
Assessment: acute enterococcal prostatitis
Plan: IV antibacterial gram positive therapy

2 CM Codes __________ __________

5. Date: 2/19/yy Location: Branton Professional Group Provider: Brent Eberhart, MD
Patient: Timothy Stelly Gender: M Age: 16
Reason for encounter: red and painful foreskin and penis with foul smelling discharge, uncircumcised
Assessment: balanitis due to E. coli
Plan: Rx antibiotics, hygiene instructions

2 CM Codes __________ __________

Female Reproductive System

6. Date: 2/19/yy Location: Branton Medical Center
Provider: Brent Eberhart, MD
Patient: Tami Boie Gender: F Age: 38
Reason for encounter: urinary incontinence (UI), difficulty with sexual encounters, feeling of pelvic heaviness
Assessment: cystocele and uterine prolapse, grade 3
Plan: schedule surgical rectocele and cystocele repair in 3 wk

Tip: Follow the cross-references in the Index.

1 CM Code __________

7. Date: 2/19/yy Location: Branton Family Practice
Provider: Kristen Conover, MD
Patient: Rena McNnitt Gender: F Age: 20
Reason for encounter: severe pelvic pain and cramps on the first day or two of her monthly period
Assessment: no specific problems except an incidental finding of **retroverted** uterus which I do not believe is the cause of the menstrual pain
Plan: patient advised to begin a daily walking program, ibuprofen or other NSAIDs to be taken 1-2 days prior to her period

2 CM Codes __________ __________

8. Date: 2/19/yy Location: Branton Family Practice
Provider: Kristen Conover, MD
Patient: Brandy Hall Gender: F Age: 22
Reason for encounter: FU on routine pap smear showing CIN II (unvaccinated for HPV)
Assessment: CIN II
Plan: schedule for Colposcopy in 2 weeks

Tip: If you are unsure whether the CIN is mild, moderate, or severe, review the inclusion notes in the Tabular List for the possible codes.

1 CM Code ___________

9. Date: 2/19/yy Location: Branton Professional Group Provider: Brent Eberhart, MD
Patient: Mildred Trawick Gender: F Age: 81
Reason for encounter: urge incontinence, bladder droops to the vaginal opening

(continued)

9. (continued)
Assessment: urge incontinence due to grade 2 cystocele on the right side
Plan: Kegel exercises, pessary, RTO in 2 months to schedule surgery if no relief

1 CM Code ___________

10. Date: 2/19/yy Location: Branton Medical Center, Outpatient Radiology Provider: Jennifer Kolb, MD
Patient: Tabitha Stelly Gender: F Age: 41
Reason for encounter: screening mammogram
Assessment: suspicious mass, right breast, and bilateral microcalcifications
Plan: schedule biopsy next week

3 CM Codes ___________ ___________ ___________

KEEP ON CODING

As a coder, you can never have too much experience. Apply everything you have learned in this chapter to code the following diagnostic statements. Use the OGCR and instructional notes in the Tabular List to help determine how many codes are required.

Instructions: Read the diagnostic statement, then use the Index and Tabular List to assign and sequence ICD-10-CM (CM) diagnosis codes. Write the code(s) on the line provided.

Urinary System

1. Hydroureter: CM Code(s) ___________
2. Cystostomy malfunction: CM Code(s) ___________
3. Carcinoma of the left kidney pelvis: CM Code(s) ___________
4. Dysuria: CM Code(s) ___________
5. Urethrocele: CM Code(s) ___________
6. Interstitial nephritis: CM Code(s) ___________
7. Trigonitis: CM Code(s) ___________
8. End stage renal disease currently receiving dialysis: CM Code(s) ___________

9. Terminal atrophy of the kidney: CM Code(s) ______________________________

10. Hypermobility of urethra with urinary stress incontinence: CM Code(s) ______________________________

11. Urinary bladder stone: CM Code(s) ______________________________

12. Ureteritis cystica: CM Code(s) ______________________________

Male Reproductive System

13. Enlarged prostate with nighttime urination: CM Code(s) ______________________________

14. Oligospermia: CM Code(s) ______________________________

15. Priapism due to trauma: CM Code(s) ______________________________

16. Infected hydrocele due to *E. coli*: CM Code(s) ______________________________

17. Cyst of tunica albuginea testes: CM Code(s) ______________________________

18. Erectile dysfunction due to type 2 diabetes: CM Code(s) ______________________________

19. Gynecomastia: CM Code(s) ______________________________

Female Reproductive System

20. Torsion of fallopian tube: CM Code(s) ______________________________

21. Decubitus ulcer of cervix: CM Code(s) ______________________________

22. Secondary amenorrhea: CM Code(s) ______________________________

23. Anteversion of uterus: CM Code(s) ______________________________

24. Endometriosis of the intestines: CM Code(s) ______________________________

25. Bartholin's gland cyst: CM Code(s) ______________________________

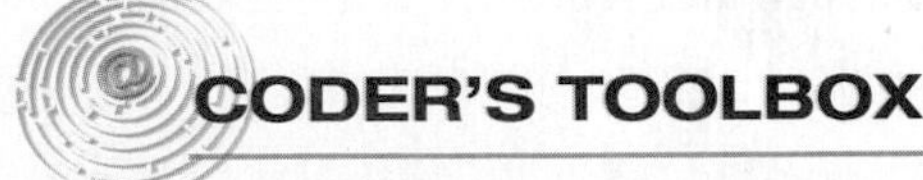

CODER'S TOOLBOX

The following resources are a starting point for learning more about diseases of the genitourinary system. The > symbol indicates a menu selection within the website in order to navigate to a specific page.

Urinary System

American Association of Kidney Patients **http://www.aakp.org/**
American Congress of Obstetricians and Gynecologists **http://www.acog.org/**
American Kidney Fund **http://www.kidneyfund.org/**
American Society of Nephrology **http://www.asn-online.org/**
American Urology Association **http://www.auanet.org/content/homepage/homepage.cfm**
Bladder Cancer Advocacy Network **http://www.bcan.org/**
CMS > Centers > End Stage Renal Disease (ESRD) Center **http://www.cms.gov/center/esrd.asp**
Home Dialysis **http://www.homedialysis.org/**
National Kidney & Urologic Diseases Information Clearinghouse (NKUDIC) **http://kidney.niddk.nih.gov/kudiseases/pubs/peritoneal/**
National Kidney Foundation **http://www.kidney.org**

Male Reproductive System

Prostate Cancer Guide **http://www.prostatecancerguide.net/**

Female Reproductive System

American Congress of Obstetricians and Gynecologists **http://www.acog.org/**
Ovarian Cancer Research Fund **http://www.ocrf.org/**
Susan G. Komen for the Cure **http://ww5.komen.org/**

23

Pregnancy, Childbirth, and the Puerperium (O00-O9A)

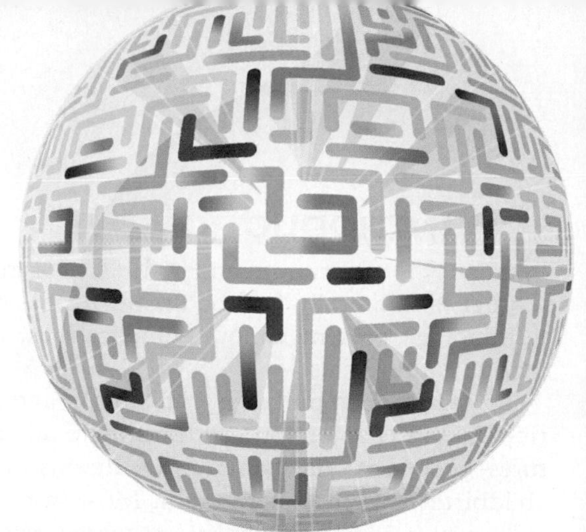

Learning Objectives

After completing this chapter, you should have the skills to:

- Spell and define the key words, medical terms, and abbreviations related to pregnancy, childbirth, and the puerperium.
- Discuss the structures, processes, and common conditions of pregnancy, childbirth, and the puerperium.
- Identify the main characteristics of coding for pregnancy, childbirth, and the puerperium.
- Abstract diagnostic information from the medical record for coding conditions of pregnancy, childbirth, and the puerperium.
- Assign codes for pregnancy, childbirth, and the puerperium.
- Arrange codes for pregnancy, childbirth, and the puerperium.
- Discuss the Official Guidelines for Coding and Reporting related to pregnancy, childbirth, and the puerperium.

Key Terms and Abbreviations

amnion
amniotic sac
antenatal
antepartum
childbirth
chorion
conception
delivery
dichorionic-diamniotic (DiDi)
ectopic
estimated date of delivery (EDD)
estimated gestational age (EGA)
fetopelvic disproportion
first trimester
gestational condition
grand multipara
gravida (G)
last menstrual period (LMP)
monoamniotic
monochorionic
multiple gestation
occipitoanterior (OA)
para (P)
partum
parturition
peripartum
placenta
postpartum
pregnancy
pregnancy induced hypertension (PIH)
prenatal
prepartum
puerperal
puerperium
second trimester
singleton
third trimester
TPAL
true labor
zygote

In addition to the key terms listed here, students should know the terms defined within tables in this chapter.

Chapter Outline

- **Obstetrics Refresher**
- **Coding Overview of Obstetrics**
- **Abstracting for Obstetrics**
- **Assigning Codes for Obstetrics**
- **Arranging Codes for Obstetrics**

ICD-10-CM codes in this chapter are from the ICD-10-CM 2014 Draft code set from the Department of Health and Human Services, Centers for Disease Control and Prevention.

INTRODUCTION

Pregnancy is a journey in and of itself, figuratively, for the mother, and literally, for the infant. It possesses unique terminology, presents unique complications, and requires unique coding skills.

In your tour of pregnancy, childbirth, and the puerperium in this chapter you will learn more about the structures, processes, and common conditions of pregnancy, childbirth, and the puerperium. Most importantly, you will practice coding for patient encounters related to pregnancy, childbirth, and the puerperium, a skill that requires you to abstract information from the medical record, assign correct codes, and arrange (sequence) the codes in the correct order.

Physicians who specialize in pregnancy and delivery are obstetrician/gynecologists (OB/GYNs). It is common for several OB/GYNs to join together in the same medical practice to provide 24/7 coverage for one another. Obstetric practices may also include a certified nurse midwife (CNM), an advanced practice nurse with specialized education in nursing and obstetrics. A CNM provides care for relatively healthy women with uncomplicated pregnancies.

For the sake of brevity, this chapter refers to pregnancy, childbirth, and the puerperium as obstetrics. As you read this chapter, open up your medical terminology book and keep a medical dictionary handy to refresh your memory of any unfamiliar obstetric terms. These are your professional resources that provide the information you need at your fingertips. It is always better to take a moment to look up details rather than guess. Also refer to the websites and organizations listed in the Coder's Toolbox at the end of the chapter for specialized information about obstetrics.

OBSTETRICS REFRESHER

Pregnancy is a normal, temporary condition that occurs within the female body, which begins at the time of **conception** (*fertilization of the female ova by the male sperm*) and ends with the birth of the fetus. The **prenatal** period is the time period from conception to the beginning of labor. It is also called the **prepartum, antepartum**, or **antenatal** period. **Childbirth,** also called **parturition,** is the period of **true labor** (*uterine contractions and dilation of the cervix*) and active **delivery** (*the expulsion of the fetus and placenta from the uterus*). The **puerperium, puerperal** period, or **postpartum** period is the six-week period following childbirth, during which time the female reproductive organs return to the prepregnant state. The **peripartum** period is the last month of pregnancy to five months postpartum.

The term (length) of a normal pregnancy is 37 to 40 weeks. The **estimated date of delivery (EDD)** is determined as 40 weeks from the **last menstrual period (LMP). Estimated gestational age (EGA)** is the number of weeks and days since the LMP. The pregnancy is divided into three trimesters, defined based on gestational age as follows:

- **first trimester**—less than 14 weeks, 0 days
- **second trimester**—14 weeks, 0 days to less than 28 weeks, 0 days
- **third trimester**—28 weeks, 0 days until delivery

SUCCESS STEP

If physician documentation of EDD or gestational age differs from the date calculated by the method shown here or another calculation method, coders should utilize the date documented by the physician.

A woman's childbearing history is described in terms of **gravida (G)** (*the number of pregnancies*) and **para (P)** (*the number of pregnancies resulting in a fetus of viable gestational age [20 weeks] regardless of whether the fetus was alive at birth*). **Grand multipara** describes a woman who has had five or more previous pregnancies resulting in a viable fetus. Pregnancies that consist of multiples, such as twins or triplets, count as *one* when describing parity. For example, a woman currently pregnant, who has had one previous pregnancy and gave birth to twins, is gravida 2 (two pregnancies including the current one) and para 1 (has had one pregnancy resulting in a viable fetus). Parity may be further described using **TPAL**, which identifies the number of term births (T), preterm births (P), spontaneous or induced abortions (A), and living children (L). TPAL is written as a four digit number. Refer to ■ FIGURE 23-1 to learn more about the various ways that childbearing history may be written.

Each structure in the pregnant uterus is labeled with its name as well as its medical terminology root/combining form in ■ FIGURE 23-2. As you learn about conditions and procedures of pregnancy, childbirth, and the puerperium, remember to apply medical terminology skills to combine word roots, prefixes, and suffixes you already know to define new terms. Refer to ■ TABLE 23-1 (page 454) for a refresher on how to build medical terms related to pregnancy, childbirth, and the puerperium.

CODING CAUTION

Be alert for medical word terms that are spelled similarly but have different meanings.

anti- (*against*) and **ante-** (*before*)

dystocia (*difficult labor*) and **dyspnea** (*difficulty breathing*)

mastalgia (*breast pain*) and **mastitis** (*inflammation of the breast*)

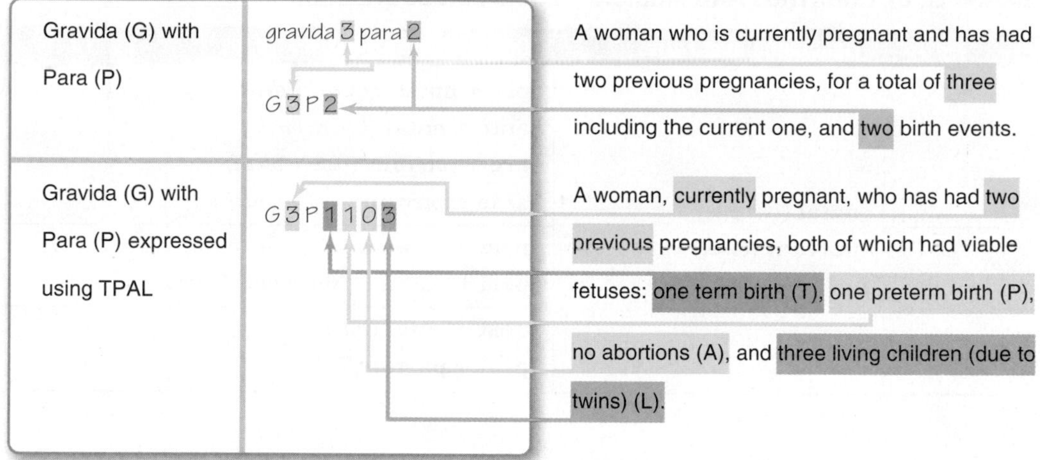

Figure 23-1 ■ Methods of Describing Childbearing History

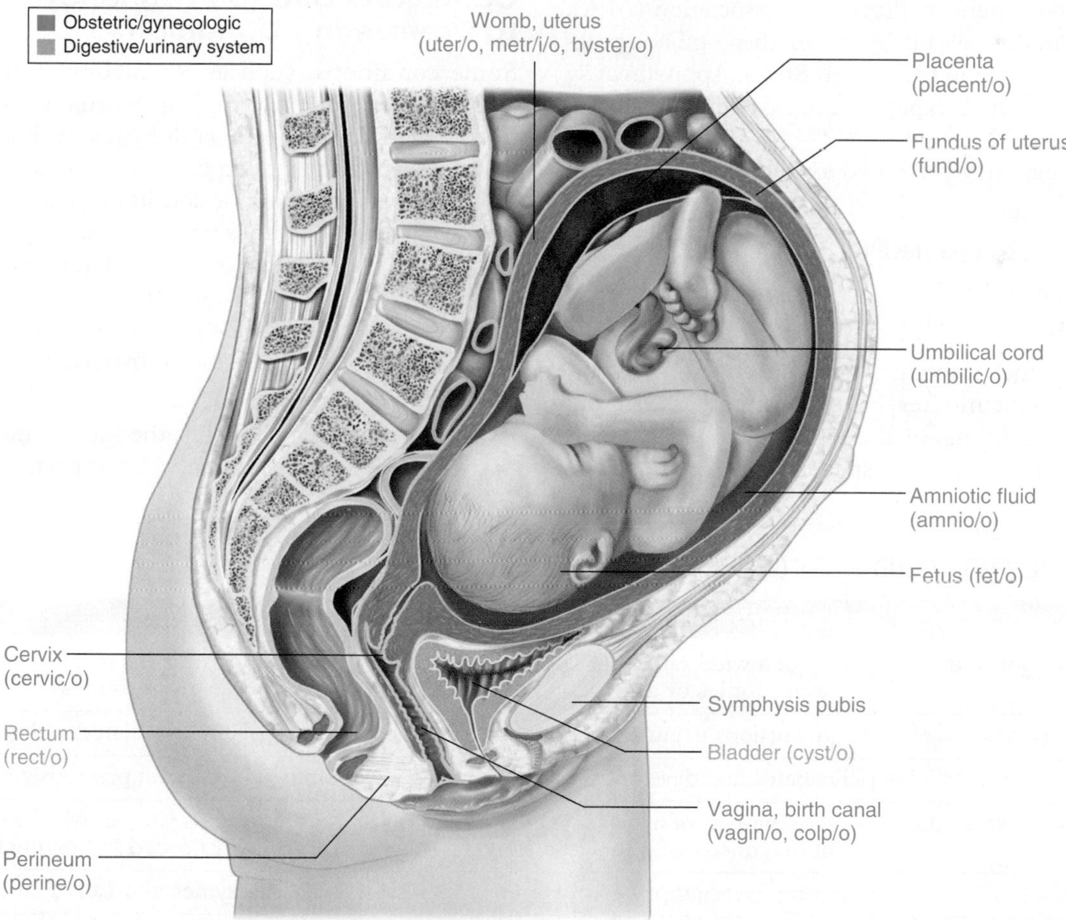

Figure 23-2 ■ Pregnant Uterus in a Full Term Pregnancy

Table 23-1 ■ **EXAMPLE OF CONSTRUCTING MEDICAL TERMS FOR OBSTETRICS**

Prefix	Root/Combining Form	Complete Medical Term
pre- (*before*) **ante-** (*before*)	**natal** (*birth*) **partum** (*birth*)	**pre + natal** (*before birth*) **ante + natal** (*before birth*) **pre + partum** (*before birth*) **ante + partum** (*before birth*)
peri- (*surrounding*)		**peri + natal** (*surrounding birth*) **peri + partum** (*surrounding birth*)
post- (*after*)		**post + natal** (*after birth*) **post + partum** (*after birth*)

In particular, coders must be familiar with the terminology related to each aspect of pregnancy, childbirth, and the puerperium.

Conditions of Pregnancy

According to the American Pregnancy Association (APA), there are over 4 million live births and another 2 million pregnancy losses every year in the United States. Approximately 20% of pregnant women experience one or more pregnancy complications.

A normal pregnancy is defined as follows:

- no preexisting conditions
- no new conditions that develop during pregnancy
- single gestation
- mother will be over age 16 and under age 35 at EDD

Disorders of the pregnancy may be due to preexisting conditions of the mother, conditions that arise during pregnancy, or conditions of the fetus or amniotic cavity. Coders use medical resources, such as reference books on diseases, to understand conditions of pregnancy, childbirth, and the puerperium, diagnostic methods, and common treatments. Refer to ■ TABLE 23-2 for a summary of conditions affecting pregnancy.

Conditions Due to Pregnancy Compared to Preexisting Conditions

Some conditions, such as Rh incompatibility and preeclampsia, occur only during pregnancy. Other conditions, such as diabetes and hypertension, may affect people at any time during life, but also have a pregnancy-related variation. When a condition has been diagnosed before a woman becomes pregnant, it is a preexisting condition. When the condition is first diagnosed during pregnancy, it is a gestational condition.

Characteristics of a gestational condition, such as gestational diabetes or gestational hypertension, include the following:

- The gestational disease has the same symptoms and signs as its non-gestational counterpart.

Table 23-2 ■ **COMMON CONDITIONS OF PREGNANCY**

Condition	Definition
Chromosomal abnormality	Any of a wide range of disorders in which a fetus has an abnormal number of chromosomes or a structural abnormality in one or more chromosomes
Eclampsia	Convulsions occurring during pregnancy or the puerperium associated with preeclampsia
Gestational diabetes	Diabetes that develops during pregnancy in a woman who did not previously have diabetes
Gestational hypertension	Development of hypertension after 20 weeks of gestation in a woman who previously was not diagnosed with hypertension; also called pregnancy induced hypertension (PIH)
HELLP syndrome	Severe preeclampsia with **H**emolysis, **E**levated **L**iver enzymes and **L**ow **P**latelet count
In vitro fertilization (IVF)	Fertilization of an ova in a laboratory dish, followed by introduction into the uterus
Preeclampsia	A metabolic disorder of pregnancy, which develops after the twentieth week, that involves gestational hypertension and proteinuria
Preexisting diabetes	Diabetes diagnosed in a woman before she becomes pregnant
Preexisting hypertension	Hypertension diagnosed in a woman before she becomes pregnant
Rhesus (Rh) incompatibility	A condition in which mother is Rh negative and develops antibodies against a fetus that is Rh positive

- The condition is not present prior to pregnancy.
- The condition usually begins after the twentieth week of pregnancy.
- The condition returns to normal when the pregnancy is over.

When diabetes or hypertension is present, coders must review the documentation carefully to determine whether it is gestational or preexisting in order to assign the correct codes.

Multiple Gestation

Multiple gestation is a pregnancy with more than one fetus, as in twins, triplets, or sextuplets, and carries greater risk for complications than **singletons** (*pregnancies with one fetus*). The rate of twin births increased over 70% from 1980 to 2004, according to the March of Dimes, and leveled off in subsequent years. The increase in multiple gestation pregnancies is due to delayed childbearing and expanding use of reproductive technology.

Coders need to be familiar with the terminology used to describe multiple gestation because it affects code assignment. Physicians describe multiple gestation pregnancies based on the number of **amnions** or **amniotic sacs**, **chorions**, and **placentas**. This is important because it directly affects the mortality risk of the fetuses. The amniotic sac is a membrane that surrounds the embryo. The chorion is an outer membrane that surrounds the amnion. The space inside the chorion and the amnion is called amniotic cavity and is filled with amniotic fluid. The amniotic cavity prevents the embryo from drying out and protects it against vibration and shocks. The placenta is the organ that allows for the exchange of oxygen, nutrients, and waste between the fetus and the mother. It attaches to the chorion and consists of chorionic material from the fetus and uterine material from the mother.

When multiple embryos each develop from separate **zygotes** (*fertilized eggs*), as happens with fraternal twins, each embryo always has its own amnion and chorion, making the pregnancy **dichorionic-diamniotic (DiDi)**.

Identical twins are created when a zygote divides to create two or more identical embryos. Normally, identical embryos are DiDi, with each embryo enclosed in its own amnion and chorion and having its own placenta. However, it is possible for more than one embryo to share a chorion or an amniotic sac. When the chorion is shared, the placenta is also shared. The sharing of the chorion and amnion is determined by how soon after fertilization the egg divides. Refer to ■ Table 23-3 to learn the possible combinations of twins and ■ Figure 23-3 to visualize the differences. **Monochorionic** (*sharing the chorion*) twins are at risk for more complications than

Table 23-3 ■ **CONFIGURATIONS OF CHORION, AMNION, AND PLACENTA OF TWINS**

Description	Number of Chorions	Number of Amnions	Number of Placentas	Division of Zygote
Monochorionic-monoamniotic (MoMo)	1	1	1	8–13 days after fertilization
Monochorionic-diamniotic (MoDi)	1	2	1	3–8 days after fertilization
Dichorionic-diamniotic (DiDi)	2	2	2	Less than 3–4 days after fertilization

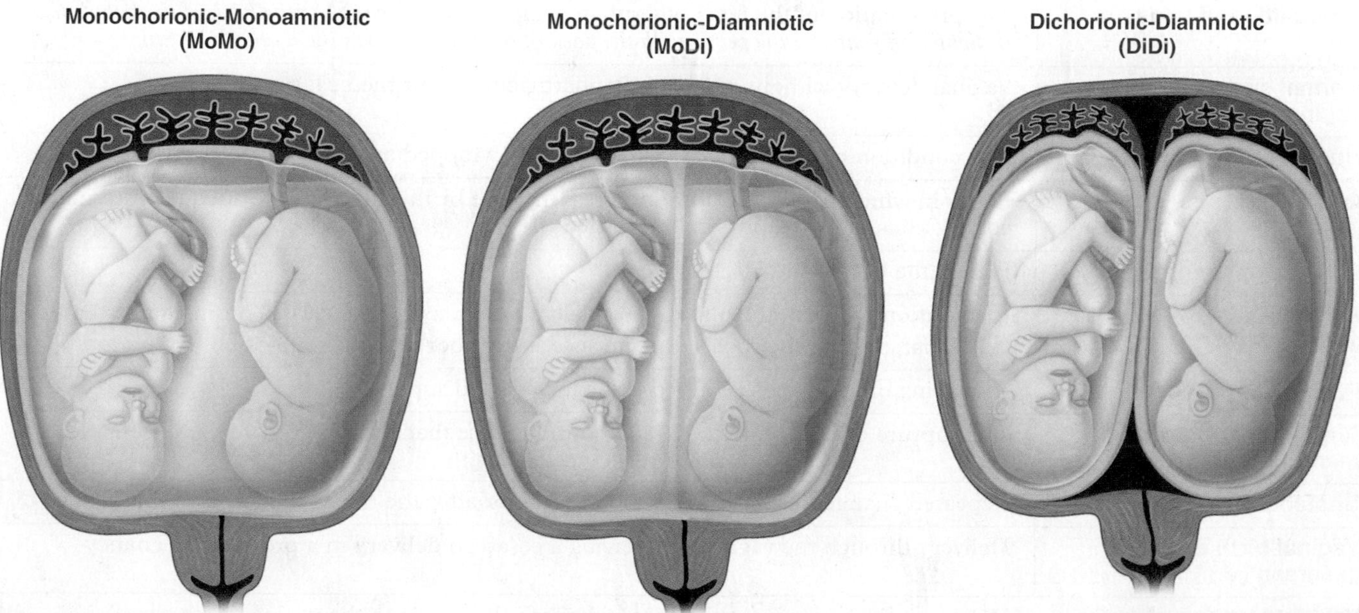

Figure 23-3 ■ Twin Configurations of the Chorion and Amnion

A

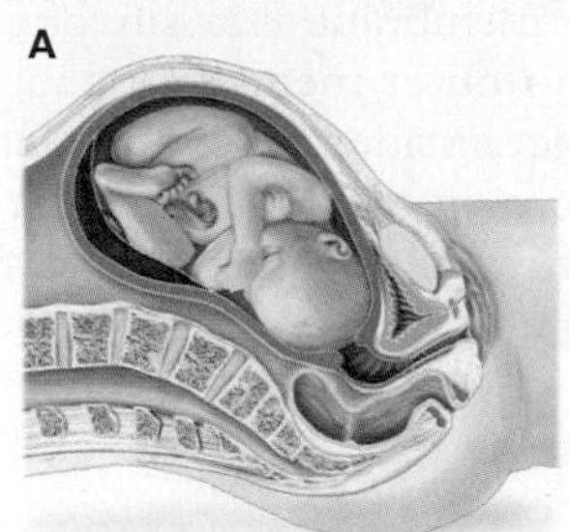

B

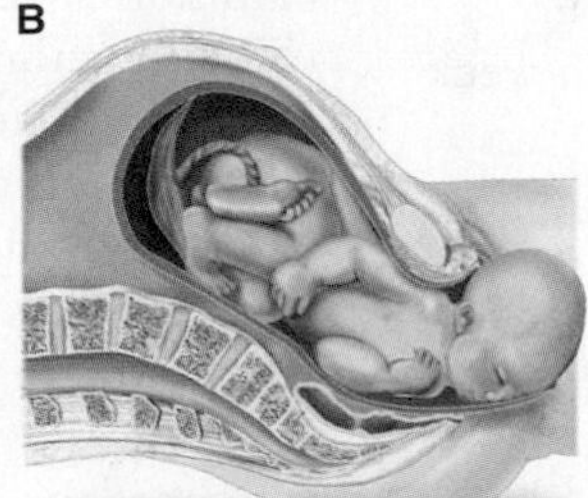

C

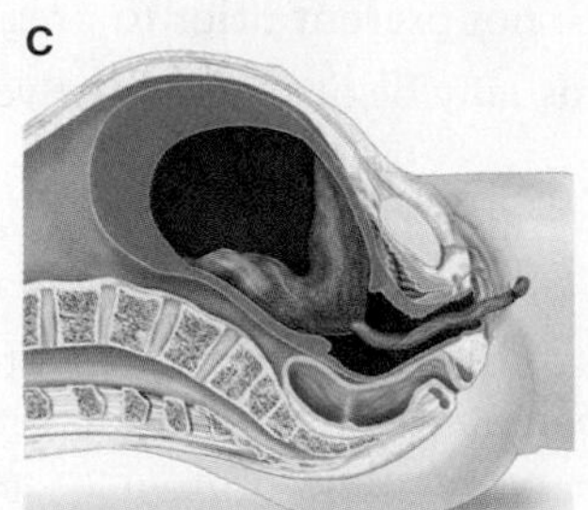

DILATION STAGE: Uterine contractions dilate cervix

EXPULSION STAGE: Birth of baby or expulsion

PLACENTAL STAGE: Delivery of placenta

Figure 23-4 ■ Three Stages of Labor and Delivery

DiDi twins; monoamniotic (*sharing the same amnion*) twins have the greatest risk of mortality.

Conditions of Childbirth

A normal delivery is defined as follows:

- single liveborn infant
- full term pregnancy
- vaginal delivery with cephalic presentation
- no induction, manipulation, or instrumentation
- no complications

Any labor and delivery that does not meet these criteria is complicated. Complications can occur during any phase of labor and delivery (■ FIGURE 23-4) and multiple complications may affect one mother. Refer to ■ TABLE 23-4 for a summary of conditions affecting labor and delivery.

Table 23-4 ■ **COMMON CONDITIONS OF CHILDBIRTH**

Condition	Definition
Assisted delivery	A delivery of the fetus using mechanical assistance, such as forceps or vacuum extractor; pharmacologic assistance, such as drugs to induce labor; or medical assistance, such as manual rotation of the fetal position
Cephalopelvic disproportion (CPD)	A cause of obstructed labor due to a mismatch between the size of the fetal head and the mother's pelvic brim; also called fetopelvic disproportion
Cesarean section (C/S, C-section)	Delivery of the fetus by making a surgical incision into the abdominal wall and uterus; also called abdominal delivery
Forceps delivery	Extraction of a fetus from the birth canal by grasping the head with forceps (tongs)
Malposition of fetus	Any presentation of the fetus other than occipitoanterior (OA) (*the back of the baby's head is slightly off center in the pelvis with the back of the head towards the mother's left thigh*)
Normal spontaneous vaginal birth (NSVB)	Vaginal delivery without mechanical, pharmacologic, or medical assistance
Nuchal cord	The condition of the umbilical cord becoming wrapped around the neck of the fetus
Obstructed labor	Labor in which the fetus cannot progress into the birth canal, despite adequate uterine contractions, due to a physical blockage
Pelvic girdle pain (PGP)	Pain at the back of the pelvis
Placenta previa	A condition in which the placenta partially or fully covers the cervix, posing a risk that it may separate from the wall of the uterus during labor (■ FIGURE 23-5)
Placental infarction	A scarring of the placenta due to inadequate blood supply
Premature rupture of membranes (PROM)	The rupture of the amniotic sac and chorion more than an hour before the onset of labor
Unstable lie	Repeated changes in the fetal position during or after the thirty-sixth week of pregnancy
Vaginal birth after cesarean (VBAC)	Delivery through the vagina after having a cesarean delivery in a previous pregnancy
Vaginal birth	Delivery of the fetus from the uterus through the cervix to the vagina (birth canal)

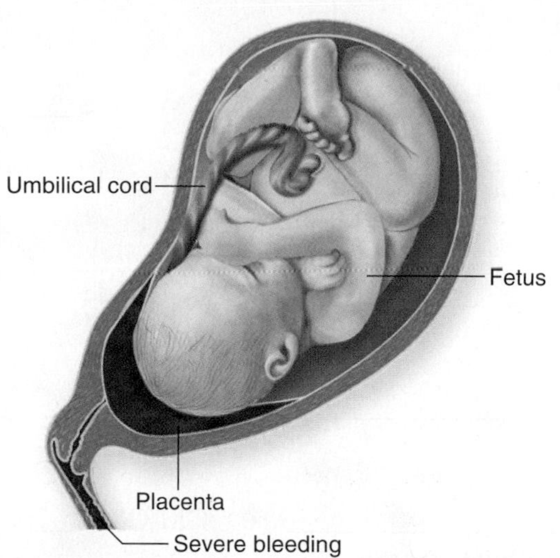

Figure 23-5 ■ Placenta Previa

Table 23-5 ■ **COMMON CONDITIONS OF THE PUERPERIUM**

Condition	Definition
Postpartum depression	Moderate to severe depression after giving birth
Postpartum hemorrhage (PPH)	Excessive bleeding following delivery
Postpartum psychosis	Sudden dramatic onset of psychotic symptoms after giving birth, often occurring in patients with bipolar disorder
Postpartum wound infection	Bacterial infection of a cesarean section wound
Puerperal mastitis	Inflammation or infection of the mammary gland in the breast during the postpartum period

Conditions of the Puerperium

Postpartum and puerperal conditions arise after delivery and are due to the post pregnancy state. Because some conditions, such as depression, can be preexisting, look for the physician's documentation that describes a condition as puerperal. Refer to ■ TABLE 23-5 for a summary of conditions affecting the puerperium.

This section provides a general reference to help understand the most common diagnoses of pregnancy, childbirth, and the puerperium, but does not list everything you need to know. Use medical terminology skills discussed earlier in this chapter to learn the meaning of unfamiliar words. Remember to keep standard reference books handy in case you get stuck. Refer to the resources in the Coder's Toolbox at the end of this chapter to learn more about conditions affecting pregnancy, childbirth, and the puerperium.

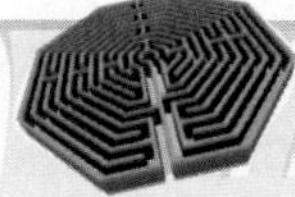

Coding Practice

Refresh your knowledge of terminology related to pregnancy, childbirth, and the puerperium. Use a medical terminology text or a website such as GlobalRph.com > Medical Terminology http://www.globalrph.com/medterm.htm to identify the meaning of word parts that may not be familiar.

Exercise 23.1 Obstetrics Refresher

Instructions: Use your medical terminology skills and resources to define the conditions, then assign the diagnosis code.

Follow these steps:

- Use slash marks "/" to break down the term in **boldface type** into its root(s) and suffix.
- Define the meaning of the word, based on the meaning of each word part.
- Assign the default diagnosis code for the condition using the Index and Tabular List.

Example: Pregnancy, complicated by, **endometritis** endo/metr/itis — Meaning: *inflammation of the lining of the uterus* — CM Code: *O86.12*

1. Pregnancy, complicated by, **hyperemesis** — Meaning __________ CM Code __________
2. Pregnancy, complicated by, **antepartum hemorrhage**, second trimester — Meaning __________ CM Code __________

(continued)

Coding Practice (continued)

3. Pregnancy, complicated by, **amnionitis**, first trimester — Meaning ______________________ CM Code __________
4. Pregnancy, complicated by, **isoimmunization** Rh, second trimester — Meaning ______________________ CM Code __________
5. Pregnancy, complicated by, **oligohydramnios**, second trimester — Meaning ______________________ CM Code __________
6. Pregnancy, complicated by, **salpingo-oophoritis**, first trimester — Meaning ______________________ CM Code __________
7. Pregnancy, **intraperitoneal** — Meaning ______________________ CM Code __________
8. Pregnancy, supervision of, high risk, older mother, **primigravida**, second trimester — Meaning ______________________ CM Code __________
9. Delivery, complicated by, **cervical dystocia**, third trimester — Meaning ______________________ CM Code __________
10. Delivery, complicated by, **abruptio placentae**, third trimester — Meaning ______________________ CM Code __________

CODING OVERVIEW OF OBSTETRICS

ICD-10-CM Chapter 15, Pregnancy, Childbirth, and the Puerperium (O00-O9A), contains nine blocks or subchapters that are divided by the phase of pregnancy and the type of condition. Review the block names and code ranges listed at the beginning of Chapter 15 in the ICD-10-CM manual to become familiar with the content and organization.

This chapter includes pregnancy with abortive outcome, complications of pregnancy, delivery and complications of delivery, and disorders arising during the postpartum period. It does not include reproductive or fertility disorders, which are classified in ICD-10-CM Chapter 14 Diseases of the Genitourinary System. An instructional note at the beginning of the chapter requires that codes in this chapter are to be used only on the mother's record, never on the newborn's record.

ICD-10-CM Chapter 15 corresponds with ICD-9-CM Chapter 11 (630-379). Numerous categories have been expanded in ICD-10-CM compared to ICD-9-CM in order to add specificity of anatomic site, time frames, and other details. In addition, some codes have new titles, while others have been combined or deleted.

Three major changes are implemented in ICD-10-CM. (1) The fifth digit required in ICD-9-CM to designate the episode of care has been eliminated. Instead, conditions are classified based on the trimester in which the condition occurs. (2) An instructional note at the beginning of the chapter directs codes to assign an additional code from category **Z3A** to identify the weeks of gestation. (3) Some codes require a seventh-character extension to identify which fetus in a multiple gestation is affected. Examples of how to assign trimester, week, and fetus identifiers are provided later in this chapter.

ICD-10-CM provides Official Guidelines for Coding and Reporting (OGCR) pregnancy, childbirth, and the puerperium in OGCR section I.C.15. OGCR provide detailed discussion of general rules for obstetric cases, selection of OB principal or first-listed diagnosis, preexisting conditions, and several specific conditions, including hypertension, diabetes, HIV, alcohol and tobacco use, normal delivery, postpartum, and abortions. OGCR regarding the use of Z codes related to pregnancy, childbirth, and the puerperium appear in OGCR I.C.21.c.11).

ABSTRACTING FOR OBSTETRICS

Because multiple complications are common during pregnancy, childbirth, and the puerperium, coders must be attentive to which complication is the reason for the encounter or admission.

Abstracting Conditions of Pregnancy

It is important to identify all the conditions affecting a pregnant woman, but coders also must identify the main reason for the specific encounter or admission, as this will determine the first-listed or principal diagnosis. Refer to ■ TABLE 23-6 for guidance on how to abstract conditions of pregnancy. In particular, coders must be attentive to distinguish between preexisting conditions and pregnancy-related conditions. They should also be familiar with the criteria for abstracting multiple gestations.

Abstracting Preexisting Conditions and Conditions Due to Pregnancy

Pregnant women may have a medical condition that must be treated in addition to caring for the pregnancy itself. Coders must determine, based on the documentation, if the condition is preexisting prior to the pregnancy or if it developed as a direct result of the pregnancy. Although the symptoms, manifestations, and complications are similar for preexisting and pregnancy-related variations of a disease, different codes are often required (OGCR I.C.15.c.). Two common conditions that fall into this category are diabetes and hypertension.

Table 23-6 ■ KEY CRITERIA FOR ABSTRACTING CONDITIONS OF PREGNANCY

- ❑ Will the patient be under age 16 or over age 35 at EDD?
- ❑ How many fetuses are there?
- ❑ What trimester is the pregnancy?
- ❑ How many weeks of gestation are completed?
- ❑ How many pregnancies has the patient had, including the current one?
- ❑ How many births has the patient had?
- ❑ What preexisting medical conditions exist?
- ❑ What complications exist?
- ❑ What is the current gestational age?
- ❑ For multiple gestations, how many chorions and amniotic sacs are present?
- ❑ For multiple gestations, which fetus is affected by the complication?
- ❑ What is the main reason for the encounter or the primary complication treated?

Prexisting and Gestational Diabetes. Preexisting diabetes should be clearly documented in the medical record and identified as type 1 or type 2. Coders should also identify any additional manifestations of diabetes and whether a type 2 diabetic is on long term use of insulin. Preexisting diabetes that is treated during pregnancy is *not* gestational diabetes. Gestational diabetes mellitus (GDM) is first diagnosed during pregnancy, usually during the second or third trimester, and usually resolves after delivery. GDM should be identified as diet-controlled or insulin-controlled. For a refresher on abstracting diabetes, refer to OGCR I.C.4.a. and Chapter 10 of this text.

> **CODING CAUTION**
>
> A patient cannot have *both* preexisting diabetes and gestational diabetes. You need to identify the condition as one or the other. If the documentation is not clear, query the physician.

Preexisting and Gestational Hypertension. Preexisting hypertension should also be clearly documented in the medical record. The type of hypertension and whether the condition involves the heart and/or kidney should also be identified. When a patient with preexisting hypertension develops preeclampsia, this combination should be noted. Gestational hypertension is first diagnosed during pregnancy and usually resolves after delivery. Coders must carefully review the documentation for gestational hypertension to determine whether it exists with significant proteinuria, which constitutes preeclampsia. Preeclampsia should be further identified as mild, moderate, severe, or HELLP syndrome. Finally, coders should note when symptoms of edema and proteinuria are documented *without* hypertension.

Abstracting Multiple Gestations

Multiple gestation is a complication of pregnancy that places both the mother and the fetuses at higher risk of developing problems. Coders must identify the number of amnions and chorions in all multiple gestation pregnancies. If the physician has documented that the number of placenta or amniotic sacs cannot be determined, this should also be noted.

Physicians identify each fetus in a multiple gestation by number, such as fetus 1, fetus 2, or fetus 3. When a fetus is affected by a prenatal or delivery complication, or the mother is affected by a condition of a fetus, coders must identify which fetus is affected (■ FIGURE 23-6, page 460).

Patient is seen in the office in week 36 with mild preeclampsia. She is pregnant with twins, DiDi, and wants to attempt vaginal delivery. Reports sporadic contractions that appear to be false labor. Fetus 2 is currently in breech position. The physician decides to admit her to the hospital for observation.

What is the current gestational age? **36 weeks**

What trimester is the pregnancy? **third**

How many fetuses exist? **two**

How many chorions are present? **two**

How many amnions are present? **two**

What complications exist? **mild preeclampsia**

What other complications exist? **breech presentation**

What fetus is affected? **fetus 2**

Figure 23-6 ■ Example of Abstracting for Multiple Gestation

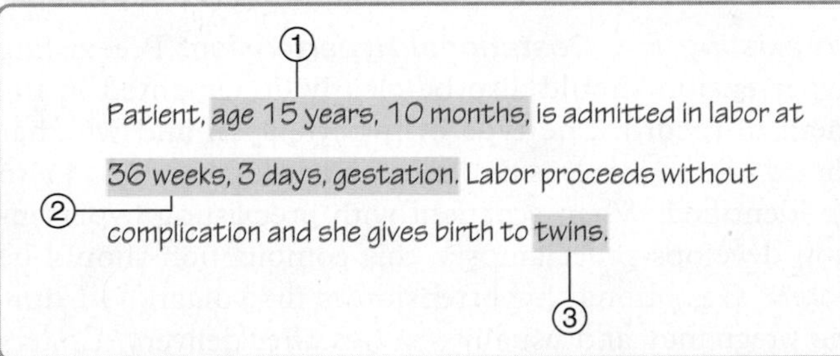

Figure 23-7 ■ Example of a Delivery with Three Complications

Abstracting Conditions of Childbirth

Any delivery that varies from the definition of a normal delivery is complicated and requires that coders identify all the complications that occurred. First, identify the main circumstance or complication of the delivery. Then, identify any additional complications. When C/S is performed, identify the main circumstance or complication that establishes the need for the C/S.

Keep in mind that certain circumstances always qualify as complications, even though they may not seem to be a specific "problem." Circumstantial complications include the following (■ FIGURE 23-7):

- age at EDD under 16 or over 35
- multiple gestation
- previous C/S
- delivery before 37 completed weeks of gestation

Table 23-7 ■ KEY CRITERIA FOR ABSTRACTING CONDITIONS OF CHILDBIRTH

- ❑ What is the reason for the admission?
- ❑ In what week of pregnancy did delivery occur?
- ❑ Is the delivery vaginal or cesarean?
- ❑ What is the reason a cesarean section was performed?
- ❑ Has the mother had a previous cesarean delivery?
- ❑ Was there a malposition of the fetus or obstructed labor?
- ❑ What other complications are present?
- ❑ How many fetuses were delivered? Were there any stillbirths?

Table 23-8 ■ KEY CRITERIA FOR ABSTRACTING CONDITIONS OF THE PUERPERIUM

- ❑ Is the encounter less than six weeks after delivery?
- ❑ What complication or condition is treated during the encounter?
- ❑ Is the condition preexisting or does it originate during the postpartum/puerperal period?

Refer to ■ TABLE 23-7 for guidance in abstracting conditions related to labor, delivery, and childbirth.

Abstracting Conditions of the Puerperium

Some conditions, such as depression or psychosis, may be preexisting, so coders need to distinguish between conditions that originate in the postpartum period and those that are preexisting. Refer to ■ TABLE 23-8 for guidance in abstracting conditions related to the puerperium.

Abstracting from Obstetric Records

Obstetric records contain unique information and abbreviations not found in other medical records. Refer to ■ FIGURE 23-8 to learn how to interpret the mini-medical-record used for obstetric cases in this text.

Guided Example of Abstracting for Obstetrics

Refer to the following example throughout this chapter to practice skills for abstracting, assigning, and sequencing pregnancy, childbirth, and the puerperium codes. Daphne Wittman, CCS-P, is a fictitious coder who guides you through the coding process.

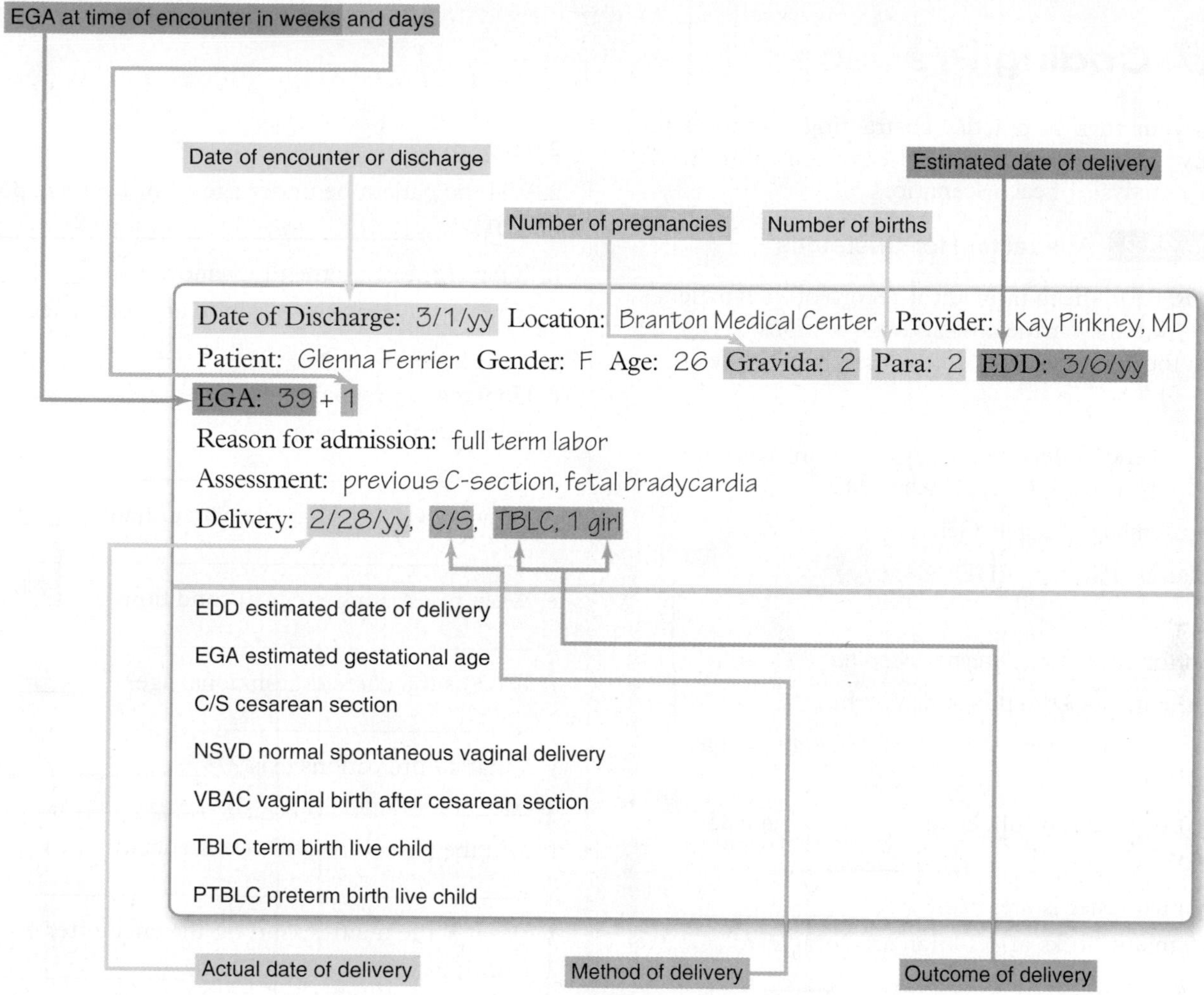

Figure 23-8 ■ Key to Interpreting the Obstetrics Mini-Medical-Record

Date of discharge: 3/1/yy Location: Branton Medical Center Provider: Kay Pinkney, MD

Patient: Glenna Ferrier Gender: F Age: 26

Gravida: 2 Para: 2 EDD: 3/6/yy

EGA: 39+1

Reason for admission: full term labor

Assessment: Attempted vaginal delivery. Labor started off well then slowed. I was concerned that prolonged labor would place the scar from the previous c/s at risk. In addition, the stress affected the fetal heart rate causing tachycardia so I proceeded with a c/s.

Delivery: 2/28/yy, C/S, TBLC, 1 girl, transferred to NICU for monitoring and management of heart rate

Follow along as Daphne Wittman, CCS-P, abstracts the diagnosis. Check off each step after you complete it.

⇨ Daphne reads through the entire record, with special attention to the reason for the admission and the final delivery data. She refers to Key Criteria for Abstracting Conditions of Childbirth (Table 23-7).

❑ *What is the reason for the admission?* full term labor

❑ *In what week of pregnancy did delivery occur?* 39+1

❑ *Is the delivery vaginal or cesarean?* C-section

❑ *What is the reason a cesarean section was performed?* previous C-section

❑ *Has the mother had a previous cesarean delivery?* Yes

❑ *How many fetuses were delivered?* 1 female

❑ *Were there any stillbirths?* No, TBLC

❑ *What other complications are present?* fetal tachycardia

⇨ At this time, Daphne does not know how many codes she will end up with. She will learn about this when she moves on to assigning codes.

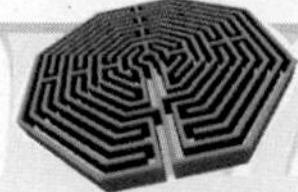

Coding Practice

Now it is your turn to practice abstracting diagnoses for pregnancy, childbirth, and the puerperium. Questions guide your analysis of each scenario.

Exercise 23.2 Abstracting for Obstetrics

Instructions: Read the mini-medical-record of each patient's encounter and answer the abstracting questions. Write the answer on the line provided. Do not assign any codes.

1. Date of encounter: 3/23/yy Location: New Life Obstetrics Provider: Kay Pinkney, MD

Patient: Kimberley Bopp Gender: F Age: 33

Gravida: 3 Para: 2 EDD: 6/30/yy

EGA: 26+2

Reason for encounter: vaginal bleeding

Assessment: placenta previa, hemorrhage

Plan: bed confinement, RTO 2 weeks, C section may be required

a. Will the patient be under age 16 or over age 35 at EDD? ______________

b. What trimester is the pregnancy? ______________
How many weeks of gestation are completed?
____

c. How many pregnancies has the patient had, including the current one? ______________
____

d. How many births has the patient had? ______________
____

e. What preexisting medical conditions exist?
____

f. What complications exist? ______________
____

2. Date of encounter: 3/23/yy Location: New Life Obstetrics Provider: Kay Pinkney, MD

Patient: Isabelle Bang Gender: F Age: 24

Gravida: 1 Para: 0 EDD: 3/23/yy

EGA: 40+2

Reason for encounter: prenatal visit

Assessment: unstable lie

Plan: C-section today at 1500

(continued)

2. (continued)

a. Will the patient be under age 16 or over age 35 at EDD? ______________

b. What trimester is the pregnancy? ______________
How many weeks of gestation are completed?
____

c. How many pregnancies has the patient had, including the current one? ______________
____

d. How many births has the patient had? ______________
____

e. What preexisting medical conditions exist?
____

f. What is the current gestational age? ______________
____

g. What complications exist? ______________
____

h. Did the patient deliver at this encounter?
____

i. What is the main reason for the encounter or the primary complication treated? ______________
____

3. Date of encounter: 3/23/yy Location: New Life Obstetrics Provider: Kay Pinkney, MD

Patient: Jayne Ditzler Gender: F Age: 35

Gravida: 1 Para: 0 EDD: 10/19/yy

EGA: 10+4

Reason for encounter: establish prenatal care

Assessment: discussed the risks of pregnancy at this age, need for BP and DM monitoring, no problems at this time

Plan: schedule amniocentesis and **chorionic villi sampling (CVS)**

a. Will the patient be under age 16 or over age 35 at EDD? ______________

b. What trimester is the pregnancy? ______________
How many weeks of gestation are completed?
____

(continued)

3. (continued)

c. How many pregnancies has the patient had, including the current one?______________________

d. How many births has the patient had?__________

e. What preexisting medical conditions exist?

f. What is the current gestational age? __________

g. What complications exist? ______________

h. What is the main reason for the encounter or the primary complication treated? __________

4. Date of encounter: 3/23/yy Location: New Life Obstetrics Provider: Kay Pinkney, MD

Patient: Summer Griner Gender: F Age: 26

Gravida: 3 Para: 2 EDD: 7/6/yy EGA: 24+6

Reason for encounter: prenatal visit, FU on gestational DM diagnosed at last visit

Assessment: GTT shows that the diabetes is being adequately controlled through diet

Plan: continue with nutritional plan and good eating habits

a. Will the patient be under age 16 or over age 35 at EDD? ______________

b. What trimester is the pregnancy?____________ How many weeks of gestation are completed?

c. How many pregnancies has the patient had, including the current one?______________________

d. How many births has the patient had?__________

e. What preexisting medical conditions exist?

f. What is the current gestational age? __________

(continued)

4. (continued)

g. What complications exist? ______________

h. What is the main reason for the encounter or the primary complication treated? __________

5. Date of encounter: 3/23/yy Location: New Life Obstetrics Provider: Kay Pinkney, MD

Patient: Helene McCarley Gender: F Age: 25

Gravida: 2 Para: 1 EDD: 6/15/yy

EGA: 28+3

Reason for encounter: routine prenatal visit

Assessment: Rhesus incompatibility

Plan: Rho(D) immune globulin treatment on Monday

a. Will the patient be under age 16 or over age 35 at EDD? ______________

b. What trimester is the pregnancy?____________ How many weeks of gestation are completed?

c. How many pregnancies has the patient had, including the current one?______________________

d. How many births has the patient had?__________

e. What preexisting medical conditions exist?

f. What is the current gestational age? __________

g. What complications exist? ______________

h. What is the main reason for the encounter or the primary complication treated? __________

6. Date of discharge: 3/24/yy Location: Branton Medical Center Provider: Kay Pinkney, MD

Patient: Lea Bloodworth Gender: F Age: 18

Gravida: 1 Para: 0 EDD: 4/6/yy EGA: 37+5

(continued)

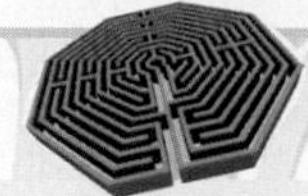

Coding Practice (continued)

6. (continued)

Reason for admission: full term labor

Assessment: placental infarction

Delivery: 3/22/yy, NSVD, stillborn, 1 girl

a. What is the reason for the admission? ________

b. In what week of pregnancy did delivery occur? ________

c. Is the delivery vaginal or cesarean? ________

d. Has the mother had a previous cesarean delivery? ________

e. Was there a malposition of the fetus or obstructed labor? ________

f. What other complications are present? ________

g. How many fetuses were delivered? ________ Were there any stillbirths? ________

7. Date of encounter: 3/24/yy Location: New Life Obstetrics Provider: Kay Pinkney, MD

Patient: Keisha Ryerson Gender: F Age: 30

Gravida: 2 Para: 1 EDD: 10/5/yy

EGA: 12+0

Reason for encounter: prenatal care, pernicious anemia

Assessment: blood work has improved, but still not where it should be

Plan: B12 injection

a. Will the patient be under age 16 or over age 35 at EDD? ________

b. What trimester is the pregnancy? ________ How many weeks of gestation are completed? ________

c. How many pregnancies has the patient had, including the current one? ________

d. How many births has the patient had? ________

(continued)

7. (continued)

e. What preexisting medical conditions exist? ________

f. What is the current gestational age? ________

g. What complications exist? ________

h. What is the main reason for the encounter or the primary complication treated? ________

8. Date of discharge: 3/24/yy Location: Branton Medical Center Provider: Kay Pinkney, MD

Patient: Jeanine Mohn Gender: F Age: 32

Gravida: 2 Para: 2 EDD: 5/18/yy

EGA: 32+2

Reason for admission: premature rupture of membranes

Assessment: severe pre-eclampsia requires c/s

Delivery: 3/22/yy, classical C/S, PTBLC, 1 girl

a. What is the reason for the admission? ________

b. In what week of pregnancy did delivery occur? ________

c. Is the delivery vaginal or cesarean? ________

d. What is the reason a cesarean section was performed? ________

e. Was there a malposition of the fetus or obstructed labor? ________

f. What other complications are present? ________

g. How many fetuses were delivered? ________ Were there any stillbirths? ________

9. Date of encounter: 3/24/yy Location: New Life Obstetrics Provider: Kay Pinkney, MD

Patient: Lily Wahlstrom Gender: F Age: 15

(continued)

9. (continued)

Birthday: 7/15 Gravida: 1 Para: 0

EDD: 6/1/yy EGA: 30+4

Reason for encounter: prenatal care, twins, MoDi

Assessment: dipstick shows new isolated gestational proteinuria

Plan: at risk for preeclampsia, RTO 4 days for repeat test.

a. Will the patient be under age 16 or over age 35 at EDD? ______

b. What trimester is the pregnancy? ______
How many weeks of gestation are completed? ______

c. How many pregnancies has the patient had, including the current one? ______

d. How many births has the patient had? ______

e. What preexisting medical conditions exist? ______

f. What is the current gestational age? ______

g. For multiple gestations, how many chorions are present? ______ How many amniotic sacs are present? ______

h. What complications exist? ______

10. Date of discharge: 3/24/yy

Location: Branton Medical Center Provider: Kay Pinkney, MD

Patient: Grace Topete Gender: F Age: 22

Gravida: 2 Para: 2 EDD: 3/16/yy

EGA: 41+3

Reason for admission: post term labor

Assessment: obstructed labor due to CPD, severe obesity mother, BMI 41

Delivery: 3/23/yy, C/S, TBLC, 1 boy

a. What is the reason for the admission? ______

b. In what week of pregnancy did delivery occur? ______

c. Is the delivery vaginal or cesarean? ______

d. Was there a malposition of the fetus or obstructed labor? ______

e. What other complications are present? ______

f. What is the reason a cesarean section was performed? ______

g. How many fetuses were delivered? ______
Were there any stillbirths? ______

ASSIGNING CODES FOR OBSTETRICS

Coders should acquaint themselves with the organization of obstetrical terms in the Index and must be attentive to distinguish between codes that apply to the mother and those that apply to the infant. In addition, they should also be familiar with how to assign codes to identify the term, the pregnancy, the trimester, and the fetus. Different rules also apply for assigning codes to prenatal visits for normal and high-risk pregnancies.

Locating Obstetrical Main Terms in the Index

The Index groups codes for pregnancy under the Main Term **Pregnancy**. The first-level subterm **complicated by** occupies most of the entry and provides second- and third-level subterms for conditions that complicate pregnancy, such as **abscess** or **placenta previa**. Other first-level subterms describe the type of pregnancy, such as **normal, ectopic,** or **multiple gestation**.

The Index groups codes for labor and delivery under the Main Term **Delivery**. The first-level subterms **cesarean for** and **complicated by** occupy most of the entry and provide second- and third-level subterms for conditions that complicate labor delivery, such as **cord, around neck, with compression** or **obstruction**. A limited number of other first-level subterms describe the type of pregnancy, such as **normal** or **forceps**.

SUCCESS STEP

Take a few minutes to review the Index entries for **Pregnancy** and **Delivery** in your ICD-10-CM manual. Highlight the beginning and end of the subterm **complicated by**.

As with any condition, most obstetrical conditions have multiple coding paths. For example, some complications of labor and delivery are also located under the Main Term **Pregnancy, complicated by**. Some conditions are also indexed under the Main Term for the name of the condition, with a subterm for pregnancy, such as **Diabetes, gestational** or **Rh, incompatibility**.

Assigning Codes for the Mother's Condition

When assigning codes for conditions related to pregnancy and childbirth, coders must recognize that although both the mother and the newborn may be affected by the same condition, they assign separate codes for each. Codes in ICD-10-CM Chapter 15 are used *only* on the mother's bill (OGCR I.C.15.a.2)). This is easy to remember because the mother's codes begin with the letter **O**.

When delivery occurs and the newborn receives medical care or occupies a bed, the baby has a separate medical record, separate bills, and separate codes. Codes for the infant begin with **P** and are assigned from ICD-10-CM Chapter 16, Certain Conditions Originating in the Perinatal Period (P00-P96). Coding for the infant is discussed in Chapter 24 of this text.

CODING CAUTION

Codes beginning with **P** should NEVER be assigned to the mother (OGCR I.C.16.a.1)).

Careful use of the Index is required in order to identify the Main Term and subterms that distinguish between the mother and the infant. A Main Term for the condition will have separate subterms for the mother and the infant. Select the subterm that corresponds to the record being coded. For example, when a mother is treated for Rh incompatibility, the code will be different than the one used when the infant is treated for the same condition (■ FIGURE 23-9).

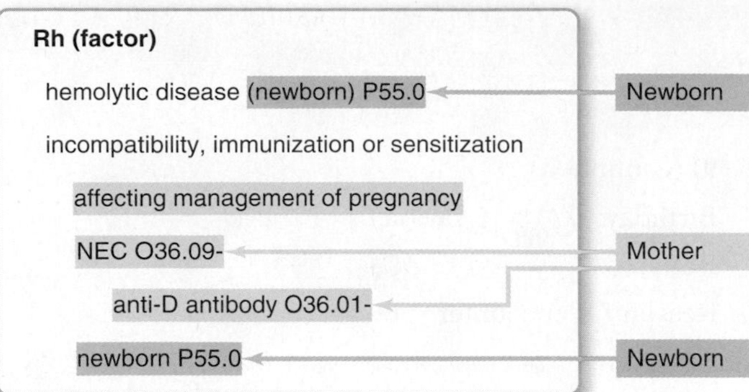

Figure 23-9 ■ Index Entry for Rh Factor, with Separate Codes for Mother and Newborn

Assigning Codes to Identify the Term of Pregnancy

Preterm labor and delivery, as well as postterm pregnancy, constitute complications and require a code. Term lengths are defined by the gestational age at the time of the encounter (■ TABLE 23-9). Codes are indexed under the Main Term **Pregnancy**, the subterm **complicated by**, and a second-level subterm for **preterm** or **postmaturity**. Alternatively, search for the Main Term **Preterm, Postterm**, or **Prolonged**, then locate the appropriate subterm for **pregnancy, labor, or delivery**.

SUCCESS STEP

Be careful to distinguish between the letter **O** (oh) that begins each code, and the number **0** (zero) that occupies other positions. When making handwritten notes, use a cursive O (with a loop at the top) for the letter; write the number zero with a slash through it Ø. By clearly distinguishing handwritten notes, you make it easier to key them in correctly. On the keyboard, use the alphabetic keys for the letter and the numeric keypad or the top row of numbers for zero. If you mix up these two similar characters, the computer in your workplace may not accept your code or, worse, the insurance company may reject your claim as unprocessable (incapable of being processed) due to an invalid code.

Assigning Codes to Identify the Trimester and Weeks

Many obstetrics codes require coders to identify the trimester and weeks of gestation. The timeframe for each trimester is defined in an instructional note at the

Table 23-9 ■ **DEFINITION OF PREGNANCY TERMS, WITH CODES**

Term	Weeks of Gestation	Code
Preterm pregnancy, delivery, or labor	Less than 37 completed weeks of gestation	O60.1-, O60.2-
Full term pregnancy	37 weeks, 0 days of gestation to 39 weeks, 6 days of gestation	No code
Postterm pregnancy	40 completed weeks to 42 completed weeks of gestation	O48.0
Prolonged pregnancy	More than 42 completed weeks of gestation	O48.1

beginning of the chapter. Trimesters are identified in the Tabular List with the fourth, fifth, or sixth character, depending on the length of the code. The symbol 4th, 5th, or 6th in front of the subcategory entry in the Tabular List indicates that an additional character is needed. The codes for each trimester are listed immediately below the subcategory heading (■ FIGURE 23-10). Conditions that only occur in one trimester, or to which the concept of trimesters does not apply, do not have a character to identify the trimester (OGCR 15.a3), 4), and 5)). For example, codes for **ectopic** pregnancy do not require a trimester designation.

Assign a code from category **Z3A Weeks of gestation** in order to identify the number of weeks of gestation completed in the pregnancy. Locate the code in the Index under the Main Term **Pregnancy** and subterm **weeks**. Category **Z3A** appears after category **Z36** in the Tabular List.

SUCCESS STEP

Experienced coders will notice that identifying the trimester is a new concept in ICD-10-CM. The trimester designation replaces the ICD-9-CM fifth digit for episode of care, which no longer applies.

CODING CAUTION

Report codes from **Z3A** for the *completed* weeks of pregnancy. Do not count partial weeks.

5th O12.0 Gestational edema

O12.00 Gestational edema, unspecified trimester

O12.01 Gestational edema, first trimester

O12.02 Gestational edema, second trimester

O12.03 Gestational edema, third trimester

Figure 23-10 ■ Tabular List Entry for Gestational Edema, Requiring a Trimester Designation

Assigning Codes to Identify the Fetus

When maternal conditions affect the fetus or fetal conditions create maternal complications, assign a seventh character to identify which fetus is involved (OGCR 15.a.6)) based on physician documentation. The applicable codes are clearly designated in the Tabular List by the symbol 7th. Seventh-character options are listed in a box at the category or subcategory level (■ FIGURE 23-11 and ■ FIGURE 23-12, page 468). Assign the seventh character of **0** in the following situations:

- for singletons
- when it is not possible for the physician to determine which fetus is affected
- when documentation does not identify the affected fetus and the coder cannot obtain clarification from the physician

SUCCESS STEP

Common sense may suggest that when there is only one fetus, you would assign the seventh character of **1**. However, the boxed instructional note directs you to assign the seventh character **0** for a singleton. The character **1** identifies *fetus number one* in a multiple gestation pregnancy.

Assigning Codes for Prenatal Visits

ICD-10-CM provides codes for routine outpatient prenatal visits, which are classified as **Supervision of pregnancy**. Different rules apply for a normal pregnancy than for high-risk patients (■ TABLE 23-10, page 468).

For routine outpatient visits with no complications present, assign a code from category **Z34 Encounter for supervision of normal pregnancy** as the only diagnosis code. Codes are divided based on whether it is the first pregnancy and also by trimester. If any complication from Chapter 15 (O00-O99) exists, the pregnancy is not classified as normal and coders should not assign a code from **Z34**. Locate the code in the Index by searching for the Main Term **Pregnancy**, the subterm **supervision of**, then

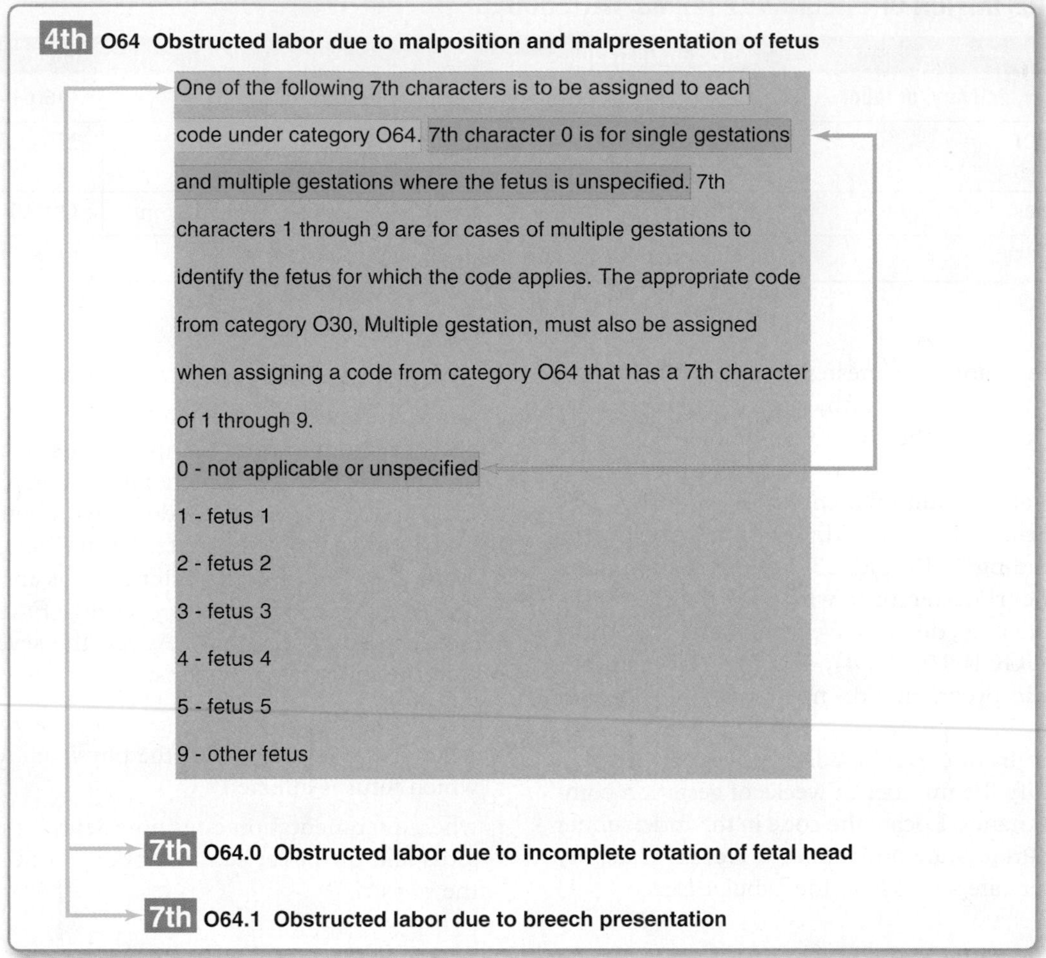

Figure 23-11 ■ Tabular List Entry for Seventh Character Identification of Fetus

Fetus 2 presents in the breech position. Physician performs a cesarean section due to obstructed labor.

O64.1XX2 Obstructed labor due to breech presentation

(Note: This example only illustrates how to identify the fetus with the seventh character and does not represent complete coding for the case.)

Figure 23-12 ■ Example of Assigning a Seventh Character to Identify the Fetus

Table 23-10 ■ CODE SEQUENCING FOR PRENATAL VISITS

Classification of Pregnancy	Code Sequencing
Normal	1. **Z34.- Encounter for supervision of normal pregnancy** Do not assign any additional codes from ICD-10-CM Chapter 15.
High risk	1. **O09.- Supervision of high-risk pregnancy** 2. Assign as many codes as needed from Chapter 15 and other chapters to identify the complication(s).

the second-level subterm **normal**. Select the third-level subterm that identifies the pregnancy as the **first** or **specified NEC** (not the first). Verify the code in the Tabular List in order to assign the correct character for the trimester.

For all other routine outpatient visits, assign a code from category **O09 Supervision of high-risk pregnancy**, as the first listed code. Assign additional codes from ICD-10-CM Chapter 15, or other chapters as needed, to describe any complications. Women who are very young—under age 15 at EDD—or older—over age 35 at EDD—are classified as high-risk pregnancies and should be assigned a corresponding code from category **O09**. Locate the code in the Index by searching for the Main Term **Pregnancy**, the subterm **supervision of**, then the second-level subterm **high risk**. Select the third-level subterm that describes the reason the pregnancy is high risk. Verify the code in the Tabular List in order to assign the correct character for the trimester (■ FIGURE 23-13).

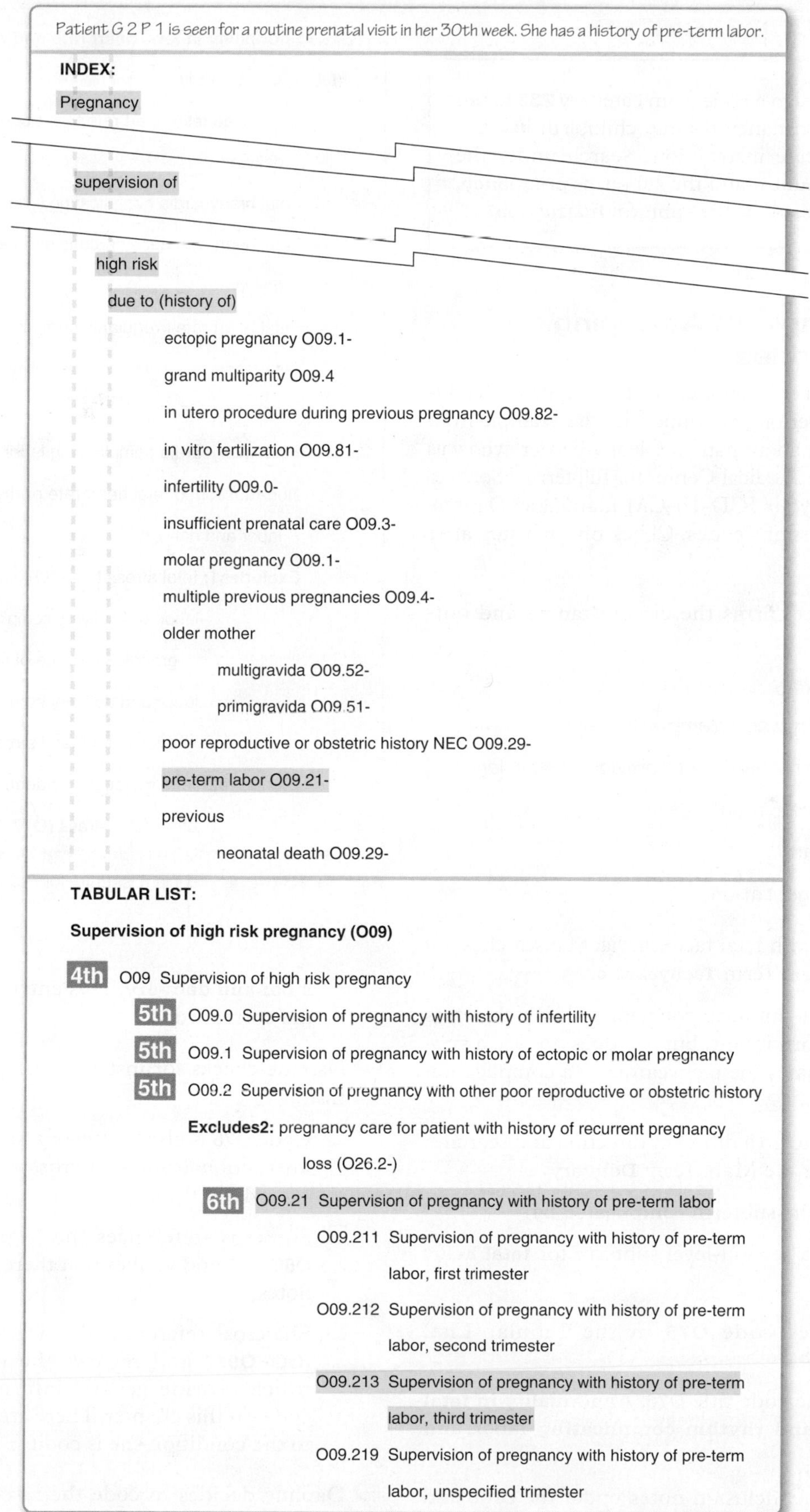

Patient G 2 P 1 is seen for a routine prenatal visit in her 30th week. She has a history of pre-term labor.

INDEX:

Pregnancy

supervision of

high risk

due to (history of)

ectopic pregnancy O09.1-

grand multiparity O09.4

in utero procedure during previous pregnancy O09.82-

in vitro fertilization O09.81-

infertility O09.0-

insufficient prenatal care O09.3-

molar pregnancy O09.1-

multiple previous pregnancies O09.4-

older mother

multigravida O09.52-

primigravida O09.51-

poor reproductive or obstetric history NEC O09.29-

pre-term labor O09.21-

previous

neonatal death O09.29-

TABULAR LIST:

Supervision of high risk pregnancy (O09)

4th O09 Supervision of high risk pregnancy

5th O09.0 Supervision of pregnancy with history of infertility

5th O09.1 Supervision of pregnancy with history of ectopic or molar pregnancy

5th O09.2 Supervision of pregnancy with other poor reproductive or obstetric history

Excludes2: pregnancy care for patient with history of recurrent pregnancy loss (O26.2-)

6th O09.21 Supervision of pregnancy with history of pre-term labor

O09.211 Supervision of pregnancy with history of pre-term labor, first trimester

O09.212 Supervision of pregnancy with history of pre-term labor, second trimester

O09.213 Supervision of pregnancy with history of pre-term labor, third trimester

O09.219 Supervision of pregnancy with history of pre-term labor, unspecified trimester

Figure 23-13 ■ Example of Selecting the First-Listed Diagnosis for Supervision of a High-Risk Pregnancy

SUCCESS STEP

Assign a code from category **Z32** for an encounter for pregnancy testing, childbirth instruction, and childcare instruction. Search under the Main Term **Encounter** and the subterms **pregnancy**, then **test**, then **result** or the subterm **instruction**.

Guided Example of Assigning Obstetrics Codes

To practice skills for assigning codes for pregnancy, childbirth, and the puerperium, continue with the example from earlier in the chapter about patient Glenna Ferrier, who was admitted to Branton Medical Center for full term labor.

Follow along in your ICD-10-CM manual as Daphne Wittman, CCS-P, assigns codes. Check off each step after you complete it.

⇨ First, Daphne confirms the circumstances and outcome of delivery:

- ❑ full term delivery
- ❑ vaginal delivery was attempted
- ❑ C-section performed due to previous C-section
- ❑ single live female infant
- ❑ fetal tachycardia
- ❑ 39 weeks of gestation

⇨ Daphne begins with fetal tachycardia. She searches the Index for the Main Term **Tachycardia**.

- ❑ She locates a subterm for neonatal, which refers to the newborn infant, but she does not see a subterm that relates the tachycardia as a complication of delivery.
- ❑ She decides to go a different direction and searches the Index for the Main Term **Delivery**.
- ❑ She locates the subterm **complicated by**.
- ❑ She locates a second-level subterm for **fetal heart rate, O76**.

⇨ Daphne verifies code **O76** in the Tabular List. (■ FIGURE 23-14).

- ❑ She reads the code title **O76, Abnormality in fetal heart rate and rhythm complicating labor and delivery**.
- ❑ She reads the inclusion notes under the code and sees the entry **Fetal tachycardia complicating labor and delivery**. This entry confirms that this is the correct code.

O76 Abnormality in fetal heart rate and rhythm complicating labor and delivery

Depressed fetal heart rate tones complicating labor and delivery
Fetal bradycardia complicating labor and delivery
Fetal heart rate decelerations complicating labor and delivery
Fetal heart rate irregularity complicating labor and delivery
Fetal heart rate abnormal variability complicating labor and delivery
Fetal tachycardia complicating labor and delivery
Non-reassuring fetal heart rate or rhythm complicating labor and delivery
Excludes1: fetal stress NOS (O77.9)
labor and delivery complicated by electrocardiographic evidence of fetal stress (O77.8)
labor and delivery complicated by ultrasonic evidence of fetal stress (O77.8)
Excludes2: fetal metabolic acidemia (O68)
other fetal stress (O77.0-O77.1)

Figure 23-14 ■ Tabular List Entry for Fetal Tachycardia

⇨ Daphne checks for instructional notes in the Tabular List.

- ❑ Code **O76** is also a category, so there are no further instructional notes to cross-references at the category level.
- ❑ She cross-references the beginning of the block **O60-O77** and verifies that there are no instructional notes.
- ❑ She cross-references the beginning of **Chapter 15 (O00-O9A)** and reviews the instructional notes, which provide general information about using codes in this chapter. There are no notes that relate to the condition she is coding.

⇨ Daphne decides to code the reason for the cesarean section next, which is the fact that the patient had a previous cesarean section. She searches the Index for the Main Term **Delivery**.

- ❑ She locates the subterm **cesarean for**.
- ❑ She locates a second-level subterm for **previous cesarean delivery O34.21**.

⇨ Daphne verifies code **O34.21** in the Tabular List.

- ❑ She reads the code title **O34.21, Maternal care for scar from previous cesarean delivery**.

⇨ Daphne checks for instructional notes in the Tabular List.

- ❑ She cross-references the beginning of the category **O34, Maternal care for abnormality of pelvic organs** and reads the instructional notes (■ FIGURE 23-15).
  - The **Includes** note describes the general purpose of this category
  - The second note states **Code first any associated obstructed labor (O65.5)**.
  - She double-checks the medical record and confirms that obstructed labor is not documented, therefore this note does not apply.
  - The third note states **Use additional code for specific condition**.
  - The specific condition is fetal tachycardia, which she has already coded. This note will also provide direction when it is time to sequence the codes.
- ❑ She cross-references the beginning of the block **O30-O48** and verifies that there are no instructional notes.
- ❑ She is already familiar with the instructional notes at the beginning of **Chapter 15 (O00-O9A)**

CODING CAUTION

Notice that Daphne did not *automatically* assign a code for obstructed labor when she read the instructional note. The expression "Code first *any*" means "Code obstructed labor, *if it is documented.*" Because obstruction is not documented, she did not assign a code for it.

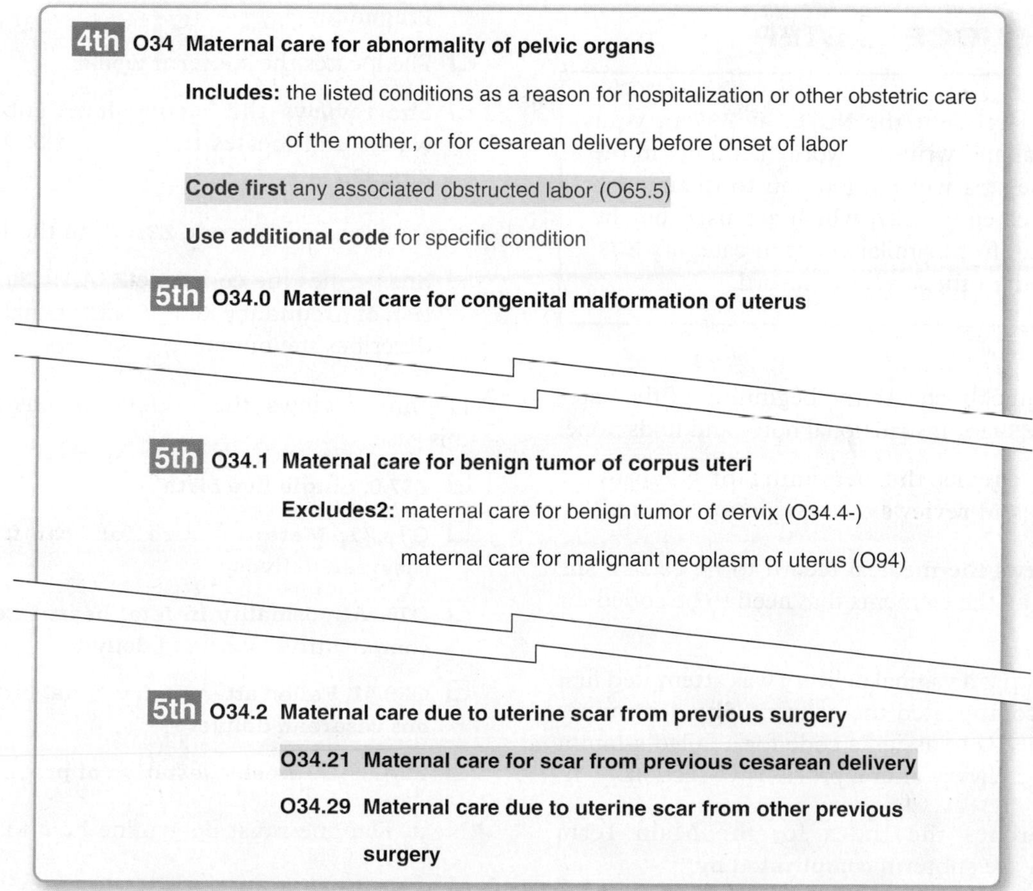

4th **O34 Maternal care for abnormality of pelvic organs**

Includes: the listed conditions as a reason for hospitalization or other obstetric care of the mother, or for cesarean delivery before onset of labor

Code first any associated obstructed labor (O65.5)

Use additional code for specific condition

5th **O34.0 Maternal care for congenital malformation of uterus**

5th **O34.1 Maternal care for benign tumor of corpus uteri**

Excludes2: maternal care for benign tumor of cervix (O34.4-)
maternal care for malignant neoplasm of uterus (O94)

5th **O34.2 Maternal care due to uterine scar from previous surgery**

O34.21 Maternal care for scar from previous cesarean delivery

O34.29 Maternal care due to uterine scar from other previous surgery

Figure 23-15 ■ Tabular List Entry Showing Instructional Notes for Code O34.21

and remembers that there are no notes that relate to the condition she is coding.

⇨ Daphne recalls that for every encounter in which a birth occurs, OGCR require coders to assign a **Z** code for outcome of the delivery (OGCR I.C.15.b.5)).

❑ She searches the Index for the Main Term **Outcome of delivery**.

❑ She locates the subterm **single**.

❑ She reviews the second-level subterms under **single** and locates **liveborn Z37.0**.

⇨ Daphne verifies the code **Z37.0** in the Tabular List.

❑ She verifies the code title **Z37.0, Single live birth** and confirms that this correctly describes the outcome.

❑ She cross-references the **NOTE:** under the category heading **Z37**, which states **This category is intended for use as an additional code to identify the outcome of delivery on the mother's record. It is not for use on the newborn record.**

❑ This note confirms that she has the correct code for the mother's record.

SUCCESS STEP

Highlight the **NOTE:** at **Z37** in your coding manual and write the word "Mother" in the margin. These tips will remind you to distinguish the codes in category **Z37**, which are used on the *mother's* record, from similar codes in category **Z38**, which are used on the *newborn's* record.

❑ Daphne quickly checks the beginning of the category **Z30-Z39** for instructional notes and finds none.

❑ She also checks the beginning of **Chapter 21 (Z00-Z99)** and reviews the instructional notes.

⇨ Daphne reviews the medical record to be certain she has captured all the elements that need to be coded for this patient.

❑ She reads that a vaginal delivery was attempted first and this complicated the delivery. She determines that she needs to assign a code for a failed attempt at vaginal delivery after a previous C-section.

⇨ Daphne searches the Index for the Main Term **Delivery** and the subterm **complicated by**.

❑ She locates a second-level subterm **failed**.

❑ She locates a third-level subterm **attempted vaginal birth after previous cesarean delivery O66.41**.

⇨ Daphne verifies code **O66.41** in the Tabular List.

❑ She reads the code title **O66.41, Failed attempted vaginal birth after previous cesarean delivery** and confirms that this describes the case.

❑ She reads the instructional note under the code that states **Code first rupture of uterus, if applicable (O71.0-, O71.1)**. She determines that the note does not apply because a uterine rupture is not documented.

❑ She has already cross-referenced the beginning of the block **O60-O77** and **Chapter 15 (O00-O9A)** for instructional notes and remembers that there are no instructions that apply to this case.

⇨ Finally, Daphne assigns a code for the weeks of gestation of the pregnancy.

❑ She checks the medical record and verifies that 39 weeks of gestation were completed.

❑ She searches the Index for the Main Term **Pregnancy**.

❑ She locates the subterm **weeks**.

❑ She reviews the second-level subterms under **weeks** and locates the subterm **39** with the code **Z3A.39**.

⇨ Daphne verifies the code **Z3A.39** in the Tabular List.

❑ She verifies the code title **Z3A.39, 39 weeks gestation of pregnancy**, and confirms that this correctly describes the outcome.

⇨ Daphne reviews the codes she has assigned for this case.

❑ **Z37.0, Single live birth**

❑ **O34.21, Maternal care for scar from previous cesarean delivery**

❑ **O76, Abnormality in fetal heart rate and rhythm complicating labor and delivery**

❑ **O66.41, Failed attempted vaginal birth after previous cesarean delivery**

❑ **Z3A.39, 39 weeks gestation of pregnancy**

⇨ Next, Daphne must determine how to sequence the codes.

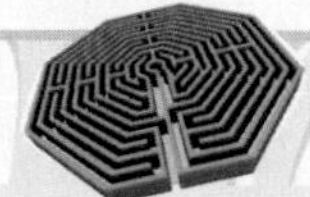

Coding Practice

Now it is your turn to practice assigning codes for pregnancy, childbirth, and the puerperium. Refer to the ***Tip*** at the end of the mini-medical-record if you need a little extra help.

Exercise 23.3 Assigning Codes for Obstetrics

Instructions: Read the mini-medical-record of each patient's encounter, review the information abstracted in Exercise 23.2, and assign ICD-10-CM diagnosis codes (CM) using the Index and Tabular List. All exercises require the second code to be from category Z3A to identify the weeks of gestation. Write the code(s) on the line provided.

1. Date of encounter: 3/23/yy Location: New Life Obstetrics Provider: Kay Pinkney, MD

Patient: Kimberley Bopp Gender: F Age: 33

Gravida: 3 Para: 2 EDD: 6/30/yy

EGA: 26+2

Reason for encounter: vaginal bleeding

Assessment: placenta previa, hemorrhage

Plan: bed confinement, RTO 2 weeks, C section may be required

2 CM Codes __________ __________

2. Date of encounter: 3/23/yy Location: New Life Obstetrics Provider: Kay Pinkney, MD

Patient: Isabelle Bang Gender: F Age: 24

Gravida: 1 Para: 0 EDD: 3/23/yy

EGA: 40+2

Reason for encounter: prenatal visit

Assessment: unstable lie

Plan: C-section today at 1500

2 CM Codes __________ __________

3. Date of encounter: 3/23/yy Location: New Life Obstetrics Provider: Kay Pinkney, MD

Patient: Jayne Ditzler Gender: F Age: 35

Gravida: 1 Para: 0 EDD: 10/19/yy

EGA: 10+4

(continued)

3. (continued)

Reason for encounter: establish prenatal care

Assessment: discussed the risks of pregnancy at this age, need for BP and DM monitoring, no problems at this time

Plan: schedule amniocentesis and **chorionic villi sampling (CVS)**

Tip: Primigravida means first pregnancy.

2 CM Codes __________ __________

4. Date of encounter: 3/23/yy Location: New Life Obstetrics Provider: Kay Pinkney, MD

Patient: Summer Griner Gender: F Age: 26

Gravida: 3 Para: 2 EDD: 7/6/yy EGA: 24+6

Reason for encounter: FU on gestational DM diagnosed at last visit

Assessment: GTT shows that the diabetes is being adequately controlled through diet

Plan: continue with nutritional plan and good eating habits

2 CM Codes __________ __________

5. Date of encounter: 3/23/yy Location: New Life Obstetrics Provider: Kay Pinkney, MD

Patient: Helene McCarley Gender: F Age: 25

Gravida: 2 Para: 1 EDD: 6/15/yy

EGA: 28+3

Reason for encounter: routine prenatal visit

Assessment: Rhesus incompatibility

Plan: Rho(D) immune globulin treatment on Monday

Tip: Select the code for the condition as it affects the mother, not the infant. Refer to OGCR I.C.15.b.2) for sequencing information.

3 CM Codes __________ __________ __________

ARRANGING CODES FOR OBSTETRICS

Coders must be attentive to selecting the principal diagnosis when a delivery occurs and to sequencing codes from Chapter 15 with codes from body system chapters. As in all coding, the principal or first-listed diagnosis is determined by the reason for the admission or encounter, OGCR, and instructional notes in the Tabular List.

Arranging Codes for When a Delivery Occurs

When a delivery occurs, a minimum of two codes are required—one for the delivery diagnosis and one for the outcome of delivery (■ TABLE 23-11). The principal diagnosis should be one of the following (OGCR I.C.15.b.4)):

- the code for normal delivery, **O80** (■ TABLE 23-12)
- the main complication of labor and delivery
- the main reason a C/S was required

Table 23-11 ■ **CODE SEQUENCING FOR THE DELIVERY ENCOUNTER**

Type of Delivery	Code Sequencing
Normal delivery	1. O80 Encounter for full-term uncomplicated delivery 2. Z37.0 Single live birth
Vaginal delivery with complications or multiple gestation	1. Main complication of labor and delivery 2. Additional complications, if any 3. Outcome of delivery Z37.-
Cesarean section	1. Main circumstance requiring C/S 2. Additional complications, if any 3. Outcome of delivery Z37.-

Table 23-12 ■ **DEFINITION OF A NORMAL DELIVERY, ICD-10-CM CODE O80**

Includes	Excludes
Minimal or no assistance	Fetal manipulation
Episiotomy	Rotation version
Spontaneous	Instrumentation/forceps
Cephalic presentation	Induced labor
Vaginal	Non-cephalic presentation
Full-term	Cesarean section
Single gestation	Preterm delivery
Live-born infant	Postterm delivery
Resolved antepartum conditions	Prolonged delivery
No other complications	Multiple gestation
	Stillbirth
	Any complication

Patient gives birth to a baby boy who makes a cephalic presentation. Aside from requesting an epidural and having an episiotomy, the patient has no problems.

(1) Index: **Delivery, normal**

Tabular List: **O80 Encounter for full-term uncomplicated delivery**

(2) Index: **Outcome of delivery, single, liveborn**

Tabular List: **Z37.0 Single live birth**

Figure 23-16 ■ Example of Sequencing Codes for a Delivery

Search the Main Term **Delivery** and subterm **complicated by** to locate the codes for complications.

The additional code is a code from category **Z37.-**, which describes the outcome of delivery in terms of the number of live infants and/or the number of still births (OGCR I.C.15.b.5)). Search the Main Term **Outcome of Delivery** for the **Z37.-** code (■ FIGURE 23-16).

SUCCESS STEP

Assign a code from **Z37.-** only during the admission in which delivery occurs. Do not assign it for subsequent admissions, even if they are for complications of delivery or for postpartum office visits. **Z37.-** is NEVER the principal or first-listed code.

Arranging Chapter 15 Codes with Codes from Other Chapters

Many complications require a code from Chapter 15 to identify the obstetric complication and an additional code from a body system chapter to describe the details of the condition. Always sequence the Chapter 15 code first (OGCR 15.a.1)) (■ TABLE 23-13). Follow this guideline regardless of whether the condition is preexisting, as in diabetes, or is specific for the postpartum period, as in postpartum thrombophlebitis (■ FIGURE 23-17). Refer to the Tabular List for instructional notes to assign additional codes (■ FIGURE 23-18).

Table 23-13 ■ **CODE SEQUENCING FOR OBSTETRIC COMPLICATIONS AND CODES FROM BODY SYSTEM CHAPTERS**

1. Code from Chapter 15 (O00-O9A)
2. Additional codes from the body system chapter(s)

Patient is seen for postpartum deep venous phlebothrombosis in the tibial vein of the left leg.

(1) Index: **Phlebothrombosis, puerperal, - see Thrombophlebitis, puerperal; Thrombophlebitis, puerperal, deep**

Tabular List: **O87.1 Deep phlebothrombosis in the puerperium**

(2) Tabular List: **Use additional code to identify the deep vein thrombosis (I82.4-, I85.5-, I82.62-, I82.72-)**

I82.442 Acute embolism and thrombosis of left tibial vein

Figure 23-17 ■ Example of Sequencing Obstetric Complications with Codes from a Body System Chapter

O87.1 Deep phlebothrombosis in the puerperium

Deep vein thrombosis, postpartum

Pelvic thrombophlebitis, postpartum

Use additional code to identify the deep vein thrombosis (I82.4-, I82.5-, I82.62-. I82.72-)

Use additional code, if applicable, for associated long-term (current) use of anticoagulants (Z79.01)

Figure 23-18 ■ Tabular List Entry for an Obstetric Complication Requiring Additional Codes from a Body System Chapter

SUCCESS STEP

The terms *thrombophlebitis* and *phlebothrombosis* are interchangeable in ICD-10-CM. Notice that both terms contain two roots, **phleb-** (*vein*) and **thromb-** (*clot*).

Guided Example of Arranging Obstetrics Codes

To practice skills for sequencing codes for pregnancy, childbirth, and the puerperium, continue with the example from earlier in the chapter about patient Glenna Ferrier, who was admitted to Branton Medical Center for full term labor.

Follow along in your ICD-10-CM manual as Daphne Wittman, CCS-P, sequences the codes. Check off each step after you complete it.

⇨ First, Daphne reviews the codes she has assigned for this case:

- ☐ **Z37.0, Single live birth**
- ☐ **O34.21, Maternal care for scar from previous cesarean delivery**
- ☐ **O76, Abnormality in fetal heart rate and rhythm complicating labor and delivery**
- ☐ **O66.41, Failed attempted vaginal birth after previous cesarean delivery**
- ☐ **Z3A.39, 39 weeks gestation of pregnancy**

⇨ To better determine the sequencing rules Daphne reads OGCR I.C.15.b.4., which states the following:

- ☐ "In cases of cesarean delivery, the selection of the principal diagnosis should be the condition established after study that was responsible for the patient's admission. If the patient was admitted with a condition that resulted in the performance of a cesarean procedure, that condition should be selected as the principal diagnosis."
- ☐ Daphne reviews the medical record and the codes she assigned. The main reason a C-section was performed was because of the scar from the previous C-section.
- ☐ Therefore, the principal diagnosis is **O34.21, Maternal care for scar from previous cesarean delivery**.
- ☐ The second code should be the next most important complication, which is the fetal tachycardia.
- ☐ The third code is failed vaginal delivery.
- ☐ The fourth code is the outcome of delivery.
- ☐ The final code is the weeks of gestation.

⇨ Daphne finalizes the codes and sequencing for this case:

(1) **O34.21, Maternal care for scar from previous cesarean delivery**

(2) **O76, Abnormality in fetal heart rate and rhythm complicating labor and delivery**

(3) **O66.41, Failed attempted vaginal birth after previous cesarean delivery**

(4) **Z37.0, Single live birth**

(5) **Z3A.39, 39 weeks gestation of pregnancy**

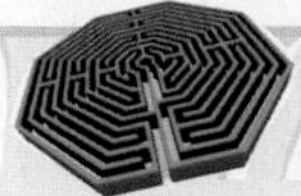

Coding Practice

Now it is your turn to practice sequencing codes for pregnancy, childbirth, and the puerperium. Refer to the ***Tip*** at the end of the mini-medical-record if you need a little extra help.

Exercise 23.4 Arranging Codes for Obstetrics

Instructions: Read the mini-medical-record of each patient's encounter, review the information abstracted in Exercise 23.2, assign ICD-10-CM diagnosis codes (CM) using the Index and Tabular List, and sequence them correctly.

1. Date of discharge: 3/24/yy Location: Branton Medical Center Provider: Kay Pinkney, MD

Patient: Lea Bloodworth Gender: F Age: 18

Gravida: 1 Para: 0 EDD: 4/6/yy EGA: 37+5

Reason for admission: full term labor

Assessment: placental infarction

Delivery: 3/22/yy, NSVD, stillborn, 1 girl

Tip: Assign a code for the placental infarction, a code for the fetal death, a code for outcome of delivery, and a code for the weeks of gestation.

4 CM Codes __________ __________ __________ __________

2. Date of encounter: 3/24/yy Location: New Life Obstetrics Provider: Kay Pinkney, MD

Patient: Keisha Ryerson Gender: F Age: 30

Gravida: 2 Para: 1 EDD: 10/5/yy

EGA: 12+0

Reason for encounter: prenatal care, pernicious anemia

Assessment: blood work has improved, but still not where it should be

Plan: B12 injection

Tip: Read the instructional notes in the Tabular List. Assign a code for the weeks of gestation

3 CM Codes __________ __________ __________

3. Date of discharge: 3/24/yy Location: Branton Medical Center Provider: Kay Pinkney, MD

Patient: Jeanine Mohn Gender: F Age: 32

Gravida: 2 Para: 2 EDD: 5/18/yy

EGA: 32+2

Reason for admission: premature rupture of membranes

Assessment: severe pre-eclampsia requires c/s

Delivery: 3/22/yy, classical C/S, PTBLC, 1 girl

Tip: Assign a code for the reason for the c/s, a code for PROM, a code for the outcome of delivery, and a code for the weeks of gestation.

4 CM Codes __________ __________ __________ __________

4. Date of encounter: 3/24/yy Location: New Life Obstetrics Provider: Kay Pinkney, MD

Patient: Lily Wahlstrom Gender: F Age: 15

Birthday: 7/15 Gravida: 1 Para: 0

EDD: 6/1/yy EGA: 30+4

Reason for encounter: prenatal care, twins, MoDi

Assessment: dipstick shows new isolated gestational proteinuria

Plan: at risk for preeclampsia, RTO 4 days for repeat test

Tip: Assign a code for the diagnosis, a code for the mother's age, a code for the twin pregnancy, and a code for the weeks of gestation

4 CM Codes __________ __________ __________ __________

5. Date of discharge: 3/24/yy Location: Branton Medical Center Provider: Kay Pinkney, MD

Patient: Grace Topete Gender: F Age: 22

Gravida: 2 Para: 2 EDD: 3/16/yy

EGA: 41+3

Reason for admission: post term labor

Assessment: obstructed labor due to CPD, severe obesity mother, BMI 41

Delivery: 3/23/yy, C/S, TBLC, 1 boy

(continued)

5. (continued)

Tip: Assign a delivery code for the obstruction, a code for postterm pregnancy, a delivery code for the obesity complication, then follow instructional notes in the Tabular List. Also assign a code for the weeks of gestation.

(continued)

5. (continued)

7 CM Codes __________ __________

__________ __________ __________

__________ __________

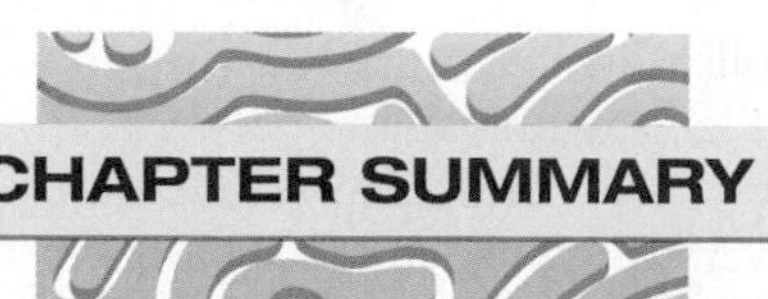

CHAPTER SUMMARY

In this chapter you learned that:

- Pregnancy is a normal, temporary condition that occurs within the female body, which begins at the time of conception and ends with the birth of the fetus.
- ICD-10-CM Chapter 15, Pregnancy, Childbirth, and the Puerperium (O00-O9A), contains nine blocks or subchapters that are divided by the phase of pregnancy and the type of condition.
- Because multiple complications are common during pregnancy, childbirth, and the puerperium, coders must be attentive to which complication is the reason for the encounter or admission.
- Coders should acquaint themselves with the organization of obstetrical terms in the Index and must be attentive to distinguish between codes that apply to the mother and those that apply to the infant.
- Coders must be attentive to selecting the principal diagnosis when a delivery occurs and to sequencing codes from Chapter 15 with codes from body system chapters.
- ICD-10-CM provides Official Guidelines for Coding and Reporting (OGCR) in section I.C.15. that cover the general rules for obstetric cases, selection of OB principal or first-listed diagnosis, preexisting conditions, and several specific conditions, including hypertension, diabetes, HIV, alcohol and tobacco use, normal delivery, postpartum, and abortions.

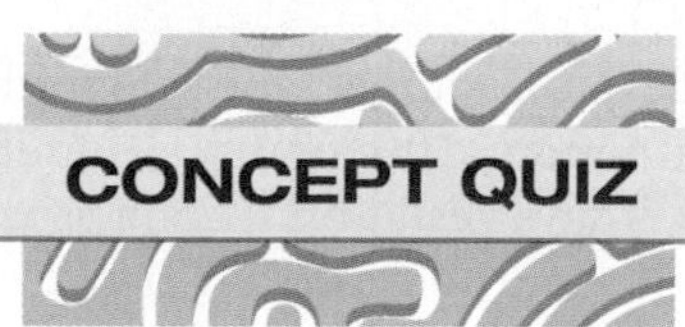

CONCEPT QUIZ

Take a moment to look back at your trip through pregnancy, childbirth, and the puerperium and solidify your skills. This is your opportunity to pull together everything you have learned.

Completion

Instructions: Write the term that answers each question based on the information you learned in this chapter. Choose from the list below. Some choices may be used more than once and some choices may not be used at all. Refer to the discussion in this chapter and the Glossary at the end of this book if you need a little extra help.

cephalic
conception
DiDi
DiMo
fetopelvic
first trimester
gestational hypertension
gravida
HELLP syndrome
last menstrual period
MoDi
MoMo
nuchal cord
occipitoanterior
para
parturition
peripartum
placenta previa
preeclampsia
prenatal
PROM
puerperium
Rhesus incompatibility
second trimester
third trimester

1. The __________________ period is the last month of pregnancy to five months postpartum.

2. The period of true labor is also called ____________________.

3. The estimated date of delivery is determined as 40 weeks from the ____________________.

4. The period from 28 weeks, 0 days until delivery is the ____________________.

5. ____________________ is the condition of the umbilical cord becoming wrapped around the neck of the fetus.

6. ____________________ is a condition in which a mother is Rh negative and develops antibodies against a fetus that is Rh positive.

7. ____________________ is a metabolic disorder of pregnancy, which develops after the twentieth week, that involves gestational hypertension and proteinuria.

8. Twin fetuses with one chorion and two amnions are ____________________.

9. Cephalopelvic disproportion is also called ____________________.

10. ____________________ is the rupture of the amniotic sac and chorion more than an hour before the onset of labor.

Multiple Choice

Instructions: Circle the letter of the best answer to each question based on the information you learned in this chapter. Refer to the discussion in this chapter and the Glossary at the end of this book if you need a little extra help.

1. Which of the following terms does NOT refer to the time period from conception to the beginning of labor?
   A. Prenatal
   B. Peripartum
   C. Antepartum
   D. Antenatal
2. A woman currently pregnant, who has had one previous pregnancy and gave birth to twins, is described as
   A. gravida 1 para 2.
   B. gravida 2 para 1.
   C. gravida 2 para 2.
   D. grand multipara.
3. A normal pregnancy includes all of the following EXCEPT
   A. no preexisting conditions.
   B. no new conditions that develop during pregnancy.
   C. single gestation.
   D. gestational diabetes.
4. What is the length of a full term pregnancy?
   A. More than 37 completed weeks of gestation
   B. 37 weeks, 0 days of gestation to 39 weeks, 6 days of gestation
   C. 40 completed weeks to 42 completed weeks of gestation
   D. More than 42 completed weeks of gestation
5. GDM is
   A. preexisitng diabetes that is treated during pregnancy.
   B. preexisitng hypertension that is treated during pregnancy.
   C. diabetes that is first diagnosed during pregnancy.
   D. hypertension that is first diagnosed during pregnancy.
6. Which of the following is a normal delivery?
   A. Induction of labor with vaginal delivery
   B. Vaginal delivery with cephalic presentation
   C. Vaginal delivery of twins
   D. Vaginal delivery at 36 weeks of gestation
7. When is a multiple gestation pregnancy coded as high risk?
   A. Only when the physician documents it as high risk
   B. Only when a cesarean section is required
   C. When there are more than two fetuses
   D. Always
8. Excessive bleeding following delivery is
   A. postpartum hemorrhage.
   B. puerperal mastitis.
   C. placenta previa.
   D. preeclampsia.
9. The seventh character of 1 identifies
   A. the first trimester.
   B. a single gestation pregnancy.
   C. fetus one in a multiple gestation pregnancy.
   D. gravida 1.
10. How many complications are documented in this case: Patient, age 15 years, 10 months, is admitted in labor at 36 weeks, 3 days gestation. Labor proceeds without complication and she gives birth to twins.
    A. None
    B. One
    C. Two
    D. Three

CODING CHALLENGE

Now it is your turn to demonstrate coding all aspects of pregnancy, childbirth, and the puerperium. Refer back to the examples and discussion in this chapter when you need a little extra help. Use your medical dictionary and anatomy references when needed.

Instructions: Read the mini-medical-record of each patient's encounter, then abstract, assign, and sequence ICD-10-CM diagnosis codes (CM) using the Index and Tabular List. Write the code(s) on the line provided.

1. Date of discharge: 3/29/yy Location: Branton Medical Center Emergency Department

Provider: Cynthia Hiatt, MD

Patient: Alisa Chalk Gender: F Age: 24

Gravida: 2 Para: 1 EDD: 9/27/yy EGA: 14+2

Reason for encounter: hurt her shoulder while lifting bags of gravel she was spreading on a walking path in the yard of her single family home, leisure status

Assessment: sprained right shoulder, does not affect pregnancy

Plan: ice and sling, FU 1 week

Tip: Remember to assign external cause codes for activity, place of occurrence, and status.

5 CM Codes __________ __________

__________ __________ __________

2. Date of encounter: 3/29/yy Location: New Life Obstetrics Provider: Kay Pinkney, MD

Patient: Jocelyn Gunning Gender: F Age: 19

Gravida: 1 Para: 0 EDD: 8/16/yy EGA: 19+6

Reason for encounter: prenatal care

Assessment: HIV positive

Plan: anti-HIV drugs beginning in second trimester, newborn to be treated within 8 hrs and for 6 months

Tip: Refer to OGCR I.C.15.f.

3 CM Codes __________ __________

____

3. Date of encounter: 3/29/yy Location: New Life Obstetrics Provider: Kay Pinkney, MD

Patient: Cathleen Gwynn Gender: F Age: 35

Gravida: 2 Para: 0 EDD: 10/25/yy

EGA: 10+0

Reason for encounter: patient presents for prenatal care after successful IVF

Assessment: previous miscarriage

Plan: schedule pre-natal visits

Tip: Assign a separate code for each risk factor.

4 CM Codes __________ __________

__________ __________

4. Date of discharge: 3/29/yy Location: Branton Medical Center Provider: Kay Pinkney, MD

Patient: Mollie Hansley Gender: F Age: 28

Gravida: 2 Para: 2 EDD: 4/5/yy EGA: 39+1

Reason for admission: labor

Assessment: cord entanglement and compression of fetus 1

Delivery: 3/28/yy, vaginal delivery converted to C/S, TBLC, 1 girl, 1 boy

Tip: By definition, twins of the opposite sex are DiDi

4 CM Codes __________ __________

__________ __________

5. Date of discharge: 3/29/yy Location: Branton Medical Center Provider: Kay Pinkney, MD

Patient: Ursula Feinberg Gender: F Age: 31

Gravida: 2 Para: 2 Date of delivery: 3/8/yy

Reason for encounter: admitted from physician office with fever of 103 degrees F and purulent discharge from operative wound

Assessment: infected C-section wound, staphylococcus

Plan: antibiotics, FU 2 weeks

2 CM Codes __________ __________

(continued)

(continued from page 479)

6. Date of discharge: 3/29/yy Location: Branton Medical Center Provider: Kay Pinkney, MD

Patient: Mayra Carra Gender: F Age: 23

Gravida: 1 Para: 1 EDD: 3/27/yy EGA: 39+4

Reason for admission: full term labor

Assessment: *obstructed labor due to prolapsed arm presentation, successfully converted to cephalic, with first degree perineal laceration*

Delivery: 3/28/yy, NSVD, TBLC, 1 girl

4 CM Codes __________ __________

__________ __________

7. Date of discharge: 3/29/yy Location: Branton Medical Center Provider: Kay Pinkney, MD

Patient: Paige Bednarz Gender: F Age: 31

Gravida: 3 Para: 2 EDD: 10/11/yy

EGA: 12+5

Reason for admission: *observation for signs of labor or other complications after failed legal abortion due to fetal chromosome abnormality*

Assessment: *no labor or other complications were noted*

Plan: RTO FU in 2 *days, supportive and genetic counseling*

Tip: Assign codes for the reason for the attempted abortion and the failed attempt.

3 CM Codes __________ __________

____

8. Date of encounter: 3/29/yy Location: New Life Obstetrics Provider: Kay Pinkney, MD

Patient: Jolene Chattin Gender: F Age: 34

Gravida: 2 Para: 2 Date of Delivery: 3/15/yy

Reason for encounter: postpartum care

Assessment: *abscess of right breast*

Plan: Rx antibiotic, RTO 2 weeks

1 CM Code __________

9. Date of encounter: 3/29/yy Location: New Life Obstetrics Provider: Kay Pinkney, MD

Patient: Shauna Meese Gender: F Age: 30

Gravida: 1 Para: 0 EDD: 10/18/yy

EGA: 11+3

Reason for encounter: prenatal visit

Assessment: *long standing essential hypertension*

Plan: antihypertensive therapy, monitor for pre-eclampsia

2 CM Codes __________ __________

10. Date of discharge: 3/29/yy Location: Branton Medical Center Provider: Kay Pinkney

Patient: Justine Stennis Gender: F Age: 21

Gravida: 2 Para: 2 EDD: 5/31/yy

EGA: 31+4

Reason for admission: premature rupture of membranes

Assessment: labor started 30 hours post admission

Delivery: 3/28/yy, VBAC, TBLC, 1 girl

4 CM Codes __________ __________

__________ __________

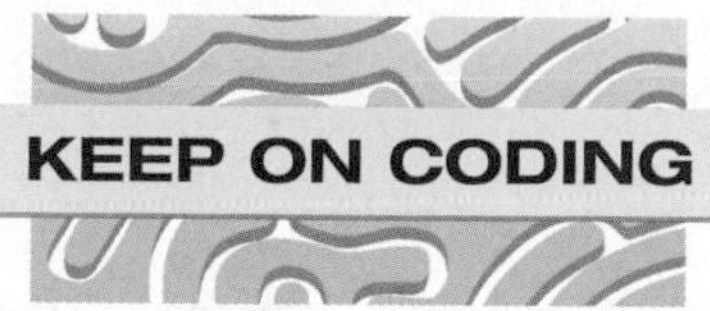

KEEP ON CODING

As a coder, you can never have too much experience. Apply everything you have learned in this chapter to code the following diagnostic statements. Use the OGCR and instructional notes in the Tabular List to help determine how many codes are required.

Instructions: Read the diagnostic statement, then use the Index and Tabular List to assign and sequence ICD-10-CM (CM) diagnosis codes. Write the code(s) on the line provided.

1. Tubal pregnancy: CM Code(s) ____________
2. Supervision of elderly primigravida, 35-week pregnancy: CM Code(s) ____________
3. Threatened abortion: CM Code(s) ____________
4. Complication of childbirth due to bariatric surgery status, 36 weeks: CM Code(s) ____________
5. Excessive weight gain during first 12 weeks of pregnancy: CM Code(s) ____________
6. Pregnancy with preexisting diabetes mellitus, type 1, in puerperium: CM Code(s) ____________
7. Pregnancy complicated by breech presentation, 39 weeks gestation: CM Code(s) ____________
8. Galactorrhea: CM Code(s) ____________
9. Postpartum thyroiditis: CM Code(s) ____________
10. Aspiration pneumonia due to anesthesia during 27th week of pregnancy (26 weeks completed): CM Code(s) ____________
11. Acute lymphoblastic leukemia complicating the pregnancy in 31st week (30 weeks completed): CM Code(s) ____________
12. Acute renal failure after an incomplete spontaneous abortion: CM Code(s) ____________
13. Herpes gestationis, 10 weeks pregnant: CM Code(s)____________
14. Fetal anemia: CM Code(s) ____________
15. Failed induction of labor by oxytocin, 40 weeks: CM Code(s) ____________
16. Triplet pregnancy delivered at 38 weeks of gestation by cesarean section, all liveborn: CM Code(s) ____________
17. Preterm labor without delivery, 33 weeks of pregnancy: CM Code(s) ____________
18. Alcohol abuse complicating pregnancy at 37 weeks: CM Code(s) ____________
19. Failed induction of labor by oxytocin, 42 weeks: CM Code(s) ____________
20. Puerperal abscess of nipple: CM Code(s) ____________
21. Abnormal glucose level complicating pregnancy, 22 weeks: CM Code(s) ____________
22. Hemorrhoids complicating pregnancy at 26 weeks: CM Code(s) ____________
23. Maternal care for incompetent cervix, 25 weeks: CM Code(s) ____________
24. Kidney infection, in 13th week of pregnancy (12 weeks completed): CM Code(s) ____________
25. Physical abuse complicating pregnancy in the 8th week (7 weeks completed): CM Code(s) ____________

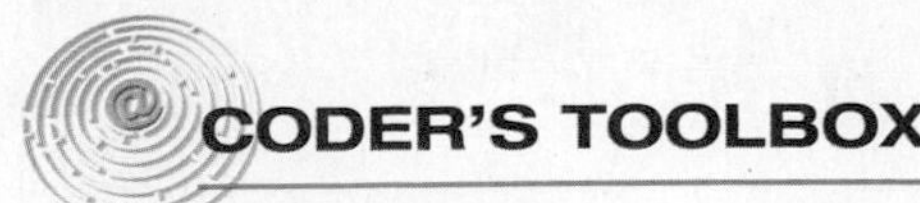

CODER'S TOOLBOX

The following resources are a starting point for learning more about pregnancy, childbirth, and the puerperium. The > symbol indicates a menu selection within the website in order to navigate to a specific page.

American Academy of Pediatrics (AAP) > Healthy Children > Teen Dating and Sex **http://www.healthychildren.org/english/ages-stages/teen/dating-sex/Pages/default.aspx**

American Academy of Pediatrics (AAP) > Healthy Children > Prenatal **http://www.healthychildren.org/English/ages-stages/prenatal/Pages/default.aspx**

American Board of Obstetrics and Gynecology **http://www.abog.org/**

American College of Nurse-Midwives **http://www.midwife.org/**

American Congress of Obstetricians and Gynecologists **http://www.acog.org/**

American Pregnancy Association **http://www.americanpregnancy.org/**

American Society for Reproductive Medicine **http://asrm.org/**

Centers for Disease Control and Prevention > Teen Pregnancy **http://www.cdc.gov/teenpregnancy/AboutTeenPreg.htm**

March of Dimes > Pregnancy > Trying to get pregnant **http://www.marchofdimes.com/Pregnancy/trying_multiples.html**

Office on Women's Health > A-Z Health Topics > Pregnancy **http://www.womenshealth.gov/pregnancy/**

Planned Parenthood > Tools for Parents **http://www.plannedparenthood.org/parents/index.htm**

Pregnancy.org **http://www.pregnancy.org/**

Society for Assistive Reproductive Technology (SART) **http://www.sart.org/**

24

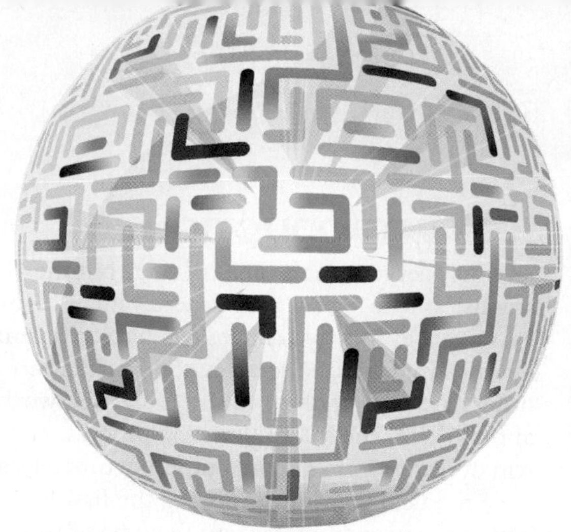

Certain Conditions Originating in the Perinatal Period (P00-P96)

Learning Objectives

After completing this chapter, you should have the skills to:

- Spell and define the key words, medical terms, and abbreviations related to conditions originating in the perinatal period.
- Discuss common conditions originating in the perinatal period.
- Identify the main characteristics of coding for conditions originating in the perinatal period.
- Abstract diagnostic information from the medical record for coding conditions originating in the perinatal period.
- Assign codes for conditions originating in the perinatal period.
- Arrange codes for conditions originating in the perinatal period.
- Discuss the Official Guidelines for Coding and Reporting related to conditions originating in the perinatal period.

Key Terms and Abbreviations

chromosomal abnormality
deformation
erythroblastosis fetalis
malformation
neonatal mortality
neonate
newborn
newborn birth status
newborn clinically significant condition
perinatal condition
perinatal period
transitory

In addition to the key terms listed here, students should know the terms defined within tables in this chapter.

Chapter Outline

- **Perinatal Refresher**
- **Coding Overview Perinatal Conditions**
- **Abstracting for Perinatal Conditions**
- **Assigning Codes for Perinatal Conditions**
- **Arranging Codes for Perinatal Conditions**

ICD-10-CM codes in this chapter are from the ICD-10-CM 2014 Draft code set from the Department of Health and Human Services, Centers for Disease Control and Prevention.

INTRODUCTION

Almost everyone is thrilled to check out the sights, sounds, smells, and feel of a brand new vehicle. However, many know that even new vehicles can have problems. Some difficulties may be due to an initial breaking-in period while others are the result of faulty materials, workmanship, or anomalies in the manufacturing process. Newborn babies win over everyone's heart but, unfortunately, some experience medical conditions during the first few weeks of life. This chapter introduces you to some of those conditions.

In your tour of the conditions originating in the perinatal period in this chapter you will learn more about the types of common perinatal conditions, why they arise, and how physicians treat them. Most importantly, you will practice coding for patient encounters related to conditions originating in the perinatal period, a skill that requires you to abstract information from the medical record, assign correct codes, and arrange (sequence) the codes in the proper order.

A pediatrician is a physician who specializes in diagnosing and treating conditions of children, including perinatal conditions. A neonatologist is a pediatric subspecialist who diagnoses and treats complex conditions of newborns. Other medical specialties also have subspecialists in pediatrics and neonatology. For example, a neonatal cardiologist specializes in diagnosing and treating heart conditions of newborns.

As you read this chapter, open up your medical terminology book and keep a medical dictionary handy to refresh your memory of any unfamiliar perinatal terms. Resourceful coders know they cannot be experts in every aspect of pathophysiology and coding, so they refer to resources to help them be accurate and efficient. This way, help is never more than an arm's length away.

PERINATAL REFRESHER

The **perinatal period** begins before birth and continues through the twenty-eighth day following birth. An infant is referred to as a **neonate** or **newborn** during the first 28 days of life (■ FIGURE 24-1). After day 28 they are classified as infants or children. **Perinatal conditions** are those that develop before birth or in the first 28 days after birth, but exclude physical **malformations** (*permanent abnormal shape of an organ or body region, resulting from arrested, delayed, or abnormal development of the embryo*), **deformations** (*a change in the size or shape of a normal structure, due to physical forces*), and **chromosomal abnormalities** (*the abnormal number or structure of chromosomes*). Perinatal conditions are often **transitory** (*temporary*), but may be long term or permanent as well.

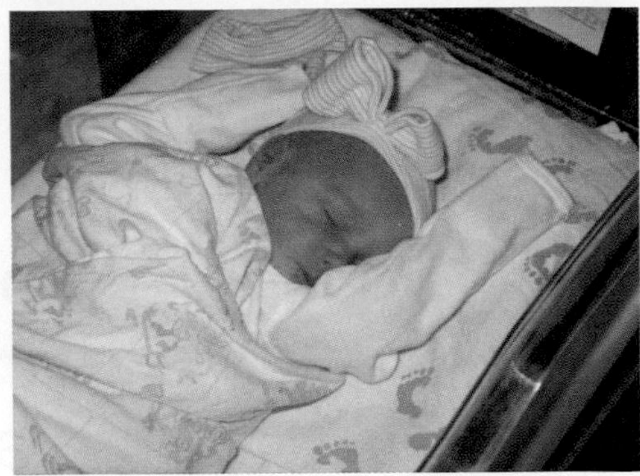

Figure 24-1 ■ A neonate or newborn is 1 to 28 days old. *Source: Bronwen Glowacki/Pearson Education.*

As you learn about perinatal conditions, remember to apply medical terminology skills to combine word roots, prefixes, and suffixes you already know to define new terms. Refer to ■ TABLE 24-1 for a refresher on how to build medical terms related to conditions originating in the perinatal period.

CODING CAUTION

Be alert for medical word roots that are spelled similarly and have different meanings.

omphal/o (*umbilicus or navel*) and **oophor/o** (*ovary*)

amni/o (*amniotic sac*), **ammon/o** (*ammonium*), and **amin/o** (*amino acid*)

Table 24-1 ■ **EXAMPLE OF CONSTRUCTING MEDICAL TERMS FOR CONDITIONS ORIGINATING IN THE PERINATAL PERIOD**

Prefix	Root/Suffix	Complete Medical Term
dys- (*abnormal, painful*)	**-pnea** (*breathing*) **-cardi/o** (*heart, heart rate*) **-rhythm/o** (*rhythm, beat*)	**dys + pnea** (*difficulty breathing*) **dys + rhythmia** (*abnormal heart beat*)
tachy- (*rapid*)		**tachy + pnea** (*rapid breathing*) **tachy + cardia** (*rapid heart rate*)
brady- (*slow*)		**brady + pnea** (*slow breathing*) **brady + cardia** (*slow heart rate*)

Conditions Originating in the Perinatal Period

Perinatal conditions are defined by the fact that they *originated* during the perinatal period, regardless of when they are diagnosed or treated. Some conditions may not be diagnosed until after the perinatal period, but because they originated during the perinatal period they are still considered perinatal conditions and are assigned codes from this ICD-10-CM chapter (■ FIGURE 24-2).

Some perinatal conditions, such as retinopathy, apnea, or tachycardia, use similar medical terms as conditions that affect adults. The condition is identified as perinatal by the use of a descriptive term, such as prematurity or newborn, in conjunction with the name of the condition. For example, retinopathy of prematurity, newborn apnea, or newborn tachycardia are perinatal conditions, while retinopathy, apnea, and tachycardia can originate at any age. Other perinatal conditions only occur in newborns, such as amnionitis or meconium aspiration syndrome. Refer to ■ TABLE 24-2 for a summary of conditions originating in the perinatal period.

In particular, coders must be aware of conditions related to neonatal birth weight.

Patient, age 15, is seen for Erb's palsy (*paralysis of the upper arm*), which resulted from damage during birth.

Patient, age 60, is seen for blindness in the left eye, which he has had since birth, as a result of retinopathy of prematurity (ROP).

Patient, age 35, is diagnosed with carcinoma of the vagina, due to exposure to diethylstibestrol (DES) which her mother took during pregnancy.

Figure 24-2 ■ Examples of Perinatal Conditions Affecting Patients Later in Life

Birth Weight

Newborn birth weight is a major indicator of newborn health and nutritional status. Both low birth weight (LBW), under 2,500 grams, and high birth weight (HBW), over 4,000 grams, are associated with health problems. Birth weight is directly tied to the estimated gestational age (EGA) at birth. The earlier infants are born, before 37 weeks gestation, the less they weigh. The longer a pregnancy continues, beyond 40 weeks, the more newborns weigh. Newborns of any EGA can be lighter or heavier in weight or smaller or larger in size compared to other infants of the same EGA. This condition is referred to by a variety of names such as small for gestational age, light-for-date, light-for-age, large-for-age, and similar.

SUCCESS STEP

Newborn birth weight is reported in grams using the metric system. A weight of 2,500 grams is equal to 5 pounds, 8 ounces.

Table 24-2 ■ COMMON CONDITIONS ORIGINATING IN THE PERINATAL PERIOD

Condition	Definition
Amnionitis	Infection or inflammation of the amniotic sac
Apgar score	An evaluation of a newborn's physical condition, performed 1 and 5 minutes after birth, to determine any immediate need for extra medical or emergency care (named after the physician who designed it, Dr. Virginia Apgar)
Appropriate for gestational age (AGA)	A fetus or newborn infant whose size is within the normal range for his or her gestational age
Birth trauma	Any physical injury to the infant during delivery
Breast engorgement	The temporary enlargement of breasts on female or male newborns, due to high levels of maternal hormones in the infant's blood
Drug withdrawal syndrome	A collection of symptoms of drug withdrawal in an infant who was exposed to narcotics in the uterus; also called neonatal abstinence syndrome (NAS)
Exceptionally large newborn	Birth weight more than 4,500 grams (9 pounds, 15 ounces)
Extremely low birth weight (ELBW)	Birth weight of less than 1,000 grams (2 pounds, 3 ounces)

(continued)

Table 24-2 ■ (continued)

Condition	Definition
Failure to thrive (FTT)	Inadequate physical growth marked by child's weight for age below the fifth percentile of the standard growth chart
Hemolytic disease of the newborn (HDN)	A blood disorder that occurs when the blood types of a mother and baby are incompatible, also called erythroblastosis fetalis
High birth weight (HBW)	Birth weight greater than 4,000 grams (8 pounds, 13 ounces)
Hyperbilirubinemia	High levels of bilirubin in the blood, which causes the infant's skin and sclera to turn yellow
Infant of diabetic mother (IDM)	An infant born to a woman who is diabetic
Intrauterine growth restriction (IUGR)	Poor growth of a baby while in the mother's womb during pregnancy. Specifically, it means the developing baby weighs less than 90% of other babies at the same gestational age.
Intraventricular hemorrhage (IVH)	Bleeding in the brain in very low birth weight premature babies, which usually resolves within a few days
Jaundice	A condition due to high bilirubin that causes the skin and parts of the eyes to turn a yellow color
Large for gestational age (LGA)	A fetus or newborn infant who is larger in size than normal for the baby's sex and gestational age, most commonly defined as a weight, length, or head circumference above the ninetieth percentile at gestational age
Low birth weight (LBW)	Birth weight less than 2,500 grams (5 pounds, 8 ounces)
Meconium aspiration syndrome (MAS)	Condition in which the newborn breathes a mixture of meconium and amniotic fluid into the lungs prior to or during delivery
Meconium peritonitis	Infection of the peritoneal cavity due to perforation of the bowel and leakage of meconium
Newborn ABO incompatibility	An infant with blood type A or B affected by comingling of type O blood from mother with blood type O
Newborn apnea	A condition in which the infant stops breathing
Newborn Rh incompatibility	Rh positive infant affected by comingling of blood with an Rh negative mother
Normal birth weight	Birth weight of 2,500 grams to 4,000 grams (5 pounds, 8 ounces to 8 pounds, 13 ounces)
Omphalitis	Infection of the umbilical stump in a newborn, usually presenting as superficial cellulitis
Respiratory distress syndrome (RDS)	A condition in which the alveolar sacs collapse due to lack of surfactant
Retinopathy of prematurity (ROP)	The abnormal growth of blood vessels in the eye that can lead to vision loss
Small for gestational age (SGA)	A fetus or newborn infant who is smaller in size than normal for the baby's sex and gestational age, most commonly defined as a weight, length, or head circumference below the tenth percentile for the gestational age
Transient tachypnea of the newborn (TTN)	Short term condition (less than 24 hours) of rapid breathing due to retained lung fluid that occurs shortly after birth in full term or near term newborns
Very low birth weight (VLBW)	Birth weight of less than 1,500 grams (3 pounds, 4 ounces)

LBW is a leading cause of neonatal mortality (*death before 29 days of age*). Although it is largely preventable in a developed country such as the United States, over 8% of infants each year are born with LBW, according to the Maternal and Child Health Bureau of the Department of Health and Human Resources, and more than six out of every 1,000 children die before one year of age. LBW is associated with failure to thrive, dehydration, and feeding disorders, as well as many chronic conditions of the digestive, pulmonary, and cardiovascular systems. Premature infants are weighed daily in the **neonatal intensive care unit (NICU)** and generally must weigh at least 1,800 grams (4 pounds) before being removed from the **incubator** (■ FIGURE 24-3). Each hospital sets its own weight standards for discharge, but the infant must be out of the incubator and steadily gaining weight before discharge.

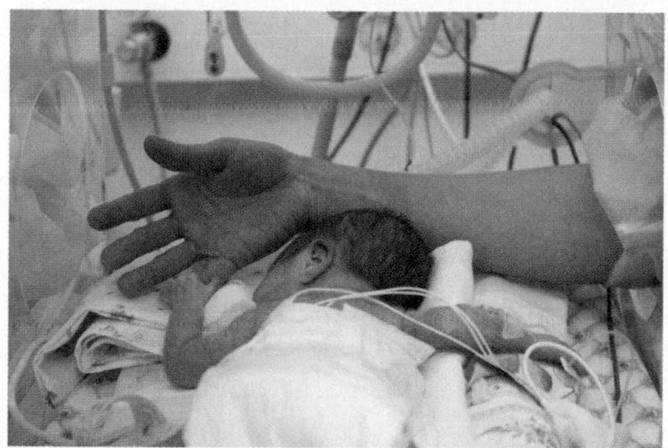

Figure 24-3 ■ Premature babies must weigh 1,800 grams before being released from an incubator. *Source: Fanfo/Fotolia.*

High birth weight is associated with diabetes and certain childhood cancers and tumors, such as leukemia and **astrocytomas**, and possibly even adult cancers, such as breast, prostate, endometrial, and colon cancer, according to the journal *Cancer Epidemiology, Biomarkers & Prevention.*

This section provides a general reference to help understand the most common conditions originating in the perinatal period, but does not list everything you need to know. Use medical terminology skills discussed earlier in this chapter to learn the meaning of unfamiliar words. Remember to keep standard reference books handy in case you get stuck. Refer to the resources in the Coder's Toolbox at the end of this chapter to learn more about conditions originating in the perinatal period.

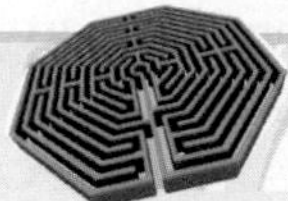

Coding Practice

Refresh your knowledge of terminology related to conditions originating in the perinatal period. Use a medical terminology text or a website such as GlobalRph.com > Medical Terminology **http://www.globalrph.com/medterm.htm** to identify the meaning of word parts that may not be familiar.

Exercise 24.1 Perinatal Refresher

Instructions: Use your medical terminology skills and resources to define the following conditions related to conditions originating in the perinatal period, then assign the default diagnosis code.

Follow these steps:

- Use slash marks "/" to break down each **boldfaced term** into its root(s) and suffix.
- Define the meaning of the **boldfaced term**, based on the meaning of each word part.
- Assign the default ICD-10-CM diagnosis code (CM) for the condition using the Index and Tabular List. Locate the Main Term Newborn, then locate the subterms in the order shown.

Example: newborn **apnea** a/pnea — Meaning: *lack of breathing* — CM Code: *P28.3*

1. Newborn, affected by, heart rate, **tachycardia** — Meaning ______ CM Code ______
2. Newborn, affected by, **intrauterine** blood loss — Meaning ______ CM Code ______
3. Newborn, **hyperbilirubinemia** — Meaning ______ CM Code ______
4. Newborn, affected by, **maternal polyhydramnios** — Meaning ______ CM Code ______
5. Newborn, infective **mastitis** — Meaning ______ CM Code ______
6. Newborn, affected by, maternal, **omphalitis** — Meaning ______ CM Code ______
7. Newborn, affected by, **hypoxic ischemic encephalopathy** — Meaning ______ CM Code ______
8. Newborn, affected by, **chorioamnionitis** — Meaning ______ CM Code ______
9. Newborn, **hyponatremia** — Meaning ______ CM Code ______
10. **erythroblastosis fetalis** — Meaning ______ CM Code ______

CODING OVERVIEW OF PERINATAL CONDITIONS

ICD-10-CM Chapter 16, Certain Conditions Originating in the Perinatal Period (P00-P96), contains 12 blocks or subchapters that are divided by anatomical site. Review the block names and code ranges listed at the beginning of Chapter 16 in the ICD-10-CM manual to become familiar with the content and organization.

This chapter includes newborn conditions that originate before birth or during the first 28 days of life and result from maternal conditions that are both related and unrelated to pregnancy, birth trauma, and underdevelopment during gestation. They also include respiratory, cardiovascular, metabolic, digestive, and hematological disorders. This chapter does not include fetal conditions that affect the mother or congenital abnormalities, both of which are classified in separate chapters. An instructional note at the beginning of the chapter requires that codes in this chapter are to be used *only* on the newborn's record, never on the mother's record.

ICD-10-CM Chapter 16 corresponds with ICD-9-CM Chapter 15 (760-779). Numerous categories have been expanded in ICD-10-CM compared to ICD-9-CM in order to add specificity to the diagnosis. Some codes have new titles, while others have been combined or deleted. ICD-10-CM defines all codes using the term *newborn* and omits the term *fetus*, which ICD-9-CM used in many code titles. Codes for the birth weight and gestational age of preterm infants have been redefined. Codes for birth trauma have greater specificity.

The sequencing of chapters in ICD-10-CM is different than in ICD-9-CM. In ICD-10-CM, this chapter, Certain Conditions Originating in the Perinatal Period (P00-P96), appears immediately after the obstetrics chapter, Pregnancy, Childbirth, and the Puerperium (O00-O9A), and is followed by Chapter 17, Congenital Malformations, Deformations and Chromosomal Abnormalities (Q00-Q99).

ICD-10-CM provides Official Guidelines for Coding and Reporting (OGCR) for conditions originating in the perinatal period in OGCR section I.C.16. OGCR provide detailed discussion of selecting the principal and additional diagnoses and how to report codes from this chapter with those from other chapters. OGCR also discuss specific coding for prematurity, low birth weight, bacterial sepsis of the newborn, and stillbirth. Additional guidelines related to assigning Z codes for newborns and infants appear in OGCR I.C.21.c.12).

ABSTRACTING FOR PERINATAL CONDITIONS

Coders must take note whether a hospitalization of a newborn includes the birth itself or whether the admission takes place after the birth episode. Abstract all **newborn clinically significant conditions**, defined as any newborn condition that meets the following criteria (OGCR I.C.16.a.6)):

- requires clinical evaluation
- requires therapeutic treatment
- requires diagnostic procedures
- extends length of hospital stay (LOS)
- increases nursing care or monitoring
- presents implications for future healthcare needs

The final criterion, conditions that present implications for future healthcare needs, is unique to newborns. Coders do not abstract and code conditions for adults that are not treated but may have implications for future needs. However, when the provider documents this information for newborns, the condition should be coded.

Abstracting birth encounter (■ Table 24-3) requires different criteria than abstracting encounters after birth (■ Table 24-4). Remember that the abstracting questions are a guide and that not every question applies to, or can be answered for, every case. For example, not all newborns are affected by a maternal condition. Also remember to abstract for symptoms and determine if they are integral to the confirmed diagnoses. After reviewing

Table 24-3 ■ **KEY CRITERIA FOR ABSTRACTING BIRTH ENCOUNTERS**

- ❑ Was the infant born in this hospital during this admission?
- ❑ Was the infant born outside the hospital, then hospitalized?
- ❑ Was the delivery vaginal or cesarean?
- ❑ What is the birth weight?
- ❑ What is the estimated gestational age at time of delivery?
- ❑ Are any conditions documented as due to prematurity?
- ❑ Did the infant suffer any birth trauma?
- ❑ What conditions of the newborn required evaluation, treatment, extended LOS, increased care, or present implications for future healthcare needs?
- ❑ Was the newborn observed for any suspected conditions not found?
- ❑ What maternal conditions affected the infant?

Table 24-4 ■ **KEY CRITERIA FOR ABSTRACTING ENCOUNTERS AFTER THE BIRTH EPISODE**

- ❑ What is the age of the patient?
- ❑ What is the reason for the encounter?
- ❑ What condition is documented?
- ❑ What is the subtype of the condition?
- ❑ What complications and comorbidities exist?
- ❑ Is the condition documented as originating in the perinatal period?

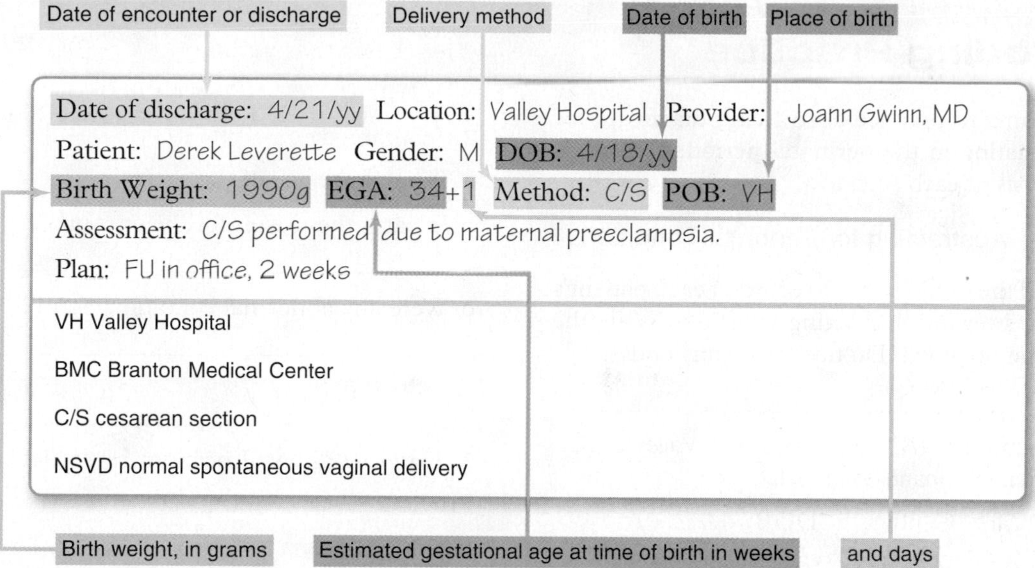

Figure 24-4 ■ Key to Interpreting the Newborn Mini-Medical-Record

the abstracting criteria, work through the guided example that follows.

Abstracting from Newborn Records

Newborn records contain unique information and abbreviations not found in other medical records. Refer to ■ FIGURE 24-4 to learn how to interpret the mini-medical-record used for newborn cases in this text.

Guided Example of Abstracting for Perinatal Conditions

Refer to the following example throughout this chapter to practice skills for abstracting, assigning, and sequencing codes for conditions originating in the perinatal period. Aaron Randell, CCS, is a fictitious coder who guides you through the process.

> Date of discharge: 4/21/yy Location: Valley Hospital (VH) Provider: Joann Gwinn, MD
>
> Patient: Derek Leverette Gender: M
>
> DOB: 4/18/yy
>
> Birth Weight: 1990g EGA: 34+1 Method: C/S
>
> Location: VH
>
> Assessment: C/S performed due to maternal preeclampsia. Infant presented with transient tachypnea (TTN) due to prematurity and was admitted to NICU. O2 and CPAP therapy were provided which restored breathing to normal within 48 hours. Patient was discharged with no symptoms.
>
> Plan: FU in office, 2 weeks

Follow along as Aaron Randell, CCS, abstracts the diagnosis. Check off each step after you complete it.

⇨ Aaron reads through the entire record, with special attention to the birth data and the final assessment.

- ❑ He notes that this record is for the birth encounter so he refers to the Key Criteria for Abstracting Birth Encounters (Table 24-3)
- ❑ *Was the infant born in this hospital during this admission?* Yes.
- ❑ *Was the delivery vaginal or cesarean?* C/S
- ❑ *What is the birth weight?* 1990 grams
- ❑ *What is the gestational age at time of delivery?* 34 weeks, 1 day
- ❑ *Are any conditions documented as due to prematurity?* transient tachypnea
- ❑ *Did the infant suffer any birth trauma?* No.
- ❑ *What conditions of the newborn required evaluation, treatment, extended LOS, increased care, or present implications for future health care needs?* transient tachypnea
- ❑ *Was the newborn observed for any suspected conditions not found?* No.
- ❑ *What maternal conditions affected the infant?* None. The mother had preeclampsia, but documentation does not state that it affected the infant.

⇨ At this time, Aaron does not know how many codes he will end up with. He will learn about this when he moves on to assigning codes.

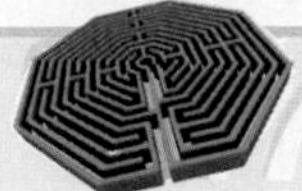

Coding Practice

Now it is your turn to practice abstracting diagnoses for conditions originating in the perinatal period. Questions guide your analysis of each scenario.

Exercise 24.2 Abstracting for Perinatal Conditions

Instructions: Read the mini-medical-record of each patient's encounter and answer the abstracting questions. Write the answer on the line provided. Do not assign any codes.

1. Date of discharge: 4/23/yy Location: Valley Hospital Provider: Joann Gwinn, MD

Patient: Dixie Dare Gender: F DOB: 4/22/yy

Birth Weight: 3521g EGA: 38+2 Type: NSVD

POB: VH

Assessment: APGARS 6, 8

Plan: FU in office, 2 weeks

a. Was the infant born in this hospital during this admission? ______

b. Was the delivery vaginal or cesarean? ______

c. What is the birth weight? ______

d. What is the estimated gestational age at time of delivery? ______

e. Are any conditions documented as due to prematurity? ______

f. Did the infant suffer any birth trauma? ______

g. What conditions of the newborn required evaluation, treatment, extended LOS, increased care, or present implications for future healthcare needs? ______

2. Date of encounter: 4/23/yy Location: Hilltop Pediatrics Provider: Joann Gwinn, MD

Patient: Estella Hockman Gender: F

DOB: 4/1/yy

Reason for encounter: routine newborn exam

Assessment: normal growth and development for age

Plan: RTO 1 month

(continued)

2. (continued)

a. What is the age of the patient? ______

b. What is the reason for the encounter? ______

c. Were any abnormal conditions found? ______

3. Date: 4/23/yy Location: Hilltop Pediatrics

Provider: Joann Gwinn, MD

Patient: Latasha Goodreau Gender: F

DOB: 4/10/yy

Reason for encounter: neonatal check up

Assessment: neonatal diabetes

Plan: Start on sulfonylurea therapy and see how she does. Insulin may not be required. RTO 2 weeks.

a. What is the age of the patient? ______

b. What is the reason for the encounter? ______

c. Were any abnormal conditions found? ______

4. Date of discharge: 4/23/yy Location: Valley Hospital Provider: Joann Gwinn, MD

Patient: Calvin Yen Gender: M DOB: 4/5/yy

Reason for encounter: admitted for observation from Emergency Department where mother stated she found the baby not breathing

Assessment: No respiratory effort for 15 seconds, resulting in slight cyanosis and bradycardia times one at home and the first hour of observation. After 6 hours of observation determined to be d/t central sleep apnea

Plan: use sleep apnea monitor and alarm

a. What is the age of the patient? ______

b. What is the reason for the encounter? ______

c. What condition is documented? ______

d. What is the subtype of the condition? ______

(continued)

4. (continued)

e. What complications and comorbidities exist? ______

f. Is the condition documented as originating in the perinatal period? ______

5. Date of discharge: 4/23/yy Location: Valley Hospital Provider: Joann Gwinn, MD

Patient: Brandon Leureux Gender: M

DOB: 4/20/yy

Birth Weight: 3200g EGA: 39+6

Type: forceps delivery POB: VH

Assessment: admitted to NICU for observation due to fetal bradycardia during labor

Plan: d/c in excellent condition, RTO 2 weeks

a. Was the infant born in this hospital during this admission? ______

b. Was the delivery vaginal or cesarean? ______

c. What is the birth weight? ______

d. What is the estimated gestational age at time of delivery? ______

e. Are any conditions documented as due to prematurity? ______

f. Did the infant suffer any birth trauma? ______

g. What conditions of the newborn required evaluation, treatment, extended LOS, increased care, or present implications for future healthcare needs? ______

h. What maternal conditions affected the infant? ______

6. Date of discharge: 4/24/yy Location: Valley Hospital Provider: Joann Gwinn, MD

Patient: Brittney Zeng Gender: F DOB: 4/21/yy

Birth Weight: 3756g EGA: 43+3 Type: NSVD

Location: born in car on way to hospital, then admitted, mother reports discolored amniotic fluid

(continued)

6. (continued)

Assessment: meconium aspiration d/t late delivery with dyspnea and tachypnea, orotracheal intubation x 1 day, O_2 x 2 days, Rx antibiotics prophylactically

Plan: d/c in good condition, RTO 2 weeks

a. Was the infant born in this hospital during this admission? ______

b. Was the infant born outside the hospital then hospitalized? ______

c. Was the delivery vaginal or cesarean? ______

d. What is the birth weight? ______

e. What is the estimated gestational age at time of delivery? ______

f. Are any conditions documented as due to prematurity? ______

g. Did the infant suffer any birth trauma? ______

h. What maternal conditions affected the infant? ______

i. What conditions of the newborn required evaluation, treatment, extended LOS, increased care, or present implications for future healthcare needs? ______

j. What is the subtype of the condition? ______

7. Date of discharge: 4/24/yy Location: Valley Hospital Provider: Joann Gwinn, MD

Patient: Janelle Mcquillen Gender: F

DOB: 4/12/yy

Birth Weight: 2016g EGA: 35+5

Type: NSVD POB: VH

Reason for admission: infant was readmitted 2 days post-discharge from physician office d/t hyperbilirubinemia of prematurity

Assessment: jaundice d/t preterm delivery, resolved with phototherapy

Plan: FU in office 2 days

(continued)

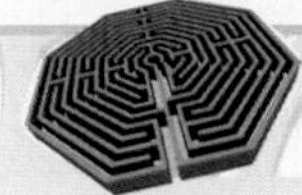

Coding Practice (continued)

7. (continued)

a. Was the infant born in this hospital during this admission? ________________

b. Was the delivery vaginal or cesarean? ________________

c. What is the birth weight? ________________

d. What is the estimated gestational age at time of delivery? ________________

e. Are any conditions documented as due to prematurity? ________________

f. Did the infant suffer any birth trauma? ________________

g. What conditions of the newborn required evaluation, treatment, extended LOS, increased care, or present implications for future healthcare needs? ________________

8. Date of discharge: 4/24/yy Location: Branton Medical Center Provider: Joann Gwinn, MD

Patient: Ebony Clawson Gender: F DOB: 4/2/yy

Birth Weight: 1923g EGA: 37+2 Type: C/S

POB: VH

Reason for admission: transferred from Valley Hospital on 4/3/yy for supervision of weight gain

Assessment: SGA and fetal growth restriction due to maternal preeclampsia and smoking during pregnancy

a. Was the infant born in this hospital during this admission? ________________

b. Was the delivery vaginal or cesarean? ________________

c. What is the birth weight? ________________

d. What is the estimated gestational age at time of delivery? ________________

e. Are any conditions documented as due to prematurity? ________________

f. Did the infant suffer any birth trauma? ________________

g. What maternal conditions affected the infant? ________________

(continued)

8. (continued)

h. What conditions of the newborn required evaluation, treatment, extended LOS, increased care, or present implications for future health care needs? ________________

9. Date of encounter: 4/24/yy Location: Hilltop Pediatrics Provider: Joann Gwinn, MD

Patient: Randal Wyche Gender: M DOB: 4/2/yy

Reason for encounter: foul smelling urine

Assessment: UTI d/t E. coli

Plan: admit to hospital for IV antibiotics

a. What is the age of the patient? ________________

b. What is the reason for the encounter? ________________

c. What condition is documented? ________________

d. What is the subtype of the condition? ________________

e. What complications and comorbidities exist? ________________

f. Is the condition documented as originating in the perinatal period? ________________

10. Date of encounter: 4/24/yy Location: Hilltop Pediatrics Provider: Joann Gwinn, MD

Patient: Theresa Sacco Gender: F DOB: 4/20/yy

Reason for encounter: first newborn check, baby was born at home with CNM in attendance

Assessment: Breast engorgement d/t maternal hormones which will resolve on its own. No problems with jaundice.

Plan: RTO 2 weeks

a. What is the age of the patient? ________________

b. What is the reason for the encounter? ________________

c. What condition is documented? ________________

d. What is the subtype of the condition? ________________

e. What complications and comorbidities exist? ________________

f. Is the condition documented as originating in the perinatal period? ________________

ASSIGNING CODES FOR PERINATAL CONDITIONS

To assign codes for newborns, coders must learn how to assign codes for birth status and for specific medical conditions. ICD-10-CM also provides separate codes for newborn medical examinations.

Assigning Codes for Newborn Birth Status

The **newborn birth status** code identifies the location of the birth, the delivery method, and the number of multiples. Assign this code to each infant only once and only when the hospital stay includes the birth episode. The exception is when an infant is born outside the hospital then hospitalized; in that instance, a birth status code should also be assigned. When a discharge includes the birth episode, assign a code from category **Z38.- Liveborn infants according to place of birth and type of delivery**. When a newborn is transferred from another hospital, the hospital where the infant was born reports a code from **Z38.-**. A birth status code should *not* be reported by the receiving hospital (OGCR I.C.16.a.2)).

Locate the newborn birth status code for singletons in the Index under the Main Term **Newborn**, subterm **born** (■ FIGURE 24-5). For multiple births, locate the Main Term **Newborn**, then the subterm for **twin**, **triplet**, **quadruplet**, or **quintuplet**. Each of these subterms has additional subterms for **born in hospital** and **by cesarean**. Always verify the code in the Tabular List.

Do not confuse category **Z38**, which is for use on the newborn record, with category **Z37 Outcome of delivery**, which is for use on the mother's record. Even though both categories appear to report similar information, they exist for different purposes. An instructional note at the beginning of each category in the Tabular List clearly defines the respective use and intended purpose.

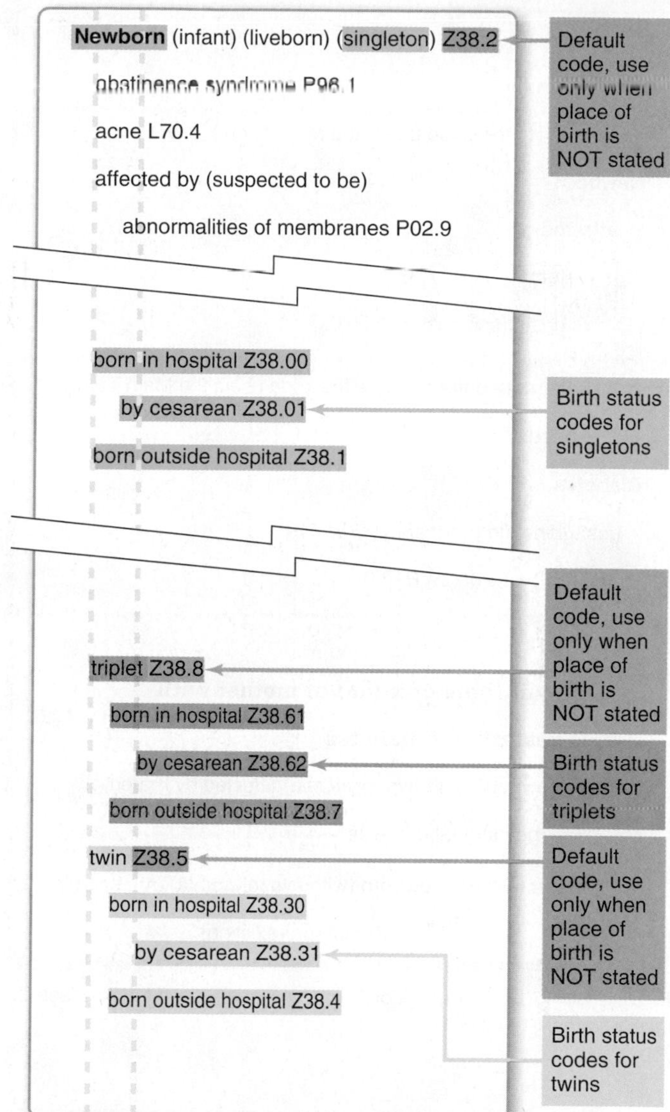

Figure 24-5 ■ Index Entries for Newborn Birth Status Codes

> **SUCCESS STEP**
>
> Highlight, flag, or draw an icon in your coding manual to remind yourself that **Z37.-** is for the mother and **Z38.-** is for the newborn. Mixing up these two code categories is a common mistake of new coders.

Assigning Codes for Conditions

Most codes for medical conditions of the newborn are indexed under the Main Term **Newborn**. The subterm **affected by** means to report the code *only* when the newborn is specifically affected by a condition. For example, when an infant is delivered with forceps assistance, assign a code only if the delivery method *affected* the infant. Do not automatically assign a code for forceps delivery to report the *fact* that forceps were used.

The subterm **maternal** describes the effect on the newborn of a condition the mother had during pregnancy, labor, or delivery. For example, when a newborn is affected by the mother's gestational diabetes (GDM), assign a code for **Newborn, affected by, maternal diabetes**. Be aware of the following distinctions among maternal and newborn codes:

- Do NOT assign code **O24.419 Gestational diabetes** to the newborn.
- Assign code **P70.0 Syndrome of infant of mother with gestational diabetes** (■ FIGURE 24-6, page 494) when the newborn is affected by maternal GDM.
- When the mother has GDM but the newborn is *not* affected by it, do not assign code **P70.0**.

When a code cannot be located under the Main Term **Newborn**, search under the name of the condition itself. Many conditions have a subterm specifically for the **newborn**, so be certain to review the subterms carefully to locate the appropriate entry (■ FIGURE 24-7, page 494).

Newborn is treated for hypoglycemia, which is due to maternal gestational diabetes.

Index: Locate the code under the Main Term **Newborn:**

Newborn
- affected by
  - maternal
    - gestational diabetes P70.0

Index (alternate entry): Locate the code using the Main Term **Diabetes:**

Diabetes
- gestational (in pregnancy) O24.419
  - affecting newborn P70.0

Tabular List:

P70.0 Syndrome of infant of mother with gestational diabetes

Newborn (with hypoglycemia) affected by maternal gestational diabetes

Excludes1: newborn (with hypoglycemia) affected by maternal (pre-existing)

Figure 24-6 ■ Example of Assigning Codes for an Infant Affected by a Maternal Condition

Newborn is treated for respiratory distress syndrome II.

Respiratory — *see also* condition
- distress syndrome (newborn) (type I) P22.0
  - type II P22.1
- syncytial virus, as cause of disease classified elsewhere B97.4

Figure 24-7 ■ Example of Locating a Newborn Code under the Main Term for the Condition

The subterm **transitory** under a newborn condition means that the condition was temporary, as many newborn conditions are.

When a condition that originated during the perinatal period is diagnosed or treated later in life, assign a perinatal code to identify the perinatal origin (OGCR I.C.16.a.4)) (■ FIGURE 24-8).

Some conditions of newborns either can be due to the birth process or be a community-acquired disease. When the documentation does not specify the cause of the condition, the default is to code it as perinatal and to assign a code from ICD-10-CM Chapter 16. When the condition is documented as community acquired, do not assign a code from Chapter 16 (OGCR I.C.16.a.5)).

Patient, age 15, is seen for Erb's palsy which resulted from damage during birth.

Index:

Erb's
- disease G71.0
- palsy, paralysis (brachial) (birth) (newborn) P14.0
  - spinal (spastic) syphilitic A52.17
- pseudohypertrophic muscular dystrophy G71.0

Tabular List:

P14.0 Erb's paralysis due to birth injury

Figure 24-8 ■ Example of Assigning a Code for a Perinatal Condition Later in Life

6th **Z00.11 Newborn health examination**

Health check for child under 29 days old

Use additional code to identify any abnormal findings

Excludes1: health check for child over 28 days old (Z00.12-)

Z00.110 Health examination for newborn under 8 days old

Health check for newborn under 8 days old

Z00.111 Health examination for newborn 8 to 28 days old

Health check for newborn 8 to 28 days old

Newborn weight check

Figure 24-9 ■ Tabular List Entry for Newborn Health Examination

Assigning Codes for Neonatal Examinations

Routine neonatal examinations are reported with **Z** codes, just as other routine physical examinations are. Search under the Main Term **Newborn** and the subterm **examination** to locate the codes in the Index. Codes are divided based on the age of the newborn (■ FIGURE 24-9).

An instructional note in the Tabular List directs coders to assign additional codes to identify any abnormal findings or conditions.

SUCCESS STEP

Routine examinations for infants over 28 days in age should be assigned a code from **Z00.12- Encounter for routine child health examination.**

Guided Example of Assigning Perinatal Codes

To practice skills for assigning codes for conditions originating in the perinatal period, continue with the example from earlier in the chapter about patient Derek Leverette, who was born at Valley Hospital.

Follow along in your ICD-10-CM manual as Aaron Randell, CCS, assigns codes. Check off each step after you complete it.

⇨ First, Aaron confirms the information he abstracted.

- ❑ This is a birth encounter of a preterm birth.
- ❑ The newborn was treated for TTN.

⇨ Aaron knows that because this is a birth encounter, he must assign a code for the birth status of the infant.

⇨ Aaron searches the Index for the Main Term **Newborn**.

- ❑ He locates the subterm **born in hospital**.
- ❑ He locates the second-level subterm **cesarean section Z38.01**

⇨ Aaron verifies code **Z38.01** in the Tabular List.

- ❑ He reads the code title for **Z38.01, Single liveborn infant, delivered by cesarean**, and confirms that this accurately describes the birth.

⇨ Aaron checks for instructional notes in the Tabular List.

- ❑ He cross-references the beginning of category **Z38** and reads the instructional note that tells him that this is the correct code for a newborn and it should never be assigned to the mother (■ FIGURE 24-10).
- ❑ He cross-references the beginning of block **Z30-Z39** and verifies that there are no instructional notes.

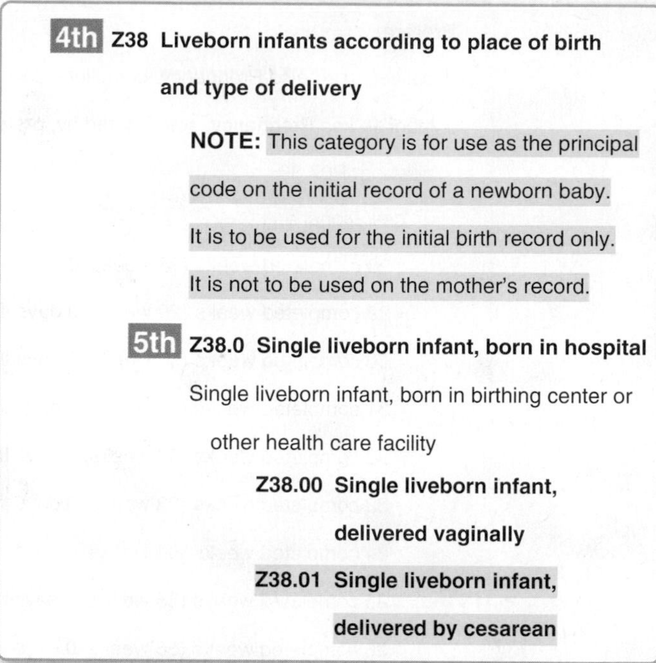

4th **Z38 Liveborn infants according to place of birth and type of delivery**

NOTE: This category is for use as the principal code on the initial record of a newborn baby. It is to be used for the initial birth record only. It is not to be used on the mother's record.

5th **Z38.0 Single liveborn infant, born in hospital**

Single liveborn infant, born in birthing center or other health care facility

Z38.00 Single liveborn infant, delivered vaginally

Z38.01 Single liveborn infant, delivered by cesarean

Figure 24-10 ■ Tabular List Instructional Note for Category Z38

- ❑ He cross-references the beginning of **Chapter 21 (Z00-Z99)** and reviews the instructional notes, which provide a general description about the use of Z codes. He determines there is no information that applies specifically to this code.

⇨ Next, Aaron decides to assign a code for TTN.

⇨ Aaron searches the Index for the Main Term **Tachypnea**.

- ❑ He locates the subterm **newborn P22.1**.

⇨ Aaron verifies code **P22.1** in the Tabular List.

- ❑ He reads the code title for **P22.1, Transient tachypnea of newborn**, and confirms that this accurately describes the diagnosis.

⇨ Aaron checks for instructional notes in the Tabular List.

- ❑ He cross-references the beginning of category **P22** and reads the **Excludes1** note. He determines that it does not apply because neither of the conditions excluded are documented for this patient.
- ❑ He cross-references the beginning of the block **P19-P29** and verifies that there are no instructional notes.
- ❑ He cross-references the beginning of **Chapter 16 (P00-P99)** and reads the instructional notes. They confirm that codes in this chapter should be used on the newborn's record.

⇨ The next code Aaron decides to assign is for the preterm birth.

Preterm

delivery (*see also* Pregnancy, complicated by, preterm labor) O60.10

labor — *see* Pregnancy, complicated by, preterm labor

newborn P07.30

gestational age

28 completed weeks (28 weeks, 0 days through 28 weeks, 6 days) P07.31

29 completed weeks (29 weeks, 0 days through 29 weeks, 6 days) P07.32

30 completed weeks (30 weeks, 0 days through 30 weeks, 6 days) P07.33

31 completed weeks (31 weeks, 0 days through 31 weeks, 6 days) P07.34

32 completed weeks (32 weeks, 0 days through 32 weeks, 6 days) P07.35

33 completed weeks (33 weeks, 0 days through 33 weeks, 6 days) P07.36

34 completed weeks (34 weeks, 0 days through 34 weeks, 6 days) P07.37

35 completed weeks (35 weeks, 0 days through 35 weeks, 6 days) P07.38

36 completed weeks (36 weeks, 0 days through 36 weeks, 6 days) P07.39

Figure 24-11 ■ Index Entry for Preterm

➩ Aaron searches the Index for the Main Term **Preterm** (■ FIGURE 24-11).

- ❑ He locates a subterm **delivery O60.10**.
- ❑ He reviews the remaining subterm and also locates subterm **newborn P07.30**.
- ❑ He notices that the codes are from different chapters because they begin with different letters. He decides to check the Tabular List for each code.
- ❑ He verifies the code title for **O60.10, Preterm labor with preterm delivery, unspecified trimester**.
- ❑ When he cross-references the beginning of the chapter, he learns that this code is from **Chapter 15 Pregnancy, Childbirth and the Puerperium (O00-O9A)**.
- ❑ He reads the instructional note in capital letters under the chapter title that states **CODES FROM THIS CHAPTER ARE FOR USE ONLY ON MATERNAL RECORDS, NEVER ON NEWBORN RECORDS**.
- ❑ This instruction tells him that he should NOT use **O60.10** because he is coding for the newborn, not the mother.
- ❑ Aaron returns to the Index to review the entries for the Main Term **Preterm**, and subterm **newborn**.
- ❑ He locates a second-level subterm **gestational age**.
- ❑ He locates the third-level subterm **34 completed weeks (34 weeks, 0 days through 34 weeks, 6 days) P07.37**. He believes this code describes the preterm newborn of gestational age *34 weeks*, which is documented in the medical record.

➩ Aaron verifies code **P07.37** in the Tabular List.

- ❑ He reads the code title for **P07.37, Preterm newborn, gestational age 34 completed weeks**, and confirms that this accurately describes the length of gestation.

➩ Aaron checks for instructional notes in the Tabular List.

- ❑ He cross-references the beginning of category **P07** and reads the instructional notes, which direct him to assign a code for birth weight in addition to gestational age. The note also provides sequencing instructions (■ FIGURE 24-12).
- ❑ He reads the code selections for low birth weight under subcategories **P07.0** and **P07.1**. He locates the code **P07.17, Other low birth weight newborn, 1750-1999 grams,** which includes the birth weight of this baby, *1790 grams*.
- ❑ He continues cross-referencing and checks the beginning of the block **P05-P08**. He verifies that there are no instructional notes for this block.
- ❑ He cross-references the beginning of **Chapter 16 (P00-P99)** and reads the instructional notes. They confirm that codes in this chapter should be used on the newborn's record.

4th P07 Disorders of newborn related to short gestation and low birth weight, not elsewhere classified

NOTE: When both birth weight and gestational age of the newborn are available, both should be coded with birth weight sequenced before gestational age

Includes: the listed conditions, without further specification, as the cause of morbidity or additional care, in newborn

Excludes1: low birth weight due to slow fetal growth and fetal malnutrition (P05.-)

5th P07.0 Extremely low birth weight newborn

Newborn birth weight 999 g. or less

5th P07.1 Other low birth weight newborn

Newborn birth weight 1000–2499 g.

P07.10 Other low birth weight newborn, unspecified weight

P07.14 Other low birth weight newborn, 1000–1249 grams

P07.15 Other low birth weight newborn, 1250–1499 grams

P07.16 Other low birth weight newborn, 1500–1749 grams

P07.17 Other low birth weight newborn, 1750–1999 grams

P07.18 Other low birth weight newborn, 2000–2499 grams

5th P07.2 Extreme immaturity of newborn

Less than 28 completed weeks (less than 196 completed days) of gestation.

5th P07.3 Preterm [premature] newborn [other]

28 completed weeks or more but less than 37 completed weeks (196 completed days but less than 259 completed days) of gestation.

Prematurity NOS

P07.30 Preterm newborn, unspecified weeks of gestation

P07.31 Preterm newborn, gestational age 28 completed weeks

Preterm newborn, gestational age 28 weeks, 0 days through 28 weeks, 6 days

P07.37 Preterm newborn, gestational age 34 completed weeks

Preterm newborn, gestational age 34 weeks, 0 days through 34 weeks, 6 days

Figure 24-12 ■ Tabular List Instructional Notes for Category P07

➩ Aaron reviews the codes he has assigned for this case.

- ❑ **P07.37, Preterm newborn, gestational age 34 completed weeks**
- ❑ **P07.17, Other low birth weight newborn, 1750-1999 grams**
- ❑ **P22.1, Transient tachypnea of newborn**
- ❑ **Z38.01, Single liveborn infant, delivered by cesarean**

➩ Next, Aaron must determine how to sequence the codes.

SUCCESS STEP

Assign codes for birth weight and gestational age *only* for preterm infants or when the physician documents their significance. Do not automatically code birth weight and gestational age for every baby.

Coding Practice

Now it is your turn to practice assigning codes for conditions originating in the perinatal period. Refer to the ***Tip*** at the end of the mini-medical-record if you need a little extra help.

Exercise 24.3 Assigning Codes for Perinatal Conditions

Instructions: Read the mini-medical-record of each patient's encounter, review the information abstracted in Exercise 24.2, and assign ICD-10-CM diagnosis codes (CM) using the Index and Tabular List. Write the code(s) on the line provided.

1. Date of discharge: 4/23/yy Location: Valley Hospital Provider: Joann Gwinn, MD

Patient: Dixie Dare Gender: F DOB: 4/22/yy

Birth Weight: 3521g EGA: 38+2 Type: NSVD

POB: VH

Assessment: APGARS 6, 8

Plan: FU in office, 2 weeks

Tip: Apgar scores of 6 (one minute after delivery) and 8 (five minutes after delivery) are considered normal.

1 CM Code __________

2. Date of encounter: 4/23/yy Location: Hilltop Pediatrics Provider: Joann Gwinn, MD

Patient: Estella Hockman Gender: F DOB: 4/1/yy

Reason for encounter: routine newborn exam

Assessment: normal growth and development for age

Plan: RTO 1 month

1 CM Code __________

3. Date of encounter: 4/23/yy Location: Hilltop Pediatrics Provider: Joann Gwinn, MD

Patient: Latasha Goodreau Gender: F

DOB: 4/10/yy

Reason for encounter: neonatal check up

Assessment: neonatal diabetes

Plan: Start on sulfonylurea therapy and see how she does. Insulin may not be required. RTO 2 weeks.

Tip: A check up is the same as an examination.

2 CM Codes __________ __________

4. Date of discharge: 4/23/yy Location: Valley Hospital Provider: Joann Gwinn, MD

Patient: Calvin Yen Gender: M DOB: 4/5/yy

Reason for encounter: admitted for observation from Emergency Department where mother stated she found the baby not breathing

Assessment: No respiratory effort for 15 seconds, resulting in slight cyanosis and bradycardia times one at home and the first hour of observation. After 6 hours of observation determined to be d/t central sleep apnea.

Plan: use sleep apnea monitor and alarm

1 CM Code __________

5. Date of discharge: 4/23/yy Location: Valley Hospital Provider: Joann Gwinn, MD

Patient: Brandon Leureux Gender: M DOB: 4/20/yy

Birth Weight: 3200g EGA: 39+6

Type: forceps delivery POB: VH

(continued)

5. (continued)

Assessment: admitted to NICU for observation due to fetal bradycardia during labor

Plan: d/c in excellent condition, RTO 2 weeks

Tip: Forceps are used only in a vaginal delivery.

2 CM Codes ____________ ____________

ARRANGING CODES FOR PERINATAL CONDITIONS

Significant perinatal sequencing guidelines relate to selecting the principal diagnosis for the birth episode, assigning codes for the weight and EGA of preterm infants, and sequencing codes for bacterial newborn sepsis.

Selecting the Principal Diagnosis for Birth Encounters

The previous section of this chapter discussed assigning a code from category **Z38** to identify the birth status on a newborn's record. This code is assigned only for hospital admissions that include the delivery or occur immediately after a birth outside the hospital. Sequence codes as follows:

1. **Z38.-** is *always* sequenced as the principal diagnosis on a newborn's record (OGCR I.C.16.a.2)). This is true regardless of any other conditions or complications that accompany the birth.
2. Sequence additional codes for any conditions that require treatment, further workup, prolong length of stay, or require resource utilization (OGCR I.C.16.c.1)). Conditions that require current treatment or workup should be sequenced based on their significance according to the provider.
3. Finally, sequence conditions documented as having implications for future healthcare needs (OGCR I.C.16.c.2)).

CODING CAUTION

Conditions not treated, but documented as having implications for future healthcare needs, should be coded *only* for newborns, never for adults.

Arranging Codes for Birth Weight and Estimated Gestational Age

A preterm infant may have difficulties due to short gestation or low birth weight. A postterm infant may be at risk for diabetes or other conditions. Assign codes that identify the birth weight and the EGA of the infant when these factors are documented to affect the infant's health status. Also assign codes for any specified conditions. For admissions that include the birth encounter, sequence the codes as follows (OGCR I.C.16.d. and e.):

1. **Z38.-** Birth status of infant, if the admission includes the birth episode
2. **P07.0-** or **P07.1-** Birth weight (Search the Index for the Main Term **Low**, subterm **birth weight**).
3. **P07.2-** or **P07.3-** Weeks of gestation (Search the Index for the Main Term **Preterm**, subterm **newborn**, second-level subterm **gestational age**).
4. Other specified conditions

For admissions that do not include the birth encounter, select the principal diagnosis based on the standard criteria in OGCR II.

SUCCESS STEP

Birth weight should always be sequenced *before* EGA, but weight does not have to be the principal diagnosis.

A full term or preterm infant may be small for its age due to slow fetal growth or malnutrition. Assign a code from **P05.- Disorders of newborn related to slow fetal growth and fetal malnutrition** in these situations.

A postterm infant may be at risk due to being large for its age. Assign a code from **P08 Disorders of newborn related to long gestation and high birth weight** in these situations.

CODING CAUTION

When you assign a code from **P05**, do *not* assign codes from **P07** for birth weight and EGA.

Arranging Codes for Bacterial Newborn Sepsis

Coding bacterial sepsis of a newborn is similar to coding any patient with sepsis, as discussed in Chapter 21 of this text and ICD-10-CM Chapter 1, Certain Infectious and Parasitic Diseases (A00-B49). One difference is that perinatal sepsis may be congenital or community acquired. When the source is not documented, the default is congenital and a newborn sepsis code should be assigned (OGCR I.C.16.f.). Category **P36 Bacterial sepsis of newborn** provides combination codes that include the most common causal organisms (■ FIGURE 24-13). If the appropriate causal organism is not included in the **P36.-** code, then assign an additional code from category **B96**. Assign and sequence codes as follows:

1. Assign a code from **P36.- Bacterial sepsis of newborn**.
2. If the causal organism is *not* provided in a combination code, assign a code from **B96 Other bacterial agents as the cause of diseases classified elsewhere**.
3. When severe sepsis or septic shock is documented, assign a code from **R65.2- Severe sepsis**.
4. Assign codes for associated acute organ dysfunction(s).

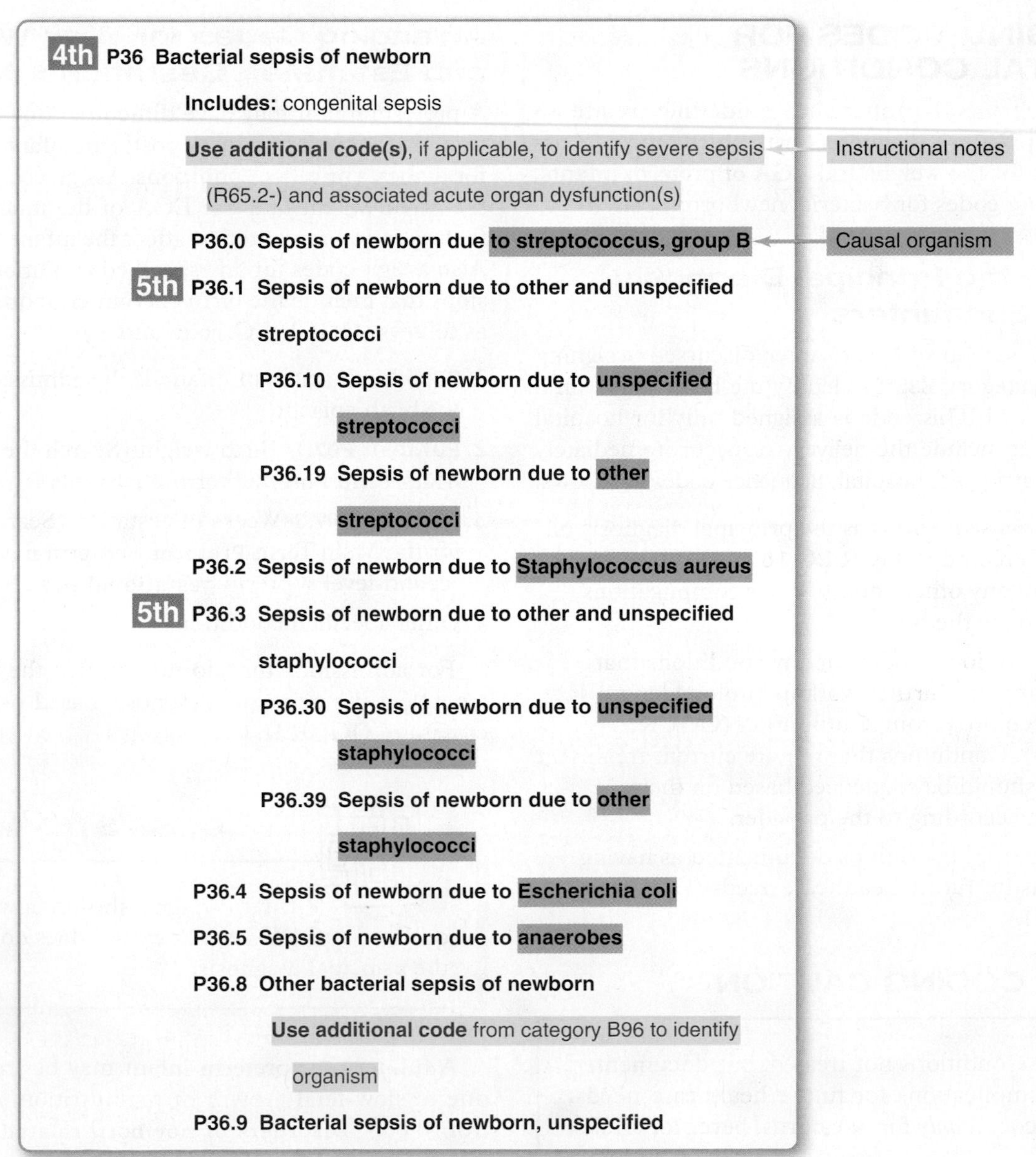

4th **P36 Bacterial sepsis of newborn**

Includes: congenital sepsis

Use additional code(s), if applicable, to identify severe sepsis (R65.2-) and associated acute organ dysfunction(s)

P36.0 Sepsis of newborn due to streptococcus, group B

5th **P36.1 Sepsis of newborn due to other and unspecified streptococci**

P36.10 Sepsis of newborn due to unspecified streptococci

P36.19 Sepsis of newborn due to other streptococci

P36.2 Sepsis of newborn due to Staphylococcus aureus

5th **P36.3 Sepsis of newborn due to other and unspecified staphylococci**

P36.30 Sepsis of newborn due to unspecified staphylococci

P36.39 Sepsis of newborn due to other staphylococci

P36.4 Sepsis of newborn due to Escherichia coli

P36.5 Sepsis of newborn due to anaerobes

P36.8 Other bacterial sepsis of newborn

Use additional code from category B96 to identify organism

P36.9 Bacterial sepsis of newborn, unspecified

Figure 24-13 ■ Tabular List Entry for Category P36 Bacterial Sepsis of Newborn

Guided Example of Arranging Perinatal Codes

To practice skills for sequencing codes for diseases of the conditions originating in the perinatal period, continue with the example from earlier in the chapter about patient Derek Leverette, who was born at Valley Hospital.

Follow along in your ICD-10-CM manual as Aaron Randell, CCS, sequences the codes. Check off each step after you complete it.

⇨First, Aaron reviews the codes he assigned.

- ❑ **P07.37, Preterm newborn, gestational age 34 completed weeks**
- ❑ **P07.17, Other low birth weight newborn, 1750-1999 grams**
- ❑ **P22.1, Transient tachypnea of newborn**
- ❑ **Z38.01, Single liveborn infant, delivered by cesarean**

⇨Aaron refers to OGCR I.C.16.a.2) Principal Diagnosis for the Birth Record.

- ❑ The OGCR states that a code from **Z38** should be the principal diagnosis for the birth episode. This enables Aaron to determine that the first code should be **Z38.01**.

⇨Aaron refers to OGCR I.C.16.d. Prematurity and Fetal Growth Retardation

- ❑ This OGCR states that codes should be assigned based on the documented birth weight and gestational age. It also states that the code for birth weight should be sequenced before the code for gestational age. He also recalls that he read an instructional note under category **P07** with the same information.
- ❑ Based on this information, Aaron determines that **P07.17** should be the second code and **P07.37** should be the third code.
- ❑ This leaves **P22.1** as the final code. Aaron checks the notes he wrote earlier to be certain that there are no instructional notes that affect the sequencing of this code.

⇨Aaron finalizes the codes and sequencing for this case:

(1) **Z38.01, Single liveborn infant, delivered by cesarean**

(2) **P07.17, Other low birth weight newborn, 1750-1999 grams**

(3) **P07.37, Preterm newborn, gestational age 34 completed weeks**

(4) **P22.1, Transient tachypnea of newborn**

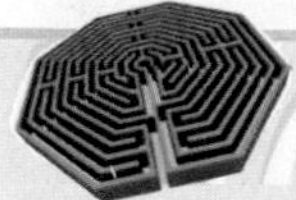

Coding Practice

Now it is your turn to practice sequencing codes for conditions originating in the perinatal period. Refer to the ***Tip*** at the end of the mini-medical-record if you need a little extra help.

Exercise 24.4 Arranging Codes for Perinatal Conditions

Instructions: Read the mini-medical-record of each patient's encounter, review the information abstracted in Exercise 24.2, assign ICD-10-CM diagnosis codes (CM) using the Index and Tabular List, and sequence them correctly.

1. Date of discharge: 4/24/yy Location: Valley Hospital Provider: Joann Gwinn, MD

Patient: Brittney Zeng Gender: F DOB: 4/21/yy

Birth Weight: 3756g EGA: 43+3 Type: NSVD

Location: born in car on way to hospital, then admitted, mother reports discolored amniotic fluid

Assessment: meconium aspiration d/t late delivery with dyspnea and tachypnea, **orotracheal intubation** x 1 day, 02 x 2 days, Rx antibiotics prophylactically

(continued)

1. (continued)

Plan: d/c in good condition, RTO 2 weeks

Tip: Meconium-related problems are most common with prolonged gestations.

3 CM Codes __________ __________ __________

2. Date of discharge: 4/24/yy Location: Valley Hospital Provider: Joann Gwinn, MD

Patient: Janelle Mcquillen Gender: F DOB: 4/12/yy

Birth Weight: 2016g EGA: 35+5 Type: NSVD

POB: VH

Reason for admission: infant was readmitted 2 days post-discharge from physician office d/t hyperbilirubinemia of prematurity

Assessment: jaundice d/t preterm delivery, resolved with phototherapy

(continued)

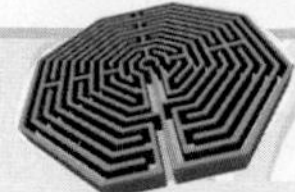

Coding Practice (continued)

2. (continued)

Plan: FU in office 2 days

3 CM Codes __________ __________

____

3. Date of discharge: 4/24/yy Location: Branton Medical Center Provider: Joann Gwinn, MD

Patient: Ebony Clawson Gender: F DOB: 4/2/yy

Birth Weight: 1923g EGA: 37+2 Type: C/S

POB: VH

Reason for admission: transferred from Valley Hospital on 4/3/yy for supervision of weight gain

Assessment: SGA and fetal growth restriction due to maternal preeclampsia and smoking during pregnancy

Tip: The term *intrauterine growth restriction* has largely replaced the older term *intrauterine growth retardation*. You also need to determine what type of condition preeclampsia is.

4 CM Codes __________ __________

__________ __________

4. Date of encounter: 4/24/yy Location: Hilltop Pediatrics Provider: Joann Gwinn, MD

Patient: Randal Wyche Gender: M DOB: 4/2/yy

Reason for encounter: foul smelling urine

Assessment: UTI d/t E. coli

Plan: admit to hospital for IV antibiotics

2 CM Codes __________ __________

5. Date of encounter: 4/24/yy Location: Hilltop Pediatrics Provider: Joann Gwinn, MD

Patient: Theresa Sacco Gender: F DOB: 4/20/yy

Reason for encounter: first newborn check, baby was born at home with CNM in attendance

Assessment: Breast engorgement d/t maternal hormones which will resolve on its own. No problems with jaundice.

Plan: RTO 2 weeks

2 CM Codes __________ __________

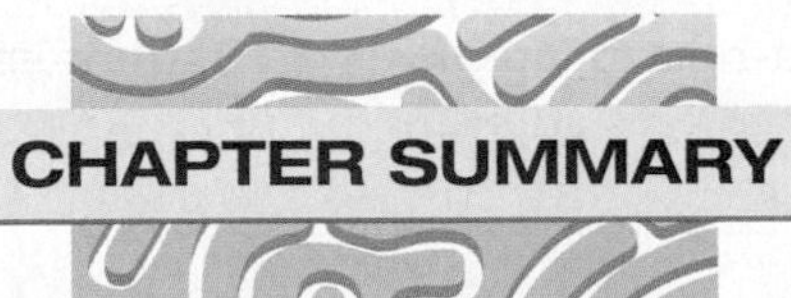

CHAPTER SUMMARY

In this chapter you learned that:

- The perinatal period begins before birth and continues through the twenty-eighth day following birth.
- ICD-10-CM Chapter 16, Certain Conditions Originating in the Perinatal Period (P00-P96), contains 12 blocks or subchapters that are divided by anatomical site.
- Coders must take note whether a hospitalization of a newborn includes the birth itself or whether the admission takes place after the birth episode.
- To assign codes for newborns, coders must learn how to assign codes for birth status, for specific medical conditions, and for newborn examinations.
- Significant sequencing guidelines relate to selecting the principal diagnosis for the birth episode, assigning codes for the weight and EGA of preterm infants, and sequencing codes for bacterial newborn sepsis.
- ICD-10-CM provides Official Guidelines for Coding and Reporting (OGCR) in OGCR I.C.16. regarding selecting the principal and additional diagnoses, and how to report codes from this chapter with those from other chapters, prematurity, low birth weight, bacterial sepsis of the newborn, and stillbirth.

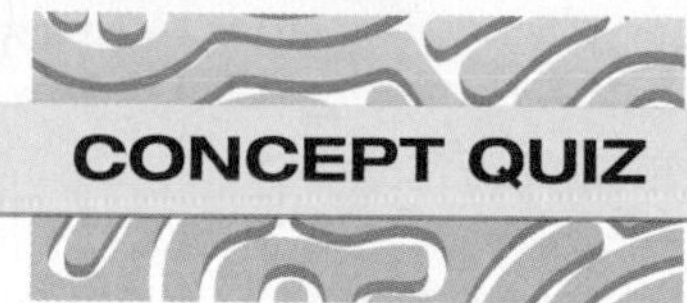

CONCEPT QUIZ

Take a moment to look back at your trip through conditions originating in the perinatal period and solidify your skills. This is your opportunity to pull together everything you have learned.

Completion

Instructions: Write the term that answers each question based on the information you learned in this chapter. Choose from the list below. Some choices may be used more than once and some choices may not be used at all. Refer to the discussion in this chapter and the Glossary at the end of this book if you need a little extra help.

1,000	Erb's palsy
1,500	LBW
2,000	LGA
2,500	MAS
4,200	meconium peritonitis
amin/o	neonate
ammon/o	omphalitis
amni/o	perinatal
amnionitis	transitory
birth trauma	VLBW

1. A newborn with a birth weight of 2,200 grams is classified as ______________.
2. Normal birth weight is defined as ______________ to ______________ grams.
3. ______________ is a condition in which the newborn breathes a mixture of meconium and amniotic fluid into the lungs prior to or during delivery.
4. A fetus or newborn infant who is larger in size than normal for the baby's sex and gestational age is classified as ______________.
5. ______________ is any physical injury to the infant during delivery.
6. Infection of the umbilical stump in a newborn is called ______________.
7. A ______________ perinatal condition is temporary.
8. An infant is referred to as a ______________ during the first 28 days of life.
9. The combining form for amniotic sac is ______________.
10. ______________ grams equals 5 pounds, 8 ounces.

Multiple Choice

Instructions: Circle the letter of the best answer to each question based on the information you learned in this chapter. Refer to the discussion in this chapter and the Glossary at the end of this book if you need a little extra help.

1. Which type of condition is NOT classified in ICD-10-CM Chapter 16 (P00-P99)?
   A. Birth trauma
   B. Conditions that result from maternal conditions
   C. Congenital abnormalities
   D. Conditions that result from underdevelopment during gestation
2. Which of the criteria for clinically significant conditions is used ONLY for newborns?
   A. A condition that requires clinical evaluation
   B. A condition that increases nursing care or monitoring
   C. A condition that extends length of hospital stay
   D. A condition that presents implications for future healthcare needs
3. A full term infant is born in the hospital with normal vaginal delivery and no complications. What code should be assigned to the newborn's birth record?
   A. O80 Encounter for full-term uncomplicated delivery
   B. Z34.03 Encounter for supervision of normal first pregnancy, third trimester
   C. Z37.0 Single live birth
   D. Z38.00 Single liveborn infant, delivered vaginally
4. Perinatal conditions are defined by the fact that they
   A. were diagnosed during the first 28 days.
   B. originated before birth or during the first 28 days.
   C. were treated during the first 28 days.
   D. result from a condition of the mother.
5. Which of the following conditions is NOT a perinatal condition?
   A. Gestational diabetes
   B. Retinopathy of prematurity
   C. Meconium aspiration syndrome
   D. Neonatal diabetes
6. The permanent abnormal shape of an organ or body region, resulting from arrested, delayed, or abnormal development of the embryo, is
   A. a deformation.
   B. a malformation.
   C. a chromosomal abnormality.
   D. Erb's palsy.

7. Perinatal codes can be used in all the following situations EXCEPT
   A. a 15-year-old with a permanent condition that originated at birth.
   B. a newborn condition that lasts only a few days.
   C. a fetal condition that affects the mother.
   D. a maternal condition that affects the newborn.
8. A birth status code from Z38 should be reported when
   A. a hospital receives a newborn from another hospital.
   B. the hospital stay includes the birth episode.
   C. a fetus is stillborn.
   D. a newborn is readmitted within 28 days of birth.
9. OGCR for Chapter 16 discuss all of the following EXCEPT
   A. selecting the principal diagnosis.
   B. low birth weight.
   C. bacterial sepsis of the newborn.
   D. neonatal diabetes.
10. A birth status code from Z38 describes the newborn's
   A. weight.
   B. gender.
   C. delivery method.
   D. gestational age.

CODING CHALLENGE

Now it is your turn to demonstrate coding all aspects of conditions originating in the perinatal period. Refer back to the examples and discussion in this chapter when you need a little extra help. Use your medical dictionary and anatomy references when needed.

Instructions: Read the mini-medical-record of each patient's encounter, then abstract, assign, and sequence ICD-10-CM diagnosis codes (CM) using the Index and Tabular List. Write the code(s) on the line provided.

1. Date of discharge: 4/29/yy Location: Valley Hospital Provider: Joann Gwinn, MD

Patient: Wendie Embree Gender: F DOB: 4/27/yy

Birth Weight: 4555g EGA: 40+4 Type: C/S

POB: VH

Assessment: LGA, watch for diabetes, otherwise healthy

Plan: FU office 2 weeks

2 CM Codes __________ __________

2. Date of discharge: 4/29/yy Location: Valley Hospital Provider: Joann Gwinn, MD

Patient: Clifford Muldowney Gender: M DOB: 4/28/yy

Birth Weight: 3010g EGA: 42+0 Type: NSVD

POB: VH

Assessment: post term, otherwise healthy

Plan: FU office 2 weeks

2 CM Codes __________ __________

3. Date of discharge: 4/29/yy Location: Branton Medical Center Provider: Joann Gwinn, MD

Patient: Josefina Houseman Gender: F

DOB: 4/22/yy

Birth Weight: 1293g EGA: 30+3 Type: C/S

POB: VH

Reason for admission: transferred from Valley Hospital on DOB due to heroin baby

Assessment: drug withdrawal syndrome complicated by prematurity with underdeveloped lungs

Plan: Weaned off heroin. RTO 3 days post discharge.

Tip: Follow the sequencing rules for poisonings.

4 CM Codes __________ __________ __________ __________

4. Date of discharge: 4/29/yy Location: Valley Hospital Provider: Joann Gwinn, MD

Patient: Lenora Ringo Gender: F DOB: 4/20/yy

Birth Weight: 3621g EGA: 39+1 Type: C/S

POB: VH

Assessment: hypoglycemia due to GDM, respiratory distress

Plan: FU weekly for first month

4 CM Codes __________ __________ __________ __________

5. Date of discharge: 4/29/yy Location: Valley Hospital Provider: Joann Gwinn, MD

Patient: Faith Mika Gender: F DOB: 4/22/yy

Birth Weight: 3489g EGA: 38+0 Type: NSVD

POB: VH

Assessment: fractured clavicle during delivery d/t prolapsed arm presentation

Plan: pin long sleeved garment to the clothes to immobilize arm if discomfort observed, lift child with care, RTO 1 week

Tip: prolapsed arm is a malpresentation

3 CM Codes __________ __________ __________

6. Date of encounter: 4/29/yy Location: Hilltop Pediatrics Provider: Joann Gwinn, MD

Patient: Tomas Nightingale Gender: M

DOB: 4/15/yy

Reason for encounter: redness, mild bleeding, and swelling of umbilical stump

Assessment: omphalitis with hemorrhage

Plan: begin 2 week regime of antimicrobial therapy, RTO in one day for reevaluation of condition

1 CM Code __________

7. Date of discharge: 4/29/yy Location: Branton Medical Center Provider: Joann Gwinn, MD

Patient: Jon Morehead Gender: M DOB: 3/29/yy

Birth Weight: 762g EGA: 28 Type: NSVD

POB: BMC

Assessment: first born of triplets with cardiomyopathy, second sibling liveborn with respiratory distress syndrome and jaundice, fetus 3 stillborn

Plan: RTO 3 days post discharge.

Tip: Each infant has its own record. Code only for the infant who is named on this record.

4 CM Codes __________ __________ __________ __________

8. Date of discharge: 4/29/yy Location: Valley Hospital Provider: Joann Gwinn, MD

Patient: William MacAulay Gender: M

DOB: 4/22/yy

Birth Weight: 3256g EGA: 40+2 Type: NSVD

POB: VH

Assessment: injury to brachial plexus and cannot move arm

Plan: Refer to physical therapist for three months. Reevaluate for reconstructive surgery if no improvement in three months.

2 CM Codes __________ __________

9. Date of discharge: 4/29/yy Location: Valley Hospital Provider: Joann Gwinn, MD

Patient: Tim Ferrigno Gender: M DOB: 4/12/yy

Reason for admission: admitted on 4/15/yy, 2 days post discharge, with acute respiratory failure d/t severe sepsis

Assessment: severe sepsis d/t staphylococcus aureus caused by amnionitis, ARF

Plan: Antibiotic therapy, careful post discharge monitoring, aggressive fluid restoration. RTO 1 week

Tip: Refer to OGCR I.C.16.f.

4 CM Codes __________ __________ __________ __________

10. Date of discharge: 4/29/yy Location: Branton Medical Center Provider: Joann Gwinn, MD

Patient: Jay Bridgewater Gender: M DOB: 4/25/yy

Birth Weight: 3185g EGA: 38+3 Type: NSVD

POB: VH

Reason for admission: transferred from Valley Hospital 6 hours after birth d/t hemolytic disease

Assessment: transfusion required for hemolytic disease due to ABO isoimmunization

Plan: FU 1 week

1 CM Code __________

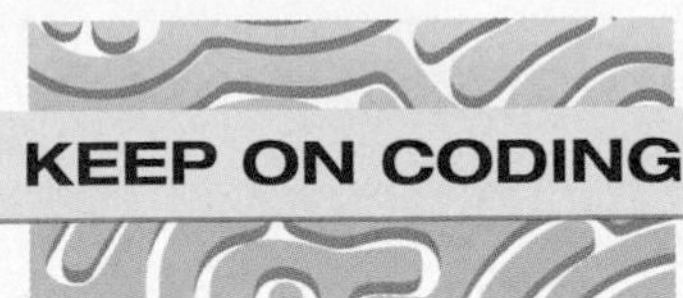

KEEP ON CODING

As a coder, you can never have too much experience. Apply everything you have learned in this chapter to code the following diagnostic statements. Use the OGCR and instructional notes in the Tabular List to help determine how many codes are required.

Instructions: Read the diagnostic statement, then use the Index and Tabular List to assign and sequence ICD-10-CM (CM) diagnosis codes. Write the code(s) on the line provided.

1. Transient neonatal myasthenia gravis: CM Code(s) ______
2. Subdural hematoma due to birth injury: CM Code(s) ______
3. Newborn small for dates, 1,150 grams: CM Code(s) ______
4. Newborn melena: CM Code(s) ______
5. Congenital pneumonia due to pseudomonas: CM Code(s) ______
6. Postterm newborn, 43 weeks gestation: CM Code(s) ______
7. Overfeeding of newborn: CM Code(s) ______
8. Neonatal jaundice due to polycythemia: CM Code(s) ______
9. Neonatal craniotabes: CM Code(s) ______
10. Atelectasis of newborn: CM Code(s) ______
11. Transitory ileus of newborn: CM Code(s) ______
12. Neonatal aspiration of blood: CM Code(s) ______
13. Phrenic nerve paralysis due to birth injury: CM Code(s) ______
14. Newborn infant of a diabetic mother: CM Code(s) ______
15. Preterm newborn, 28 completed weeks: CM Code(s) ______
16. Noninfective neonatal diarrhea: CM Code(s) ______
17. Newborn affected by mother's type 1 diabetes during pregnancy: CM Code(s) ______
18. Neonatal goiter: CM Code(s) ______
19. Anemia of prematurity: CM Code(s) ______
20. Congenital hydrocele: CM Code(s) ______
21. Rh isoimmunization of newborn: CM Code(s) ______
22. Neonatal coma: CM Code(s) ______
23. Cardiac arrest of newborn: CM Code(s) ______
24. Massive umbilical hemorrhage of newborn: CM Code(s) ______
25. Transitory neonatal neutropenia: CM Code(s) ______

CODER'S TOOLBOX

The following resources are a starting point for learning more about conditions originating in the perinatal period. The > symbol indicates a menu selection within the website in order to navigate to a specific page.

American Academy of Pediatrics **http://www.aap.org/**

Brachial Plexus Palsy Foundation (BPPF) **http://www.brachialplexuspalsyfoundation.org/**

Cancer Epidemiology, Biomarkers & Prevention (CEBP), October 2011, High Birthweight and Cancer: Evidence and Implications **http://cebp.aacrjournals.org/content/15/1/1.full**

Community Connect to Research > High-Quality Health Information > Health Topics > Congenital and Neonatal Conditions **http://www.connecttoresearch.org/topics/1300005**

March of Dimes **http://www.marchofdimes.com/**

Maternal and Child Health > Child Health USA **http://mchb.hrsa.gov/chusa11**
http://www.pennmedicine.org/obgyn/health_info/neo/conditions.html

Penn Medicine (University of Pennsylvania Health System) > Departments and Services > Health Information > Neonatology The United Brachial Plexus Network (UBPN) **http://www.ubpn.org/**

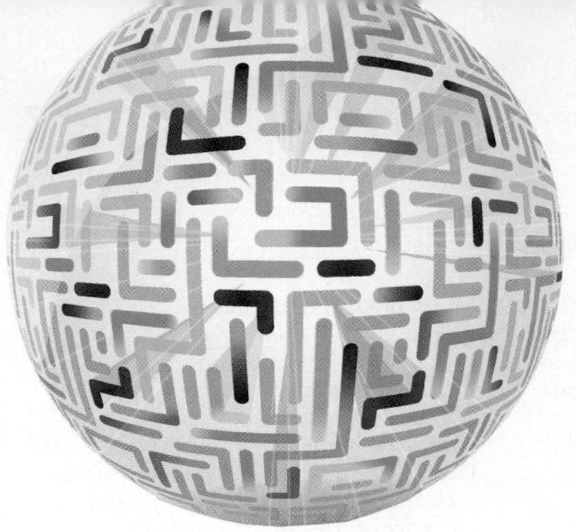

25

Congenital Malformations, Deformations, and Chromosomal Abnormalities (Q00-Q99)

Learning Objectives

After completing this chapter, you should have the skills to:

- Spell and define the key words, medical terms, and abbreviations related to congenital malformations, deformations, and chromosomal abnormalities.
- Discuss common congenital malformations, deformations, and chromosomal abnormalities.
- Identify the main characteristics of coding for congenital malformations, deformations, and chromosomal abnormalities.
- Abstract diagnostic information from the medical record for coding congenital malformations, deformations, and chromosomal abnormalities.
- Assign codes for congenital malformations, deformations, and chromosomal abnormalities.
- Arrange codes for congenital malformations, deformations, and chromosomal abnormalities.
- Discuss the Official Guidelines for Coding and Reporting related to congenital malformations, deformations, and chromosomal abnormalities.

Key Terms and Abbreviations

abnormal development
anomaly
arrested development
congenital abnormality
delayed development

In addition to the key terms listed here, students should know the terms defined within tables in this chapter.

Chapter Outline

ICD-10-CM codes in this chapter are from the ICD-10-CM 2014 Draft code set from the Department of Health and Human Services, Centers for Disease Control and Prevention.

INTRODUCTION

Two types of problems with a new vehicle are those due to faulty manufacturing materials and those due to poor workmanship or assemblage. Some may be correctable and some may not. Congenital conditions can be thought of in a similar way. Conditions can result from abnormal development of the embryo or physical damage to an anatomical part that developed normally.

In your tour of the congenital malformations, deformations, and chromosomal abnormalities in this chapter you will learn more about the types of congenital malformations, deformations, and chromosomal abnormalities, why they arise, and how physicians treat these conditions. Most importantly, you will practice coding for patient encounters related to congenital malformations, deformations, and chromosomal abnormalities, a skill that requires you to abstract information from the medical record, assign correct codes, and arrange (sequence) the codes in the proper order. For the sake of brevity, this text refers to congenital malformations, deformations, and chromosomal abnormalities as congenital abnormalities.

Physicians of any specialty may treat congenital conditions, based on the body system affected.

As you read this chapter, open up your medical terminology book and keep a medical dictionary handy to refresh your memory of any unfamiliar terms related to congenital abnormalities. These are your professional resources that provide the information you need at your fingertips.

CONGENITAL ABNORMALITIES REFRESHER

Congenital abnormalities are specific types of perinatal conditions. Both congenital and perinatal conditions originate during pregnancy or the first 28 days of life. Both types of conditions may be diagnosed and treated **in utero**, during the first 28 days, or at any time later in life. In common usage, the terms are frequently used interchangeably.

In ICD-10-CM, congenital abnormalities include physical malformations, deformations, and chromosomal abnormalities. Conditions that do not meet these definitions are classified as perinatal conditions. A congenital malformation or **anomaly** is a permanent abnormal shape of an organ or body region, which is due to problems of embryonic development. Malformations may be the result of **arrested development**, in which embryonic development of a structure stopped before it should have; **delayed development**, in which embryonic development of a structure started late or progressed slowly; or **abnormal development**, in which embryonic development of a structure occurred on schedule but took an uncommon physical variation in the womb. Examples of malformations are transposition of the great vessels (aorta and pulmonary artery) and spina bifida.

A deformation or deformity is a change in the size or shape of a normal structure, due to extrinsic physical forces, such as intrauterine compression. Examples of deformities are dislocation of the hip and rotational deformities.

A chromosomal abnormality is the abnormal number or structure of chromosomes. Examples are Down syndrome and Prader-Willi syndrome.

SUCCESS STEP

Although many eponyms end with a possessive, such as Alzheimer's disease, this is not the case with Down syndrome. The current terminology is Down syndrome, not Down**'s** syndrome. This does not affect your coding, but proper use of terminology demonstrates your professionalism. Also remember that only the first word of an eponym is capitalized.

As you learn about congenital abnormalities, remember to apply medical terminology skills to combine word roots, prefixes, and suffixes you already know to define new terms. Refer to ■ TABLE 25-1 (page 510) for a refresher on how to build medical terms related to congenital malformations, deformations, and chromosomal abnormalities.

CODING CAUTION

Be alert for medical terms that are spelled similarly and have different meanings.

hydrocele (*bulge of fluid*) and **hydrocephalus** (*water or fluid in the head/brain*)

polydactyly (*many fingers or toes*) and **syndactyly** (*webbed fingers or toes*)

Conditions Related to Congenital Abnormalities

Congenital abnormalities are the leading cause of infant mortality, according to the Centers for Disease Control and Prevention (CDC). Over 4,000 congenital abnormalities have been identified by physicians. According to the March of Dimes, the most common congenital abnormalities are heart defects, cleft lip or cleft palate, and Down syndrome. Certain conditions reflect multiple abnormalities that occur together. For example, tetralogy of Fallot and Shone's syndrome are each a combination of

Table 25-1 ■ **EXAMPLE OF CONSTRUCTING MEDICAL TERMS FOR CONGENITAL ABNORMALITIES**

Prefix/Suffix	Combining Form	Complete Medical Term
a/an- (*lacking*) **en-** (*within*)	**cephal/o** (*head/brain*) **hydr/o** (*water*)	**an + en + cephaly** (*lack of part of the brain*) **a + tresia** (*lack of an opening*)
micro- (*small*)		**micro + cephaly** (*small head*) **hydro + cephaly** (*water or fluid in the head/brain*)
-cele (*hernia, bulge*) **-tresia** (*opening*)		**hydro + cele** (*bulge of fluid*) **en + cephalo + cele** (*hernia in the brain*)

Table 25-2 ■ **COMMON CONGENITAL ABNORMALITIES**

Condition	Definition
Aortic coarctation	A narrowing of the aorta
Cleft lip or palate	A notch or division of the upper lip or roof of the mouth
Developmental dysplasia of the hip (DDH)	Disruption in the normal relationship between the head of the femur and the acetabulum (hip socket)
Down syndrome	A genetic condition in which a person has 47 chromosomes instead of the usual 46, also called Trisomy 21 (■ FIGURE 25-1)
Esophageal ring	An abnormal ring of tissue around the esophagus
Hydrocephalus	A buildup of fluid inside the skull
Hydronephrosis	Excessive collection of urine in the kidneys
Hypospadias	A congenital condition in which the opening of the urethra is on the underside, rather than the end, of the penile shaft, and may be located as far down as in the scrotum or perineum
Marfan syndrome	A genetic disorder of connective tissue characterized by elongated bones and ocular and circulatory defects
Meckel's diverticulum	A congenital bulge in the intestine caused by a remnant of the embryonic yolk stalk
Patent foramen ovale	An opening in the septum between the two atria of the heart
Prader-Willi syndrome	A genetic disorder due to a deletion of paternal chromosome 15 characterized by short stature, intellectual disability, muscle weakness, abnormally small hands and feet, non-functioning gonads, and uncontrolled appetite leading to extreme obesity
Rotational deformities	Abnormal position of the femur or tibia
Spina bifida	A birth defect in which the backbone and spinal canal do not close before birth
Tetralogy of Fallot	A congenital heart defect consisting of four malformations: pulmonary stenosis (obstructed outflow of blood from the right ventricle to the lungs), ventricle septal defect (VSD) (an opening between the ventricles), dextraposition or overriding aorta (blood from the aorta flowing into both the left and right ventricles), and hypertrophy (enlargement) of the right ventricle
Tongue tie	A condition in which the bottom of the tongue is attached to the floor of the mouth by a band of tissue called the lingual frenulum
Transposition of the great vessels	A congenital heart defect in which the aorta and pulmonary artery are switched, preventing pulmonary circulation
Trisomy	A genetic disorder in which a person has three copies, rather than two, of genetic material
Shone's syndrome	A set of four congenital heart defects: a supravalve mitral membrane (SVMM), parachute mitral valve, subaortic stenosis, and coarctation of the aorta

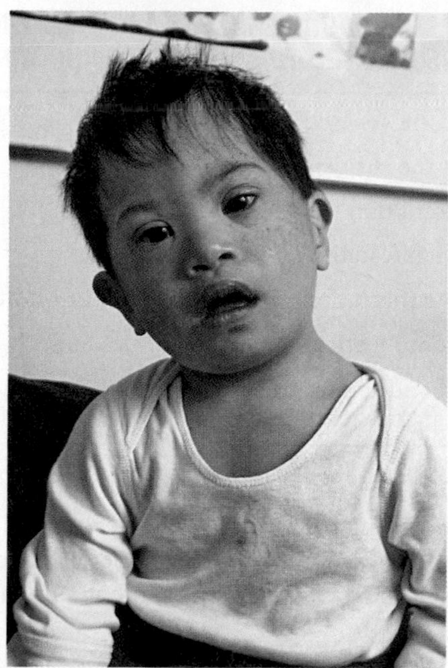

Figure 25-1 ■ A Patient with Down Syndrome. *Source: George Dodson/Pearson Education/PH College.*

four specific heart abnormalities, but the the specific abnormalities are different for each. Although certain congenital abnormalities are known to be caused by genetics, environment, or a combination of both, the cause of the vast majority is unknown. Refer to ■ TABLE 25-2 for a summary of congenital abnormalities.

This section provides a general reference to help understand the most common congenital abnormalities, but does not list everything you need to know. Use medical terminology skills discussed earlier in this chapter to learn the meaning of unfamiliar words. Remember to keep standard reference books handy in case you get stuck. Refer to the resources in the Coder's Toolbox at the end of this chapter to learn more about conditions related to congenital malformations, deformations, and chromosomal abnormalities.

Coding Practice

Refresh your knowledge of terminology related to congenital malformations, deformations, and chromosomal abnormalities. Use a medical terminology text or a website such as GlobalRph.com > Medical Terminology **http://www.globalrph.com/medterm.htm** to identify the meaning of word parts that may not be familiar.

Exercise 25.1 Congenital Abnormalities Refresher

Instructions: Use your medical terminology skills and resources to define the following conditions related to congenital malformations, deformations, and chromosomal abnormalities, then assign the default diagnosis code.

Follow these steps:

- Use slash marks "/" to break down each term into its root(s) and suffix.
- Define the meaning of the word, based on the meaning of each word part. When multiple words are listed, define the meaning of the **boldfaced** word.
- Assign the default ICD-10-CM diagnosis code (CM) for the condition using the Index and Tabular List.

Example: microgastria micro/gastr/ia Meaning: *condition of a very small stomach* CM Code: *Q40.2*

1. ichthyosis Meaning ______________ CM Code ________
2. left renal **agenesis** Meaning ______________ CM Code ________
3. frontal **encephalocele** Meaning ______________ CM Code ________
4. macrotia Meaning ______________ CM Code ________
5. vaginal **atresia** Meaning ______________ CM Code ________
6. cryptorchidism Meaning ______________ CM Code ________
7. polydactyl Meaning ______________ CM Code ________
8. **polycystic** kidney disease Meaning ______________ CM Code ________
9. **bicornuate** uterus Meaning ______________ CM Code ________
10. pseudohermaphroditism Meaning ______________ CM Code ________

CODING OVERVIEW OF CONGENITAL ABNORMALITIES

ICD-10-CM Chapter 17, Congenital Malformations, Deformations, and Chromosomal Abnormalities (Q00-Q99), contains 11 blocks or subchapters that are divided by organ system. Review the block names and code ranges listed at the beginning of Chapter 17 in the ICD-10-CM manual to become familiar with the content and organization.

This ICD-10-CM chapter compares to ICD-9-CM Chapter 14 (740-759) and appears in a different sequence within the coding manual than it did in ICD-9-CM. Numerous conditions contain more codes for greater specificity and laterality than in ICD-9-CM. Codes for cleft palate are divided by anatomic site rather than bilateral or unilateral and complete or incomplete. Codes for reduction defects of the upper and lower limbs are significantly restructured. Codes for chromosomal abnormalities have been expanded to identify the specific genetic abnormality.

This chapter includes congenital physical and chromosomal abnormalities. It does not include acquired variations of conditions that may be either congenital or acquired, which are classified in the corresponding body system chapter. It also does not include conditions originating during the birth process, which are classified in ICD-10-CM Chapter 16, Certain Conditions Originating in the Perinatal Period (P00-P96).

ICD-10-CM provides Official Guidelines for Coding and Reporting (OGCR) for congenital malformations, deformations, and chromosomal abnormalities in OGCR section I.C.17. OGCR provide discussion of sequencing codes from this chapter, multiple coding, and use of these codes throughout the patient lifespan. An instructional note at the beginning of Chapter 17 in the Tabular List states that codes from this chapter should not be used on records of mothers or unborn fetuses.

ABSTRACTING FOR CONGENITAL ABNORMALITIES

Coders must identify whether a condition is congenital and what manifestations exist. In addition, coders should follow abstracting guidelines for the body system(s) affected.

Many conditions may be either congenital or acquired. Therefore, the coder must identify the documentation regarding when the condition originated. Chromosomal abnormalities and other conditions that are, by definition, congenital, do not require explicit documentation regarding the congenital nature.

Coders should review all manifestations of the congenital condition and identify those that are integral to the condition and those that are not. When a specific code exists for a condition, coders should report only the manifestations that are related but *not integral* to the condition. When congenital conditions do not have a unique code, assign a nonspecific code and report all manifestations.

Table 25-3 ■ KEY CRITERIA FOR ABSTRACTING CONDITIONS RELATED TO CONGENITAL ABNORMALITIES

- ❑ What is the specific condition?
- ❑ What is the subtype?
- ❑ Is the condition clearly congenital?
- ❑ What manifestations are present?
- ❑ What manifestations are integral to the condition?
- ❑ What complications or comorbidities exist?
- ❑ Which condition or manifestation is the main reason for the encounter?

Age is not a factor when reporting congenital conditions. Unless a congenital defect can be repaired, congenital conditions exist throughout a patient's life and may be reported at any time.

Refer to ■ Table 25-3 for guidance on how to abstract conditions related to congenital malformations, deformations, and chromosomal abnormalities, then work through the detailed example that follows. Remember that the abstracting questions are a guide and that not every question applies to, or can be answered for, every case. Also remember to consult key criteria for abstracting specific body system conditions. For example, to code for a congenital condition in a newborn, follow the key criteria listed here, as well as key criteria for abstracting birth encounters.

Guided Example of Abstracting Congenital Abnormalities

Refer to the following example throughout this chapter to practice skills for abstracting, assigning, and sequencing codes related to congenital malformations, deformations, and chromosomal abnormalities. Geneva Deckard, CPC, is a fictitious coder who guides you through the coding process.

Date: 5/21/yy Location: Branton Medical Center

Provider: Matthew Bunker, MD

Patient: Lucia Ovalle Gender: F Age: 9 months

Reason for encounter: cyanosis, tachypnea, difficulty feeding, failure to thrive

Assessment: blood work and imaging studies reveal tetralogy of Fallot (TOF); congenital atrial septal defect (ASD) is also present and can be corrected at the same time as TOF surgery, if parents consent

Plan: corrective surgery

Follow along as Geneva Deckard, CPC, abstracts the diagnosis. Check off each step after you complete it.

➪ Geneva reads through the entire record, with special attention to the reason for the encounter and the final assessment. She refers to the Key Criteria for Abstracting Conditions Related to Congenital Abnormalities (Table 25-3)

- ❑ *What is the specific condition?* tetralogy of Fallot
- ❑ *What is the subtype?* Not applicable.
- ❑ *Is the condition clearly congenital?* Yes, the condition is congenital by definition.
- ❑ *What manifestations are present?* cyanosis, tachypnea, difficulty feeding, failure to thrive
- ❑ *What manifestations are integral to the condition?* All manifestations listed are common with TOF.
- ❑ *What complications or comorbidities exist?* congenital atrial septal defect
- ❑ *Which condition or manifestation is the main reason for the encounter?* tetralogy of Fallot

➪ At this time, Geneva does not know which of these conditions may need to be coded, nor how many codes she will end up with. She will learn about this when she moves on to assigning codes.

Coding Practice

Now it is your turn to practice abstracting diagnoses for congenital malformations, deformations, and chromosomal abnormalities. Questions guide your analysis of each scenario.

Exercise 25.2 Abstracting for Congenital Abnormalities

Instructions: Read the mini-medical-record of each patient's encounter and answer the abstracting questions. Write the answer on the line provided. Do not assign any codes.

1. Date: 5/23/yy Location: Branton Medical Center Provider: Matthew Bunker, MD

Patient: Marvin Janssen Gender: M Age: 32

Reason for admission: mitral valve replacement

Assessment: mitral valve prolapse d/t congenital Marfan's syndrome

Plan: valve replacement was successful, FU office 2 weeks

a. What is the specific condition? ______________

b. What is the subtype? ______________

c. Is the condition clearly congenital? ______________

____

d. What manifestations are present? ______________

e. What manifestations are integral to the condition? ______________

f. What complications or comorbidities exist?

____

g. Which condition or manifestation is the main reason for the encounter? ______________

2. Date: 5/23/yy Location: Branton Medical Center Provider: Ann Colyer, MD

Patient: Stanley Reilly Gender: M DOB: 4/26/yy

Reason for admission: removal of a renal cyst

Assessment: congenital renal cyst, congenital hydronephrosis

Plan: RTO 2 weeks

a. What is the specific condition? ______________

b. What is the subtype? ______________

c. Is the condition clearly congenital? ______________

____

d. What manifestations are present? ______________

____

e. What manifestations are integral to the condition?

____

f. What complications or comorbidities exist?

____

g. Which condition or manifestation is the main reason for the encounter? ______________

3. Date: 5/23/yy Location: New Life Obstetrics Provider: Kay Pinkney, MD

Patient: Crystal Muniz Gender: F Age: 16

Reason for encounter: referred by family physician for gynecological consult on amenorrhea

Assessment: ultrasound reveals missing uterus, which has not been surgically removed

(continued)

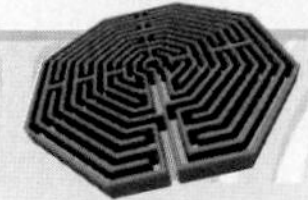

Coding Practice (continued)

3. (continued)

a. What is the specific condition? ______________

b. What is the subtype? ______________

c. Is the condition clearly congenital? ______________

____

d. What manifestations are present? ______________

e. What manifestations are integral to the condition? ______________

f. What complications or comorbidities exist?

____

g. Which condition or manifestation is the main reason for the encounter? ______________

4. Date: 5/23/yy Location: Branton Gastroenterology Provider: Stanley Garrett, MD

Patient: Hazel Brookshire Gender: F

DOB: 4/23/yy

Reason for encounter: FU on endoscopy after referral from pediatrician because infant is constantly spitting up

Assessment: congenital Schatzki esophageal ring

Plan: we attempted to dilate the ring and will evaluate for surgery if that is unsuccessful

a. What is the specific condition? ______________

b. What is the subtype? ______________

c. Is the condition clearly congenital? ______________

____

d. What manifestations are present? ______________

e. What manifestations are integral to the condition? ______________

f. What complications or comorbidities exist?

____

g. Which condition or manifestation is the main reason for the encounter? ______________

5. Date: 5/24/yy Location: Branton Medical Center Outpatient Procedure Center

Provider: Bruce Prentice, MD

Patient: Jere McClung Gender: F Age: 1 year

Reason for encounter: surgical correction of polydactyly

Assessment: accessory thumb of right hand

Plan: FU office 1 week

a. What is the specific condition? ______________

b. What is the subtype? ______________

c. Is the condition clearly congenital? ______________

____

d. What manifestations are present? ______________

e. What manifestations are integral to the condition? ______________

f. What complications or comorbidities exist?

____

g. Which condition or manifestation is the main reason for the encounter? ______________

6. Date: 5/23/yy Location: Hilltop Pediatrics

Provider: Joann Gwinn, MD

Patient: Brandi Mosier Gender: F DOB: 4/26/yy

Reason for encounter: management of Down syndrome and FU on genetic testing

Assessment: Down syndrome, nonmosaic type, hypotonia, obstructive sleep apnea d/t hypertrophy of tonsils and adenoids, ASD

Plan: FU with cardiologist and neurologist

a. What is the specific condition? ______________

b. What is the subtype? ______________

c. Is the condition clearly congenital? ______________

____

d. What manifestations are present? ______________

e. What manifestations are integral to the condition? ______________

f. What complications or comorbidities exist?

____

g. Which condition or manifestation is the main reason for the encounter? ______________

7. Date of discharge: 5/24/yy Location: Branton Medical Center Provider: Jeremy Abernethy, MD

Patient: Mark Chevalier Gender: M DOB: 5/18/yy

Birth Weight: 2169g EGA: 38+4 Type: NSVD

POB: BMC

Assessment: SGA, the blood test FISH (fluorescent in situ hybridization) is positive for Prader-Willi syndrome. Hypotonia and abnormally small testes which cannot be detected within the scrotal sac, secondary to Prader-Willi.

Plan: follow feeding plan, evaluate for supplemental growth hormone in 1 month

a. What is the specific condition? ______________

b. What is the subtype? ______________

c. Is the condition clearly congenital? ______________

____

d. What manifestations are present? ______________

____

e. What manifestations are integral to the condition?

____

f. What complications or comorbidities exist?

____

g. Which condition or manifestation is the main reason for the encounter? ______________

8. Date: 5/24/yy Location: Hilltop Pediatrics

Provider: Joann Gwinn, MD

Patient: Frank Jorge Gender: M DOB: 4/24/yy

Reason for encounter: routine examination

Assessment: infant was born with microgastria and now has failure to thrive

Plan: refer to nutritionist for feeding guidance, WU for vitamin, mineral, and hormone deficiencies

a. What is the specific condition? ______________

b. What is the subtype? ______________

(continued)

8. (continued)

c. Is the condition clearly congenital? ______________

____

d. What manifestations are present? ______________

e. What manifestations are integral to the condition? ______________

f. What complications or comorbidities exist?

____

g. Which condition or manifestation is the main reason for the encounter? ______________

9. Date of discharge: 5/24/yy Location: Valley Hospital Provider: Joann Gwinn, MD

Patient: Dennis Daughtry Gender: M

DOB: 5/14/yy

Birth Weight: 3216g EGA: 38+2 Type: C/S

POB: VH

Assessment: Meckel's diverticulum and congenital pyloric stenosis with vomiting

Plan: Evaluate effectiveness of pyloric balloon dilation that was performed. If unsuccessful, consider surgery to correct stenosis. Surgery is not needed for Meckel's unless bleeding occurs.

a. What is the specific condition? ______________

b. What is the subtype? ______________

c. Is the condition clearly congenital? ______________

____

d. What manifestations are present? ______________

e. What manifestations are integral to the condition?

____

f. What complications or comorbidities exist?

____

g. Which condition or manifestation is the main reason for the encounter? ______________

(continued)

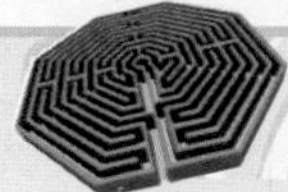

Coding Practice (continued)

10. Date: 5/24/yy Location: City Center Cardiology

Provider: Matthew Bunker, MD

Patient: Eva Abel Gender: F Age: 3 months

Reason for encounter: referred by pediatrician due to heart murmur

Assessment: patent foramen ovale and congenital VSD

Plan: treat VSD medically, postpone surgery if symptoms increase, no treatment needed for patent foramen ovale at this time, RTO 3 months

a. What is the specific condition? ______________

(continued)

10. (continued)

b. What is the subtype? ______________

c. Is the condition clearly congenital? ______________

d. What manifestations are present? ______________

e. What manifestations are integral to the condition? ______________

f. What complications or comorbidities exist? ______________

g. Which condition or manifestation is the main reason for the encounter? ______________

ASSIGNING CODES FOR CONGENITAL ABNORMALITIES

ICD-10-CM distinguishes between conditions that can be either congenital in origin or acquired. For some conditions, the default code in the Index is for congenital origin, with the acquired version appearing as a subterm. For other conditions, the default code is for the acquired version, with the congenital origin appearing as a subterm. Coders can determine which variation is identified by the default code in the Index by reading the nonessential modifiers that appear in parentheses after the Main Term. When either of these terms, congenital or acquired, appears as a nonessential modifier, the other term usually appears as a subterm. Refer to ■ FIGURE 25-2 for the Main Term **Deformity** to compare the difference between the subterm **bone**, for which the default is **(acquired)**, and the subterm **brain**, for which the default code is **(congenital)**. Notice that the code for the congenital variation is from ICD-10-CM Chapter 17 and begins with Q, while the code for the acquired version does not begin with Q, but rather, the letter from the corresponding body system chapter.

SUCCESS STEP

When the documentation does not specify either congenital or acquired, assign the default code. Remember that the nonessential modifier in parentheses does *not* have to be present in the documentation in order to assign the code.

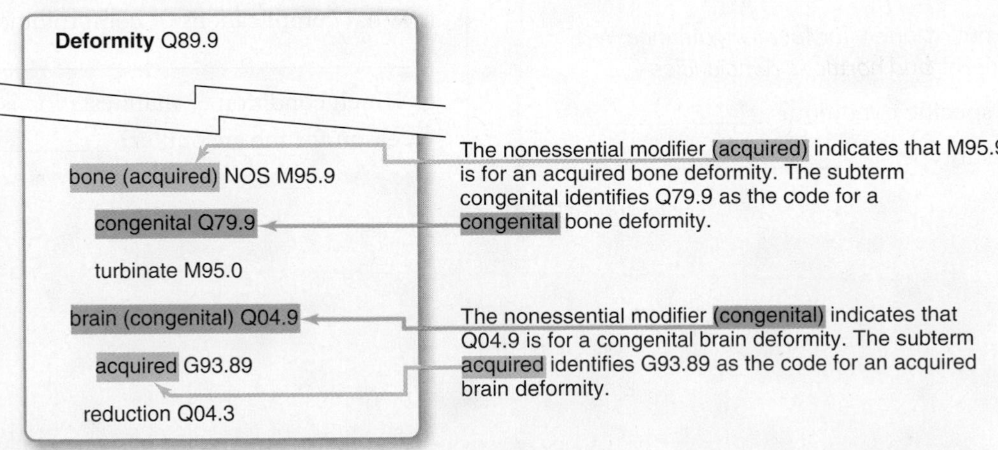

Figure 25-2 ■ Index Entry Showing Acquired and Congential as Nonessential Modifiers and Subterms

Some conditions are congenital by definition and do not have an acquired form. When this is the case, the Index does not provide an alternative subterm for acquired and all code options begin with Q (■ FIGURE 25-3). Subterms describe variations of the congenital condition.

When a congenital abnormality has been corrected, assign a personal history code to identify the history of the condition (OGCR I.C.17.). Search under the Main Term **History**, subterm **personal**, and the second-level subterm for the name of the condition. When the specific condition does not appear as a subterm, search under the Main Term **History**, subterm **personal**, the second-level subterm **congenital malformation**, and a third-level subterm for the body system involved (■ FIGURE 25-4).

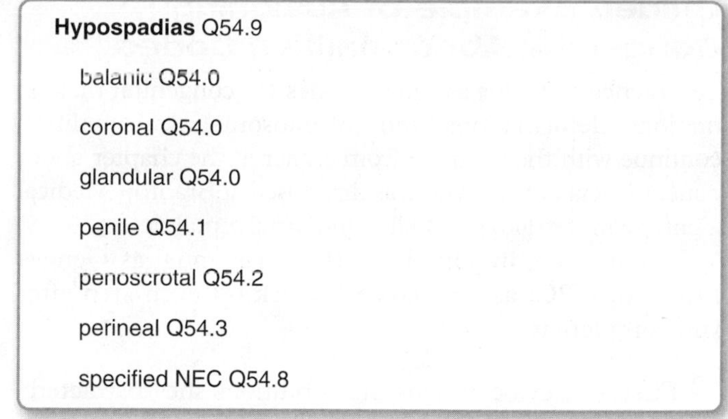

Hypospadias Q54.9
- balanic Q54.0
- coronal Q54.0
- glandular Q54.0
- penile Q54.1
- penoscrotal Q54.2
- perineal Q54.3
- specified NEC Q54.8

Figure 25-3 ■ Index Main Term for a Condition That Is Only Congenital in Origin

History

- personal
  - cleft lip (corrected) Z87.730
  - cleft palate (corrected) Z87.730
  - collapsed vertebra (healed) Z87.311
    - due to osteoporosis Z87.310
  - combat and operational stress reaction Z86.51
  - congenital malformation (corrected) Z87.798
    - circulatory system (corrected) Z87.74
    - digestive system (corrected) NEC Z87.738
    - ear (corrected) Z87.720
    - eye (corrected) Z87.721
    - face and neck (corrected) Z87.790
    - genitourinary system (corrected) NEC Z87.718
    - heart (corrected) Z87.74
    - integument (corrected) Z87.76
    - limb(s) (corrected) Z87.76
    - musculoskeletal system (corrected) Z87.76
    - neck (corrected) Z87.790
    - nervous system (corrected) NEC Z87.728
    - respiratory system (corrected) Z87.75
    - sense organs (corrected) NEC Z87.728
    - specified NEC Z87.798

Subterms for specific congenital conditions

Subterms for congenital malformation by body system

Figure 25-4 ■ Index Entry for Personal History of Congenital Conditions

Guided Example of Assigning Congenital Abnormalities Codes

To practice skills for assigning codes for congenital malformations, deformations, and chromosomal abnormalities, continue with the example from earlier in the chapter about patient Lucia Ovalle, who was diagnosed at Branton Medical Center with tetralogy of Fallot and atrial septal defect.

Follow along in your ICD-10-CM manual as Geneva Deckard, CPC, assigns codes. Check off each step after you complete it.

⇨ First, Geneva confirms the conditions she abstracted:

- ❑ *tetralogy of Fallot*
- ❑ *congenital atrial septal defect*

⇨ Geneva searches the Index for the Main Term **Tetralogy**.

- ❑ She locates the entry **Tetralogy of Fallot Q21.3**.
- ❑ There are no subterms.

⇨ Geneva verifies code **Q21.3** in the Tabular List.

- ❑ She reads the code title for **Q21.3, Tetralogy of Fallot**, and confirms that this accurately describes the diagnosis.

⇨ Geneva checks for instructional notes in the Tabular List.

- ❑ She cross-references the beginning of category **Q21** and reads the **Excludes1** instructional note that directs her to *not* use this code if the cardiac septal defect is *acquired*.
- ❑ She determines that this note does not apply because her patient's condition is congenital.
- ❑ She cross-references the beginning of the block **Q20-Q28** and verifies that there are no instructional notes.
- ❑ She cross-references the beginning of **Chapter 17 (Q00-Q99)** and reviews the instructional notes. She determines that the **NOTE:** does not apply to this case because the patient is not a mother or a fetus. She determines that the **Excludes1** note does not apply because the condition is not an inborn error of metabolism.

⇨ Next, Geneva works on the code for *congenital atrial septal defect*.

⇨ Geneva searches the Index for the Main Term **Defect**.

- ❑ She locates the subterm **septal (heart) NOS**.
- ❑ She reads the subterms and notices that there is not a subterm for congenital. However, there is a separate subterm for **acquired**, which she knows she does *not* want.
- ❑ She locates the second-level subterm **atrial Q21.1** and notices that it is a Q code from ICD-10-CM Chapter 17 on congenital abnormalities.
- ❑ The third-level subterms under **atrial** relate to myocardial infarction, which does not apply to this patient.

⇨ Geneva verifies the code **Q21.1** in the Tabular List.

- ❑ She reads the code title for **Q21.1, Atrial septal defect**, and confirms that this accurately describes the diagnosis.

⇨ Geneva checks for instructional notes in the Tabular List.

- ❑ She notices that this code is in the same category that code **Q21.3, Tetralogy of Fallot**, was.
- ❑ She believes that she remembers what the instructional notes stated for the category, block, and chapter, but does a quick double check to be certain.

⇨ Geneva reviews the codes she has assigned for this case.

- ❑ **Q21.1, Atrial septal defect**
- ❑ **Q21.3, Tetralogy of Fallot**

⇨ Next, Geneva must determine how to sequence the codes.

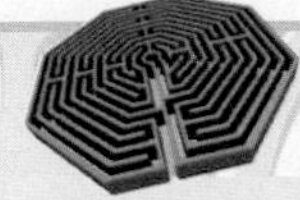

Coding Practice

Now it is your turn to practice assigning codes for congenital malformations, deformations, and chromosomal abnormalities.

Exercise 25.3 Assigning Codes for Congenital Abnormalities

Instructions: Read the mini-medical-record of each patient's encounter, review the information abstracted in Exercise 25.2, and assign ICD-10-CM diagnosis codes (CM) using the Index and Tabular List. Write the code(s) on the line provided.

1. Date: 5/23/yy Location: Branton Medical Center Provider: Matthew Bunker, MD

Patient: Marvin Janssen Gender: M Age: 32

Reason for admission: mitral valve replacement

Assessment: mitral valve prolapse d/t congenital Marfan's syndrome

Plan: valve replacement was successful, FU office 2 weeks

1 CM Code ___________

2. Date: 5/23/yy Location: Branton Medical Center Provider: Ann Colyer, MD
Patient: Stanley Reilly Gender: M DOB: 4/26/yy
Reason for admission: removal of a renal cyst
Assessment: congenital renal cyst, congenital hydronephrosis
Plan: RTO 2 weeks
2 CM Codes __________ __________

3. Date: 5/23/yy Location: New Life Obstetrics
Provider: Kay Pinkney, MD
Patient: Crystal Muniz Gender: F Age: 16
Reason for encounter: referred by family physician for gynecological consult on amenorrhea
Assessment: ultrasound reveals missing uterus, which has not been surgically removed
1 CM Code __________

4. Date: 5/23/yy Location: Branton Gastroenterology Provider: Stanley Garrett, MD
Patient: Hazel Brookshire Gender: F
DOB: 4/23/yy
Reason for encounter: FU on endoscopy after referral from pediatrician because infant is constantly spitting up
Assessment: congenital Schatzki esophageal ring
Plan: we attempted to dilate the ring and will evaluate for surgery if that is unsuccessful
1 CM Code __________

5. Date: 5/24/yy Location: Branton Medical Center Outpatient Procedure Center
Provider: Bruce Prentice, MD
Patient: Jere McClung Gender: F Age: 1 year
Reason for encounter: surgical correction of polydactyly
Assessment: accessory thumb of right hand successfully removed
Plan: FU office 1 week
1 CM Code __________

ARRANGING CODES FOR CONGENITAL ABNORMALITIES

Codes for congenital abnormalities may be either a principal/first-listed diagnosis or a secondary diagnosis, based on the circumstances of the encounter and the definition of principal diagnosis in OGCR I.C.II (OGCR I.C.17.). When a patient has multiple congenital abnormalities, which is not unusual, sequence the codes based on the circumstances of the encounter. Although this chapter does not have many instructional notes in the Tabular List, remember to always look for them and follow their direction for multiple coding and sequencing.

When coding for Down syndrome (**Q90.-**), an instructional note in the Tabular List states **Use additional code(s) to identify any associated physical conditions and the degree of intellectual disabilities (F70-F79)** (■ FIGURE 25-5).

Patient who has moderate mental retardation is seen for nonmosaicism Down syndrome. Patient also has associated hypothyroidism and celiac disease.

(1) **Q90.0 Trisomy 21, nonmosaicism (meiotic nondisjunction)**

(2) **F71 Moderate intellectual disabilities**

(3) **E03.9 Hypothyroidism, unspecified**

(4) **K90.0 Celiac disease**

Figure 25-5 ■ Example of Arranging Codes for Down Syndrome

SUCCESS STEP

When congenital abnormalities are diagnosed as part of the birth episode, assign a code from category **Z38.**- to describe the birth status of the infant. Always sequence the **Z38** code first, followed by codes for congenital or any other conditions.

SUCCESS STEP

Non-mosaic Down syndrome occurs when there is an extra copy of chromosome 21 in every cell of the body. It accounts for the majority of Down cases.

Guided Example of Arranging Congenital Abnormalities Codes

To practice skills for sequencing codes for congenital malformations, deformations, and chromosomal abnormalities, continue with the example from earlier in the chapter about patient Lucia Ovalle, who was diagnosed at Branton Medical Center with tetralogy of Fallot and atrial septal defect.

Follow along in your ICD-10-CM manual as Geneva Deckard, CPC, sequences the codes. Check off each step after you complete it.

⇨ First, Geneva confirms the codes she assigned:

❑ **Q21.1, Atrial septal defect**

❑ **Q21.3, Tetralogy of Fallot**

⇨ Geneva reviews the medical record to determine which code is the principal diagnosis.

❑ The workup and studies found both conditions, and TOF is the more serious condition because it consists of four malformations. ASD is secondary to TOF.

⇨ Geneva finalizes the codes and sequencing for this case:

(1) **Q21.3, Tetralogy of Fallot**

(2) **Q21.1, Atrial septal defect**

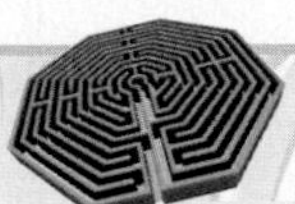

Coding Practice

Now it is your turn to practice sequencing codes for congenital malformations, deformations, and chromosomal abnormalities. Refer to the ***Tip*** at the end of the mini-medical-record if you need a little extra help.

Exercise 25.4 Arranging Codes for Congenital Abnormalities

Instructions: Read the mini-medical-record of each patient's encounter, review the information abstracted in Exercise 25.2, assign ICD-10-CM diagnosis codes (CM) using the Index and Tabular List, and sequence them correctly.

1. Date: 5/23/yy Location: Hilltop Pediatrics

Provider: Joann Gwinn, MD

Patient: Brandi Mosier Gender: F DOB: 4/26/yy

Reason for encounter: management of Down syndrome and FU on genetic testing

Assessment: Down syndrome, nonmosaic type, hypotonia, obstructive sleep apnea due to hypertrophy of tonsils and adenoids, ASD

Plan: FU with cardiologist and neurologist

(continued)

1. (continued)

***Tip*:** Nonmosaicism is also called meiotic nondisjunction. Be careful to read any Excludes1 notes you encounter.

3 CM Codes ________ ________ ________

2. Date of discharge: 5/24/yy Location: Branton Medical Center Provider: Jeremy Abernethy, MD

Patient: Mark Chevalier Gender: M

DOB: 5/18/yy

Birth Weight: 2169g EGA: 38+4

Type: NSVD POB: BMC

Assessment: SGA, the blood test FISH (fluorescent in situ hybridization) is positive for Prader-Willi syndrome. Hypotonia and abnormally small testes (**hypoplasia**) which cannot be detected within the scrotal sac, secondary to Prader-Willi

4 CM Codes ________ ________ ________ ________

3. Date: 5/24/yy Location: Hilltop Pediatrics

Provider: Joann Gwinn, MD

Patient: Frank Jorge Gender: M DOB: 4/24/yy

Reason for encounter: routine examination

Assessment: infant was born with microgastria and now has failure to thrive

Plan: refer to nutritionist for feeding guidance, WU for vitamin, mineral, and hormone deficiencies

Tip: Be sure to check the age of the patient.

3 CM Codes __________ __________ __________

4. Date of discharge: 5/24/yy Location: Valley Hospital Provider: Joann Gwinn, MD

Patient: Dennis Daughtry Gender: M

DOB: 5/14/yy

Birth Weight: 3216g EGA: 38+2

Type: C/S POB: VH

(continued)

4. (continued)

Assessment: Meckel's diverticulum and congenital pyloric stenosis with vomiting

Plan: Evaluate effectiveness of pyloric balloon dilation that was performed. If unsuccessful, consider surgery to correct stenosis. Surgery is not needed for Meckel's unless bleeding occurs.

3 CM Codes __________ __________ __________

5. Date: 5/24/yy Location: City Center Cardiology

Provider: Matthew Bunker, MD

Patient: Eva Abel Gender: F Age: 3 months

Reason for encounter: referred by pediatrician due to heart murmur

Assessment: patent foramen ovale and congenital VSD

Plan: treat VSD medically, postpone surgery if symptoms increase, no treatment needed for patent foramen ovale at this time, RTO 3 months

2 CM Codes __________ __________

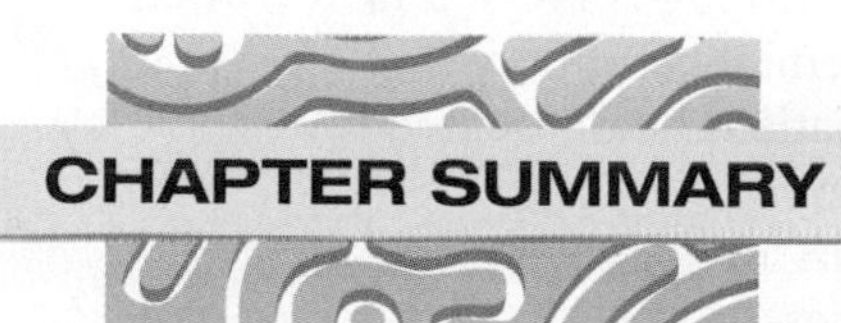

CHAPTER SUMMARY

In this chapter you learned that:

- Congenital abnormalities are specific types of perinatal conditions, which include physical malformations, deformations, and chromosomal abnormalities.
- ICD-10-CM Chapter 17, Congenital Malformations, Deformations, and Chromosomal Abnormalities (Q00-Q99), contains 11 blocks or subchapters that are divided by organ system.
- Coders must identify whether a condition is congenital and what manifestations exist.
- Coders can determine whether a condition identified by the default code in the Index is the congenital variation or the acquired variation by reading the nonessential modifiers that appear in parentheses after the Main Term.
- Codes for congenital abnormalities may be either a principal/first-listed diagnosis or a secondary diagnosis, based on the circumstances of the encounter.
- ICD-10-CM provides Official Guidelines for Coding and Reporting (OGCR) in OGCR section I.C.17., which discuss sequencing codes from this chapter, multiple coding, and use of these codes throughout the patient lifespan.

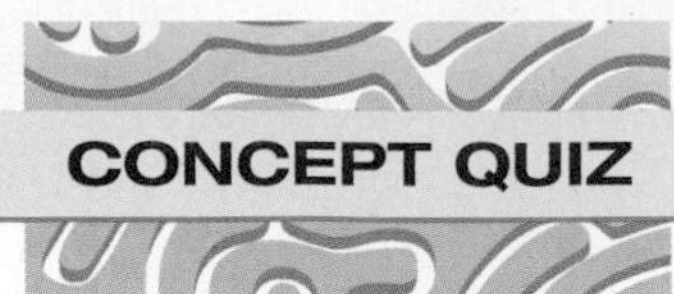

CONCEPT QUIZ

Take a moment to look back at your trip through congenital malformations, deformations, and chromosomal abnormalities and solidify your skills. This is your opportunity to pull together everything you have learned.

Completion

Instructions: Write the term that answers each question based on the information you learned in this chapter. Choose from the list below. Some choices may be used more than once and some choices may not be used at all. Refer to the discussion in this chapter and the Glossary at the end of this book if you need a little extra help.

adults	Marfan syndrome
aortic coarctation	mothers
chromosomal abnormality	newborns
cleft palate	patent foramen ovale
deformity	Prader-Willi syndrome
Down syndrome	spina bifida
hydrocephalus	transposition of the great vessels
hydronephrosis	Turner syndrome
hypospadias	
malformation	

1. Down syndrome is an example of a ____________________.
2. Dislocation of the hip is an example of a ____________________.
3. ____________________ is a notch or division of the roof of the mouth.
4. ____________________ is the excessive collection of urine in the kidneys.
5. ____________________ is a congenital heart defect in which the aorta and pulmonary artery are switched, preventing pulmonary circulation.
6. An instructional note at the beginning of Chapter 17 in the Tabular List states that codes from this chapter should not be used on records of ____________________.
7. ____________________ is a congenital condition in which the opening of the urethra is on the underside of the penile shaft.
8. ____________________ is a genetic disorder of connective tissue characterized by elongated bones and ocular and circulatory defects.
9. ____________________ is a genetic condition in which a person has 47 chromosomes instead of the usual 46.
10. ____________________ is a chromosomal defect in females in which they are missing all or part of one X chromosome.

Multiple Choice

Instructions: Circle the letter of the best answer to each question based on the information you learned in this chapter. Refer to the discussion in this chapter and the Glossary at the end of this book if you need a little extra help.

1. Which condition is NOT part of tetralogy of Fallot?
   A. Pulmonary stenosis
   B. Atrial septal defect
   C. Overriding aorta
   D. Hypertrophy of the right ventricle
2. Prader-Willi syndrome is characterized by all of the following EXCEPT
   A. circulatory defects.
   B. short stature.
   C. muscle weakness.
   D. non-functioning gonads.
3. Chapter 17 (Q00-Q99) classifies
   A. acquired conditions.
   B. perinatal conditions.
   C. chromosomal abnormalities.
   D. conditions of unborn fetuses.
4. Which of the following is NOT a factor when reporting congenital conditions?
   A. Age of the patient being treated
   B. Manifestations
   C. Congenital nature of condition
   D. Comorbidities
5. Which of the following is NOT a common manifestation of tetralogy of Fallot?
   A. Blue skin
   B. Rapid breathing
   C. Rapid heart rate
   D. Difficulty feeding
6. The correct code for a congenital bone deformity is
   A. M95.9.
   B. Q79.9.
   C. Q04.9.
   D. M95.0.

7. When the documentation does not specify either congenital or acquired, what should the coder do?
   A. Assign a code for congenital.
   B. Assign a code for acquired.
   C. Assign a code for NOS.
   D. Assign the default code.
8. When a congenital abnormality has been corrected, what code should you assign?
   A. Continue to code the congenital condition.
   B. Assign a code for personal history of the condition.
   C. Assign the default code.
   D. Do not assign any code.
9. When congenital abnormalities are diagnosed as part of the birth episode, the principal diagnosis should be
   A. determined according to the circumstances of admission.
   B. the most serious congenital condition.
   C. any birth trauma.
   D. the birth status of the infant.
10. A patient has an intellectual disability, Down syndrome, hypothyroidism, and celiac disease. What is the principal diagnosis?
   A. Intellectual disability
   B. Down syndrome
   C. Hypothyroidism
   D. Celiac disease

CODING CHALLENGE

Now it is your turn to demonstrate coding all aspects of congenital malformations, deformations, and chromosomal abnormalities. Refer back to the examples and discussion in this chapter when you need a little extra help. Use your medical dictionary and anatomy references when needed.

Instructions: Read the mini-medical-record of each patient's encounter, then abstract, assign, and sequence ICD-10-CM diagnosis codes (CM) using the Index and Tabular List. Write the code(s) on the line provided.

1. Date of discharge: 5/29/yy Location: Branton Medical Center Provider: Joann Gwinn, MD

Patient: Adam Haddad Gender: M DOB: 5/14/yy

Birth Weight: 3421g EGA: 39+0 Type: NSVD

POB: BMC

Assessment: unilateral cleft lip on left side, with cleft palate, hard

Plan: Detailed review of estimated repair protocol with parents. Visiting nurse to supervise feeding for 2 days. RTO 3 days.

2 CM Codes __________ __________

2. Date: 5/29/yy Location: Branton Medical Center Provider: Cynthia Hiatt, MD

Patient: Amy Schick Gender: F Age: 50

Reason for encounter: patient was attempting to adjust her office chair when the mechanism gave and caught and crushed her finger

Assessment: finger crush injury of right hand, congenital deficiency of the development of hands and fingers, bilaterally, complicates the repair

Plan: Arm and hand loosely wrapped in splint, elevate hand above elbow. RTO in one day, schedule reconstruction after swelling has abated.

Tip: There is not a specific external cause code for this accident. Code as exposure to inanimate mechanical forces.

4 CM Codes __________ __________ __________ __________

(*continued*)

(continued from page 523)

3. Date: 5/29/yy Location: Branton Medical Center Provider: Matthew Bunker, MD

Patient: Kelli Burdette Gender: F Age: 2

Reason for encounter: reconstructive heart surgery

Assessment: congenital Shone's syndrome with aortic stenosis, subaortic stenosis, aortic coarctation, bicuspid aortic valve

Plan: FU in office 3 days

4 CM Codes __________ __________ __________ __________

4. Date of encounter: 5/29/yy Location: Branton Medical Center Provider: Lorene Garman, MD

Patient: Roger Ranson Gender: M

DOB: 5/28/yy

Birth Weight: 2421g EGA: 36+0 Type: c/s

POB: BMC

Reason for encounter: spina bifida suspected at second trimester screening and confirmed by ultrasound and at birth

Assessment: spina bifida of the thoracic region

Plan: surgical repair recommended

***Tip*:** **This is an inpatient consultation with the pediatric neurologist. When coding for the physician, do not report the birth status of the infant, which is reported only on the inpatient record.**

1 CM Code __________

5. Date: 5/29/yy Location: Neurology Associates Provider: Lorene Garman, MD

Patient: Edward Blythe Gender: M Age: 2

Reason for encounter: Referral from neurologist

Assessment: lingual frenum extending toward the tip of tongue, which is fused to mouth floor and affects speech

Plan: refer for speech therapy

1 CM Code __________

6. Date: 5/29/yy Location: Branton Gastroenterology Provider: Stanley Garrett, MD

Patient: Wayne Brewer Gender: M Age: 5

Reason for encounter: referred by pediatrician for dysphagia

Assessment: congenital esophageal web with esophageal spasm and reflux esophagitis

Plan: schedule balloon dilatation and electrocauterization

3 CM Codes __________ __________ __________

7. Date: 5/29/yy Location: Branton Professional Group Provider: Brent Eberhart, MD

Patient: Marcus Fish Gender: M Age: 1 year

Reason for encounter: preoperative exam for cryptorchism repair tomorrow

Assessment: cleared for surgery, bilateral perineal cryptorchism

Plan: surgery tomorrow at 11:00 am

***Tip*:** **Assign a Z code for the preoperative exam.**

2 CM Codes __________ __________

8. Date: 5/29/yy Location: Northwest Orthopedics Provider: Bruce Prentice, MD

Patient: Andre Vasques Gender: M

Age: 1 month

Reason for encounter: fitting of knee braces, bilateral

Assessment: congenital genu recurvatum

Plan: instruct parents on daily passive physical therapy, schedule pt treatments x 12 on weekly basis

***Tip*:** **Assign a Z code for the fitting of the braces. Genu recurvatum is a minor backward curving of knee joints causing bowed legs.**

2 CM Codes __________ __________

9. Date of discharge: 5/29/yy Location: Branton Medical Center Provider: Joann Gwinn, MD

Patient: Carlos Moll Gender: M DOB: 5/28/yy

Birth Weight: 3011g EGA: 38+0 Type: NSVD

POB: BMC

Assessment: penoscrotal hypospadias

Plan: we will keep an eye on the hypospadias to see if treatment is necessary or if it will correct independently, FU in office 2 days for jaundice check

2 CM Codes ___________ ___________

10. Date: 5/29/yy Location: Branton Medical Center Provider: Maria Buena, MD

Patient: Shawn Pfeifer Gender: F DOB: 5/20/yy

Birth Weight: 3011g EGA: 38+0 Type: C/S

POB: BMC

Reason for encounter: open heart surgery

Assessment: transposition of great vessels

Plan: will follow in hospital until d/c

Tip: This is an inpatient procedure by the neonatal cardiothoracic surgeon. When coding for the physician, do not report the birth status of the infant, which is reported only on the inpatient record.

1 CM Code ___________

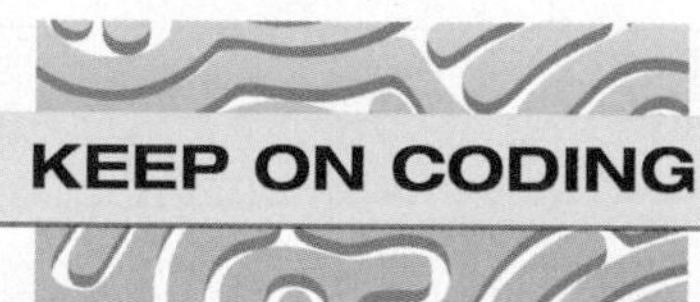

KEEP ON CODING

As a coder, you can never have too much experience. Apply everything you have learned in this chapter to code the following diagnostic statements. Use the OGCR and instructional notes in the Tabular List to help determine how many codes are required.

Instructions: Read the diagnostic statement, then use the Index and Tabular List to assign and sequence ICD-10-CM (CM) diagnosis codes. Write the code(s) on the line provided.

1. Congenital glaucoma: CM Code(s) ___________
2. Accessory ovary: CM Code(s) ___________
3. Karyotype 45, X: CM Code(s) ___________
4. Schwannomatosis: CM Code(s) ___________
5. Lobster-claw, left hand: CM Code(s) ___________
6. Congenital clawfoot: CM Code(s) ___________
7. Congenital cyst of the pancreas: CM Code(s) ___________
8. Anomaly of the aqueduct of Sylvius: CM Code(s) ___________
9. Ectopic kidney: CM Code(s) ___________
10. Supernumerary nipple: CM Code(s) ___________
11. Laryngocele: CM Code(s) ___________
12. Cleft lip, median: CM Code(s) ___________
13. Low-set ears: CM Code(s) ___________

14. Anencephaly: CM Code(s) ____________

15. Arnold-Chiari syndrome with hydrocephalus: CM Code(s) ____________

16. Plagiocephaly: CM Code(s) ____________

17. Marfan's syndrome: CM Code(s) ____________

18. Blue sclera: CM Code(s) ____________

19. Ebstein's anomaly: CM Code(s) ____________

20. Atresia of the aorta: CM Code(s) ____________

21. Short rib syndrome: CM Code(s) ____________

22. Congenital spondylolysis: CM Code(s) ____________

23. Strawberry nevus: CM Code(s) ____________

24. Epidermolysis bullosa letalis: CM Code(s) ____________

25. Congenital hiatal hernia: CM Code(s) ____________

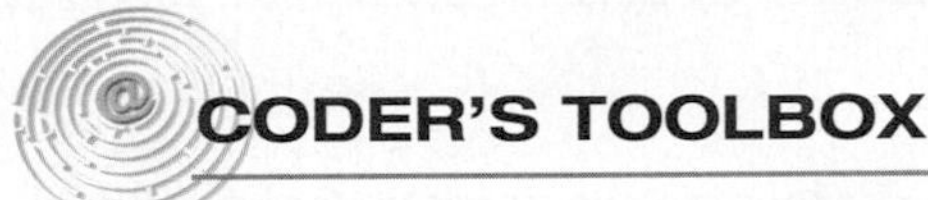

CODER'S TOOLBOX

The following resources are a starting point for learning more about congenital malformations, deformations, and chromosomal abnormalities. In addition to these sites which specifically discuss congenital conditions, refer to general resources for the body system involved. The > symbol indicates a menu selection within the website in order to navigate to a specific page.

American Heart Association > Conditions > Congenital Defects Children & Adults **http://www.heart.org/HEARTORG/Conditions/CongenitalHeartDefects/Congenital-Heart-Defects_UCM_001090_SubHomePage.jsp**

eOrthopod > Children's > Patient Guides > Rotational deformities in children **http://www.eorthopod.com/content/rotational-deformities-in-children**

March of Dimes **http://www.marchofdimes.com/**

National Down Syndrome Society **http://www.ndss.org/**

The Fetal Care Center > Fetal Conditions **http://www.fetalcare.org/fetal-conditions**

SECTION THREE

Inpatient Procedure Coding

Section Three: Inpatient Procedure Coding guides you through the steps of hospital procedure coding for each type of procedure. You will learn how to apply the three skills of an "Ace" coder—abstract, assign, and arrange—for a broad variety of patient encounters.

PROFESSIONAL PROFILE
MEET...

Karen Weiss, RHIA, Lead Coder
Avera Queen of Peace Hospital and Health Services

I have been in coding for over 30 years. When I started, healthcare was just rolling out ICD-9-CM. Now, here we are again, rolling out ICD-10-CM/PCS. Hopefully the industry will be able to use what it learned when implementing ICD-9-CM to create a more successful transition to ICD-10-CM/PCS.

My education includes a B.S. in health information administration, and my first coding position began after a one-month management internship with Marion Health Center in Sioux City, Iowa. After learning all of the basic processes and work flow in the department, I was educated in the management of those processes and other departmental responsibilities. Upon receiving my degree, I accepted a coding and abstracting position with Marion Health Center while my husband finished his course studies. Six months later, I accepted a position as Medical Record (Health Information) Department Director at a 120-bed acute care hospital.

In my current position as a Lead Coder, I am responsible for staffing, work flow analysis, auditing, and education. I also assist with inpatient and emergency department coding. I enjoy the variety in coding, because no two patients are alike. I feel like I am helping the patient by being thorough in recording their health history; helping the physician by meeting documentation standards; and helping the hospital by obtaining the maximum accurate reimbursement. The challenges are staying abreast of the multitude of changes in the healthcare industry, educating physicians, and feeling like hospital administration does not always truly understand coders' role and the true impact coders have on facility reimbursement.

My advice to coding students is to learn the Official Guidelines for Coding and Reporting (OGCR); they are the foundation of the coding classification and reimbursement systems. Be able to cite, apply, and communicate those guidelines to other professionals to ensure appropriate documentation to support reimbursement.

The transition to ICD-10-CM/PCS will be difficult and very expensive for hospitals and all affiliated providers. The expense is not only the cost of training and software, but also the loss of productivity. Studies from other countries, which implemented less complex versions of ICD-10 than the United States, reveal that productivity took a significant downturn after implementation and did not return to the same level, even five years later.

This is similar to what we experienced after ICD-9-CM was implemented in 1980, which was followed by the implementation of the inpatient prospective payment system (IPPS) and diagnosis related groups (DRGs) in 1983. The codes were new to us; coding as a profession was not as well-defined as it is today; and many coders were not fully trained. Consequently, the data used for rate setting was not accurate and payment rates for inpatient hospital services were severely impacted. It took nearly five years after implementation to get the reimbursement calculations reset to more appropriate levels so that providers were accurately reimbursed for their services. Using what we learned from the previous experience, CMS, AHIMA, and AAPC are guiding providers to undertake appropriate planning and training for ICD-10-CM/PCS well in advance in order minimize the impacts on productivity and reimbursement.

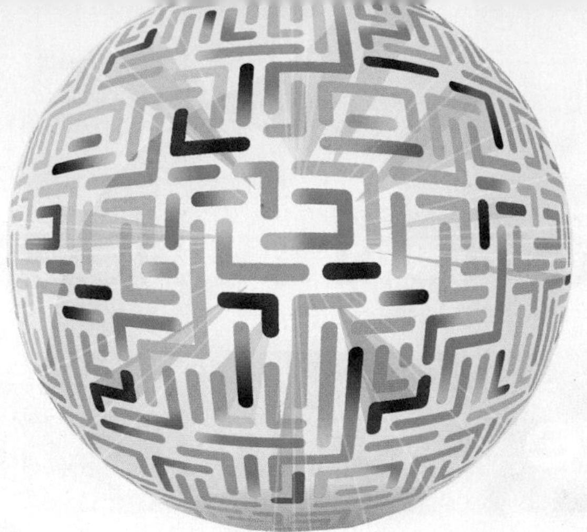

26

ICD-10-PCS Procedure Coding

Learning Objectives

After completing this chapter, you should have the skills to:

- Spell and define the key words, medical terms, and abbreviations related to ICD-10-PCS coding.
- Identify the purpose of ICD-10-PCS.
- Outline the organization of the ICD-10-PCS manual.
- Explain the ICD-10-PCS code structure.
- Discuss ICD-10-PCS Coding Guidelines.
- Describe the basic ICD-10-PCS procedure coding process.

Key Terms and Abbreviations

Approach
Body Part
Body System
build a code
character
CMS-1500 form
Completeness
Device
expandability
granular
ICD-10-PCS Coding Guidelines
multiaxial nature
principal procedure
Qualifier
Root Operation
Section
significant procedure
standardized terminology
structural integrity
Table
UB form
value

In addition to the key terms listed here, students should know the terms defined within tables in this chapter.

Chapter Outline

- **The Purpose of ICD-10-PCS**
- **ICD-10-PCS Coding Manual Organization**
- **ICD-10-PCS Code Structure**
- **ICD-10-PCS Coding Guidelines**
- **Introduction to the Steps of ICD-10-PCS Procedure Coding**

ICD-10-PCS codes in this chapter are from the ICD-10-PCS 2014 Draft code set from the Department of Health and Human Services, Centers for Medicare and Medicaid Services.

INTRODUCTION

When a new interchange opens on a road you are familiar with, it can be confusing and frustrating. The old road got you where you wanted to go, and you probably wish they had left it alone. Now you have to think about a trip that once was automatic. Coding is much the same way. While ICD-10-CM diagnosis coding represents a new interchange, ICD-10-PCS procedure coding is an entirely new road, from the dirt, to the substrate, to the top coat. Not only is it different from the inpatient procedure coding system that experienced coders are familiar with, it is also different from every other coding system that new coders learn, including ICD-10-CM diagnosis coding and CPT® coding. However, just as you eventually realize that a new road or new interchange is efficient and faster, you will also appreciate the new procedure coding system's ease, consistency, and logic.

In your tour of ICD-10-PCS in this chapter, you will learn about why a new inpatient procedure coding system was developed, how it is structured, and how to use it. Most importantly, you will practice locating basic information in the ICD-10-PCS coding manual.

As you read this chapter, open up your medical terminology book and keep a medical dictionary handy to refresh your memory of any unfamiliar terms. These are your professional resources that provide the information you need at your fingertips. It is always better to take a moment to look up details, rather than guess. Also refer to the websites and organizations listed in Coder's Toolbox at the end of the chapter for specialized information about procedure coding.

THE PURPOSE OF ICD-10-PCS

ICD-10-PCS (referred to as PCS in this text) is a new coding system used by hospitals for coding inpatient procedures. Unlike ICD-10-CM, which parallels ICD-9-CM in its overall structure, ICD-10-PCS is an entirely new system designed from scratch, for use in the United States. It was developed to overcome the limitations of other coding systems, with specific goals and usability criteria.

History of the ICD-10-PCS Code Set

Because procedural technology has advanced considerably since ICD-9-CM procedure codes were adopted in 1979, procedure codes are now extremely outdated. In addition, the four-digit format of ICD-9-CM procedure codes limited the total number of codes that could exist, and consequently, limited the ability to add new codes as technology progressed. As a result, CMS funded a project in 1992 to design a complete replacement for ICD-9-CM Volume 3. In 1995, CMS awarded a three-year contract to 3M Health Information Systems (3M) to develop a new inpatient procedure coding system, which was completed in 1998. CMS updates the system annually to incorporate new technologies and procedures. ICD-10-PCS was developed by the United States solely for use in the United States. ICD-10-PCS is not used by other countries.

CODING CAUTION

Although ICD-10-PCS has a similar name and is being implemented at the same time as ICD-10-CM, the two systems are completely separate. They were developed by different parties with distinct structures and unique guidelines.

Characteristics of ICD-10-PCS

The goal in developing ICD-10-PCS was to incorporate several specific attributes (characteristics): completeness, unique definitions, expandability, multiaxial nature, standardized terminology, and structural integrity. Understanding these characteristics helps coders appreciate the benefits of the system.

Completeness

Completeness means that there should be a unique code for every procedure that is significantly different in body part, approach, or method. In ICD-9-CM Volume 3, the same code was sometimes used to describe procedures on different body parts, with different approaches, or different methods, which created confusion due to lack of detail.

Unique Definitions

ICD-10-PCS codes are constructed of seven characters, or positions, each with a distinct purpose and meaning. The description of a code is based on the meaning of each value in the code, so the description is unique and cannot change. New codes are created by adding a new value for one of the positions. By design, an entire code cannot be redefined or reused, as can happen in other medical coding systems.

Expandability

Expandability means that the structure of the code set allows new procedures to be easily incorporated. In ICD-9-CM Volume 3, sometimes all of the codes in a specific numeric grouping were already used, making it impossible to add a new code for a new procedure in the same grouping. New codes were often added in an illogical place, with unrelated codes.

Multiaxial Nature

The multiaxial nature of PCS codes means that each position or character within a code number has a designated meaning or purpose. Each position should be used for that meaning for all related codes and, to the extent possible, for all codes in the manual. For example, in the Medical and Surgical Section, the fourth character of the code represents the body part on which the physician performed the procedure. So regardless of what kind of procedure is done, or in what body system, the fourth character identifies the body part.

SUCCESS STEP

ICD-10-PCS has more than 71,000 codes compared to less than 4,000 in ICD-9-CM Volume 3 and approximately 7,800 in CPT. As a result, ICD-10-PCS codes have greater specificity than ICD-9-CM or CPT codes do.

Standardized Terminology

Standardized terminology means that the code set includes definitions of the terminology it uses; each term must have only one meaning. This is in contrast to the use, in other coding systems, of eponyms and Latin-based medical terms, both of which can be interpreted with a wide range of meanings. ICD-10-PCS includes English definitions for 31 different types of medical and surgical procedures to ensure consistent reporting. Examples of the benefits of this approach include the following:

- ICD-10-PCS defines the specific meaning of each procedure so that all users apply it in the same way. In CPT and ICD-9-CM, a Latin-based medical term, such as *arthroplasty*, can refer to the repair of a joint, replacement of part of a joint, or replacement of the entire joint. ICD-10-PCS uses common English words to describe procedures, such as **Repair** or **Replacement**, and each has a specific definition. **Repair** is officially defined as *restoring a body part to its normal structure*. **Replacement** is officially defined as *putting in a device that replaces a body part*. Every user of ICD-10-PCS applies these definitions.
- ICD-10-PCS eliminates the use of eponyms to describe procedures. For example, the Whipple procedure, a pancreaticoduodenectomy, is a complex surgical procedure that involves the pancreas, as well as portions of the stomach, duodenum, common bile duct, and gallbladder. The specific organs, and portions of the organs, removed depends on the patient's needs and the surgeon. ICD-9-CM provided one code for the Whipple procedure, regardless of what was done. ICD-10-PCS breaks the procedure down into its component parts, with each organ receiving its own code, resulting in as many as five codes to report the procedure. This detail provides accurate and consistent reporting.
- ICD-10-PCS limits the use of combination codes, which describe two or more procedures with a single code. Instead, separate codes are reported for each separate procedure performed. This gives a full and accurate report of exactly what was done for each patient.

Structural Integrity

Structural integrity means that ICD-10-PCS can easily be expanded without disrupting the structure of the system. The values of the seven characters that make up a code can be assigned as needed. The system can evolve as medical technology and clinical practice progress, with much greater room for expansion than other medical coding systems. For example, in CPT, some sections of the book are running out of numbers, requiring that numbers be borrowed from other sections and then be resequenced out of numerical order. This cannot happen in ICD-10-PCS.

A coding system that is internally consistent, logically constructed, and adaptable to new technology enables coders to use it more consistently, resulting in data that is more granular (*specific*), reliable (reported in the same way by all users), and valid (accurately describes what it is intended to describe).

Hospital Use of ICD-10-PCS

According to the Uniform Hospital Data Discharge Set (UHDDS) inpatient hospitals must report all significant procedures. Significant procedures are those that are surgical in nature, carry a procedural risk, carry an anesthetic risk, or require specialized training.

The principal procedure is one that was performed for definitive treatment, rather than one performed for diagnostic or exploratory purposes, or was necessary to take care of a complication. If there appear to be two procedures that meet these criteria, then the one most related to the principal diagnosis should be selected as the principal procedure.

Hospitals use ICD-10-PCS procedure codes to identify the resources hospitals use in performing procedures when billing the patient's insurance. Hospital resources include the following:

- hospital staff, such as nurses, surgical technicians, nurse aides, and ancillary personnel
- space, equipment, and supplies, such as operating rooms, surgical instruments, X-ray, MRI, and CT equipment, surgical supplies, and linens
- overhead, such as utilities, operating expenses, and general administration

Hospital resources do not include the physician. In most cases, physicians own their own practices or are members of a group practice. The hospital does not employ them. The physician's practice bills the patient's insurance for the professional service performed by the physician. The hospital bills the patient's insurance for resources the hospital used.

Hospitals assign ICD-10-PCS codes for the procedures performed, not for each staff member, supply item, or other resource used. The diagnoses and procedures performed determine the diagnosis related group (MS-DRG), used by Medicare and many other payers for reimbursement. Payment is a predetermined amount based on the average amount of staff, supplies, and other resources used for patients in that MS-DRG.

SUCCESS STEP

PCS is used only when a hospital or other inpatient facility bills for inpatient services. Hospital outpatient services and physicians use CPT and HCPCS codes. However, some states may require that ICD-10-PCS codes be included when reporting statistics for outpatient hospital services.

Guided Example of the Use of ICD-10-PCS

Refer to the following example throughout this chapter to learn about ICD-10-PCS codes.

Date of procedure: 8/26/yy Location: Branton Medical Center Surgeon: Tanya Schmitt, MD

Anesthesiologist: Reginald Pincus, MD

Patient: Michael Longo Gender: M Age: 52

Preprocedure diagnosis: Crohn's disease with abscess

Procedure description: Temporary loop ileostomy. Made incision in right abdominal wall. Opened anterior wall of ileum loop and brought through to the skin, then closed the wound around the exposed ileum. Patient tolerated px (*procedure*) well.

Postprocedure diagnosis: Crohn's disease of large intestine with abscess

Follow this patient's surgical procedure and bill through the hospital, physician's office, and anesthesiologist's office to understand the difference between inpatient procedure codes and physician procedure codes.

- Tanya Schmitt, MD, who is part of Branton Professional Group, uses the operating rooms, surgical instruments, equipment, supplies, and nursing staff at Branton Medical Center to perform the procedure.
- Reginald Pincus, MD, who is part of Branton Anesthesiology Providers, administers the anesthesia using Branton Medical Center's anesthesia equipment and supplies; monitors the patient during and after the procedure; and assures that the patient wakes up without complications.
- After surgery, Mr. Longo is transferred to a medical-surgical floor. Dr. Schmitt checks on Mr. Longo each day and discharges him six days after surgery.
- Mr. Longo's insurance will receive three separate bills for services from the following organizations, for the amounts listed:

  1. Branton Medical Center, $12,500.00
  2. Branton Professional Group, $1,027.00
  3. Branton Anesthesiology Providers, $485.00

- Review the information outlined below to better understand why there are three bills.

  1. **Branton Medical Center** bills Mr. Longo's insurance for his entire length of stay, including room and board, the technical component of laboratory tests, and operating room resources. The cost is $12,500.00.
     - ❑ Branton Medical Center's coder, Marcy Elwood, CCS, assigns the ICD-10-CM diagnosis code, **K50.114, Crohn's disease of large intestine with abscess**, as the principal diagnosis. The coder assigns an ICD-10-PCS procedure code, **0D1B0Z4, Bypass Ileum to Cutaneous, Open Approach**, as the principal procedure. (You will learn how to assign PCS codes in the next chapter.)
     - ❑ The hospital's biller prepares the UB form (*Uniform Bill, the standard hospital billing form*), or its electronic equivalent. The biller enters **K50.114** in the block for the principal diagnosis, ICD-10-PCS code **0D1B0Z4** in the principal procedure block, and the date of surgery, 8/26/yy. In the block for operating physician, Dr. Schmitt's name and National Provider Number (NPI) are entered. Total charges are entered as $12,500.00. The facility is Branton Medical Center. Payment will be made to Branton Medical Center.
  2. **Branton Professional Group** bills Mr. Longo's insurance for Dr. Schmitt's services, which include admitting him, performing the procedure, making the follow-up visits, and discharging him. The surgeon's fee is $1,027.00.
     - ❑ Branton Professional Group's coder, Chrystal Crago, CCA, assigns the same ICD-10-CM diagnosis code, **K50.114** that the hospital did, but assigns a CPT surgical code (**44310 Ileostomy or jejunostomy, non-tube**) for the procedure.
     - ❑ Branton Professional Group's biller prepares a claim on the CMS-1500 form (*the standard physician billing form*) or its electronic equivalent. The biller lists the ICD-10-CM code **K50.114** in the diagnosis block, the date of the procedure, 8/26/yy, CPT surgical code 44310 in the services block. The charge for the surgeon is $1,027.00. Branton Medical Center is listed as the service facility. The billing provider is Branton Professional Group. Payment will be made to Branton Professional Group.

3. **Branton Anesthesiology Providers** bills Mr. Longo's insurance for the anesthesia management by Dr. Pincus. The anesthesiologist's fee is $485.00.

 - ❑ Branton Anesthesiology Providers' coder, Lance Staiger, CPC, assigns the same ICD-10-CM diagnosis code, **K50.114**, but assigns a CPT anesthesia code **(00840-P1 Anesthesia for intraperitoneal procedures in lower abdomen including laparoscopy; not otherwise specified - normal healthy patient)** for the anesthesiologist's services.
 - ❑ The Branton Anesthesiology Providers biller prepares a claim on the CMS-1500 form or its electronic equivalent. The biller enters the ICD-10-CM code **K50.114** as the diagnosis, the date of the procedure, 8/26/yy, and the CPT anesthesia code **00840-P1** in the services block. The charge for the anesthesiologist is $485.00. Branton Medical Center is listed as the service facility. The billing provider is Branton Anesthesiology Providers. Payment will be made to Branton Anesthesiology Providers.

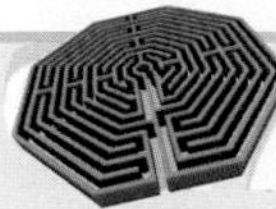

Coding Practice

Review the terminology and concepts in this section regarding the purpose of ICD-10-PCS.

Exercise 26.1 The Purpose of ICD-10-PCS

Instructions: Fill in each blank with the correct term(s) from this section of the chapter.

1. ____________ means that there should be a unique code for every procedure that is significantly different in body part, approach, or methods.
2. ____________ means that each position or character within a code number has a designated meaning or purpose and should be used for that meaning for all related codes.
3. ____________ means that the code set includes definitions of the terminology it uses and each term must have only one meaning.
4. Data that is granular is ____________.
5. ____________ are those that are surgical in nature, carry a procedural risk, carry an anesthetic risk, or require specialized training.
6. The ____________ is one that was performed for definitive treatment, rather than one performed for diagnostic or exploratory purposes, or was necessary to take care of a complication.
7. Hospitals use ICD-10-PCS procedure codes to describe and bill the patient's insurance for the ____________ hospital's use in performing procedures.
8. What are the three entities who will submit bills after a patient has an inpatient hospital surgical procedure performed?

 ____

 ____

 ____
9. Of the three entities listed in question 8, which one(s) bill using ICD-10-CM diagnosis codes?

 ____
10. Of the three entities listed in question 8, which one(s) bill using ICD-10-PCS procedure codes?

 ____

ICD-10-PCS CODING MANUAL ORGANIZATION

Open the ICD-10-PCS manual and follow along with the information outlined next, which describes the overall organization of the manual. The ICD-10-PCS manual has the following major sections:

- **Introduction**—The Introduction describes the history of ICD-10-PCS and gives detailed instructions on how use the manual. It provides reference material that lists the character definitions and values for each section of the manual.
- **ICD-10-PCS Coding Guidelines**—This section consists of A. Conventions, B. Medical and Surgical Section Guidelines, and C. Obstetrics Section Guidelines.
- **Index**—This section is an alphabetical listing of procedures, which identifies the correct reference table to use to build the code.
- **Tables**—This section contains reference tables or grids used to build each ICD-10-PCS code. Tables appear in alphanumeric order based on the first three characters of the code (■ FIGURE 26-1).
- **Appendices**—This section contains several appendices with additional reference material (■ TABLE 26-1). Coders should become familiar with the appendices because they contain valuable information that makes coding easier and more accurate.

0 Medical and Surgical
F Hepatobiliary System and Pancreas
9 Drainage Taking or letting out fluids and/or gases from a body part

Body Part Character 4	*Approach Character 5*	*Device Character 6*	*Qualifier Character 7*
0 Liver 1 Liver, Right Lobe 2 Liver, Left Lobe 4 Gallbladder G Pancreas	0 Open 3 Percutaneous 4 Percutaneous Endoscopic	0 Drainage Device	Z No Qualifier
0 Liver 1 Liver, Right Lobe 2 Liver, Left Lobe 4 Gallbladder G Pancreas	0 Open 3 Percutaneous 4 Percutaneous Endoscopic	Z No Device	X Diagnostic Z No Qualifier

Figure 26-1 ■ Example of a PCS Table

Table 26-1 ■ **ICD-10-PCS CODING MANUAL APPENDICES**

Appendix Title	Contents	Use
Body Part Key	Crosswalk between anatomical terms and the PCS Body Part description.	Determine what Body Part value corresponds with a specific anatomic site, such as a blood vessel, tendon, or nerve.
Character Meanings	Lists all possible values and meanings for Character 3 through Character 7. Organized by Section, then Body System, in the same order as the Tables.	Interpret the meaning of codes already assigned.
Comparison of Medical and Surgical Root Operations	Organizes Medical and Surgical Root Operations into nine groups with similar objectives.	Help determine the appropriate Root Operation.
Components of the Medical and Surgical Approach Definitions	Defines all Approaches (Character 5) for the Medical and Surgical Section.	Identify the official definition of surgical Approaches.
Device Aggregation Table	Defines the operation, body system, and general Device value for each specific device.	Determine the appropriate operations, body systems, and PCS device value for each class of devices.
Device Key	Crosswalk from device brand names and common names to the PCS Device description.	Determine what Device value to use for a specific product.
Root Operation Definitions	Defines all Root Operations in Sections 0 Medical and Surgical, and Sections 1 through 9, Medical and Surgical-Related. Organized by Section.	Identify the official definition of Root Operations.
Type and Type Qualifier Definitions Sections B-H	Defines all Types (Character 3) and Type Qualifiers (Character 5) for Ancillary Sections, B through H. Organized by Character and Section.	Identify the official definition of Types and Type Qualifiers.

SUCCESS STEP

The order of the sections and specific content may vary based on the manual's publisher or based on yearly updates, so it is helpful to review the organization of your particular manual. Apply self-adhesive tabs on the pages to identify each appendix.

In addition to the supplemental information contained within the ICD-10-PCS coding manual, CMS also publishes a separate electronic *ICD-10-PCS Reference Manual* (■ TABLE 26-2, page 534). The Reference Manual is updated annually and can be downloaded from the CMS website free of charge. This document provides detailed background on ICD-10-PCS, explanations of all Sections and Root Operations, tables of all character values, and many case examples.

Table 26-2 ■ **ICD-10-PCS REFERENCE MANUAL CONTENTS**

Chapter	Title	Contents
1	Overview	Includes a general introduction to ICD-10-PCS, a brief history of its development, and a presentation of the code structure, organization, and characteristics. The first part of the overview contains basic information; the second and third parts discuss structure, characteristics, and applications in more detail.
2	Procedures in the Medical and Surgical Section	Provides reference material for each root operation in the Medical and Surgical section (0), with the full definition, additional explanation as needed, a code example, and coding exercises for each root operation.
3	Procedures in the Medical and Surgical-Related Sections	Provides reference material for each of the Medical and Surgical-related sections (1 through 9), with definitions, additional explanation as needed, a code example, and coding exercises for each section.
4	Procedures in the Ancillary Sections	Provides reference material for each of the ancillary sections (B through H), with definitions, additional explanation as needed, a code example, and coding exercises for each section.
Appendix A	ICD-10-PCS Definitions	Tables listing the full definitions of all root operations and approaches in the Medical and Surgical section.
Appendix B	ICD-10-PCS Coding Guidelines	Contains guidelines for coding procedures with ICD-10-PCS.

The ICD-10-PCS Reference Manual can be downloaded at CMS > Medicare > ICD 10 > Downloads > 2012 ICD-10-PCS Reference Manual and Slides **http://www.cms.gov/ICD10/Downloads/2012_pcs_ref_manual.pdf.**

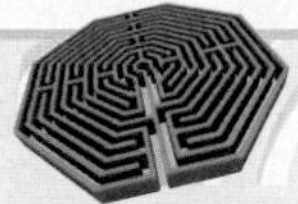

Coding Practice

Review the terminology and concepts in this section regarding the organization of the ICD-10-PCS coding manual and the *ICD-10-PCS Reference Manual.*

Exercise 26.2 ICD-10-PCS Coding Manual Organization

Instructions: Fill in each blank with the correct term(s) from this section of the chapter.

Part A

Name the section of the ICD-10-PCS coding manual coders use to locate the following information:

1. Conventions ____________
2. An alphabetical listing of procedures that identifies the correct reference table to use to build the code ____________
3. Reference material that lists the character definitions and values for each section of the manual ____________

Part B

Refer to Table 26-1 and name the title of the appendix in the ICD-10-PCS coding manual coders use to locate the following information:

4. Identify the official definition of Root Operations ____________
5. Determine what Body Part value corresponds with a specific anatomic site ____________
6. Determine what Device value to use for a specific product ____________
7. The electronic *ICD-10-PCS Reference Manual* can be downloaded for free from what organization's website? ____________

Part C

Name the chapter of the *ICD-10-PCS Reference Manual* coders use to locate the following information:

8. Definitions, additional explanation as needed, a code example, and coding exercises for the ancillary Sections B through H ____________
9. A general introduction to ICD-10-PCS, a brief history of its development, and a presentation of the code structure, organization, and characteristics ____________
10. Reference material for each root operation in the Medical and Surgical section (0) ____________

ICD-10-PCS CODE STRUCTURE

ICD-10-PCS codes have a logical, consistent structure that contains seven alphanumeric positions, called characters. An ICD-10-PCS code is best understood as the result of a process in which coders build a code. The process consists of assigning values to each character, based on specific characteristics of the procedure the physician performs. The ICD-10-PCS manual uses Tables, which are reference grids used to select the body part, operative approach, and other characteristics of the procedure.

ICD-10-PCS codes consist of seven positions or characters, each with a designated purpose, which creates consistency across codes. Coders select individual letters and numbers, called values, in a standard order to occupy the seven characters of the code. Each character represents a specific aspect of the procedure and can have up to 34 different values, consisting of the ten digits, 0 to 9, and 24 letters, A to H, J to N, and P to Z. Not every character uses all 34 values. For some sections and some characters, only a few values are used while in others, most of the values are used. Each Section of the manual designates how each character of the code is used within that Section. The definition of each value, for example **1** or **A**, is based on the position it occupies. Examples are provided in the discussion that follows.

SUCCESS STEP

ICD-10-PCS values do not use the letters I and O in order to avoid confusion with the numbers 0 and 1. This is different from ICD-10-CM, which *does* use both the letters I and O and the numbers 1 and 0.

The options and values for a character vary based on the first character of the code, which identifies the Section. The largest Section is Medical and Surgical, which is used as an example to introduce PCS codes in the remainder of this chapter. Characters in the Medical and Surgical Section are defined as follows:

- Character 1 defines the Section, or broad procedure category where the code is found.
- Character 2 defines the Body System in which the procedure is performed.
- Character 3 defines the Root Operation, or the objective of the procedure.
- Character 4 defines the Body Part, or specific anatomical site where the physician performed the procedure.
- Character 5 defines the Approach, or the surgical technique used to reach the procedure site.
- Character 6 defines the Device left in place at the end of the procedure.
- Character 7 defines a Qualifier for the code, which describes additional information about the procedure.

The Introduction in the ICD-10-PCS coding manual identifies the character meanings for each Section. An appendix in most ICD-10-PCS manuals provides a complete listing of all the Characters for all Sections. Refer to the Introduction and the appendix Character Meanings to become familiar with information needed to fully understand and assign ICD-10-PCS codes.

The following discussion identifies the purpose of each character and gives examples of how it is used. Chapters 27 and 28 of this text discuss how to use the Index and Tables to arrive at a code.

Character 1: Section

The first character in all PCS codes describes the Section, or the broad procedure category, where the code is found (■ TABLE 26-3). The largest Section is Medical and Surgical. Other Sections classify medical and surgical-related procedures, such as Obstetrics or Chiropractic, and ancillary services, such as Nuclear Medicine or Mental Health.

Table 26-3 ■ **CHARACTER 1: SECTION**

Value	Section Name
0	Medical and Surgical
Medical and Surgical-Related Procedures	
1	Obstetrics
2	Placement
3	Administration
4	Measurement and Monitoring
5	Extracorporeal Assistance and Performance
6	Extracorporeal Therapies
7	Osteopathic
8	Other Procedures
9	Chiropractic
Ancillary Procedures	
B	Imaging
C	Nuclear Medicine
D	Radiation Oncology
F	Physical Rehabilitation and Diagnostic Audiology
G	Mental Health
H	Substance Abuse Treatment

Adapted from http://www.cms.gov/ICD10/Downloads/2012_pcs_ref_manual.pdf

Character 2: Body System

The second character in the Medical and Surgical Section identifies the Body System, the general physiological system or anatomical region involved, such as central nervous system or endocrine system. The Medical and Surgical Section has 31 possible values for the Body System. The Body System values do not always correlate to the commonly defined organ systems. Large systems may have multiple values in Character 2. For example, the skeletal system has five Body System values, each referring to a specific component (■ TABLE 26-4). Because within each PCS Body System there can be up to 34 values for Body Part, codes can be more specific when large systems are divided into multiple values. This enables the skeletal system, for example, to have up to 170 Body Part values. If the Skeletal System were defined with only one value, then the number of Body Part values would be limited to 34.

Many Sections other than Medical and Surgical also use Character 2 to describe Body System, but may also use it for other purposes. The Placement Section (Section value 2) uses Character 2 for Anatomical Orifice. The Physical Rehabilitation and Diagnostic Audiology Section (Section value F) uses Character 2 for Section Qualifier, which is a broad type of service such as Rehabilitation.

CODING CAUTION

The Body System values in PCS are not related to the letters used in ICD-10-CM diagnosis codes. For example, in diagnosis coding, codes for the gastrointestinal system begin with **K**. In PCS coding, the gastrointestinal system has a Body System value of **D**.

Character 3: Root Operation

The third character in the Medical and Surgical Section, and most other Sections, defines the Root Operation, which describes the objective of the procedure (excision, destruction, extraction). The options and values for Character 3 vary from one Section to the next and from one Body Part value to the next within a Section. Root Operations are Main Terms in the Index, so coders must be familiar with their names and definitions. The names and definitions of Character 3 appear at the top of each Table in the ICD-10-PCS manual. In addition, an appendix in most ICD-10-PCS manuals defines the all Root Operations for the Medical and Surgical Section, provides expanded explanations, and gives examples.

For example, a Latin-based medical term such as *gastrectomy* can mean removing all or part of the stomach. The definitions of the words *excision* and *resection* are sometimes used interchangeably in common medical usage, such as stomach excision or stomach resection, and can mean that either all of the stomach or part of the stomach is removed. Without referring to the operative report, the extent of the procedure is unclear. ICD-10-PCS defines these terms in specific ways. **Excision** is defined as *cutting off a portion of a body part without replacement* while **Resection** is defined as *cutting off all of a body part without replacement*. Therefore, cutting out a portion of the stomach is coded as the Root Operation **Excision** (value **B**), while cutting out all of the stomach is coded as the Root Operation **Resection** (value **T**).

The 31 Medical and Surgical Root Operations are organized into nine groups, based on the overall objective of the procedure. An appendix in most ICD-10-PCS manuals provides a useful breakdown of the nine groups, which makes it easier to locate a desired Root Operation. The nine groups are not part of the final code; they are simply an organizational tool for coders.

Table 26-4 ■ **BODY SYSTEM VALUES FOR THE SKELETAL SYSTEM**

Value	Description
N	Head and Facial Bones
P	Upper Bones
Q	Lower Bones
R	Upper Joints
S	Lower Joints

CODING CAUTION

Coders are required to follow the definitions in the ICD-10-PCS manual, but physicians are not expected to change the words they use in documentation. Regardless of what word the physician uses to describe a procedure, coders are required to assign the Root Operation based on the official ICD-10-PCS definition (Guideline A11).

Character 4: Body Part

The fourth character in the Medical and Surgical Section identifies the Body Part, or specific anatomical site, where the physician performed the procedure. The Body System (Character 2) provides a general indication of the procedure location. The Body Part and Body System values together provide a precise description of the procedure site.

Most Sections use Character 2 for Body System and Character 4 for Body Part. However, some Sections use Character 2 for a different purpose. Sections that do not define Body System in Character 2 may use Character 4 for Body System.

The definition of each Body Part value in the Medical and Surgical Section is unique to each Body System. For

Table 26-5 ■ **EXAMPLE OF MULTIPLE BODY PART VALUES FOR A SINGLE ORGAN: THE LARGE INTESTINE**

Excerpt from Table 0BD, Excision, Gastrointestinal System: Character 4, Body Part	
Value	**Description**
E	Large Intestine
F	Large Intestine, Right
G	Large Intestine, Left
H	Cecum
J	Appendix
K	Ascending Colon
L	Transverse Colon
M	Descending Colon
N	Sigmoid Colon
P	Rectum

example, in Character 2 (Body System), value **5** identifies the upper veins and the Body Part value of **B** refers to the **right basilic vein**. When the Character 2 (Body System) value is **7** for the **lymphatic and hemic systems**, the Body Part Value **B** refers to the mesenteric lymphatic system. Review the appendix to see how the same value represents different information in different Body System tables.

When selecting the Body Part for a particular Root Operation, coders must refer to the appropriate Table and identify how that Table defines Body Part. Some organs and anatomical areas are divided into multiple Body Parts for coding purposes. For example, the large intestine is a single organ, but ICD-10-PCS assigns multiple Body Part values (■ TABLE 26-5). Coders should match the most specific Body Part value with the most specific Root Operation value. For example, when surgeons cut out the entire descending colon, they are taking out *part* of the organ, the large intestine, but *all* of the PCS Body Part value **M Descending Colon**. Therefore, coders select the Root Operation **T Resection**, defined as *cutting out, without replacement, all of a body part* and match it with the Body Part value **M Descending Colon**. Do not assign the Root Operation **B Excision**, which is defined as *cutting out, without replacement, a portion of a body part*, and match it with the less specific Body Part value **E Large Intestine** (■ FIGURE 26-2).

Character 5: Approach

The fifth character in the Medical and Surgical Section defines the Approach, or the surgical technique used to reach the procedure site, such as open, endoscopic, or external. Each Table in the ICD-10-PCS manual lists the acceptable Approaches for each Root Operation value and Body Part value. Definitions for each Approach appear in the appendix and are further discussed in Chapter 27.

Sections other than Medical and Surgical use Character 5 for a wide range of purposes. For example, the Extracorporeal Therapies Section (Section value 6) uses Character 5 for Duration and the Imaging Section (Section value **B**) uses Character 5 for **Contrast**.

Character 6: Device

The sixth character in the Medical and Surgical Section defines the Device left in place at the end of the procedure for those procedures that involve a device. Device values fall into four basic categories: grafts and prostheses, implants, simple or mechanical appliances, electronic appliances. Each Table in the ICD-10-PCS manual lists the acceptable devices for each Root Operation value and Device value.

Procedure description: Partial colectomy. Excised the entire descending colon.

CORRECT

Root Operation: **T - Resection,** *cutting out, without replacement, all of a body part*

Body Part: **M - Descending Colon**

INCORRECT

Root Operation: **B - Excision,** *cutting out, without replacement, a portion of a body part*

Body Part: **E - Large Intestine**

Explanation: Select the most specific Body Part value **(Descending Colon (M))** and match it with the most specific Root Operation **(Resection (T)).** Also notice that you should not select the Root Operation **Excision (B)** based on the physician's use of the word "excised." Select the Root Operation based on the PCS definition.

Figure 26-2 ■ Example of Matching the Root Operation with the Body Part

Sections other than Medical and Surgical use Character 6 for a variety of purposes, including **Method** (Osteopathic section) and **Isotope** (Radiation Oncology section). When no device applies, the Table lists the value **Z No Device** for Character 6.

Character 7: Qualifier

The seventh character in the Medical and Surgical Section defines a Qualifier for the code. A Qualifier specifies an additional attribute of the procedure, if applicable. Examples of Medical and Surgical Qualifiers are the type of adhesive used on a replacement joint, such as cemented or uncemented, and the direction of the surgical approach, such as anterior or posterior. Each Table in the ICD-10-PCS manual lists the acceptable Qualifier values for each Approach value. When no qualifier applies, the Table lists the value **Z No Qualifier** for Character 7.

CODING CAUTION

In ICD-10-CM, the seventh character is called an extension and is only used on *selected* codes. In ICD-10-PCS, the seventh character is called a Qualifier and is required on *all* codes.

Guided Example of Building a PCS Code

Continue with the example of Michael Longo who had an ileostomy, to learn the meaning of an ICD-10-PCS code.

Follow along as Marcy Elwood, CCS, the coder at Branton Medical Center, assigns the ICD-10-PCS code **0D1B0Z4**.

➪ Refer to the Build-A-Code Table (■ TABLE 26-6) to understand how a PCS code is structured. You will learn how Marcy used the Index and Tables to arrive at this code in Chapters 27 and 28.

Table 26-6 ■ **BUILD-A-CODE 0D1B0Z4 BYPASS ILEUM TO CUTANEOUS, OPEN APPROACH**

Character (Position)	Name	Value	Description
1	Section	0	Medical and Surgical
2	Body System	D	Gastrointestinal
3	Root Operation	1	Bypass
4	Body Part	B	Ileum
5	Approach	0	Open
6	Device	Z	No Device
7	Qualifier	4	Cutaneous

- ❑ The value **0** for Character 1 identifies that the procedure is from the Medical and Surgical Section.
- ❑ The value **D** for Character 2 identifies that the Body System is **Gastrointestinal**.
- ❑ The value **1** for Character 3 identifies that the Root Operation is **Bypass**. PCS defines **Bypass** as *altering the route of passage of the contents of a tubular body part.*
- ❑ The value **B** for Character 4 identifies that the Body Part is **Ileum**.
- ❑ The value **0** for Character 5 identifies that the Approach is **Open**.
- ❑ The value **Z** for Character 6 identifies that the Device is **No Device** because the PCS Table does not provide any options for this character.
- ❑ The value **4** for Character 7 identifies that the Qualifier is **Cutaneous** because in the Root Operation **Bypass**, PCS uses the Qualifier to identify the end site of the bypass.

➪ Now you can see the entire meaning of the code **0D1B0Z4, Bypass Ileum to Cutaneous, Open Approach**. You will learn how to use the Index and Tables to arrive at this code in later chapters of this text.

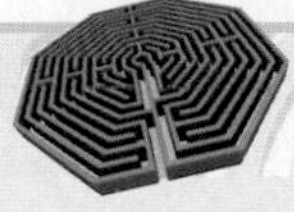

Coding Practice

Review the terminology and concepts in this section regarding ICD-10-PCS code structure.

Exercise 26.3 ICD-10-PCS Code Structure

Instructions: Fill in each blank with the correct term(s) from this section of the chapter.

1. ______________ are reference grids used to select the body part, operative approach, and other characteristics of the procedure.
2. Coders select individual letters and numbers, called ______________, in a standard order to occupy the seven characters of the code.
3. ICD-10-PCS values do not use the letters ______________ and ______________ in order to avoid confusion with numbers.

Provide the Character number (1 through 7) and name for the following:

4. Character ______________, called the ______________, has the value of 0 for all Medical and Surgical procedures.
5. Character ______________, called the ______________, identifies the technique used to reach the procedure site in the Medical and Surgical Section.
6. Character ______________, called the ______________, identifies the specific anatomical site where the physician performed the procedure, in the Medical and Surgical Section.
7. Resection is an example of Character ______________, called the ______________, in the Medical and Surgical Section.
8. The direction of the surgical approach, such as anterior or posterior, is an example of Character ______________, called the ______________, in the Medical and Surgical Section.
9. Character ______________, called the ______________, identifies the general physiological system or anatomical region involved, such as central nervous system or endocrine system in the Medical and Surgical Section.
10. Values for Character ______________, called the ______________, fall into four basic categories: grafts and prostheses, implants, simple or mechanical appliances, electronic appliances.

ICD-10-PCS CODING GUIDELINES

ICD-10-PCS provides Coding Guidelines at the front of the ICD-10-PCS manual. Guidelines are divided into three sections: A-Conventions; B-Medical and Surgical Section Guidelines; and C-Obstetric Section Guidelines. Throughout this text, information from the Coding Guidelines section will be cross-referenced as *Guideline*, followed by the specific reference number, such as Guideline A6 or Guideline B3.6a. Follow along in the ICD-10-PCS manual to become acquainted with each section of the Coding Guidelines.

A—Conventions

Conventions describe how ICD-10-PCS codes are constructed and the basic rules of using ICD-10-PCS. Examples are presented for many specific guidelines. The most important guidelines to memorize while learning PCS include the following. This provides an overview. The details will be discussed later in this chapter and other PCS chapters.

- A6. The purpose of the alphabetic index is to locate the appropriate table that contains all information necessary to construct a procedure code. The PCS Tables should always be consulted to find the most appropriate valid code.
- A8. All seven characters must be specified to be a valid code. If the documentation is incomplete for coding purposes, query the physician for the necessary information.
- A9. Within a PCS table, valid codes include all combinations of choices in Characters 4 through 7 contained in the same row of the table.
- A11. Many of the terms used to construct PCS codes are defined within the system. It is the coder's responsibility to determine what the documentation in the medical record equates to in the PCS definitions.

B—Medical and Surgical Section Guidelines (Section 0)

Medical and Surgical Section Guidelines apply specifically to ICD-10-PCS in the Medical and Surgical Section (value **0**). The organization of this section correlates with each character in the Medical and Surgical Codes, as follows:

- B2. Body System
- B3. Root Operation
- B4. Body Part
- B5. Approach
- B6. Device
- B7. Qualifier

Each of these subsections contains *General guidelines*, which apply to the Medical and Surgical Section as a whole, and also provides additional guidelines that apply to specific Root Operations, Approaches, and other elements. Specific guidelines from this section will be discussed later in this text.

C—Obstetric Section Guidelines (Section 1)

Obstetrics is the only Section besides Medical and Surgical that has specific guidelines. There are only a few guidelines, which will be discussed in detail in Chapter 28 of this text.

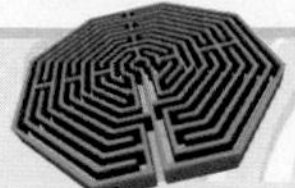

Coding Practice

Review the terminology and concepts in this section regarding ICD-10-PCS coding guidelines.

Exercise 26.4 ICD-10-PCS Coding Guidelines

Instructions: Fill in each blank with the correct term(s) from this section of the chapter.

1. ______________ describe how ICD-10-PCS codes are constructed and the basic rules of using ICD-10-PCS.
2. Guideline ______________ states that all seven characters must be specified to be a valid code.
3. Within a PCS table, valid codes include all combinations of choices in Characters 4 through 7 contained in the same ______________ the table.
4. Who is responsible to determine what the documentation in the medical record equates to in the PCS definitions? ______________.
5. ______________ is the only Section besides Medical and Surgical that has specific guidelines.

INTRODUCTION TO THE STEPS OF ICD-10-PCS PROCEDURE CODING

The three skills of an ace coder apply to coding procedures, but the mechanics are different than sequencing diagnoses because the code set is different. Follow these steps:

1. **Abstract** procedures from the medical record, beginning with PCS definitions of the Root Operation.
2. **Assign**, or build, the PCS code values using the Index and Tables.
3. **Arrange**, or sequence, PCS codes based on the definition of the principal procedure.

An overview of these skills is provided next. Chapters 27 and 28 of this text discuss these skills in detail and provide examples.

Abstract Procedures from the Medical Record

The key to accurate abstracting in PCS is to read the information provided in the procedure report and interpret it in a manner consistent with ICD-10-PCS definitions of the Root Operation or Root Type. The Root Operation or Root Type also functions as the Main Term in the Index and directs coders to the correct Table. The Introduction of the ICD-10-PCS manual provides the definition for each Root Operation and Root Type, which are divided by Section.

SUCCESS STEP

The appendix provides Root Operation definitions for Section **0**, Medical and Surgical, and Sections **1** through **9**, Medical and Surgical-Related. The appendix also provides Root Type definitions for Sections **B** through **H**, Ancillary.

Coders must read the procedure report and *interpret* what was done based on the definitions of the Root Operations or Root Types. Physicians are not required or expected to document using ICD-10-PCS definitions, but may document using the terminology they are most comfortable and familiar with. Coders will not find Root Operations described in the procedure report using the exact PCS words (■ FIGURE 26-3). Even when physicians use words that are similar to Root Operations, such as excision, resection, or removal, the coder is obligated to interpret the physician's description in light of the PCS definitions. Guideline A11 states the following:

> **Many of the terms used to construct PCS codes are defined within the system. It is the coder's responsibility to determine what the documentation in the medical record equates to in the PCS definitions. The physician is not expected to use the terms used in PCS code descriptions, nor is the coder required to query the physician when the correlation between the documentation and the defined PCS terms is clear.**

SUCCESS STEP

Although you do not need to memorize specific codes or character values, you should plan to memorize the *definitions* of the most commonly used Root Operations and Root Types. While in the learning stage, ALWAYS verify the definition of the Root Operation in the PCS manual.

Assign ICD-10-PCS Codes

Assigning PCS codes requires coders to locate the Root Operation in the Index then refer to a Table to build the code.

Procedure description: Appendectomy. Removed entire appendix laparoscopically.

CORRECT

Root Operation: **T - Resection** *cutting off all of a body part, without replacement*

INCORRECT

Root Operation: **P - Removal** *taking out or off a device from a body part*

Explanation: Even though the documentation uses the word *removed*, do not use the Root Operation **Removal** because the PCS definition does not describe the procedure performed. The Root Operation **Removal** applies only to taking devices out of the body. The Root Operation **Resection** describes cutting off a body part, such as the appendix.

Figure 26-3 ■ Example of Abstracting a Root Operation

ICD-10-PCS Index

The Index uses two types of Main Terms for the Medical and Surgical Section:

- the name of the Root Operation, such as Excision
- the common procedure name, excluding eponyms, such as appendectomy

Under the Main Term are indented subterms that describe the anatomical sites or other variations of the Root Operation. Following the subterm is the partial code, which provides the first three to five characters of the code. The first *three* characters of the partial code identify the appropriate Table to use.

ICD-10-PCS Tables

After locating the appropriate procedure in the Index and identifying the first three characters of the partial code, cross-reference the appropriate Table to build the rest of the code. Follow three steps to look up a PCS code in the tables:

1. Locate the Table using the first three characters of the partial code provided in the Index.
2. Build the code by locating the row in the Table that contains the appropriate Body Part value for Character 4. Then select the appropriate values for Characters 4, 5, 6, and 7 from within the same row of the Table.
3. Verify the character values by comparing the values selected against the documentation.

Arrange ICD-10-PCS Codes

Sequencing procedure codes is generally easier than sequencing diagnosis codes because there are fewer sequencing rules. When multiple procedures are performed, follow these general sequencing guidelines:

- Sequence as the first procedure the one most closely related to the principal diagnosis.
- When a procedure is required to care for a complication, sequence it before other procedures.
- When a diagnostic or exploratory procedure is followed by a definitive treatment, sequence the definitive procedure first and the diagnostic or exploratory procedure second.

ICD-10-PCS Medical and Surgical Section Guidelines provide guidance on coding multiple procedures. The Guidelines are discussed further in Chapter 28 of this text.

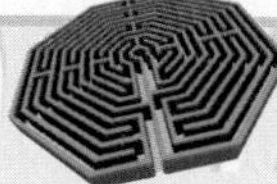

Coding Practice

Review the terminology and concepts in this section regarding PCS procedure coding.

Exercise 26.5 Introduction to the Steps of PCS Procedure Coding

Instructions: Fill in each blank with the correct term(s) from this section of the chapter.

1. The ______________ functions as the Main Term in the Index and directs coders to the correct Table.
2. Coders ______________ find Root Operations described in the procedure report using the exact PCS words.
3. Coders must read the procedure report and ______________ what was done based on the definitions of the Root Operations

(continued)

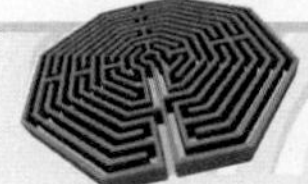

Coding Practice (continued)

4. Coders should plan to memorize the ______________ of the most commonly used Root Operations and Root Types.
5. In the Medical and Surgical Section, the Index uses what two types of Main Terms? ______________ ______________
6. The anatomical site is a ______________ in the Index.
7. The first ______________ characters of the partial code identify the appropriate Table to use.
8. Build the code by locating the row in the Table that contains ______________.
9. Select the appropriate values for Characters ______________ from within the same row of the Table.
10. The first sequenced procedure should be one most closely related to the ______________.

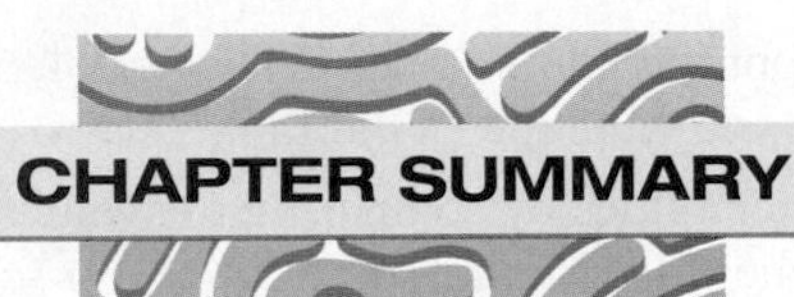

CHAPTER SUMMARY

In this chapter you learned that:

- ICD-10-PCS is a new coding system to be used by hospitals for coding inpatient procedures.
- The ICD-10-PCS manual contains the Introduction, ICD-10-PCS Coding Guidelines, Index, Tables, and Appendices.
- ICD-10-PCS codes have a logical, consistent structure that contains seven alphanumeric positions, called characters.
- ICD-10-PCS Coding Guidelines are divided into three sections: Conventions, which are labeled beginning with the letter A; Medical and Surgical Section Guidelines, which are labeled beginning with the letter B; and Obstetric Section Guidelines, which are labeled beginning with the letter C.
- The three skills of an ace coder—abstract, assign, and arrange—apply to coding procedures in ICD-10-PCS, but the mechanics are somewhat different from sequencing diagnoses because the code set is different.

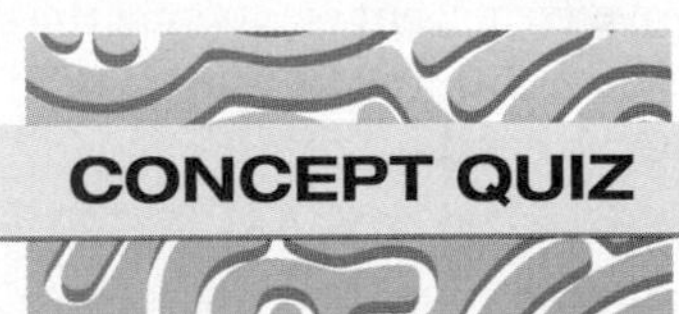

CONCEPT QUIZ

Take a moment to look back at your trip through ICD-10-PCS and solidify your skills. This is your opportunity to pull together everything you have learned.

Completion

Instructions: Write the term that answers each question based on the information you learned in this chapter. Choose from the list below. Some choices may be used more than once and some choices may not be used at all. Refer to the discussion in this chapter and the Glossary at the end of this book if you need a little extra help.

Approach(es)	Body System(s)
Body Part(s)	Character(s)
Device(s)	Root Operation(s)
expandability	Section(s)
multiaxial	standardized terminology
Qualifier(s)	value(s)

1. ICD-10-PCS codes are constructed of seven ______________ or positions, each with a distinct purpose and meaning.
2. ______________ means that the structure of the code set allows new procedures to be easily incorporated.
3. ______________ means that the code set includes definitions of the terminology it uses and each term must have only one meaning.

4. To build a PCS code, coders assign ______________________ to each character, based on specific characteristics of the procedure the physician performs.
5. Each Section of the manual designates how each ______________________ of the code is used within that Section.
6. The Medical and Surgical Section has 31 possible values for the ______________________.
7. P, Upper Bones is a ______________________ value with the skeletal system.
8. The ______________________ describes the objective of the procedure.
9. Character 5 in the Medical and Surgical Section provides definitions for the ______________________.
10. Assign value Z when there is no ______________________.

Multiple Choice

Instructions: Circle the letter of the best answer to each question based on the information you learned in this chapter. Refer to the discussion in this chapter and the Glossary at the end of this book if you need a little extra help.

1. ICD-10-PCS does NOT include
   A. eponyms.
   B. standardized terminology.
   C. definitions.
   D. granularity.
2. Hospital resources include all of the following EXCEPT
   A. nurses.
   B. physicians.
   C. surgical technicians.
   D. equipment.
3. ICD-10-PCS is used for billing of
   A. physician services.
   B. hospital outpatient services.
   C. hospital inpatient services.
   D. all of the above.
4. Tables are reference grids that appear in alphanumeric order based on which character(s) of the code?
   A. The first character
   B. The first two characters
   C. The first three characters
   D. The first four characters
5. What Root Operation is defined as *cutting off a portion of a body part without replacement*?
   A. Excision
   B. Resection
   C. Removal
   D. Bypass
6. Ileostomy is an example of what Root Operation?
   A. Excision
   B. Resection
   C. Removal
   D. Bypass
7. When coding an ileostomy, the Body Part is
   A. gastrointestinal.
   B. small intestine.
   C. ilium.
   D. ileum.
8. Abstract procedures from the medical record, *beginning* with PCS definitions of the
   A. Body System.
   B. Root Operation.
   C. Body Part.
   D. Approach.
9. Assign the PCS code values using
   A. only the Index.
   B. the Index and Tables.
   C. the appendix.
   D. Section descriptors.
10. Which of the following should be sequenced before any other procedures?
    A. A diagnostic or exploratory procedure
    B. The first procedure performed
    C. A procedure required to care for a complication
    D. Eponyms

CODING CHALLENGE

Now it is your turn to demonstrate the ability to locate information in the ICD-10-PCS manual. Refer back to the examples and discussion in this chapter when you need a little extra help.

Part A

Instructions: Using the PCS Index, look up the Root Operation and subterms listed. Write the partial code provided in the Index in the space provided.

(*continued*)

(continued from page 543)

Example: Alteration, Abdominal Wall
Partial Code: OWOF

1. Bypass, Duct, Hepatic, Left: Partial Code ____________
2. Excision, Disc, Lumbosacral: Partial Code ____________
3. Fusion, Metacarpophalangeal, Right: Partial Code ____________
4. Release, Pulmonary Trunk: Partial Code ____________
5. Supplement, Tendon, Foot, Left: Partial Code ____________

Part B

Instructions: Look up the Table represented by the three-character partial code. Write out the values represented by the Section, Body System, and Root Operation.

Example: Table **021**
Character 1, Section: 0 Medical and Surgical
Character 2, Body System: 2 Heart and Great Vessels
Character 3, Root Operation: 1 Bypass

(continued)

(continued)

6. Table **B51**
   Character 1, Section: ____________
   Character 2, Body System: ____________
   Character 3, Root Operation: ____________
7. Table **0H9**
   Character 1, Section: ____________
   Character 2, Body System: ____________
   Character 3, Root Operation: ____________
8. Table **0KS**
   Character 1, Section: ____________
   Character 2, Body System: ____________
   Character 3, Root Operation: ____________
9. Table **07L**
   Character 1, Section: ____________
   Character 2, Body System: ____________
   Character 3, Root Operation: ____________
10. Table **04R**
    Character 1, Section: ____________
    Character 2, Body System: ____________
    Character 3, Root Operation: ____________

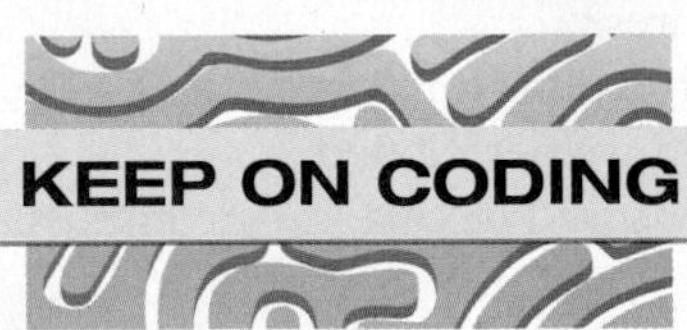

KEEP ON CODING

Part A

Instructions: Using the PCS Index, look up the Root Operation and subterms listed. Write the partial code provided in the Index in the space provided.

Example: Alteration, Abdominal Wall: Partial Code OWOF

1. Alteration, Nose: Partial Code ____________
2. Change Diaphragm: Partial Code ____________
3. Creation, Male: Partial Code ____________
4. Destruction, Cervix: Partial Code ____________
5. Dilation, Esophagus: Partial Code ____________

6. Extirpation, Anus: Partial Code ______

7. Fragmentation, Trachea: Partial Code ______

8. Inspection, Fallopian Tube: Partial Code ______

9. Map, Brain: Partial Code ______

10. Occlusion, Urethra: Partial Code ______

11. Reattachment, Tooth, Upper: Partial Code ______

12. Release, Nerve, Trigeminal: Partial Code ______

13. Repair, Jejunum: Partial Code ______

14. Supplement, Larynx: Partial Code ______

15. Transfer, Tendon, Head and Neck: Partial Code ______

Part B

Instructions: Look up the Table represented by the three-character partial code. Write out the values represented by the Section, Body System, and Root Operation.

Example: Table **021**

Character 1, Section: *0 Medical and Surgical*

Character 2, Body System: *2 Heart and Great Vessels*

Character 3, Root Operation: *1 Bypass*

16. Table **0CR**

Character 1, Section: ______

Character 2, Body System: ______

Character 3, Root Operation: ______

17. Table **0JH**

Character 1, Section: ______

Character 2, Body System: ______

Character 3, Root Operation: ______

18. Table **0N9**

Character 1, Section: ______

Character 2, Body System: ______

Character 3, Root Operation: ______

19. Table **0PT**

Character 1, Section: ______

Character 2, Body System: ______

Character 3, Root Operation: ______

20. Table **10E**

Character 1, Section: ______

Character 2, Body System: ______

Character 3, Root Operation: ______

21. Table **2W3**

Character 1, Section: ______

Character 2, Anatomical Region: ______

Character 3, Root Operation: ______

22. Table **BV2**

Character 1, Section: ______

Character 2, Body System: ______

Character 3, Root Type: ______

23. Table **F07**

Character 1, Section: ______

Character 2, Section Qualifier: ______

Character 3, Root Type: ______

24. Table **GZJ**

Character 1, Section: ______

Character 2, Body System: ______

Character 3, Root Type: ______

25. Table **HZ4**

Character 1, Section: ______

Character 2, Body System: ______

Character 3, Root Type: ______

CODER'S TOOLBOX

The following resources are a starting point for learning more about ICD-10-PCS. The > symbol indicates a menu selection within the website in order to navigate to a specific page.

The following ICD-10-PCS files are available on the CMS website:

CMS > Medicare > ICD10 > 2012 ICD-10-PCS and GEMs > Downloads
http://www.cms.gov/ICD10/11b15_2012_ICD10PCS.asp#TopOfPage

- 2012 Code Tables and Index
- 2012 Official ICD-10-PCS Coding Guidelines
- 2012 ICD-10-PCS Reference Manual and Slides
- 2012 Addendum
- 2012 Code Descriptions—Long and Abbreviated Titles and README files

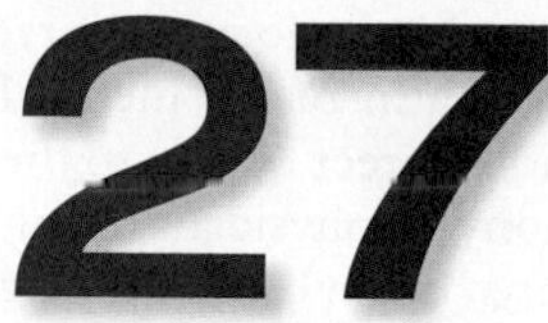

27 Medical and Surgical Procedures (Section 0), Part 1

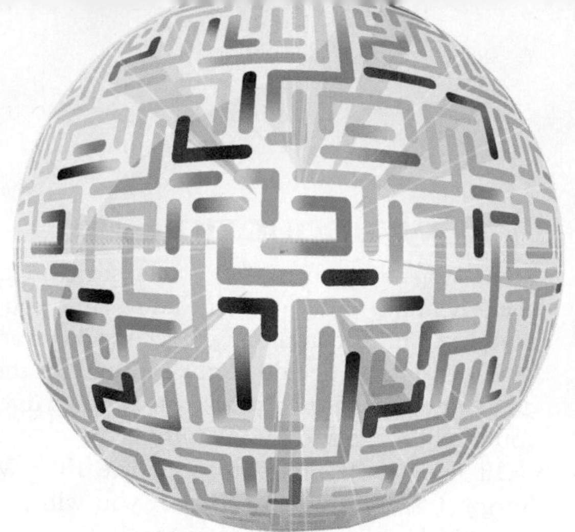

Learning Objectives

After completing this chapter, you should have the skills to:

- Spell and define the key words, medical terms, and abbreviations related to medical and surgical procedures.
- Discuss common Medical and Surgical procedures.
- Identify the main characteristics of coding Medical and Surgical procedures.
- Discuss PCS Guidelines for Medical and Surgical procedures.

Key Terms and Abbreviations

Device
diagnostic procedure
divided
External
Open
Percutaneous
Percutaneous Endoscopic
surgical approach
therapeutic procedure
Via Natural or Artificial Opening
Via Natural or Artificial Opening Endoscopic
Via Natural or Artificial Opening Endoscopic with Percutaneous Endoscopic Assistance

In addition to the key terms listed here, students should know the terms defined within tables in this chapter.

Chapter Outline

- **Medical and Surgical Refresher**
- **Coding Overview of Medical and Surgical Procedures**

ICD-10-PCS codes in this chapter are from the ICD-10-PCS 2014 Draft code set from the Department of Health and Human Services, Centers for Medicare and Medicaid Services.

INTRODUCTION

Some stops on your road trip may seem so large they are overwhelming and you don't know how you will see everything. This is common with theme parks and large museums. You may decide to take in part of the venue one day and come back for more on another day. Even then, you might not get to see everything.

In your preliminary tour of the PCS Medical and Surgical Section in this chapter you will become familiar with the largest section in the PCS manual, how it is structured, and how to use it. Most importantly, you learn many of the definitions that are the cornerstone of ICD-10-PCS and are essential to accurate code assignment. This is your get-acquainted tour, which will be continued in Chapter 28 with more detailed information.

As you read this chapter, open up your medical terminology book and keep a medical dictionary handy to refresh your memory of any unfamiliar terms. These are your professional resources that provide the information you need at your fingertips. Also refer to the websites and organizations listed in Coder's Toolbox at the end of the chapter for specialized information about procedure coding.

MEDICAL AND SURGICAL REFRESHER

Physicians perform a wide range of procedures on any body part. Because no coder can be familiar with every possible procedure, it is important to apply medical terminology skills to combine familiar word roots, prefixes, and suffixes to define new procedural terms. Procedural terms combine the word root(s) for one or more body parts, such as *gastr/o* with a suffix that describes the type of procedure, such as *-ectomy*.

Although PCS establishes its own terminology and definitions of Root Operations, physicians will continue to use traditional Latin-based medical terms, such as *gastrectomy*, and eponyms, such as the Whipple procedure, which is one type of gastrectomy. Latin-based medical terms appear in the PCS Index and redirect coders to the most likely Root Operations. To convert physician terminology to Root Operation definitions, begin by identifying the meaning of medical terms. As you learn about procedures that physicians perform, refer to ■ TABLE 27-1 for a refresher on how to build medical terms.

CODING CAUTION

Be alert for procedural suffixes that are spelled similarly and have different meanings.

-tomy (*cut into*), **-ectomy** (*cut out*), and **-stomy** (*create a new mouth*)

-centesis (*surgical puncture to remove fluid*), **-lysis** (*removal, separation*), and **-desis** (*to bind together*)

Coders need to know the difference between a treatment and a diagnostic procedure; they also need to know the types of surgical approaches to a procedure.

Treatment and Diagnostic Procedures

Physicians may order procedures for either therapeutic or diagnostic purposes. A therapeutic procedure is performed in order to treat a disease or condition. Examples are a cholecystectomy due to gallbladder disease, a coronary artery bypass to treat atherosclerosis, or removal of a skin lesion that is cancerous. A diagnostic procedure is performed to obtain information needed to make a diagnosis and treatment plan. Examples are performing a biopsy of a tumor in order to determine if it is malignant or performing amniocentesis to determine if a fetus has chromosomal abnormalities.

Table 27-1 ■ **EXAMPLE OF CONSTRUCTING MEDICAL TERMS FOR PROCEDURES**

Combining Form	Suffix	Complete Medical Term
gastr/o (*stomach*)	**-ectomy** (*cutting out*) **-scopy** (*visual examination*) **-plication** (*folding*)	**gastro + ectomy** (*cutting out the stomach*) **duodeno + ectomy** (*cutting out the duodenum*) **gastro + duoden + ectomy** (*cutting out the stomach and duodenum*)
duoden/o (*duodenum, first section of small intestine*)		**gastro + scopy** (*visual examination of the stomach*) **duodeno + scopy** (*visual examination of the duodenum*) **gastro + duodeno + scopy** (*visual examination of the stomach and duodenum*)
		gastro + plication (*folding the stomach*)

Surgical Approaches

The surgical approach describes how the surgeon accessed the operative site. A variety of methods may be used for most procedures. The surgeon's decision is based on the reason the procedure is being done, the circumstances of the patient, the proven effectiveness of one approach over others, and other factors.

In some cases, the surgeon may plan to use one approach, then need to change to another approach due to complicating factors. For example, the surgeon may plan to perform an endoscopic cholecystectomy, but due to adhesions must change to an open approach. PCS definitions of surgical approaches follow.

Open

An Open procedure is one in which an incision is made through the skin and subcutaneous tissue. Fascia and muscles are divided (*separated*) and the organ, body cavity, or region is directly visualized with the naked eye by the surgeon. All steps to access the procedure site, including the initial incision on the skin, subsequent divisions to reach the surgical site, and layered closure, are part of the procedure. An open approach is the most invasive and carries the highest risk to the patient. Surgeons will generally opt for a less invasive approach whenever possible. Examples of the open approach are an abdominal hysterectomy and an open coronary artery bypass graft (CABG).

Percutaneous

In a Percutaneous procedure, the skin is punctured or a very small incision made to access the site, but a full length incision is not made. An example is a needle biopsy of any joint or organ.

Percutaneous Endoscopic

In a Percutaneous Endoscopic procedure, the surgeon makes several, usually two to four, small incisions, approximately one-half to one inch in length. A fiber optic camera is inserted through one incision and surgical instruments are inserted through the other openings. The camera transmits an image of the operative site to a television monitor. Examples of the percutaneous endoscopic approach are a laparoscopic cholecystectomy and arthroscopic repair of a joint.

SUCCESS STEP

Endoscopy is a generic name for any procedure using a fiber optic viewing scope. The procedure may also carry the name of the site accessed, such as colonoscopy, laparoscopy, or gastroscopy.

Via Natural or Artificial Opening

In the approach Via Natural or Artificial Opening, the surgeon accesses the surgical site through a body opening that already exists, such as the mouth, nose, ear, anus, or vagina. Artificially made openings, such as a tracheotomy or colostomy mouth, may also be used. In either situation, a new incision is not required. Examples are insertion of an endotracheal tube through the oral cavity and placement of a Foley catheter through the urinary tract.

Via Natural or Artificial Opening Endoscopic

In the approach Via Natural or Artificial Opening Endoscopic, the surgeon inserts an endoscope through an existing natural or artificial opening. Examples are a colonoscopy, in which the endoscope is inserted through the anus, and an endoscopic examination of the esophagus, in which the endoscope is inserted through the mouth.

Via Natural or Artificial Opening Endoscopic with Percutaneous Endoscopic Assistance

In the approach Via Natural or Artificial Opening Endoscopic with Percutaneous Endoscopic Assistance, two endoscopes are used: one through a natural or artificial opening and the second one through percutaneous access. Surgeons choose this approach when they cannot perform the entire procedure through the natural or artificial opening. An example is vaginal hysterectomy performed with laparoscopic assistance (LAVH).

External

When the entire treatment is performed on the skin or mucous membranes, the approach is External. Examples of the external approach are a tonsillectomy and removal of a skin lesion. Another method for an external approach is applying direct or indirect pressure. An example is a closed fracture reduction.

The surgical approach is always documented in the procedure note, but it is not necessarily stated with the PCS terms listed here. For example, when using an open approach, the surgeon describes the initial incision, each subsequent division, and the layered closure, but may not use the word "open." When accessing the site through a natural or artificial opening, the documentation names the opening, such as vagina, but does state "via natural opening." Coders are responsible for interpreting the documentation and assigning the correct PCS value based on PCS definitions.

In addition to the surgical approach, some procedures also identify the directional approach. For example, procedures on the spine may be performed from a posterior or anterior approach and, in some cases, both. When the directional approach is not explicitly stated, the coder can determine it based on the location of the incision.

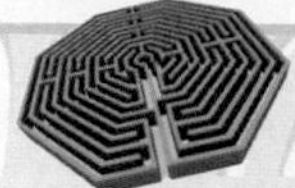

Coding Practice

Refresh your knowledge of terminology related to Medical and Surgical procedures. Use a medical terminology text or a website such as GlobalRph.com > Medical Terminology **http://www.globalrph.com/medterm.htm** to identify the meaning of word parts that may not be familiar to you.

Exercise 27.1 Medical and Surgical Refresher

Instructions: Use your medical terminology skills and resources to define the following terms, then look them up in the ICD-10-PCS Index.

Follow these steps:

- Use slash marks "/" to break down each term into its root(s) and suffix.
- Define the meaning of the word, based on the meaning of each word part.
- Look up the term in the ICD-10-PCS Index, and write down the **name(s)** of Root Operation(s) the Index cross references you to.
- Do not assign any codes.

Example: gastrectomy gastr/ectomy Meaning: *excision of the stomach* Root Operation(s): *Excision, Resection*

1. angioplasty Meaning ______ Root Operation(s) ______
2. hysterectomy Meaning ______ Root Operation(s) ______
3. ovariocentesis Meaning ______ Root Operation(s) ______
4. arthrodesis Meaning ______ Root Operation(s) ______
5. herniorrhaphy Meaning ______ Root Operation(s) ______
6. adhesiolysis Meaning ______ Root Operation(s) ______
7. colostomy Meaning ______ Root Operation(s) ______
8. tracheotomy Meaning ______ Root Operation(s) ______
9. esophagoplication Meaning ______ Root Operation(s) ______
10. cholecystopexy Meaning ______ Root Operation(s) ______

CODING OVERVIEW OF MEDICAL AND SURGICAL PROCEDURES

The Medical and Surgical Section is the largest Section of ICD-10-PCS, containing 31 Body Systems and 31 Root Operations. ICD-10-PCS provides Guidelines for Medical and Surgical codes in section B of the Guidelines. Six subdivisions of the Guidelines, B2 through B7 correspond to each character within a Medical and Surgical code.

CODING CAUTION

If you are already familiar with CPT® coding for physicians, be careful to not confuse CPT guidelines with PCS guidelines. The two are not comparable and, sometimes, are contradictory.

The Section value for Medical and Surgical is **0**. The characters of Medical and Surgical procedure codes are shown in ■ TABLE 27-2. Chapter 26 provided an overview of the general purpose of the characters in the Medical and Surgical Section. In the following sections, additional coding requirements for Characters 2 through 7 are highlighted.

Character 2: Medical and Surgical Body System

The second character in the Medical and Surgical Section defines the Body System, the general physiological system or anatomical region. PCS divides most organ systems into multiple Body System values in order to achieve greater granularity (■ TABLE 27-3).

Values **W**, **X**, and **Y** describe Anatomic Regions, which are used when a procedure is performed on an area that is larger than a specific Body Part (Guideline B2.1a). Examples include the following types of procedures:

- control of postprocedural bleeding in an extremity
- amputation of all or part of an extremity
- drainage of a body cavity

The Index is organized by Root Operation with the first-level subterm often being the Body System. Coders must select the most specific Body System value available. Search for a subterm that identifies the specific Body System before selecting a subterm for an anatomic region.

Table 27-2 ■ **SEVEN CHARACTERS OF MEDICAL AND SURGICAL PROCEDURES**

1	2	3	4	5	6	7
Section 0	Body System	Root Operation	Body Part	Approach	Device	Qualifier

Table 27-3 ■ **MEDICAL AND SURGICAL CHARACTER 2: BODY SYSTEM VALUES WITH ORGAN SYSTEM**

Value	PCS Body System Description	Traditional Organ System
0	Central Nervous System	Nervous system
1	Peripheral Nervous System	
2	Heart and Great Vessels	Cardiovascular system
3	Upper Arteries	
4	Lower Arteries	
5	Upper Veins	
6	Lower Veins	
7	Lymphatic and Hemic System	Blood and immune system
8	Eye	Special senses
9	Ear, Nose, Sinus	Special senses (Ear) and Respiratory system
B	Respiratory System	
C	Mouth and Throat	Digestive system
D	Gastrointestinal System	
F	Hepatobiliary System and Pancreas	
G	Endocrine System	Endocrine system
H	Skin and Breast	Integumentary system
J	Subcutaneous Tissue and Fascia	
K	Muscles	Muscular system
L	Tendons	
M	Bursae and Ligaments	
N	Head and Facial Bones	Skeletal system
P	Upper Bones	
Q	Lower Bones	
R	Upper Joints	
S	Lower Joints	
T	Urinary System	Genitourinary system
U	Female Reproductive System	
V	Male Reproductive System	
W	Anatomical Regions, General	Body areas
X	Anatomical Regions, Upper Extremities	
Y	Anatomical Regions, Lower Extremities	

Adapted from: Department of Health and Human Services, Centers for Medicare and Medicaid Services, accessed: http://www.cms.gov/ICD10/Downloads/2012_Code_Tables_and_Index.zip/pcs_2012.pdf

Character 3: Medical and Surgical Root Operation

The Medical and Surgical Section has 31 Root Operations, the most of any Section. Root Operations are the core of PCS coding because they serve as Main Terms in the Index. Coders cannot assign a Root Operation based on the common meaning of a word such as removal or excision; they must apply the full definition that PCS provides in the Tables (Guideline B3.1a).

The PCS definition of all Root Operations appears in the appendix of most ICD-10-PCS coding manuals (■ TABLE 27-4). Root Operations are divided into groups

(text continued on page 555)

Table 27-4 ■ **ROOT OPERATION DEFINITIONS IN ALPHABETICAL ORDER, WITH EXPLANATIONS AND EXAMPLES**

Value	Root Operation	Description
0	Alteration	**Definition:** Modifying the anatomic structure of a body part without affecting the function of the body part. **Explanation:** Principal purpose is to improve appearance. **Includes/Examples:** Face lift, breast augmentation
1	Bypass	**Definition:** Altering the route of passage of the contents of a tubular body part. **Explanation:** Rerouting contents of a body part to a downstream area of the normal route, to a similar route and body part, or to an abnormal route and dissimilar body part. Includes one or more anastomoses, with or without the use of a device. **Includes/Examples:** Coronary artery bypass, colostomy formation
2	Change	**Definition:** Taking out or off a device from a body part and putting back an identical or similar device in or on the same body part without cutting or puncturing the skin or a mucous membrane. **Explanation:** All CHANGE procedures are coded using the approach EXTERNAL. **Includes/Examples:** Urinary catheter change, gastrostomy tube change
3	Control	**Definition:** Stopping, or attempting to stop, postprocedural bleeding. **Explanation:** The site of the bleeding is coded as an anatomical region and not to a specific body part. **Includes/Examples:** Control of post-prostatectomy hemorrhage, control of post-tonsillectomy hemorrhage
4	Creation	**Definition:** Making a new genital structure that does not take over the function of a body part. **Explanation:** Used only for sex change operations. **Includes/Examples:** Creation of vagina in a male, creation of penis in a female
5	Destruction	**Definition:** Physical eradication of all or a portion of a body part by the direct use of energy, force, or a destructive agent. **Explanation:** None of the body part is physically taken out. **Includes/Examples:** Fulguration of rectal polyp, cautery of skin lesion
6	Detachment	**Definition:** Cutting off all or a portion of the upper or lower extremities. **Explanation:** The body part value is the site of the detachment, with a qualifier if applicable to further specify the level where the extremity was detached. **Includes/Examples:** Below knee amputation, disarticulation of shoulder
7	Dilation	**Definition:** Expanding an orifice or the lumen of a tubular body part. **Explanation:** The orifice can be a natural orifice or an artificially created orifice. Accomplished by stretching a tubular body part using intraluminal pressure or by cutting part of the orifice or wall of the tubular body part. **Includes/Examples:** Percutaneous transluminal angioplasty, pyloromyotomy
8	Division	**Definition:** Cutting into a body part without draining fluids and/or gases from the body part in order to separate or transect a body part. **Explanation:** All or a portion of the body part is separated into two or more portions. **Includes/Examples:** Spinal cordotomy, osteotomy.
9	Drainage	**Definition:** Taking or letting out fluids and/or gases from a body part. **Explanation:** The qualifier DIAGNOSTIC is used to identify drainage procedures that are biopsies. **Includes/Examples:** Thoracentesis, incision and drainage

Table 27-4 ■ (continued)

Value	Root Operation	Description
B	Excision	**Definition:** Cutting out or off, without replacement, a portion of a body part. **Explanation:** The qualifier DIAGNOSTIC is used to identify excision procedures that are biopsies. **Includes/Examples:** Partial nephrectomy, liver biopsy
C	Extirpation	**Definition:** Taking or cutting out solid matter from a body part. **Explanation:** The solid matter may be an abnormal byproduct of a biological function or a foreign body; it may be imbedded in a body part or in the lumen of a tubular body part. The solid matter may or may not have been previously broken into pieces. **Includes/Examples:** Thrombectomy, choledocholithotomy
D	Extraction	**Definition:** Pulling or stripping out or off all or a portion of a body part by the use of force. **Explanation:** The qualifier DIAGNOSTIC is used to identify extraction procedures that are biopsies. **Includes/Examples:** Dilation and curettage, vein stripping
F	Fragmentation	**Definition:** Breaking solid matter in a body part into pieces. **Explanation:** Physical force (e.g., manual, ultrasonic) applied directly or indirectly is used to break the solid matter into pieces. The solid matter may be an abnormal byproduct of a biological function or a foreign body. The pieces of solid matter are not taken out. **Includes/Examples:** Extracorporeal shockwave lithotripsy, transurethral lithotripsy
G	Fusion	**Definition:** Joining together portions of an articular body part rendering the articular body part immobile. **Explanation:** The body part is joined together by fixation device, bone graft, or other means. **Includes/Examples:** Spinal fusion, ankle arthrodesis
H	Insertion	**Definition:** Putting in a nonbiological appliance that monitors, assists, performs, or prevents a physiological function but does not physically take the place of a body part. **Includes/Examples:** Insertion of radioactive implant, insertion of central venous catheter
J	Inspection	**Definition:** Visually and/or manually exploring a body part. **Explanation:** Visual exploration may be performed with or without optical instrumentation. Manual exploration may be performed directly or through intervening body layers. **Includes/Examples:** Diagnostic arthroscopy, exploratory laparotomy
K	Map	**Definition:** Locating the route of passage of electrical impulses and/or locating functional areas in a body part. **Explanation:** Applicable only to the cardiac conduction mechanism and the central nervous system. **Includes/Examples:** Cardiac mapping, cortical mapping
L	Occlusion	**Definition:** Completely closing an orifice or the lumen of a tubular body part. **Explanation:** The orifice can be a natural orifice or an artificially created orifice. **Includes/Examples:** Fallopian tube ligation, ligation of inferior vena cava
M	Reattachment	**Definition:** Putting back in or on all or a portion of a separated body part to its normal location or other suitable location. **Explanation:** Vascular circulation and nervous pathways may or may not be reestablished. **Includes/Examples:** Reattachment of hand, reattachment of avulsed kidney
N	Release	**Definition:** Freeing a body part from an abnormal physical constraint by cutting or by the use of force. **Explanation:** Some of the restraining tissue may be taken out but none of the body part is taken out. **Includes/Examples:** Adhesiolysis, carpal tunnel release
P	Removal	**Definition:** Taking out or off a device from a body part. **Explanation:** If a device is taken out and a similar device put in without cutting or puncturing the skin or mucous membrane, the procedure is coded to the root operation CHANGE. Otherwise, the procedure for taking out a device is coded to the root operation REMOVAL. **Includes/Examples:** Drainage tube removal, cardiac pacemaker removal

(continued)

Table 27-4 ■ (continued)

Value	Root Operation	Description
Q	Repair	**Definition:** Restoring, to the extent possible, a body part to its normal anatomic structure and function. **Explanation:** Used only when the method to accomplish the repair is not one of the other root operations. **Includes/Examples:** Colostomy takedown, suture of laceration
R	Replacement	**Definition:** Putting in or on biological or synthetic material that physically takes the place and/or function of all or a portion of a body part. **Explanation:** The body part may have been taken out or replaced, or may be taken out, physically eradicated, or rendered nonfunctional during the Replacement procedure. A Removal procedure is coded for taking out the device used in a previous replacement procedure. **Includes/Examples:** Total hip replacement, bone graft, free skin graft
S	Reposition	**Definition:** Moving to its normal location, or other suitable location, all or a portion of a body part. **Explanation:** The body part is moved to a new location from an abnormal location, or from a normal location where it is not functioning correctly. The body part may or may not be cut out or off to be moved to the new location. **Includes/Examples:** Reposition of undescended testicle, fracture reduction
T	Resection	**Definition:** Cutting out or off, without replacement, all of a body part. **Includes/Examples:** Total nephrectomy, total lobectomy of lung
V	Restriction	**Definition:** Partially closing an orifice or the lumen of a tubular body part. **Explanation:** The orifice can be a natural orifice or an artificially created orifice. **Includes/Examples:** Esophagogastric fundoplication, cervical cerclage
W	Revision	**Definition:** Correcting, to the extent possible, a portion of a malfunctioning device or the position of a displaced device. **Explanation:** Revision can include correcting a malfunctioning or displaced device by taking out or putting in components of the device such as a screw or pin. **Includes/Examples:** Adjustment of position of pacemaker lead, recementing of hip prosthesis
U	Supplement	**Definition:** Putting in or on biological or synthetic material that physically reinforces and/or augments the function of a portion of a body part. **Explanation:** The biological material is non-living, or is living and from the same individual. The body part may have been previously replaced, and the Supplement procedure is performed to physically reinforce and/or augment the function of the replaced body part. **Includes/Examples:** Herniorrhaphy using mesh, free nerve graft, mitral valve ring annuloplasty, put a new acetabular liner in a previous hip replacement
X	Transfer	**Definition:** Moving, without taking out, all or a portion of a body part to another location to take over the function of all or a portion of a body part. **Explanation:** The body part transferred remains connected to its vascular and nervous supply. **Includes/Examples:** Tendon transfer, skin pedicle flap transfer
Y	Transplantation	**Definition:** Putting in or on all or a portion of a living body part taken from another individual or animal to physically take the place and/or function of all or a portion of a similar body part. **Explanation:** The native body part may or may not be taken out, and the transplanted body part may take over all or a portion of its function. **Includes/Examples:** Kidney transplant, heart transplant

Source: Department of Health and Human Services, Centers for Medicare and Medicaid Services, accessed: http://www.cms.gov/ICD10/Downloads/2012_Code_Tables_and_Index.zip/pcs_2012.pdf

of procedures with similar objectives in a separate appendix (■ TABLE 27-5). Use these tables when abstracting Medical and Surgical procedures.

SUCCESS STEP

The fact that PCS provides standard, official definitions for all parts of the code makes it unique among medical coding systems. Although it may feel intimidating to memorize definitions, they are a feature that makes the system user-friendly and logical.

Easily Confused Root Operations

Coders must distinguish between Root Operation definitions that sound similar. The following information highlights the differences between easily confused Root Operations. Refer back to Table 27-4 and Table 27-5 to review Root Operation definitions and examples.

Excision (B) and Resection (T). **Excision (B)** is cutting off a *portion* of a Body Part, as defined by PCS, and **Resection (T)** is cutting off *all* of a Body Part defined by PCS. The key to determining which Root Operation to use is to identify the Body Part values that a Root Operation Table provides. This may require that the coder review both the Table for **Excision** and the Table for **Resection** for a given Body System, in order to determine which Root Operation to use (Guideline B3.8).

The Body Part values determine if all or part of a Body Part was cut out. For example, each lobe of the lung has a separate Body Part value. When one entire lobe is cut out, use **Resection** to describe that the entire *lobe* was removed. Do not use **Excision** to describe that a portion of the entire organ, the *lung*, was removed, because a more specific Body Part is provided (■ FIGURE 27-1).

Occlusion (L) and Restriction (V). In an embolization procedure, the surgeon seeks to narrow or close a vessel. When the objective is to completely close the vessel, as in a tumor embolization, the Root Operation is **Occlusion (L)**, *completely closing an orifice or the lumen of a tubular body part*. The objective is to completely close off the blood supply.

When the objective is to narrow the vessel, as when treating an aneurysm, the Root Operation is **Restriction (V)**, *partially closing an orifice or the lumen of a tubular body part.* The objective is to narrow the diameter of the vessel at a point where it is abnormally wide (Guideline B3.12).

Destruction (5) and Fragmentation (F). The Root Operations **Destruction** and **Fragmentation** obliterate solid matter. **Destruction (5)** is *physical eradication of all or a portion of a body part by the direct use of energy, force, or a destructive agent*, and is directed toward an anatomical body part. None of the body part is physically taken out. Examples are fulguration of a rectal polyp or cautery of a skin lesion.

The target of **Fragmentation (F)** (*breaking solid matter in a body part into pieces*) is solid matter within a body part, such as a foreign body or an abnormal byproduct. The most common example is calculus, which can be destroyed using a number of different methods.

Insertion (H) and Supplement (U). The Root Operations Insertion and Supplement both place objects into the body. **Insertion (H)** is *putting in a nonbiological appliance that monitors, assists, performs, or prevents a physiological function but does not physically take the place of a body part.* Examples are insertion of a central venous catheter or a radioactive implant. These devices help the body perform its functions.

Supplement (U) is *putting in or on biological or synthetic material that physically reinforces and/or augments the function of a portion of a body part.* Examples are repairing a hernia with mesh or putting a new liner in a previous joint replacement. These devices provide physical reinforcement or strengthening. When coding either Insertion or Supplement, the device is specified in Character 6, Device. These Root Operations include accessing the site, performing the repair, if any, and placing the device. Do not code the incision or repair with an additional Root Operation.

Character 4: Medical and Surgical Body Part

The fourth character in the Medical and Surgical Section defines the Body Part, or specific anatomical site, where the physician performed the procedure. The definition of each Body Part value in the Medical and Surgical Section is unique to each Body System. For example, in Body System **8 Eye**, the Body Part value **1** is **Left Eye**. In Body System **L Tendons**, the Body Part value **1** is **Right Shoulder Tendon**. Body Parts appear as first- or second-level subterms in the Index. In most cases, the partial code in the Index directs coders not only to the correct Table, but also to the correct Character 4 value.

Table 27-5 ■ **ROOT OPERATION GROUPS, WITH PROCEDURE OBJECTIVE, SITE, AND EXAMPLES**

Root Operations That Take Out Some or All of a Body Part				
Root Operation	**Value**	**Objective of Procedure**	**Procedure Site**	**Example**
Excision	B	Cutting out/off without replacement	Some of a body part	Breast lumpectomy
Resection	T	Cutting out/off without replacement	All of a body part	Total mastectomy
Detachment	6	Cutting out/off without replacement	Extremity only, any level	Amputation above elbow
Destruction	5	Eradicating without replacement	Some/all of a body part	Fulguration of endometrium
Extraction	D	Pulling out/off without replacement	Some/all of a body part	Suction D&C
Root Operations That Take Out Solids/Fluids/Gases from a Body Part				
Root Operation	**Value**	**Objective of Procedure**	**Procedure Site**	**Example**
Drainage	9	Taking/letting out fluids/gases	Within a body part	Incision and drainage
Extirpation	C	Taking/cutting out solid matter	Within a body part	Thrombectomy
Fragmentation	F	Breaking solid matter into pieces	Within a body part	Lithotripsy
Root Operations Involving Cutting or Separation Only				
Root Operation	**Value**	**Objective of Procedure**	**Procedure Site**	**Example**
Division	8	Cutting into/separating a body part	Within a body part	Neurotomy
Release	N	Freeing a body part from constraint	Around a body part	Adhesiolysis
Root Operations That Put In/Put Back or Move Some/All of a Body Part				
Root Operation	**Value**	**Objective of Procedure**	**Procedure Site**	**Example**
Transplantation	Y	Putting in a living body part from a person/animal	Some/all of a body part	Kidney transplant
Reattachment	M	Putting back a detached body part	Some/all of a body part	Reattach finger
Transfer	X	Moving a body part to function for a similar body part	Some/all of a body part	Skin transfer flap
Reposition	S	Moving a body part to normal or other suitable location	Some/all of a body part	Move undescended testicle
Root Operations That Alter the Diameter/Route of a Tubular Body Part				
Root Operation	**Value**	**Objective of Procedure**	**Procedure Site**	**Example**
Restriction	V	Partially closing orifice/lumen	Tubular body part	Gastroesophageal fundoplication
Occlusion	L	Completely closing orifice/lumen	Tubular body part	Fallopian tube ligation
Dilation	7	Expanding orifice/lumen	Tubular body part	Percutaneous transluminal coronary angioplasty (PTCA)
Bypass	1	Altering route of passage	Tubular body part	Coronary artery bypass graft (CABG)
Root Operations That Always Involve a Device				
Root Operation	**Value**	**Objective of Procedure**	**Procedure Site**	**Example**
Insertion	H	Putting in non-biological device	In/on a body part	Central line insertion
Replacement	R	Putting in device that replaces a body part	Some/all of a body part	Total hip replacement
Supplement	U	Putting in device that reinforces or augments a body part	In/on a body part	Abdominal wall herniorrhaphy using mesh
Change	2	Exchanging device w/out cutting/ puncturing	In/on a body part	Drainage tube change

Table 27-5 ■ (continued)

Root Operations That Always Involve a Device				
Root Operation	**Value**	**Objective of Procedure**	**Procedure Site**	**Example**
Removal	P	Taking out device	In/on a body part	Central line removal
Revision	W	Correcting a malfunctioning/ displaced device	In/on a body part	Revision of pacemaker insertion
Root Operations Involving Examination Only				
Root Operation	**Value**	**Objective of Procedure**	**Procedure Site**	**Example**
Inspection	J	Visual/manual exploration	Some/all of a body part	Diagnostic cystoscopy
Map	K	Location electrical impulses/ functional areas	Brain/cardiac conduction mechanism	Cardiac electrophysiological study
Root Operations That Define Other Repairs				
Root Operation	**Value**	**Objective of Procedure**	**Procedure Site**	**Example**
Control	3	Stopping/attempting to stop postprocedural bleed	Anatomical region	Post-prostatectomy bleeding control
Repair	Q	Restoring body part to its normal structure	Some/all of a body part	Suture laceration
Root Operations That Define Other Objectives				
Root Operation	**Value**	**Objective of Procedure**	**Procedure Site**	**Example**
Fusion	G	Rendering joint immobile	Joint	Spinal fusion
Alteration	0	Modifying body part for cosmetic purposes without affecting function	Some/all of a body part	Face lift
Creation	4	Making new structure for sex change operation	Perineum	Artificial vagina/penis

Source: Department of Health and Human Services, Centers for Medicare and Medicaid Services, accessed: http://www.cms.gov/ICD10/Downloads/2012_pcs_ref_manual.pdf

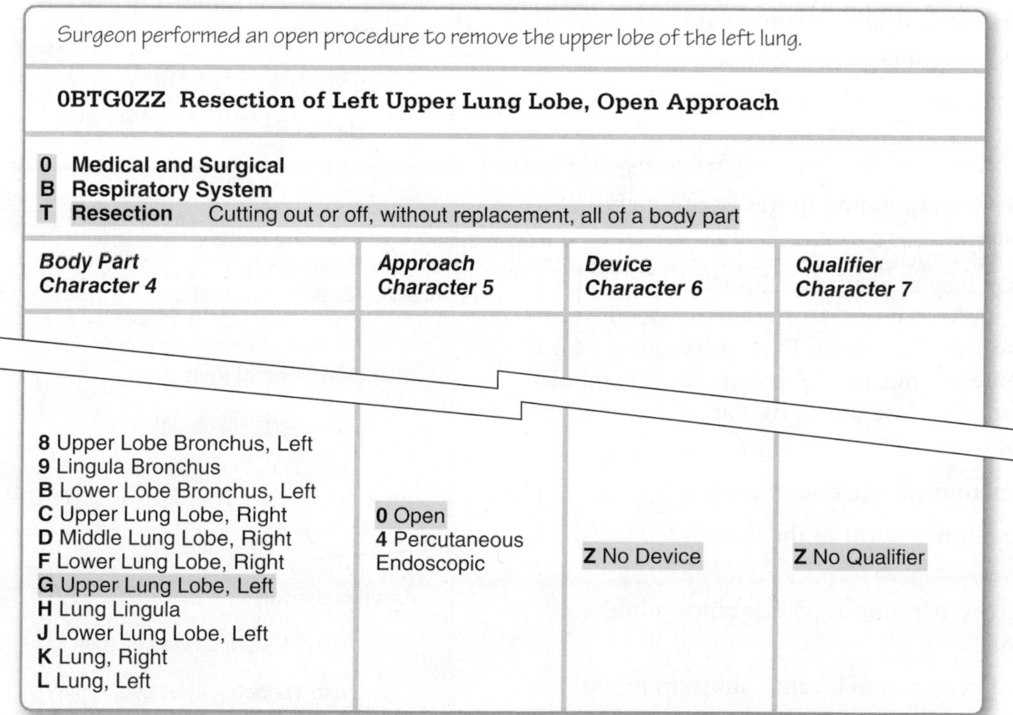

Figure 27-1 ■ Example of Coding Resection Instead of Excision

The challenge for coders is matching the documented anatomical site to the most specific PCS Body System and Body Part value. For example, under the Root Operation **Reposition**, PCS provides Body System and Body Part values for the following sites in the upper arm:

- muscles of the upper arm
- tendons of the upper arm
- head of the humerus
- shaft of the humerus
- acrominoclavicular joint

Each of these is a separate Index entry (■ FIGURE 27-2) under Root Operation **Reposition (S)**. The Body System and Body Part values differ. It would be easy to miss the entry, **humeral head**, and focus instead on the entry for **upper arm** without noticing the previous level subterm which identifies the Body System as **Muscle, Tendon,** or **Joint.**

Another challenge with Body Parts is that the site documented in the medical record may be more specific, or use a different term, than what PCS provides. Guideline B4 specifies how to code Body Parts for various Body Systems. Assign a code for the closest body part, branch, or region for which PCS provides a value.

The Index includes entries for many anatomical sites that direct coders to the PCS Body Part to use. Anatomical site entries do not provide a partial code or Table number; they simply identify the PCS Body Part (■ FIGURE 27-3). Coders still need to locate the corresponding Root Operation as an Index Main Term in order to identify the correct Table, as follows:

1. Identify the anatomical site documented.
2. Locate the anatomical term in the Index.
3. Identify the corresponding PCS Body Part description which appears after the word *use*.
4. Use the PCS description to select the Body Part value from the Table corresponding to the Root Operation and Body System.

The Body Part Key appendix of the PCS manual provides a helpful table that cross-references specific anatomical terms to the PCS Body Part (■ TABLE 27-6). If an anatomical site cannot be located in the Index, also refer to this appendix . Use the Body Part Key as follows (■ FIGURE 27-4):

1. Identify the anatomical site documented.
2. Locate the anatomical term in the first column.
3. Identify the corresponding PCS description in the second column.
4. Use the PCS description to locate a subterm in the Index, or select the Body Part value from the Table corresponding to the Root Operation and Body System.

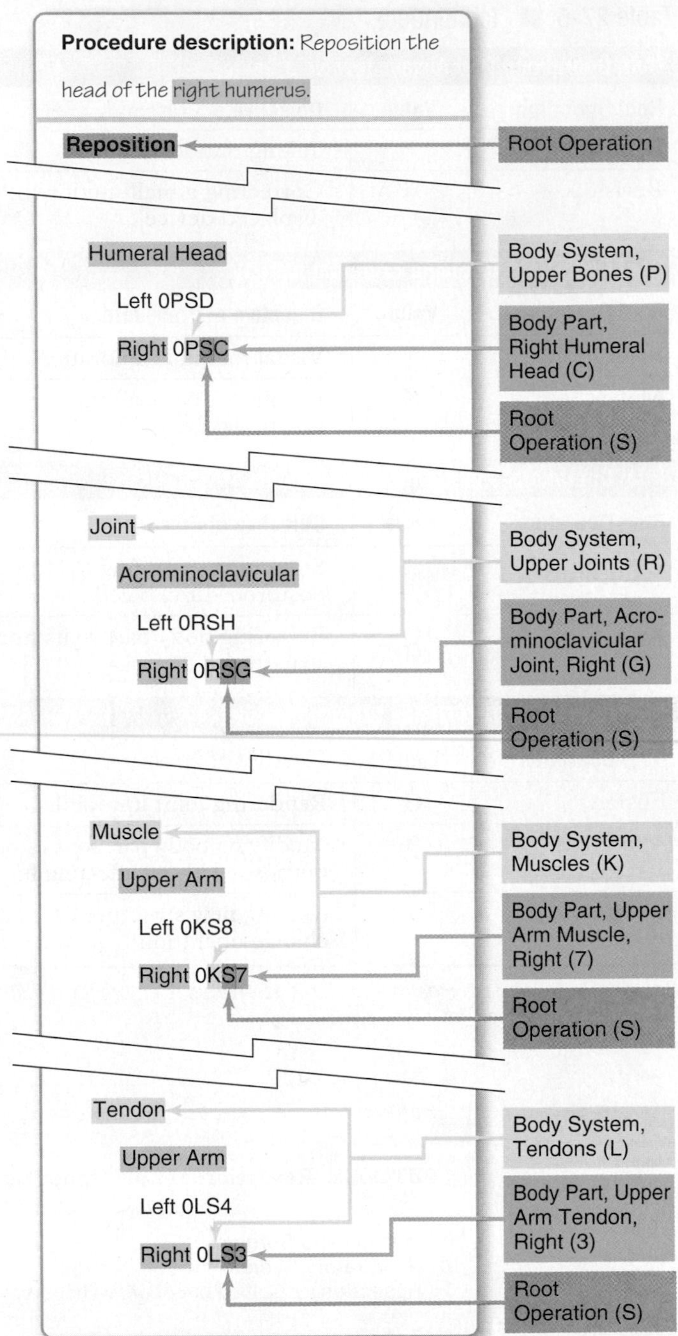

Figure 27-2 ■ Example of Locating the Correct Body Part in the Index

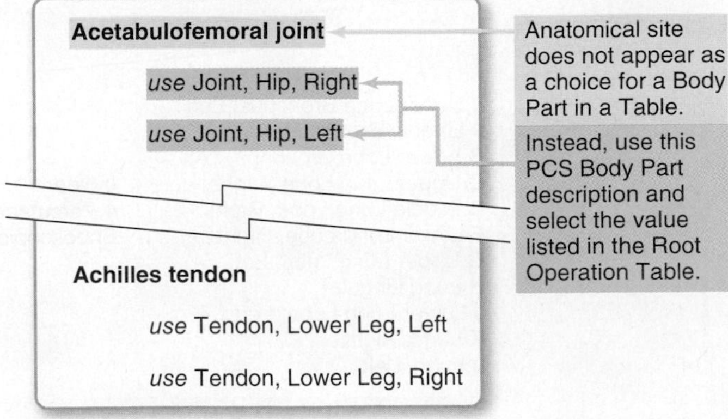

Figure 27-3 ■ Index Entry for an Anatomical Site with Cross-Reference to PCS Body Part

Table 27-6 ■ **EXCERPT FROM PCS BODY PART KEY APPENDIX**

Anatomical Term	PCS Description
Acetabulofemoral joint	Hip Joint, Right Hip Joint, Left
Achilles tendon	Lower Leg Tendon, Right Lower Leg Tendon, Left
Alveolar process of maxilla	Maxilla, Right Maxilla, Left
Aortic intercostal artery	Thoracic Aorta

Source: Department of Health and Human Services, Centers for Medicare and Medicaid Services, accessed: http://www.cms.gov/ICD10/Downloads/2012_Code_Tables_and_Index.zip/pcs_2012.pdf

Character 5: Medical and Surgical Approach

The Medical and Surgical Section uses seven different values to define the Approach (■ TABLE 27-7, page 560). An appendix in most ICD-10-PCS manuals defines each Approach, which was also defined earlier in this chapter of the text. Guideline B5 discusses specific coding situations related to an open approach with percutaneous endoscopic assistance, the external approach, and percutaneous procedures performed with a device such as fragmentation of kidney stones performed via percutaneous nephrostomy.

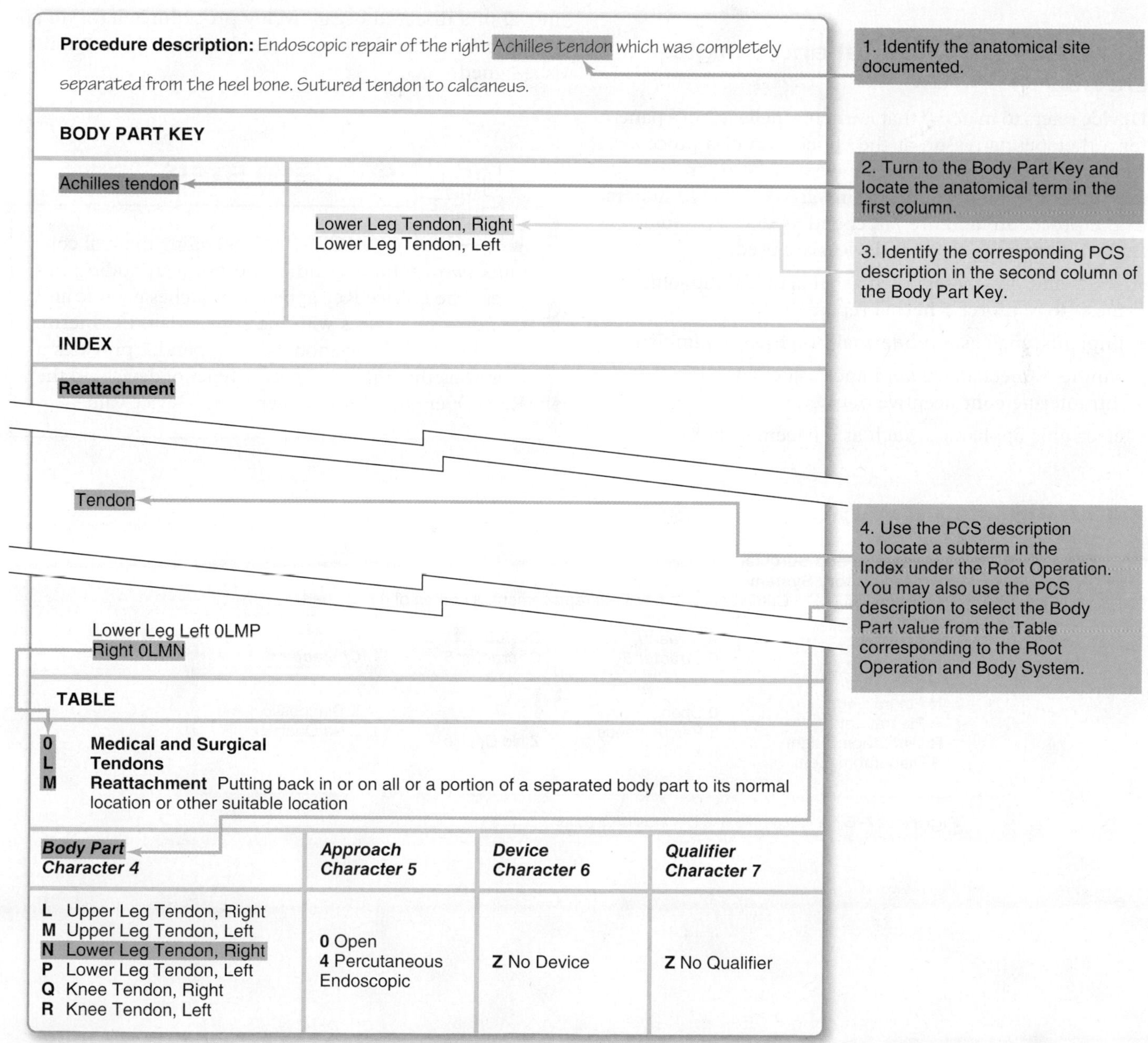

Figure 27-4 ■ Example of Using the Body Part Key Appendix to PCS Body Part

Table 27-7 ■ **VALUES FOR MEDICAL AND SURGICAL APPROACH**

Value	Approach
0	Open
3	Percutaneous
4	Percutaneous Endoscopic
7	Via Natural or Artificial Opening
8	Via Natural or Artificial Opening Endoscopic
F	Via Natural or Artificial Opening Endoscopic with Percutaneous Endoscopic Assistance
X	External

Source: Department of Health and Human Services, Centers for Medicare and Medicaid Services, accessed: http://www.cms.gov/ICD10/Downloads/2012_pcs_ref_manual.pdf

Character 6: Medical and Surgical Device

Device refers to material that is intentionally left in a patient for a therapeutic reason at the conclusion of a procedure. Material such as sutures, radiological markers, and temporary post-operative wound drains are considered integral to the procedure and are *not* coded as devices (Guideline B6.1b). Four basic types of devices are used:

- grafts and prostheses, such as an artificial hip joint or mesh to reinforce a hernia repair
- implants, such as a subdermal progesterone implant
- simple or mechanical appliances, such as an intrauterine contraceptive device
- electronic appliances, such as a pacemaker

Refer to the Character 6 column in the Table for a Root Operation to identify the Device values that are available for each procedure. Frequently, no device is used, so assign **Z No Device** for Character 6. Device guidelines appear in Guideline B6.

Character 7: Medical and Surgical Qualifier

The Qualifier character describes a wide range of additional attributes that may be applicable to a procedure. One of the most common Qualifier values is **X Diagnostic** (■ Figure 27-5). Some procedures may be done either to help diagnose a disease or to treat it. For example, an excisional biopsy is coded as the Root Operation **Excision (B)** with the Qualifier **Diagnostic (X)**. Excision may also be performed for treatment purposes, such as removal of a diseased organ. Many procedures have no applicable Qualifier, in which case the value **Z No Qualifier** is assigned.

SUCCESS STEP

The ICD-10-PCS coding manual contains two useful appendices to assist in coding devices. The Device Key appendix matches generic and brand name devices with the appropriate PCS term. The Device Aggregation Table appendix provides a crosswalk that matches specific types of devices to the Root Operation, Body System, and Device value.

0 Medical and Surgical
B Respiratory System
B Excision Cutting out or off, without replacement, a portion of a body part

Body Part Character 4	*Approach Character 5*	*Device Character 6*	*Qualifier Character 6*
N Pleura, Right P Pleura, Left R Diaphragm, Right S Diaphragm, Left	0 Open 3 Percutaneous 4 Percutaneous Endoscopic	Z No Device	X Diagnostic Z No Qualifier

Figure 27-5 ■ Example of a Diagnostic Qualifier

Coding Practice

Take this opportunity to become familiar with Root Operation definitions and values.

Exercise 27.2 Coding Overview of Medical and Surgical Procedures

Instructions: Use the appendix Root Operation Definitions in the ICD-10-PCS manual to identify the following Medical and Surgical Root Operations. Write the name and character value on the lines provided.

Example: Cutting out or off, without replacement, a portion of a body part — Root Operation: *Excision* — Value: *B*

1. Cutting into a body part, without draining fluids and/or gases from the body part, in order to separate or transect a body part — Root Operation ________ Value ________
2. Putting in a non-biological appliance that monitors, assists, performs, or prevents a physiological function but does not physically take the place of a body part — Root Operation ________ Value ________
3. Pulling or stripping out or off all or a portion of a body part by the use of force — Root Operation ________ Value ________
4. Stopping, or attempting to stop, postprocedural bleeding — Root Operation ________ Value ________
5. Taking out or off a device from a body part — Root Operation ________ Value ________
6. Putting in or on biological or synthetic material that physically reinforces and/or augments the function of a portion of a body part — Root Operation ________ Value ________
7. Expanding an orifice or the lumen of a tubular body part — Root Operation ________ Value ________
8. Physical eradication of all or a portion of a body part by the direct use of energy, force, or a destructive agent — Root Operation ________ Value ________
9. Restoring, to the extent possible, a body part to its normal anatomic structure and function — Root Operation ________ Value ________
10. Expanding an orifice or the lumen of a tubular body part — Root Operation ________ Value ________

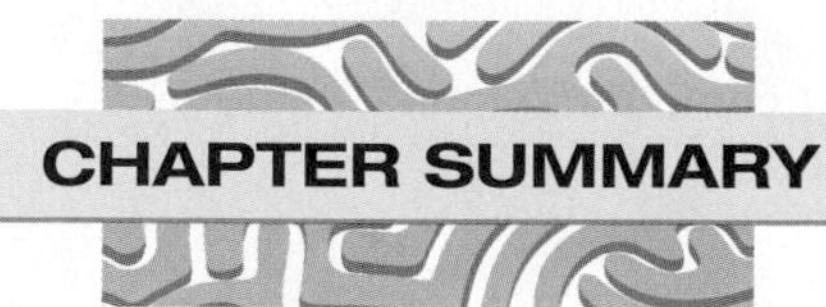

CHAPTER SUMMARY

In this chapter you learned that:

- Coders need to understand the difference between treatments and diagnostic procedures as well as the description of various surgical approaches.
- The Medical and Surgical Section is the largest Section of ICD-10-PCS, containing 31 Body Systems and 31 Root Operations.
- ICD-10-PCS provides Guidelines for Medical and Surgical codes in section B of the Guidelines, which contains six subdivisions corresponding to each character within a Medical and Surgical code.

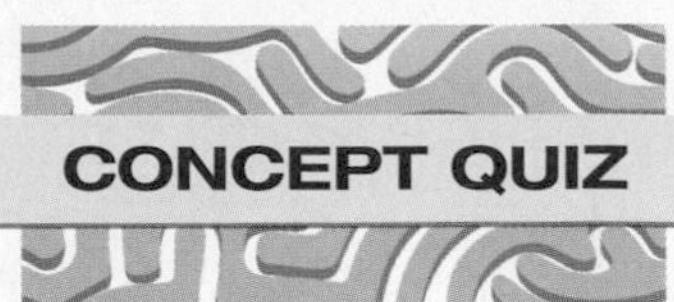

CONCEPT QUIZ

Take a moment to look back at your trip through Medical and Surgical procedures and solidify your skills. This is your opportunity to pull together everything you have learned.

Completion

Instructions: Use the Body Part Key appendix in the ICD-10-PCS manual to identify the PCS description for each anatomical term. Search for the anatomical term in the left column of the Body Part Key, then write down the PCS description from the right column. Some choices may be used more than once and some choices may not be used at all. Refer to the discussion in this chapter if you need a little extra help.

Example: Achilles tendon Lower Leg Tendon

Ampulla of Vater	Pelvic Bone
Basal Ganglia	Pelvic Bone
Colic Vein	Pons
Common Bile Duct	Prepuce
External Iliac Artery	Pulmonary Artery, Left
Facial Muscle	Small Intestine
Greater Omentum	Trigeminal Nerve
Greater Saphenous Vein	Uterine Supporting Structure
Intracranial Vein	Vas Deferens
Pancreatic Duct	

1. Anterior cerebral vein ____________
2. Duct of Wirsung ____________
3. Gasserian ganglion ____________
4. Basis pontis ____________
5. Broad ligament ____________
6. Hepatopancreatic ampulla ____________
7. Botallo's duct ____________
8. Glans penis ____________
9. External pudendal vein ____________
10. Iliac crest ____________

Multiple Choice

Instructions: Circle the letter of the best answer to each question based on the information you learned in this chapter. Refer to the discussion in this chapter and the Glossary at the end of this book if you need a little extra help.

1. What Approach is used for a procedure in which an incision is made through the skin and subcutaneous tissue?
   A. Open
   B. Percutaneous
   C. Percutaneous Endoscopic
   D. External
2. What Approach is used for a procedure in which the endoscope is inserted through the anus?
   A. Percutaneous Endoscopic
   B. Via Natural or Artificial Opening
   C. External
   D. Via Natural or Artificial Opening Endoscopic
3. Which of the following is a Body System in ICD-10-PCS?
   A. Digestive System
   B. Skeletal System
   C. Upper Bones
   D. Cardiovascular System
4. Destruction of calculus is an example of which Root Operation?
   A. Excision
   B. Destruction
   C. Fragmentation
   D. Removal
5. Tumor embolization is an example of which Root Operation?
   A. Resection
   B. Occlusion
   C. Destruction
   D. Restriction
6. What Root Operation is used when the procedure involves cutting out the left upper lobe of the lung?
   A. Repair
   B. Resection
   C. Removal
   D. Excision
7. One of the most common Qualifier values is
   A. T Therapeutic.
   B. X Diagnostic.
   C. 0 Open.
   D. R Bilateral.
8. A procedure that leaves a drainage device in the patient is by definition
   A. therapeutic.
   B. diagnostic.
   C. exploratory.
   D. supplemental.

9. Which of the following Root Operations takes out solids/fluids/gases from a Body Part?
   A. Alteration
   B. Dilation
   C. Extirpation
   D. Extraction

10. Which of the following Root Operations always involves a device?
   A. Change
   B. Drainage
   C. Occlusion
   D. Reposition

CODING CHALLENGE

Now it is your turn to demonstrate your understanding of Root Operations for Medical and Surgical procedures. Refer back to the examples and discussion in this chapter when you need a little extra help. Use your medical dictionary and anatomy references when needed.

Instructions: Determine the Root Operation for each procedure listed. Use the Index to look up the Root Operation and the corresponding Body Part. Write the partial code in the blank. **Do not assign the entire code**.

Example: Removed the entire descending colon — Root Operation: Resection — Partial Code: ODTM

1. Sigmoidoscopy with removal of a sigmoid polyp — Root Operation ____________ Partial Code ________
2. Open reduction of left tibial fracture — Root Operation ____________ Partial Code ________
3. Cystoscopy with dilation of constricted bladder neck — Root Operation ____________ Partial Code ________
4. Cautery of a nosebleed — Root Operation ____________ Partial Code ________
5. Amputation of right leg at the knee — Root Operation ____________ Partial Code ________
6. Laparoscopic cholecystectomy — Root Operation ____________ Partial Code ________
7. Pulling out the nail of right index finger — Root Operation ____________ Partial Code ________
8. Removal of metal shards from the left upper eyelid with tweezers — Root Operation ____________ Partial Code ________
9. Cervical cerclage performed transvaginally — Root Operation ____________ Partial Code ________
10. Taking out a cardiac pacemaker from the chest wall — Root Operation ____________ Partial Code ________

KEEP ON CODING

Instructions: Determine the Root Operation for each procedure listed. Use the Index to look up the Root Operation and the corresponding Body Part. Write the partial code in the blank. **Do not assign the entire code.**

Example: Removed the entire descending colon — Root Operation: Resection — Partial Code: ODTM

1. Drainage of fluid, left knee joint — Root Operation ____________ Partial Code ________
2. Change of Foley catheter — Root Operation ____________ Partial Code ________

3. Right carpal tunnel release Root Operation ______________________ Partial Code ________
4. Reduction of fractured left wrist Root Operation ______________________ Partial Code ________
5. Tonsillectomy Root Operation ______________________ Partial Code ________
6. Varicose vein stripping, left lower leg Root Operation ______________________ Partial Code ________
7. Left inguinal hernia repair Root Operation ______________________ Partial Code ________
8. Extracorporeal shockwave lithotripsy (EWSL), right kidney Root Operation ______________________ Partial Code ________
9. Rhinoplasty of acquired deformity Root Operation ______________________ Partial Code ________
10. Colostomy of ascending colon Root Operation ______________________ Partial Code ________
11. Total thyroidectomy Root Operation ______________________ Partial Code ________
12. Post partum bilateral fallopian tube ligation Root Operation ______________________ Partial Code ________
13. Biopsy of the ileum Root Operation ______________________ Partial Code ________
14. Amputation of right forearm Root Operation ______________________ Partial Code ________
15. Facelift Root Operation ______________________ Partial Code ________
16. Left knee replacement Root Operation ______________________ Partial Code ________
17. Hernia repair, left, with mesh reinforcement Root Operation ______________________ Partial Code ________
18. Heart transplant Root Operation ______________________ Partial Code ________
19. Cystoscopy for hematuria Root Operation ______________________ Partial Code ________
20. Endotracheal intubation Root Operation ______________________ Partial Code ________
21. Removal of a drainage tube from the gallbladder Root Operation ______________________ Partial Code ________
22. Clipping of right femoral aneurysm Root Operation ______________________ Partial Code ________
23. Control of post operative bleeding of the esophagus Root Operation ______________________ Partial Code ________
24. Fusion of right ankle joint Root Operation ______________________ Partial Code ________
25. Transfer of the hypoglossal nerve Root Operation ______________________ Partial Code ________

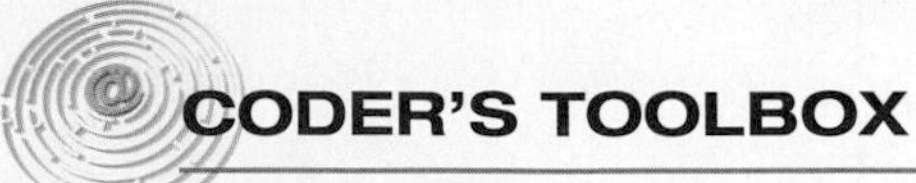

CODER'S TOOLBOX

The following resources are a starting point for learning more about medical and surgical procedures. The > symbol indicates a menu selection within the website in order to navigate to a specific page.

American Cancer Society > Treatments and Side Effects > Treatment Types > Surgery http://www.cancer.org/Treatment/TreatmentsandSideEffects/TreatmentTypes/Surgery/surgery-treatment-toc

Encyclopedia of Surgery http://www.surgeryencyclopedia.com/

Society of American Gastrointestinal and Endoscopic Surgeons (SAGES) http://www.sages.org/publication/id/PI11/

Web MD > A to Z Guides > Health Features > Surgery Lite > Understanding Endoscopic Surgery http://www.webmd.com/a-to-z-guides/features/understanding-endoscopic-surgery

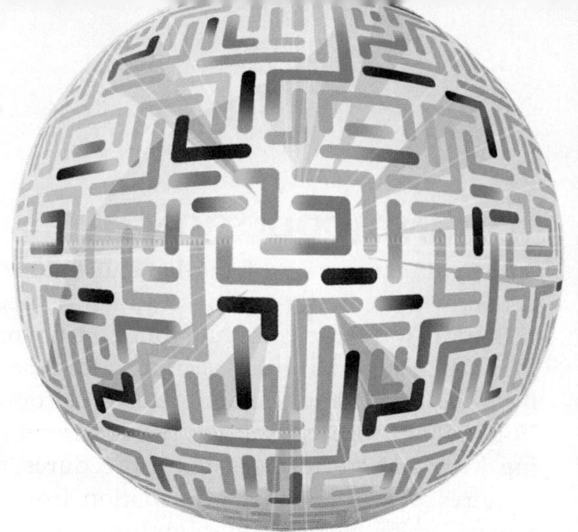

28

Medical and Surgical Procedures (Section 0), Part 2

Learning Objectives

After completing this chapter, you should have the skills to:

- Spell and define the key words, medical terms, and abbreviations related to Medical and Surgical procedure coding.
- Abstract information from the medical record for Medical and Surgical Root Operations and procedures.
- Assign codes for Medical and Surgical procedures.
- Arrange codes for Medical and Surgical procedures.
- Discuss PCS Guidelines for Medical and Surgical procedures.

Key Terms and Abbreviations

operative report   procedure report

In addition to the key terms listed here, students should know the terms defined within tables in this chapter.

Chapter Outline

- **Abstracting Medical and Surgical Procedures**
- **Assigning Medical and Surgical Procedure Codes**
- **Arranging Medical and Surgical Procedure Codes**

ICD-10-PCS codes in this chapter are from the ICD-10-PCS 2014 Draft code set from the Department of Health and Human Services, Centers for Medicare and Medicaid Services.

INTRODUCTION

After you get the lay-of-the-land in a large sightseeing venue, you are better equipped to enjoy specific parts of it that are most appealing. In your continuing tour of the PCS Medical and Surgical section in this chapter, you will have the opportunity to sink your teeth into the details. You will practice coding for patient encounters involving Medical and Surgical PCS procedures, a skill which requires you to abstract information from the medical record, assign correct codes, and arrange (sequence) the codes in the proper order.

As you read this chapter, open up your medical terminology book and keep a medical dictionary handy to refresh your memory of any unfamiliar terms. These are your resources that provide the information you need to be successful. A hallmark of a professional coder is someone who is always learning and referring to resources to increase their knowledge and skills. Also refer to the websites and organizations listed in Coder's Toolbox at the end of the chapter for specialized information about procedure coding.

ABSTRACTING MEDICAL AND SURGICAL PROCEDURES

Because identifying the correct Root Operation is the basis of ICD-10-PCS coding, coders must learn the differences between similar Root Operations. This enables them to abstract appropriately. Physicians are not expected to use PCS terminology when documenting. Coders must read what physicians document and equate it to the definitions provided by PCS (Guideline A11). Refer to Guideline B3, which provides further details on Root Operations. Then, follow key criteria for abstracting Medical and Surgical procedures in order to identify the correct Root Operation.

Key Criteria for Abstracting Medical and Surgical Procedures

In order to abstract for Medical and Surgical procedures, coders need to determine what procedures were performed and what approach was used. After reading the procedure report, use the abstracting table (■ TABLE 28-1) as follows:

1. Answer the General Questions in order to get a basic understanding of the procedure.
2. Answer the Root Operation Questions. One question should be answered *Yes*, the rest should be answered *No*.
3. For the Root Operation Question that was answered *Yes*, refer to the right-hand column to identify the Root Operations that could apply.
4. Look up the definition of each of the applicable Root Operations in the ICD-10-PCS coding manual appendix, Root Operation Definitions, or, Comparison of Medical and Surgical Root Operations.
5. Identify the one Root Operation that matches the procedure documented. This Root Operation will be the Main Term when you use the Index.
6. Repeat the abstracting process for each procedure that was performed.

Abstracting criteria for Medical and Surgical-Related procedures and Ancillary procedures are presented in later chapters.

CODING CAUTION

In order to assign a Root Operation, its full definition in the PCS manual must be applied (Guideline B3.1a). If the full definition is not applicable, continue searching for another Root Operation.

SUCCESS STEP

Each of the Root Operation questions in Table 28-1 correlates with one of the nine Root Operation groups in the Comparison of Medical and Surgical Root Operations appendix of the ICD-10-PCS manual. The first question relates to the first group in this appendix, the second question relates to the second group in this appendix, and so forth.

Abstracting Procedure Reports

After completing a procedure, physicians prepare a **procedure report** or **operative report** that describes the details of what was done. The format varies with each physician or hospital, but must include the following information:

- date of procedure
- name of procedure performed
- names of the surgeon and all assistants
- preprocedure or provisional diagnosis
- a detailed description of the procedure, such as patient preparation, anesthesia, instruments and supplies used, incisions made, visualized structures, findings, alterations performed, tissue removed, estimated blood loss, closing process, and patient status
- postprocedure diagnosis

The procedure report may be dictated, then transcribed, or entered directly into an electronic medical record (EMR). The procedure report is maintained in a

Table 28-1 ■ **KEY CRITERIA FOR ABSTRACTING MEDICAL AND SURGICAL PROCEDURES**

General Questions	
❑ What is the stated procedure?	
❑ What organ or body part is involved?	
❑ Is the procedure description what you would expect based on the name of the procedure?	
❑ What surgical approach is used?	
❑ Was more than one procedure, or a combined procedure, performed?	
Root Operation Questions	**Root Operation (Value)**
❑ Did the procedure take out some or all of a body part without replacement?	Destruction (5) Detachment (6) Excision (B) Extraction (D) Resection (T)
❑ Did the procedure take out solids, fluids, or gases from a body part?	Drainage (9) Extirpation (C) Fragmentation (F)
❑ Did the procedure involve cutting or separation only, within or around a body part?	Division (8) Release (N)
❑ Did the procedure put in, put back, or move some or all of a body part?	Reattachment (M) Reposition (S) Transfer (X) Transplantation (Y)
❑ Did the procedure alter the diameter or route of a tubular body part?	Bypass (1) Dilation (7) Occlusion (L) Restriction (V)
❑ Did the procedure involve an external device left in place in, on, or in replacement of a body part?	Change (2) Insertion (H) Removal (P) Replacement (R) Revision (W) Supplement (U)
❑ Did the procedure involve examination only?	Inspection (J) Map (K)
Operations Involving Other Repairs	
❑ Did the procedure stop or attempt to stop postprocedural bleeding?	Control (3)
❑ Did the procedure restore a body part to its normal structure?	Repair (Q)
Operations Involving Other Objectives	
❑ Did the procedure render a joint immobile?	Fusion (G)
❑ Was the procedure for cosmetic purposes only, without affecting the function of the body part?	Alteration (0)
❑ Was the procedure a sex change operation?	Creation (4)

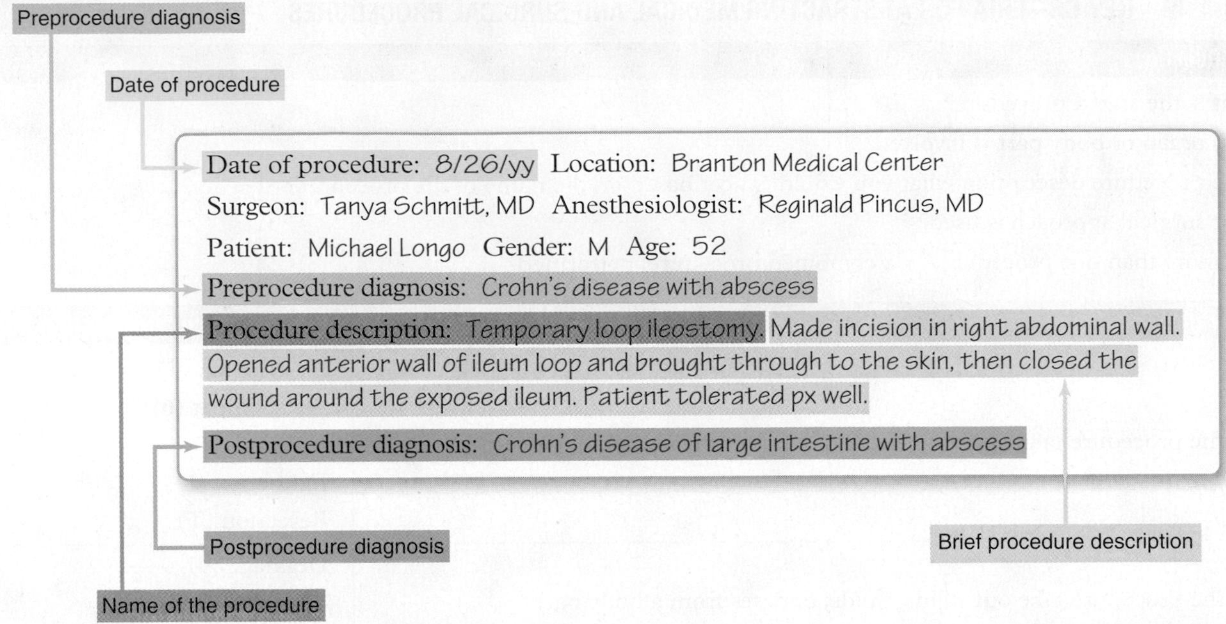

Figure 28-1 ■ Key to Interpreting the Procedure Report Mini-Medical-Record

designated section of the patient's overall medical record. The mini-medical-record used for procedure cases in this text provides a limited snapshot of the most pertinent information. Refer to ■ FIGURE 28-1 to learn how to interpret the mini-medical-record used for procedure reports.

Guided Example of Abstracting Procedures

To practice skills for abstracting procedures, refer to the following the example of Michael Longo, who had an ileostomy at Branton Medical Center, which will be used throughout this chapter. Marcy Elwood, CCS, is the fictitious coder at the hospital who guides you through the coding process.

> Date of procedure: 8/26/yy Location: Branton Medical Center Surgeon: Tanya Schmitt, MD
>
> Anesthesiologist: Reginald Pincus, MD
>
> Patient: Michael Longo Gender: M Age: 52
>
> Preprocedure diagnosis: Crohn's disease with abscess
>
> Procedure description: Temporary loop ileostomy. Made incision in right abdominal wall. Opened anterior wall of ileum loop and brought through to the skin, then closed the wound around the exposed ileum. Patient tolerated px (*procedure*) well.
>
> Postprocedure diagnosis: Crohn's disease of large intestine with abscess

Follow along as Marcy Elwood, CCS, abstracts the Root Operation from the medical record. Check off each step after you complete it.

⇨ Marcy reads through the procedure report, with special attention to the preprocedure diagnosis, the procedure name and description, and the postprocedure diagnosis.

⇨ Marcy refers to Key Criteria for Abstracting Medical and Surgical Procedures (Table 28-1).

- ☐ *What is the procedure?* temporary loop ileostomy (■ FIGURE 28-2)
- ☐ *What organ or body part is involved?* the ileum
- ☐ *Is the procedure description what you would expect based on the name of the procedure?* Yes, the ileum was divided

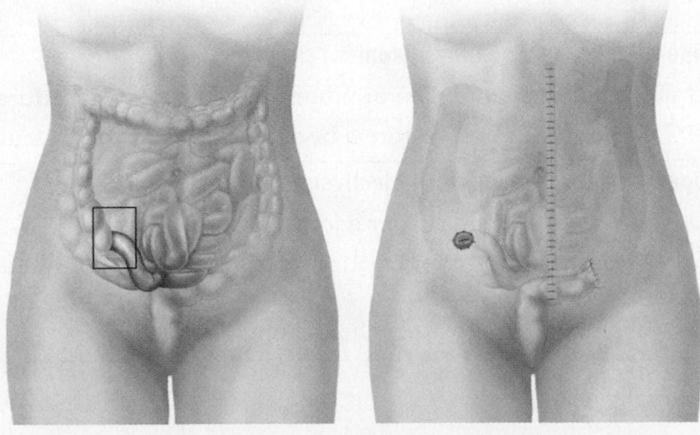

Figure 28-2 ■ A loop ileostomy re-routes the contents of the small intestine in order to bypass the large intestine.

and the free end was brought through the right abdominal wall to the skin. This created a new route to evacuate the contents of the small intestine.

- ❑ *What surgical approach is used?* open
- ❑ *Was more than one procedure, or a combined procedure, performed?* No.
- ❑ She reads the abstracting questions and answers **Yes** to the question: *Did the procedure alter the diameter or route of a tubular body part?*

⇨ The Key Criteria for Abstracting Medical and Surgical Procedures directs Marcy to review the definitions of four Root Operations.

⇨ She turns to to the appendix Comparison of Medical and Surgical Root Operations in the ICD-10-PCS coding manual.

- ❑ She locates the group titled Procedures That Alter the Diameter/Route of a Tubular Body Part and reads the definition of each Root Operation.
- ❑ After reading the definitions, she believes that **Bypass (1)** best describes the ileostomy.

⇨ Next, Marcy turns to the appendix Root Operation Definitions in the ICD-10-PCS manual.

- ❑ She locates the entry for **1 Bypass**.
- ❑ She reads the Definition, Explanation, and Examples listed and concludes that **Bypass** is the correct Root Operation because this operation altered the route of a tubular body part, the ileum.

⇨ At this time, Marcy has abstracted the procedure and determined that the Root Operation is **Bypass**. Next, she will build the PCS code.

Coding Practice

Now it is your turn to practice abstracting diagnoses for Medical and Surgical procedures. Questions guide your analysis of each scenario.

Exercise 28.1 Abstracting Medical and Surgical Procedures

Instructions: Read the mini-medical-record of each patient's encounter and answer the abstracting questions. Write the answer on the line provided. Do not assign any codes.

1. Date of procedure: 3/28/yy Location: Branton Medical Center Surgeon: Tanya Schmitt, MD

Anesthesiologist: Reginald Pincus, MD

Patient: Maribeth Crape Gender: F Age: 83

Preprocedure diagnosis: pressure ulcer, left hip

Procedure description: Open excisional debridement of left hip. Used scissors to cut out necrosis and devitalized tissue, through full epidermis and subcutaneous tissue, 1 cm beyond the wound margin.

Postprocedure diagnosis: healing stage III pressure ulcer, left hip

a. What is the stated procedure?________________

____

b. What organ or body part is involved? ________________

____

(continued)

1. (continued)

c. Is the procedure description what you would expect based on the name of the procedure?

____

d. What surgical approach is used? ________________

____

e. Was more than one procedure, or a combined procedure, performed?________________

____

f. Review the Root Operation Questions. To which question did you answer yes? ________________

____

g. Review the definitions of the Root Operations that answer this question. Which Root Operation correctly describes this procedure? ________________

____

2. Date of procedure: 3/28/yy Location: Branton Medical Center Surgeon: Tanya Schmitt, MD

Anesthesiologist: Reginald Pincus, MD

Patient: Cherise Tremel Gender: F Age: 48

Preprocedure diagnosis: mass in left breast

(continued)

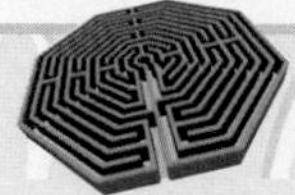

Coding Practice (continued)

2. (continued)

Procedure description: Needle biopsy. Using a needle, took out a tissue sample from the left breast that was previously marked with a wire.

Postprocedure diagnosis: benign neoplasm, breast per pathology report

a. What is the stated procedure? ____________

b. What organ or body part is involved? ____________

c. Is the procedure description what you would expect based on the name of the procedure? ____________

d. What surgical approach is used? ____________

e. Was more than one procedure, or a combined procedure, performed? ____________

f. Review the Root Operation Questions. To which question did you answer yes? ____________

g. Review the definitions of the Root Operations that answer this question. Which Root Operation correctly describes this procedure? ____________

h. Was the procedure diagnostic or therapeutic? ____________

3. Date of procedure: 3/28/yy Location: Branton Medical Center Surgeon: Stanley Garrett, MD

Anesthesiologist: Reginald Pincus, MD

Patient: Greg Allen Gender: M Age: 15

Preprocedure assessment: presented to ED with vomiting, acute abdominal pain, RLQ tenderness, T 101 degrees

Procedure description: Appendectomy. Made three small umbilical incisions and placed laparoscope. Expanded abdominal cavity with carbon dioxide to aid visualization. Grasped appendix and divided with stapler. Cauterized appendiceal stump. Removed appendix, irrigated and suctioned abdominal cavity.

(continued)

3. (continued)

Removed instruments and closed incision. Patient tolerated procedure well, no complications.

Postprocedure diagnosis: acute appendicitis with rupture

a. What is the stated procedure? ____________

b. What organ or body part is involved? ____________

c. Is the procedure description what you would expect based on the name of the procedure? ____________

d. What surgical approach is used? ____________

e. Was more than one procedure, or a combined procedure, performed? ____________

f. Review the Root Operation Questions. To which question did you answer yes? ____________

g. Review the definitions of the Root Operations that answer this question. Which Root Operation correctly describes this procedure? ____________

4. Date of procedure: 3/28/yy Location: Branton Medical Center Surgeon: Bruce Prentice, MD

Anesthesiologist: Julianne Paiz, MD

Patient: Stella Tyrrell Gender: F Age: 61

Preprocedure diagnosis: gangrene in left great toe, due to non-healing plantar (*sole of foot*) ulcer

Procedure description: mid-level amputation of L great toe at interphalangeal joint

Postprocedure diagnosis: diabetes with gangrene

a. What is the stated procedure? ____________

b. What organ or body part is involved? ____________

c. Is the procedure description what you would expect based on the name of the procedure? ____________

(continued)

4. (continued)

d. What surgical approach is used? ____________

____

e. Was more than one procedure, or a combined procedure, performed?____________

____

f. Review the Root Operation Questions. To which question did you answer yes? ____________

____

g. Review the definitions of the Root Operations that answer this question. Which Root Operation correctly describes this procedure? ____________

____

5. Date of procedure: 3/28/yy Location: Branton Medical Center Surgeon: Kay Pinkey, MD

Anesthesiologist: Julianne Paiz, MD

Patient: Beth Mcafee Gender: F Age: 23

Preprocedure: hypermenorrhea

Procedure description: Transvaginal dilation and curettage. Inserted speculum to hold the vagina open. Progressively dilated cervix and uterus with os dilator. Inserted curette and scraped endometrial wall. Tissue sent to lab for analysis.

Postprocedure diagnosis: hypermenorrhea

***Tip*:** Scraping (curretage) is classified as removal by force.

a. What is the stated procedure? ____________

____

b. What organ or body part is involved? ____________

____

c. Is the procedure description what you would expect based on the name of the procedure?____

____

d. What surgical approach is used? ____________

____

e. Was more than one procedure, or a combined procedure, performed?____________

____

(continued)

5. (continued)

f. Review the Root Operation Questions. To which question did you answer yes? ____________

____

g. Review the definitions of the Root Operations that answer this question. Which Root Operation correctly describes this procedure? ____________

____

h. Was the procedure diagnostic or therapeutic?

____

6. Date of procedure: 4/28/yy Location: Branton Medical Center Surgeon: Kay Pinkey, MD

Anesthesiologist: Julianne Paiz, MD

Patient: Joann Lindeman Gender: F Age: 52

Preprocedure diagnosis: endometriosis

Procedure description: Ablation of ovaries and endometrium. Inserted the endoscope through the vagina into the uterus to cauterize the endometrium (lining of uterus). When that was successfully completed, withdrew the scope, applied a new tip. Made three incisions on the lower abdomen and inserted endoscope to treat each ovary.

Postprocedure diagnosis: endometriosis

***Tip*:** Code multiple procedures when the same root operation is performed on different Body Parts as defined by distinct values of the Body Part character (Guideline B3.2a).

a. What is the stated procedure? ____________

____

b. What organ or body part is involved? ____________

____

c. Is the procedure description what you would expect based on the name of the procedure?____

____

d. What surgical approach is used? ____________

____

e. Was more than one procedure, or a combined procedure, performed?____________

____

(continued)

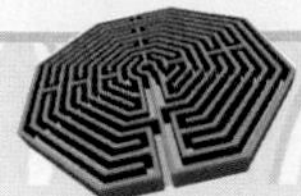

Coding Practice (continued)

6. (continued)

f. Review the Root Operation Questions. To which question did you answer yes? ______________

g. Review the definitions of the Root Operations that answer this question. Which Root Operation correctly describes this procedure? ______________

h. Repeat the abstracting process for each procedure that was performed.

7. Date of procedure: 4/28/yy Location: Branton Medical Center Surgeon: Tanya Schmitt, MD

Anesthesiologist: Reginald Pincus, MD

Patient: Megan Brandt Gender: F Age: 52

Preprocedure diagnosis: pain RUQ, T 102 degrees, vomiting, acute cholecystitis with calculi in the common bile duct causing obstruction. Extensive known abdominal adhesions prevent a laparoscopic approach.

Procedure description: Cholecystectomy. Made subcostal incision and isolated gallbladder from surrounding structures with laparotomy packs. Excised entire gallbladder and common bile duct. Hemostasis was achieved. Closed operative wound. Patient tolerated procedure well.

Postprocedure diagnosis: acute cholecystitis with calculi in the common bile duct causing obstruction

***Tip*:** Code multiple procedures when the same root operation is performed on different Body Parts as defined by distinct values of the Body Part character (Guideline B3.2a).

a. What is the stated procedure? ______________

b. What organ or body part is involved? ______________

c. Is the procedure description what you would expect based on the name of the procedure? ______________

(continued)

7. (continued)

d. What surgical approach is used? ______________

e. Was more than one procedure, or a combined procedure, performed? ______________

f. Review the Root Operation Questions. To which question did you answer yes? ______________

g. Review the definitions of the Root Operations that answer this question. Which Root Operation correctly describes this procedure? ______________

h. Repeat the abstracting process for each procedure that was performed.

8. Date of procedure: 4/28/yy Location: Branton Medical Center Surgeon: Margo Bittinger, MD

Anesthesiologist: Reginald Pincus, MD

Patient: Nelson Hummer Gender: M Age: 43

Preprocedure diagnosis: detached R retina

Procedure description: Trans pars plana vitrectomy (TPPV) with synthetic scleral buckle. Made incision in pars plana and used vitreous cutter to suction out all vitreous. Injected balanced saline solution (BSS) to replace vitreous. Sutured scleral buckle which effectively closed the break. Pt tolerated px well.

Postprocedure diagnosis: detached R retina

a. What is the stated procedure? ______________

b. What organ or body part is involved? ______________

c. Is the procedure description what you would expect based on the name of the procedure? ______________

d. What surgical approach is used? ______________

(continued)

8. (continued)

e. Was more than one procedure, or a combined procedure, performed?____________________

f. Review the Root Operation Questions. To which question did you answer yes? ____________________

g. Review the definitions of the Root Operations that answer this question. Which Root Operation correctly describes this procedure? ____________________

h. Repeat the abstracting process for each procedure that was performed.

9. Date of procedure: 4/28/yy Location: Branton Medical Center Surgeon: Margo Bittinger, MD Anesthesiologist: Reginald Pincus, MD

Patient: Ted Wey Gender: M Age: 75

Preprocedure diagnosis: blepharoptosis obscuring vision

Procedure description: Bilateral upper blepharoplasty. Cut out a crescent of skin and subcutaneous tissue from fold of R eyelid, sutured to restore normal position of eyelid. Repeated on left side.

Postprocedure diagnosis: blepharoptosis obscuring vision

a. What is the stated procedure? ____________________

b. What organ or body part is involved? ____________________

c. Is the procedure description what you would expect based on the name of the procedure?____________________

d. What surgical approach is used? ____________________

e. Was more than one procedure, or a combined procedure, performed?____________________

f. Review the Root Operation Questions. To which question did you answer yes? ____________________

(continued)

9. (continued)

g. Review the definitions of the Root Operations that answer this question. Which Root Operation correctly describes this procedure? ____________________

h. Repeat the abstracting process for each procedure that was performed.

10. Date of procedure: 4/28/yy Location: Branton Medical Center Surgeon: Bruce Prentice, MD Anesthesiologist: Julianne Paiz, MD

Patient: Darcy Sease Gender: F Age: 23

Preprocedure diagnosis: fractured R tibia and R humerus

Procedure description: Open reduction, R tibia with internal fixations device. Closed reduction, percutaneous internal fixation. Applied cast to right humerus.

Postprocedure diagnosis: fractured R tibia, fractured R humerus shaft

a. What is the stated procedure? ____________________

b. What organ or body part is involved? ____________________

c. Is the procedure description what you would expect based on the name of the procedure? ____________________

d. What surgical approach is used? ____________________

e. Was more than one procedure, or a combined procedure, performed?____________________

f. Review the Root Operation Questions. To which question did you answer yes? ____________________

g. Review the definitions of the Root Operations that answer this question. Which Root Operation correctly describes this procedure? ____________________

h. Repeat the abstracting process for each procedure that was performed.

ASSIGNING MEDICAL AND SURGICAL PROCEDURE CODES

Assigning PCS codes requires coders to locate the Root Operation in the Index, then refer to a Table to build the code. PCS does not contain any modifiers. The Tables do not contain any instructional notes.

ICD-10-PCS Index

The Index uses two types of Main Terms for the Medical and Surgical Section:

- the name of the Root Operation
- the common procedure name

ICD-10-PCS does *not* use eponyms as Main Terms or procedure names. The most direct way to locate a code is to use the Root Operation. However, when the Root Operation is difficult to determine, locate a Main Term for the common procedure name, such as *colectomy*, then follow the cross-references to the appropriate Main Term(s) and Table(s) (■ FIGURE 28-3). The Index may provide more than one cross-reference because the common procedure names can be ambiguous. For example, a colectomy may involve any of the following procedures:

- cutting out the entire colon, which is a **Resection**
- cutting out one complete segment of the colon, which is also a **Resection**, because each segment has a separate Body Part value
- cutting out a portion of one segment, which is an **Excision**, because a portion of a defined Body Part is cut out

Under the Main Term are indented subterms that describe the anatomical site or other variation of the Root Operation. Following the subterm is the partial code, which provides the first three to five characters of the code. The first *three* characters of the partial code identify the appropriate Table to use.

CODING CAUTION

When the Index provides more than one cross-reference, it does NOT mean that you can use any of the options listed for any procedure. It is your responsibility as a coder to determine which specific Root Operation describes the procedure you are coding.

Colectomy

see Excision, Gastrointestinal System 0DB

see Resection, Gastrointestinal System 0DT

Figure 28-3 ■ Example of Index Entry for a Common Procedure Name, with Cross-References to Multiple Root Operations

Guided Example of Using the PCS Index

To practice skills for using the PCS Index, continue with the example from earlier in the chapter of Michael Longo, who had an ileostomy at Branton Medical Center.

Follow along as Marcy Elwood, CCS, searches the Index for the Root Operation. Check off each step after you complete it.

➪ First, Marcy confirms the procedure and Root Operation she abstracted.

- ❑ The Root Operation is **Bypass (1)**.
- ❑ The anatomic site is the ileum.
- ❑ The procedure is ileostomy.

➪ Marcy searches the Index for the Main Term **Bypass** and locates it (■ FIGURE 28-4).

- ❑ She locates the subterm **Ileum 0D1B**.
- ❑ She notes **0D1B** is the partial code.
- ❑ She determines that she needs Table **0D1**, which is the first three letters of the partial code.

➪ Marcy demonstrates an alternative way to locate the code, in case you are unsure of the Root Operation.

- ❑ She locates the Main Term **Ileostomy**.
- ❑ Under the **Ileostomy**, the Index provides two subterm entries with cross-references to the Root Operations (■ FIGURE 28-5).
  - ***see* Bypass, Ileum 0D1B**
  - ***see* Drainage, Ileum 0D9B**
- ❑ These cross-references direct her to two possible Root Operations.
  - She reviews the PCS definition of each Root Operation and determines that **Bypass** is the correct Root Operation based on the objective of the procedure.

➪ Next, Marcy will locate the Table and build the code.

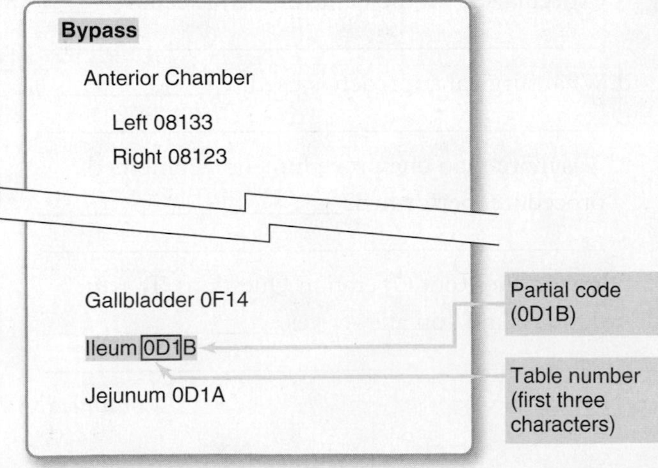

Figure 28-4 ■ Index Entry for Main Term Bypass and Subterm Ileum

Ileostomy

see Bypass, Ileum 0D1B

see Drainage, Ileum 0D9B

Figure 28-5 ■ Index Entry for Main Term Ileostomy

ICD-10-PCS Tables

After locating the appropriate procedure in the Index and identifying the first three characters of the partial code, cross-reference the appropriate Table to build the rest of the code. Follow three steps to look up a PCS code in the tables:

1. Locate the Table.
2. Build the code.
3. Verify the character values.

CODING CAUTION

Never assign a code based on the Index alone. You must always refer to the Table to build all seven characters of the code. The Index rarely lists more than three or four characters. Even when the Index provides a seven character code, you must still verify the values using the Table to be certain it accurately describes the documented procedure.

1. Locate the Table

Locate the Table that matches the first *three* letters of the partial code. The Tables are organized in alphanumeric order by the Section, the first character of a code. Tables beginning with numbers **0** through **9** appear first, followed by Tables beginning with a letter, **B** through **Z**. Within each Section, Tables are sequentially arranged according to the value of the second character, Body System.

For example, Tables that begin with **001** through **09Z** appear before Tables that begin with **0B1** through **0ZZ**. The first three letters of the code and the definition of each letter are listed at the top of the Table.

SUCCESS STEP

To locate Tables quickly, use small adhesive tabs. Within the Medical and Surgical Section, create tabs for the first two characters of the Table numbers, such as 00, 01, and so on through 0Y.

2. Build the Code

The three characters of the partial code that identify the Table are the first three characters of the code, representing the Section (**0** for Medical and Surgical), the Body System, and the Root Operation. The Table consists of a grid that lists the available options for characters 4 through 7 (■ FIGURE 28-6). To build the rest of the

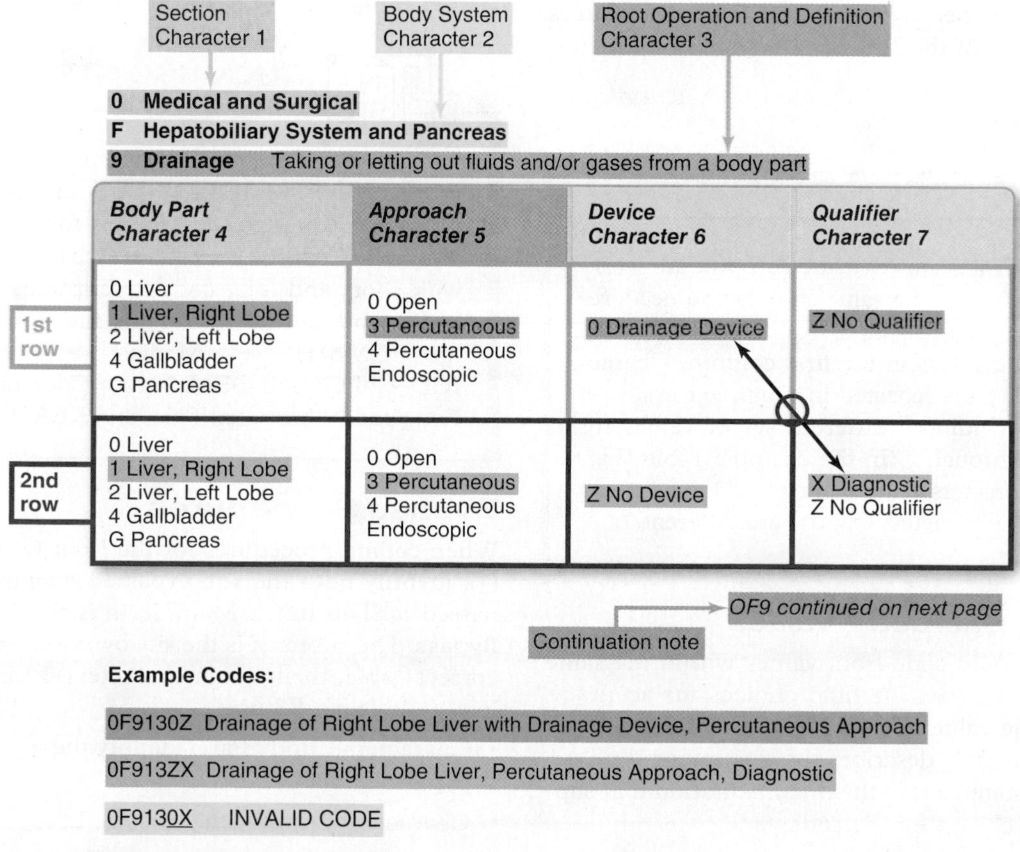

Body Part Character 4	Approach Character 5	Device Character 6	Qualifier Character 7
0 Liver 1 Liver, Right Lobe 2 Liver, Left Lobe 4 Gallbladder G Pancreas	0 Open 3 Percutaneous 4 Percutaneous Endoscopic	0 Drainage Device	Z No Qualifier
0 Liver 1 Liver, Right Lobe 2 Liver, Left Lobe 4 Gallbladder G Pancreas	0 Open 3 Percutaneous 4 Percutaneous Endoscopic	Z No Device	X Diagnostic Z No Qualifier

Example Codes:

0F9130Z Drainage of Right Lobe Liver with Drainage Device, Percutaneous Approach

0F913ZX Drainage of Right Lobe Liver, Percutaneous Approach, Diagnostic

0F9130X INVALID CODE

Figure 28-6 ■ Annotated PCS Table

code, select one value from each column to describe the procedure. The first column of the grid is for Body Part (Character 4); the second column is for Approach (Character 5); the third column is for Device (Character 6); and the final column is for Qualifier (Character 7). Select one, and only one, value from each column, staying within the same row.

Each row is mutually exclusive of other rows in the same Table. All values for a code must be taken from the *same* boxed row within the Table. Review the sample codes shown at the bottom of Figure 28-6 and note the following:

- Code **0F9130Z** is a valid code that is built from values in the first row of the table.
- Code **0F913ZX** is a valid code that is built from values in the second row of the table.
- Code **0F9130X** is NOT a valid code because it mixes a value from the first row for Character 6 with a value from the second row for Character 7.

The differences between the first and second rows of this Table are as follows:

- The first row contains a value for Character 6 for **0 Drainage Device** and the second row does not.
- The second row contains a value for Character 7 for **X Diagnostic** and the first row does not.

A procedure that leaves a drainage device in the patient is therapeutic by definition, not diagnostic. Therefore the values for Character 6, Device, **0 Drainage**, and Character 7, Qualifier, **X Diagnostic,** are mutually exclusive and cannot be used together. By choosing all character values from the same row of the Table, coders are able to construct valid codes.

SUCCESS STEP

If it seems that the row you are working from does not list the value choices you need, review the rest of the Table to see if another row applies. Sometimes, the values in the first column, Character 4, Body Part, are repeated in multiple rows, with other rows providing a different set of values for Characters 5 through 7. In the example Table (Figure 28-6), Characters 4 and 5 are exactly the same in both rows, but Characters 6 and 7 are different.

3. Verify the Character Values

After building a valid code from values within the same row of the Table, review the final choices for accuracy. Double-check the value of each character of the code to verify that it accurately describes the documented procedure. Identify a statement in the documentation that supports each value chosen for the code.

CODING CAUTION

Always be careful to double-check your work for accuracy when writing or entering a code into software. Because ICD-10-PCS codes are alphanumeric, it is easy to transpose characters, which results in an incorrect code. It is also easy to confuse a hastily written number **2** with the letter **Z** or the number **5** with the letter ***S***.

Tips for Using Tables

Certain formatting and layout elements of a Table affect the ability to build an accurate code. Be alert for the following items:

- Pages may contain more than one grid. Be careful to select the grid that *exactly* matches the first three code characters listed in the Index.
- Tables may be subdivided into rows, which are separated with solid lines. In order to build a valid code, all values must come from the same row within the Table. Do not combine values from different rows or different Tables. Doing so will result in an invalid code.
- Long Tables may span more than one page. If you cannot find what you need, even though you are confident that you have selected the correct three-character Table, look to see if it continues on the next page. When a Table is continued on the next page, a note stating ***continued on next page*** appears below the Table.

SUCCESS STEP

Due to the large number of ICD-10-PCS codes, the ICD-10-PCS manual does not provide a complete description for the final code. However, CMS does post a searchable electronic file with short and long code descriptions for all valid codes. You can download the file from **www.cms.gov**, CMS Home > Medicare > ICD-10 > 2012 ICD-10-PCS and GEMs2012 > Code Descriptions - Long and Abbreviated Titles and README files.

Bypass Procedures

When coding procedures for the Root Operation **Bypass (1)**, identify both the site bypassed *from* and the site bypassed *to*. The Index Main Term is the Root Operation **Bypass**. The subterm is the site bypassed *from*. Locate the correct Table, then assign characters 4 through 7 as follows (Guideline B3.6a):

- Character 4, Body Part: Identify the anatomical site bypassed *from*.
- Character 5, Approach.

- Character 6, Device: Identify the material used for the bypass. If existing material is used, select **Z No Device**.
- Character 7, Qualifier: Identify the anatomical site bypassed *to*.

CODING CAUTION

Coding coronary artery bypass grafts (CABG) follows a different protocol than coding bypass procedures on other parts of the body (Guideline B3.6b). For CABG, Character 4 identifies the *number* of sites; Character 7 identifies the site bypassed *from*.

Guided Example of Using PCS Tables

To practice skills for building a code using the PCS Tables, continue with the example from earlier in the chapter of Michael Longo, who had an ileostomy at Branton Medical Center.

Follow along as Marcy Elwood, CCS, builds the code for the ileostomy. Check off each step after you complete it.

⇨ Marcy searches the Tables for Table **0D1** (■ FIGURE 28-7).

- ❑ She verifies the identifying information at the top of the Table to be certain she has the correct Table.
  - Section **0 Medical and Surgical**
  - Body System **D Gastrointestinal System**
  - Operation **1 Bypass**: Altering the route of passage of the contents of a tubular body part
- ❑ She notes that **0D1** are the first three characters of the code.

⇨ Marcy now needs to assign the value for Character 4, Body Part.

- ❑ She searches the first column of the Table until she locates the entry for **B Ileum**.
- ❑ **Ileum** occupies only one row of the Table, so she determines that this is the correct row to use.
- ❑ The value for Character 4 is **B**.
- ❑ The code is now **0D1B**, which matches the partial code that was in the Index.

⇨ Next, Marcy needs to assign the value for Character 5, Approach.

- ❑ She re-reads the procedure description in the medical record and identifies that the surgeon used an open approach.
- ❑ In row **B Ileum** of the Table, she reads the values in the second column for Approach.
- ❑ She locates the entry for **0 Open** and determines that it is consistent with the documentation.
- ❑ Marcy now has five characters in the code: **0D1B0**.

0 Medical and Surgical
D Gastrointestinal System
1 Bypass: Altering the route of passage of the contents of a tubular body part

Body Part Character 4	*Approach Character 5*	*Device Character 6*	*Qualifier Character 7*
1 Esophagus, Upper 2 Esophagus, Middle 3 Esophagus, Lower 5 Esophagus	0 Open 4 Percutaneous Endoscopic 8 Via Natural or Artificial Opening Endoscopic	7 Autologous Tissue Substitute J Synthetic Substitute K Nonautologous Tissue Substitute Z No Device	4 Cutaneous 6 Stomach 9 Duodenum A Jejunum B Ileum
B Ileum	0 Open 4 Percutaneous Endoscopic 8 Via Natural or Artificial Opening Endoscopic	7 Autologous Tissue Substitute J Synthetic Substitute K Nonautologous Tissue Substitute Z No Device	4 Cutaneous B Ileum H Cecum K Ascending Colon L Transverse Colon M Descending Colon N Sigmoid Colon P Rectum Q Anus

Figure 28-7 ■ Table 0D1, Code 0D1B0Z4

➩ Next, Marcy needs to assign the value for Character 6, Device.

- ❑ She re-reads the procedure description in the medical record and determines that no device was used.
- ❑ In row **B Ileum** of the Table, she reads the values in the third column for Device.
- ❑ She locates the entry for **Z No Device** and determines that it is consistent with the documentation.
- ❑ Marcy now has six characters in the code: **0D1B0Z.**

➩ Finally, Marcy needs to assign the value for Character 7, Qualifier.

- ❑ She refers to Guideline B3.6a, which states: **Bypass procedures are coded by identifying the body part bypassed 'from' and the body part bypassed 'to.' The fourth character body part specifies the body part bypassed from, and the <u>qualifier specifies the body part bypassed to</u>.**
- ❑ She re-reads the procedure description in the medical record and determines that the body part bypassed *to* was the skin.
- ❑ In row **B Ileum** of the Table, she reads the values in the fourth column for Qualifier.
- ❑ She locates the entry for **4 Cutaneous** and determines that it is consistent with the documentation.

Table 28-2 ■ **BUILD-A-CODE 0D1B0Z4**

Character (Position)	Name	Value	Description
1	Section	0	Medical and Surgical
2	Body System	D	Gastrointestinal
3	Root Operation	1	Bypass
4	Body Part	B	Ileum
5	Approach	0	Open
6	Device	Z	No Device
7	Qualifier	4	Cutaneous

- ❑ Marcy now has all seven characters in the code: **0D1B0Z4.**

➩ Marcy double-checks each value in the code for accuracy.

- ❑ She writes each code value into her Build-A-Code table (■ TABLE 28-2).
- ❑ She compares each value with the documentation and identifies the specific statement in the document to support each value.

➩ Marcy's final code is **0D1B0Z4,** which means **Bypass Ileum to Cutaneous, Open Approach.**

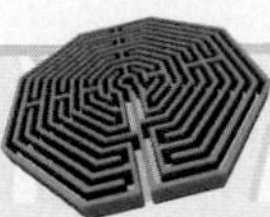

Coding Practice

Now it is your turn to practice assigning codes for Medical and Surgical procedures. Refer to the ***Tip*** at the end of the mini-medical-record if you need a little extra help.

Exercise 28.2 Assigning Medical and Surgical Procedure Codes

Instruction: Read the mini-medical-record of each patient's encounter, review the information abstracted in Exercise 28.1, assign ICD-10-PCS procedure codes (PCS) using the Index and Tables.

1. Date of procedure: 3/28/yy Location: Branton Medical Center Surgeon: Tanya Schmitt, MD

Anesthesiologist: Reginald Pincus, MD

Patient: Maribeth Crape Gender: F Age: 83

Preprocedure diagnosis: pressure ulcer, left hip

Procedure description: Open excisional debridement of left hip. Used scissors to cut out necrosis

(continued)

1. (continued)

and devitalized tissue, through full epidermis and subcutaneous tissue, 1 cm beyond the wound margin.

Postprocedure diagnosis: healing stage III pressure ulcer, left hip

Tip: Use the Body Part Key appendix of the ICD-10-PCS manual to determine how to classify the hip.

1 PCS Code ___________

2. Date of procedure: 3/28/yy Location: Branton Medical Center Surgeon: Tanya Schmitt, MD

Anesthesiologist: Reginald Pincus, MD

Patient: Cherise Tremel Gender: F Age: 48

Preprocedure diagnosis: mass in left breast

(continued)

2. (continued)

Procedure description: Needle biopsy. Using a needle, took out a tissue sample from the left breast that was previously marked with a wire.

Postprocedure diagnosis: benign neoplasm, breast per pathology report

1 PCS Code __________

3. Date of procedure: 3/28/yy Location: Branton Medical Center Surgeon: Stanley Garrett, MD

Anesthesiologist: Reginald Pincus, MD

Patient: Greg Allen Gender: M Age: 15

Preprocedure assessment: presented to ED with vomiting, acute abdominal pain, RLQ tenderness, T 101 degrees

Procedure description: Appendectomy. Made three small umbilical incisions and placed laparoscope. Expanded abdominal cavity with carbon dioxide to aid visualization. Grasped appendix and divided with stapler. Cauterized appendiceal stump. Removed appendix, irrigated and suctioned abdominal cavity. Removed instruments and closed incision. Patient tolerated procedure well, no complications.

Postprocedure diagnosis: acute appendicitis with rupture

1 PCS Code __________

4. Date of procedure: 3/28/yy Location: Branton Medical Center Surgeon: Bruce Prentice, MD

Anesthesiologist: Julianne Paiz, MD

Patient: Stella Tyrrell Gender: F Age: 61

Preprocedure diagnosis: gangrene in left great toe, due to non-healing plantar (*sole of foot*) ulcer

Procedure description: mid-level amputation of L great toe at interphalangeal joint

Postprocedure diagnosis: diabetes with gangrene

1 PCS Code __________

5. Date of procedure: 3/28/yy Location: Branton Medical Center Surgeon: Kay Pinkey, MD

Anesthesiologist: Julianne Paiz, MD

Patient: Beth Mcafee Gender: F Age: 23

Preprocedure: hypermenorrhea

Procedure description: Transvaginal dilation and curettage. Inserted speculum to hold the vagina open. Progressively dilated cervix and uterus with os dilator. Inserted curette and scraped endometrial wall. Tissue sent to lab for analysis.

Postprocedure diagnosis: hypermenorrhea

***Tip*:** Hypermenorrhea is abnormally heavy menstrual flow. Dilation is a procedural step necessary to reach the operative site (uterus) so it does not get a separate code (Guideline B3.1b).

1 PCS Code __________

ARRANGING MEDICAL AND SURGICAL PROCEDURE CODES

The prerequisite to sequencing PCS codes is to determine when multiple codes are required. Guideline B3.2 provides specific information about coding multiple procedures. Additional guidelines within B3 provide further direction relating to specific Root Operations. A summary of multiple procedure guidelines follows.

Components of a Procedure

Do not assign separate codes to integral components of a Root Operation (Guideline B3.1b). The procedural steps required to open the operative field, reach the operative site, and close the operative wound are included in the Root Operation and are not coded separately (■ FIGURE 28-8). A Root Operation definition that includes multiple steps should be assigned a single code (■ FIGURE 28-9, page 580).

Surgeon performed a laparotomy to reach the site of an open liver biopsy, excised tissue from the right lobe of the liver, and performed a layered closure

0FB10ZX Excision of Right Lobe Liver, Open Approach, Diagnostic

Figure 28-8 ■ Example of a Single Code That Includes the Incision, Excision, and Layered Closure

Surgeon performed a laparoscopic repair of a left inguinal hernia and inserted a mesh panel for reinforcement.

0YU64JZ Supplement Left Inguinal Region with Synthetic Substitute, Percutaneous Endoscopic Approach

Figure 28-9 ■ Example of a Single Code That Includes Multiple Components

Multiple Body Parts

When the same Root Operation is performed on different Body Parts with distinct values, assign separate codes for each Body Part character (Guideline B3.2a). Sequence first the procedure most closely related to the principal diagnosis. If both procedures are equally related to the principal diagnosis, either may be sequenced first (■ FIGURE 28-10).

Multiple Body Sites the Same Body Part Value

When the same Root Operation is performed on two different sites, but they both share the same Body Part value, assign a separate code for each procedure (Guideline B3.2b). Both codes will be exactly the same (■ FIGURE 28-11).

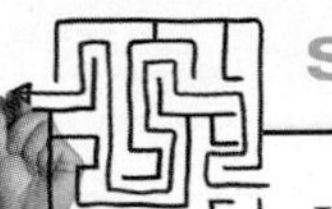

SUCCESS STEP

ICD-10-PCS does NOT require any modifiers to indicate that multiple procedures were performed.

Surgeon performed excisional biopsies of the liver and the pancreas.

0FB10ZX Excision of Right Lobe Liver, Open Approach, Diagnostic

0FBG0ZX Excision of Pancreas, Open Approach, Diagnostic

TABLE

0 Medical and Surgical
F Hepatobiliary System and Pancreas
B Excision Cutting out or off, without replacement, a portion of a body part

Body Part Character 4	*Approach Character 5*	*Device Character 6*	*Qualifier Character 6*
0 Liver 1 Liver, Right Lobe 2 Liver, Left Lobe 4 Gallbladder G Pancreas	0 Open 3 Percutaneous 4 Percutaneous Endoscopic	Z No Device	X Diagnostic Z No Qualifier

0 Medical and Surgical
F Hepatobiliary System and Pancreas
B Excision Cutting out or off, without replacement, a portion of a body part

Body Part Character 4	*Approach Character 5*	*Device Character 6*	*Qualifier Character 6*
0 Liver 1 Liver, Right Lobe 2 Liver, Left Lobe 4 Gallbladder G Pancreas	0 Open 3 Percutaneous 4 Percutaneous Endoscopic	Z No Device	X Diagnostic Z No Qualifier

EXPLANATION

Both procedures use the same Table, and all Character values are the same in both codes, except Character 4. Therefore, assign a separate code for each Body Part value. **Do NOT try to combine both Body Part values into the same code.** A code such as **0FB1G0ZX** is invalid because it contains eight characters, not seven. Each Character can have only one value in each code.

Figure 28-10 ■ Example of a Multiple Coding of the Same Root Operation and Different Body Part Values

Surgeon performed percutaneous excisional biopsies on the sartorius muscle and gracilis muscle of the right leg.

BODY PART KEY

Anatomical Site	PCS Description
Gracilis muscle	Upper Leg Muscle, Right Upper Leg Muscle, Left
Sartorius muscle	Upper Leg Muscle, Right Upper Leg Muscle, Left

0KBQ3ZX Excision of Right Upper Leg Muscle, Percutaneous Approach, Diagnostic

0KBQ3ZX Excision of Right Upper Leg Muscle, Percutaneous Approach, Diagnostic

Figure 28-11 ■ Example of Multiple Coding for Separate Sites with the Same Body Part Value

Multiple Root Operations on the Same Body Part

When more than one Root Operation, each with a distinct objective, is performed on the same Body Part value, assign a separate code to each procedure. Use a separate Root Operation Table for each procedure (Guideline 2b.3c). For example, assign separate codes for **Destruction** of sigmoid lesion (Table **0D5**) and **Bypass** of sigmoid colon (Table **0D1**) performed at the same operative session.

Root Operation Is Converted

When an intended Root Operation is attempted using one Approach, but is converted to a different approach, assign separate codes for each approach (Guideline 2b.3d). For example, when a laparoscopic cholecystectomy is converted to an open cholecystectomy, code the laparoscopic approach as percutaneous endoscopic **Inspection (0FJ44ZZ)**, because **Inspection** describes the first procedure that was performed using the percutaneous endoscopic approach. Code the open procedure as open **Resection (0FT40ZZ)**, because the cutting out of the body part was performed using the open approach. Sequence the code for the approach that was converted *to* (**Resection**) first and the approach that was converted *from* (**Inspection**) second.

Discontinued Procedures

When the intended procedure is discontinued, code the procedure to the Root Operation performed (Guideline B3.3). If a procedure is discontinued before any other Root Operation is performed, code the root operation **Inspection (J)** of the body part or anatomical region inspected. For example, a planned aortic valve replacement procedure is discontinued after the initial thoracotomy and before any incision is made in the heart muscle, when the patient becomes hemodynamically unstable. This procedure is coded as an open **Inspection** of the mediastinum (**0WJC0ZZ**).

Biopsy Followed by More Definitive Treatment

Biopsies and therapeutic treatments may use the same Root Operations. When the procedure is stated to be diagnostic, assign Character 7 Qualifier as **X Diagnostic.** When a diagnostic **Excision (B)**, **Extraction (D)**, or **Drainage (9)** is followed by a definitive treatment, such as **Destruction (5)**, **Excision (B)**, or **Resection (T)** at the same procedure site, code *both* the biopsy and the definitive treatment (Guideline B3.4) (■ FIGURE 28-12). The definitive treatment is the procedure most closely related to the principal diagnosis, so sequence the definitive procedure first, followed by the diagnostic procedure.

Surgeon performed a needle biopsy from a suspicious area of the left breast and sent to pathology for an intraoperative frozen section. The pathologist called back that the tissue was malignant, so an open partial mastectomy was performed.

(1) **0HBU0ZZ Excision of Left Breast, Open Approach**

(2) **0HBU3ZX Excision of Left Breast, Percutaneous Approach, Diagnostic**

Figure 28-12 ■ Example of Coding Biopsy Followed by Definitive Treatment

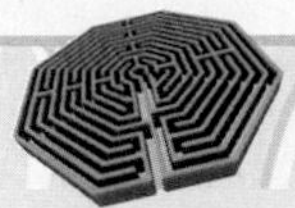

Coding Practice

Now it is your turn to practice arranging codes for Medical and Surgical procedures. Refer to the ***Tip*** at the end of the mini-medical-record if you need a little extra help.

Exercise 28.3 Arranging Medical and Surgical Procedure Codes

Instructions: Read the mini-medical-record of each patient's encounter, review the information abstracted in Exercise 28.1, assign ICD-10-PCS procedure codes (PCS) using the Index and Tables, and arrange them correctly.

1. Date of procedure: 4/28/yy Location: Branton Medical Center Surgeon: Kay Pinkey, MD

Anesthesiologist: Julianne Paiz, MD

Patient: Joann Lindeman Gender: F Age: 52

Preprocedure diagnosis: endometriosis

Procedure description: Ablation of ovaries and endometrium. Inserted the endoscope through the vagina into the uterus to cauterize the endometrium (lining of uterus). When that was successfully completed, withdrew the scope, applied a new tip. Made three incisions on the lower abdomen and inserted endoscope to treat each ovary.

Postprocedure diagnosis: endometriosis

Tip: This procedure describes endoscopic ablation of endometriosis in the endometrium and ovaries. Assign one code for each site.

2 PCS Codes __________ __________

2. Date of procedure: 4/28/yy Location: Branton Medical Center Surgeon: Tanya Schmitt, MD

Anesthesiologist: Reginald Pincus, MD

Patient: Megan Brandt Gender: F Age: 52

Preprocedure diagnosis: Pain RUQ, T 102 degrees, vomiting, acute cholecystitis with calculi in the common bile duct causing obstruction. Extensive known abdominal adhesions prevent a laparoscopic approach.

Procedure description: Cholecystectomy. Made subcostal incision and isolated gallbladder from surrounding structures with laparotomy packs. Excised entire gallbladder and common bile duct. Hemostasis was achieved. Closed operative wound. Patient tolerated procedure well.

Postprocedure diagnosis: acute cholecystitis with calculi in the common bile duct causing obstruction

2 PCS Codes __________ __________

3. Date of procedure: 4/28/yy Location: Branton Medical Center Surgeon: Margo Bittinger, MD

Anesthesiologist: Reginald Pincus, MD

Patient: Nelson Hummer Gender: M Age: 43

Preprocedure diagnosis: detached R retina

Procedure description: Trans pars plana vitrectomy (TPPV) with synthetic scleral buckle. Made incision in pars plana and used vitreous cutter to suction out all vitreous. Injected balanced saline solution (BSS) to replace vitreous. Sutured scleral buckle which effectively closed the break. Pt tolerated px well.

Postprocedure diagnosis: detached R retina

2 PCS Codes __________ __________

4. Date of procedure: 4/28/yy Location: Branton Medical Center Surgeon: Margo Bittinger, MD

Anesthesiologist: Reginald Pincus, MD

Patient: Ted Wey Gender: M Age: 75

Preprocedure diagnosis: blepharoptosis obscuring vision

Procedure description: Bilateral upper blepharoplasty. Cut out a crescent of skin and subcutaneous tissue from fold of R eyelid, sutured to restore normal position of eyelid. Repeated on left side.

Postprocedure diagnosis: blepharoptosis obscuring vision

2 PCS Codes __________ __________

5. Date of procedure: 4/28/yy Location: Branton Medical Center Surgeon: Bruce Prentice, MD

Anesthesiologist: Julianne Paiz, MD

Patient: Darcy Sease Gender: F Age: 23

Preprocedure diagnosis: fractured R tibia and R humerus

Procedure description: Open reduction, R tibia with internal fixations device. Closed reduction, percutaneous internal fixation. Applied cast to right humerus

Postprocedure diagnosis: fractured R tibia, fractured R humerus shaft

Tip: Refer to Guideline B3.15.

2 PCS Codes __________ __________

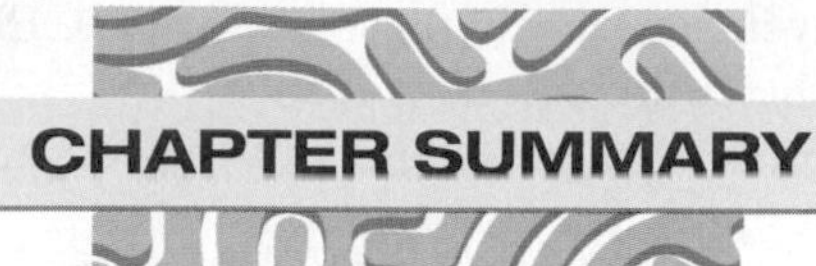

CHAPTER SUMMARY

In this chapter you learned that:

- Because identifying the correct Root Operation is the basis of ICD-10-PCS coding, coders must learn the differences between similar Root Operations in order to abstract appropriately.
- Assigning PCS codes requires coders to locate the Root Operation in the Index, then refer to a Table to build the code.
- The prerequisite to sequencing PCS codes is to determine when multiple codes are required, which is discussed in Guideline B3.2.

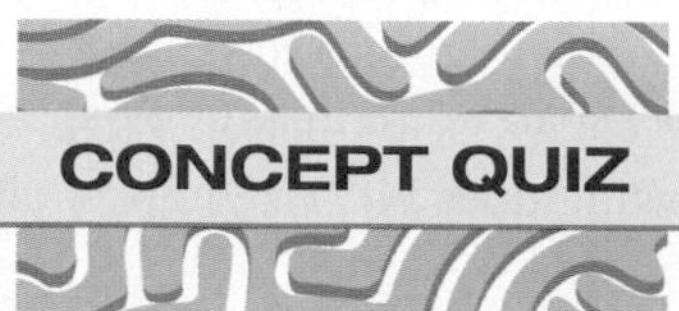

CONCEPT QUIZ

Take a moment to look back at your trip through Medical and Surgical procedures and solidify your skills. This is your opportunity to pull together everything you have learned.

Completion

Instructions: Write the term that answers each question based on the information you learned in this chapter. Choose from the list below. Some choices may be used more than once and some choices may not be used at all. Refer to the discussion in this chapter if you need a little extra help. When the question provides a pair of terms in parentheses, choose the correct answer from one of the two word choices.

does	Removal
does NOT	Resection
Excision	to
from	two
one	

1. When coding an ileostomy, Character 7 identifies the site bypassed (to/from)_______________.
2. When a diagnostic procedure is followed by a definitive treatment at the same procedure site, assign _______________ code(s).
3. ICD-10-PCS (does/does NOT) _______________ require modifiers to indicate that multiple procedures were performed.
4. When coding CABG, Character 7 identifies the site bypassed (to/from) _______________.
5. When dilation is a procedural step necessary to reach the operative site, it (does/does NOT) _______________ get a separate code.
6. Endoscopic ablation of endometriosis in the endometrium and ovaries is assigned _______________ code(s).
7. Taking out a lymph node chain is assigned to the Root Operation _______________.
8. A PCS Table (does/does NOT) _______________ contain instructional notes.
9. When coding a colostomy, Character 4 identifies the site bypassed (to/from) _______________.
10. When the Index provides more than one cross-reference, it (does/does NOT) _______________ mean that you can choose any of the options listed for any procedure.

Multiple Choice

Instructions: Circle the letter of the best answer to each question based on the information you learned in this chapter. Refer to the discussion in this chapter and the Glossary at the end of this book if you need a little extra help.

1. Coders must read what physicians document and
   A. assign codes that use the exact same words.
   B. refer to ICD-10-PCS manual Body Part Key appendix to identify the Root Operation.
   C. locate the Approach as the Main Term in the Index.
   D. equate it to the definitions provided by PCS.
2. The basis of ICD-10-PCS coding is identifying the correct
   A. Section.
   B. Root Operation.
   C. Approach.
   D. Qualifier.

3. Which Root Operation should NOT be used when the procedure takes out some or all of a body part without replacement?
   A. Removal (P)
   B. Destruction (5)
   C. Extraction (D)
   D. Resection (T)
4. Which Root Operation SHOULD be used when the procedure restores a body part to its normal structure?
   A. Resection (T)
   B. Revision (W)
   C. Alteration (0)
   D. Repair (Q)
5. Which Root Operation should NOT be used when the procedure alters the diameter or route of a tubular body part?
   A. Bypass (1)
   B. Change (2)
   C. Dilation (7)
   D. Restriction (V)
6. Which of the following items does NOT normally appear on a procedure report?
   A. Date of admission
   B. Date of procedure
   C. Estimated blood loss
   D. Postprocedure diagnosis
7. A colectomy may include any of the following EXCEPT
   A. cutting out the entire colon.
   B. cutting out one complete segment of the colon.
   C. cutting out a portion of one segment.
   D. creating a new outlet for the colon contents.
8. Which of the following Tables appears first in the ICD-10-PCS manual?
   A. 09Z
   B. 0D1
   C. 102
   D. 0XX
9. Which characteristic is NOT true of PCS Tables?
   A. Pages may contain more than one grid.
   B. Tables may contain more than one Root Operation.
   C. Tables may be subdivided into rows.
   D. Long Tables may span more than one page.
10. Which of the following does NOT require multiple codes?
    A. The physician performs the same Root Operation on different Body Parts.
    B. The physician performs the same Root Operation on two different sites.
    C. The physician performs a layered closure when using the Open Approach.
    D. The physician performs more than one Root Operation, each with a distinct objective, on the same Body Part value.

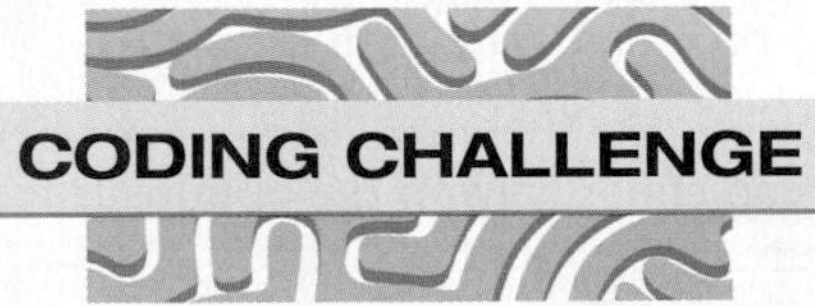

CODING CHALLENGE

Now it is your turn to demonstrate coding both diagnoses and procedures for Medical and Surgical procedures. Refer back to the examples and discussion in this chapter when you need a little extra help. Use your medical dictionary and anatomy references when needed.

Instructions: Read the mini-medical-record of each patient's encounter. First, abstract, assign, and arrange ICD-10-CM diagnosis codes (CM) using the Index and Tabular List. Then abstract, assign, and arrange ICD-10-PCS procedure codes (PCS) using the Index and Tables. Write the code(s) on the lines provided.

1. Date of procedure: 9/28/yy Location: Branton Medical Center Surgeon: Kay Pinkey, MD

Anesthesiologist: Julianne Paiz, MD

Patient: Shirlee Kazanowski Gender: F Age: 26

Preprocedure diagnosis: polycystic ovaries

Procedure description: Oophorectomy. Approached transvaginally with laparoscopic assistance. Located and removed entirety of both ovaries.

Postprocedure diagnosis: polycystic ovaries

Tip: Transvaginally means the surgeon approached through (*trans*) the vagina.

1 CM Code ___________

1 PCS Code ___________

2. Date of procedure: 9/28/yy Location: Branton Medical Center Surgeon: Tanya Schmitt, MD

Anesthesiologist: Reginald Pincus, MD

Patient: Patient: Sheri Wiggs Gender: F Age: 48

Preprocedure: metastatic breast cancer

Procedure description: Lymphadenectomy. Open left axillary total lymphadenectomy and percutaneous left cervical lymphadenectomy of the first node only.

Postprocedure diagnosis: left breast cancer with metastasis to lymph nodes

Tip: Assign diagnosis codes for both the primary and metastatic cancer. Sequence the reason for the treatment first. Taking out a single lymph node is an Excision and taking out the entire (total) chain is a Resection.

3 CM Codes __________ __________ __________

2 PCS Codes __________ __________

3. Date: 9/28/yy Location: Branton Medical Center Surgeon: Bruce Prentice, MD

Anesthesiologist: Julianne Paiz, MD

Patient: Alan Chadwell Gender: M Age: 26

Preprocedure diagnosis: necrosis and spreading infection after injury 1 month ago with potential for sepsis

Procedure description: Amputation. Detached 5th phalanges and entire metacarpal, right hand

Postprocedure diagnosis: infection, subcutaneous tissue, right hand, organism unknown

Tip: A ray of the hand includes the finger (phalanges) and metacarpal.

1 CM Code __________

1 PCS Code __________

4. Date of procedure: 9/28/yy Location: Branton Medical Center Surgeon: Bruce Prentice, MD

Anesthesiologist: Julianne Paiz, MD

Patient: Roxanne Halsted Gender: F Age: 68

Preprocedure diagnosis: primary degenerative osteoarthritis localized to the knee, extreme difficulty walking

(continued)

4. (continued)

Procedure description: Total L knee replacement. Made midline incision 10 cm above L patella, entered joint capsule medially, and exposed tibiofemoral joint. Resected tibia and femur, then sized for prosthetic. Inserted synthetic knee prosthesis, cemented in place, and closed operative wound. Minimal blood loss. Pt tolerated px well.

Postprocedure diagnosis: primary degenerative osteoarthritis

1 CM Code __________

1 PCS Code __________

5. Date of procedure: 9/28/yy Location: Branton Medical Center Surgeon: Tanya Schmitt, MD

Anesthesiologist: Reginald Pincus, MD

Patient: Edwina Becerril Gender: F Age: 71

Preprocedure diagnosis: subacute intracranial hemorrhage

Procedure description: Hematoma drainage. Made craniotomy incision and retracted skin flap and muscle layer. Drilled burr hole, evacuated hematoma, and inserted drain.

Postprocedure diagnosis: subacute subdural hemorrhage

1 CM Code __________

1 PCS Code __________

6. Date of procedure: 9/28/yy Location: Branton Medical Center Surgeon: Kay Pinkney, MD

Anesthesiologist: Julianne Paiz, MD

Patient: Louisa Giardina Gender: F Age: 18

Preprocedure diagnosis: abdominal aortic aneurysm (AAA)

Procedure description: EVAR (*endovascular aneurysm repair*) with synthetic graft. Made incision into femoral artery. With fluoroscopic guidance, guided delivery catheter with compressed graft into abdominal aorta to site of aneurysm. Inflated balloon to expand graft and affix it to vessel wall. Withdrew catheter and closed incision.

Postprocedure diagnosis: AAA

(continued)

(continued from page 585)

6. (continued)

Tip: An endovascular graft is placed inside the vessel and physically takes over the function, rendering the original vessel nonfunctional. Do not assign an additional code for the fluoroscopy portion of the procedure because it is not a Medical and Surgical procedure from Section 0.

1 CM Code __________

1 PCS Code __________

7. Date of procedure: 9/28/yy Location: Branton Medical Center Surgeon: Lorene Garman, MD

Anesthesiologist: Reginald Pincus, MD

Patient: Ernest Elias Gender: M Age: 18

Preprocedure diagnosis: spinal cord lesions

Procedure description: Electrocauterization. Made two 1.5 cm incisions at T7 and inserted endoscope and electrocautery. Cauterized single lesion. Withdrew instruments and closed wounds. Proceeded to make two 1.5 cm incisions at L3 and inserted endoscope and electrocautery. Cauterized two lesions. Withdrew instruments and closed wounds.

Postprocedure diagnosis: benign neoplasm, spinal cord, lumbar and thoracic

Tip: When the same Root Operation is performed at two distinct Body Part sites, assign separate codes (Guideline B3.2a).

1 CM Code __________

2 PCS Codes __________ __________

8. Date of procedure: 9/28/yy Location: Branton Medical Center Surgeon: Kay Pinkey, MD

Anesthesiologist: Julianne Paiz, MD

Patient: Kelly Shenk Gender: F Age: 35

Preprocedure diagnosis: sterilization following delivery

Procedure description: Tubal ligation. Laparoscopic bilateral occlusion of fallopian tubes with extraluminal clips.

Postprocedure diagnosis: sterilization

Tip: Code only for the sterilization in this exercise. Do not code for the delivery because the delivery is not coded from Medical and Surgical Section 0.

1 CM Code __________

1 PCS Code __________

9. Date of procedure: 9/28/yy Location: Branton Medical Center Surgeon: Tanya Schmitt, MD

Anesthesiologist: Reginald Pincus, MD

Patient: Lance Kaczmarski Gender: M Age: 58

Preprocedure diagnosis: change in bowel habits, rectal bleeding, family history of colon cancer

Procedure description: colonoscopy

Postprocedure diagnosis: first degree internal hemorrhoids, r/o CA colon, idiopathic change in bowel habits

3 CM Codes __________ __________ __________

1 PCS Code __________

10. Date of procedure: 9/28/yy Location: Branton Medical Center Surgeon: Tanya Schmitt, MD

Anesthesiologist: Reginald Pincus, MD

Patient: Bernice Duff Gender: F Age: 17

Preprocedure: second debridement for extensive burns on both arms

Procedure description: Excisional debridement and graft. Cut out necrotic subcutaneous tissue and fascia and applied autologous skin substitute on both lower arms and nonautologous tissue substitute on both upper arms.

Postprocedure diagnosis: second and third degree burns to anterior and posterior of right and left upper and lower arms, 18% TBSA (total body surface area) with burns, 9% TBSA third degree burns

Tip: Each portion (upper and lower) of each arm is coded as a separate body area for the diagnosis and procedure. Refer to OGCR I.C.19.a. to review the use of ICD-10-CM code extensions. Do not code external cause, source, or intent of burns.

5 CM Codes __________ __________ __________ __________ __________

4 PCS Codes __________ __________ __________ __________

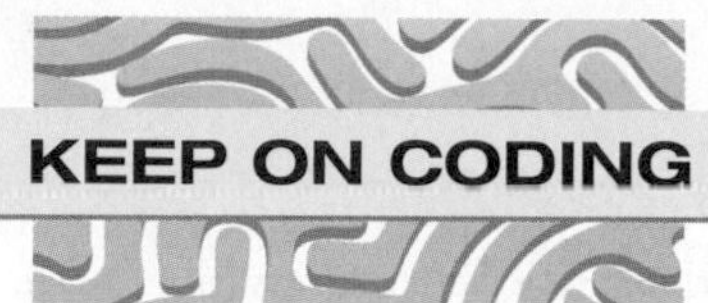

KEEP ON CODING

As a coder, you can never have too much experience. Apply everything you have learned in this chapter to code the following procedural statements. Use the Guidelines to help determine how many codes are required.

Instructions: Read the procedural statement, then use the Index and Tables to assign and sequence ICD-10-PCS (PCS) procedure codes. Write the code(s) on the line provided.

1. Bypass ileum to skin, open: PCS Code(s) ____________
2. Left first toe amputation, complete: PCS Code(s) ____________
3. Tarsal tunnel release, right, endoscopic: PCS Code(s) ____________
4. Right total knee replacement with cemented implant: PCS Code(s) ____________
5. Open biopsy of left extraocular muscle: PCS Code(s) ____________
6. Reattachment of right index finger: PCS Code(s) ____________
7. Endoscopic dilation of ileocecal valve: PCS Code(s) ____________
8. Control of post-operative tonsillectomy bleeding: PCS Code(s) ____________
9. Removal of drainage tube from gallbladder: PCS Code(s) ____________
10. Open clipping of cerebral aneurysm: PCS Code(s) ____________
11. Open pancreas transplant from organ donation: PCS Code(s) ____________
12. Open reduction left humeral head with internal fixation device: PCS Code(s) ____________
13. Diagnostic dilatation and curettage (D&C): PCS Code(s) ____________
14. Open revision of left hip replacement liner: PCS Code(s) ____________
15. Laparoscopic excision of the sigmoid colon: PCS Code(s) ____________
16. Drainage of right knee fluid, percutaneous: PCS Code(s) ____________
17. Suture of laceration of skin of back: PCS Code(s) ____________
18. Endoscopic facial nerve transfer: PCS Code(s) ____________
19. Open bilateral breast augmentation with silicone implants: PCS Code(s) ____________
20. Endoscopic left internal carotid endarterectomy: PCS Code(s) ____________
21. Cauterization of skin of right upper leg: PCS Code(s) ____________
22. Arthroscopic examination of left ankle: PCS Code(s) ____________
23. Open fusion of right finger phalangeal joint with internal fixation: PCS Code(s) ____________
24. Cataract extraction, right eye: PCS Code(s) ____________
25. Endoscopic bilateral vasectomy: PCS Code(s) ____________

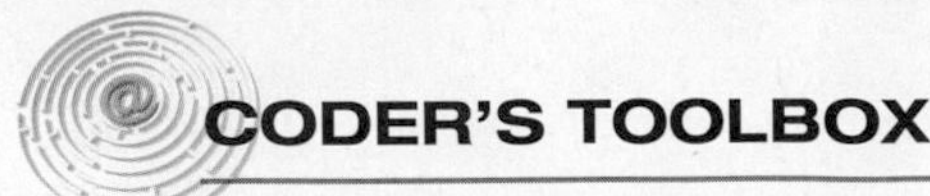

CODER'S TOOLBOX

The following resources are a starting point for learning more about specific medical and surgical procedures. The > symbol indicates a menu selection within the website in order to navigate to a specific page.

Mayo Clinic > Departments > Colon and Rectal Surgery http://www.mayoclinic.org/colon-rectal-surgery/

OR-Live http://www.orlive.com/

Society of American Gastrointestinal and Endoscopic Surgeons (SAGES) http://www.sages.org/publication/id/PI11/

Web MD > A to Z Guides > Health Features > Surgery Lite > Understanding Endoscopic Surgery http://www.webmd.com/a-to-z-guides/features/understanding-endoscopic-surgery

EdHeads > Activities > Virtual Knee Replacement surgery http://www.edheads.org/activities/knee/index.shtml

You Tube > Heart Surgery 101(video) http://www.youtube.com/watch?v=41DR5i3XFaY

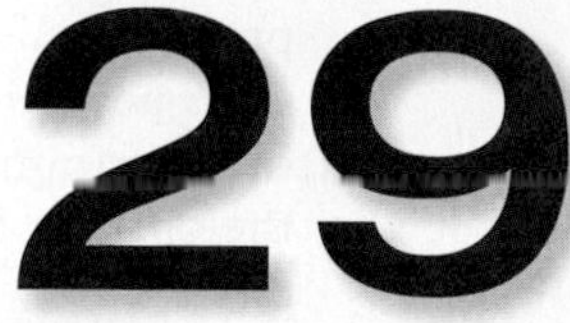

29

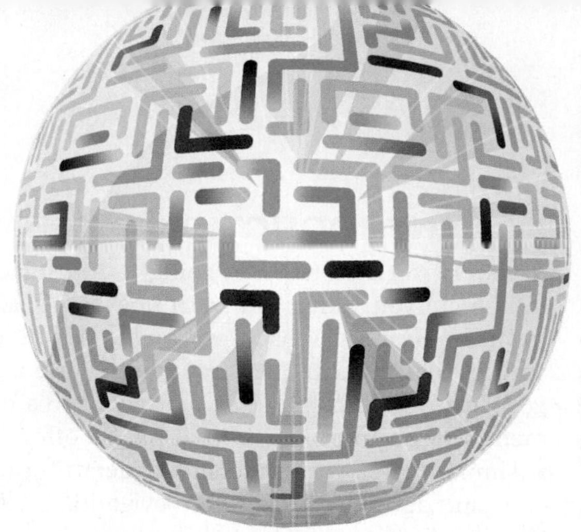

Medical and Surgical-Related (Sections 1-9) and Ancillary Procedure Coding (Sections B-D, F-H)

Learning Objectives

After completing this chapter, you should have the skills to:

- Spell and define the key words, medical terms, and abbreviations related to Medical and Surgical-Related procedures.
- Discuss common Medical and Surgical-Related procedures.
- Identify the main characteristics of coding Medical and Surgical-Related procedures.
- Abstract, assign, and arrange codes for Medical and Surgical-Related procedures.
- Discuss PCS Guidelines for Obstetric procedures.
- Spell and define the key words, medical terms, and abbreviations related to Ancillary procedures.
- Discuss common Ancillary procedures.
- Identify the main characteristics of coding Ancillary procedures.
- Abstract, assign, and arrange codes for Ancillary procedures.

Key Terms and Abbreviations

allopathic
anatomical imaging
cardioversion
doctor of osteopathy (DO)
extracorporeal
functional imaging
hyperbaric oxygen therapy (HBOT)
products of conception

In addition to the key terms listed here, students should know the terms defined within tables in this chapter.

Chapter Outline

- **Terminology Refresher**
- **Coding Overview**
- **Abstracting, Assigning, and Arranging Codes**

ICD-10-PCS codes in this chapter are from the ICD-10-PCS 2014 Draft code set from the Department of Health and Human Services, Centers for Medicare and Medicaid Services.

INTRODUCTION

If you are an avid traveler, going to new places does not intimidate you. After you learn how to get around a few towns or even a few backcountry areas, you learn certain strategies and techniques that you can use anywhere you go. Thus, you are able to quickly adapt to a new environment and begin seeing what it has to offer. PCS coding is similar. After you understand the structure of a PCS code and develop the skills for navigating the Medical and Surgical Section, you can apply those skills to learn how to code procedures in other Sections.

In this chapter, you will take a helicopter tour of the remaining Sections of PCS, which are divided into Medical and Surgical-Related procedures and Ancillary procedures. You will learn how codes in these Sections are structured, how Root Operations are defined, and other unique characteristics. Most importantly, you will practice coding for patient encounters involving Medical and Surgical-Related procedures and Ancillary procedures, a skill that requires you to abstract information from the medical record, assign correct codes, and arrange (sequence) the codes in the proper order.

As you read this chapter, open up your medical terminology book and keep a medical dictionary handy to refresh your memory of any unfamiliar terms. Your professional resources help you stay on track and minimize potential frustration. Also refer to the websites and organizations listed in Coder's Toolbox at the end of the chapter for specialized information about procedure coding.

TERMINOLOGY REFRESHER

Medical terms for Medical and Surgical-Related and Ancillary procedures use different suffixes than those in the Medical and Surgical Section. Familiar suffixes such as *-ectomy* and *-plasty* do not appear because procedures in these Sections do not cut out or repair body parts. Some procedure names do not use Latin forms at all. As you learn about procedures that physicians perform, refer to ■ TABLE 29-1 for a refresher on how to build medical terms.

CODING CAUTION

Be alert for medical terms that are spelled similarly and have different meanings.

pyel/o (*renal pelvis*) and **pyl/e** (*portal vein*)

-desis (*to tie, bind together*) and **-pheresis** (*removal*)

Table 29-1 ■ **EXAMPLE OF CONSTRUCTING MEDICAL TERMS FOR MEDICAL AND SURGICAL-RELATED PROCEDURES**

Root/Combining Form	Prefix/Suffix	Complete Medical Term
cardi/o (*heart*) **electr/o** (*electricity*)	**echo-** (*reflected sound*) **-graphy** (*process of recording*) **-therapy** (*treatment*)	**cardio + graphy** (*a recording of the heart*) **echo + cardio + graphy** (*a recording of the heart using reflected sound*) **electro + cardio + graphy** (*a recording of the heart using electricity*)
plasma- (*clear fluid*)	**-pheresis** (*to remove*) **a-** (*lack of*)	**plasma + pheresis** (*to remove the clear fluid from the blood*) **a + pheresis** (*to remove blood from the body*)

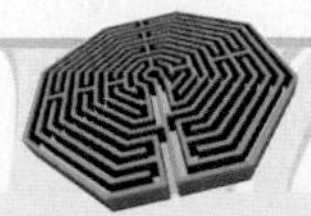

Coding Practice

Refresh your knowledge of terminology-related procedures in this chapter. Use a medical terminology text or a website such as GlobalRph.com > Medical Terminology **http://www.globalrph.com/medterm.htm** to identify the meaning of word parts that may not be familiar to you.

Exercise 29.1 Terminology Refresher

Instructions: Use your medical terminology skills and resources to define the following terms, then look them up in the ICD-10-PCS Index.

Follow these steps:

- Use slash marks "/" to break down each term into its root(s) and suffix.
- Define the meaning of the word, based on the meaning of each word part.
- Look up the term in the ICD-10-PCS Index, and write down the name(s) of Root Operation(s) the Index cross-references you to.
- Do not assign any codes.

Example: discography disco/graphy — Meaning: make a recording of an intervertebral disc — Root Operation(s): Plain Radiography, Fluoroscopy

1. audiometry Meaning ______ Root Operation(s) ______
2. pyelography Meaning ______ Root Operation(s) ______
3. chemoembolization Meaning ______ Root Operation(s) ______
4. amniotomy Meaning ______ Root Operation(s) ______
5. cholangiogram Meaning ______ Root Operation(s) ______
6. pleurodesis, chemical injection Meaning ______ Root Operation(s) ______
7. myleogram Meaning ______ Root Operation(s) ______
8. venography Meaning ______ Root Operation(s) ______
9. oximetry, fetal Meaning ______ Root Operation(s) N/A
10. electroencephalogram Meaning ______ Root Operation(s) ______

CODING OVERVIEW

PCS Sections other than Medical and Surgical are grouped into two general categories: Medical and Surgical-Related Procedures and Ancillary Procedures. These names are descriptive titles that summarize PCS Sections, but they do not occupy a Character within the code itself. Codes in these sections have seven Characters that are used differently than in the Medical and Surgical Section in order to reflect the specific types of procedures classified in each Section.

Overview of Medical and Surgical-Related Procedures

Medical and Surgical-Related procedures (Sections 1 to 9) include obstetrical procedures, administration of substances, measurement and monitoring of body functions, and extracorporeal therapies. Refer to ■ TABLE 29-2 as a guide to the Medical and Surgical-Related Sections.

In Sections **1 Obstetrics** and **2 Placement,** all seven Characters are defined in the same way as they are in the Medical and Surgical Section. In Sections 3 through 9, Character 6 is used for new purposes, not defined in Medical and Surgical, as follows:

- Section **3 Administration** defines Character 6 as **Substance.**
- Section **4 Measurement and Monitoring** and **5 Extracorporeal Assistance and Performance** define Character 6 as **Function.**
- Sections **7 Osteopathic, 8 Other Procedures,** and **9 Chiropractic** define Character 6 as **Method.**

Overview of Ancillary Procedures

Ancillary procedures (Sections B to D and F to H) include six PCS Sections consisting of imaging, nuclear medicine, radiation oncology, physical therapy and rehabilitation, mental health, and substance abuse treatment.

Table 29-2 ■ SEVEN CHARACTERS OF MEDICAL AND SURGICAL-RELATED PROCEDURES

Character: 1	2	3	4	5	6	7
Obstetrics **1**	Body System	Root Operation	Body Part	Approach	Device	Qualifier
Placement **2**	Body System	Root Operation	Body Region	Approach	Device	Qualifier
Administration **3**	Body System	Root Operation	Body Region	Approach	Substance	Qualifier
Measurement and Monitoring **4**	Body System	Root Operation	Body Region	Approach	Function	Qualifier
Extracorporeal Assistance and Performance **5**	Body System	Root Operation	Body System	Duration	Function	Qualifier
Extracorporeal Therapies **6**	Body System	Root Operation	Body System	Duration	Qualifier	Qualifier
Osteopathic **7**	Body System	Root Operation	Body Region	Approach	Method	Qualifier
Other Procedures **8**	Body System	Root Operation	Body Region	Approach	Method	Qualifier
Chiropractic **9**	Body System	Root Operation	Body Region	Approach	Method	Qualifier

Table 29-3 ■ **SEVEN CHARACTERS OF ANCILLARY PROCEDURES**

Character: 1	2	3	4	5	6	7
Imaging **B**	Body System	Root Type	Body Part	Contrast	Qualifier	Qualifier
Nuclear Medicine **C**	Body System	Root Type	Body Part	Radionuclide	Qualifier	Qualifier
Radiation Oncology **D**	Body System	Root Type	Body Part	Modality Qualifier	Isotope	Qualifier
Physical Rehabilitation and Diagnostic Audiology **F**	Section Qualifier	Root Type	Body System & Region	Qualifier	Equipment	Qualifier
Mental Health **G**	Body System	Root Type	Type Qualifier	Qualifier	Qualifier	Qualifier
Substance Abuse Treatment **H**	Body System	Root Type	Type Qualifier	Qualifier	Qualifier	Qualifier

Refer to ■ TABLE 29-3 as a guide to the Ancillary Sections. The definitions of some Characters in the Ancillary Sections differ from those seen in previous Sections because they vary according to the specific type of service provided. Character 3 is defined as Root Type, rather than Root Operation. Other differences include the following:

- Section **B Imaging** defines Character 5 as **Contrast** and Character 6 as **Qualifier**.
- Section **C Nuclear Medicine** defines Character 5 as **Radionuclide.**
- Section **D Radiation Oncology** defines Character 5 as **Modality Qualifier** and Character 6 as **Isotope.**
- Section **F Physical Rehabilitation and Diagnostic Audiology** defines Character 4 as **Body System and Region,** rather than **Body Part.** It defines Character 5 **Type Qualifier** and Character 6 as **Equipment.**
- Sections **G Mental Health** and **H Substance Abuse** define Character 4 as **Type Qualifier**. Characters 5 through 7 are **Qualifiers,** which are not used.

ABSTRACTING, ASSIGNING, AND ARRANGING CODES

The following discussion provides basic definitions and information to help identify and distinguish the broad range of Medical and Surgical-Related and Ancillary procedures. Refer to the *ICD-10-PCS Reference Manual*, which can be downloaded free of charge from the CMS website (www.cms.gov) for additional details on all procedures discussed in this chapter.

Coding for Medical and Surgical-Related Procedures

Medical and Surgical-Related procedures in Sections **1** through **9** are usually performed in conjunction with Medical and Surgical (Section **0**) procedures, but are not operative procedures in and of themselves. Key Criteria for abstracting Medical and Surgical-Related procedures (■ TABLE 29-4) aid in identifying which Section's Root

Table 29-4 ■ **KEY CRITERIA FOR ABSTRACTING MEDICAL AND SURGICAL-RELATED PROCEDURES**

General Questions

- ❑ What is the stated procedure?
- ❑ What body region or body part is involved?
- ❑ What approach is used?
- ❑ Is the procedure description what you would expect based on the name of the procedure?
- ❑ Was more than one procedure, or a combined procedure, performed?

Specific Questions	Refer to Root Operations in This Section
(Answer *Yes* to one question)	
❑ Does the procedure involve a fetus?	Section 1 Obstetric
❑ Does the procedure place an object in or on the patient without cutting or puncturing the skin or mucous membrane?	Section 2 Placement
❑ Is a diagnostic or therapeutic substance given to the patient?	Section 3 Administration
❑ Does the procedure involve measurement or monitoring?	Section 4 Measurement and Monitoring
❑ Does the procedure use equipment to support a critical physiological function?	Section 5 Extracorporeal Assistance and Performance

Table 29-4 ■ (continued)

Specific Questions	Refer to Root Operations in This Section
❑ Does the procedure involve other extracorporeal procedures?	Section 6 Extracorporeal Therapies
❑ Is the procedure osteopathic or chiropractic manipulation?	Section 7 Osteopathic or Section 9 Chiropractic
❑ Does the procedure involve another methodology in attempt to remediate or cure a disorder or disease?	Section 8 Other Procedures

Operations should be used. After reading the procedure report, use the abstracting table as follows:

1. Answer the General Questions in order to get a basic understanding of the procedure.
2. Answer the Specific Questions. One question should be answered *Yes*; the rest should be answered *No*.
3. For the Specific Question that was answered *Yes*, refer to the Section identified in the second column and review the Root Operations available in this Section.
4. Look up the definition of each of the applicable Root Operations in the appendix of the ICD-10-PCS coding manual.
5. Identify the one Root Operation that matches the procedure documented. This Root Operation will be the Main Term when you use the Index.
6. Repeat the abstracting process for each procedure that was performed.

The Root Operations and other key information for each Medical and Surgical-Related Section follow.

Section 1 Obstetrics

Section **1 Obstetrics** is the only Section besides Medical and Surgical that has Guidelines, which appear in section C of the Guidelines. The only procedures coded in the Obstetrics section are those performed on the products of conception (*embryo or fetus*). However, not all procedures on the fetus or embryo appear in the Obstetrics Section. Some appear in other Sections as well. Follow the guidance in the Index regarding which Section to use. Procedures performed on the pregnant female, other than the products of conception, are coded with the appropriate Root Operation in the Medical and Surgical Section (Guideline C1).

Codes in Section **1 Obstetrics** have the same structure as codes in the Medical and Surgical Section, with all seven characters retaining the same meaning. Obstetrics has only one Body System, **Pregnancy (0)** for Character 2 and only three Body Part values for Character 4 as follows:

- **Products of Conception (0)**
- **Products of Conception, Retained (1)**
- **Products of Conception, Ectopic (2)**

This Section has 12 Root Operations, ten of which are also found in Medical and Surgical Section. Refer to the ICD-10-PCS appendices for a complete list of Root Operations with definitions, explanations, and examples. The two Root Operations unique to Obstetrics are:

- **Abortion (A)**, Artificially terminating a pregnancy
- **Delivery (E)**, Assisting the passage of the products of conception from the genital canal

Identify the type of delivery as follows:

- For cesarean section deliveries and forceps-assisted vaginal deliveries, use the Root Operation **Extraction (D)** (■ FIGURE 29-1).
- For manually-assisted vaginal deliveries, use Root Operation **Delivery (E)**.

For procedures performed following a delivery or abortion, involving curettage of the endometrium or evacuation of retained products of conception, use the Root Operation **Extraction (D)** and the Body Part **Products of Conception, Retained (0)**.

For diagnostic or therapeutic dilation and curettage performed during times *other* than the postpartum or post-abortion period use Section **0 Medical and Surgical**, Root Operation **D Extraction**, and the Body Part **B Endometrium** (Guideline C2).

SUCCESS STEP

When coding procedures performed for pregnant women, use ICD-10-PCS procedure codes from any Section of the manual. However, when coding diagnoses for pregnant women, a code from the ICD-10-CM obstetrics chapter is necessary even if the condition was not caused by the pregnancy, such as preexisting diabetes or hypertension.

Patient delivers one liveborn infant with a low cervical cesarean section.

10D00Z1 Extraction, Products of Conception, Low Cervical

Figure 29-1 ■ Example of PCS Coding for Obstetrics Section, Root Operation Extraction (Low Cervical Cesarean Section)

Table 29-5 ■ **SECTION 2, PLACEMENT, CHARACTER 3, ROOT OPERATION DEFINITIONS**

Value	Description	Definition
0	Change	Taking out or off a device from a body region and putting back an identical or similar device in or on the same body region without cutting or puncturing the skin or a mucous membrane
1	Compression	Putting pressure on a body region
2	Dressing	Putting material on a body region for protection
3	Immobilization	Limiting or preventing motion of a body region
4	Packing	Putting material in a body region
5	Removal	Taking out or off a device from a body region
6	Traction	Exerting a pulling force on a body region in a distal direction

Section 2 Placement

The Root Operations in Section **2 Placement** include only those procedures performed without making an incision or a puncture (■ TABLE 29-5, page 594). Refer to the ICD-10-PCS appendix for a complete list of Root Operations with definitions, explanations, and examples. Coders need to make distinctions between procedures in Section **2 Placement** and procedures in Section **F Physical Rehabilitation and Diagnostic Audiology**.

The Root Operation **Immobilization (3)** in this Section applies to the fitting of devices, such as splints and braces, in inpatient settings *other than rehabilitation* (■ FIGURE 29-2, page 594). When these services are provided in a rehabilitation setting, use Section **F Physical Rehabilitation and Diagnostic Audiology**.

The Root Operation **Traction (6)** in this section applies to the use of **mechanical traction** apparatus. When **manual traction** is performed by a physical therapist, use the Root Type Qualifier (Character 5) **Manual Therapy Techniques (5)** in Section **F Physical Rehabilitation and Diagnostic Audiology** (■ FIGURE 29-3, page 594).

Physician places a cast on the right tibia of an inpatient hospital patient.

2W3QX2Z Immobilization, Leg, Lower, Right, Cast, No Qualifier

Figure 29-2 ■ Example of PCS Coding for Placement Section, Root Operation Immobilization (Cast for a Hospital Inpatient)

Section 3 Administration

Section **3 Administration** includes infusions, injections, and transfusions, as well as other related procedures, such as irrigation and tattooing. All codes in this Section define procedures in which a diagnostic or therapeutic substance is given to the patient. Refer to the ICD-10-PCS appendices for a complete list of Root Operations with definitions, explanations, and examples. Root Operations in this Section are classified according to

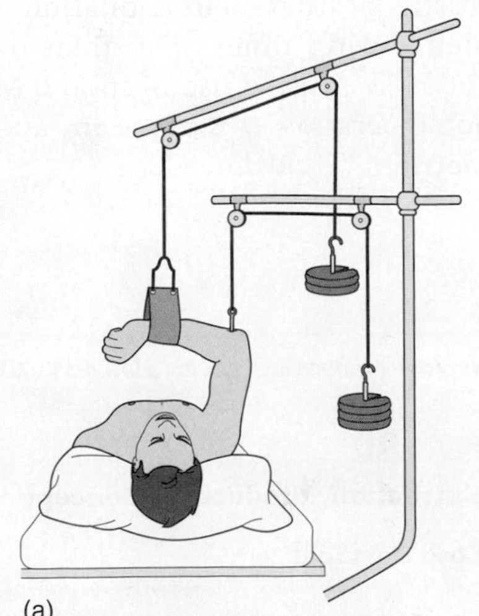

(a)

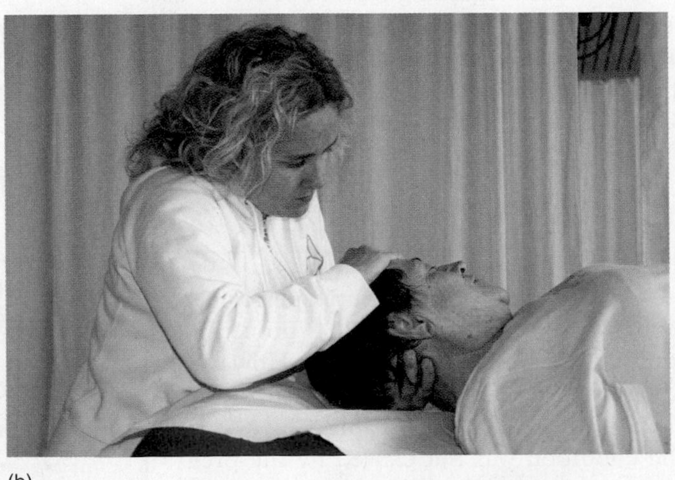

(b)

Figure 29-3 ■ (a) Mechanical traction uses equipment to apply a pulling force. (b) Manual traction is performed with the hands.
Source: Fahrner78/Dreamstime.

Table 29-6 ■ **SECTION 3, ADMINISTRATION, CHARACTER 3, ROOT OPERATION DEFINITIONS**

Value	Description	Definition
0	Introduction	Putting in or on a therapeutic, diagnostic, nutritional, physiological, or prophylactic substance except blood or blood products
1	Irrigation	Putting in or on a cleansing substance
2	Transfusion	Putting in blood or blood products

Physician implants a donor egg which was fertilized in-vitro into the recipient, transabdominally.

3E0P3Q1 Introduction, Reproductive, Female, Ovum, Fertilized, Percutaneous, Nonautologous

Figure 29-4 ■ Example of PCS Coding for Administration Section, Root Operation Introduction (In-Vitro Fertilization Implant)

the broad category of substance administered as follows (■ TABLE 29-6):

- When a blood product is administered, use the Root Operation **Transfusion (2)**.
- When a cleansing substance is administered, use the Root Operation **Irrigation (1)**.
- When all other substances are administered, such as anti-neoplastic substances, use the Root Operation **Introduction (0)** (■ FIGURE 29-4).

Section 4 Measurement and Monitoring

This Section has only two Root Operations, which differ in one respect:

- **Measurement (0)** defines one procedure or a single level taken at a point in time, such as single EKG reading.
- **Monitoring (1)** defines a series of procedures or a series of levels obtained repetitively, over a period of time, such as ambulatory Holter monitoring (■ FIGURE 29-5).

Character 6 **Function** defines the physiological function being tested. Refer to the ICD-10-PCS appendices for a complete list of Root Operations with definitions, explanations, and examples.

SUCCESS STEP

Monitoring the fetal heart rate is an example of a procedure performed on the products of conception that is coded from a Section other than Obstetrics (Figure 29-5).

The heart rate of a fetus was monitored continuously during labor.

4A1HXCZ Monitoring, Products of Conception, Cardiac, Rate, External, Rate, No Qualifier

Figure 29-5 ■ Example of PCS Coding for Measurement and Monitoring Section, Root Operation (Fetal Heart Rate)

Section 5 Extracorporeal Assistance and Performance

Section **5 Extracorporeal Assistance and Performance** includes procedures performed in a critical care setting that use equipment to support a physiological function in some way, such as breathing, circulating the blood, or restoring the natural rhythm of the heart. Extracorporeal refers to procedures or processes that take place outside of the body. Examples of procedures in this Section are mechanical ventilation, cardioversion (*application of an electric shock in order to restore normal heartbeat*), hyperbaric oxygen therapy (HBOT) (*breathing 100% oxygen under increased atmospheric pressure*), and hemodialysis.

This section has two Root Operations, **Assistance (0)** and **Performance (1)**, both of which describe the same kinds of procedures. They vary only in the degree of control exercised over the physiological function. **Assistance** defines procedures that support a physiological function but *do not take complete control* of it, such as an intra-aortic balloon pump used to support cardiac output and hyperbaric oxygen treatment. **Performance** defines procedures where *complete control* is exercised over a physiological function, such as total mechanical ventilation, cardiac pacing, and cardiopulmonary bypass (■ FIGURE 29-6).

Character 5 **Duration** describes the duration of the procedure. Character 6 **Function** describes the body function being acted upon.

Section 6 Extracorporeal Therapies

Section **6 Extracorporeal Therapies** describes other extracorporeal procedures that are not defined by **Assistance** and **Performance** in Section 5. Examples are ultraviolet phototherapy, apheresis, and whole body hypothermia.

Patient undergoing a CABG was placed on a cardiopulmonary bypass machine.

(1) **5A1221Z Performance, Cardiac, Continuous, Output**

(2) **5A1935Z Performance, Respiratory, Less than 24 Consecutive Hours, Ventilation**

Figure 29-6 ■ Example of PCS Coding for Extracorporeal Assistance and Performance Section, Root Operation Performance (Cardiopulmonary Bypass Machine)

Table 29-7 ■ **SECTION 6, EXTRACORPOREAL THERAPIES, CHARACTER 3, ROOT OPERATION DEFINITIONS**

Value	Description	Definition
0	Atmospheric Control	Extracorporeal control of atmospheric pressure and composition
1	Decompression	Extracorporeal elimination of undissolved gas from body fluids
2	Electromagnetic Therapy	Extracorporeal treatment by electromagnetic rays
3	Hyperthermia	Extracorporeal raising of body temperature
4	Hypothermia	Extracorporeal lowering of body temperature
5	Pheresis	Extracorporeal separation of blood products
6	Phototherapy	Extracorporeal treatment by light rays
7	Ultrasound Therapy	Extracorporeal treatment by ultrasound
8	Ultraviolet Light Therapy	Extracorporeal treatment by ultraviolet light
9	Shock Wave Therapy	Extracorporeal treatment by shock waves

Although the definitions of most Root Operations in this Section are consistent with the term as used in the medical community, coders should still refer to the PCS definition of each procedure (■ TABLE 29-7). For example, **Decompression (1)** (*extracorporeal elimination of undissolved gas from body fluids*) and **Hyperthermia (4)** (*extracorporeal lowering of body temperature*) have more specialized meanings in PCS than in the medical community in general.

The Root Operation **Pheresis (5)** (*extracorporeal separation of blood products*) is used to treat diseases where too much of a blood component is produced, such as leukemia, or to remove a blood product, such as platelets from a donor, for transfusion into a patient who needs it.

Section 7 Osteopathic

Section **7 Osteopathic** is one of the smallest sections in ICD-10-PCS. It contains one Body System, **Anatomical Regions (W)**, one Root Operation, **Treatment (0)**, and one Approach, **External (X)**. The methods listed for Character 6 are not explicitly defined in ICD-10-PCS, but rely on the standard definitions used in this specialty. A doctor of osteopathy (DO) is a licensed physician who has the same licensing, training, and qualifications as a doctor of medicine (MD), also called allopathic physicians. Osteopathic physicians receive an additional 300 to 500 hours in the musculoskeletal system and study of hands-on manual manipulation. The codes in this Section are specifically for osteopathic manual manipulation. Assign codes from any PCS section for other services provided by an osteopath.

Section 8 Other Procedures

Section **8 Other Procedures** contains codes for procedures not included in the other Medical and Surgical-Related Sections. This Section has one Root Operation, **Other Procedures (0)**, defined as methodologies that attempt to remediate or cure a disorder or disease. There are relatively few procedure codes in this section, including holistic therapies such as acupuncture and meditation; the fertilization portion of an in-vitro fertilization procedure; and computer- and robotic-assisted procedures.

Section 9 Chiropractic

The Chiropractic Section consists of one Body System, **Anatomical Regions (W)**, and one Root Operation, **Manipulation (B)**, which is defined as manual procedures that involve a direct thrust to move a joint past the physiological range of motion, without exceeding the anatomical limit.

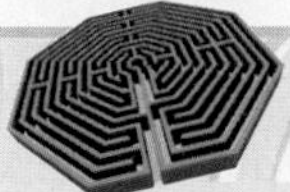

Coding Practice

Now it is your turn to practice assigning codes for Medical and Surgical-Related Procedures. Refer to Table 29-4 Key Criteria for Abstracting Medical and Surgical-Related Procedures and the ***Tip*** at the end of the mini-medical-record if you need a little extra help.

Instructions: Read the mini-medical-record of each patient's encounter and assign ICD-10-PCS procedure codes (PCS) using the Index and Tables. Write the code(s) on the line provided. Do not assign diagnosis codes in this exercise.

Exercise 29.2 Coding for Medical and Surgical-Related Procedures (Sections 1 to 9)

1. Date of discharge: 2/29/yy Location: Branton Medical Center Provider: Kay Pinkney, MD

Patient: Isabelle Landman Gender: F Age: 22

Gravida: 2 Para: 2 EDD: 4/18/yy EGA: 33+2

Reason for admission: premature rupture of membranes

Assessment: severe pre-eclampsia requires c/s

Delivery: 2/29/yy low C/S, PTBLC, 1 girl

Tip**:** PTBLC (Preterm birth, live child)

1 PCS Code __________

2. Date of procedure: 2/29/yy Location: Branton Medical Center Provider: Matthew Bunker, MD

Patient: Dean Defranco Gender: M Age: 47

Indication: angina pectoris

Procedure description: cardiac stress test to measure total activity, single measurement, followed by ECC of the right and left heart

Tip**:** The Root Operation Measurement is a single reading. The Root Operation Monitoring is a continuous reading.

2 PCS Codes __________ __________

3. Date of procedure: 2/29/yy Location: Branton Medical Center Provider: Kay Pinkney, MD

Patient: Daphne Scheid Gender: F Age: 33

Gravida: 2 Para: 2 EDD: 2/28/yy

EGA: 39+1

(continued)

3. (continued)

Assessment: fetal bradycardia

Procedure description: mid forceps delivery

Delivery: 2/29/yy TBLC, 1 girl

Tip**:** TBLC (Term birth, live child)

1 PCS Code __________

4. Date of procedure: 2/29/yy Location: Branton Medical Center Provider: Lorene Garman, MD

Patient: Brent Gadbois Gender: M Age: 32

Indication: peripheral neuritis, left arm

Procedure description: nerve block injection to the median nerve using a regional anesthetic

Tip**:** The median nerve is in the arm. An injection is the Root Operation Introduction.

1 PCS Code __________

5. Date of procedure: 2/29/yy Location: Branton Medical Center Provider: Bruce Prentice, MD

Patient: Tamika Krikorian Gender: F Age: 15

Indication: fractured R radius

Procedure description: application of short arm cast

Tip**:** The Root Operation Immobilization (3) in Section 2 Placement applies to the fitting of devices in inpatient settings other than rehabilitation.

1 PCS Code __________

Coding for Ancillary Procedures

Ancillary procedures in Sections B to D and F to H include all aspects of diagnostic and therapeutic radiology, nuclear medicine, physical rehabilitation, and behavioral health. Character 3 is Root Type rather than Root Operation, as it is in previous Sections. Each of these Sections introduces characters and definitions unique to its procedures. When a particular character is not used for a specific purpose, it is labeled as a Qualifier with the default value **Z None**. All codes must contain seven characters. Refer to the ICD-10-PCS appendix Type and Type Qualifier Definitions Sections B-H for detailed definitions used in these Sections.

Key abstracting criteria aid in identifying what Section of Root Operations should be used (■ TABLE 29-8, page 598). After reading the procedure report, use the abstracting table as follows:

1. Answer the General Questions in order to get a basic understanding of the procedure.
2. Answer the Section Questions. One question should be answered *Yes*; the rest should be answered *No*.
3. For the Section Question that was answered *Yes*, refer to the Section identified to review the Root Types that could apply.

Table 29-8 ■ **KEY CRITERIA FOR ABSTRACTING ANCILLARY PROCEDURES**

General Questions
❑ What is the stated procedure?
❑ What body region or body part is involved?
❑ What approach is used?
❑ Is the procedure description what you would expect based on the name of the procedure?
❑ Was more than one procedure, or a combined procedure, performed?

Specific Questions (Answer *Yes* to one question)	Refer to Root Types in This Section
❑ Does the procedure involve imaging/radiography?	Section B Imaging
❑ Does the procedure involve nuclear medicine?	Section C Nuclear Medicine
❑ Does the procedure involve radiation therapy?	Section D Radiation Therapy
❑ Does the procedure involve physical rehabilitation in a rehabilitation facility or diagnostic audiology?	Section F Physical Rehabilitation and Diagnostic Audiology
❑ Is the procedure related to behavioral health?	Section G Mental Health
❑ Is the procedure related to substance abuse treatment?	Section 6 Substance Abuse Treatment

4. Look up the definition of each of the applicable Root Types in the appendix of the ICD-10-PCS coding manual.
5. Identify the one Root Type that matches the procedure documented. This Root Operation will be the Main Term when you use the Index.
6. Repeat the abstracting process for each procedure that was performed.

Root Types and other key information for each Ancillary Section follow.

Physician uses fluoroscopic guidance to perform a percutaneous transluminal angioplasty (PTA) of left common femoral artery using low osmolar contrast.

B41G1ZZ Fluoroscopy, Lower Arteries, Lower Extremity Arteries, Left, Low Osmolar, None

Figure 29-7 ■ Example of PCS Coding for Imaging Section, Root Operation Fluoroscopy (PTA Guidance)

Section B Imaging

Section **B Imaging** includes diagnostic radiology and its branches, each of which is a Root Type (■ TABLE 29-9). Characters are defined as follows (■ FIGURE 29-7):

- Character 5 **Contrast** identifies the type of contrast medium used, if any. Because X-ray beams pass through soft tissue, the use of a contrast dye makes soft structures more readily visible.
- Character 6 **Qualifier**, value **0 Unenhanced and Enhanced** identifies an image taken without contrast followed by one with contrast. Otherwise, assign **Z None**.

Table 29-9 ■ **SECTION B, IMAGING, CHARACTER 3, ROOT TYPE DEFINITIONS**

Value	Description	Definition
0	Plain Radiography	Planar display of an image developed from the capture of external ionizing radiation on photographic or photoconductive plate (■ FIGURE 29-8(a))
1	Fluoroscopy	Single plane or bi-plane real time display of an image developed from the capture of external ionizing radiation on a fluorescent screen; may also be stored by either digital or analog means
2	Computerized Tomography (CT scan)	Computer reformatted digital display of multiplanar images developed from the capture of multiple exposures of external ionizing radiation (■ FIGURE 29-8(b))
3	Magnetic Resonance Imaging (MRI)	Computer reformatted digital display of multiplanar images developed from the capture of radio-frequency signals emitted by nuclei in a body site excited within a magnetic field (■ FIGURE 29-8(c))
4	Ultrasonography	Real time display of images of anatomy or flow information developed from the capture of reflected and attenuated high-frequency sound waves

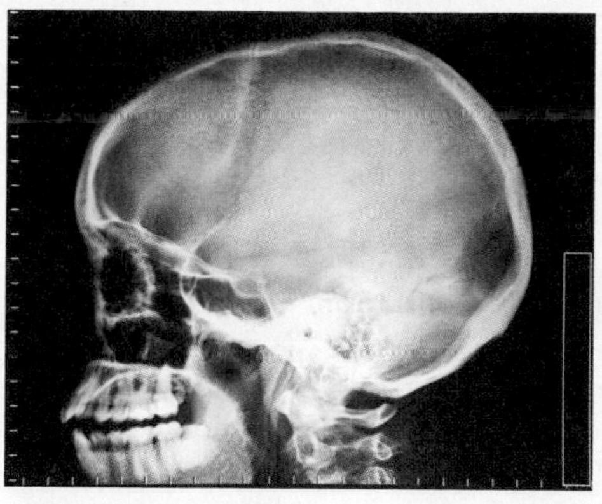

(a) Plain Radiography

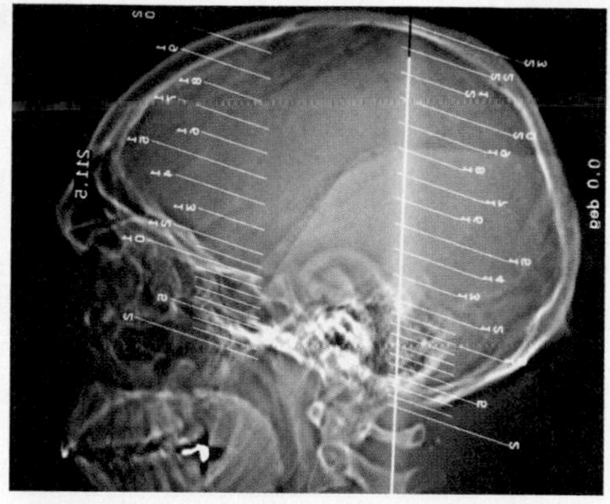

(b) CT

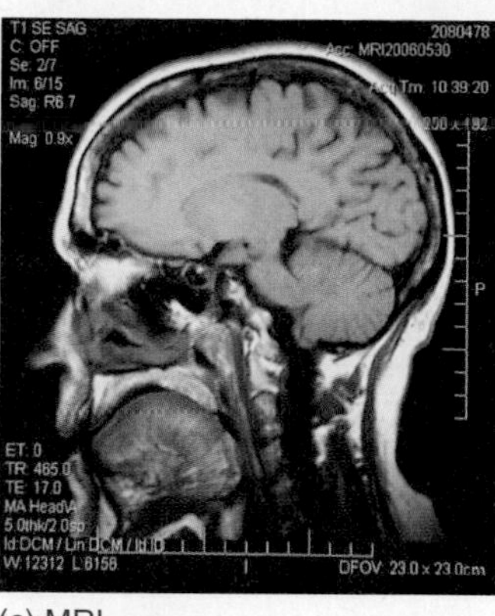

(c) MRI

Figure 29-8 ■ Images of the Head Made Using (a) Plain Radiography (b) CT and (c) MRI. *Sources: (a) ©Gualtiero Boffi/Dreamstime.com (b) ©Andesign101/Dreamstime.com (c) ©Katrina Brown/Dreamstime.com.*

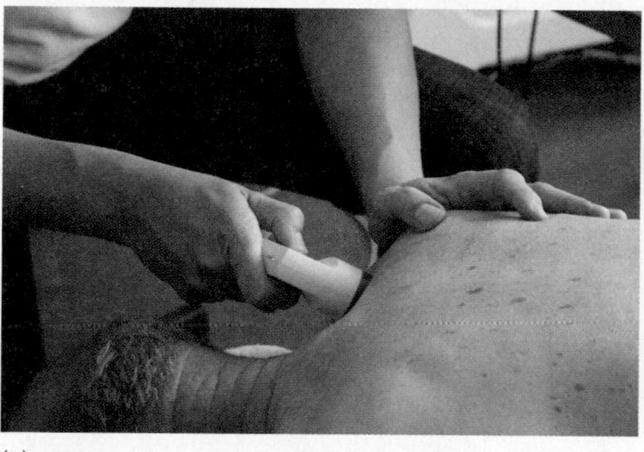

(a)

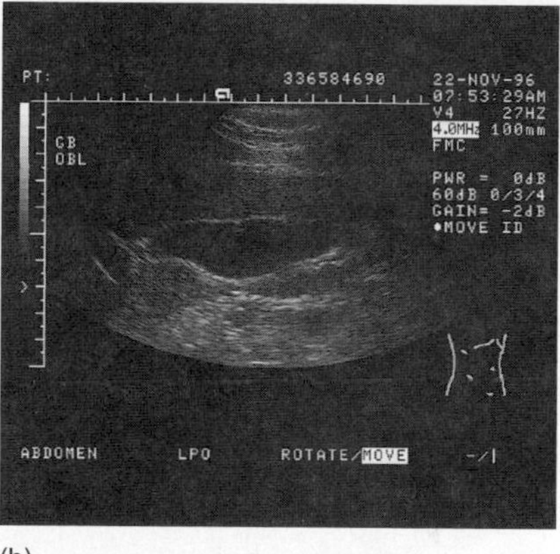

(b)

Figure 29-9 ■ (a) Ultrasound therapy uses sound waves to stimulate tissue. (b) Ultrasound imaging uses sound waves to create an image. *Sources: (a) Patricia Hofmeeste/Dreamstime (b) Teresa Resch*

- Character 7 **Qualifier** has only one value, **Z None**, which should be assigned for all codes.

SUCCESS STEP

Ultrasound is energy created by high-frequency sound waves, which can be used for therapy, such as stimulating muscle and nerve tissue, or for imaging purposes. When you see a reference to ultrasound, remember to determine whether it is therapeutic ultrasound or ultrasound imaging, also called ultrasonography or sonogram, so you can select the correct Root Operation (■ FIGURE 29-9).

Section C Nuclear Medicine

Root Types for Section **C Nuclear Medicine** identify the methods used (■ TABLE 29-10, page 600). Nuclear medicine is a specialized branch of radiology that provides functional imaging, which allows the physician to observe organ function in real time. Patients take a very small amount of radioactive material, also called radiopharmaceuticals, internally and imaging equipment detects the resulting gamma rays. This is in contrast to anatomical imaging of traditional radiology, which captures a static image of an anatomical part.

The Nuclear Medicine Section is organized similarly to the Imaging Section with the following differences:

- Character 5 **Radionuclide** defines the radiation source used in the procedure. Choices are applicable for the root procedure type.
- Character 6 **Qualifier** and Character 7 **Qualifier** have only one value, **Z None**, which should be assigned for all codes in both positions.

CODING CAUTION

Do not confuse the Root Type Tomographic (Tomo) Nuclear Medicine Imaging with the Root Type Computerized Tomography (CT). Read the procedure report carefully to determine which method is documented.

Table 29-10 ■ **SECTION C, NUCLEAR MEDICINE, CHARACTER 3, ROOT TYPE DEFINITIONS**

Value	Description	Definition
1	Planar Nuclear Medicine Imaging	Introduction of radioactive materials into the body for single plane display of images developed from the capture of radioactive emissions
2	Tomographic (Tomo) Nuclear Medicine Imaging	Introduction of radioactive materials into the body for three-dimensional display of images developed from the capture of radioactive emissions
3	Positron Emission Tomography (PET)	Introduction of radioactive materials into the body for three-dimensional display of images developed from the simultaneous capture, 180 degrees apart, of radioactive emissions
4	Nonimaging Nuclear Medicine Uptake	Introduction of radioactive materials into the body for measurements of organ function, from the detection of radioactive emissions
5	Nonimaging Nuclear Medicine Probe	Introduction of radioactive materials into the body for the study of distribution and fate of certain substances by the detection of radioactive emissions from an external source
6	Nonimaging Nuclear Medicine Assay	Introduction of radioactive materials into the body for the study of body fluids and blood elements by the detection of radioactive emissions
7	Systemic Nuclear Medicine Therapy	Introduction of unsealed radioactive materials into the body for treatment

Section D Radiation Therapy

Section **D Radiation Therapy** contains therapeutic radiology procedures performed for cancer treatment. Character meanings are described below.

- Character 3 **Root Type** identifies the modality:
  - **Beam radiation (0)**
  - **Brachytherapy (1)**
  - **Stereotactic radiosurgery (2)**
  - **Other radiation (Y)**
- Character 4 **Treatment Site** is the anatomical location treated.
- Character 5 **Modality Qualifier** further specifies treatment modality.
- Character 6 **Isotope** defines the radioactive isotope used, if applicable.
- Character 7 **Qualifier** has only one value, **Z None**, which should be assigned for all codes.

CODING CAUTION

PCS codes for radiation therapy are reported once per treatment. Do not confuse these with CPT codes for physician radiation treatment management, which are reported once for every five fractions or treatment sessions.

Section F Physical Rehabilitation and Diagnostic Audiology

The Character definitions in this Section are disctinct from any other PCS Sections, as follows:

- Character 2 is **Section Qualifier**, rather than **Body System**, and specifies whether the procedure is **Rehabilitation (0)** or **Diagnostic Audiology (1)**.
- Character 3 **Root Type** defines the general type of procedure (■ TABLE 29-11).
- Character 4 **Body System and Region** defines the body system and body region combined, where applicable.
- Character 5 **Qualifier** further specifies the procedure type.
- Character 6 **Equipment** specifies the equipment used, if any.
- Character 7 **Qualifier** has only one value, **Z None**, which should be assigned for all codes.

The Root Type **Device Fitting (D)** is for use by inpatient rehabilitation facilities. All other inpatient facilities should assign codes for the Root Operation **Immobilization (3)** from Section **2 Placement** (■ FIGURE 29-10).

Patient in a rehabilitation facility is fitted for a short arm cast.

F0DZ7EZ Device Fitting, None, Static Orthosis, Orthosis, None

Figure 29-10 ■ Example of PCS Coding for Physical Rehabilitation Section, Root Type Device Fitting (Short Arm Cast)

Table 29-11 ■ **SECTION F, PHYSICAL REHABILITATION AND DIAGNOSTIC AUDIOLOGY, CHARACTER 3, ROOT TYPE DEFINITIONS**

Value	Description	Definition
0	Speech Assessment	Measurement of speech and related functions
1	Motor and/or Nerve Function Assessment	Measurement of motor, nerve, and related functions
2	Activities of Daily Living Assessment	Measurement of functional level for activities of daily living
3	Hearing Assessment	Measurement of hearing and related functions
4	Hearing Aid Assessment	Measurement of the appropriateness and/or effectiveness of a hearing device
5	Vestibular Assessment	Measurement of the vestibular system and related functions
6	Speech Treatment	Application of techniques to improve, augment, or compensate for speech and related functional impairment
7	Motor Treatment	Exercise or activities to increase or facilitate motor function
8	Activities of Daily Living Treatment	Exercise or activities to facilitate functional competence for activities of daily living
9	Hearing Treatment	Application of techniques to improve, augment, or compensate for hearing and related functional impairment
B	Hearing Aid Treatment	Application of techniques to improve the communication abilities of individuals with cochlear implant
C	Vestibular Treatment	Application of techniques to improve, augment, or compensate for vestibular and related functional impairment
D	Device Fitting	Fitting of a device designed to facilitate or support achievement of a higher level of function
F	Caregiver Training	Training in activities to support patient's optimal level of function

Section G Mental Health

Section **G Mental Health** uses Character 3 **Root Type** (■ TABLE 29-12) and Character 4 **Type Qualifier**. Characters 2, 5, 6, and 7 are placeholders only and should be assigned the value **Z None** for all codes.

Table 29-12 ■ **SECTION G, MENTAL HEALTH, CHARACTER 3, ROOT TYPE DEFINITIONS**

Value	Description
1	Psychological Tests
2	Crisis Intervention
5	Individual Psychotherapy
6	Counseling
7	Family Psychotherapy
B	Electroconvulsive Therapy
C	Biofeedback
F	Hypnosis
G	Narcosynthesis
H	Group Therapy
J	Light Therapy

Section H Substance Abuse Treatment

Section **H Substance Abuse Treatment** is organized similarly to Mental Health and has seven Root Types (■ TABLE 29-13). Root Type **2 Detoxification Services** does not provide values for Characters 4 through 7. Root Types **3** through **6** use Character 4 for Type Qualifier, which describes the type of counseling provided. Root Types **8 Medication Management** and **9 Pharmacotherapy** use the Type Qualifier to identify the medication.

Table 29-13 ■ **SECTION H, SUBSTANCE ABUSE TREATMENT, CHARACTER 3, ROOT TYPE DEFINITIONS**

Value	Description
2	Detoxification Services
3	Individual Counseling
4	Group Counseling
5	Individual Psychotherapy
6	Family Counseling
8	Medication Management
9	Pharmacotherapy

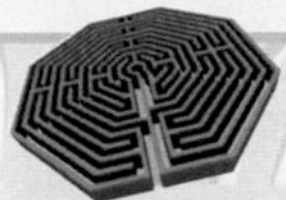

Coding Practice

Now it is your turn to practice assigning codes for Ancillary Procedures. Refer to Table 29-8 Key Criteria for Abstracting Ancillary Procedures and the ***Tip*** at the end of the mini-medical-record if you need a little extra help.

Exercise 29.3 Coding for Ancillary Procedures (Sections B to D, F to H)

Instructions: Read the mini-medical-record of each patient's encounter and assign ICD-10-PCS procedure codes (PCS) using the Index and Tables. Write the code(s) on the line provided. Do not assign diagnosis codes in this exercise.

1. Date of procedure: 3/29/yy Location: Branton Medical Center Provider: Jennifer Kolb, MD

Patient: Tamika Krikorian Gender: F Age: 15

Indication: injured R radius

Procedure description: X-ray of the right radius

Findings: fractured R radius

Tip: X-ray cross-references you to the Root Operation Plain Radiography.

1 PCS Code __________

2. Date of procedure: 3/29/yy Location: Branton Medical Center Provider: Jennifer Kolb, MD

Patient: Rick Puskar Gender: M Age: 57

Indication: cirrhosis, r/o hepatocellular carcinoma

Procedure description: CT scan of liver with and without contrast

Findings: enlarged liver as expected but no tumors identified

Tip: Contrast dye is used to help certain areas show up better.

1 PCS Code __________

3. Date of procedure: 3/29/yy Location: Branton Medical Center Provider: Richard Blackford, MD

Patient: Lewis Bourland Gender: M Age: 61

Diagnosis: prostate cancer

Procedure description: low dose rate (LDR) brachytherapy of prostate using Iridium 192

Tip: Iridium 192 is the isotope used.

1 PCS Code __________

4. Date of procedure: 3/29/yy Location: Branton Rehabilitation Center Provider: Kristen Conover, MD

Patient: Lacey Cranston Gender: F Age: 81

Indication: status post-hip replacement, left hip

Procedure description: range of motion and joint mobility exercises for the left hip with walker

Tip: A walker is assistive equipment.

1 PCS Code __________

5. Date of procedure: 3/29/yy Location: Branton Medical Center Provider: Brett Camden, MD

Patient: Derrick Amsler Gender: M Age: 26

Indication: severe depression

Procedure description: electroconvulsive therapy (ECT) bilateral, single seizure

Tip: The aim of ECT is to induce a therapeutic seizure in which the person loses consciousness and has convulsions lasting for at least 15 seconds.

1 PCS Code __________

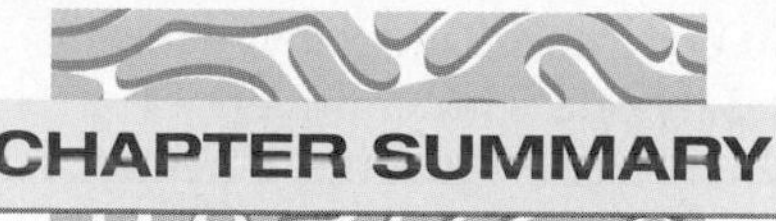

CHAPTER SUMMARY

In this chapter you learned that:

- Medical terms used in the Medical and Surgical-Related and Ancillary Procedures Sections use different suffixes than those in the Medical and Surgical Section.
- Medical and Surgical-Related procedures include obstetrical procedures, administration of substances, measurement and monitoring of body functions, and extracorporeal therapies.
- Ancillary Procedures includes six PCS Sections consisting of imaging procedures, nuclear medicine, radiation oncology, physical therapy and rehabilitation, mental health, and substance abuse treatment.
- Key abstracting criteria aid in identifying what Section of Root Operations should be used.
- ICD-10-PCS provides Guidelines for the Obstetrics Section.

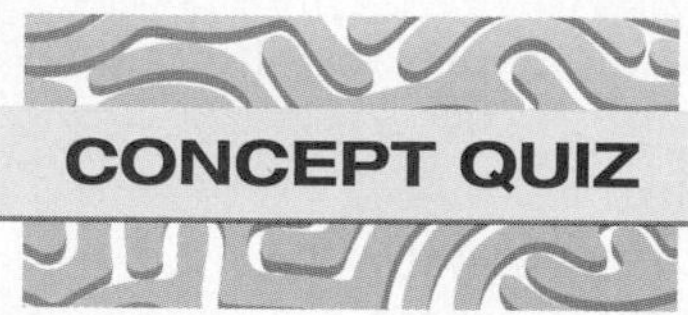

CONCEPT QUIZ

Take a moment to look back at your trip through Medical and Surgical-Related and Ancillary procedures and solidify your skills. This is your opportunity to pull together everything you have learned.

Completion

Instructions: Identify the Root Operation or Root Type described by each definition. Write the answer on the line. Choose from the list below. Some choices may be used more than once and some choices may not be used at all. Refer to the discussion in this chapter and the appendices in the ICD-10-PCS manual if you need a little extra help.

Abortion	Immobilization
Assistance	Introduction
Change	Measurement
Compression	Monitoring
Computerized Tomography	Removal
Delivery	Tomographic Nuclear Medicine Imaging
Device Fitting	Traction
Hearing Aid Assessment	Ultrasonography
Hearing Assessment	Ultrasound Therapy
Hearing Treatment	

1. ______________________ Putting in or on a therapeutic, diagnostic, nutritional, physiological, or prophylactic substance except blood or blood products
2. ______________________ Application of techniques to improve, augment, or compensate for hearing and related functional impairment
3. ______________________ Assisting the passage of the products of conception from the genital canal
4. ______________________ Procedures that support a physiological function but do not take complete control of it
5. ______________________ Extracorporeal treatment by ultrasound
6. ______________________ Limiting or preventing motion of a body region
7. ______________________ Fitting of a device designed to facilitate or support achievement of a higher level of function
8. ______________________ Real time display of images of anatomy or flow information developed from the capture of reflected and attenuated high-frequency sound waves
9. ______________________ Exerting a pulling force on a body region in a distal direction
10. ______________________ Introduction of radioactive materials into the body for three-dimensional display of images developed from the capture of radioactive emissions

Multiple Choice

Instructions: Circle the letter of the best answer to each question based on the information you learned in this chapter. Refer to the discussion in this chapter and the Glossary at the end of this book if you need a little extra help.

1. Codes from the Obstetrics Section (1) describe
   A. procedures for any pregnancy-related condition.
   B. all procedures for pregnant women.
   C. procedures for pregnant women and newborns.
   D. procedures on the embryo or fetus.
2. Products of Conception is a
   A. Body System.
   B. Body Part.
   C. Root Operation.
   D. Qualifier.
3. Codes for procedures where a diagnostic or therapeutic substance is given to the patient are located in what Section?
   A. Placement
   B. Administration
   C. Extracorporeal Assistance and Performance
   D. Other Procedures
4. What Root Operation should be used when a physician implants a donor egg that was fertilized in-vitro into the recipient?
   A. Introduction
   B. Placement
   C. Transfusion
   D. Assistance
5. The use of a cardiopulmonary bypass machine during a CABG operation is coded with what Root Operation?
   A. Bypass
   B. Pheresis
   C. Assistance
   D. Performance
6. How should you code an image taken without contrast followed by one with contrast?
   A. Assign the Character 6 Qualifier Unenhanced and Enhanced.
   B. Assign two codes, one for the Root Operation Without Contrast and one for the Root Operation With Contrast.
   C. Assign the Root Operation Fluoroscopy.
   D. Assign the Root Operation CT Scan.
7. Which Section uses Character 6 to identify equipment?
   A. Obstetrics (1)
   B. Measurement and Monitoring (4)
   C. Imaging (B)
   D. Physical Rehabilitation and Diagnostic Audiology (F)
8. Which type of radiology provides functional imaging?
   A. Ultrasonography
   B. Computerized Tomography
   C. Nuclear Medicine
   D. Radiation Therapy
9. Which of the following is NOT a Root Type in Section G Mental Health?
   A. Crisis Intervention
   B. Group Counseling
   C. Electroconvulsive Therapy
   D. Hypnosis
10. Which Root Operation is a method of radiation therapy?
   A. Stereotactic radiosurgery
   B. Vestibular treatment
   C. Systemic Nuclear Medicine Therapy
   D. Pheresis

CODING CHALLENGE

Now it is your turn to demonstrate coding all aspects of Medical and Surgical-Related and Ancillary procedures. Refer back to the examples and discussion in this chapter when you need a little extra help. Use your medical dictionary and anatomy references when needed.

Instructions: Read the mini-medical-record of each patient's encounter, then abstract, assign, and sequence ICD-10-CM diagnosis codes (CM) *and* ICD-10-PCS procedure codes (PCS) using the Index and Tables. Write the code(s) on the line provided.

1. Date of discharge: 9/29/yy Location: Branton Medical Center Provider: Kay Pinkey, MD

Patient: Elisabeth Arnette Gender: F Age: 27
Gravida: 1 Para: 0 EDD: 10/6/yy EGA: 37+5

Reason for admission: full term labor

Delivery: 9/28/yy, NSVD, liveborn born, 1 girl

Tip: NSVD (Normal, spontaneous, vaginal delivery)

2 CM Codes __________ __________

1 PCS Code __________

2. Date of procedure: 9/29/yy Location: Branton Medical Center Provider: Matthew Bunker, MD

Patient: Clyde Campion Gender: M Age: 53

Indication: Suspected ventricular tachycardia following an episode of syncope. Transient heart arrhythmias and transient cardiac ischemia.

Procedure description: Holter monitor 24 hours

Plan: ventricular tachycardia confirmed. Patient to receive implantable defibrillator

1 CM Code ___________

1 PCS Code ___________

3. Date of procedure: 9/29/yy Location: Branton Medical Center Provider: Debora Ridgley, DO

Patient: Greg Mcquade Gender: M Age: 31

Diagnosis: Postpolio syndrome (PPS). Severe neck pain and weakness. Had polio at age 5 when living overseas.

Procedure description: osteopathic myofascial release of the neck

Plan: oxygen therapy, physical therapy to affected muscles daily and on outpatient basis post-discharge

2 CM Codes ___________ ___________

1 PCS Code ___________

4. Date of procedure: 9/29/yy Location: Branton Medical Center Provider: Jennifer Kolb, MD (Radiologist), Matthew Bunker, MD (Cardiologist)

Patient: Louisa Giardina Gender: F Age: 18

Preprocedure diagnosis: AAA

Procedure description: EVAR (*endovascular aneurysm repair*) with synthetic graft. Made incision into femoral artery. With low osmolar fluoroscopic guidance, guided delivery catheter with compressed graft into abdominal aorta to site of aneurysm. Inflated balloon to expand graft and affix it to vessel wall. Withdrew catheter and closed incision.

Postprocedure diagnosis: AAA

Tip: You previously coded the repair and the graft. Now code the entire procedure, including the fluoroscopy.

1 CM Code ___________

2 PCS Codes ___________ ___________

5. Date of procedure: 9/29/yy Location: Branton Rehabilitation Center Provider: Bruce Prentice, MD

Patient: Trudy Fuhrman Gender: F Age: 78

Diagnosis: left hip fracture following a fall

Procedure description: placement of intermittent pneumatic compression (IPC) device covering both calves to prevent deep vein thrombosis (DVT)

Plan: continue nighttime use of IPC during one week of rehab for post surgery mobility

Tip: Do not assign an external cause code for the fall.

1 CM Code ___________

2 PCS Codes ___________ ___________

6. Date of procedure: 9/29/yy Location: Branton Medical Center Provider: Jennifer Kolb, MD

Patient: Candy Winkelman Gender: F Age: 48

Diagnosis: pancreatic cancer with liver metastases

Procedure description: photon beam radiation >10MeV treatment of pancreas and heavy particle radiation treatment of liver

Tip: 10MeV describes the strength of the radiation.

2 CM Codes ___________ ___________

2 PCS Codes ___________ ___________

7. Date of procedure: 9/29/yy Location: Branton Medical Center Provider: Brett Camden, MD

Patient: Brent Burciaga Gender: M Age: 25

Diagnosis: Patient found running naked down the street in the night. Previously diagnosed with Bipolar Personality Disorder. Parents report that he recently stopped his meds because he "felt cured."

Procedure description: Crisis intervention. Placed on 72 hour hold, lithium (gluconate) resumed plus antipsychotic meds

Plan: Begin psychotherapy and medication regimen to stabilize patient. Family session scheduled to discuss OP tx plan and medication review.

Tip: Assign external cause codes using the Table of Drugs and Chemicals.

3 CM Codes ___________ ___________ ___________

1 PCS Code ___________

(*continued*)

(continued from page 605)

8. Date of procedure: 9/29/yy Location: Branton Medical Center Provider: Brett Camden, MD

Patient: Timothy Petties Gender: M Age: 57

Diagnosis: alcohol addiction with delirium tremens

Procedure description: antabuse therapy

Plan: Continue detox within a stimulus free environment, liver function tests. Admit to inpatient alcohol rehab.

1 CM Code __________

1 PCS Code __________

9. Date of procedure: 6/15/yy Location: Branton Medical Center Provider: Kay Pinkney, MD

Patient: Cathleen Gwynn Gender: F Age: 35

Gravida: 1 Para: 0 EDD: 10/25/yy EGA: 19+5

Reason for encounter: Threatened spontaneous abortion. Spotting.

Procedure description: routine fetal ultrasound, twin gestation

(continued)

9. (continued)

Findings: Fetal movement recorded, fetus a: 12 oz., fetus b: 11.5 oz., cardiac heart rate noted. Mother on bed rest, monitor cervix with vaginal ultrasound.

2 CM Codes __________ __________

1 PCS Code __________

10. Date of procedure: 9/29/yy Location: Branton Medical Center

Provider: Jennifer Kolb, MD (Radiologist), Matthew Bunker, MD (Cardiologist)

Patient: Dan Bechtold Gender: M Age: 52

Indication: Unabated angina. Left ventricle failure.

Procedure description: PET scan of myocardium using Fluorine 18 to assess myocardial viability and patient's candidacy for a revascularization procedure

Findings: Viable heart muscle. Schedule Transmyocardial revascularization (TMR) using laser to produce channels directly into the heart muscle.

1 CM Code __________

1 PCS Code __________

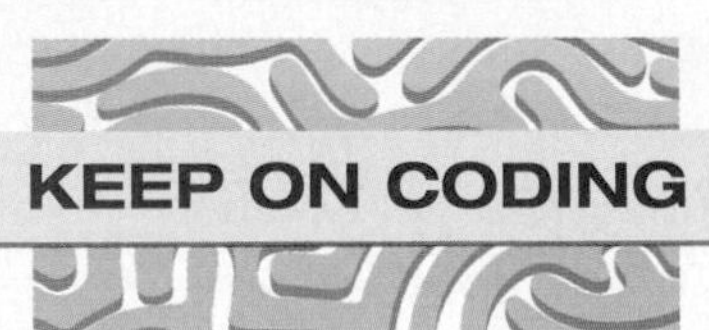

KEEP ON CODING

As a coder, you can never have too much experience. Apply everything you have learned in this chapter to code the following procedural statements. Use the Guidelines to help determine how many codes are required.

Instructions: Read the procedural statement, then use the Index and Tables to assign and sequence ICD-10-PCS (PCS) procedure codes. Write the code(s) on the line provided.

1. Abortion using laminaria: PCS Code(s) __________
2. Classical cesarean section: PCS Code(s) __________
3. Traction for fracture of right upper leg: PCS Code(s) __________
4. Splinting of left hand: PCS Code(s) __________
5. Pain nerve block injection in the spine: PCS Code(s) __________
6. Transfusion of non-autologous frozen red blood cells via peripheral vein: PCS Code(s) __________
7. Esophageal motility study, via endoscope: PCS Code(s) __________

8. Electroencephalogram (EEG): PCS Code(s) ______

9. Intermittent Positive Airway Pressure (IPAP) respiratory ventilation for 36 hours. PCS Code(s) ______

10. Hyperbaric oxygen treatment for non-healing ulcer, left ankle: PCS Code(s) ______

11. Phototherapy of the skin, multiple treatments: PCS Code(s) ______

12. Osteopathic treatment of the neck using general mobilization: PCS Code(s) ______

13. Collection of sperm for fertility study: PCS Code(s) ______

14. Chiropractic manipulation of the lumbar spine using mechanically assisted technique: PCS Code(s) ______

15. Magnetic Resonance Imaging (MRI) of the brain without contrast: PCS Code(s) ______

16. Ultrasound of the gallbladder: PCS Code(s) ______

17. Whole body positron Emission Tomography (PET) scan of heart: PCS Code(s) ______

18. Stereotactic radiosurgery of the prostate using Gamma beam: PCS Code(s) ______

19. Fitting of left prosthetic leg: PCS Code(s) ______

20. Hearing screening assessment in a sound booth: PCS Code(s) ______

21. Mobility training using a wheelchair: PCS Code(s) ______

22. Biofeedback: PCS Code(s) ______

23. Individual interactive mental health psychotherapy services: PCS Code(s) ______

24. Alcohol detoxification: PCS Code(s) ______

25. Methadone maintenance for heroin addiction: PCS Code(s) ______

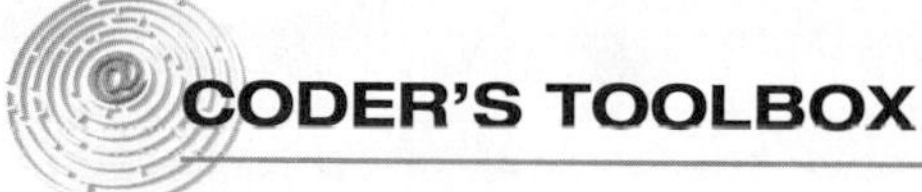

CODER'S TOOLBOX

The following resources are a starting point for learning more about procedures in this chapter.

American College of Radiology (ACR) **http://www.acr.org/**

American Society for Radiation Oncology (ASTRO) **http://www. astro.org**

Radiological Society of North America (RSNA) **http://www.rsna.org/**

Society of Radiologists in Ultrasound (SRU) **http://www.sru.org/**

SECTION FOUR

Putting It All Together

Section Four: Putting It All Together pulls together what you have learned and launches you toward the next steps in your coding career. You will learn how to make the transition to coding from full chart notes and operative reports, as well as how developments in health information technology will enhance your role.

PROFESSIONAL PROFILE MEET...

Marie Schanbacher, HIM Coder
Virginia Gay Hospital, Clinics, Home Health & Nursing and Rehab

I recently completed my Associates Degree in billing and coding and was hired as an HIM coder a few months before I finished my degree. My education was a big part of preparing me for my career because I was able to take what I learned and apply it to my position as an HIM coder. I needed very little assistance from my HIM Director or my co-workers to get started. Next, I plan on becoming AHIMA certified and possibly going back for my BS in Healthcare Management. Receiving my degrees and certification are very important for my career as a coder because it shows that I have the educational background for the position and the know-how to accurately do my job.

This is my first job in billing and coding. I told the nurse at my doctor's office what I was going to school for and she told me to fill out an application. When a position opened in the HIM Department, she called me and let me know about it. She and my doctor put in a good word for me. As a part of the interview process, I was asked to translate a dictation and then code the diagnoses, which I was able to accomplish very quickly. I also told the HIM Director that even though I had not received my degree or certification at that time, I would be willing to sign a letter of confidentiality for HIPAA purposes. She was impressed and, even though she had more qualified applicants, she hired me.

I code superbills for three clinics, outpatient records, radiology, and lab reports. I also transcribe dictation reports, pull medical records for Release of Information, file, and assist the HIM Director when she needs help. Once I become efficient with these responsibilities, I will be assigned more responsibilities. The most challenging part of my job is making sure that the codes I assign are 100% accurate. Our facility does not yet have an encoder, but I know that the more comfortable I become with coding, the more accurate I will be. After I received my degree, I received a \$0.50 increase over my beginning wage; after I receive my AHIMA certification, I will receive an additional \$0.50 per hour.

To be successful in medical billing and coding it is important that, as a student, you learn everything you possibly can about the field. Get a good education. Complete all school assignments. Ask for assistance on codes that you are not sure of and practice reworking the codes that you miss on assignments. Once you receive your degree and certification, keep on top of all updates and any additional learning that may be needed.

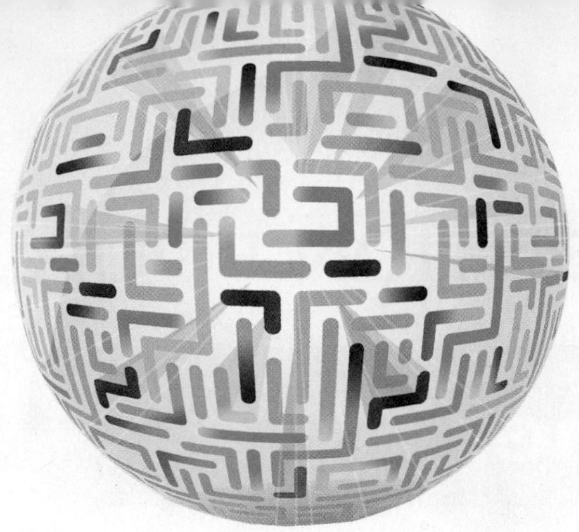

30

Advanced Coding and Health Information Technology

Learning Objectives

After completing this chapter, you should have the skills to:

- Spell and define the key words, medical terms, and abbreviations related to chart notes, operative reports, and health information technology.
- Demonstrate how to locate coding information in chart notes.
- Demonstrate how to locate coding information in operative reports.
- Discuss the impact of health information technology on coding.

Key Terms and Abbreviations

American Recovery and Reinvestment Act of 2009 (ARRA)
assessment
certified EHR technology
chief complaint (CC)
computer-assisted coding (CAC)
consultation
edit check
electronic health record (EHR)
electronic medical record (EMR)
encoder
Health Information Technology for Economic and Clinical Health Act (HITECH)
history of present illness (HPI)
meaningful use
natural language programming (NLP)
past medical history (PMH)
physical examination (PE or PX)
plan
reason for encounter
recommendations
structured input

In addition to the key terms listed here, students should know the terms defined within tables in this chapter.

Chapter Outline

- **Coding from Chart Notes**
- **Coding from Operative Reports**
- **Health Information Technology**

ICD-10-CM codes in this chapter are from the ICD-10-CM 2014 Draft code set from the Department of Health and Human Services, Centers for Disease Control and Prevention.

ICD-10-PCS codes in this chapter are from the ICD-10-PCS 2014 Draft code set from the Department of Health and Human Services, Centers for Medicare and Medicaid Services.

INTRODUCTION

When you return home after an extended road trip, it is fun to look back through all the maps, brochures, souvenirs, and photographs you collected along the way. You are amazed by all the places you visited, the activities you enjoyed, and the people you met, and you are eager to share your adventure with others. Thus the Thanksgiving Day-slide show was born, when all the relatives gathered after dinner and relived your travels with you. Of course, the slide projector has been replaced in recent years by digital photos, online albums, and social media. But you still want to share your experiences with others. At the same time, you are already planning your next trip: where you will go, who will go with you, and what new experiences you anticipate.

In this final chapter of your ICD-10-CM/PCS tour, you will look back on where you have been, consider how to plan the next phase of your trip, and preview destinations that are on the coding horizon. Most importantly, you will practice coding for patient encounters from expanded medical records using both ICD-10-CM and ICD-10-PCS, a skill which requires you to abstract information, assign correct codes, and arrange (sequence) the codes in the proper order.

As you read this chapter, open up your medical terminology book and keep a medical dictionary handy. Because coders frequently encounter unfamiliar terms, these professional resources provide the information needed, so you can complete your task quickly and efficiently.

CODING FROM CHART NOTES

Physicians document each patient encounter in a chart note or progress note. Coders must read through all the details of the encounter, abstract the relevant information, then assign and sequence codes. A variety of documentation formats are used, depending on physician preference, organizational protocols, and electronic health record (EHR) systems in use, but in all cases, coders need to read, locate, and interpret information in order to assign codes. The mini-medical-record used in this text encapsulates the essential nuggets from documentation. After coders master basic coding, they continue to learn in order to develop advanced skills in sorting through all of the information contained in a piece of documentation. This section highlights how to locate the needed coding information in a typical physician chart note. The chart notes contain sections with headings similar to the following:

- Chief Complaint (CC)/ Reason for Encounter/ Consultation—the patient's stated reason for the visit or, for consultations, the reason stated in the referral request for the specialist to examine the patient.
- History of Present Illness (HPI)—a statement of how the patient's current condition began and how it has progressed.
- Past Medical History (PMH)—a review of the patient's past conditions, which may or may not be resolved, and past surgical procedures. It also includes any current problems that are not included in the reason for the encounter or referral.
- Physical Examination (PE or PX)—the physician's examination and factual findings, results of tests performed or reviewed.
- Assessment—the physician's diagnostic statement.
- Plan/Recommendations—planned treatments, prescriptions, patient instructions, and recommended treatments.

Annotated Example of Coding from Chart Notes

When coding from an actual chart note, coders must read the documentation several times and aggregate details from various sections of the report in order to form a complete picture of the encounter and determine the diagnoses to code. To code from a chart note, follow these steps and cross-reference the examples of each in ■ Figure 30-1 (pages 612–613) using the numbers provided in parentheses:

- Read the patient's stated reason for the encounter (1) and the physician's assessment (5). Determine if these are consistent with each other and/or add any details that may be required.
- Refer to the key criteria for abstracting for the body system(s) related to the diagnostic statement. Read through the entire record, noting what items support or modify the stated diagnosis.
- Identify the symptoms (2) and signs (4). Determine if they are consistent with the assessment (5) and/or add any details that may be required by the codes.
- Identify any statement of personal disease history (3a), family disease history (3b), or risk factors (3c) that may contribute information to the diagnosis.
- Review the examination findings (4) and identify any additional risk factors or findings that contribute to the diagnosis.
- Review the plan (6) to identify any additional risk factors or symptoms the physician considers significant and to identify all conditions treated during the encounter.
- Do not assign codes for scheduled treatments (6) because they were not provided during the encounter.
- Re-read the assessment (5). Identify all confirmed diagnoses. Compare the diagnoses to the symptoms identified earlier (2) to determine which are integral to

the condition and which may not be. In the outpatient setting, do not assign codes for uncertain or rule-out diagnoses (OGCR IV.D. and H.). Do not assign diagnosis codes for conditions not managed or not stated as significant to the current problem.

- Sequence the diagnoses according the problem chiefly responsible for the services provided (OGCR IV.G.).

CODING CAUTION

Do not assign diagnosis codes solely from the Chief Complaint or Assessment sections of the chart note. You need to read the entire chart note to identify any additional details or variations.

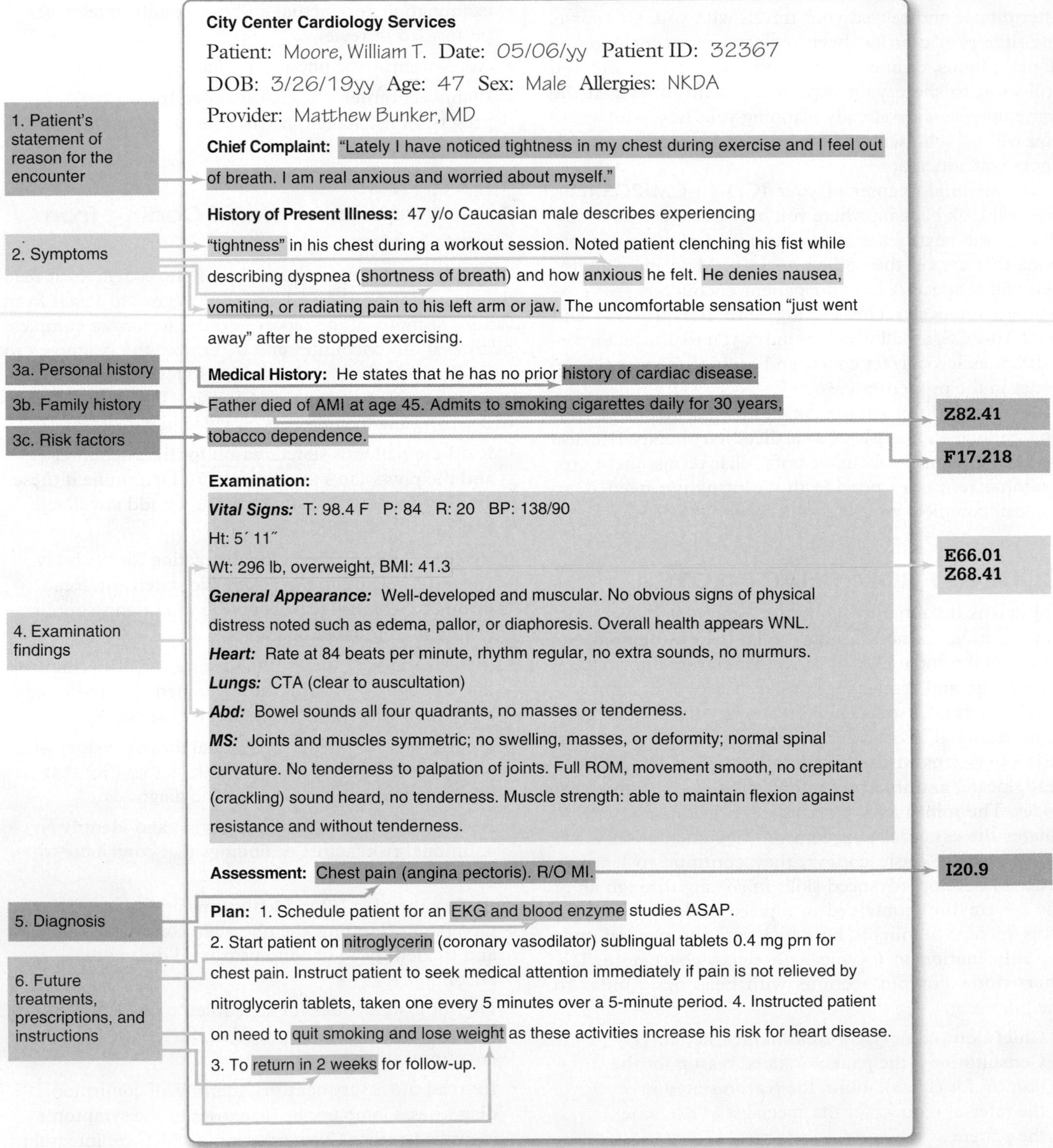

City Center Cardiology Services

Patient: Moore, William T. Date: 05/06/yy Patient ID: 32367

DOB: 3/26/19yy Age: 47 Sex: Male Allergies: NKDA

Provider: Matthew Bunker, MD

Chief Complaint: "Lately I have noticed tightness in my chest during exercise and I feel out of breath. I am real anxious and worried about myself."

History of Present Illness: 47 y/o Caucasian male describes experiencing "tightness" in his chest during a workout session. Noted patient clenching his fist while describing dyspnea (shortness of breath) and how anxious he felt. He denies nausea, vomiting, or radiating pain to his left arm or jaw. The uncomfortable sensation "just went away" after he stopped exercising.

Medical History: He states that he has no prior history of cardiac disease. Father died of AMI at age 45. Admits to smoking cigarettes daily for 30 years, tobacco dependence.

Examination:

Vital Signs: T: 98.4 F P: 84 R: 20 BP: 138/90

Ht: 5´ 11˝

Wt: 296 lb, overweight, BMI: 41.3

General Appearance: Well-developed and muscular. No obvious signs of physical distress noted such as edema, pallor, or diaphoresis. Overall health appears WNL.

Heart: Rate at 84 beats per minute, rhythm regular, no extra sounds, no murmurs.

Lungs: CTA (clear to auscultation)

Abd: Bowel sounds all four quadrants, no masses or tenderness.

MS: Joints and muscles symmetric; no swelling, masses, or deformity; normal spinal curvature. No tenderness to palpation of joints. Full ROM, movement smooth, no crepitant (crackling) sound heard, no tenderness. Muscle strength: able to maintain flexion against resistance and without tenderness.

Assessment: Chest pain (angina pectoris). R/O MI.

Plan: 1. Schedule patient for an EKG and blood enzyme studies ASAP.

2. Start patient on nitroglycerin (coronary vasodilator) sublingual tablets 0.4 mg prn for chest pain. Instruct patient to seek medical attention immediately if pain is not relieved by nitroglycerin tablets, taken one every 5 minutes over a 5-minute period. 4. Instructed patient on need to quit smoking and lose weight as these activities increase his risk for heart disease.

3. To return in 2 weeks for follow-up.

Figure 30-1a ■ Example of a Cardiology Chart Note. *Source: Adapted from Rice, Jane,* Medical Terminology: A Word-Building Approach, *6th Ed., ©2008. Reprinted and electronically reproduced by permission of Pearson Education, Inc., Upper Saddle River, New Jersey.*

ICD-10-CM Codes:

(1) **I20.9 Angina pectoris**

(2) **F17.218 Nicotine dependence, cigarettes, with other nicotine-induced disorders**

(3) **Z82.41 Family history of sudden cardiac death**

(4) **E66.01 Morbid (severe) obesity due to excess calories**

(5) **Z68.41 Body mass index (BMI) 40.0-44.9, adult**

Note: The coder assigns a CPT code for the office visit.

Figure 30-1b ■ Coding for Cardiology Chart Note

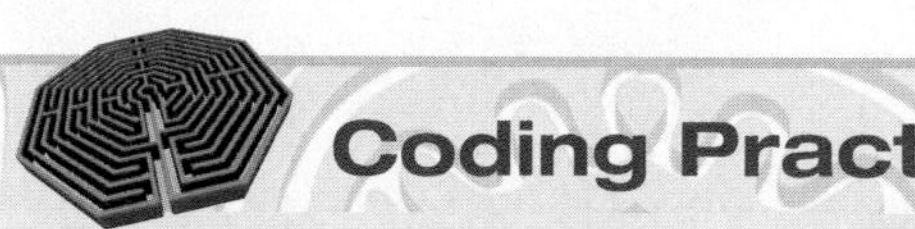

Coding Practice

Now it is your turn to demonstrate your understanding of coding from chart notes. Try to answer the questions from memory first, then refer back to the information in this section if you need a little extra help.

Exercise 30.1 Coding from Chart Notes

Part 1

Instructions: Write the abbreviation(s) that answer(s) each question based on the information you learned in this section. Choose from the list below.

CC	PE	assessment
HPI	PMH	plan

1. Begin analyzing a chart note by reading the ______________ and ______________.
2. Symptoms are usually documented in the ______________ or ______________.
3. Information about past diseases, family diseases, and risk factors are located in the ______________.
4. Additional risk factors, signs, or contributing factors may be found in the ______________.
5. Do not code for future treatments, which appear in the ______________.

Part 2

Instructions: Define what the following abbreviations represent. Write your answers on the lines.

6. HTN ______________________________
7. LBP ______________________________
8. BP ______________________________
9. CTA ______________________________
10. BPH ______________________________

(continued)

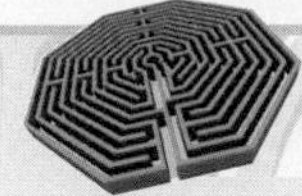

Coding Practice (continued)

Part 3

Instructions: Abstract, assign, and sequence ICD-10-CM codes for the following chart notes.

11. Review the annotated chart note from a gastroenterology consultation in FIGURE 30-2.

Assign ICD-10-CM codes where indicated, then sequence them correctly.

5 CM Codes ________ ________ ________ ________ ________

11. Branton Gastroenterology

Patient: Jeff Flannery Date: 01/30/yy DOB: 9/30/19yy Age: 56
Sex: Male Allergies: NKDA Provider: Stanley Garrett, MD
Referred by: Kristen Conover, MD (Branton Family Practice)

1. Reason for the referral to gastroenterologist

Reason for Consultation:
Evaluation of recurrent epigastric and LUQ pain.

History of Present Illness:

2. Symptoms

Patient is a 56 year old male. He reports a long history of mild dyspepsia, characterized by burning epigastric pain, especially when his stomach is empty. This pain has been relieved by OTC antacids. Approximately two weeks ago, the pain became significantly worse. He is also nauseated and has vomited several times.

Past Medical History:

3a. Medical history

3b. Current problem not treated here

3c. Risk factor

Patient's history is not significant for other digestive system disorders. He had a tonsillectomy at age 8. He sustained a compound fracture of the left ankle in a bicycle accident at age 11 that required surgical fixation. More recently, he has been diagnosed with an enlarged prostate gland and surgery has been recommended. However, he would like to resolve this epigastric pain before going forward with the TURP. He also has long standing problems with alcohol dependence. ________

Assign Codes

Results of Physical Examination:

4. Examination findings and test results

CBC indicates anemia and a fecal occult blood test is positive for blood in the feces. ________
A blood test for *Helicobacter pylori* is positive. Erosion in the gastric lining was visualized on an upper GI. Follow-up gastroscopy found evidence of mild reflux esophagitis and an ulcerated lesion in the lining of the pyloric section of the stomach. The ulcer is 1.5 cm in diameter and deep, with evidence of bleeding. ________
Multiple biopsies were negative for gastric ca. ________

Assessment:

5. Diagnosis

Acute peptic ulcer. Gastric cancer has been ruled out in light of negative biopsies. ________

Recommendations:

6. Future treatments, prescriptions, and instructions

A gastrectomy to remove the ulcerated portion of the stomach is indicated because the ulcer is already bleeding. Patient started on Tagamet to reduce stomach acid. Added Keflex to treat the bacterial infection and iron pills to reverse anemia. Patient was instructed to eat frequent small meals and avoid alcohol and irritating foods. ________

Figure 30-2 ■ Exercise 30.1, Question 11, Gastroenterology Chart Note. *Source: Adapted from Fremgen, Bonnie, F.; Frucht, Suzanne S., Medical Terminology: A Living Language, 4th Ed., © 2009. Reprinted and electronically reproduced by permission of Pearson Education, Inc., Upper Saddle River, New Jersey.*

12. Review the chart note from a urology consultation in ■ FIGURE 30-3. Use a highlighter and analyze it following the process used in the previous chart notes in this chapter. Abstract the chart note to determine how many ICD-10-CM diagnosis codes are required. Then assign and sequence the codes.

CM Codes ____________________

12. Branton Professional Group—Urology Clinic

Patient: Peter Mock Date: 03/30/yy DOB: 7/13/19yy Age: 60 Sex: Male Allergies: NKDA
Provider: Brent Eberhart, MD Referred by: Kristen Conover, MD (Branton Family Practice)

Reason for Encounter:
Has been "using the restroom a lot. I always need to go and feel like I cannot wait, but not much comes out."

History of Present Illness:
This "has been happening for awhile, but has gotten to be a problem within the last month or two." Frequency, urgency, decrease in amount and force of urinary stream.

Past Medical History:
Rotator cuff repair 20 years ago. Had physical therapy about a year ago for LBP but it is "not bothering him lately." Currently takes Lisinopril for HTN.

Results of Physical Examination:
Vital signs: T: 98.8F P: 82 R: 20 BP: 146/89
Ht: 6'1" Wt: 191 lb.
General appearance: Healthy 60 year old male. Appears uncomfortable. Hesitant in talking about symptoms.
Heart: Regular rate and rhythm. No murmurs, gallops, or rubs.
Lungs: CTA.
Abd: Bowel sounds all 4 quadrants. No masses or tenderness. No distention of bladder or renal tenderness
Prostate: DRE revealed enlarged prostate, approximately 5.5 cm, projecting 1.5 cm into the rectum. Smooth without normal central groove, no nodules or indurations, tender, firm to rubbery consistency.

Assessment: BPH

Plan: urinalysis and PSA test. Rx finasteride 5 mg PO once a day for 6 months for BPH. FU 6 months

Figure 30-3 ■ Exercise 30.1, Question 12, Urology Chart Note. *Source: Adapted from Rice, Jane,* Medical Terminology: A Word-Building Approach, *6th Ed., © 2008. Reprinted and electronically reproduced by permission of Pearson Education, Inc., Upper Saddle River, New Jersey.*

CODING FROM OPERATIVE REPORTS

Physicians document surgical operations and procedures with operative reports, which provide the details of exactly how the procedure was performed. Coders must read through all the details of the procedure, abstract the relevant information, then assign and sequence codes. This can be challenging and overwhelming because many of the details reported—such as the anesthetic, instruments, sutures, and other supplies—are not required in order to assign diagnosis and procedure codes. All of the information for a code is not concisely listed in one spot. Coders must read the report several times until they have identified all the details necessary to assign codes. The mini-medical-record used in this text encapsulates the essential nuggets from operative reports. After coders master basic coding, they need to develop advanced skills to sort through all of the details in an operative report in order to locate the essential coding information. A typical operative report contains sections with headings similar to the following. The format varies with each physician or hospital but must include the following information:

- date of procedure
- name of procedure performed
- names of the surgeon and assistants
- preoperative or provisional diagnosis
- a detailed description of the procedure, such as patient preparation, anesthetic, instruments and supplies used, incisions made, visualized structures, findings, alterations performed, tissue removed, estimated blood loss, closing process, and patient status
- postoperative diagnosis

The operative report usually specifies the instruments the surgeon used (■ TABLE 30-1 and ■ FIGURE 30-4, page 616). Instruments may carry a generic name, such as scalpel, or an eponym, such as Mayo-Hegar (needle holder) or Metzenbaum (scissors). A number indicates the size, such as a #10 blade or 5-0 Vicryl sutures.

SUCCESS STEP

In general, codes are not assigned for specific instruments. However, the instruments used can help determine the operative approach and other details. For example, when an endoscope is used, you know that at least one aspect of the approach is endoscopic. When the report describes an incision several centimeters long, then describes dividing and retracting subsequent layers, you know that an open approach is being used.

Table 30-1 ■ **INSTRUMENTS USED BY SURGEONS**

Purpose	Types
Absorption	Sponge, towel, dressing
Cutting	Knife, scalpel, scissors, electrocautery, bone saw, wire, snare, stapler
Drainage	T-tube, drain, catheter, hemovac, chest tube, water seal
Grasping, holding	Forceps, clamp, hemostat
Occlusion	Ligature (sutures), clips, clamps
Viewing	Retractor, speculum, endoscope, microscope
Wound closure	Needle holder, sutures (catgut, Vicryl, silk, nylon), stapler

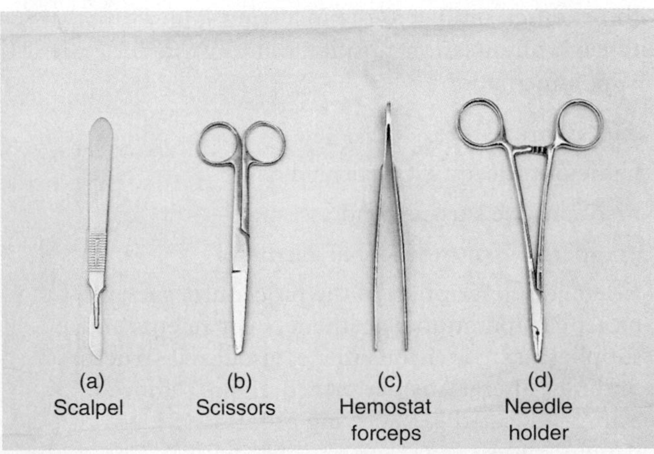

Figure 30-4 ■ The operative report identifies the instruments the surgeon uses. *Source: Michal Heron/Pearson Education.*

Annotated Example of Coding from Operative Reports

To code from an operative report, follow these steps and cross-reference the examples of each in ■ FIGURE 30-5 (pages 617–618) using the numbers in parentheses:

- Read the preoperative and postoperative diagnoses (1). Determine if these are consistent with each other and/or add any details that may be required.
- Read the name of the procedure(s) performed as stated by the surgeon (2).
- Refer to the key criteria for abstracting for the body system(s) related to the diagnostic statement. Read through the entire record, noting what items support or modify the stated diagnosis.
- Identify the indications, symptoms, and signs (3). Determine if they are consistent with the postoperative diagnosis and/or add any details that may be required by the codes (3a, 3c, 3d, 3e).
- Identify any comorbidities (3a) or complications that create an operative risk.
- Refer to the key criteria for abstracting procedures for the procedures related to the procedural description. Read through the entire record, noting what items support or modify the stated procedure.
- Refer to ICD-10-PCS Guidelines to determine when multiple procedures should be coded.
- Identify the following for each procedure:
  - operative approach (4) (The same operative approach may be applicable to more than one procedure.)
  - objective of the procedure as it relates to the Root Operation definition (6, 7, 8, 9)
  - anatomical site (5, 6, 8)
  - devices (9)
  - other details required by the specific procedure
- Re-read the entire report to confirm that all diagnoses and procedures are identified. Be certain to identify a diagnosis to support each procedure.
- Sequence the diagnoses according the problem chiefly responsible for the services provided (OGCR IV.G.).
- Sequence the principal procedure followed by additional procedures.

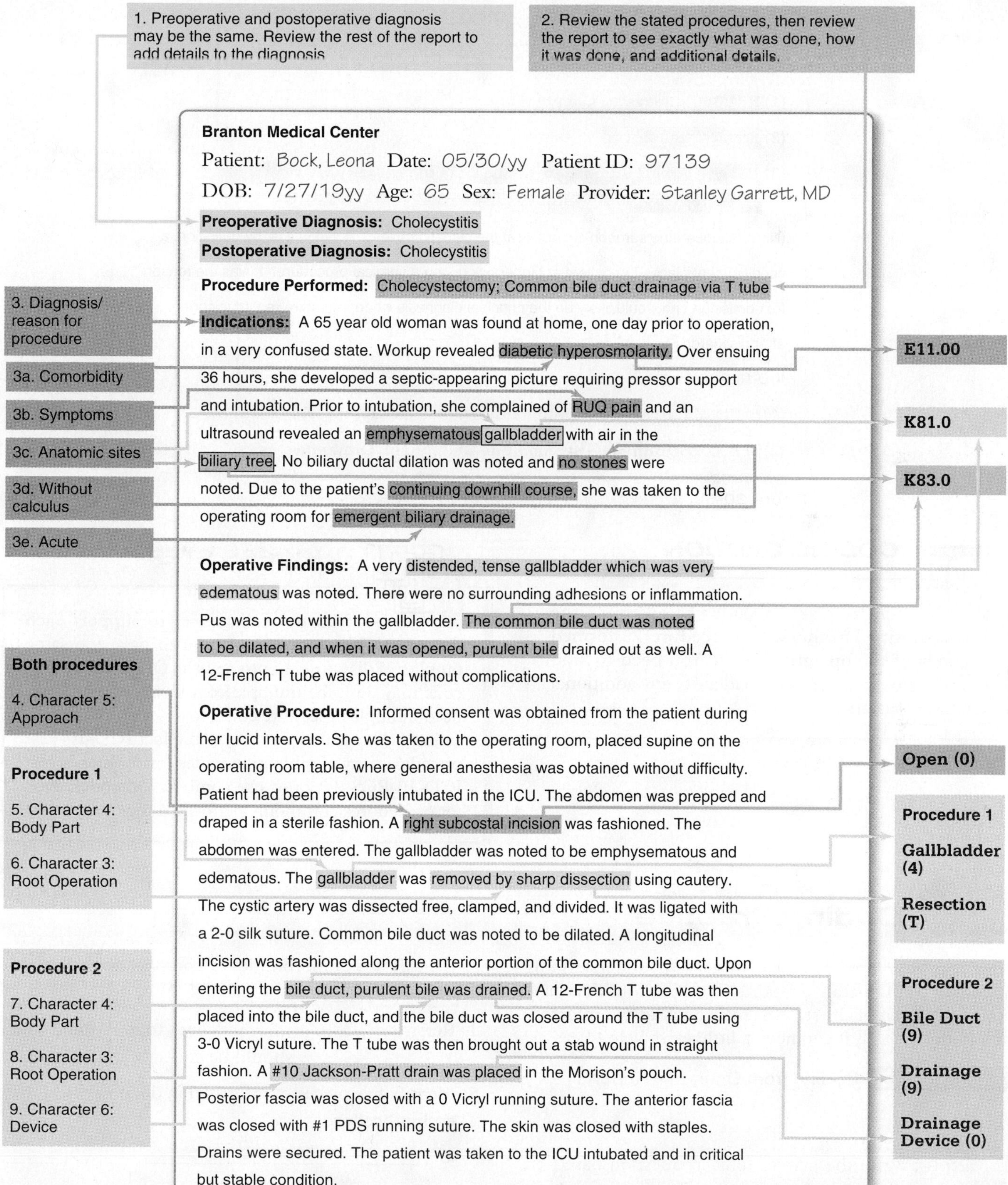

Branton Medical Center

Patient: Bock, Leona Date: 05/30/yy Patient ID: 97139

DOB: 7/27/19yy Age: 65 Sex: Female Provider: Stanley Garrett, MD

Preoperative Diagnosis: Cholecystitis

Postoperative Diagnosis: Cholecystitis

Procedure Performed: Cholecystectomy; Common bile duct drainage via T tube

Indications: A 65 year old woman was found at home, one day prior to operation, in a very confused state. Workup revealed diabetic hyperosmolarity. Over ensuing 36 hours, she developed a septic-appearing picture requiring pressor support and intubation. Prior to intubation, she complained of RUQ pain and an ultrasound revealed an emphysematous gallbladder with air in the biliary tree. No biliary ductal dilation was noted and no stones were noted. Due to the patient's continuing downhill course, she was taken to the operating room for emergent biliary drainage.

Operative Findings: A very distended, tense gallbladder which was very edematous was noted. There were no surrounding adhesions or inflammation. Pus was noted within the gallbladder. The common bile duct was noted to be dilated, and when it was opened, purulent bile drained out as well. A 12-French T tube was placed without complications.

Operative Procedure: Informed consent was obtained from the patient during her lucid intervals. She was taken to the operating room, placed supine on the operating room table, where general anesthesia was obtained without difficulty. Patient had been previously intubated in the ICU. The abdomen was prepped and draped in a sterile fashion. A right subcostal incision was fashioned. The abdomen was entered. The gallbladder was noted to be emphysematous and edematous. The gallbladder was removed by sharp dissection using cautery. The cystic artery was dissected free, clamped, and divided. It was ligated with a 2-0 silk suture. Common bile duct was noted to be dilated. A longitudinal incision was fashioned along the anterior portion of the common bile duct. Upon entering the bile duct, purulent bile was drained. A 12-French T tube was then placed into the bile duct, and the bile duct was closed around the T tube using 3-0 Vicryl suture. The T tube was then brought out a stab wound in straight fashion. A #10 Jackson-Pratt drain was placed in the Morison's pouch. Posterior fascia was closed with a 0 Vicryl running suture. The anterior fascia was closed with #1 PDS running suture. The skin was closed with staples. Drains were secured. The patient was taken to the ICU intubated and in critical but stable condition.

Figure 30-5a ■ Example of a Gastroenterology Operative Report. *Source: Adapted with permission from Health Professions Institute,* Medical Transcription: Fundamentals and Practice, *3rd Ed., © 2007. Reprinted and electronically reproduced by permission of Pearson Education, Inc., Upper Saddle River, New Jersey.*

(continued on next page)

(continued from page 617)

ICD-10-CM Codes:

(1) **K81.0 Cholecystitis, acute**

(2) **K83.0 Cholangitis**

(3) **E11.00 Type 2 diabetes mellitus with hyperosmolarity without nonketotic hyperglycemic-hyperosmolar coma (NKHHC)**

(Note: Although the surgeon did not treat the diabetic hyperosmolarity, it is, by definition, a condition that places the patient at higher risk during a surgical procedure. It was the reason for admission and would likely be the principal diagnosis when the entire record is coded after discharge.)

ICD-10-PCS Codes:

(1) **0FT40ZZ Resection, Gallbladder, Open, No Device, No Qualifier**

(2) **0F9900Z Drainage, Common Bile Duct, Open, Drainage Device, No Qualifier**

Figure 30-5b ■ Coding for Gastroenterology Operative Report

CODING CAUTION

Do not assign codes solely from the Postoperative Diagnosis or Procedure Performed sections of the operative report. You need to read the entire operative report to identify any additional details or variations.

SUCCESS STEP

You need diagnoses to support each procedure, but you do not have to have the same number of diagnoses as procedures. One combination code may describe multiple conditions, but you may need multiple procedure codes to describe all the procedures. This is due, in part, to the fact ICD-10-CM provides many combination codes for diagnoses, but ICD-10-PCS does not use combination codes, even for procedures commonly performed together.

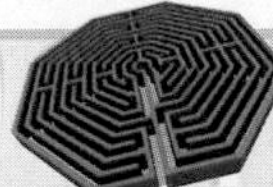

Coding Practice

Now it is your turn to demonstrate your understanding of coding from operative reports. Try to answer the questions from memory first, then refer back to the information in this section if you need a little extra help.

Exercise 30.2 Coding from Operative Reports

Part 1

Instructions: Write the answer to each question based on the information you learned in this section.

1. Begin analyzing an operative report by reading the ________________.
2. Determine the symptoms and signs are consistent with the postoperative diagnosis and add any ________________ that may be required by the codes.
3. Identify any comorbidities or complications that create an ________________.
4. Refer to ICD-10-PCS Guidelines to determine when ________________ should be coded.
5. Identify five pieces of information documented for each procedure.

   a. ________________________________

   b. ________________________________

   c. ________________________________

   d. ________________________________

   e. ________________________________

Part 2

Instructions: State the purpose of each of the following surgical instruments.

6. electrocautery ______________________
7. retractor ______________________
8. hemostat ______________________
9. catgut ______________________
10. wire ______________________

Part 3

Instructions: Assign ICD-10-CM and ICD-10-PCS codes for the following operative reports.

11. Review the annotated operative report from an orthopedics procedure in ■ FIGURE 30-6. Assign ICD-10-CM and ICD-10-PCS codes and sequence them correctly.

    2 CM Codes ____________ ____________

    4 PCS Codes ____________ ____________

    ____________ ____________

11. Branton Medical Center

Patient: Cabrera, Brandee Date: 05/30/yy Patient ID: 57321

DOB: 10/2/19yy Age: 19 Sex: Female Provider: Bruce Prentice, MD

Preoperative Diagnosis: Herniated disk C7-T1 and osteophyte C7

Postoperative Diagnosis: Herniated disk C7-T1 and osteophyte C7

Operation:

Anterior excision, cervical disk and spur, C7-T1

Cloward fusion, C7-T1, using bone bank

Anesthesia: General

Indications: This patient was having progressive weakness of her extremities and some feelings of numbness. Studies showed a rather prominent herniated disk at C7-T1 and associated spur at C7 that was compressing the spinal cord. It was decided to remove this disk and spur.

Procedure: The patient was given adequate endotracheal general anesthesia and placed on the operating table in the supine position. The anterior neck was prepared and draped in a sterile manner, and a skin incision was made beginning at the midline and extending lateralward for approximately 5 cm. The incision was carried down through deeper layers and the C7-T1disk space was identified. Verification as to localization was performed using x-ray of cervical spine. Using the Cloward instruments, a 12 mm hole was then drilled at the C7-T1disk space. The disk space was cleansed as well as possible of all the disk material as well as posterior protruding C7spur. A 14 mm bone plug was then selected from the bone bank bone, and was carefully inserted into the C7-T1disk space. Hemostasis was acquired and the wound was closed with absorbable sutures. No complications were noted during the operation. Blood loss was approximately 200mL. None was given for replacement.

Figure 30-6 ■ Exercise 30.2, Question 11, Orthopedics Operative Report. *Source: Adapted with permission from Health Professions Institute*, Medical Transcription: Fundamentals and Practice, *3rd Ed., © 2007. Reprinted and electronically reproduced by permission of Pearson Education, Inc., Upper Saddle River, New Jersey.*

(continued)

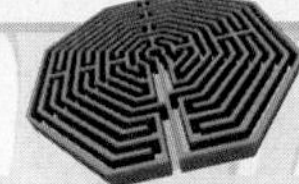

Coding Practice (continued)

12. Review the annotated operative report for a neurology procedure in ■ FIGURE 30-7. Abstract the report to determine how many ICD-10-CM and ICD-10-PCS codes are required. Then assign and sequence the codes.

CM Codes ______________________

PCS Codes ______________________

12. Branton Medical Center

Patient: Cassity, Janet Date: 05/30/yy Patient ID: 64197

DOB: 4/16/19yy Age: 61 Sex: Female Provider: Stanley Garrett, MD

Preoperative Diagnosis: Subacute subdural hemorrhage on the right

Postoperative Diagnosis: Subacute subdural hemorrhage on the right

Operation: Craniotomy and excision of subacute subdural hematoma on the right

Anesthesia: General

Indications: The patient was suffering from headaches and at time had a slowed pulse. Studies showed a rather extensive chronic or subacute subdural hematoma on the right. It was decided to excise this hematoma.

Procedure: The patient was given adequate endotracheal general anesthesia and placed on the operating table in the supine position with her head turned toward the left. The scalp was prepared and draped in a sterile manner, and a linear skin incision was made, beginning in front of the ear and extending over the top of the head. The scalp was retracted and a free bone flap was turned in the right frontoparietal region. The dura was opened, and subdural fluid was noted approximately 1 cm or so in depth, which was covering the right cerebral hemisphere. This subdural was evacuated in all directions, carefully. Hemostasis was acquired, and the dura was again closed. The bone flap was plated into position and the scalp was closed in two layers. No complications were noted during the operation. Blood loss was approximately 100 milliliter.

Figure 30-7 ■ Exercise 30.2, Question 12, Neurology Operative Report. *Source: Adapted with permission from Health Professions Institute,* Medical Transcription: Fundamentals and Practice, *3rd Ed., © 2007. Reprinted and electronically reproduced by permission of Pearson Education, Inc., Upper Saddle River, New Jersey.*

HEALTH INFORMATION TECHNOLOGY

Hospitals, physicians, and other providers are using health information technology (HIT) advancements to streamline decades-old methods of capturing, storing, and using healthcare data. Health information management (HIM) and coding departments are at the center of this slowly emerging transformation. Proactive coders embrace new technology that increasingly uses computers to perform predictable, repetitive work, positioning themselves to accomplish more complex coding and data analysis tasks and, thus, adding value to an organization. Three HIT applications that coders interface with are encoders, EHR, and computer-assisted coding (CAC).

Encoders

Encoders are enhanced electronic coding manuals. They were first introduced in the 1980s and have helped improve the productivity and accuracy of coders. This software allows coders to input key words, such as the Main Term, and access hot links to potential codes.

Table 30-2 ■ **EXAMPLES OF ENCODER EDIT CHECKS**

- ❑ Code first
- ❑ Diagnosis-procedure mismatch
- ❑ Invalid characters (I and O in PCS)
- ❑ Manifestation codes
- ❑ Medicare medical necessity
- ❑ Mutually exclusive diagnoses
- ❑ Mutually exclusive procedures
- ❑ Patient age
- ❑ Patient gender
- ❑ Seven characters required (PCS)
- ❑ Unacceptable principal diagnosis
- ❑ Use additional code
- ❑ Use additional digit(s)

Coders can then review the code options and select the one that accurately matches the documentation.

Encoders provide edit checks based on OGCR, instructional notes, and payer rules. An edit check is a feature built into software that alerts users to, or prevents, certain errors, based on rules that are programmed into the system (■ TABLE 30-2). An edit check may be as simple as requiring that a patient record have a female gender in order to assign an obstetrics code or as complicated as alerting users when codes are sequenced incorrectly.

An encoder may also cross-reference or hot-link users to reference information, such as the following:

- OGCR
- PCS Guidelines
- *Coding Clinic* newsletter, published by the American Hospital Association
- *CPT Assistant* newsletter, published by the American Medical Association
- medical dictionary
- anatomical diagrams
- Medicare manual

Encoders are easily updated when quarterly and annual code updates are published; they can create reports that track service utilization and trends, and provide other valuable information to the provider.

Many companies design and sell encoder programs, but the basic functions of all are similar. Menus may be configured differently and the add-on reference tools may vary. Some products interface with other systems in a facility, such as a billing or EHR system; others are standalone programs that can run on any computer. Once coders learn one brand of software, it is usually easy to adapt to others.

SUCCESS STEP

When you learn an encoder in school, make screen shots of two or three commonly used screens and include them in your professional portfolio. This enables you to demonstrate your skills to potential employers.

CODING CAUTION

An encoder is not a substitute or shortcut to learning how to use the coding manuals. You must still master the basics of abstracting, assigning, and sequencing codes. Coders need to understand what information they must give the software in order for it to provide accurate feedback. An untrained user can make coding errors with an encoder, just as they would using the physical manuals.

Electronic Health Records

An electronic health record (EHR), also called an electronic medical record (EMR), is an electronic version of a patient's medical history, which is maintained by a provider over time.

Benefits of EHR Systems

At their simplest, EHRs are computerized versions of patients' charts, but when fully implemented, they are real-time, patient-centered records that enable authorized providers to immediately access medical information from remote locations. Key capabilities include the following:

- contains all of the key administrative clinical data relevant to a person's care under a particular provider, including demographics, progress notes, problem list, medications, vital signs, past medical history, immunizations, laboratory data and radiology reports
- streamlines the clinician's workflow by sending information to the appropriate parties, such as the pharmacy or a consulting provider, and reducing paperwork and documentation time for providers
- supports other care-related activities, including evidence-based decision support, quality management, and outcomes reporting
- improves privacy and security of patient records compared to paper-based systems

One of the key features of an EHR system is that it can be created, managed, and consulted by authorized providers and staff across multiple healthcare organizations (■ FIGURE 30-8, page 622). A single EHR system can bring together information from current and past doctors, emergency facilities, school and workplace clinics,

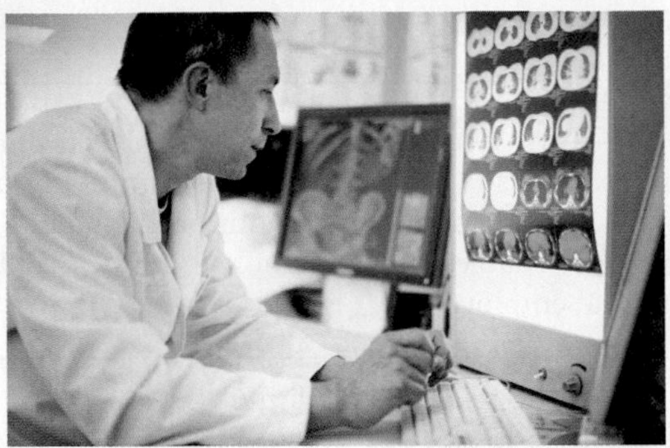

Figure 30-8 ■ EHR systems enable providers to view patient records across organizations. *Source: Logoboom/Dreamstime.*

pharmacies, laboratories, and medical imaging facilities. For example:

- A physician can view medications prescribed by other providers to avoid duplication or medication interactions.
- An emergency department can view a patient's medical history to more quickly identify a problem or risk factor.
- A provider can view imaging studies electronically, which may help to understand the progression of a patient's condition.

Funding Incentives for EHR Systems

The Health Information Technology for Economic and Clinical Health Act (HITECH), which is part of the American Recovery and Reinvestment Act of 2009 (ARRA), includes financial incentives for providers who adopt EHR systems and demonstrate use in ways that can improve quality, safety, and effectiveness of care. The goal behind the funding is to encourage providers to adopt EHR systems sooner than they otherwise would, because Congress believes EHR systems can help improve quality of care and reduce costs.

Despite much talk about streamlining healthcare delivery over the past several decades, HITECH is the first time that substantial federal money has been allocated to help providers improve care delivery. CMS states that, according to current estimates, as much as $27 billion will be paid to providers over ten years to support EHR adoption. The Office of the National Coordinator for Health Information Technology (ONC), CMS, and other agencies within the Department of Health and Human Services (DHHS) are working together to establish the criteria for the funding of EHR systems.

Meaningful Use

Under the incentive program, eligible Medicare providers can receive as much as $44,000 over a five-year period; eligible Medicaid providers can receive as much as $63,750 over six years. Medicaid providers receive the first year incentive payment when they adopt, implement, or upgrade certified EHR technology. In subsequent years, they must demonstrate meaningful use in order to qualify for additional payments. Meaningful use means providers must show they are using certified EHR technology in ways that can be measured. In order to qualify for meaningful use, an EHR system must allow:

- e-prescribing
- electronic exchange of health information to improve quality of health care
- submission of information on clinical quality measures

Certified EHR Technology

Certified EHR technology gives assurance to purchasers that a specific EHR system provides the necessary features to meet the meaningful use criteria. Certification also helps providers and patients be confident that the electronic health IT products and systems they use are secure, can maintain data confidentially, and can work with other systems to share information. A certified EHR system meets the following criteria:

- includes patient demographic and clinical health information, such as medical history and problem list
- provides clinical decision support
- supports physician order entry
- captures and queries information relevant to healthcare quality
- exchanges electronic health information with, and integrates such information from, other sources

Congressional Budget Office Analysis

The **Congressional Budget Office (CBO)** expects that accelerating the implementation of health IT will reduce healthcare spending by decreasing the following costs:

- the number of inappropriate tests and procedures
- paperwork and administrative overhead
- the number of adverse events resulting from medical errors

CBO also believes that improved technology will improve the quality of care provided to patients for several reasons. It should:

- improve the information available to clinicians at the time of treatment;
- encourage the use of evidence-based medicine; and
- help physicians manage patients with complex, chronic conditions.

The purpose of the incentive payments is to accelerate the adoption of HIT. The CBO anticipates that approximately 90% of doctors and 70% of hospitals will be using comprehensive EHR systems by 2019. It estimates that the accelerated adoption will reduce service utilization by eliminating redundant services and tests, thus saving Medicare $4.4 billion from 2011 to 2019. CBO estimates that, during the same time period, the HITECH Act will save the government approximately $12 billon on direct spending in the Medicare, Medicaid, and Federal Employee Health Benefits programs.

Computer-Assisted Coding

The move to adopt EHRs and create a national health information infrastructure has spawned numerous additional technology initiatives, including computer-assisted coding (CAC). CAC is the use of computer software that automatically generates a set of medical codes for review, validation, and use based upon clinical documentation provided by healthcare practitioners. It differs from an EHR in that an EHR stores and tracks clinical information, but does not convert it into codes. CAC differs from encoders in that encoders require people to conduct an electronic search for each individual code to be assigned, whereas CAC automatically generates codes based on documentation. CAC does not eliminate coders; it transforms their jobs from repetitive production-oriented tasks into ones of critical thinking, analysis, and auditing.

Impacts of CAC

Two key issues create incentives to adopt CAC: reimbursement and fraud. Reimbursement is directly impacted by both the speed and accuracy of coding. Every day that a patient account is delayed before billing increases an organization's accounts receivable (money owed to the organization) and reduces cash flow (the amount of cash coming in the door). This can potentially create the need to borrow cash to keep operating which, in turn, incurs additional expenses. In addition, coding errors and inconsistencies can cause payment to be denied or further delayed while payers suspend the claim, research it, and request supporting documentation. CAC and other forms of electronic coding help address both the speed and accuracy of coding.

Accuracy and consistency of coding also help organizations avoid potentially fraudulent practices, intentional or unintentional. OGCR, PCS Guidelines, and payer rules can be incorporated into the intelligence underlying the software to help ensure compliance. Software can create an audit trail that automatically documents changes made to codes and the reason for the changes. CAC helps relieve coders of time-consuming repetitive tasks and allows them more time to focus on reviewing exceptions and complex cases.

Technology Alternatives

CAC can be incorporated using two different technologies: structured input or natural language programming (NLP). Structured input, also known as codified input, uses menus that contain clinical terms. As physicians document, they select a series of menu items that create the narrative text within the documentation. These same menu choices are directly linked to codes that are automatically generated based on the documentation. Structured input differs from a pick-list in that it automatically generates the code based on the clinical term selected; it does not require a person to manually select the code.

For example, a structured input menu has a menu item such as *Personal medical history*. Subsequent menus prompt the physician to select the condition, *Cancer*; the organ, *Colon*; the site, *Descending*; and the behavior, *Primary*. The field for personal medical history is filled with *Personal history of cancer, descending colon, primary malignant* and the ICD-10-CM code **Z85.038** is displayed automatically for the coder to validate.

NLP, also known as computational linguistics, uses artificial intelligence to extract pertinent data and terms from a text-based document, analyze them, and convert them into the most likely applicable codes. Coders review the output using an application that displays the codes and clinical documentation side-by-side. Coders also validate the codes against local and national coverage guidelines, edit discrepancies, and finalize the codes. NLP differs from structured input in that structured input requires human intervention to select the condition and the associated clinical details, whereas NLP does so automatically.

For example, a natural language processor scans the documentation and identifies the phrase *history of cancer*. It then analyzes the context and semantics of the sentence to determine whether one of several options is present:

- personal history of colon cancer
- no history of colon cancer
- family history of colon cancer

The CAC displays the code that matches the result, then the coder verifies the code against the documentation to be certain the software interpreted it correctly.

Barriers to CAC

No system is without its drawbacks and challenges (■ Table 30-3). The benefits of CAC must outweigh the considerable cost of purchasing, designing, customizing,

Table 30-3 ■ COMPUTER-ASSISTED CODING ADVANTAGES AND BARRIERS

Advantages of CAC	Barriers to CAC
❑ Increased coding productivity	❑ Cost of CAC hardware and software
❑ Increased efficiency; frees professional from mundane tasks	❑ Complexity, quality, and format of health record documentation
❑ Comprehensive code assignment	❑ User resistance to change
❑ Consistent application of rules	❑ Technological limitations
❑ Electronic coding audit trail	❑ Potential increase in errors in the coding process
	❑ Lack of industry standards

Source: AHIMA e-HIM™ Work Group on Computer-Assisted Coding. "Delving into Computer-assisted Coding" (AHIMA Practice Brief). Journal of AHIMA 75, no.10 (Nov-Dec 2004): 48A-H (with web extras).

implementing, and training. The time required to define the customized inputs and coding links for each provider is significant. This, and the time required for coders to review the codes created by CAC for each case, must be less than the time coders currently spend coding the cases using an encoder in order for a system to be cost-effective. In addition, if a programming error creates an incorrect code link that is not identified, the error may be repeated an infinite number of times, thus negatively impacting reimbursement and fraud alerts, rather than improving them.

CAC works best within environments that have a limited number of diagnoses and procedures, a limited number of source documents, a limited number of users, and fewer coding guidelines because these limitations make programming easier. The complexity of programming increases exponentially as the number of variations that must be incorporated increase. As a result, CAC and other forms of electronic documentation are currently implemented primarily in outpatient settings, such as the physician office, radiology, pathology, emergency department, and other hospital outpatient departments. Developing CAC for hospital inpatient use involves a broader range of diagnoses and procedures, more users, more forms, and more extensive coding guidelines and, as a result, is more time consuming and costly. Of course, the potential benefits are also greater. Coders in any setting embrace technology because it elevates their professionalism and enables them to focus on tasks requiring judgment and critical thinking, while computers assist them with the repetitive tasks.

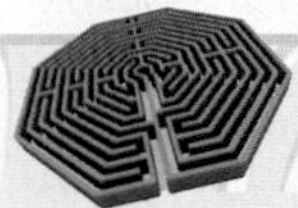

Coding Practice

Now it is your turn to demonstrate your understanding of health information technology. Try to answer the questions from memory first, then refer back to the information in this section if you need a little extra help.

Exercise 30.3 Health Information Technology

Instructions: Write your answers to the following questions on the line(s) provided.

1. What is the purpose of edit checks?

____

2. List five examples of edit checks.

____

____

____

____

3. Respond to this scenario: A classmate tells you she does not see the need to look up codes in the physical manual because she will be able to use an encoder in her job. What do you tell her?

____

____

____

4. Describe one example of using the EHR across organizations.

____

____

____

5. What piece of legislation includes financial incentives for providers who adopt EHR systems and demonstrate use in ways that can improve quality, safety, and effectiveness of care?

____

6. In order to qualify for meaningful use, an EHR system must allow what three activities?

____

____

____

7. Name three ways that the CBO believes EHR systems will help reduce costs.

____

____

____

8. Explain the difference between CAC and encoders.

____

____

____

9. Why are CACs and other forms of electronic documentation currently implemented primarily in outpatient settings?

____

____

____

10. Respond to this scenario: A classmate tells you that she is considering switching majors because all coding will be taken over by computers in the near future. What do you tell her? ______________________ ______________________ ______________________

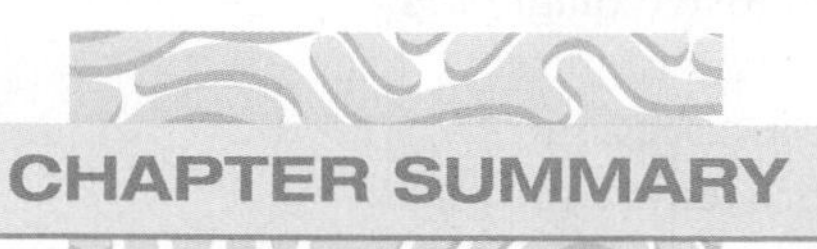

CHAPTER SUMMARY

In this chapter you learned that:

- After coders master basic coding, they need to develop advanced skills in sorting through all of the information contained in a typical physician chart note.
- Coding from an operative report can be challenging and overwhelming because coders must distinguish between coding-related information and details that are not required in order to assign diagnosis and procedure codes, such as the anesthetic, instruments, sutures, and other supplies.
- Proactive coders embrace new technology, such as encoders, electronic health records, and computer-assisted coding that perform predictable, repetitive work, and position themselves to accomplish more complex coding and data analysis tasks, which adds value to an organization.

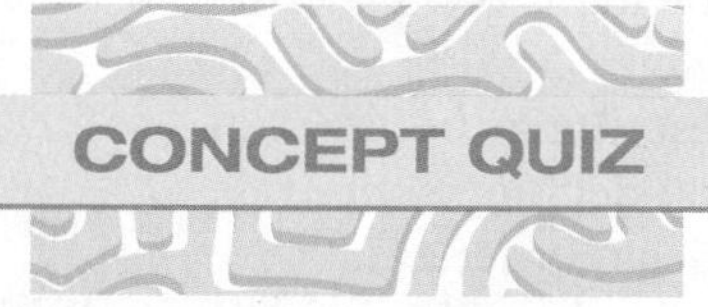

CONCEPT QUIZ

Take a moment to look back at your trip through this chapter and solidify your skills. This is your opportunity to pull together everything you have learned.

Completion

Instructions: Write the term that answers each question based on the information you learned in this chapter. Choose from the list below. Some choices may be used more than once and some choices may not be used at all. Refer to the discussion in this chapter and the Glossary at the end of this book if you need a little extra help.

ARRA	HITECH
CAC	HPI
NLP	indications
CC	meaningful use
certified EHR technology	PMH
EHR	postoperative diagnosis
encoder	structured input
HIT	

1. ______________________ is the patient's stated reason for the visit.
2. ______________________ is a review of the patient's past conditions, which may or may not be resolved, and past surgical procedures.
3. The ______________________ of an operative report contains symptoms, signs, and comorbidities.
4. Do not assign codes directly from the ______________________ section of the operative report.
5. ______________________ requires that systems are able to exchange electronic health information with, and integrate such information from, other sources.
6. ______________________ uses artificial intelligence to extract pertinent data and terms from a text-based document, analyze them, and convert them into the most likely applicable codes.
7. The purpose of the incentive payments is to accelerate the adoption of ______________________.
8. ______________________ is the first substantial commitment of federal resources to help providers improve care delivery.

9. ____________________ means that providers must show they are using EHR technology in ways that can be measured.
10. A ____________________ system uses menu choices made by physicians to automatically generate the associated codes.

Multiple Choice

Instructions: Circle the letter of the best answer to each question based on the information you learned in this chapter. Refer to the discussion in this chapter and the Glossary at the end of this book if you need a little extra help.

1. A patient sees a gastroenterologist for epigastric pain, nausea, and vomiting, which are due to a peptic ulcer. The patient is also seeing a urologist for BPH. What diagnoses should the gastroenterologist assign?
   A. BPH and peptic ulcer
   B. Epigastric pain, nausea, and vomiting
   C. BPH, peptic ulcer, epigastric pain, nausea, and vomiting
   D. Peptic ulcer
2. A patient sees a urologist for polyuria, nocturia, and oliguria due to BPH. What diagnoses should be assigned?
   A. Polyuria
   B. Polyuria, nocturia, and oliguria
   C. BPH, polyuria, nocturia, and oliguria
   D. BPH
3. Assign diagnosis codes for
   A. all conditions and symptoms mentioned in the chart note.
   B. information reported in the chief complaint only.
   C. symptoms that are integral to the condition.
   D. conditions stated as significant or treated by the physician.
4. Cholangitis is
   A. inflammation of the blood vessels.
   B. inflammation of the gallbladder.
   C. inflammation of the common bile duct.
   D. inflammation of the gallbladder and common bile duct.
5. Software that allows coders to input key words, such as the Main Term, and access hot links to potential codes is a (an)
   A. encoder.
   B. EHR.
   C. CAC.
   D. NLP.
6. Which of the following is NOT an edit check in an encoder?
   A. Mutually exclusive diagnoses
   B. Seven characters required
   C. Medication interaction
   D. Diagnosis-procedure mismatch
7. An electronic health record (EHR) is also referred to as a(an)
   A. CAC.
   B. EMR.
   C. NLP.
   D. HIT.
8. Incentive funding for EHR adoption is made possible by
   A. HIPAA.
   B. HITECH.
   C. CAC.
   D. COB.
9. Which of the following is NOT a criterion for a certified EHR system?
   A. Supports e-prescribing
   B. Provides clinical decision support
   C. Supports physician order entry
   D. Exchanges electronic health information with, and integrates such information from, other sources
10. Which of the following is NOT an advantage of CAC?
    A. Increased coding productivity
    B. Consistent application of rules
    C. Electronic coding audit trail
    D. Complexity, quality, and format of health record documentation

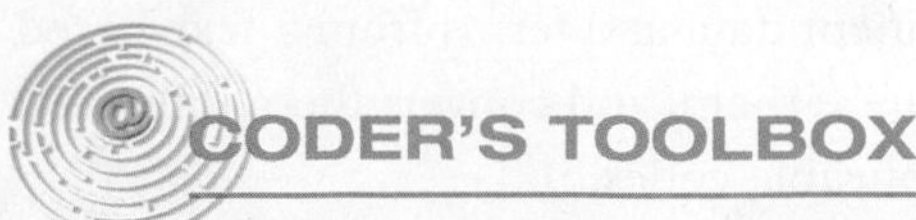

The following resources are a starting point for learning more about the topics in this chapter. The > symbol indicates a menu selection within the website in order to navigate to a specific page.

Surgical Procedures

Medscape > Reference > Procedures
http://emedicine.medscape.com/clinical_procedures

Medscape > Search > Sutures and Needles
http://emedicine.medscape.com/article/884838-overview

Health Information Technology

AHIMA > Resources > Body of Knowledge > Practice Briefs > Automated Coding Workflow and CAC Practice Guidance. (Journal of AHIMA 81, no.7 (July 2010): 51-56). http://library.ahima.org/xpedio/groups/public/documents/ahima/bok1_047691.hcsp?dDocName=bok1_047691

AHIMA > Resources > Body of Knowledge > Practice Briefs > e-HIM Practice Transformation (Updated) (Journal of AHIMA 81, no.8 (August 2010): 52-55). http://library.ahima.org/xpedio/groups/public/documents/ahima/bok1_047862.hcsp?dDocName=bok1_047862

American Medical Association > Physician Resources > HIT Resources http://www.ama-assn.org/ama/pub/physician-resources/health-information-technology.page?

American Society for Gastrointestinal Endoscopy (ASGE) > Search > Financial Incentives Available in 2011 for Physicians and Hospitals Adopting Electronic Health Records (4-3-2009) http://www.asge.org/uploadedFiles/Members_Only/Advocacy/HITECH%20ACT%2004-01-2009%20v2.pdf

Certification Commission for Health Information Technology (CCHIT) http://www.cchit.org

CMS Home > Regulations and Guidance > EHR Incentive Programs https://www.cms.gov/ehrincentiveprograms/

Department of Health and Human Services, Office of the National Coordinator (ONC) for Health Information Technology http://healthit.hhs.gov/portal/server.pt/community/healthit_hhs_gov__home/1204

General Accountability Office > GAO High Risk and Other Major Government Challenges > Governmental Management Challenges > Furthering the Exchange of Electronic Patient Health Information http://www.gao.gov/highrisk/challenges/information_technology/furthering_exchange.php

Health Information and Management Systems Society > Topics and Tools > Electronic Health Record http://www.himss.org/ASP/topics_ehr.asp

National e-Health Collaborative http://www.nationalehealth.org

The American Recovery and Reinvestment Act (H.R. 1) (To locate the content of ARRA, perform an Internet search for *The American Recovery and Reinvestment Act (H.R. 1)* and select the following or similar link from the Government Printing Office (GPO)). http://frwebgate.access.gpo.gov/cgibin/getdoc.cgi?dbname=111_cong_bills&docid=f:h1enr.pdf

APPENDIX

ANSWER KEY TO CODING PRACTICE EXERCISES (Odd-numbered questions)

The words in parentheses ( ) following a code provide the Index entries for the Main Term and subterms of one coding path. Selections for additional characters in the Tabular List are also after the subterms. Coding answers are based on the 2012 Draft ICD-10-CM/PCS code sets.

CHAPTER 1: YOUR CAREER AND CODING

Exercise 1.1 What Is Coding?

1. Coding is the process of accurately assigning codes to verbal descriptions of patients' conditions and the healthcare services provided to treat those conditions.
3. Abstract—determine which elements of the visit require codes
   Assign—determine the codes that describe the patient's condition and services
   Arrange—sequence the codes in proper order

Exercise 1.2 Understanding Patient Encounters

1. after an encounter is completed
3. history, examination, testing

Exercise 1.3 Certification

1. Certification is a voluntary achievement that documents that a coder has attained a certain level of proficiency by passing a rigorous examination.
3. CCS—hospital inpatient and outpatient coding
   CCS-P—physician office coding
   CCA—apprentice coder

Exercise 1.4 Coding Careers

1. Student answers will vary, so any item from Table 1-3 is acceptable.
3. 30 to 40 words per minute (wpm) or 9,000 to 12,000 keystrokes per hour (ksph)

CHAPTER 2: CODING AND REIMBURSEMENT

Exercise 2.1 Healthcare Payers

1. most people age 65 and over, people of any age with end stage renal disease (ESRD), and people with disabilities
3. group, self-insured, individual

Exercise 2.2 Documentation

1. establishing the medical need for services
3. The medical record is the comprehensive collection of all information on a patient at a particular facility. Progress notes are the record of a specific patient encounter.

Exercise 2.3 Life Cycle of an Insurance Claim

1. It is the time when providers begin collecting insurance information.
3. Student answers will vary and should include three of the following:
   - Characters in a code are mistyped, creating an invalid code.
   - Codes have too many or too few characters.
   - Diagnosis does not match the procedure.
   - Codes are sequenced incorrectly.
   - Additional codes required by the Guidelines or Instructional Notes are missing.
   - Patient gender does not match the diagnosis or procedure.
   - Patient age does not match the diagnosis or procedure.

Exercise 2.4 Federal Compliance

1. When providers are overpaid they are legally obligated to report the overpayment to Medicare, to refund the money, and may even have to pay interest on it.
3. False Claims Act (FCA)

CHAPTER 3: THE TRANSITION TO ICD-10-CM/PCS

Exercise 3.1 History of ICD-10-CM/PCS

1. October 1, 2013
3. Inpatient hospitals

Exercise 3.2 Overview of the Transition Process

1. The first rule specified the compliance date for mandatory use of ICD-10-CM/PCS as October 1, 2013. The second rule updated the HIPAA transaction standards.
3. Student answers will vary and may include any of the following:
   - The number of codes has increased from 14,000 in ICD-9-CM to 68,000+ in ICD-10-CM.
   - The length of codes has increased from three to five characters in ICD-9-CM to three to seven characters in ICD-10-CM.
   - Code structure has changed from primarily numeric in ICD-9-CM (except for V and E codes) to all codes being alphanumeric in ICD-10-CM.
   - Code formats have been added in ICD-10-CM to include seventh-digit extensions to describe particular circumstances.
   - ICD-10-CM terminology and disease classifications were updated to be consistent with current clinical practice.
   - ICD-10-CM codes describe greater levels of clinical detail and specificity than may have been described by a single code in ICD-9-CM.
   - ICD-10-CM contains more combination codes that describe multiple related conditions with a single code.

Exercise 3.3 Impact on Healthcare Information Systems

1. Claims, encounter, and payment information
   - Coordination of Benefits
   - Eligibility for a health plan
   - Referrals
   - Non-HIPAA mandated formats for Medicare Fee-for-Service (FFS)
3. Student answers will vary and may include any of the following:
   - Modify field sizes to accommodate the longer codes.
   - Change data type of fields from primarily numeric (with the exception of V and E for the first character) to completely alphanumeric for every character.
   - Add a new field as a version indicator to distinguish between ICD-9-CM and ICD-10-CM/PCS codes.
   - Increase the number of diagnosis codes allowed on a claim.
   - Implement detailed rules to improve the explanations of claim corrections, reversals, recoupment of payments, and the processing of refunds.

Exercise 3.4 Impact on Medical Providers

1. Student answers will vary and may include any of the following:
   - They are responsible for implementing the impacts on information systems.
   - They need to make sure the coders they employ receive adequate training.

- They need to ensure that their own medical documentation provides the additional level of specificity needed under ICD-10-CM/PCS.
- Providers who personally assign some or all diagnostic codes themselves also need to learn the coding guidelines for ICD-10-CM.
- They must accomplish all of these changes while continuing to maintain a high patient load.

3. Schedulers often select the reason or purpose for patients' planned visits from a list that is ultimately tied to diagnosis codes.

Exercise 3.5 Impact on Medical Coders

1. a. Code the trimester of pregnancy rather than the episode of care.
   b. Has codes for approximately 100 types of falls. Has three extensions for the episode of care as initial, subsequent, or for sequela.
   c. Most bilateral sites have codes for laterality.
3. Coders should not use GEMs to assign codes for specific patient encounters.

CHAPTER 4: INTRODUCTION TO ICD-10-CM DIAGNOSIS CODING

Exercise 4.1 Organization of ICD-10-CM

1. category
3. block
5. code
7. category
9. block

Exercise 4.2 Conventions: Exclusion Notes

1. Do not use together
3. OK
5. OK
7. OK
9. Do not use together

Exercise 4.3 Conventions: Use Additional Characters, Extensions, and Placeholders

1. Correct
3. **G43.101**
5. **O31.01X1**
7. **S71.151S**
9. **S72.022K**

Exercise 4.4 Locating the Main Term

1. Wound
3. Infection
5. Fever
7. Malaria
9. Failure

Exercise 4.5 How to Code Diagnoses

1. a. Syndrome
   b. toxic shock
   c. A48.3
   d. no
   e. Use additional code to identify the organism (B95, B96)
   f. streptococcus A
   g. no
   h. Includes: diseases generally recognized as communicable or transmissible
   i. no
   j. B95
   k. B95.0
   l. yes
   m. A48.3
   n. B95.0

CHAPTER 5: NEOPLASMS (C00-D49)

Exercise 5.1 Neoplasm Refresher

1. osteo/sarc/oma malignant neoplasm of bone and connective tissue
3. lip/oma neoplasm of fatty tissue
5. aden/oma neoplasm of a gland
7. oste/oma neoplasm of bone
9. neuro/blast/oma neoplasm of immature nerve cells

Exercise 5.2 Abstracting for Neoplasms

1. a. right breast, lower outer quadrant
   b. yes, brain
   c. no
   d. chemotherapy
3. a. stomach
   b. the top portion of the curve
   c. no
   d. no
   e. review results of biopsy and CT scan
5. a. classical lymphocyte depleted Hodgkin lymphoma
   b. no
   c. anemia
   d. anemia

Exercise 5.3 Assigning Codes for Neoplasms

1. **D25.1** (Leiomyoma, uterus, intramural)
3. **C16.1** (Table of Neoplasms, stomach, fundus, malignant primary)

Exercise 5.4 Arranging Codes for Neoplasms

1. **Z51.11** (Chemotherapy, neoplasm)
   C50.511 (Table of Neoplasms, breast, lower outer quadrant, right, malignant primary)
   C79.31 (Table of Neoplasms, brain, overlapping lesion, malignant secondary)
3. **C81.30** (Lymphoma, Hodgkin, classical, lymphocyte depleted, unspecified site)
   D63.0 (Anemia, in, neoplastic disease)

CHAPTER 6: SYMPTOMS, SIGNS, AND ABNORMAL CLINICAL AND LABORATORY FINDINGS, NOT ELSEWHERE CLASSIFIED (R00-R99)

Exercise 6.1 Symptoms and Signs Refresher

1. dys/pnea difficulty breathing, R06.00
3. a/phagia unable to swallow, R13.0
5. lymph/adeno/pathy abnormal condition of lymph nodes, R59.1
7. hyp/ox/emia low oxygen in the blood, R09.02
9. glycos/uria sugar in urine, R81

Exercise 6.2 Abstracting Symptoms and Signs

1. a. no
   b. abnormal laboratory test
   c. abnormal
3. a. no
   b. seizures
   c. seizures
5. a. extreme nervousness and irritability
   b. uncertain condition the physician wants to try and eliminate
   c. no
   d. yes, hyperthyroidism
   e. nervousness and irritability

Exercise 6.3 Assigning Codes for Symptoms and Signs

1. **R94.5** (Abnormal, function studies, liver)
3. **R56.9** (Seizures)

Exercise 6.4 Arranging Codes for Symptoms and Signs

1. **E11.9** (Diabetes, type 2)
   G47.9 (Sleep, disorder or disturbance)
3. **R10.13** (Pain, epigastric)
   K85.9 (Pancreatitis, acute)
   K83.0 (Cholangitis)

CHAPTER 7: FACTORS INFLUENCING HEALTH STATUS AND CONTACT WITH HEALTH SERVICES (Z00-Z99)

Exercise 7.1 Introduction to Z Codes

1. Student answers will vary and may include any of the following:
   - aftercare
   - counseling
   - follow up
   - immunizations
   - observation
   - obstetrics
   - routine or administrative examinations (pre-employment, annual check-up)
   - screening examinations (colonoscopy, mammogram).
3. a. Screening
   b. Donor
   c. Non-specific
   d. History

Exercise 7.2 Abstracting for Z Codes

1. a. annual medical examination
   b. no
3. a. adjustment of cardiac pacemaker
   b. no
5. a. 6-month follow up for malignant neoplasm of prostate
   b. no
   c. malignant neoplasm of prostate
   d. personal history
   e. prostate

Exercise 7.3 Assigning Z Codes

1. **Z00.00** (Examination, annual)
3. **Z45.018** (Fitting and adjustment of, pacemaker)

Exercise 7.4 Arranging Z Codes

1. **Z12.31** (Screening, disease, neoplasm, breast, routine mammogram)
   Z85.3 (History, personal, malignant neoplasm, breast)
3. **I20.0** (Angina, unstable)
   Z72.0 (Tobacco, use)

CHAPTER 8: EXTERNAL CAUSES OF MORBIDITY (V01-Y99)

Exercise 8.1 Abstracting for External Causes

1. a. 3 cm laceration on forehead
   b. fell off toilet and hit her head on the sink
   c. initial
3. a. malunion of non-displaced comminuted fracture, left femur shaft
   b. assault by handgun
   c. subsequent
5. a. fractured scapula, left side
   b. traffic accident, while driving a van
   c. subsequent
   d. unknown
   e. driving
   f. van
   g. driver
   h. pickup truck
   i. volunteer

Exercise 8.2 Assigning Codes for External Causes

1. **S01.81XA** (Laceration, forehead, initial encounter)
   Index to External Causes:
   W18.12XA (Fall, off toilet, with subsequent striking against object, initial encounter)
3. **S72.352P** (Fracture, femur, shaft, comminuted, left, subsequent, closed, malunion)
   Index to External Causes:
   X93.XXXD (Assault, firearm, subsequent encounter)

Exercise 8.3 Arranging Codes for External Causes

1. **I21.3** (Infarction, myocardium)
   Index to External Causes:
   X37.2XXA (Exposure to forces of nature, blizzard, initial encounter)
   Y92.014 (Place, residence, house, driveway)
   Y93.H1 (Activity, snow, shoveling)
   Y99.8 (Status, Other)
3. **S81.832A** (Puncture, leg, lower, left, initial encounter)
   Index to External Causes:
   W54.0XXA (Bite, dog)
   Y92.480 (Place, sidewalk)
   Y93.01 (Activity, walking)
   Y99.0 (Status, civilian activity done for pay)

CHAPTER 9: DISEASES OF THE DIGESTIVE SYSTEM (K00-K94)

Exercise 9.1 Digestive System Refresher

1. ile/us pertaining to the ileum K56.7
3. gingiv/itis inflammation of the gums K05.10
5. stomat/itis inflammation of the mouth K12.1
7. diverticul/itis inflammation of diverticula K57.92
9. proct/itis inflammation of the anus and rectum K62.89

Exercise 9.2 Abstracting for the Digestive System

1. a. indigestion
   b. stomach
   c. perforation, bleeding
   d. chronic
   e. no, indigestion is integral to a perforated ulcer
   f. chronic perforated peptic ulcer in stomach with bleeding
3. a. GI series
   b. no, it is a procedure
   c. ulcerative
   d. fistula
   e. ulcerative colitis with fistula
5. a. hematemesis
   b. present, cirrhosis is not curable
   c. portal hypertension
   d. portal hypertensive gastropathy
   e. no, they are integral to the condition
   f. yes, it is coexisting condition that the physician documents
   g. portal hypertension

Exercise 9.3 Assigning Codes for the Digestive System

1. **K25.6** (Ulcer, stomach, chronic, with hemorrhage, and perforation)
3. **K51.913** (Colitis, ulcerative, with, complication, fistula)
5. **K57.53** (Diverticulitis, intestine, large, with, small, with bleeding)

Exercise 9.4 Arranging Codes for the Digestive System

1. **K70.31** (Cirrhosis, liver, alcoholic, with ascites)
   F10.20 (Alcohol, addiction)
3. **K94.02** (Infection, colostomy)
   L03.311 (Cellulitis, abdominal wall)
   B95.61 (Infection, bacterial, as cause of disease classified elsewhere, staphylococcus, aureus)
5. **K02.52** (Caries, dental, pit and fissure, penetrating into dentin)
   K02.51 (Caries, dental, pit and fissure, limited to enamel)

Exercise 9.5 Coding Neoplasms of the Digestive System

1. **D12.5** (Poylp, colon, sigmoid, benign)
   Z86.010 (History, personal, neoplasm, benign, colon polyp)
   Z80.0 (History, family, malignant neoplasm, gastrointestinal tract)
3. **C22.0** (Cancer, hepatocellular)
   F10.20 (Dependence, alcohol)
   B18.2 (Hepatitis, C, chronic)
5. **C25.9** (Table of Neoplasms, pancreas, primary)
   C78.7 (Table of Neoplasms, liver, secondary)
   C77.9 (Table of Neoplasms, lymph, secondary)

CHAPTER 10: ENDOCRINE, NUTRITIONAL, AND METABOLIC DISEASES (E00-E89)

Exercise 10.1 Endocrine System Refresher

1. thyro/toxic/osis condition of thyroid poisoning E05.90
3. thyro/megaly enlargement of the thyroid E01.0
5. hyper/glyc/emia elevated blood sugar R73.9
7. pan/hypo/pituitary/ism deficiency in all hormones of the pituitary E23.0
9. hypo/para/thyroid/ism pertaining to a low parathyroid gland E20.9

Exercise 10.2 Abstracting for the Endocrine System

1. a. diabetes monitoring
   b. type 2
   c. none
   d. none
3. a. ketoacidosis
   b. type 1
   c. ketoacidosis
   d. weakness, shortness of breath, severe abdominal pain with vomiting
   e. no, they are integral to ketoacidosis
   f. no, insulin is always used with type 1 diabetes
5. a. neuropathy
   b. type 2
   c. no, documentation does not stated due to
   d. peripheral autonomic neuropathy
   e. type 2 diabetes

Exercise 10.3 Assigning Codes for the Endocrine System

1. **E11.9** (Diabetes, type 2)
3. **E10.10** (Diabetes, type 1, with, ketoacidosis)

Exercise 10.4 Arranging Codes for the Endocrine System

1. **K86.1** (Pancreatitis, chronic)
   E08.649 (Diabetes, due to underlying condition, with hypoglycemia, without coma)
   Z79.4 (Long term drug therapy, insulin)
3. **E24.0** (Cushing's syndrome, pituitary dependent)
   D35.2 (Table of Neoplasms, pituitary, benign)

Exercise 10.5 Coding Neoplasms of the Endocrine System

1. **C73** (Carcinoma, papillary, serous, see Table of Neoplasms, thyroid, malignant primary)
3. **D15.0** (Thymoma)
5. **Z51.11** (Chemotherapy, neoplasm)
   C25.9 (Table of Neoplasms, pancreas, malignant primary)
   C79.9 (Table of Neoplasms, malignant secondary)

CHAPTER 11: DISEASES OF THE SKIN AND SUBCUTANEOUS TISSUE (L00-L99)

Exercise 11.1 Integumentary System Refresher

1. pachy/derma thick skin L85.9
3. peri/follicul/itis inflammation around a hair follicle L01.02
5. erythro/derma red skin L53.9
7. onycho/crypt/osis condition of a hidden (ingrown) nail L60.0
9. hidr/aen/itis inflammation of sweat gland L73.2

Exercise 11.2 Abstracting for the Integumentary System

1. a. was at the beach all day and did not have sunscreen applied
   b. sun, ultraviolet rays
   c. 2nd
   d. blistering
3. a. red and tender area on the left great toe
   b. ingrown nail
   c. no, the symptoms are integral to the condition
5. a. erythema multiforme minor
   b. stomatitis
   c. herpes simplex virus
   d. falling off of layers of skin
   e. 15%

Exercise 11.3 Assigning Codes for the Integumentary System

1. **L55.1** (Sunburn, second degree)
3. **L60.0** (Ingrowing, nail)

Exercise 11.4 Arranging Codes for the Integumentary System

1. **L03.116** (Cellulitis, lower limb, left lower)
   B95.0 (streptococcus, A, as cause of disease classified elsewhere)
3. **I87.011** (Postphlebitic syndrome, *see* Syndrome, postthrombotic, with ulcer, lower right extremity)
   L97.212 (Ulcer, lower limb, calf, right, exposed fat layer)

Exercise 11.5 Coding Neoplasms of the Integumentary System

1. **C44.399** (Table of Neoplasms, skin, eyebrow, chin)
   C44.01 (Table of Neoplasms, skin, lip, basal cell)
3. **Z51.12** (Immunotherapy, antineoplastic)
   C43.59 (Melanoma, skin, back)
   C79.9 (Melanoma, metastatic, NOS)

5. **C4A.62** (Carcinoma, Merkel cell, upper limb, including shoulder, left)
Z94.0 (Transplant, kidney)

CHAPTER 12: DISEASES OF THE MUSCULOSKELETAL SYSTEM AND CONNECTIVE TISSUE (M00-M99)

Exercise 12.1 Musculoskeletal Refresher

1. arthro/pathy abnormal condition of the joint M12.9
3. fibro/my/algia pain of muscle fiber M79.7
5. chondro/calcin/osis condition of calcium salt in cartilage M11.20
7. chondro/malacia softening of cartilage M94.20
9. teno/synov/itis inflammation of tendon sheath M65.9

Exercise 12.2 Abstracting for the Musculoskeletal System

1. a. pain in lower back and hips
b. fibromyalgia
c. no, the symptoms are integral to the condition
d. no, physical therapy was not provided during this encounter
3. a. acute hip pain
b. fracture of ilium
c. osteoporosis
d. pathologic
e. no, it is integral to the fracture
5. a. knee pain
b. no, it is integral to the injury
c. sequela
d. anterior horn of the medial meniscus
e. left
f. tackle in football
g. no, only code the activity of the external cause for the initial encounter

Exercise 12.3 Assigning Codes for the Musculoskeletal System

1. **M79.7** (Fibromyalgia)
3. **M80.059A** (Osteoporosis, age related, with current pathological fracture, ilium, unspecified)

Exercise 12.4 Arranging Codes for the Musculoskeletal System

1. **M84.58XA** (Fracture, pathological, due to, neoplastic disease, vertebra, initial encounter)
C79.51 (Table of Neoplasms, bone, vertebra, secondary)
C61 (Table of Neoplasms, prostate, primary)
3. **M11.841** (Arthritis, in, crystals, due to dicalcium phosphate, *see* specified type, hand joint, right hand)
E21.0 (Hyperparathyroidism, primary)

Exercise 12.5 Coding Neoplasms of the Musculoskeletal System

1. **C40.21** (Table of Neoplasms, bone, patella, right)
3. **Z51.11** (Chemotherapy, cancer)
C91.00 (Leukemia, acute lymphoblastic, NOS)
5. **C40.22** (Table of Neoplasms, bone, primary, femur, left)
Z51.11 (Chemotherapy, cancer)

CHAPTER 13: INJURY, POISONING, AND CERTAIN OTHER CONSEQUENCES OF EXTERNAL CAUSES (S00-T88)

Exercise 13.1 Injury and Poisoning Refresher

1. displaced fracture
3. perforation
5. Gustilo
7. poisoning
9. adverse effect

Exercise 13.2 Abstracting for Injury and Poisoning

1. a. tibia, right
b. growth plate at the upper end
c. Salter Harris
d. Type III
e. pain, tenderness, swelling, and distortion on right knee
f. no, they are integral to the fracture
g. initial
h. tackle in sports
i. accidental
j. school
k. recreation
l. football
3. a. laceration, wound
b. index finger, right
c. remove sutures
d. subsequent
e. cut with knife
f. no, OGCR I.C.19.a.) instructs coders to NOT assign an aftercare code, but to assign an injury code with the extension for subsequent care
5. a. Flunitrazepam
b. assault
c. examination
d. rape, sexual assault
e. initial
f. boyfriend
g. yes, the abuse is confirmed

Exercise 13.3 Assigning Codes for Injury and Poisoning

1. **S89.031A** (Fracture, tibia, upper end, physeal, Salter Harris Type III, right, initial)
3. **S61.200D** (Wound, finger, index, right, subsequent)

Exercise 13.4 Arranging Codes for Injury and Poisoning

1. **I48.91** (Fibrillation, atrial)
T46.0X5A (Table of Drugs and Chemicals: Digitalis, adverse effect, initial)
N18.2 (Disease, kidney, chronic, stage 2)
3. **T54.2X1A** (Table of Drugs and Chemicals: Sulfuric, acid, accidental, initial encounter)
T26.61XA (Corrosion, cornea, right eye, initial encounter)
T26.51XA (Corrosion, eyelid, right)
T26.52XA (Corrosion, eyelid, left)
T20.66XA (Corrosion, cheek/forehead, second degree)
Index to External Causes:
Y92.014 (Place of occurrence, residence, house, driveway)
Y99.8 (Activity, leisure activity)

CHAPTER 14: DISEASES OF THE CIRCULATORY SYSTEM (I00-I99)

Exercise 14.1 Circulatory System Refresher

1. hyper/tension abnormally high (blood) pressure I10
3. cardio/myo/pathy abnormal condition of the heart muscle I42.9
5. arterio/scler/osis hardening of arteries I70.90
7. lympho/cele a swelling containing lymph I89.8
9. thrombo/angi/itis inflammation of the lining of a blood vessel with a clot I73.1

Exercise 14.2 Abstracting for the Circulatory System

1. a. an infarction that affects only a small portion of the heart wall, usually due to a decreased, but not totally occluded, blood supply

b. same as a.
c. Infarct

3. a. between the right atrium and the right ventricle
b. The patient's mitral valve was replaced with a valve from a pig
c. The mitral valve has does not close properly and is allowing blood to flow backwards into the atrium.

5. a. shortness of breath, hypertension, congestive heart failure, atrial fibrillation
b. CHF
c. no causal relationship is stated or implied
d. CHF, it is the cause of the increased symptoms
e. anticoagulant
f. antiplatelet

6. a. stroke
b. embolus
c. a particle or clot that has travelled from another location
d. within
e. cerebral atherosclerosis, hypertension
f. history of tobacco use
g. The clot was surgically removed.

Exercise 14.3 Assigning Codes for the Circulatory System

1. **I21.4** (Infarct, myocardium, nontransmural)
3. **I34.0** (Insufficiency, mitral valve)
5. **I83.811** (Varix, leg, right, with pain)

Exercise 14.4 Arranging Codes for the Circulatory System

1. **I21.11** (Infarction, myocardial, STEMI, involving right coronary artery)
I25.2 (Infarction, myocardial, old)
Z86.73 (History, personal, transient ischemic attack)
3. **I63.411** (Infarction, cerebral, due to, embolism, cerebral arteries, right middle cerebral artery)
I67.2 (Arteriosclerosis, cerebral)
I10 (Hypertension)
Z92.82 (Status, administration of tPA)
Z72.0 (History, personal, tobacco use)
5. **I26.99** (Embolism, pulmonary)
I82.512 (Thrombosis, vein, femoral, chronic, left)

CHAPTER 15: DISEASES OF THE BLOOD AND BLOOD-FORMING ORGANS AND CERTAIN DISORDERS INVOLVING THE IMMUNE MECHANISM (D50-D89)

Exercise 15.1 Refresher on the Blood

1. hemo/philia blood attraction D66
3. thrombo/cyto/penia deficiency of platelet cells D69.6
5. eosino/philia accumulation of eosinophils D72.1
7. pan/hemato/penia deficiency of all types of blood cells D61.9
9. erythro/blasto/phthi/sis wasting away of immature red blood cells D61.09

Exercise 15.2 Abstracting for the Blood

1. a. reduction in lymphocyte count
b. lymphocytopenia
c. no, a definitive diagnosis was made

3. a. pain and swelling in LUQ
b. enlargement of the spleen
c. inflammation of the spleen
d. removal of the spleen
e. LUQ
f. splenitis

5. a. tachycardia, headaches, fatigue
b. anemia due to CKD
c. yes
d. CKD
e. stage 3 CKD
f. anemia in chronic disease

Exercise 15.3 Assigning Codes for the Blood

1. **D72.810** (Lymphocytopenia)
3. **D73.89** (Splenitis)

Exercise 15.4 Arranging Codes for the Blood

1. **C18.9** (Table of Neoplasms, colon, malignant primary)
C79.9 (Table of Neoplasms, malignant secondary)
D64.81 (Anemia antineoplastic chemotherapy induced)
3. **R73.09** (Pre-diabetes)
D50.9 (Anemia, iron deficiency)

Exercise 15.5 Coding Malignancies of the Blood

1. **Z51.11** (Chemotherapy, cancer)
C94.20 (Leukemia, acute myeloid, M7, not having achieved remission)
3. **C91.01** (Leukemia, acute lymphoblastic, in remission)
5. **Z51.0** (Radiation, therapy)
C82.18 (Lymphoma, follicular, grade 2, multiple sites)

CHAPTER 16: DISEASES OF THE RESPIRATORY SYSTEM (J00-J99)

Exercise 16.1 Respiratory System Refresher

1. pneumato/cele hernia or swelling in the lung J98.4
3. pneumo/hemo/thorax air and blood in the chest J94.2
5. naso/pharyng/itis inflammation of the nose and throat J00
7. laryngo/plegia paralysis of the voice box J38.00
9. tracheo/stenosis narrowing of the trachea J39.8

Exercise 16.2 Abstracting for the Respiratory System

1. a. extrinsic asthma
b. coughing, wheezing, and SOB
c. acute exacerbation
d. none
e. mild intermittent

3. a. COPD
b. declining spirometry, SOB
c. no
d. no, they are integral to the disease process
e. yes, it is the reason for services provided
f. no, they are COPD

5. a. acute bronchitis
b. COPD, chronic bronchitis
c. acute bronchitis is an exacerbation of the COPD
d. yes, it is the reason for admission
e. no, it is part of COPD
f. tobacco dependence

Exercise 16.3 Assigning Codes for the Respiratory System

1. **J45.21** (Asthma, intermittent (mild), with, acute exacerbation)
3. **J44.9** (Disease, lung, obstructive)

Exercise 16.4 Arranging Codes for the Respiratory System

1. **J15.7** (Pneumonia, lobular, *see* Pneumonia, broncho, Mycoplasma pneumoniae)
J20.0 (Bronchitis, acute, due to Mycoplasma pneumoniae)

I50.9 (Failure, heart)
Z99.81 (Dependence on, oxygen)

3. **J61** (Asbestosis)
   J45.30 (Asthma, mild persistent)
   R68.3 (Clubfinger)

Exercise 16.5 Coding Neoplasms of the Respiratory System

1. **C34.12** (Table of Neoplasms, lung, upper lobe, malignant primary, left)
   Z51.0 (Radiotherapy)
   Z72.0 (Tobacco, use)
3. **C77.0** (Table of Neoplasms, lymph, gland, cervical malignant secondary)
   C14.0 (Table of Neoplasms, pharynx, malignant primary)
   F10.20 (Dependence, alcohol)
   Z87.891 (History, personal, nicotine dependence)
5. **C31.0** (Table of Neoplasms, sinus, maxillary, primary malignant)

CHAPTER 17: DISEASES OF THE NERVOUS SYSTEM AND SENSE ORGANS (G00-G99)

Exercise 17.1 Nervous System Refresher

1. neur/oma tumor on a nerve D36.10
3. encephalo/myelo/radicul/itis inflammation of the spinal cord and nerve roots in the head G61.0
5. neuro/myo/tonia contraction of the nerves and muscles G71.19
7. hemi/chorea jerky movements on one side of the body G25.5
9. my/asthenia lack of strength in the muscles G70.9

Exercise 17.2 Abstracting for the Nervous System

1. a. pharmacoresistant migraine
   b. yes, pharmacoresistant means intractable
   c. no
   d. yes
   e. no, only 48 hours
   f. no
3. a. tremors, difficulty walking
   b. Parkinson's disease
   c. no, they are integral to the disease
   d. primary
   e. no
5. a. generalized weakness
   b. hyponatremia
   c. early onset
   d. she could wander off
   e. yes, hallucinations and wandering
   f. hyponatremia
   g. AD and dementia with behavioral disturbance, they created an elopement risk

Exercise 17.3 Assigning Codes for the Nervous System

1. **G43.119** (Migraine, with aura, intractable, without status migrainosus)
3. **G20** (Parkinsonism)

Exercise 17.4 Arranging Codes for the Nervous System

1. **G89.21** (Pain, chronic, due to trauma)
   M51.26 (Displacement, intervertebral, lumbar)
3. **G43.611** (Migraine, with aura, persistent, with cerebral infarction, intractable, with status migrainosus)
   I63.541 (Infarction, cerebral, due to, stenosis, cerebral arteries, right cerebellar artery)
   I10 (Hypertension)

Exercise 17.5 Coding Neoplasms of the Nervous System

1. **D33.0** (Table of Neoplasms, Hypothalmus, benign)
3. **G89.3** (Pain, due to cancer)
   C83.38 (Lymphoma, diffuse large cell, B cell, multiple sites)
   G55 (Compression, nerve, root, neoplastic disease)
5. **D64.81** (Anemia, due to, antineoplastic chemotherapy)
   T45.1X5A (Table of Drugs and Chemicals: Antineoplastic, adverse effect, initial)
   G89.3 (Pain, due to cancer)
   C56.2 (Table of Neoplasms, ovary, malignant primary, left)
   C79.31 (Table of Neoplasms, Brain, malignant secondary)

CHAPTER 18: MENTAL, BEHAVIORAL, AND NEURODEVELOPMENTAL DISORDERS (F01–F99)

Exercise 18.1 Psychiatry Refresher

1. agora/phobia fear of the marketplace F40.00
3. tricho/tillo/mania preoccupation with pulling hair F63.3
5. pedo/philia attraction towards children F65.4
7. dys/morpho/phobia fear of abnormal body shape F45.22
9. para/phrenic near or beside the mind (a disorder between paranoia and schizophrenia) F20.0

Exercise 18.2 Abstracting for Psychiatry

1. a. hyperactivity, short attention span, and irritability
   b. attention deficit hyperactive disorder
   c. predominately hyperactive type
   d. none, they are due to the main disorder
3. a. medical management, prescription renewal
   b. schizophrenia
   c. paranoid
   d. no
5. a. gastritis with hemorrhaging
   b. alcohol
   c. yes, states it is alcohol-induced
   d. dependence
   e. yes
   f. 0.09%, 90 mg per 100 ml
   g. no
   h. cocaine

Exercise 18.3 Assigning Codes for Psychiatry

1. **F90.1** (Disorder, attention-deficit hyperactivity, hyperactive type)
3. **Z76.0** (Issue of, repeat prescription)
   F20.0 (Schizophrenia, paranoid)

Exercise 18.4 Arranging Codes for Psychiatry

1. **F64.2** (Disorder, gender identity, childhood)
   F84.0 (Disorder, autistic)
3. **F31.4** (Disorder, bipolar, severe depression)
   K70.31 (Cirrhosis, liver, alcoholic, with ascites)
   F10.20 (Dependence, alcohol)

CHAPTER 19: DISEASES OF THE EYE AND ADNEXA (H00-H59)

Exercise 19.1 Eye Refresher

1. photo/kerat/itis inflammation of the cornea due to light H16.131
3. lago/pthalmos inability of the eye to close H02.209
5. dacryo/aden/itis inflammation of the tear gland H04.001

7. retino/schisis splitting of the retina H33.102
9. irido/cycl/itis inflammation of the iris and ciliary body H20.9

Exercise 19.2 Abstracting for the Eye

1. a. use ultrasonic vibrations to liquefy the lens and suck it out, followed by implanting an artificial lens
   b. cataract
   c. age related, nuclear
   d. left
3. a. blepharitis
   b. nonulcerative
   c. bilateral
   d. upper, upper
5. a. anterior uveitis
   b. bilateral
   c. cataracts
   d. neovascularization
   e. left
   f. yes
   g. arthritis
   h. rheumatoid, juvenile

Exercise 19.3 Assigning Codes for the Eye

1. **H25.12** (Cataract, senile, nuclear, left)
3. Either code can be sequenced first.
   H01.004 (Blepharitis, left, upper)
   H01.001 (Blepharitis, right, upper)

Exercise 19.4 Arranging Codes for the Eye

1. **Z01.01** (Examination, vision, with abnormal findings)
   E11.339 (Diabetes, type 2, with retinopathy, nonproliferative, moderate)
3. **H18.003** (Deposit, cornea, bilateral)
   H11.113 (Deposit, conjunctiva, bilateral)
   N18.6 (Disease, kidney, chronic, stage 5)
   Z99.2 (Status, hemodialysis)

Exercise 19.5 Coding Neoplasms of the Eye

1. **C69.21** (Retinoblastoma, right)
3. **C79.49** (Table of Neoplasms, choroid, malignant secondary)
   Z85.3 (History, personal, malignant neoplasm, breast)
   Z90.11 (Status, mastectomy, right)
5. **C88.4** (Lymphoma, mucosa associated lymphoid tissue)

CHAPTER 20: DISEASES OF THE EAR AND MASTOID PROCESS (H60-H95)

Exercise 20.1 Ear Refresher

1. labyrinth/itis inflammation of the labyrinth H83.03
3. cholesteat/oma mass of fat (cholesterol, cells) H71.92
5. presby/cusis old (age) hearing H91.13
7. oto/rrhagia bleeding from the ear H92.22
9. mastoid/algia pain in the mastoid bone H70.91

Exercise 20.2 Abstracting for the Ear

1. a. repair of the eardrum
   b. otitis media
   c. nonsuppurtive (serous)
   d. bilateral
   e. chronic
3. a. ringing, buzzing, difficulty hearing
   b. no, they are integral to tinnitus
   c. objective tinnitus, observable by the physician
   d. right
5. a. left earache, fever, head congestion
   b. otitis media
   c. suppurative
   d. acute
   e. yes
   f. earache, fever because it is suppurative and antibiotics were prescribed
   g. left
   h. sinusitis
   i. acute
   j. yes
   k. head congestion, possibly fever
   l. otitis media, because it is an infection
   m. yes, mother smokes cigarettes in the house

Exercise 20.3 Assigning Codes for the Ear

1. **H65.23** (Otitis, media, nonsuppurative, chronic, serous, bilateral)
3. **H93.11** (Tinnitus, *see* category H93.1, right)

Exercise 20.4 Arranging Codes for the Ear

1. **H80.03** (Otosclerosis involving oval window, nonobliterative, bilateral)
   H90.0 (Deafness, conductive, bilateral)
3. **H83.01** (Labyrinthitis, right)
   M54.5 (Pain, low back)

CHAPTER 21: CERTAIN INFECTIOUS AND PARASITIC DISEASES (A00-B99)

Exercise 21.1 Infectious Disease Refresher

1. candida, inflammation of the bronchus due to candida, B37.1
3. herpes, eyelid affected by the herpes virus, B02.30
5. amoeba, condition of the skin due to an amoeba, A06.7
7. rickettsia (not rickets), an eruptive disease caused by rickettsia, A79.1
9. tuberculus, condition of the anus due to tuberculus, A18.32

Exercise 21.2 Abstracting for Infectious Diseases

1. a. lack of energy, fatigue, loss of appetite, fever, and chills
   b. confirmed by blood test
   c. mononucleosis
   d. no, they are integral to the condition
3. a. *Staphylococcus aureus*
   b. yes, *Staphylococcus*
   c. yes
5. a. *Staphylococcus aureus*
   b. yes
   c. no
   d. no
   e. no
7. a. toe pain
   b. great toe
   c. right
   d. initial
   e. yes
   f. yes
   g. no
9. a. dysuria, weakness, and fever
   b. urosepsis or urinary tract infection
   c. *Eschericha coli* (non-Shiga toxin-producing)
   d. no
   e. yes
   f. no
   g. urosepsis

Exercise 21.3 Assigning Codes for Infectious Diseases

1. **B27.00** (Mononucleosis, Epstein-Barr)
3. **Z21** (Human, immunodeficiency virus, asymptomatic)
   Z71.7 (Human, immunodeficiency virus, counseling)
5. **A41.01** (Sepsis, Staphylococcus, aureus)

Exercise 21.4 Arranging Codes for Infectious Diseases

1. **B20** (Acquired, immunodeficiency syndrome)
   C46.0 (Kaposi's, sarcoma, skin)
3. **J15.211** (Pneumonia, Staphylococcus, aureus, Methicillin susceptible)
5. **A41.02** (Sepsis, staphyloccus aureus, methicillin resistant)
   R65.21 (Sepsis, severe, with septic shock)
   I50.9 (Failure, heart)

CHAPTER 22: DISEASES OF THE GENITOURINARY SYSTEM (N00-N99)

Exercise 22.1 Genitourinary System Refresher

1. a/meno/rrhea lack of menstrual flow N91.2
3. dys/pareunia painful sexual intercourse N94.1
5. cysto/ptosis prolapse or sagging of the bladder N32.89
7. urethro/rrhagia bleeding from the urethra N36.8
9. uretero/cele hernia of the ureter N28.89

Exercise 22.2 Abstracting for the Genitourinary System

1. a. female reproductive
   b. endometriosis
   c. uterus
   d. no, endometriosis is not caused by an infectious organism
3. a. urinary
   b. occasional excruciating low back pain
   c. calculi
   d. yes
   e. kidney and ureter
   f. no
   g. no
5. a. female reproductive
   b. vaginal discharge, burning, redness in perineal area
   c. vaginitis
   d. bacterial
   e. staphylococcus
   f. no, it is treatable

Exercise 22.3 Assigning Codes for Genitourinary System

1. **N80.0** (Endometriosis, uterus)
3. **N20.2** (Calculus, kidney, with calculus, ureter)

Exercise 22.4 Arranging Codes for the Genitourinary System

1. **N40.1** (Enlarged prostate, with lower urinary tract symptoms)
   N13.8 (Obstruction, urinary)
   R33.8 (Retention, urinary)
3. **N39.0** (Infection, urinary tract)
   B96.29 (Escherichia coli, as cause of disease classified elsewhere, non-Shiga toxin-producing)
   Z87.440 (History, personal, urinary tract infection)

Exercise 22.5 Coding Neoplasms of the Genitourinary System

1. **C61** (Table of Neoplasms, prostate, malignant primary)
3. **N30.41** (Cystitis, irradiation, with hematuria)
   C56.9 (Table of Neoplasms, ovary, malignant primary, unspecified laterality)
   C79.9 (Table of Neoplasms, malignant secondary)
   Index to External Causes:
   Y84.2 (Radiation, complication of or abnormal reaction to)
5. **C50.212** (Table of Neoplasms, breast, upper inner quadrant, left)

CHAPTER 23: PREGNANCY, CHILDBIRTH, AND THE PUERPERIUM (O00-O9A)

Exercise 23.1 Obstetrics Refresher

1. hyper/emesis excessive vomiting O21.0
3. amnion/itis inflammation of the amnion O41.1210
5. oligo/hydr/amnios little water in the amnion O41.02X0
7. intra/peritoneal within the peritoneum O00.0
9. cervical dys/tocia difficult labor due to the cervix O62.2

Exercise 23.2 Abstracting for Obstetrics

1. a. no
   b. 2nd trimester, 26 weeks
   c. 3
   d. 2
   e. none
   f. placenta previa, hemorrhage
3. a. yes, over age 35
   b. 1st trimester, 10 weeks
   c. 1
   d. 0
   e. none
   f. 10 weeks, 4 days
   g. the patient's age is a complication
   h. prenatal encounter for high risk pregnancy
5. a. no
   b. 3rd trimester, 28 weeks
   c. 2
   d. 1
   e. none
   f. 28 weeks, 3 days
   g. Rhesus incompatibility
   h. Rhesus incompatibility
7. a. no
   b. 1st trimester, 12 weeks
   c. 2
   d. 1
   e. none
   f. 12 weeks, 0 days
   g. pernicious anemia
   h. pernicious anemia
9. a. yes, under age 15
   b. 3rd trimester, 30 weeks
   c. 1
   d. 0
   e. none
   f. 30 weeks, 4 days
   g. 1 chorion, 2 amnions
   h. gestational proteinuria

Exercise 23.3 Assigning Codes for Obstetrics

1. **O44.12** (Pregnancy, complicated by, placenta, previa with hemorrhage, second trimester)
   Z3A.26 (Pregnancy, weeks of gestation, 26 weeks)

3. **O09.511** (Pregnancy, supervision, older mother, primigravida, first trimester)
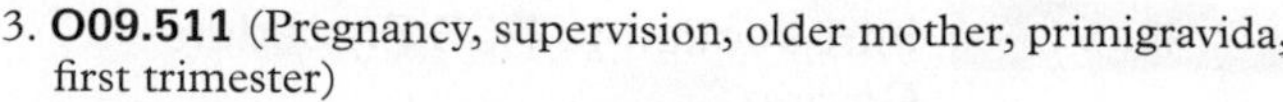
Z3A.10 (Pregnancy, weeks of gestation, 10 weeks)

5. **O09.899** (Pregnancy, supervision, high risk, due to, specified, NEC, third trimester)
O36.0130 (Rh, incompatibility affecting management of pregnancy, anti-D antibody, third trimester, single gestation)
Z3A.28 (Pregnancy, weeks of gestation, 28 weeks)

Exercise 23.4 Arranging Codes for Obstetrics

1. **O43.813** (Infarction, placenta, third trimester)
O36.4XX0 (Pregnancy, complicated by, death of fetus, single gestation)
Z37.1 (Outcome of delivery, single, stillborn)
Z3A.37 (Pregnancy, weeks of gestation, 37 weeks)

3. **O14.13** (Delivery, cesarean, pre-eclampsia, severe, third trimester)
O42.913 (Delivery, complicated, premature rupture of membranes, unspecified length of time between rupture and onset of labor, third trimester)
Z37.0 (Outcome of delivery, single, liveborn)
Z3A.32 (Pregnancy, weeks of gestation, 32 weeks)

5. **O65.4** (Delivery, complicated by, obstruction, fetopelvic disproportion,)
O48.0 (Pregnancy, post-term)
O99.214 (Delivery, complicated by, obesity, complicating pregnancy)
E66.01 (Obesity, severe)
Z68.41 (BMI, 40.0-44.9)
Z37.0 (Outcome of delivery, single, liveborn)
Z3A.41 (Pregnancy, weeks of gestation, 41 weeks)

CHAPTER 24: CERTAIN CONDITIONS ORIGINATING IN THE PERINATAL PERIOD (P00-P96)

Exercise 24.1 Perinatal Refresher

1. tachy/cardia pertaining to rapid heart rate P29.11
3. hyper/bilirubin/emia excessive bilirubin in the blood P59.9
5. mast/itis inflammation of the breast P39.0
7. hyp/oxic low oxygen, ischem/ic lack of blood supply, en/cephalo/pathy abormal condition inside the head P91.60
9. hypo/natr/emia low sodium in the blood P74.2

Exercise 24.2 Abstracting for Perinatal Conditions

1. a. yes
   b. vaginal
   c. 3,521 grams
   d. 38 weeks, 2 days
   e. no
   f. no
   g. none
3. a. 13 days
   b. neonatal check up
   c. yes, neonatal diabetes
5. a. yes
   b. vaginal
   c. 3,200 grams
   d. 39 weeks, 6 days
   e. no
   f. no
   g. bradycardia during labor
   h. none, the bradycardia is a condition of the infant, not the mother
7. a. no, this is a readmission
   b. vaginal
   c. 2,016 grams
   d. 35 weeks, 6 days
   e. yes, jaundice
   f. no
   g. jaundice
9. a. 22 days
   b. foul smelling urine
   c. urinary tract infection
   d. due to *E. coli*
   e. none
   f. yes, based on the age

Exercise 24.3 Assigning Codes for Perinatal Conditions

1. **Z38.00** (Newborn, single, born in hospital)
3. **Z00.111** (Newborn, examination, 8 to 28 days)
P70.2 (Diabetes, neonatal)
5. **Z38.00** (Newborn, single, born in hospital)
P03.811 (Newborn, affected by, heart rate abnormalities, intrauterine, during labor)

Exercise 24.4 Arranging Codes for Perinatal Conditions

1. **Z38.1** (Newborn, born outside hospital)
P08.22 (Prolonged, gestation, newborn)
P24.01 (Aspiration, meconium, with respiratory symptoms)
3. **P05.17** (Small for dates, 1750-1999)
P05.9 (Newborn, affected by, fetal, growth retardation)
P00.0 (Newborn, affected by, maternal, condition, hypertensive disorder)
P04.2 (Newborn, affected by, tobacco)
5. **Z00.110** (Newborn, Examination, under 8 days old)
P83.4 (Engorgement, breast, newborn)

CHAPTER 25: CONGENITAL MALFORMATIONS, DEFORMATIONS, AND CHROMOSOMAL ABNORMALITIES (Q00-Q99)

Exercise 25.1 Congenital Abnormalities Refresher

1. ichthy/osis abnormal condition of scaliness Q80.9
3. en/cephalo/cele hernia of the brain Q01.0
5. a/tresia lack of opening Q52.4
7. poly/dactyl many fingers or toes Q69.9
9. bi/cornate two horns or heart shaped Q51.3

Exercise 25.2 Abstracting for Congenital Abnormalities

1. a. Marfan's syndrome
   b. not applicable
   c. yes
   d. mitral valve prolapse
   e. MVP is not integral to Marfan's syndrome
   f. no others
   g. MVP
3. a. lack of a uterus
   b. none
   c. yes, it is congenital by definition
   d. amenorrhea
   e. amenorrhea
   f. none
   g. lack of a uterus
5. a. polydactyl
   b. accessory thumb of right hand
   c. yes, it is congenital by definition
   d. none

e. none
f. none
g. accessory thumb of right hand

7. a. Prader-Willi
b. none
c. yes
d. hypotonia, hypogonadism
e. hypotonia
f. small for gestational age
g. birth

9. a. pyloric stenosis
b. not applicable
c. yes
d. vomiting
e. vomiting
f. Meckel's diverticulum
g. birth; pyloric stenosis was treated during the admission

Exercise 25.3 Assigning Codes for Congenital Abnormalities

1. **Q87.418** (Syndrome, Marfan's, with cardiovascular manifestations)
3. **Q51.0** (Absence, uterus, congenital)
5. **Q69.1** (Accessory, thumb)

Exercise 25.4 Arranging Codes for Congenital Abnormalities

1. **Q90.0** (Down syndrome, nonmosaicism)
Q21.1 (Defect, septal, atrial)
Q34.8 (Deformity, respiratory system, specified)
3. **Z00.121** (Examination, child over 28 days, with abnormal findings)
Q40.2 (Microgastria)
R62.51 (Failure to thrive, child over 28 days old)
5. **Q21.0** (Defect, septal, ventricular)
Q21.1 (Patent, foramen ovale)

CHAPTER 26: ICD-10-PCS PROCEDURE CODING

Exercise 26.1 The Purpose of ICD-10-PCS

1. Completeness
3. Standardized terminology
5. Significant procedures
7. resources
9. all of them: the hospital, the surgeon, the anesthesiologist

Exercise 26.2 ICD-10-PCS Coding Manual Organization

1. ICD-10-PCS Coding Guidelines
3. Introduction
5. Body Part Key
7. CMS
9. 1

Exercise 26.3 ICD-10-PCS Code Structure

1. Tables
3. I, O
5. 5, Approach
7. 3, Root Operation
9. 2, Body System

Exercise 26.4 ICD-10-PCS Coding Guidelines

1. Conventions
3. row
5. Obstetrics

Exercise 26.5 Introduction to PCS Procedure Coding

1. Root Operation
3. interpret
5. Root Operation, common procedure name
7. 3
9. 4, 5, 6, and 7

CHAPTER 27: MEDICAL AND SURGICAL PROCEDURES (SECTION 0), PART 1

Exercise 27.1 Medical and Surgical Refresher

1. angi/oplasty surgical repair of a vessel; Dilation, Repair, Replacement, Supplement
3. ovario/centesis surgical puncture of the ovary to remove fluid; Drainage
5. hernio/rrhaphy suturing of a hernia; Repair, Supplement
7. colo/stomy creating a new mouth/opening in the colon; Bypass, Drainage
9. esophago/plication folding of the esophagus; Restriction

Exercise 27.2 Coding Overview of Medical and Surgical Procedures

1. Division 8
3. Extraction D
5. Removal P
7. Detachment 6
9. Repair Q

CHAPTER 28: MEDICAL AND SURGICAL PROCEDURES (SECTION 0), PART 2

Exercise 28.1 Abstracting Medical and Surgical Procedures

1. a. excisional debridement
b. skin and subcutaneous tissue of the hip
c. yes
d. open
e. no
f. Did the procedure take out some or all of a body part without replacement?
g. Excision

3. a. appendectomy
b. appendix
c. yes
d. laparoscopic
e. no
f. Did the procedure take out some or all of a body part without replacement?
g. Resection

5. a. dilation and curettage
b. uterus
c. yes
d. via natural opening
e. no, dilation is a procedural step necessary to reach the operative site (uterus) so it does not get a separate code
f. Did the procedure take out some or all of a body part without replacement?
g. Extraction
h. therapeutic

7. a. cholecystectomy/choledochectomy
b. gallbladder/common bile duct
c. no, a choledochectomy was also performed
d. open/open
e. yes, two sites removed

f. Did the procedure take out some or all of a body part without replacement? for both
g. Resection/Resection

9. a. blepharoplasty
b. eyelid
c. yes
d. Open
e. two procedures, one on each eye
f. Did the procedure restore a body part to its normal structure?
g. Repair

Exercise 28.2 Assigning Medical and Surgical Procedure Codes

1. **0JBM0ZZ** (Excision, Subcutaneous tissue, Upper Leg, Open, No Device, No Qualifier)
3. **0DTJ4ZZ** (Resection, Appendix, Percutaneous Endoscopic, No Device, No Qualifier)
5. **0UDB7ZZ** (Extraction, Endometrium, Via Natural or Artificial Opening, No Device, No Qualifier)

Exercise 28.3 Arranging Medical and Surgical Procedure Codes

1. **0U5B8ZZ** (Destruction, Endometrium, Via Natural or Artificial Opening Endoscopic, No Device, No Qualifier)
0U524ZZ (Destruction, Ovary, Bilateral, Percutaneous Endoscopic, No Device, No Qualifier)
3. **08T43ZZ** (Vitrectomy, Resection, Vitreous Right, Percutaneous, No Device, No Qualifier)
08U03JZ (Buckling, scleral with implant, OR Supplement, Eye, Right, Percutaneous, Synthetic Substitute, No Qualifier)
5. **0QSG04Z** (Reposition, Lower Bones, Tibia Right, Open, Internal Fixation Device, No Qualifier)
0PSF34Z (Reposition, Upper Bones, Humeral Shaft Right, Percutaneous, Internal Fixation Device, No Qualifier)

CHAPTER 29: MEDICAL AND SURGICAL-RELATED (SECTIONS 1-9) AND ANCILLARY PROCEDURE CODING (SECTIONS B-D, F-H)

Exercise 29.1 Terminology Refresher

1. audio/metry measurement of hearing; Hearing Assessment
3. chemo/embolization blocking a vessel with a chemical agent; Introduction
5. chol/angio/gram a record of gall bladder vessels/duct; Plain Radiography, Fluoroscopy
7. myleo/gram record of spinal cord or bone marrow; CT, MRI
9. oxi/metry measurement of oxygen; no other Root Operation listed

Exercise 29.2 Coding for Medical and Surgical-Related Procedures (Sections 1 to 9)

1. **10D00Z1** (Extraction, products of conception, low cervical)
3. **10D07Z4** (Extraction, products of conception, mid forceps)
5. **2W3CX2Z** (Immobilization, Arm, Lower, Right, External, Cast, No Qualifier)

Exercise 29.3 Coding for Ancillary Procedures (Sections B to D, F to H)

1. **BP0JZZZ** (Plain Radiography, Forearm, Right)
3. **DV10B8Z** (Brachytherapy, Prostate, Low Dose Rate, Iridium 192, None)
5. **GZB2ZZZ** (Electroconvulsive Therapy, Bilateral, Single Seizure, None, None, None)

CHAPTER 30: ADVANCED CODING AND HEALTH INFORMATION TECHNOLOGY

Exercise 30.1 Coding from Chart Notes

1. CC, Assessment
3. PMH
5. Plan
7. low back pain
9. clear to auscultation
11. Gastroenterology Chart Note
K25.0 (Ulcer, stomach, acute, with hemorrhage)
D50.9 (Anemia, deficiency, iron)
K21.0 (Reflux, gastroesophageal, with esophagitis)
B96.81 (Infection, Helicobacter pylori, as the cause of diseases classified elsewhere)
F10.288 (Dependence, alcohol with specified disorder)

Exercise 30.2 Coding from Operative Reports

1. preoperative and postoperative diagnoses
3. operative risk
5. a. operative approach
b. objective of the procedure as it relates to the Root Operation definition
c. anatomical site
d. devices
e. other details required by the specific procedure
7. viewing
9. suturing
11. Orthopedics Operative Report
CM:
M50.23 (Displacement, intervertebral disc, cervicothoracic)
M25.78 (Osteophyte, vertebrae)
PCS:
0RT40ZZ (Resection, Disc, Cervicothoracic Vertebral, Open, No Device, No Qualifier)
0PB30ZZ (Excision, Vertebra, Cervical, Open, No Device, No Qualifier)
0RG40K0 (Fusion, Cervicothoracic Vertebral, Open, Nonautologous Tissue Substitute, Anterior Approach, Anterior Column)
BR00ZZZ (Plain Radiography, Cervical Spine, None, None, None)

Exercise 30.3 Health Information Technology

1. Edit checks alert users to, or prevent, certain errors.
3. Student answers will vary but should include the concept that coders need to understand what information they must give the software in order for it to provide accurate feedback. An untrained user can make coding errors with an encoder, just as they would using the physical manuals.
5. Health Information Technology for Economic and Clinical Health Act (HITECH), which is part of the American Recovery and Reinvestment Act of 2009 (ARRA)
7. Reduce the number of inappropriate tests and procedures, paperwork and administrative overhead, and the number of adverse events resulting from medical errors.
9. CAC works best within environments that have a limited number of diagnoses and procedures, a limited number of source documents, a limited number of users, and fewer coding guidelines because these limitations make programming easier.

Glossary

The glossary provides defintions for key terms, supplemental terms, and abbreviations. The number in brackets [ ] indiciates the chapter in which the term is first discussed.

A

AAPC a professional organization for coders founded in 1988, formerly known as the American Academy of Professional Coders [1]
abnormal development embryonic development of a structure that occurred on schedule but took on an uncommon physical variation or development in the womb [25]
abnormal finding a laboratory test or clinical finding in which the readings are not within the normal average range established for that particular test [6]
absence seizure see petit mal seizure [17]
abstract read the medical record and determine which elements of the encounter require codes [1]
abuse mistakenly accepting payment for items or services that should not be paid for by Medicare [2]; the physical, emotional, or sexual mistreatment by one person toward another [13]; a usage pattern of a substance in a quantity or frequency that creates legal, employment, social, or family problems, or places the individual at physical risk, without causing physical dependence [18]
accessory organ an organ that assists an organ system carry out its functions but does not fulfill a major function of the system [9]
Accredited Standards Committee (ASC) X12N Version 4010 an electronic transaction standard used with ICD-9-CM [3]
Accredited Standards Committee (ASC) X12N Version 5010 the revised set of HIPAA transaction standards adopted to coincide with ICD-10-CM [3]
acoustic neuroma see vestibular schwannoma [20]
acquired immunodeficiency syndrome (AIDS) a disease caused by the HIV virus, which weakens and paralyzes the immune system [21]
actinic keratosis a precancerous lesion [11]
activity what the person was doing at the time of the event [8]
acute exacerbation a sudden increase in the intensity or type of symptoms, such as shortness of breath, wheezing, and chest tightness; commonly called an asthma attack [16]
acute kidney failure the rapid loss of kidney function over a period of days or weeks [22]
acute myocardial infarction (AMI) a myocardial infarction (heart attack) that has occured within the past four weeks; also called a current myocardial infarction [14]
acute rhinitis a common cold that affects the upper respiratory tract [16]
acute tubular necrosis the damage to the renal tubules due to reduced blood flow or toxins in the urine [22]
addiction a usage pattern that involves compulsive reliance on the substance to the extent that is physically or psychologically difficult to stop, despite the significant problems it creates; also called dependence [18]
additional diagnosis any diagnosis that is not the principal or first-listed; also called secondary [4]
adenocarcinoma cancerous tumor of a gland [5]
adenoma tumor of a gland [5]
adjustment disorder an abnormal difficulty in responding to life changes [18]
adjuvant the additional treatments when more than one type of treatment is used [5]
admitting privileges an agreement between a physician and hospital that gives the physician authority to admit a patient to the hospital [1]
adnexa the associated anatomic structures of the eye, which includes the ocular muscles, eyelids, and conjunctiva [19]
advanced level job a job obtained after several year of experience that may include management of others or focus on a specialized area of technical expertise [1]
adverse effect an undesired physical response to a medication that was correctly prescribed and properly administered [8]
aerosol therapy a medication used to treat respiratory diseases that is suspended in a mist that is inhaled [16]
Aftercare a Z code category used for the initial treatment of a disease that has been performed and in which the patient requires continued care during the healing or recovery phase, or for the long-term consequences of the disease [7]
AHIMA American Health Information Management Association [1]
airway obstruction a reduction in the amount of inhaled air in each breath, most commonly caused by a reduction in the diameter of the bronchioles due to inflammation [16]
alimentary cana a continuous tube, approximately 30 feet in length, which begins at the mouth; continues through the esophagus, stomach, small intestine, large intestine; and exits the body at the rectum and anus [9]
allergic a hypersensitivity to a substance that is usually harmless [20]
allergic rhinitis a condition of hay fever that affects the upper respiratory tract [16]
allograft the tissue from another person [11]
alopecia a condition of hair loss resulting in baldness [11]
alphanumeric a combination of letters and numbers [1]
alveoli the small air sacs where the bronchioles end [16]
Alzheimer's disease (AD) a progressive degenerative brain disease [17]
ambulatory surgery a surgical procedure that does not require an overnight stay in the hospital [1]
amelogenesis imperfecta a tooth development disorder in which the teeth are covered with thin, abnormally formed enamel and are easily damaged [9]
American Health Information Management Association (AHIMA) a professional organization for coders founded in 1928 [1]
American Recovery and Reinvestment Act of 2009 (ARRA) an economic stimulus package that was signed into law in February 2009 [30]
amnion see amniotic sac [23]
amnionitis an infection or inflammation of the amniotic sac [24]
amniotic sac a membrane that surrounds the embryo; also called the amnion [23]
amyotrophic lateral sclerosis (ALS) a chronic, terminal neurological disease characterized by a progressive loss of motor neurons and muscle atrophy; also called Lou Gehrig disease [17]
anatomical imaging a type of traditional radiology that captures a static image of an anatomical part [29]
ancillary services provided in addition to medical care, such as laboratory, radiology, or physical therapy [1]
and a preposition physicians use to indicate that two conditions are present in the same patient, but one condition does not cause the other [10]
anemia a blood disorder characterized by a reduction in the number of red blood cells, which results in less oxygen reaching the tissues [15]
aneurysm a bulge in the wall of an artery due to weakening, most commonly occurring in the abdominal aorta and cerebral arteries [14]

angina intense pain and spasms [14]
angiography an imaging study of the circulatory system in which X-rays are taken after an opaque dye is injected into a blood vessel [14]
angioplasty the insertion of an inflatable catheter in a blood vessel and expanding it to compress plaque against the wall of the vessel [14]
anomaly a permanent abnormal shape of an organ or body region, resulting from arrested, delayed, or abnormal development of the embryo; also called a malformation [25]
antenatal see prenatal [23]
antepartum see prenatal [23]
antiarrythmic a drug used to treat heart rhythm disorders by slowing the electrical impulses in the heart so it can resume a regular rhythm [15]
antihypertensive a drug used to treat high blood pressure [15]
anxiety disorder an abnormal activity that interferes with normal activities [18]
aorta the first artery leading out of the heart to the body, which then repeatedly subdivides into smaller arteries that lead to each body region and anatomic site [14]
aortic coarctation a narrowing of the aorta [25]
aortic valve the valve that controls the blood flow from the left ventricle to the aorta [14]
Apgar score an evaluation of a newborn's physical condition that is performed 1 and 5 minutes after birth to determine any immediate need for extra medical or emergency care [24]
aplastic anemia an anemia that is due to a loss of red bone marrow [15]
appendicitis inflammation and possible rupture of the appendix [9]
appendicular skeleton a division of the skeleton that contains 126 bones and consists of the arms, shoulders, wrists, hands, legs, hips, ankles, and feet [12]
Approach the fifth character in a PCS Medical and Surgical code that identifies the surgical technique, defined by PCS, used to reach the procedure site [26]
appropriate for gestational age (AGA) a fetus or newborn infant whose size is within the normal range for his or her gestational age [24]
arrange place codes in the order dictated by the guidelines and instructional notes (sequence) [1]
arrested development embryonic development of a structure that stopped before it should have [25]
arrhythmia an abnormal heartbeat [14]
arteries the large, thick-walled vessels that carry blood away from the heart [14]
arteriole a small artery [14]
arteriosclerotic heart disease (ASHD) the formation of plaque in the coronary arteries; also called ischemic heart disease and coronary heart disease (CHD) [14]
arthralgia a pain in a joint [12]
arthritis the damage or inflammation of a joint [12]
ASHD arteriosclerotic heart disease [14]
aspiration inhalation of a foreign substance into the respiratory tract [16]
assessment the diagnostic statement; the cause of the patient's current symptoms [2]
assign determine codes that accurately describe the patient's condition, reflect the highest level of specificity possible, and contain the correct number of characters for that code [1]
assisted delivery a delivery of the fetus using mechanical, pharmacologic, or medical assistance [23]
astrocytoma a tumor of the brain or spinal cord that is composed of astrocytes [24]
asymptomatic a patient who has no symptoms [6]
atherosclerosis the formation of plaque on the inner walls of arteries in the heart [14]
atonic a seizure characterized by a brief loss of muscle tone [17]
atopic asthma due to allergens; also called extrinsic [16]
atria plural for atrium, two of the four chambers of the heart that receive blood from the body and the lungs [14]
atrial fibrillation (A-fib) an irregular heartbeat in the atria characterized by an abnormal quivering of heart fibers [14]
atrioventricular (AV) node an electrical relay station between the atria and the ventricles [14]
atrioventricular (AV) valve valve that controls the flow of blood from the atria to the ventricles [14]
atrioventricular bundle a group of cardiac muscle fibers that connect the atria with the ventricles; also called bundle of His [14]
attending physician the physician who oversees and coordinates all aspects of the patient's inpatient care [1]
audit an investigation of the provider's billing and coding practices [2]
auditory canal the part of the external ear that funnels the sound waves [20]
aura a sensation of voices or colored light [17]
auricle the visible part of the ear, which collects sound waves; also called pinna [20]
autograft the tissue from a patient [11]
autoimmune a condition in which the body's immune system attacks and destroys healthy body tissue [10]
autologous a grafted vessel from the patient [14]
automatic adjudication the process in which a computer automatically determines which procedure codes are covered and how much the insurance company is obligated to pay, then triggers the payment [2]
autonomic nervous system the system that controls the sensory impulses from the blood vessels, the heart, and organs in the chest, abdomen, and pelvis, through nerves, to the brain [14]
AV atrioventricular [14]
avascular necrosis of bone the death of bone tissue due to a lack of blood [12]
axial skeleton a division of the skeleton that contains 60 bones that are basically stationary and make up the skull, sternum, ribs, and vertebrae [12]

B

bacteria a one-celled germ that multiplies quickly and may release toxins creating illnesses [21]
barium enema injection of a chalky substance into the colon through the anus to make organs visible on an X-ray; also called lower GI series [9]
barium swallow swallowing of a chalky substance and viewing it on an X-ray; also called upper GI series [9]
Barlow's syndrome see mitral valve prolapse (MVP) [14]
Bartholin's gland a gland that secretes mucus [22]
basal cell carcinoma (BCC) a cancer appearing in the lowest layer of the epidermis, which accounts for 75% of new skin cancer cases [11]
BBB bundle branch block [14]; blood-brain barrier [17]
behavior a classification of neoplasms that is categorized as malignant or benign [5]
behavioral disorder a manifestation of mental disturbances that result in extreme or disruptive conduct, such as rage, withdrawal, or substance abuse [18]
behavioral disturbance an action that includes aggression, wandering, depression, delusion or hallucinations, sleep disturbances, or poor eating habits [18]
Bell's palsy the inflammation of the seventh (VII) cranial nerve, which is the facial nerve [17]
benign not life threatening [5]
benign prostatic hyperplasia (BPH) see benign prostatic hypertrophy (BPH) [22]
benign prostatic hypertrophy (BPH) the abnormal growth of epithelial cells of the prostate, causing compression or obstruction of the urethra; also called benign prostatic hyperplasia (BPH) or enlarged prostate (EP) [22]
biopsy the scraping, punching, or cutting a piece of tissue in order to examine it under a microscope [5] [11]
birth trauma any physical injury to the infant during delivery [24]
blepharitis an inflammation and infection of hair follicles and glands at the margins of the eyelids, due to virus, bacteria, allergic response, or exposure to irritants [19]
block in ICD-10-CM, a contiguous range of codes within a chapter that is comparable to a section in ICD-9-CM; also called a subchapter [4]
blood the bodily fluid that transports and passes nutrients, oxygen, carbon dioxide, water, proteins, and hormones to cells and

transports waste products to excretory oxygen; also called the hemic system [15]
blood alcohol concentration (BAC) see blood alcohol level (BAL) [18]
blood alcohol content see blood alcohol level (BAL) [18]
blood alcohol level (BAL) a measurement of the amount of alcohol present in the blood; also called blood alcohol content or blood alcohol concentration (BAC) [18]
blood-brain barrier (BBB) a naturally occurring barrier of vessels and capillaries that filters blood flowing to the brain and prevents certain toxic substances from infiltrating brain tissue and the central nervous system [17]
blood creatinine a blood test used to determine the amount of creatinine present; an abnormal result would suggest renal dysfunction [22]
body the main portion of the muscle [12]
Body Part a specific anatomical site, defined by the PCS system, where the procedure was performed [26]
Body System the general body system, defined by the PCS system, where the procedure was performed [26]
bone marrow the connective tissue in the cavities of bones [15]
bone saw a saw used to cut bone [28]
BP blood pressure
BPH benign prostatic hyperplasia or hypertrophy [22]
brain the body part that governs perception of the senses, emotions, consciousness, memory, and voluntary movements [17]
breast engorgement the temporary enlargement of breasts on female or male newborns, due to high levels of maternal hormones in the infant's blood [24]
bronchi the plural of bronchus, bronchial tubes [16]
bronchial tree the configuration of bronchi subdividing into smaller and smaller branches [16]
bronchioles the smallest bronchi in the bronchial tree, which do not contain rings of cartilage [16]
bronchiolitis inflammation of the bronchiole [16]
bronchitis inflammation of the bronchus [16]
bronchodilator a medication used to treat respiratory diseases that relaxes muscle spasms in bronchial tubes [16]
bronchogenic lung cancer that begins in the cells that line the bronchi [16]
bronchospasm a contraction of smooth muscle in the walls of the bronchi and bronchioles, causing narrowing of the lumen [16]
brushing using a tool with soft hair-like tufts to remove tiny bits of tissue [28]
buccal pertaining to the cheek [28]
build a code the process of assigning values to each character based on specific characteristics of the procedure the physician performed [26]
bulbo-urethral gland the gland that provides a mucous secretion before ejaculation, which becomes part of the semen [22]
bulla a blister [11]
bundle branch a division of the bundle of His [14]
bundle branch block (BBB) the blockage of the conduction of electrical impulse through the branches of the atrioventricular bundle [14]
bundle of His see atrioventricular bundle [14]
burns the damage to skin by heat, electricity, or radiation [13]
bursitis the inflammation of fluid around a joint [12]
bypass graft the creation of a new route around a blockage in a blood vessel using a vessel from another part of the body, another person, or a synthetic substitute [14]

C

CA carcinoma, cancer [5]
CA in situ cells that have begun to change but are contained within the epithelial layer [5]
CABG coronary artery bypass graft [14]
CAD coronary artery disease [14]
calculi hard balls of cholesterol (fat); also called stones [9]
cancer a malignant tumor of epithelial cells, which line body cavities and organs; synonymous with carcinoma [5]
candida, candidiasis a yeast fungi [21]
capillary the very thin-walled membrane at the end of the arterioles that allow blood to diffuse into body tissues and receive waste products from the tissues to send back into the bloodstream [14]
carbuncle a skin infection that involves a group of hair follicles [11]
carcinoid a benign or malignant tumor arising from the mucosa of the gastrointestinal tract [10]
carcinoid syndrome a collection of symptoms caused by carcinoid tumors, characterized by flushing, cyanosis, abdominal cramps, diarrhea, and heart valve disease; see also carcinoid [10]
carcinoma a malignant tumor of epithelial cells, which line body cavities and organs; synonymous with cancer [5]
carcinoma of unknown primary (CUP) a neoplasm diagnosed at a late stage after it has metastasized and the physician is unable to determine the site of origin [5]
cardiac catheterization a cardiac function test in which a thin tub is passed through a blood vessel to the heart to visualize the structure, collect blood samples, and determine the blood pressure of the heart [14]
cardiac function test a measurement of the capacity of the heart in real time; tests include cardiac catheterization, electrocardiography, Holter monitor, and stress testing [14]
cardiac scan an imaging study of the circulatory system in which a scan is taken of the heart after the patient receives radioactive thallium intravenously [14]
cardiac sphincter the valve between the esophagus and the stomach [9]
cardiology lab a testing center to evaluate a heart problem [1]
cardiovascular (CV) system the body system that distributes blood throughout the body and includes the heart and blood vessels; also called the circulatory system [14]
cardioversion an application of an electric shock in order to restore a normal heartbeat [29]
career path the progression of jobs and responsibilities throughout one's working life [1]
cartilage the fibrous tissue found at the end of bones [12]
case production the number of cases a coder codes each day while maintaining high accuracy [1]
cataract a cloudiness of the lens that usually develops slowly over time due to aging [19]
category three characters in length [4]
causal relationship one disease caused by another [10]
cause/causal event a description of how an injury or health condition happened [8]
CBC complete blood count
CC chief complaint [2]
CCA Certified Coding Apprentice [1]
CCS Certified Coding Specialist [1]
CCS-P Certified Coding Specialist – Physician [1]
CDC Centers for Disease Control and Prevention [4]
celiac disease an abnormal immune reaction to gluten and poor absorption of nutrients [9]
cell type a classification of neoplasms that is based on the characteristics or appearance of the cell [5]
cellulitis an inflammation under the skin [11]
central nervous system (CNS) the control center for the nervous system, which processes information and provides short term control over other organ systems; consists of the brain and spinal cord [17]
cephalopelvic disproportion (CPD) a cause of obstructed labor due to a mismatch between the size of the fetal head and the mother's pelvic brim; also called fetopelvic disproportion [23]
cerebral an object located within the brain [14]
cerebral palsy a functional disorder of the brain manifested by motor impairment [17]
cerebrovascular accident (CVA) a sudden drop in blood supply to the brain; also called stroke [14]
certification a voluntary achievement that documents that a coder has attained a certain level of proficiency by passing a rigorous examination [1]

certified EHR technology proof that a specific EHR system provides the necessary features to meet the meaningful use criteria [30]

cerumen the earwax that protects and lubricates the ear [20]

ceruminoma an excessive accumulation of ear wax; also called impacted cerumen [20]

cervical dysplasia an abnormal change in the cells on the surface of the cervix that may lead to cancer if not treated [22]

cervical intraepithelial neoplasia (CIN) the condition cervical dysplasia seen on a cervical biopsy, classified as mild dysplasia (CIN 1), moderate to marked dysplasia (CIN II), and severe dysplasia to cancer in situ (CIN III) [22]

cesarean section (c/s, C/S, C-section) the delivery of the fetus by making a surgical incision into the abdominal wall and uterus; also called an abdominal delivery [23]

chalazion a small hard cyst on the eyelid caused by blockage of a gland on the eyelid [19]

chapter a subdivision of ICD-10-CM that contains codes for a body system or related conditions [4]

character one of the seven positions that make up the ICD-10-PCS codes [26]

CHD coronary heart disease [14]

CHF congestive heart failure [14]

chief complaint (CC) the problem that has brought the patient to see the doctor or other reason for the visit [2]

childbirth the period of true labor and active delivery; also called parturition [23]

chlamydia a sexually transmitted disease [21]

cholecystitis inflammation of the gall bladder [9]

choledocholithiasis calculi in the common bile duct [9]

cholelithiasis calculi in the gall bladder [9]

cholesteatoma a cyst or benign tumor consisting of epithelial cells and fat [20]

chorion the outer membrane that surrounds the amnion [23]

chorionic villi sampling (CVS) the removal of a small piece of the chorion for genetic analysis [23]

choroid the opaque middle layer that supplies blood to the eye [19]

chromosomal abnormality the abnormal number or structure of chromosomes [23]

chronic bronchitis an inflammation of the bronchi with a productive cough for three months, in two consecutive years [16]

chronic kidney disease (CKD) the slow loss of kidney function over a period of months or years [14]

chronic obstructive pulmonary disease (COPD) the combination of chronic bronchitis and emphysema as comorbidities [16]

chronic pain syndrome (CPS) a collection of pain conditions lasting more than six months and unresponsive to treatment [17]

CIN cervical intraepithelial neoplasia [22]

circulatory system the body system that distributes blood throughout the body and includes the heart, and blood vessels; also called the cardiovascular (CV) system [14]

circumstances of admission facts, signs, and symptoms that require the admission [4]

cirrhosis scarring of liver tissue that blocks the normal flow of blood through the liver [9]

CKD chronic kidney disease [14, 22]

clavicle the collar bone [13]

clean claims insurance claims that pass the front-end edit checks and have no missing or invalid information [2]

cleft lip or palate a notch or division of the upper lip or roof of the mouth [25]

click murmur syndrome see mitral valve prolapse (MVP) [14]

clinically significant condition a condition that coexists at the time of admission, develops subsequently, or affects the treatment received and/or the length of stay; also called relevant condition [4]

clinically significant condition (newborn) a condition of newborns that requires clinical evaluation, therapeutic treatment, diagnostic procedures, extended length of hospital stay (LOS), increase in nursing care or monitoring, or presents implications for future healthcare needs [24]

clitoris a part of the female genital system that is a small sensitive protrusion [22]

clonic a seizure characterized by a series of muscle contractions and relaxations on both sides of the body [17]

closed fracture a type of fracture in which the bone does not break the skin [13]

cluster headache a unilateral pain in the eye or temple, affecting primarily men [17]

CM Clinical Modification; used in this text as shorthand for ICD-10-CM [3]

CMS Centers for Medicare and Medicaid Services [2]

CMS-1500 form the standard physician billing form [26]

CNS central nervous system [17]

c/o complains of [4]

cochlea a snail-shaped organ that makes hearing possible [20]

code the final level of subdivision and may be three, four, five, six, or seven characters in length [4]

code set a distinct system of medical codes [1]

Codes on Dental Procedures and Nomenclature (CDT®) the HIPAA-mandated code set for dental services [1]

coding path the sequence of Main Terms and subterms the coder must search in the Index in order to locate the code [4]

coding the process of accurately assigning codes to verbal descriptions of patients' conditions and the healthcare services provided to treat those conditions [1]

cognitive disorder a failure to develop or deterioration of mental comprehension [18]

colloid the gelatin-like or mucous substance found in tissues [19]

combination code a single code that describes two or more conditions [4]

computer-assisted coding (CAC) the use of computer software that automatically generates a set of medical codes for review, validation, and use based upon clinical documentation provided by healthcare practitioners [30]

comorbidity a condition or disease that exists at the same time, but usually independent of, another disease in the same patient [9]

completeness a PCS characteristic meaning there is a unique code for every procedure that is significantly different in body part, approach, or methods [26]

complex partial a seizure that is associated with both sides of the cerebrum and causes a change in or loss of consciousness; also called a psychomotor seizure [17]

complex regional pain syndrome see reflex sympathetic dystrophy (RSD) [17]

compliance following the rules [2]

complication an abnormal medical reaction that results from a medical or surgical procedure [8]

conception the fertilization of the female ova by the male sperm [23]

cone a photoreceptor cell of the retina that is sensitive to bright light and color vision [19]

confirmed a diagnostic statement that the physician is confident of [4]

congenital a condition that appears at birth [10]

congenital abnormality a specific type of perinatal condition that originates during pregnancy or the first 28 days of life [25]

congestive heart failure (CHF) the inability of the heart to maintain circulation [14]

Congressional Budget Office (CBO) a federal agency that provides economic data to Congress [30]

conjunctiva the membrane that lines the eyelids [19]

conjunctivitis a viral or bacterial inflammation and infection of the conjunctiva [19]

Contact/Exposure a Z code category used for patients who do not show any sign or symptom of a disease but are suspected to have been exposed to it by close personal contact with an infected individual or are in an area where a disease is epidemic [7]

continuous positive airway pressure (CPAP) device a ventilation device that blows a stream of air into the nose during sleep in order to keep the airway open [17]

contusion a bruise [13]

conventions the use of symbols, typeface, and layout features to succinctly convey interpretive information [4]

Coordination and Maintenance Committee a federal interdepartmental committee comprised of the four cooperating parties (representatives from the Centers for Medicare and Medicaid Services (CMS), the Centers for Disease Control and Prevention's (CDC) National Center for Health Statistics (NCHS), the American Hospital Association (AHA), and the American Health Information Management Association (AHIMA)) that oversees all changes of the ICD-10-CM, which must be consistent with WHO's ICD-10 [4]

COPD chronic obstructive pulmonary disease [16]

cornea the clear hard portion of the sclera that protects the lends [19]

coronary artery bypass graft (CABG) an open heart surgery procedure to create a bypass around a blocked coronary artery [14]

coronary artery disease (CAD) an insufficient blood supply to the heart due to an obstruction of one or more coronary arteries [14]

coronary circulation the section of the circulatory system that occurs within the heart and carries blood from the aorta to the tissues of the heart in order to maintain the function of the heart itself [14]

coronary heart disease (CHD) see arteriosclerotic heart disease (ASHD) [14]

corrosion the damage of skin due to chemicals [13]

Counseling a Z code category used for a patient or family member who receives assistance in the aftermath of an illness or injury, or when support is required in coping with family or social problems [7]

covered entity an organization that sends or receives electronic healthcare transactions [1]

CPC Certified Professional Coder [1]

CPC-H Certified Professional Coder – Hospital [1]

CPS chronic pain syndrome [17]

CPT® Current Procedural Terminology [1]

cranial nerve II the nerve that transmits visual information from the external environment to the brain; also called the optic nerve [19]

Crohn's disease an inflammatory bowel disease (IBD) with inflammation and ulcers in the alimentary tract characterized by a thickening of the mucous membrane [9]

cryotherapy application of cold; also called freezing [28]

c/s, C/S cesarean section [23]

culture a test used to identify the microorganism that is causing an infection [11]

culture and sensitivity a lab test of secretions, such as sputum, to observe bacterial growth and test to determine antibiotic effectiveness [16]

CUP carcinoma of unknown primary [14]

curet spoon-shaped instrument [28]

curettage using a curet to scrape away material [28]

current MI see acute myocardial infarction (AMI) [14]

Current Procedural Terminology (CPT®) the HIPAA-mandated code set for hospital outpatient and physician procedure coding [1]

CV cardiovascular

CVA cerebrovascular accident [14]

cystitis see urinary tract infection (UTI) [22]

D

decubitus ulcer a pressure ulcer or bed sore [11]

deep vein thrombosis (DVT) the formation of a thrombus within a deep vein, usually in the leg or pelvis [14]

default code a code number immediately following a Main Term or subterm that represents the condition most commonly associated with the entry, or the unspecified code for the condition [4]

deformation see deformity [24]

deformity a change in the size or shape of a normal structure, due to extrinsic physical forces; also called a deformation [25]

degeneration the breakdown of bone or tissue [12]

degenerative neural disease a class of diseases marked by degeneration of nerves and brain tissue, resulting in abnormalities in muscle and sensory functions [17]

degree the depth of a burn or corrosion [13]

delayed a patient who is waiting to seek care [12]

delayed development the embryonic development of a structure that is started late or progresses slowly [25]

delirium a state of confusion, restlessness, and incoherence [18]

delivery the expulsion of the fetus and placenta from the uterus [23]

deltoid triangular in shape [4]

delusion a false belief that hinders the ability to function [18]

dementia a loss of brain function that affects memory, thinking, language, judgment, and behavior [17]

denied a claim that was processed and found to be ineligible for payment [2]

dependence see addiction [18]

dermatitis herpetiformis (DH) an extremely itchy, blistering skin rash [11]

Destruction the PCS Root Operation defined as physical eradication of all or a portion of a body part by the direct use of energy, force, or a destructive agent [28]

Detachment the PCS Root Operation defined as cutting off all or part of the upper or lower extremities [28]

developmental dysplasia of the hip (DDH) a disruption in the normal relationship between the head of the femur and the acetabulum (hip socket) [25]

Device character six of a PCS Medical and Surgical code that identifies the material that is intentionally left in a patient for a therapeutic reason at the conclusion of a procedure [26]

DHHS Department of Health and Human Services [2]

diabetes mellitus (DM) a common disease of the endocrine system resulting in elevated glucose levels over an extended period of time and excess excretion of urine, usually due to malfunction of the pancreas [10]

diabetic ketoacidosis (DKA) a high level of ketones that has accumulated in the blood and turns acidic [10]

diabetic nephropathy the accumulated damage to the glomerulus capillaries due to chronic high blood sugar [22]

diabetic retinopathy the abnormal expression of blood vessels and hemorrhaging in the vessels of the retina, caused by diabetes [19]

diagnosis patient illness, disease, condition, injury, or other reason for seeking healthcare services [1]

diagnostic procedure a procedure performed to obtain information needed to make a diagnosis and treatment plan [27]

diagnostic radiology imaging services to evaluate or diagnose a health problem [1]

dialysis a treatment that filters the blood to remove waste, excess salt, and water [22]

dialysis-related amyloidosis (DRA) a deposit of a starchy substance amyloid in the joints due to dialysis [22]

diaphysis the long narrow part of the long bone; also called the shaft [12]

diastole the time during the heart cycle when the chamber relaxes as it fills with blood [14]

dichorionic-diamniotic (DiDi) two embryos developed from separate zygotes, resulting in each embryo having its own amnion and chorion [23]

digestive system the body system that receives nutrients, breaks them down, absorbs them into the blood to be used by the body, and eliminates solid waste products; also called the gastrointestinal GI system [9]

digital rectal examination (DRE) physical examination of the rectum using the fingers [9]

disarticulation an amputation that occurs at a joint [28]

dislocation a condition in which two bones are out of place at the joint [12]

displaced a condition in which the fragments of bone move out of alignment due to a traumatic fracture [13]

dissociative disorder a disruption in consciousness, memory, identity, or perception [18]

distal epiphysis the rounded end of a long bone that is furthest from the trunk [12]

distributed seizure a seizure that is the result of abnormal activity on both sides of the brain; also called a generalized seizure [17]

diverticula pouches formed when the lining of the intestine pushes through the intestinal muscle layer [9]

diverticular disease the presence and/or inflammation of diverticula [9]

diverticulitis a bacterial infection of diverticula [9]

diverticulosis the presence of diverticula [9]

divided separation [27]

DM diabetes mellitus [10]

doctor of osteopathy (DO) a licensed physician who has the same licensing, training, and qualifications as a doctor of medicine (MD) plus an additional 300 to 500 hours in the musculoskeletal system and study of hands-on manual manipulation [29]

document the act of recording the reason a physician saw the patient, the diagnostic techniques used, tests or treatments planned, and the overall assessment of the patient [1]

documentation the written or electronic record of medical care and services provided [2]

dominance the side of the body an individual favors [17]

Donor a Z code category used for living individuals who are donating blood or other body tissue [7]

doppler ultrasonography an imaging study of the circulatory system in which an image is created by measuring sound-wave echoes off of tissues and organs [14]

Down syndrome a genetic condition in which a person has 47 chromosomes instead of the usual 46; also called Trisomy 21 [25]

drug withdrawal syndrome a collection of symptoms of drug withdrawal in an infant who was exposed to narcotics in the uterus; also called neonatal abstinence syndrome (NAS) [24]

ductal a cancer which starts in the milk ducts of the breast [22]

due to a preposition physicians use to indicate that one condition is caused by or is a manifestation of another condition [10]

DVT deep vein thrombosis [14]

dyspnea a patient experiencing difficulty breathing [23]

dystocia a patient experiencing a difficult labor [23]

dystonia the erratic jerky movements due to improperly functioning muscle tension [17]

E

E. coli *Escherichia coli*

eardrum see tympanum [20]

early onset AD Alzheimer's disease that is diagnosed before age 65 [17]

eating disorder a serious disturbance in eating behavior [18]

ECC echocardiogram [14]

ECG electrocardiogram; see also EKG [14]

echocardiography (ECC) an imaging study of the circulatory system in which a non-invasive ultrasound procedure is done to visualize internal cardiac structures [14]

eclampsia the presence of convulsions occurring during pregnancy or the puerperium associated with preeclampsia [23]

ectopic outside of the uterus [23]

EDD estimated date of delivery [23]

edit check a feature built into software that alerts users to, or prevents, certain errors based on rules that are programmed into the system [30]

EGA estimated gestational age [23]

EGD esophagogastroduodenoscopy [9]

EKG electrocardiogram [14]

electrocardiogram, electrocardiography (ECG, EKG) a cardiac function test resulting in a graphical recording of the electrical activity of the heart [14]

electrocautery an instrument with disposable tips that uses heat generated by an electrical current to cut or destroy tissue [28]

electroconvulsive therapy a procedure in which electric currents are passed through the brain deliberately triggering a brief seizure; can reverse symptoms of certain mental illnesses [18]

electrolyte a chemical compound that separates into charged particles in a solution [22]

electronic health record (EHR) an electronic version of a patient's medical history, which is maintained by a provider over time; also called electronic medical record (EMR) [30]

electronic medical record (EMR), see electronic health record (EHR) [30]

embolectomy the removal of a clot from a blood vessel [14]

embolus an abnormal particle circulating in the blood, such as an air bubble or thrombus that has broken loose from its point of origin [14]

emergency department an organized department of an acute care hospital that provides treatment of an injury or health problem that cannot be delayed without harm to the patient [1]

empyema pus in a body cavity [16]

emphysema an enlargement and rupture of alveolar sacs at the end of the bronchioles, causing an abnormal accumulation of air in the tissue [16]

emulsification milking or sucking out [28]

encephalitis a viral inflammation of the brain and meninges [17]

encoder an enhanced electronic coding manual that was first introduced in the 1980s, which improved the productivity and accuracy of coders [30]

encounter a specific interaction between a patient and healthcare provider [1]

Encounter for Obstetrical and Reproductive Services a Z code category used for obstetric or reproductive encounters when none of the problems or complications included in the codes from the obstetrics chapter exist [7]

endarterectomy the removal of the disease or damaged inner lining of an artery [14]

endocarditis an inflammation in the lining of the heart or valves, due to bacteria or another disease [14]

endocardium the smooth inner layer that reduces the friction as the blood flows through the heart [14]

endocrine system the body system that produces, stores, and releases hormones [10]

endometriosis the growth of endometrial tissue in any area other than the uterus [22]

endoscopic retrograde cholangiopancreatography (ERCP) use of a combination of fluoroscopy and endoscopy to visually examine or treat a condition of liver, gallbladder, bile ducts, and pancreas [9]

endoscopic ultrasound (EUS) an ultrasound examination performed by installing the ultrasonic transducer transmitter on the end of an endoscope [9]

endotracheal intubation the placement of a tube through the mouth and glottis into the trachea to create a viable airway [16]

enlarged prostate (EP) see benign prostatic hypertrophy (BPH) [22]

entitlement programs healthcare payment program for which recipients qualify based on specific criteria [2]

entry-level job a job upon graduation in order to gain basic skills, become familiar with the healthcare field, and establish excellent work habits [1]

EOB explanation of benefits [2]

EP enlarged prostate [22]

epicardium the inner layer of the pericardium; also called a visceral pericardium [14]

epilepsy a brain disorder in which neurons signal abnormally, causing seizures and/or unconsciousness [17]

eponym named after a person [4]

equilibrium a sense of balance [20]

Erb's palsy the paralysis of the upper arm [24]

ERCP endoscopic retrograde cholangiopancreatography [9]

erectile dysfunction (ED) the chronic inability to achieve or maintain a penile erection until ejaculation; also called impotence [22]

erythema multiforme a red fluid-filled lesion that can cause layers of skin to fall off [11]

erythroblastosis fetalis a blood disorder that occurs when the blood types of a mother and baby are incompatible; also called hemolytic disease of the newborn (HDN) [24]

erythrocyte a red blood cell (RBC) [15]

Escherichia coli the *E. coli* bacteria that can cause serious food poisoning [21]

esophageal ring an abnormal ring of tissue around the esophagus [25]

esophagitis irritation of the esophagus caused by acid reflux and weak cardiac sphincter [9]

esophagogastroduodenoscopy (EGD) endoscopic examination of the esophagus, stomach, and duodenum [9]

estimated date of delivery (EDD) a number determined by counting 40 weeks from the last menstrual period (LMP) [23]

estimated gestational age (EGA) the number of weeks and days since the last menstrual period [23]

etiology cause [4]

EUS endoscopic ultrasound [9]

Eustachian tube the connection between the ear and the nasopharynx [22]

exceptionally large newborn a birth weight more than 4,500 grams (9 pounds, 15 ounces) [24]
exchange the process of obtaining oxygen from the air and delivering it to the lung and blood for distribution to tissue cells, and to removing the gaseous waste product, carbon dioxide, from the blood and lungs and expelling it [16]
Excision the PCS Root Operation defined as cutting out or off, without replacement, a portion of a body part
Excludes1 a convention indicating the condition represented by the code and the condition listed as excluded are mutually exclusive and should not be coded together [4]
Excludes2 a convention indicating the condition excluded is not part of the condition represented by the code, but the patient may have both conditions at the same time [4]
exfoliation the falling off in scales or layers [11]
exocrine a secretion externally via a duct [10]
exostectomy removal of bony bump [28]
expandability a PCS characteristic that means the structure of the code set allows new procedures to be easily incorporated [26]
explanation of benefits (EOB) a statement from the insurance company that lists all the services the provider billed, which ones were accepted for payment, how much the insurance company will pay, how much the patient owes, and how much will not be paid [2]
extension the seventh character of a code that must appear in that position regardless of the length of the code [4]
External a PCS value for the Approach that identifies that the entire treatment is performed on the skin or mucous membranes [27]
external cause an event such as an accident, force of nature, assault, or situation that causes an injury [8]
external ear a section of the ear that consists of the auricle or pinna, the auditory canal, and the tympanic membrane [20]
external job a job with a company different than the one where the employee currently works [1]
external radiotherapy directs precise doses of X-ray beams at specific sites in order to kill or shrink tumors and cancerous cells [5]
extracorporeal the procedures or processes that take place outside of the body [29]
extremely low birth weight (ELBW) a birth weight of less than 1,000 grams (2 pounds, 3 ounces) [24]
extrinsic asthma due to allergens; also called atopic [16]

F

failure to thrive (FTT) inadequate physical growth marked by child's weight for age below the fifth percentile of the standard growth chart [24]
fallopian tube the tube through which eggs are transported for fertilization and implantation in the uterus [22]
False Claims Act (FCA) a federal law that imposes penalties on individuals and companies who defraud government programs [2]
family history a condition that a patient's family member had in the past or currently has that causes the patient to be at higher risk of also contracting the disease [5]
fascia the fibrous tissue that connects muscle to muscle [12]
fatigue fracture see stress fracture [12]
fat-plug tympanoplasty a procedure done to treat eardrum perforations [20]
FCA False Claims Act [2]
Federal Register the official daily publication for rules, proposed rules, and notices of federal agencies and organizations, as well as executive orders and other presidential documents [3]
female factor infertility a problem in the female genital system that diminishes reproduction [21]
femur the thigh bone [12]
fetopelvic disproportion see cephalopelvic disproportion (CPD) [23]
fibrocystic breast disease a lump of benign fibrous tissue in the breast [22]
final rule a legally required notice of final regulations, which is published in the Federal Register [3]
first-listed diagnosis the diagnosis, condition, problem, or other reason for the encounter visit shown in the medical record to be chiefly responsible for the services provided in outpatient settings [4]
first trimester the time in a pregnancy when the gestational age is less than 14 weeks, 0 days [23]
fistula an abnormal connection between an organ, vessel, or intestine and another structure [9]
focal seizure a seizure that occurs in one part of the brain; also called a partial or localized seizure [17]
folic acid a B-complex vitamin needed by the body to manufacture red blood cells [15]
folic acid deficiency anemia an anemia due to a lack of folic acid [15]
folliculitis an inflammation of space around the hair root [11]
Follow-up a Z code category used for continuing surveillance following completed treatment of a disease, condition, or injury when the condition has been fully treated and no longer exists [7]
forceps a tweezers-type of instrument with two blades, and sometimes a handle, for compressing or grasping tissues [28]
forceps delivery the extraction of a fetus from the birth canal by grasping the head with forceps (tongs) [23]
foreign body an object that does not belong in the body [13]
formed element a blood cell [15]
four cooperating parties the organizations that oversee the development of ICD-ICD-10-PCS-CM: the Centers for Medicare and Medicaid Services (CMS), the Centers for Disease Control and Prevention's (CDC) National Center for Health Statistics (NCHS), the American Hospital Association (AHA), and the American Health Information Management Association (AHIMA) [3]
fracture a broken bone [12]
fragility fracture see pathologic fracture [12]
fraud knowingly billing for services that were never given or billing for a service that has a higher reimbursement than the service produced [2]
front-end edit check a computerized scan of insurance claims for valid data, performed by the payer [2]
FU follow up
fulguration destruction of living tissue using electrical sparks (direct) or electrode (indirect) [28]
full term pregnancy a pregnancy that is between 38 weeks, 0 days to 39 weeks, 6 days of gestation [23]
functional imaging a type of nuclear medicine that allows the physician to observe organ function in real time [29]
functional quadriplegia complete immobility due to a severe physical disability or frailty [6]
fundoplication wrapping stitches around the upper part of the stomach and lower part of the esophagus to increase pressure [9]
fungi primitive vegetables that reproduce through spores [21]
furuncle a skin infection involving an entire hair follicle and the surrounding skin tissue [11]

G

gangrene the decay or death of tissue in the body caused by a lack of blood supply [10]
gastritis inflammation of stomach lining [9]
gastroenteritis bacterial or viral infection of the stomach and intestines [9]
gastroesophageal reflux disease (GERD) backward flow of stomach contents into the esophagus [9]
gastrointestinal (GI) system digestive system [9]
General Equivalence Mappings (GEMs) a crosswalk between ICD-10-CM/PCS codes and ICD-9-CM codes, which is the authoritative source for comparing codes between the two code sets [3]
generalized seizure see distributed seizure [17]
genital prolapse downward displacement of the uterus or vagina to an abnormal position [21]
genitourinary (GU) system the body system that includes the urinary and genital system [22]
gestational age the number of weeks and days since the last menstrual period (LMP) [23]

gestational condition a condition that is first diagnosed during pregnancy [23]
gestational diabetes (GDM) a condition in which elevated glucose levels are diagnosed during pregnancy in women with no prior history of diabetes [10]
gestational hypertension the development of hypertension after 20 weeks gestation in a woman who previously was not diagnosed with hypertension; also called pregnancy induced hypertension (PIH) [23]
GI gastrointestinal [9]
giardia an intestinal tract infection caused by a protozoa [21]
glaucoma an increased fluid pressure within the eye that damages the optic nerve and can cause blindness [19]
glomerular filtration rate (GFR) a method used to measure kidney function and to determine the stage of kidney disease [22]
glomerulonephritis the inflammation of the glomerulus of the kidney, allowing protein and blood into the urine [22]
glomerulus a cluster of capillaries that separates the urinary space from the blood [22]
glucagon a hormone produced in the pancreas [10]
glucose tolerance test (GTT) a diagnostic measure to evaluate how the body breaks down sugar [10]
glycouria sugar in the urine [10]
goiter an enlargement of the thyroid gland that is not cancer [10]
grand mal seizure a seizure characterized by a sudden loss of consciousness and falling to the floor and affects the entire brain; also called tonic-clonic [17]
grand multipara a woman who has had five or more previous pregnancies resulting in a viable fetus [23]
granular, granularity detailed [3]
Graves disease overproduction by the thyroid gland due to an autoimmune condition in which autoantibodies are directed against the thyroid-stimulating hormone (TSH) receptor [10]
gravida (G) the number of pregnancies a woman has had [23]
group health plan insurance coverage offered through an employer or union [2]
gustatory the sense of taste [17]
Gustilo classification system a system that classifies open fractures into three major categories depending on the method of injury, soft tissue damage, and degree of skeletal involvement [13]

H

H. pylori *Helicobacter pylori*
hallucination a false visual, auditory, olfactory, or tactile perception [18]
hallux valgus bunion [28]
HbA1c a blood test that measures the glucose attached to hemoglobin [10]
Health Care Common Procedure Coding System (HCPCS) the HIPAA-mandated code set for supplies, items, and services not included in CPT [1]
Health Information Technology for Economic and Clinical Health Act (HITECH) an act that provides the financial incentives for providers who adopt EHR systems and demonstrate how the use of an EHR can improve quality, safety, and effectiveness of care [30]
Health Insurance Portability and Accountability Act (HIPAA) a federal law passed in 1996 that has numerous provisions relating to consumer health insurance and electronic health transactions [1]
healthcare administrators individuals in each healthcare organization responsible for managing the organization [3]
hearing loss—conductive a hearing loss due to abnormal formation of the external or middle ear [20]
hearing loss—sensorineural a hearing loss due to abnormal formation of the cochlea or cochlear nerve [20]
heartburn burning chest pain [9]
Helicobacter pylori (H. pylori) a bacteria that causes gastrointestinal ulcers [9]
HELLP syndrome a severe form of preeclampsia with hemolysis, elevated liver enzymes, and low platelet count [23]
helminth see parasite [21]
hematuria blood in the urine [22]
hemic system the method to transport and pass nutrients, oxygen, carbon dioxide, water, proteins, and hormones to cells and transport waste products to excretory oxygen; also called blood [15]
hemiplegia the paralysis of one side of the body [17]
hemodialysis (HD) a method for removing waste from the blood in which blood is processed through a machine when the kidneys cease to function [22]
hemoglobin (Hb) the oxygen-carrying component of erythrocytes [15]
hemolytic anemia an anemia that is due to excessive loss of erythrocytes [15]
hemolytic disease of the newborn (HDN) see erythroblastosis fetalis [24]
hemophilia a genetic disorder in which blood takes too long to clot [15]
hemostasis the stopping of bleeding or hemorrhage [15]
hepatitis inflammation of the liver due to viruses named A, B, or C [9]
hernia protrusion of an organ through a weakened area in a muscle [9]
herpes the shingles virus [21]
herpes zoster a painful, blistering skin rash due to the varicella-zoster virus that causes chickenpox; also causes shingles [21]
hiatal hernia protrusion of the stomach through a weakened area in the diaphragm [9]
high birth weight (HBW) birth weight greater than 4,000 grams (8 pounds, 13 ounces) [24]
HIPAA Health Insurance Portability and Accountability Act [1]
histology a classification of neoplasms that is based on the type of tissue [5]
History (of) a Z code category used for personal history codes to explain a patient's past medical condition that no longer exists and is not receiving any treatment, but that has the potential for recurrence [7]
history of the present illness (HPI) an interview of the patient regarding symptoms related to the chief complaint and how the problem has progressed [2]
HIV human immunodeficiency virus
Holter monitor a cardiac function test that involves a portable ECG worn by the patient for an extended period of hours or days to measure heart activity in a variety of situations [14]
homeostasis the maintenance of a stable internal physical state [17]
hordeolum a bacterial inflammation of a sebaceous gland on the edge or lining of the eyelid; also called a stye [19]
hormones chemical messengers that regulate many body functions including growth, development, metabolism, sexual function, reproduction, and mood [10]
hospital acquired condition (HAC) a serious condition that develops after admission [16]
HPV human papilloma virus, which causes cervical cancer [21]
human immunodeficiency virus (HIV) a virus that infects and destroys helper T cells of the immune system and causes AIDS [21]
human papilloma virus (HPV) a virus that causes cervical cancer [21]
Huntington's chorea an inherited progressive, degenerative disease involving loss of muscle control and personality changes [17]
hydrocele a bulge of fluid [25]
hydrocephalus an excess of cerebrospinal fluid trapped in the brain [17]
hydronephrosis the distention of the renal pelvis due to excessive urine collection in the kidney [22]
hyperbaric oxygen therapy (HBOT) provision of 100% oxygen under increased atmospheric pressure [29]
hyperbilirubinemia a high level of bilirubin in the blood, which causes the infant's skin and sclera to turn yellow [24]
hypercapnia a high carbon dioxide level [16]
hyperglycemia a severely elevated blood sugar level due to a lack or deficiency of insulin [10]
hyperosmolarity hyperglycemic nonketotic syndrome (HHNS) an elevated glucose level without ketoacidosis, usually occuring in elderly type 2 diabetics with other conditions [10]
hypertension (HTN) an abnormally high arterial blood pressure [14]
hyperthyroidism an inappropriately elevated thyroid function [10]
hypogammaglobulinemia a deficiency of gamma globulins and antibodies in the blood [15]

hypoglycemia an abnormally low blood sugar level often due to excessive use of insulin or other glucose-lowering medications [10]
hypospadias a congenital condition in which the opening of the urethra is on the underside, rather than the end of the penile shaft, and may be located as far down as the scrotum or perineum [25]
hypothyroidism a deficiency of thyroid hormone, usually due to lack of production by the thyroid or inadequate secretion of hormones by the pituitary gland or hypothalamus [10]
hypoxemia a low level of oxygen [16]

I

ICD-10-PCS Coding Guidelines a section of the ICD-10-PCS manual that consists of conventions and provides the official rules to be used when coding from ICD-10-PCS [26]
ICD-9-CM Procedure Codes a HIPAA-mandated code set for hospital inpatient procedure coding, effective until September 30, 2013 [1]
idiopathic of unknown cause [17]
ileoanal anastomosis procedure in which the surgeon removes the colon and attaches the ileum to the inside of the rectum allowing for normal passage of waste [9]
ileum small intestine [9]
ileus a condition in which the bowel does not work correctly but there is no structural problem [9] [13]
ilium the pelvic bone [12]
impairment the degree to which an individual's normal abilities are limited [18]
implantable cardioverter-defibrillator a small electronic device that is implanted in the chest to correct arrhythmia by speeding up, slowing down, smoothing out, or coordinating the heart; also called a pacemaker [14]
impotence see erectile dysfunction (ED) [22]
impression an effect produced on the mind by outside stimuli [6]
impulse-control disorder an extreme difficulty in controlling impulses, despite the negative consequences [18]
in a preposition physicians use to indicate that one condition is caused by or is a manifestation of another condition [10] [23]
inconclusive HIV a test result that means the antibody test was neither positive nor negative; also called indeterminate HIV [21]
incontinence the inability to control the bladder muscles [22]
incubator a medical device that allows a newborn to be in an environment where the temperature, humidity, and oxygen concentration can be controlled [24]
incus the anvil-shaped bone in the middle ear that receives vibrations from the malleus and transmits them to the stapes [20]
indeterminate HIV see inconclusive HIV [21]
Index an alphabetical list of diseases and injuries, reasons for encounters, and external causes, which coders must always reference when searching for a code [4]
individual health insurance a health insurance plan that people purchase directly from a health insurance company [2]
infant of diabetic mother (IDM) an infant born to a woman who is diabetic [24]
infection inflammation due to an infectious agent [12]
inferior vena cava one of the largest veins that carry deoxygenated blood back to the right ventricle [14]
inflammatory bowel disease (IBD) a group of disorders in which the intestines become red and swollen, probably as a result of an immune reaction of the body against its own intestinal tissue; includes Crohn's disease and ulcerative colitis [9]
inguinal hernia protrusion of the colon through a weakened area in a groin muscle [9]
initial encounter in ICD-10-CM, an encounter in which an injury or illness receives active treatment [4]
inner ear see labyrinth [20]
Inoculations and Vaccinations a Z code category used for encounters for prophylactic inoculations and vaccinations against a disease [7]
inpatient encounters physician interactions with patients who have been formally admitted to a healthcare facility [1]
INR international normalized ratio, a test that measures the time it takes blood to clot and compares it to an average [14]
insertion the point where the muscle attaches to a bone that moves [12]
instructional note an official coding direction in the ICD-10-CM manual, which coders are required to follow in order to abstract, assign, and sequence codes accurately [4]
insulin a hormone made by the pancreas that controls the level of sugar glucose in the blood [10]
insulin pump a small implantable device that dispenses small doses of rapid-acting insulin [10]
integral a routine finding, symptom, or sign [6]
integumentary pertaining to a covering [11]
intellectual disability the modern term for mental retardation [18]
intent the purpose of an injury: accidental, assault, legal intervention or military operation, medical procedure, or self-harm [8]
internal job a job within the same organization where the employee currently works [1]
internal mammary artery (IMA) the blood vessel located on the inside of the chest cavity, which is resistant to cholesterol buildup; often used in a coronary artery bypass graft [14]
internal radiotherapy treatment that uses radioactive pellets or containers within a body cavity to target the malignant area [5]
International Classification of Diseases, 10th Revision (ICD-10) a worldwide reporting system developed by the World Health Organization (WHO) for classifying epidemiological and mortality data [3]
International Classification of Diseases, 10th Revision, Clinical Modification (ICD-10-CM) a HIPAA-mandated code set for diagnosis coding, effective October 1, 2013 [1]
International Classification of Diseases, 10th Revision, Procedure Classification System (ICD-10-PCS) a HIPAA-mandated code set for hospital inpatient procedure coding, effective October 1, 2013 [1]
International Classification of Diseases, 9th Revision, Clinical Modification (ICD-9-CM) a HIPAA-mandated code set for diagnosis coding, effective until September 30, 2013 [1]
intestinal obstruction a physical blockage of the intestine that prevents waste from passing through [9]
intoxication a state in which a person has consumed more of a substance than they can physically tolerate, resulting in behavioral or physical abnormalities [18]
intractable migraine a migraine that is resistant to treatment; also be called pharmacoresistant [17]
intrauterine growth restriction (IUGR) the poor growth of a baby while in the mother's womb during pregnancy [24]
intraventricular hemorrhage (IVH) bleeding in the brain in very low birth weight premature babies, which usually resolves within a few days [24]
intrinsic asthma that is not due to allergens; also called non-atopic [16]
in utero within the uterus [25]
in vitro fertilization (IVF) the fertilization of an ova in a laboratory dish, followed by introduction into the uterus
involuntary muscle a muscle controlled by a subconscious part of the brain [12]
iron deficiency anemia an anemia due to insufficient iron to manufacture hemoglobin [15]
irritable bowel syndrome (IBS) a combination of symptoms such as cramping, abdominal pain, bloating, constipation, diarrhea [9]
ischemia see arteriosclerotic heart disease [14]
IV intravenous

J

jaundice a condition due to high bilirubin that causes the skin and parts of the eyes to turn a yellow color [24]
joint the place where two or more bones meet [12]

K

keratin the horny tissues found in the epidermis, hair, and nails [19]
keratitis the inflammation and ulceration of the surface of the cornea [19]

keratosis an overgrowth of horny tissue [11]
kidney the part of the urinary system that produces urine and regulates the level of electrolytes and body fluid [22]
kleptomania the urge to steal items that a person generally does not need, and usually has little value to them [18]
knife a non-disposable cutting instrument consisting of a handle and permanently attached blade [28]

L

labia major the folds of flesh that surround and protect the opening to the vagina [22]
labia minor the fold of flesh that surrounds and protects the urethra [22]
laboratory a department or organization that analyzes biological specimens [1]
labyrinth a fluid-filled cavity in the temporal bone that contains the cochlea; also called the inner ear [20]
labyrinthitis a viral or bacterial inflammation or infection of the semi-circular canals of the inner ear [20]
laceration a torn or jagged wound [13]
LAD left anterior descending coronary artery [14]
large for gestational age (LGA) a fetus or newborn infant who is larger in size than normal for the baby's sex and gestational age [24]
laryngitis irritated vocal cords that affect the upper respiratory tract [16]
larynx the voice box [16]
laser destruction using heat and power from an intense beam of radiation created from light [28]
last menstrual period (LMP) the last menstrual period that a woman has before becoming pregnant, which is used to determine the estimated date of delivery (EDD) [23]
late effect problem after the active healing is completed (sequela) [4]
late onset AD Alzheimer Disease that is diagnosed after age 65 [17]
left anterior descending coronary artery (LAD) the artery that travels down the anterior portion of the heart, positioned between the right and left ventricles [14]
left atrium the upper left chamber of the heart, which receives blood from the lungs [14]
left ventricle the lower left chamber of the hears, which ejects blood to the body [14]
lens the clear part of the front of the eye that focuses light rays on the retina [19]
leprosy a chronic bacterial disease characterized by the formation of nodules on the surface of the body [21]
leukemia a malignant disease of the blood forming organs, which does not produce tumors [5]
leukocyte a white blood cell (WBC) [15]
Lewy body disease a condition in which patients have abnormal protein structures in certain areas of the brain [18]
lichen an eruption of flat papules [11]
ligament the fibrous tissue that connect bones to bones [12]
LLQ left lower quadrant
lobar pneumonia bacterial pneumonia that primarily affects one lobe of the lung [16]
lobes the segments of the lungs [16]
lobular breast cancer a breast cancer that starts in the lobules that produce milk [22]
lobular pneumonia pneumonia that primarily affects the bronchi and lobules (clusters of alveoli that surround each bronchial branch); also called bronchopneumonia [16]
localized disease a disease that primarily affects a single organ or body system [21]
localized seizure see focal seizure [17]
Lou Gehrig disease see amyotrophic lateral sclerosis (ALS) [17]
low birth weight (LBW) a birth weight less than 2,500 grams (5 pounds, 8 ounces) [24]
lower GI series see barium enema [9]
lower respiratory tract a part of the respiratory system that consists of the trachea, bronchi, and lungs [16]
lower urinary tract symptoms (LUTS) a nonspecific term referring to symptoms related to urine storage and voiding disturbances [22]
lumen passageway [28]
lung a respiratory organ composed of the spongy tissue that receives deoxygenated blood from the heart through the pulmonary artery, re-oxygenates it, and sends it back to the heart through the pulmonary vein [16]
LUTS lower urinary tract symptoms
LUQ left upper quadrant

M

macular degeneration the gradual loss of central vision due to aging, with no cure [19]
magnetic resonance cholangiopancreatography (MRCP) use of MRI to examine liver, gallbladder, bile ducts, pancreas, and pancreatic duct [9]
Main Term the primary index entry [4]
malaria an acute or chronic disease caused by parasites and characterized by high fevers, shaking chills, flu-like symptoms, and anemia [21]
male factor infertility a problem in the male genital system that diminishes reproduction [21]
malformation a permanent abnormal shape of an organ or body region, resulting from arrested, delayed, or abnormal development of the embryo [24]
malignant life threatening [5]
malignant neoplasm life-threatening tumor commonly referred to as cancer [5]
malleus the hammer shaped bone in the middle ear that transmits vibrations to the incus [20]
malposition of fetus any presentation of the fetus other than occipitoanterior (OA) [23]
malunion a condition in which the end of a fractured bone segment did not heal with proper alignment [12]
managed care companies that attempt to control the cost of healthcare while providing better outcomes through contracts with providers and health insurance companies [2]
manifestation signs and symptoms [4]
manometry a test to measure the pressure of a valve [9]
manual review analysis of an insurance claim in which the claim is suspended from an automatic process and processed by a claims analyst [2]
manual traction a procedure in which a physical therapist uses his/her hands to hold or stretch a body part [29]
march fracture see stress fracture [12]
Marfan syndrome a genetic disorder of connective tissue characterized by elongated bones, ocular, and circulatory defects [25]
mastalgia a pain in the breast [23]
mastitis the inflammation of the breast [23]
mastoid process the portion of the temporal bone of the skull that juts forward behind the ear [20]
mastoiditis a serious infection of the mastoid process that carries the risk of infecting the brain [20]
MDRO multiple drug resistant organism [21]
meaningful use evidence from providers that they are using certified EHR technology in ways that can be measured [30]
mechanical traction a procedure in which equipment is used to apply a pulling force on a body part [29]
Meckel's diverticulum a congenital bulge in the intestine caused by a remnant of the embryonic yolk stalk [25]
meconium aspiration syndrome (MAS) a condition in which the newborn breathes a mixture of meconium and amniotic fluid into the lungs prior to or during delivery [24]
meconium peritonitis an infection of the peritoneal cavity due to perforation of the bowel and leakage of meconium [24]
Medicaid (MCD) a healthcare payment program for low income families that is funded two-thirds by the federal government and one-third by state governments [2]
medical necessity establishing the medical need for services [2]
medical payment coverage included in automobile insurance that pays for medical expenses incurred during an automobile accident [2]
medical record the comprehensive collection of all information on a patient at a particular facility [2]
medical review a department in the insurance company in that a nurse, physician, or other clinician investigates the claim for medical necessity [2]

Medicare (MCR) a federal government program that pays for healthcare services for most people age 65 and over or people of any age with end stage renal disease (ESRD) [2]

Medicare Administrative Carriers (MAC) private companies that process Medicare Part A and Part B claims [2]

Medicare Advantage Part C Medicare [2]

Medigap Medicare supplement insurance policy sold by private insurance companies to fill "gaps" in Part A and Part B coverage [2]

melanoma a tumor of melanocytes [11]

Meniere's disease an abnormality of the fluid of the inner ear that can lead to a progressive hearing loss [20]

meningitis a contagious, acute inflammation of the pia matter and the arachnoid mater in the brain [17]

menorrhea menstrual flow [6]

mental disorder a psychological or physical condition that disrupts an individual's personality, mind, and emotions in such a way that they affect the ability to function and interact with others [18]

metabolism the processes of digestion, elimination, breathing, blood circulation, and maintaining body temperature [10]

metastasize the action of neoplasms to spread and invade organs [5]

metastatic bone disease (MBD) the invasion of the bone by cancer that begins in another organ [12]

methicillin susceptible Staphylococcus aureus (MSSA) a type of staph bacteria that responds to commonly used antibiotics [21]

methicillin-resistant Staphylococcus aureus infection (MRSA) a type of staph bacteria that does not respond to commonly used antibiotics [21]

MI myocardial infarction [14]

microincision a tiny cut into the skin [28]

middle ear a small air-filled cavity in the temporal bone that contains the ossicles [20]

mid-level job a job obtained after two or three years of experience [1]

migraine headache a severe, debilitating headache caused by vasodilation [17]

misadventure an error during a medical or surgical procedure [8]

Miscellaneous a Z code category used for additional codes that provide useful information on circumstances that may affect a patient's care and treatment [7]

mitral valve prolapse (MVP) a disorder in which the two leaflets that comprise the valve fall backward into the left atrium, which results in regurgitation; also called click murmur syndrome or Barlow's syndrome [14]

mitral valve the valve that controls the blood flow from the left atrium to the left ventricle [14]

MMR measles, mumps, and rubella vaccine

modifier a word or words in a diagnostic statement that limit the meaning of another; also called a qualifier [6]

monoamniotic multiple fetuses sharing the same amnion [23]

monochorionic multiple fetuses sharing the same chorion [23]

monochorionic-diamniotic (MoDi) two embryos sharing the same chorion and placenta but with separate amnions [23]

monochorionic-monoamniotic (MoMo) multiple embryos sharing the same chorion, amnion, and placenta [23]

mononucleosis a viral infection causing fever, sore throat, and swollen lymph glands [21]

monoplegia the paralysis of one limb [17]

mood disorder an instability of mood; also called affective disorder [18]

morbidity causes of disease and illness [3]

MRSA methicillin-resistant *Staphylococcus aureus* [21]

MS musculoskeletal [12]

MSSA methicillin-susceptible *Staphylococcus aureus* [21]

mucoid pertaining to a sticky fluid secreted by the mucous membrane [20]

mucosa mucous membrane [28]

multiaxial nature a PCS characteristic meaning that each character of the code has a designated meaning or purpose [26]

multiple coding assigning more than one code to fully describe a condition [4]

multiple drug resistant organism (MDRO) a bacteria that survives exposure to many different antibiotics [21]

multiple gestation a pregnancy that involves more than one fetus [23]

multiple sclerosis a chronic, progressive disorder of the CNS characterized by muscle impairment due to patches of hardened tissue in the brain or spinal cord [17]

muscular system provides for movement of the body as well as the operation of individual organs, maintenance of body posture, and production of heat [12]

musculoskeletal (MS) system the skeletal and muscular systems of the body that support the body, protect internal organs, produce blood cells, store minerals, provide movement to the body, maintain body posture, and production of heat [12]

myalgia a muscle pain [12]

myasthenia a weakness in the muscle [12]

myocardial infarction (MI) is the death of heart tissue caused by an interruption to the blood supply; commonly known as a heart attack [14]

myocardium the thick muscular inner layers that contract to pump blood [14]

myoclonic seizure a seizure characterized by jerking and twitching of the upper body, arms, or legs [17]

myosarcoma a malignant tumor in the muscle [12]

myositis inflammation of a muscle [12]

N

Na sodium

narcolepsy a condition characterized by brief sudden attacks of deep sleep [17]

nasogastric nose to stomach [9]

National Center for Health Statistics (NCHS) the organization that adapted ICD-10 for use in the United States [3]

National Drug Codes (NDC) a HIPAA-mandated code set that identifies the manufacturer, product, and package size of all drugs and biologics recognized by the Food and Drug Administration (FDA) [1]

native vessel the patient's original blood vessel [14]

natural language programming (NLP) artificial intelligence that extracts pertinent data and terms from a text-based document, analyzes them, and converts them into the most likely applicable codes [30]

NCPDP National Council for Prescription Drug Programs [3]

neck of a long bone the area between the proximal epiphysis and the shaft [12]

needle aspiration using a needle to suction tissue or fluid from the body [28]

neonatal intensive care unit (NICU) a section of the hospital that treats newborns with serious conditions [24]

neonatal mortality the death of a newborn before 28 days of age [24]

neonate an infant during the first 28 days of life; also called a newborn [24]

neoplasm abnormal growth of new tissue [5]

neoplastic fracture a fragility fracture due to a neoplastic disease [12]

nephritic syndrome a collection of disorders affecting the kidneys characterized by nonpurulent inflammatory glomerular disorders that allow proteins and red blood cells to pass into the urine [22]

nephrons the functioning part of each kidney that filters waste from the blood [22]

nephropathy a disease of the kidneys [10]

nephroptosis the downward placement of the kidney from its normal location [22]

nephrotic syndrome a collection of disorders affecting the kidneys, characterized by proteinuria, but not hematuria [22]

nervous system the body system that directs the body's response to internal and external stimuli and coordinates the activities of other organ systems [17]

networking building professional relationships with others [1]

neurodevelopmental disorder a condition that results from impaired development of the nervous system during infancy or childhood [17]

neuron a cluster of nerve cells [17]

neuropathy a disease of the nerves [10]

neutropenia a decrease in neutrophils [15]

newborn see neonate [24]

newborn ABO incompatibility an infant with blood type A or B affected by comingling of blood from a mother with blood type O [24]

newborn apnea a condition in which the infant stops breathing [24]

newborn birth status a code that identifies the location of the birth, the delivery method, and the number of multiples [24]

newborn clinically significant condition a condition of newborns that requires clinical evaluation, therapeutic treatment, diagnostic procedures, extended length of hospital stay (LOS), increase in nursing care or monitoring, or presents implications for future healthcare needs [24]

newborn Rh incompatibility an Rh positive infant affected by comingling of blood with an Rh negative mother [24]

Newborns and Infants a Z code category used for health supervision and care of foundling, routine child health examination, and classification of birth status of liveborn infants [7]

non-atopic asthma see intrinsic asthma [16]

nonautologous a grafted vessel from a source other than the patient, such as a cadaver or animal [14]

nonbiological a grafted vessel from a synthetic source [14]

nondisplaced a traumatic fracture in which the fragments of bone remain properly aligned [13]

nonessential modifiers the words in parentheses after a Main Term or subterm, which are included in the default description of the code and do not need to be present in the medical record in order to use the code [4]

non-excisional debridement removing contaminated or dead tissue without cutting, such as with a curet or brush [28]

Non-specific a Z code category used in an outpatient setting when there is no further documentation to permit more precise coding [7]

non-ST elevation MI (NSTEMI) a myocardial infarction in which the ST segment on an EKG is not elevated, indicating that a vessel is only partially blocked [14]

non-toxic goiter an enlargement of the thyroid that is not associated with overproduction of thyroid hormone or malignancy [10]

nontransmural infarction see subendocardial infarction [14]

nontraumatic not due to an accident or injury [28]

nonunion the failure of the ends of the fractured bone segments to reunite [12]

normal birth weight a birth weight of 2,500 grams (5 pounds, 8 ounces) to 4,200 grams (9 pounds, 4 ounces) [24]

normal spontaneous vaginal birth (NSVB) a vaginal delivery without mechanical, pharmacologic, or medical assistance [23]

nosocomial any hospital-acquired infection [21]

novel influenza A a class of viruses that normally circulate in animals and may infect humans, such as avian flu and H1N1[21]

NSTEMI non-ST elevation myocardial infarction [14]

NSVB normal spontaneous vaginal birth [23]

NSVD normal spontaneous vaginal delivery [23]

nuchal cord the condition of the umbilical cord becoming wrapped around the neck of the fetus [23]

nutritional anemia an anemia that is due to malabsorption or poor dietary intake [15]

O

O_2 oxygen

Observation extended monitoring, which may require an overnight stay but does not meet the requirements for a formal inpatient admission [1]; a Z code category used for a person who is being observed for a suspected condition that is ruled out [7]

obstructed labor a labor in which the fetus cannot progress into the birth canal, despite adequate uterine contractions, due to a physical blockage [23]

occipitoanterior (OA) the presentation of the fetus in which the back of the baby's head is slightly off center in the pelvis with the back of the head towards the mother's left thigh [23]

occlusion a blockage [14]

ocular globe the eyeball [19]

Office of the Inspector General (OIG) a division of the Department of Health and Human Services (HHS) that investigates fraud, abuse, and other noncompliance matters in the Medicare and Medicaid programs [2]

old MI a myocardial infarction that is more than four weeks old [14]

olfactory the sense of smell [17]

omphalitis an infection of the umbilical stump in a newborn, usually presenting as superficial cellulitis [24]

oncologist physician who specializes in the diagnosis and treatment of tumors [5]

Open a PCS value for the Approach in which an incision is made through the skin and subcutaneous tissue [27]

open fracture a fracture in which the bone breaks through the skin [13]

open wound a wound in which the underlying tissue is exposed to the air [13]

operative report a description of the surgical procedure done by the physician that is completed after the procedure [28]

opportunistic infection a disease that attacks those with weakened immune systems but does not develop in those with healthy immune systems [21]

optic nerve see cranial nerve II [19]

orbital cavity the bony structure that is around the eye; commonly known as the eye socket [19]

origin the point at which the muscle is attached [12]

Original Medicare Part A Medicare [2]

orotracheal intubation the placement of a tube through the mouth into the respiratory or gastrointestinal tract [24]

osseous pertaining to a bone [12]

ossicles a part of the middle ear that amplifies vibrations and transmits them to the inner ear [20]

osteoarthritis an inflammation of a bone and joint [12]

osteoporosis the thinning of bone tissue and loss of bone density [12]

osteoporosis fracture a fragility fracture in a person with osteoporosis [12]

osteosarcoma a malignant tumor in the bone [12]

ostomy an artificial opening between a hollow organ and the skin [7]

OTC over the counter; a medication patients can purchase without a prescription [4]

otitis externa an inflammation of the external ear (pinna) [20]

otitis media (OM) an infection of the middle ear [20]

otitis media (OM)-nonsuppurative an inflammation of the middle ear that does not produce pus [20]

otitis media (OM)-serous a subtype of nonsuppurative otitis media involving clear fluid in the middle ear [20]

otitis media (OM)-suppurative an infection of the middle ear, usually bacterial, involving the discharge of pus; also called purulent otitis media [20]

otosclerosis a loss of mobility of the stapes bone [20]

outpatient encounter an interaction with a patient who has not been formally admitted to a healthcare institution [1]

oval window a thin membrane that covers the opening to the inner ear and passes vibrations to the cochlea [20]

ovary the gland in which eggs are produced in females [22]

overcoding coding for a more complex diagnosis or procedure than is documented [2]

overlapping lesion contiguous site where a tumor continues from one site to the adjacent one without interruption [5]

P

P pulse; see also para and TPAL

P. aeruginosa *Pseudomonas aeruginosa*

pacemaker a small electronic device that is implanted in the chest to correct arrhythmia; also called an implantable cardioverter-defibrillator [14]

pancreatitis inflammation of the pancreas [9]

pancytopenia an abnormal reduction in the number of all types of blood cells: red, white, and platelets [15]

pandemic a disease outbreak that spreads to multiple continents [21]

PAP a diagnostic procedure that screens for precancerous cervical dysplasia and cervical cancer [22]

papule a firm bump [11]

para (P) the number of pregnancies resulting in a fetus of viable gestational age (20 weeks) regardless of whether the fetus was alive at birth [23]

paracentesis a procedure to take out the fluid that has collected in a body cavity, most commonly the peritoneal cavity in the abdomen [5]

paranoia a mental condition of delusions of persecution [18]

parasite a plant or animal that lives in or on another living organism, or host, and often causes damage to the host; also called helminth [21]
parietal pericardium the outer layer of the pericardium [14]
Parkinson's disease (PD) a degenerative disease that affects muscle control and coordination [17]
Parkinsonian see Parkinsonism [17]
Parkinsonism a combination of conditions in which dementia is diagnosed at first, followed at a later time with an additional diagnosis of Parkinson's disease; also called Parkinsonian dementia [17]
Part A Medicare hospital insurance that covers a specific list of services for inpatient hospital care, skilled nursing facilities, hospice, and home healthcare; also called Original Medicare [2]
Part B Medicare coverage for a specific list of physician services, outpatient hospital care, and home healthcare; also known as supplemental medical insurance (SMI) [2]
Part C an optional replacement of Part A and Part B, which is offered by private health insurance companies [2]
Part D Medicare prescription drug coverage [2]
partial code the first three to five characters of the PCS code [26]
partial seizure see focal seizure [17]
parturition see childbirth [23]
patch testing a test in which an allergen is applied to the skin to observe the reaction [11]
patent foramen ovale an opening in the septum between the two atria of the heart [25]
pathologic fracture a fracture that is caused by a disease rather than trauma; also called a fragility fracture [12]
pathologist a physician who identifies diseases by studying cells under a microscope [5]
past medical history (PMH) a review of the patient's past conditions, which may or may not be resolved, and past surgical procedures; also includes any current problems that are not included in the reason for the encounter or referral [30]
payers insurance companies or public programs that pay for healthcare services [1]
PCP primary care physician
PCS Procedure Coding System; used in this text as shorthand for ICD-10-PCS [3]
pelvic girdle pain (PGP) a pain at the back of the pelvis [23]
pelvic inflammatory disease (PID) inflammation of the female reproductive tract above the cervix [21]
pemphigus an autoimmune disease that erupts in blisters [11]
penetrating wound see puncture wound [13]
penis the external male organ that carries urine and semen out of the body [22]
perceptual disturbance a misinterpretation of surroundings or events [18]
Percutaneous a PCS value for the Approach that identifies a procedure in which the skin is punctured or a small incision is made to access the site, but a full depth incision is not made [27]
Percutaneous Endoscopic a PCS value for the Approach that identifies a procedure in which a surgeon makes several, usually two to four, incisions so a fiber optic camera can be inserted through one incision and surgical instruments can be inserted into the other openings [27]
perforation the cutting or puncturing of the wall or membrane of an internal organ or structure [13]
pericarditis an inflammation of the pericardial sac that surrounds the heart [14]
pericardium a double-walled sac filled with fluid, which is the outer layer [14]
perinatal condition a condition that develops before birth or in the first 28 days after birth, but excludes malformations, deformations, and chromosomal abnormalities [24]
perinatal period the time before birth and continues through the twenty-eighth day following birth [24]
peripartum the period that is the last month of pregnancy to five months postpartum [23]
peripheral artery disease (PAD) the damage to arteries outside the heart resulting in decreased blood flow to the limbs [10] [14]
peripheral nervous system (PNS) consists of the 12 nerves that radiate out from the brain and the 31 pairs of nerves that radiate from the spinal cord to all other areas of the body [17]
peritoneal dialysis (PD) a type of dialysis in which the peritoneal membrane is used to filter the blood [22]
peritoneal membrane the lining of the abdomen [22]
pernicious anemia an anemia due to insufficient absorption of Vitamin B12 [15]
personal history a condition the patient had in the past, was resolved, and is no longer being treated, but has the potential for recurrence, and therefore may require continued monitoring [5]
personal injury protection (PIP) coverage included in automobile insurance that pays for medical expenses incurred during an automobile accident [2]
personality disorder a persistent inflexible patterns of behavior that affects interpersonal relationships [18]
petit mal seizure a seizure characterized by muscle twitching or jerking for several seconds; also called an absence seizure [17]
phacoemulsification use of ultrasonic vibrations to fragment the lens of the eye and suction it out [28]
phalanx one bony segment of a finger [28]
pharmacoresistant resistant to medication [17]
pharyngitis a sore throat [16]
pharynx the throat [16]
physical examination (PE) a hands-on evaluation of a patient's vital signs, physical functions, and organ systems relevant to the chief complaint; physician's examination and factual findings, results of tests performed or reviewed [2] [30]
physical therapy non-invasive treatments to correct a musculoskeletal problem [1]
physician office an outpatient clinic at which physicians evaluate and manage new or existing health problems and provide preventive care services [1]
physis the growth plate near end of a long bone [13]
pinna the visible part of the ear that collects sound waves; also called auricle [20]
pityriasis a rough, dry scale [11]
place the location where the event occurred [8]
placenta the organ that allows for the exchange of oxygen, nutrients, and waste between the fetus and mother [23]
placenta previa a condition in which the placenta partially or fully covers the cervix [23]
placental infarction a scarring of the placenta due to an inadequate blood supply [23]
plan planned treatments, prescriptions, patient instructions, and recommended treatments [30]
plaque a semi-hardened accumulation of substances from fluids [14]
plasma a clear fluid [15]
pleural effusion an abnormal amount of fluid found around the lung [16]
pneumothorax air in the chest [16]
poisoning the improper use of a medication that causes an undesired physical response [13]
polycystic kidney disease a condition in which numerous cysts occupy much of the kidney tissue [22]
polycythemia an abnormal increase in the number of circulating red blood cells [15]
polydactyly the presence of many fingers or toes [25]
polynephritis see pyelonephritis [22]
portal hypertension increase in blood pressure in the portal vein [9]
postpartum see puerperium [23]
postpartum depression a moderate to severe depression after giving birth [23]
postpartum hemorrhage (PPH) an excessive amount of bleeding following delivery [23]
postpartum psychosis a sudden dramatic onset of psychotic symptoms after giving birth, often occurring in patients with bipolar disorder [23]
postpartum wound infection a bacterial infection of a cesarean section wound [23]
postterm pregnancy a pregnancy with between 40 and 42 completed weeks of gestation [23]
Prader-Willi syndrome a genetic disorder due to a deletion of paternal chromosome 15 characterized by short stature, mental retardation, muscle weakness, abnormally small hands and feet, non-functioning

gonads, and uncontrolled appetite leading to extreme obesity [25]

precerebral located outside of the brain [14]

prediabetes blood glucose levels are higher than normal but not yet high enough to be diagnosed as diabetes [10]

preeclampsia a metabolic disorder of pregnancy, which develops after the twentieth week, that involves gestational hypertension and proteinuria [23]

preexisting diabetes diabetes that is diagnosed in a woman before she becomes pregnant [23]

preexisting hypertension hypertension that is diagnosed in a woman before she becomes pregnant [23]

preferred providers an exclusive network of providers, which patients are encouraged to use through lower out-of-pocket costs for deductibles, coinsurance, and copayments [2]

pregnancy a normal, temporary condition that occurs in the female body, which begins at the time of conception and ends with the birth of the fetus [23]

pregnancy induced hypertension (PIH) see gestational hypertension [23]

premature rupture of membranes (PROM) the rupture of the amniotic sac and chorion more than an hour before the onset of labor [23]

prenatal the time period from conception to the beginning of labor; also called prepartum, antepartum, or antenatal period [23]

prepartum see prenatal [23]

preterm pregnancy, delivery, or labor a pregnancy with less than 37 completed weeks of gestation [23]

prevalence the percentage of a population affected with a disease at a point in time [21]

primary neoplasm a tumor in which malignant cells break through the epithelial membrane into the organ [5]

principal diagnosis the condition established after study to be chiefly responsible for occasioning the admission of the patient to the hospital for care [4]

principal procedure a procedure that is performed for definitive treatment, rather than one performed for diagnostic or exploratory purposes, or was necessary to take care of a complication [26]

private health insurance coverage for healthcare services offered by private corporations [2]

PRN as needed; abbreviation for the Latin phrase *pro re nata* [4]

procedure a service healthcare professionals provide to patients [1]

procedure report a description of a nonsurgical procedure done by the physician that is completed after the procedure [28]

productive cough a cough with sputum [16]

products of conception the embryo or fetus [29]

professional organization an organization that promotes a standard of skill and ethical behavior within a certain field or profession [1]

prognosis future knowledge; the expected course of the disease [5]

progress notes the record of a specific patient encounter [2]

prolonged pregnancy a pregnancy with more than 42 completed weeks of gestation [23]

prompt pay state laws that require insurance companies to process claims within a specific period of time [2]

prophylactic prevention of the spread of disease or infection [7]

prostate the part of the male genital system that secretes fluid to nourish the sperm [22]

prostate specific antigen (PSA) a blood test used to screen for prostate cancer [22]

prostatic intraepithelial neoplasia (PIN) neoplastic changes in the epithelial cells of the prostate ducts showing some features of cancer, but not invasive [21]

protection a function of the integumentary system that helps prevent invasion by pathogens, mechanical harm, and loss of fluids and electrolytes [11]

protein fraction a deficiency of gamma globulins [15]

proteinemia protein in the blood [10]

proteinuria protein in the urine [10]

protozoa a one-celled being that is more complex than bacteria and uses other living things as a source of food and a place to live [21]

proximal epiphysis the rounded end of a long bone closest to the trunk [12]

Pseudomonas aeruginosa the *P. aeruginosa* bacteria [21]

psoriasis a round red patch covered with white scales [11]

psychoactive substance a substance that has the ability to alter behavior, impair judgment, or create medical problems [18]

psychomotor seizure see complex partial seizure [17]

psychotherapy a method of using non-physical techniques, such as talking, interpreting, listening, rewarding, and role playing, to treat disorders [18]

psychotic disorders delusions and hallucinations [18]

pt (lower case abbreviation) patient

PT (upper case abbreviation) physical therapy

PTBLC preterm birth live child [23]

puerperal see puerperium [23]

puerperal mastitis the inflammation or infection of the mammary gland in the breast during the postpartum period [23]

puerperium the six-week period following childbirth in which the female reproductive organs return to the prepregnant state; also called the puerperal period or postpartum period [23]

pulmonary circulation the section of the circulatory system that occurs between the heart and lungs [14]

pulmonary function test a diagnostic test that gives information regarding air flow in and out of the lungs, lung volumes, and gas exchange between the lungs and bloodstream [16]

pulmonary valve the valve that controls the blood flow from the right ventricle to the pulmonary artery [14]

puncture wound a wound caused by a sharp-pointed object passing through the skin into the underlying tissues; also called a penetrating wound [13]

pupil the black central part of the eye that opens and closes in response to light [19]

Purkinje fibers the cardiac muscles that rapidly transmit impulses from the atrioventricular node to the ventricles [14]

purpura a small hemorrhage in the skin [15]

purulent otitis media see otitis media (OM)-suppurative [20]

px procedure

pyelonephritis an acute or chronic infection of the renal medulla and upper urinary tract as a result of untreated cystitis; also called polynephritis [22]

pyogenic arthritis an infectious arthritis in which pus is formed during the disease process [12]

pyothorax pus in the chest [16]

pyromania an impulsive desire to start fires [18]

Q

quadriplegia the paralysis of all limbs [17]

qualified diagnosis a diagnosis that is limited or uncertain [6]

qualifier a word or words in a diagnostic statement that limit the meaning of another; also called a modifier [6]

Qualifier the seventh character of a PCS code that describes additional information about the procedure [26]

query to ask [1]

Qui Tam a provision in the False Claims Act that includes a financial reward to those who turn in violators [2]

R

R respiration

radiofrequency ablation low-frequency electromagnetic waves targeted at a small area [28]

reconcile comparison of the EOB to the original bill to verify that each service billed was paid in the amount expected [2]

Recovery Audit Contractor (RAC) a program authorized by the Tax Relief and Health Care Act of 2006 to identify Medicare overpayments and underpayments to healthcare providers and suppliers [2]

reflex sympathetic dystrophy (RSD) a chronic pain syndrome in which an extremity experiences intense burning pain and changes in skin texture and temperature; also called complex regional pain syndrome [17]

reflux nephropathy a disease of the kidneys that results from a backward flow of urine into the kidneys [22]

refractory resistant to treatment [17]

regulation a function of the integumentary system that raises and lowers body temperature through constriction and dilation of blood vessels and sweat glands [11]
regurgitation the backward leakage of blood through the opening of the left atrium [14]
rejected claim an insurance claim with missing or invalid data that is not accepted into the insurance company's computer system for processing [2]
relapse the return of the disease after remission [15]
related a symptom, finding, or sign that is connected to a disease, but is not integral [6]
relevant condition see clinically significant condition [4]
remission (alcohol or drug dependence) a usage pattern in which a patient has a history of past drug or alcohol dependence that has been documented by the physician [18]
remission (leukemia) a state in which the blood counts return to normal and bone marrow samples show no sign of disease [15]
renal pelvis the portion of the kidney where urine collects [22]
reproductive duct a part of the internal genital organs of the male reproductive system [22]
Resection the PCS Root Operation defined as cutting out or off, without replacement, all of a body part [28]
respiratory distress syndrome (RDS) a condition in which the alveolar sacs collapse due to lack of surfactant [24]
respiratory system the system that obtains oxygen from the air and delivers it to the lungs and blood for distribution to tissue cells and removes the gaseous waste product carbon dioxide from the blood and lungs and expels it [16]
retina the innermost layer that contains sensory receptor cells [19]
retinal detachment the separation of the retina from the choroid layer of the eye [19]
retinopathy of prematurity (ROP) the abnormal growth of blood vessels in the eye that can lead to vision loss [24]
Rhesus (Rh) incompatibility a condition in which the mother is Rh negative and develops antibodies against a fetus that is Rh positive [23]
right atrium the right upper chamber of the heart, which receives blood from the body [14]
right ventricle the right lower chamber of the heart, which ejects blood to the lungs [14]
RLQ right lower quadrant
rod a photoreceptor cell of the retina that is sensitive to dim light and used for night vision [19]
Root Operation the third character of a PCS Medical and Surgical code, which identifies the objective of the procedure [26]
rotational deformity an abnormal position of the femur or tibia [25]
Routine and Administrative Examination a Z code category used for routine examinations or administrative purposes [7]
RTO return to office [7]
Rule of Nines the division of the body into areas, each of which comprises 9% of the total body surface area [13]
ruptured tympanic membrane see tympanic membrane perforation (TMP) [20]
RUQ right upper quadrant
Rx prescription

S

saccule a membranous pouch containing serum fluid of the inner ear [20]
salpingitis the inflammation of a tube [22]
Salter-Harris classification a system that classifies epiphysis fractures in order to identify involvement of the growth plate and estimate the prognosis and potential for growth disturbance [13]
sarcoidosis a formation of nodules in the lymph nodes, lungs, bone, and skin [15]
scalpel a two-part cutting instrument consisting of a reusable handle and a disposable blade [28]
schizoaffective disorder a condition characterized by an extended period in which schizophrenia is accompanied by major depressive, manic, or mixed episodes [18]
schizoid of childhood a condition characterized by severe and sustained impairment in social interactions, and restricted, repetitive patterns of behaviors, interests, and activities; also called Asperger's Syndrome [18]
schizoid personality disorder a condition characterized by a persistent withdrawal from social relationships and lack of emotional responsiveness in most situations [18]
schizophrenia a condition characterized by the inability to distinguish between thoughts and reality, think logically, and have normal emotional and social relationships [18]
schizophreniform disorder a condition that is identical to schizophrenia except that the total duration is greater than one month but less than six months; impaired social or occupational functioning may not be present [18]
schizothymia a mild form of schizophrenia [18]
schizotypal personality disorder a condition characterized by trouble with relationships and disturbances in thought patterns, appearance, and behavior [18]
scissors a cutting instrument with two blades that bypass each other [28]
sclera the hard white outer layer of the eye [19]
sclerotherapy injection of a chemical irritant such as alcohol or talc to cause inflammation and eventual obliteration of the lumen [28]
Screening a test to detect the potential existence of a disease at an early stage in a patient who has no symptoms [5]; a Z code category used for testing for disease or disease precursors in seemingly well individuals so that early detection and treatment can be provided for those who test positive for the disease [7]
sebaceous pertaining to oil [11]
second trimester the time in a pregnancy when the gestational age is between 14 weeks, 0 days and less than 28 weeks, 0 days [23]
secondary diabetes a condition in which glucose levels are elevated due to an external factor, such as medication, surgery, pancreatic disease, or other illness [10]
secondary diagnosis any diagnosis that is not the principal or first-listed; also called additional [4]
secondary neoplasm the sites or metastases where a neoplasm spreads to [5]
secondary Parkinsonism a Parkinson-type abnormal movement that is caused by medication or another condition [17]
secondary to a preposition physicians use to indicate that one condition is caused by or is a manifestation of another condition [10]
secretion a function of the integumentary system that gives off perspiration for temperature control and sebum to protect from dehydration and penetration by harmful substances [11]
secretory pertaining to the release of fluid [20]
Section the first character of a PCS code that identifies the broad procedure category where the code is found [26]
self-insured health plans health plans offered by large employers or unions who set aside money in a reserve fund and pay for employees, medical expenses from the fund [2]
semicircular canals the superior, posterior, and inferior canals in the ear that contain endolymph [20]
sensation a function of the integumentary system that contains sensory receptors for pain, touch, heat, cold, and pressure [11]
sepsis a severe, life-threatening, system-wide reaction to infection caused by disease-causing organisms, especially bacteria, in the blood or tissues [21]
septic shock a life-threatening low blood pressure due to sepsis [21]
septicemia a systemic disease associated with the presence and persistence of bacteria, viruses, fungi or other organisms or toxins in the blood [21]
sequela a problem after the active healing is completed (late effect) [4]
sequence to place codes in the order dictated by the guidelines and instructional notes [1]
serology a blood test used to diagnose diseases [21]
seromucinous pertaining to secretions of the mucus and serous layers [20]
serum assay a lab test that measures the presence and quantity of a substance in the blood [10]

severe sepsis acute or multiple organ dysfunction (MOD) due to sepsis [21]
sexual disorders a repetitive and prolonged sexual activity and sexual dysfunction that interferes with normal relationships or daily activities [18]
shaft the long narrow part of the long bone; also called the diaphysis [12]
Shone's syndrome a set of four congenital heart defects: a supravalve mitral membrane, parachute mitral valve, subaoritc stenosis, and coarctation of the aorta [25]
sickle cell anemia a genetic disorder in which red blood cells take on a sickle shape and lead to hemolytic anemia [15]
sickle cell crisis a pain caused because blood vessels have become blocked or the defective red blood cells damage organs in the body [15]
sign objective evidence of a disease or condition, usually observed by the physician [4]
significant procedure a procedure that is surgical in nature, carries a procedural risk, carries an anesthetic risk, or requires specialized training [26]
simple partial seizure a seizure that affects only a small region of the brain and does not cause loss of consciousness [17]
singleton a pregnancy with one fetus [23]
sinoatrial (SA) node the location where the electrical impulses of the heart begin [14]
sinusitis a sinus infection [16]
site of origin a classification of neoplasms that is based on the anatomic site where the growth begins; also called topography [5]
skeletal system supports the body, protects internal organs, produces blood cells, stores minerals, and serves as a point of attachment for the skeletal muscles [12]
sleeping disorder an abnormal sleep problem [18]
small for gestational age (SGA) a fetus or newborn infant who is smaller in size than normal for the baby's sex and gestational age [24]
smallpox an infectious disease with the last known case in 1977 [21]
snare a wire loop on a handle used to encircle and cut through the base of lesions [28]
SO sudden onset
SOB shortness of breath
somatoform a physical symptom that is not explained by medical conditions [18]
spermatocele benign cystic swelling of sperm in the ducts of the epididymis [21]
sphincterotomy making a surgical cut into a circular muscle that functions as a valve [9]
spina bifida a congenital neural tube defect disorder in which vertebrae do not fuse [17]
spinal cord the body part that relays information to and from the brain [17]
sprain an overstretching, bruise, or tear of a ligament [12]
squamous cell carcinoma (SCC) cancer found in the flat squamous cells [11]
squamous intraepithelial lesion (SIL) a cervical dyplasia seen on a PAP smear, graded as low-grade (LSIL), high-grade (HSIL), and possibly cancerous or malignant [22]
ST elevation MI (STEMI) a myocardial infarction in which the ST segment of an EKG is elevated, indicating that the MI completely occludes a vessel [14]
stage 1 pressure ulcer skin redness due to prolonged pressure that does not go away [11]
stage 2 pressure ulcer skin damage to the epidermis due to prolonged pressure that extends into the dermis [11]
stage 3 pressure ulcer skin damage through the full thickness of the dermis and into the subcutaneous tissue due to prolonged pressure [11]
stage 4 pressure ulcer skin damage extending into the muscle, tendon, or bone due to prolonged pressure [11]
staging the process of determining how far a cancer has spread [5]
stain the coloring of blood cells during lab testing to better see their characteristics [15]
standardized terminology a PCS characteristic meaning the code set includes definitions of the terminology, but each term must have only one meaning [26]
stapes, stapedes the stirrup shaped bone in the middle ear that receives vibrations from the incus [20]
State Children's Health Insurance Program (SCHIP) a federal government program to provide health insurance to children in families with incomes below 200% of the federal poverty level [2]
Status a Z code category used for a patient who is either a carrier of a disease or has the sequela or residual of a past disease or condition [7]; the nature of employment at the time of an external cause of injury: civilian employment, military, volunteer, or recreational/leisure [8]
status asthmaticus an acute exacerbation that does not respond to the standard treatments of bronchodilators and steroids [16]
status epilepticus an epileptic seizure that lasts more than 30 minutes or is a near-constant state of seizures [17]
status migrainosus a migraine that lasts more than 72 hours [17]
STEMI ST elevation myocardial infarction [14]
stenosis a narrowing of a valve or vessel [14]
stent insertion the placement of a mesh tube in a blood vessel to keep it open, due to atherosclerosis [14]
steroid a type of medication used to reduce inflammation [16]
stomatitis redness, ulcers, and/or bleeding of the mouth due to bacteria, viruses, or fungi [9]
strain an overstretching, bruise, or tear of a bone or tendon [12]
stress fracture a fracture of a bone that has been subjected to repeated use or impact; also called a march fracture or fatigue fracture [12]
stress testing a cardiac function test that measure ECG and oxygen levels as a patient performs an increasing level of exercises on a treadmill or stationary bicycle [14]
stripping making tiny incisions, grasping tissue, and pulling it out [28]
structural integrity a PCS characteristic meaning the system can be expanded without disrupting the structure of the system [26]
structured input uses menus that contain clinical terms to create the narrative text within a document [30]
subcategory a level of subdivision after a category and before a code that has four or five characters [4]
subchapter in ICD-10-CM, a contiguous range of codes within a chapter that is comparable to a section in ICD-9-CM; also called a block [4]
subcutaneous under the skin [11]
subendocardial infarction the death of heart tissue that affects only a small portion of the heart wall, usually due to a decreased, but not totally occluded, blood supply; also called a nontransmural infarction [14]
subluxation the partial dislocation of bones in a joint [12]
subQ subcutaneous
subsequent encounter a healthcare encounter during the healing phase of an injury [4]
subsequent MI a MI that occurs within four weeks of a previous AMI [14]
substance disorder drug and alcohol use, abuse, and addiction [18]
subterm a word indented under each Main Term that further describes the Main Term in greater detail [4]
suction sucking out with a flexible plastic tube hooked up to a vacuum machine or system [28]
sudoriferous pertaining to sweat [11]
superficial injury an injury to the surface of the skin, such as an abrasion, blister, contusion, constriction, insect bite, or superficial foreign body [13]
superior vena cava one of the largest veins that carry deoxygenated blood back to the right ventricle [14]
supplementary medical insurance (SMI) Medicare Part B [2]
suppurative discharging pus [28]
surgical approach the description of how the surgeon accessed the operative site [27]
suspended claims that are removed from the automatic process for manual review [2]
symptom subjective evidence of a disease or condition, usually reported by the patient [4]
syndactyly the presence of webbed fingers or toes [25]
synthetic tissue that is manmade [11]
syphilis a sexually transmitted disease (STD) caused by bacteria, which produces chancres, rashes, and systemic lesions [21]

systemic affecting the entire body [21]
systemic circulation the section of the circulatory system that occurs between the heart and the rest of the body [14]
systemic inflammatory response syndrome (SIRS) an acute system-wide inflammatory reaction with at least two manifestations: fever, tachycardia, tachypnea, leukocytosis, or leukopenia [6] [21]
systole the time during the heart cycle when the chamber contracts as it ejects blood [14]

T

T temperature
T&A tonsillectomy and adenoidectomy
Table PCS reference tables or grids used to build each code [26]
Table of Drugs and Chemicals the section of the ICD-10-CM manual used to assign codes for poisoning, adverse effects, toxic effects, and underdosing [13]
Tabular List a numerical listing in ICD-10-CM of diseases and injuries, reasons for encounters, and external causes [4]
tactile the sense of touch [18]
target organ the organ receiving hormones or treatment [10]
TBLC term birth live child [23]
TBSA total body surface area [13]
tendon the fibrous tissue that connects bones to muscles [12]
tendonitis the inflammation of a tendon [12]
terrorism an event involving weapons of mass destruction or specific terrorism-related offenses [8]
testis the part of the male genital system that provides the male sex hormone, testosterone [22]
tetralogy of Fallot a congenital heart defect consisting of four malformations: pulmonary stenosis, ventricle septal defect, dextraposition or overriding aorta, and hypertrophy of the right ventricle [25]
thalessemia a genetic disorder that results in defective formation of hemoglobin [15]
therapeutic procedure a procedure performed in order to treat a disease or condition [27]
therapeutic radiology treatments using radiation [1]
third-party administrator (TPA) a private company that processes claims for self-insured health plans [2]
third-party payer an entity other than the patient or physician who pays for healthcare services [2]
third trimester the time in a pregnancy when the gestational age is between 28 weeks, 0 days and delivery [23]
thoracentesis a procedure to remove fluid from the space between the lining of the outside of the lungs and the wall of the chest [5] [16]
thrombocyte a platelet [15]
thrombophilia a tendency to create blood clots [15]
thrombus a clot of blood formed within a blood vessel that remains attached to its point of origin [14]
thyrotoxicosis an excessive quantity of circulating thyroid hormone due to overproduction by the thyroid gland originating from outside the thyroid, or from loss of storage function and leakage from the gland [10]
tinnitus a ringing of the ear that may be subjective or objective [20]
tolerate the amount of a substance a person can absorb before resulting in behavioral or physical abnormalities [18]
tongue tied a condition in which the bottom of the tongue is attached to the floor of the mouth by a band of tissue called the lingual frenulum [25]
tonic-clonic seizure see grand mal [17]
tonic seizure a seizure characterized by prolonged muscle contractions or a stiffening [17]
topography a classification of neoplasms that is based on the anatomic site at which the growth begins; also called site of origin [5]
Tourette syndrome a condition that causes people to make repeated, quick movements or sounds, which they have no control over [17]
toxic effect a harmful substance that is ingested or comes into contact with a person and causes and undesired physical response [13]
toxoplasmosis an infection due to the parasite *Toxoplasma gondii*, usually affecting the brain, lung, heart, eyes, or liver [21]
TPAL a description of parity that identifies the number of term births (T), preterm births (P), spontaneous or induced abortions (A), and living children (L) [23]
trachea the windpipe [10]
tracheal cartilage the part of the body that keeps the trachea and bronchi open [16]
tracheostomy tube a surgical opening in the neck leading to the trachea [16]
transaction standards programming specifications [3]
transient ischemic attack (TIA) a brief episode of cerebral ischemia [14]
transient tachypnea of the newborn (TTN) a short-term condition of rapid breathing due to retained lung fluid that occurs shortly after birth in full term or near term newborns [24]
transitory temporary [24]
transmural MI the death of heart tissue that extends through the entire thickness of the heart muscle [14]
transposition of the great vessels a congenital heart defect in which the aorta and pulmonary artery are switched, preventing pulmonary circulation [25]
traumatic an acute current injury that results from an accident [12]
traumatic amputation the severing of a body part accidentally [13]
Tricare (TC) health insurance coverage for family members of active duty personnel and for retired military personnel and their families [2]
trichinosis a roundworm infection caused by eating raw pork or certain other meats [21]
trichomoniasis a sexually transmitted disease [21]
tricuspid valve the valve that controls the blood flow from the right atrium to the right ventricle [14]
trisomy a genetic disorder in which a person has three copies, rather than two, of genetic material [25]
true labor the period during which the uterine contracts and the cervix dilates [23]
tuberculosis (TB) a contagious bacterial infection that involves the lungs, but may spread to other organs [21]
tympanic membrane see tympanum [16] [20]
tympanic membrane perforation (TMP) a hole or break in the eardrum; also called a ruptured tympanic membrane [20]
tympanum the part of the external ear that separates it from the middle ear; also called the tympanic membrane or eardrum [20]
type 1 diabetes a condition in which the body's immune system attacks pancreatic beta cells, so that the pancreas does not produce insulin; previously called insulin-dependent diabetes mellitus (IDDM) or juvenile-onset diabetes [10]
type 2 diabetes a condition in which the pancreas produces insulin, but the body does not use it properly; previously called non-insulin-dependent diabetes mellitus (NIDDM) or adult-onset diabetes [10]

U

UB form Uniform Bill, the standard hospital billing form [26]
UHDDS Uniform Hospital Data Discharge Set [4]
ulcer a sore on the lining of the stomach (gastric ulcer) or duodenum (peptic ulcer) [9]; an open sore on the skin with loss of surface tissue and degeneration of underlying tissue [11]
ulcerative colitis an inflammatory bowel disease (IBD) with inflammation and sores, called ulcers, in the lining of the rectum and colon [9]
uncertain diagnosis a condition preceded by the words probable, possible, suspected, questionable, rule out, working diagnosis, or a similar word [4]
underdosing taking less of a medication than is prescribed by a provider or a manufacturer's instruction [3] [13]
Uniform Hospital Data Discharge Set (UHDDS) a list of data elements and definitions prepared by the Centers for Disease Control and Prevention and used by hospitals for inpatient discharge data collection [4]
unique definition a PCS characteristic meaning each code is constructed of seven characters so the description is one of a kind and cannot be changed [26]

unrelated a symptom, sign, or abnormal finding not connected to a disease [6]
unstable lie the repeated changes in the fetal position during or after the thirty-sixth week of pregnancy [23]
unstageable pressure ulcer skin damage due to prolonged pressure that cannot be visually assessed due to dead cells, eschar, or wound exudate [11]
upper GI series see barium swallow [9]
upper respiratory tract a part of the respiratory system that consists of the nose, pharynx, and larynx [16]
uremia a toxic blood condition due to the inability of the kidneys to remove nitrogenous substances from the body [22]
ureter a tube that drains each kidney [22]
urethra the tube that carries urine out of the body [22]
urinary bladder a muscular sac that holds urine until it is expelled through the urethra [22]
urinary tract infection (UTI) a bacterial infection of the urinary bladder; also called cystitis [22]
urticaria the presence of hives [11]
use (substance) a usage pattern that involves consuming a substance in moderate amounts that do not create significant legal, social, employment, family, or medical problems [18]
uterus a hollow muscular organ in females that provides for the development of the fetus; also called the womb [22]
UTI urinary tract infection
utricle a small, saclike structure of the labyrinth of the inner ear [20]
uvea the middle layer of the eye consisting of the iris, ciliary body, and choroid [19]
uvula a pendant fleshy lobe, most commonly referred to as one in the back of the mouth [19]

V

vagina the birth canal [22]
vaginal birth the delivery of the fetus from the uterus through cervix to the vagina [23]
vaginal birth after cesarean (VBAC) the delivery through the vagina after having a cesarean delivery in a previous pregnancy [23]
value individual letters and numbers that make up the seven characters of a PCS code [26]
valve repair the correction of a physical defect in a heart valve [14]
valve replacement the replacement of a heart valve with a synthetic or porcine (pig) valve [14]
valvular disorder a condition characterized by damage to or a defect in one of the four heart valves [14]
varicella the chicken pox virus [21]
vascular dementia dementia due to many small strokes [18]
vasodilation the enlargement of the blood vessels [17]
vasoocclusive crisis a form of sickle cell crisis in which the patient experiences severe pain due to infarctions, which may occur in nearly any location [15]
VBAC vaginal birth after cesarean [23]
vein the mechanism that carries blood from the capillaries back to the heart in successively larger veins leading to the superior vena cava and inferior vena cava [14]
venography an imaging study of the circulatory system in which X-rays are taken of the veins by tracing the venous pulse [14]
ventilation-perfusion scan a nuclear medicine test useful in identifying pulmonary emboli by showing if blood is flowing to all parts of the lung [16]
ventilator a machine that assists in breathing [16]
ventilator associated pneumonia (VAP) pneumonia that develops 48 hours or more after mechanical ventilation is given using an endotracheal tube or tracheostomy tube [16]
ventricle one of the lower heart chambers, which ejects blood to the lungs and the body [14]
ventricular fibrillation (V-fib) an irregular heartbeat in the ventricles, characterized by an abnormal quivering of heart fibers [14]
venule a small vein [14]
vertebra one of the bony segments of the spine [12]
vertigo a sensation of motion or dizziness [20]
very low birth weight (VLBW) a birth weight less than 1,500 grams (3 pounds, 4 ounces) [24]
vestibular schwannoma a benign tumor of the vestibular cochlear nerve; also called an acoustic neuroma [20]
vestibulocochlear nerve the transmission of the sounds waves from the brain to the cranial nerve VIII to make hearing possible [20]
Veteran Health Administration (VHA) an integrated healthcare delivery system with more than 1,400 sites of care to provide health services to veterans with service-related disabilities [2]
Via Natural or Artificial Opening a PCS value for the Approach that identifies access to a surgical site through a body opening that already exists or through an artificially made opening [27]
Via Natural or Artificial Opening Endoscopic a PCS value for the Approach that identifies a procedure using a natural or artificial opening for endoscopic access [27]
Via Natural or Artificial Opening Endoscopic with Percutaneous Endoscopic Assistance a PCS value for the Approach that identifies a procedure in which two endoscopes are used: one through a natural or artificial opening and the second through percutaneous access [27]
virus a capsule that contains genetic material and uses the body's own cells to multiply [21]
visceral pericardium see epicardium [14]
vitiligo the loss of pigmentation [11]
vitreous body the transparent jelly that fills the eyeball and is surrounded by a membrane [19]
voluntary muscles the muscles a person can choose to contract and relax [12]
volvulus twisting of a portion of the small or large intestine or stomach into a loop, which obstructs the passage of digestive material [9]
Von Willebrand's disease a genetic disorder marked by bleeding of the mucosa [15]
vulvovaginitis the inflammation of the vulva and vagina [22]

W

WBC white blood cell; white blood cell count
whistleblower an individual who reports violators of the False Claims Act [2]
white blood cell disorder a condition that diminishes the body's immune response and increases the risk of infection [15]
wire a slender, flexible length of stranded metal used to cut bone or tissue [28]
with a preposition physicians use to indicate that two conditions are interrelated [10]
workers compensation (WC) programs required by each state to pay for medical costs due to employment-related injuries or illnesses [2]
wound a cut or opening in the skin or mucous membrane [13]
WU work up

X

xenograft the tissue from an animal [11]

Z

Z code a code used for encounters and in healthcare settings when the reason for the encounter is not a disease, injury, or external cause that is classified in the preceding ICD-10-CM chapters for body systems (A00 to Y89); comparable to ICD-9-CM V codes [7]
zygote a fertilized egg [23]

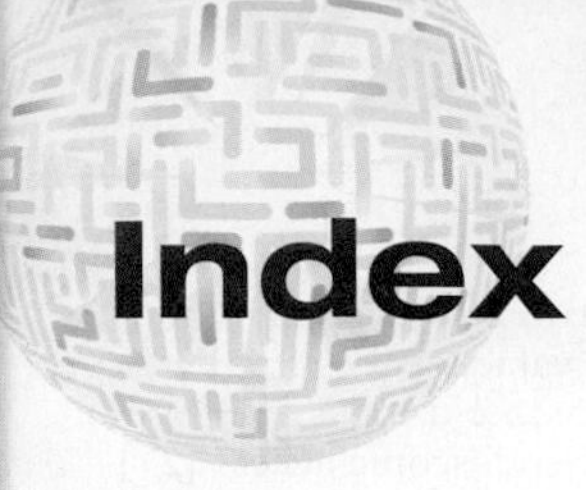

Index

References are to pages. Pages followed by "f" indicate figures; "t" tables.

A

B

C

D

E

H

I

J

N

O

P

Q

R

S

T

U